Botanical Dermatology

Plants and Plant Products Injurious to The Skin

John Mitchell
M.D., F.R.C.P., F.R.C.P. (C), F.A.C.P.
Division of Dermatology
The University of British Columbia
Vancouver, Canada

and

Arthur Rook
M.A., M.D., F.R.C.P.
Department of Dermatology
Addenbrooke's Hospital
Cambridge, England

With a foreword by

Marion B. Sulzberger, M.D., San Francisco

and contributions by

Niels hjorth, Copenhagen
Alexander Fisher, New York
Veikko Pirilä, Helsinki
Bjorn Hausen, Hamburg

1979 Vancouver
Greengrass

ISBN 0-88978-047-1

Greenglass Ltd.
691 W. 28th Avenue,
Vancouver, British Columbia
Canada V5H 2H4

MANUFACTURED IN CANADA BY SCRIVENERS' PULP PRESS LTD.

Canadian Cataloguing in Publication Data

Mitchell, John, 1923-
Botanical dermatology

Bibliography: p.
Includes Index.

1. Poisonous plants - Toxicology.
2. Contact dermatitis. I. Rook, Arthur J.
II. Title.
RA1250.M58 615.9'52 C78-002156-8

Acknowledgments

To the Division of Dermatology (Wm. D. Stewart, M. D., Head), Faculty of Medicine, and the staff of the Woodward Biomedical Library, The University of British Columbia.

In this book, the description of a plant family, its number of genera and species and geographical distribution: the description of a genus, its number of species and geographical distribution and other pertinent information have been recorded from the Dictionary of the Flowering Plants and Ferns (The late J. C. Willis) revised by H. K. Airy Shaw, Cambridge University Press, Seventh edition (1966) and mostly revised according to the Eighth Edition of the Dictionary (1973). We thank Dr. Airy Shaw, Royal Botanic Gardens, Kew, Surrey, England and Mrs. Kathleen Aversano Subsidiary Rights Department, Cambridge University Press, American Branch, 32 East 57th Street, New York, N. Y. 10022 for permission to record the information from the Dictionary in this book.

'Diagnosis of contact dermatitis from plants' is reprinted from a paper published in The International Journal of Dermatology by permission of J. B. Lippincott Co., East Washington Square, Philadelphia, Pa. 19106 and Dr. L. C. Parish, executive editor of the Journal, 1601 Walnut St., Philadelphia, Pa. 19102, U. S. A.

Professor Niels Hjorth and Dr. S. Karger have given permission for reprinting of the section on Primula dermatitis from the valuable series 'Current Problems in Dermatology' published by S. Karger, Basel. (Vol. 3. 1970, pp. 31-50).

'Patch testing with perfume ingredients' is reprinted from the journal Contact Dermatitis (1975: 1, 166) by permission of Dr. A. A. Fisher, author, Dr. C. D. Calnan, editor, and Munksgaard, 35 Norre Sogade, DK-1016 Copenhagen K. Denmark, publishers.

To Veikko Pirilä, Department of Dermatology, University Central Hospital, Helsinki, Finland and Bjorn Hausen, Laboratory for Experimental Allergology, University Hospital, Hamburg, West Germany for personal communications.

To members of the North American Contact Dermatitis Group, Howard Maibach, chairman — physician, biologist, friend.

Contents

Foreword

It is not the naked savage in the tropical rain-forest who has the greatest exposure to plants and plant products. With the growing industrialization and increasing complexity of modern life, man's encounters with plants and their products grow ever more numerous. Often the exposed individual is unaware of the occurrence or the nature of the exposure. Inevitably, as the number of exposures to plants and their products increases, the number of injuries keeps pace.

With the possible exception of organs exposed to plants by ingestion, the skin is the organ most frequently and intimately exposed to plants and their products. Consequently, skin injuries from plants are exceedingly common and of growing concern.

At first glance, it seems astonishing that until now no text has dealt comprehensively and authoritatively with this important field. However, on closer scrutiny, one finds many reasons for this delay. First, as pointed out in the authors' preface, until the last decade or so an accurate compilation was almost impossible because botanical, phytochemical and medical information was not sufficiently precise in many of the reports of plant skin injuries.

In addition to this valid reason, on studying this monumental text by Drs. John C. Mitchell and Arthur Rook one sees other forceful reasons why no one has attempted before now to write a definitive work on skin injuries by plants. A subject so vast, so multifaceted, so demanding of countless hours of search and research, requires a combination of qualities possessed by few authors.

First and foremost, no non-dermatologist could do the job; for correct description, diagnosis and classification of the various skin lesions produced by plants are essential. In addition, the authors had to know considerable botany, not a little phytochemistry, a substantial amount of immunology and toxicology, and a good deal about pharmacy, perfumery, dyeing, painting, forestry, woodworking, farming, gardening, and a host of other processes and activities too numerous to recite here.

Because of the quantity and complexity of the material, the writing of this treatise has demanded enormous dedication and sacrifice of time by the authors during the past ten years.

Some idea of the dimension of the subject can be gained by noting that the authors have found and analyzed reports of skin injuries by 248 families of plants, comprising some 1405 genera and thousands of species.

The complexities of the subject matter are truly formidable. Every plant produces a large number of different chemicals. Two hundred different amino acids can be found in plants, in mammals only thirty. Moreover, the same plant will produce different quantities and kinds of chemicals when growing under different conditions. Think of any wine grape and how it differs according to season, region and vineyard. Many of the injurious allergenic chemicals in plants will cross react immunologically with chemicals in entirely different plants and with allergens of non-plant provenance.

Numerous other variables influence the production and form of a skin injury by a plant. Some of the variables are the rate and manner in which the injurious chemicals are transferred from plant to skin; the partition coefficient between plant surface and skin surface; the amount of friction, wetness and heat attending the exposure; variations in the skin's susceptibility from individual to individual, from site to site and from time to time in the same individual.

I need not go on with this listing for I am certain that no one will doubt the magnitude and difficulty of the task that Drs. Mitchell and Rook have accomplished. Nor can anyone doubt the value of the service they have rendered to dermatologists, to other physicians, phytochemists, cosmetologists, perfumers, the patients themselves, and all the many others who are in any way concerned with the injurious effects of plants and plant products upon the human skin.

This encyclopedic and authenticated reference work will save all concerned persons many hours of tedious and often vain searching of the literature in the attempt to identify offending plants and chemicals; to recognize the skin lesions they produce; to discover in what guises and manner they are encountered and to learn to avoid them.

BOTANICAL DERMATOLOGY will almost certainly go into numerous printings and editions, for it satisfies a crying need and will continue to be invaluable for years to come.

Marion B. Sulzberger, M. D.

PREFACE

Man's primitive ancestors must have had experience of dermatitis caused by plants, and have learned to recognize and avoid species which harmed them. They must have noticed that whilst some plants were harmful to everyone who handled them, others produced ill effects in only a few, and they must have wondered why this was so.

At a later stage our ancestors began to extract from plants substances which they applied to their skins to colour them, or with therapeutic intent. In each stage of man's development the pattern of his contact with plants and their products has changed, but the frequency and variety of contacts have increased to such a degree that even the desk-bound city-dweller is exposed to numerous species, either as house plants in his home or office, or as sophisticated aroma chemicals in his food, drink and cosmetics. Dermatitis caused by living plants or by plant products is now an important clinical problem in almost all countries.

The authors of this book have been interested for many years in dermatitis caused by plants. The problem differs in many respects from those presented by contact dermatitis of any other origin. A living plant is a complex chemical factory. The chemical composition of a single species may vary quantitively with the season and the conditions of cultivation. The association in a single species of sensitizing substances and of irritants, may complicate the detection of reactions to the former. The distribution of the offending chemicals within the plant and the ease with which they are released play a large part in determining the clinical pattern of dermatitis to which they give rise. Some knowledge of botany is therefore needed by the dermatologist who is effectively to investigate plant dermatitis.

The growth of medical knowledge of plant dermatitis is summarized on pp. 1 - 25 . This historical survey carries a number of lessons for the contemporary dermatologist. The first is that accurate identification of the offending plant is essential; the second is that, once actually identified, the plant must be referred to by its scientific name. We have had occasion to discard numerous published case reports as valueless because one or both of these lessons had been ignored. Consequently the literature on plant dermatitis, extensive though it is, has often been misleadingly anecdotal, and it is only during the past decade that a sufficiently large volume of publications, acceptable as reliable both botanically and medically, has accumulated to make it possible to complete a meaningful account of the plant dermatitis problem.

The immunological mechanisms involved in allergic reactions of the skin have been the subject of intensive research, particularly in the last ten years. Our increased knowledge of these mechanisms has of course materially enhanced our understanding of some of the ways in which plant chemicals can injure the skin.

Finally the past decade has seen an immense expansion of phytochemical research, some of it designed to discover new chemicals with pharmaceutical or industrial applications, but much of it pure research undertaken in the interests of chemical taxonomy. Although there are many thousands of species which have not yet been studied, the chemical composition of a very large number of plants has been reported, and hundreds of others are under active investigation.

The authors considered that the state of progress of our knowledge of the clinical syndromes, the pathological mechanisms and the chemical agents had reached the point at which a comprehensive review could be of great value to those concerned with the clinical care of patients with dermatitis caused by plants or plant products, or with the broader aspects of environmental health. They hope that this compilation will serve to introduce such physicians to the phytochemical literature, and that the phytochemists will find in the clinical problems a challenge, to the solution of which they will wish to contribute.

John Mitchell

Arthur Rook

Mailing address:

John C. Mitchell, M. D.
Dermatology Laboratory,
Shaughnessy Hospital,
4500 Oak Street,
Vancouver, B. C., Canada
V6H 3N1

Toxic plants - Associated disorders

The literature of hayfever (allergic rhinitis), oro-nasal and respiratory irritation, allergic alveolitis and lung disorders from inhalation of plants, adverse effects on the eyes, and systemic effects and death from contact with plants has been briefly included in this review. Such topics have been noted and indexed but they have not been exhaustively reviewed. The scope of this book has been deliberately restricted to adverse reactions to skin contact with plants and plant products, the literature on which is in itself extensive and widely scattered. For the same reason allergic and toxic reactions following the injection of plant and plant products have not been listed; a number of readily accessible publications cover this subject comprehensively. The authors, who are neither botanists or phytochemists, will be grateful if readers will bring to their notice any errors or omissions.

CONTACT DERMATITIS FROM PLANTS

Two forms of contact dermatitis are recognized:

Irritant contact dermatitis, which can result from exposure of the skin to plants such as *Euphorbia* spp. or *Ranunculus* spp., affects all individuals if the amount and duration of the exposure is sufficient. In lay terms, irritant contact dermatitis is a chemical burn affecting anyone close enough to a hot enough 'fire'.

Allergic contact dermatitis, from exposure of the skin to *Toxicodendron* spp., *Primula obconica*, etc., affects only some individuals, who acquire a specific altered capacity to react to the plants. Such a capacity is not present at birth but is acquired by postnatal exposure, is specific for the chemical compounds responsible, such as pentadecylcatechol (*Toxicodendron*, Anacardiaceae), or the quinone, primin (*Primula*, Primulaceae), depends upon an altered immunological status of the individual, is mediated by sensitized lymphocytes rather than by antibody and is therefore designated 'cell mediated hypersensitivity', and is presented clinically as a skin

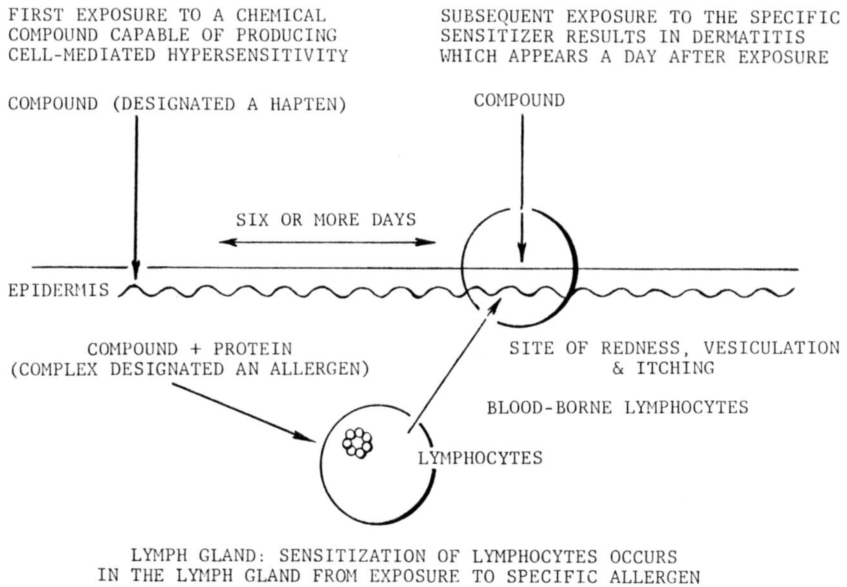

Pathogenetic mechanisms of allergic contact dermatitis.

reaction manifested by redness, vesiculation (small blisters within the epidermis) and itching.

Pathogenesis of Allergic Contact Dermatitis

Following initial contact with a chemical compound which is capable of producing 'cell-mediated hypersensitivity', a process of sensitization occurs in some individuals and, during the course of a minimum of six days, lymphocytes located in lymph glands become sensitized and are released into the blood stream. Following subsequent exposure to the specific sensitizer, circulating lymphocytes accumulate at the site and dermatitis becomes manifest one or two days later at the skin site of re-exposure. Such delay in the appearance of dermatitis at the site of re-exposure is indicated by an alternative term for the reaction, namely 'delayed hypersensitivity'.

Delayed hypersensitivity may be detected by means of a 'patch test'; a chemical compound is applied to the skin, by necessity in a non-irritant dose, and the skin site is examined 48 hours later; a positive patch test reaction, provided non-specific irritancy is excluded, indicates a state of delayed hypersensitivity and is a deliberate elicitation, under controlled conditions, of allergic contact dermatitis as part of the clinical investigation of affected patients.

Immunochemistry of Contact Dermatitis

In the pathogenesis of allergic contact dermatitis, small molecular weight chemical compounds, designated haptens, become bound to skin protein to form higher molecular weight complexes, designated allergens or antigens, which induce sensitization of lymphocytes. The means and the site of attachment of compounds derived from plants to skin proteins are thus of interest to dermatologists and the immunochemical requisites of some compounds have been clarified by phytochemical studies. Two such examples are

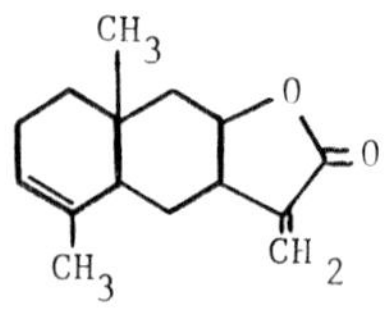

I

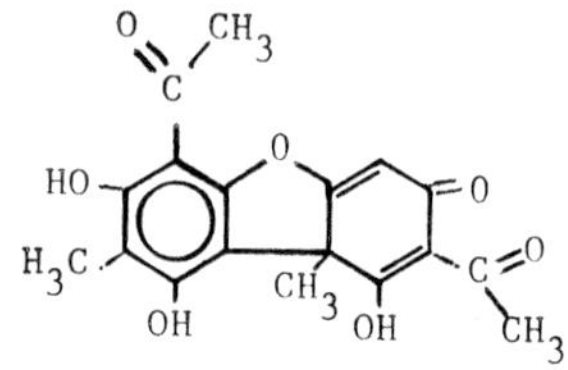

II

as follows: The main functional group of sesquiterpene lactones, e.g. alantolactone (I), derived from Composite species such as Inula is an α-methylene group attached to the γ-lactone; reduction of this group renders the compounds inactive for contact allergy. d-Usnic acid (II), from lichens, is a sensitizer whereas ℓ-Usnic acid is inactive; the specificity can thus extend to stereochemical configurations and exemplifies the remarkable capacity of sensitized lymphocytes to distinguish between related compounds. Relatively few plant sensitizers have been identified, and include

(III, α-methylene-γ-butyrolactone
Tulipa, Liliaceae),

(IV, δ-3-carene
Pinus, Pinaceae),

(V, allylisothiocyanate
Cruciferae spp.),

(VI, 4-methoxydalbergione
Dalbergia spp:, Leguminosae),

(VII, oxyayanin
Distemonanthus, Leguminosae),

(VIII, anthothecol
Khaya, Meliaceae),

(IX, lapachol
Tectona, Verbenaceae),

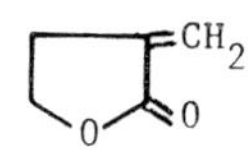

III

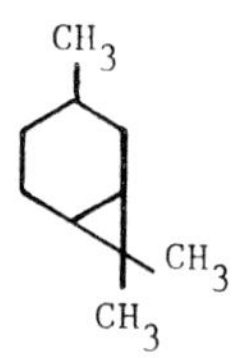

IV

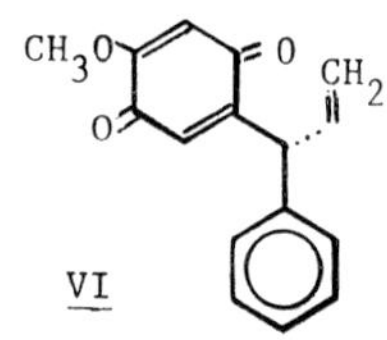

VI

$CH_2=CH-CH_2-N=C=S$

V

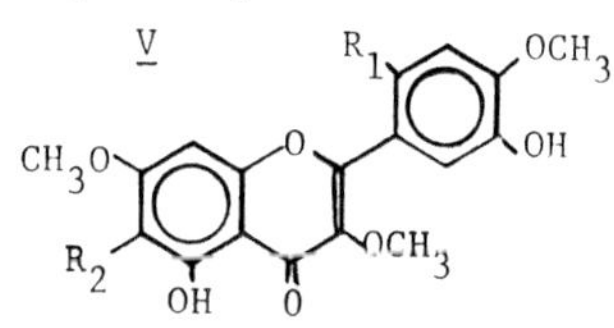

A $R_1=OH$; $R_2=H$

B $R_1=H$; $R_2=OH$

VII

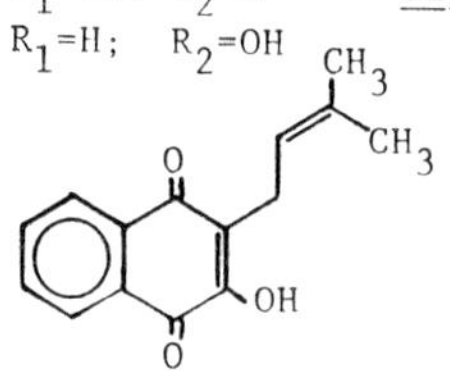

IX

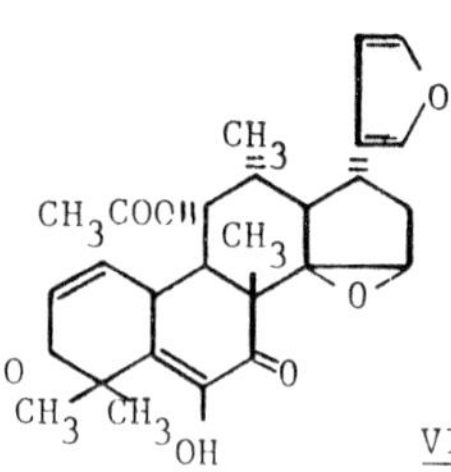

VIII

(X, chlorophorin *Chlorophora*, Moraceae),

(XI, thymoquinone *Libocedrus*, Cupressaceae)

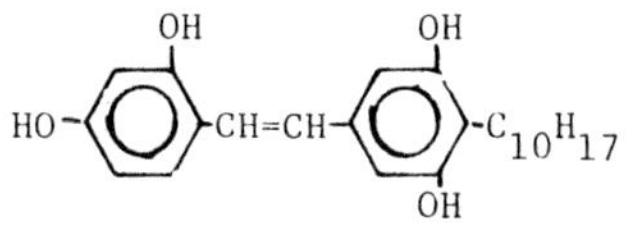

X

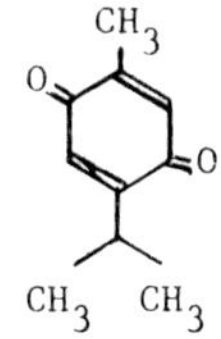

XI

Cross-Sensitivity in Allergic Contact Dermatitis

An individual may become specifically sensitized to unrelated materials such as turpentine and nickel and is then said to exhibit 'multiple specific sensitivity'. Cross-sensitivity patterns are also observed; thus an individual may become sensitized to alantolactone and subsequently show positive patch test reactions to numerous related sesquiterpene lactones derived from various plants of the Composite family. When there is no evidence of prior exposure to such plants, 'cross-sensitivity' is implied.

At the botanical level, apparently anomalous cross-sensitivity patterns have been observed. Thus our interest in plants of the family Compositae was aroused by the finding that one of some fifty forest-workers in British Columbia who had allergic contact dermatitis from the liverwort *Frullania* (Jubulaceae) was also contact-sensitive to *Chrysanthemum* x *morifolium* (Compositae). The patient actually found this out himself when he was obliged to retire from forest-work because of severe recurrent occupational dermatitis and took up growing chrysanthemums as a retirement hobby. Cross-sensitivity between a lowly bryophyte and a botanically unrelated composite, which is considered to be higher on the evolutionary scale, was found to be explicable in phytochemical terms, viz. the presence of frullanolide, a sesquiterpene lactone in *Frullania* related to lactones of *Chrysanthemum*.

Atopy

The genetically determined state known as atopy may become manifest as hayfever, allergic asthma and atopic dermatitis. 'Immediate hypersensitivity' is a feature of atopy and may be detected by a 'scratch' test of the skin. A wheal reaction appears within a few minutes of re-exposure to some allergens and is mediated by circulating antibody (immunoglobulin).

HISTORY OF DERMATITIS VENENATA (CONTACT DERMATITIS) FROM PLANTS AND OF EPICUTANEOUS TESTING.

'Quod cibus est aliis, aliis est venenum'
'One man's food is another man's poison'
Lucretius, De Rerum Natura: On the Nature of Things First Century B.C.

About 4000 years ago, a paste of Castor oil bean (Ricinus) was rubbed on the scalp as an irritant to promote hair growth; the anonymous compiler of the Herbal was then citing from an ancient book. An Assyrian Herbal written 1000 years before Hippocrates, the Father of Medicine (c. 400 B.C.), contained about 250 medicaments of plant origin and more than 700 drugs can be found in the Papyrus Ebers which was written about 1500 B.C. These evidently summarised prescriptions of a long tradition before them (Dawson 1929); seventy-four prescriptions pertained to hair washes, dyes, oils and depilatories. The use of Psoralea in India for a pigmenting effect was recorded about 1400 B.C. and the psoralen plant, Ammi, in Egypt in the 13th Century A.D.

The great Materia Medica of Dioscorides in the 1st Century A.D. which contained many descriptions of untoward reactions of the skin to plants, was the text-book of the Western World for over 1000 years.

Dioscorides was critical of some other observers, writing "But they have transmitted the powers of medicines and their examination cursorily, not estimating their efficacy by experience, but by vain prating about the cause, having lifted up each medicine to a heap of controversy: and besides this they have recorded one thing by mistake for another ... And in the face of plain evidence (one writer) sets down many such falsehoods, which are tokens that he acquired his information not by his own observation, but had it only from the false relation of hearsay."

In the Nineteenth Century there were many observations of the ill-effects by plants applied to diseased skin for the purpose of treatment. Unjustifiably, many such plants have been listed from book to book as hazards in the garden.

Aetius (Sixth Century A.D.) wrote on cutaneous diseases and is said to have introduced the term eczema (lit. 'out boiling'), (Wright 1940). In the Seventh Century A.D. dermatitis from the Japanese Lacquer Tree (Rhus verniciflua) was described, one of the earliest skin diseases to be reported in the Orient (Toyama 1918). Irritant effects of plants were recognized by Al-Samarqandi in early medieval Arabian Medicine (Levey and Al-Khaledy 1967).

The opening of the New World led to the recognition by Valdes (1535) (cited by Pardo-Castello 1923) of the irritant effects of Hippomane, (Manchineel): "In this island Hispaniola on the coast of the setting sun ... there are innumerable mancanillos ... And it has been proved by many, and at many times, that in lying down to sleep carelessly under these trees, on getting up it is with great headache and swelling of the eyes, eyebrows and cheeks. And even in the case that dew from this tree touches the face, it acts like fire and burns the skin as far as it reaches, and should it enter the eyes, it blinds them and may endanger the eyesight."

He also wrote of skin reactions to anacardiaceous plants, Comocladia and Metopium (Guao):

"Guao is a tree rather than a plant, I have seen it so tall. The leaves look like those of the acebo or holly-tree of Spain, but the guao leaf is very green and curly ... it is a powerful caustic in such a manner that the white milk that exudes and even the dew from the tree, falling on a man's face or any other part of his body, burns it, raising blebs, and the skin swells - all of which is very marvellous."

Other anacardiaceous trees (Lithraea and Gluta) were early recognized as capable of producing dermatitis.

Feuillée, who visited the coast of Chile in 1702-1712, related that some of his seamen suffered severely as the result of cutting down some Lithi trees (Lithraea caustica). By the following day their heads had swollen to an extraordinary size and their features had become indistinguishable so that they might have been taken for monsters rather than men. Molina in 1809 wrote that "the effluvium from this tree, especially in summer, produces painful pustules and swellings on the hands and face of those who stop beneath its shade. The effect is various, however, with various persons; there are some who are very little, if at all, incommoded by it, while others are severely affected." The author, who elsewhere was described as "one of the most pernicious blunderers who have brought confusion into Natural History", was close to the truth on this occasion (Sprague 1921).

In 1750 Rumphius noted that "The exhalations of a tree, Gluta renghas, are considered noxious, and the people of Macassar ... entertain such dread of it, that they dare not remain long under it, much less repose beneath its shade; they say that whoever receives the droppings from it will have his body swell and be affected with malignant sores" (Sprague 1921).

The recorded history of dermatitis from the New World Toxicodendron (syn. Rhus) (poison ivy) dates from 1609 (McNair 1923). Subsequent observations led to a crisp Latin summary in the first North American Materia Medica (Schoepf 1787) which emphasized that not all those who were exposed became affected: "... pustulas acres, tumores doloresque in corpore (non omni) pariunt".

The English herbalists Gerard (1597) and Culpeper (1653) recorded skin reactions to many plants. Gerard himself experienced the irritant effect of an Euphorbia (Spurge) and his companion was also affected: ...'Some write by report of others, that it enflameth exceedingly, but myselfe speak by experience ... I tooke but one drop of it into my mouth; which neverthelesse did so inflame and swell in my throte that I hardly escaped with my life.'

Euphorbia (spurge) has a colourful history, named for Euphorbus, physician to King Juba of Numidia. Theophrastus in the 4th century B.C. noted that the juice of the spurge could blind animals, or even a man. Dioscorides (First century A.D.) and Pliny (23-79 A.D.) described the method of collecting the juice so as to prevent irritation of the hands and face. Gum Euphorbia was formerly used as an officinal ingredient of a rubefacient plaster. In India, the plant juices were used by criminals to destroy the eyes of domestic animals and planted as a cattle fence, the spiny forms used to be a formidable obstacle to cavalry. Planted around African kraals, Euphorbia acted as a deterrent to marauders and on graves discouraged browsing animals. Culpeper (1652) wrote of the irritant effect of spurges which "abound with a hot and acrid juice, which when applied outwardly, eats away warts and other excrescences". An Euphorbia is said to have been the active ingredient of the slow acting poison employed by Catarina Sforza (1463-1509). The plants which were used for their juice to brand horses in Texas and can yield poisonous honey are no longer officially medicinal but serve to make an anti-fouling paint for ship's bottoms. Recently their use for actinic keratoses has been revived.

Herbals were succeeded in one direction by Floras and in another by books of medicinal plants (Nissen 1958) and scientific toxicology began with Orfila (1814-15). Some 1,500 books and pamphlets of medicinal plants, from all parts of the world, were collected in a bibliography by de Laszlo (1958).

Herbals have been published in modern times (Wren 1968, Grieve 1970), and Herbal Medicine survives and in China, receives official encouragement. Some forty plants and plant products were listed as present in 114 proprietary skin remedies by Underwood and Gaul in 1948. They deplored the use of such products for treating plant dermatitis but went on to recommend oatmeal baths in therapy.

Kaempfer, in 1712, was the first to describe what was definitely an occupational dermatitis, from lacquer varnish (Rhus) (Noojin 1954).

Plenck (1776) classified diseases of the skin adopting a binominal method like that used for plants by Linnaeus of whom he was an admirer and possibly a student (Lane 1933).

Piffard (1881) and Morrow (1887) reviewed the adverse effects of plant products applied to the skin as topical therapeutic agents. Croton oil (Croton tiglium) known as irritant since the 28th Century B.C., was used in the 19th Century A.D. as a counter-irritant by pricking it into the skin for pulmonary disease. This process called "Bauncheitismus" fell into disuse. Over 5000 pounds were imported into the United States in 1878 but in 1883, only 300 pounds (White 1887).

Doctors were not overworked (Dulake 1977). Medicine was simpler because nearly all serious illness was fatal, thus shortening attendance and reducing the workload. The sickness of the well-to-do was aggravated by bleeding, purgatives, emetics, blisters, cupping, leeches, cauterization and medication with traditional, empirical remedies. Treatment relied on the antiphlogistic theory designed to weaken the patient and draw away the mythical substance phlogiston, some surviving in spite of their treatment, and not, as was thought, because of it. The sick poor made do with herbal remedies, which were often innocuous. Today, iatrogenic disease is as common but, in the West, the poor are not spared. In 1887, White recorded the cutaneous effects of about 100 plant species. In 1911, Pammel published a book on poisonous plants and noted skin effects from many of them; he drew on 1,097 references in the literature to that date.

Epicutaneous testing to plants and plant products

A record of an epicutaneous test to a plant (Rosa) dates from 1645 (Macalpine and Hunter (1956). An anonymous investigator applied a rose to the cheek of a woman 'while she was asleep, to try if her antipathy against that flower were so great as she used to pretend.' A positive result (consisting of 'blisters') was observed. Malten (1972) accepts this report as the first recorded epicutaneous test and one carried out with proper psychological precautions. There is doubt, however, about the veracity of the reporter, Digby, (Pepys 1660-1669).

In 1795, Fontana applied a cut leaf of Toxicodendron (poison ivy) to the back of his own hand and, three days later, developed dermatitis of the hands and face. He found that the period of latency before development of dermatitis was three, four or six days.

In 1798 Horsfield, a medical student at the University of Pennsylvania, found that dermatitis was produced by application of the juice of the plant to the skin.

Possibly the next recorded epicutaneous test to a plant was carried out during explorations by Leichhardt and his party in Australia: 'John Murphy having no pockets in his trousers, put the seeds which he found into his bosom, close to the skin, where he had already deposited a great number of Sterculia, and was much inconvenienced by starry prickles which surround the seeds. Afterwards, finding the drooping Grevillea in fruit, he gathered some capsules and placed them as before stated. Upon arriving at the camp he felt great pain and, on examining the place, he saw, to his greatest horror, that the whole of the skin of the epigastric region was coloured black and raised into a great number of painful blisters. Upon his showing it to me, I thought that it was caused by the Sterculia prickles having irritated the skin and rendered it more sensitive to the sharp properties of the exudation of the seed vessels of Grevillea. Brown, however, merely touched the skin of his arm with the matter when blisters immediately rose, showing clearly its properties. The discoloration of the skin was like the effects of nitrate of silver',

(Leichhardt 1847).

McNair (1923) and Rostenberg (1955) recorded the early history of experiments in poison-ivy (Toxicodendron) dermatitis.

The chief causes of various infectious diseases were formerly thought to be gaseous and the word malaria is derived from that concept. Van Mons in 1797 had his brother expose the hand to gas from the plant with conflicting results (McNair 1923).

In 1798, Horsfield recorded tests with blister fluid of skin affected by poison ivy; he applied the blister fluid to susceptible individuals and observed no positive reactions. Busey in 1873, and White in 1873, and others recorded negative tests with blister fluid (Rostenberg 1955).

In 1865 Maisch observed that after suffering an attack of Rhus dermatitis, he transferred the poisonous effects to some other persons merely by shaking hands with them. He applied distilled aqueous extracts of the plant to several persons and eruptions were produced in several instances. By his method of preparation, the extract was probably acetic acid contaminated with urushiol. Pfaff (1897) carried out many experiments upon himself and others with an oily extract of the Rhus; he found that 0.001mg. of plant oil applied in olive oil was active.

Primula obconica was botanically described by Hance (1880) and dermatitis from it recognized by White (1888) in America. Ferguson (1890) referred to a case of dermatitis from P. obconica observed in 1889 in England and suggested the hairs of the plant as the cause rather than a fungus implicated by Lee (1890). Now it is known that the allergenic quinone, primin, is indeed present in the hairs (trichomes).

Contact reactions to P. obconica were named erysipelas (Pooley 1893, Southern 1891) and contact urticaria (Southern 1891), and vesicular contact dermatitis was named herpes (Mackintosh 1885).

Kirk (1889) carried out tests with Primula obconica and, in order to obtain sensitisation, he employed repeated application of the plant to irritated skin under occlusion. Ferguson (1890) tested a gardener and his own skin with a leaf of the plant with positive results. Contact reactions to ophthalmic alkaloids were recognized early and a patch test to atropine (Atropa) was carried out by Collins (1888). The introduction of patch testing to Dermatology is credited to Jadassohn (1895, 1904). At about the same time (1895), Fabre was carrying out patch tests with caterpillar hairs (Rostenberg and Solomon 1968). In 1906, von Pirquet defined the concept of allergy. Nestler's work (1900-1920) confirmed sensitization to Primula but irritancy and allergic effects were not distinguished. Open epicutaneous tests with an ether extract of the leaves of P. obconica were carried out by Foerster (1910). Simpson (1917) obtained positive patch test reactions with an alcoholic extract of the leaves in sensitized patients and negative reactions in controls. Cash (1911) clearly distinguished irritant from allergic effects on the skin, described an incubation period, delayed hypersensitivity reactions, the spontaneous flare up phenomenon (although he did not use so awkward a phrase), different levels of sensitivity in different individuals, different degrees of reactivity of various skin sites for patch testing, dissemination of dermatitis after patch testing and flares of positive patch test sites following patch testing. He applied measured quantities of an allergenic alkaloid, chloroxylonine (from Chloroxylon swietenia, East Indian Satinwood) to measured areas of skin in aqueous and oily vehicles and carried out quantitative patch testing, finding that 0.0000165gm. of the chemical would elicit a reaction in a sensitized individual.

He also discussed 'hardening', although he did not use that controversial term. It was to be a generation later that patch testing became an office procedure for investigation of allergic contact dermatitis.

The patch test was first used

in the United States (in animals) by Markley (1920). During the 1920's, Bloch developed the technique using Primula obconica and he introduced the use of a standard series of seven test substances which included P. obconica, tincture of arnica (Arnica), quinine (Cinchona) and turpentine (Pinus), (Bloch 1924, 1929). In 1923, Jadassohn described 'hardening', or hyposensitisation. In 1926, Oppenheim described 'meadow dermatitis', later found to be evoked by plants yielding linear furanocoumarins and ultraviolet light and named phytophotodermatitis (Klaber 1942). Cummer (1927) obtained a positive patch test reaction with diluted Balsam of Peru (Myroxylon). In North America, the patch test was introduced as an office investigative procedure by Sulzberger and Wise (1931). Lists of patch test substances in non-irritant concentrations were provided by Kesten and Laszlo (1931) and by Rostenberg and Sulzberger (1939). Shelmire (1939, 1940) described the manufacture and use of plant extracts for patch testing.

A notable feature of the history of patch testing with plants has been application by non-medical individuals of offending plants to their own skins (Munz 1932) in order to assist their physicians (Ackland 1893, Senear 1933). Ackland's patient found that it was not necessary for the juice of the leaves to be applied to the skin; if the fingers, after handling the plant, touched the face, the eruption was produced there as well: "A strange feature was the fact that there was no effect until after the lapse of so many (twelve) hours".

Patch-testing was slow to achieve recognition as a useful diagnostic tool. At least one reason was puzzlement that a patch test applied to a skin site did not necessarily reproduce any dermatitis at the original site. Heroic measures were employed in attempts to produce a focal flare (Hall 1921, Hunt 1931). The spontaneous flare phenomenon, that is dermatitis occurring at a site as long as several weeks after application of a plant derivative, (Cash 1911) now known to represent active sensitization by patch testing, possibly did little credit to the novel diagnostic test as a 'rational' tool (Levin 1924, 1933). The still-unsolved problem of a ready distinction between irritancy and allergic effects posed difficulties then and now.

Alleged epidemic contact dermatitis from Primula farinosa without any patch testing (Sharpe 1912) and epidemic patch test dermatitis from an irritant plant Clematis based on inadequate clinical data (Lancaster 1937) represent some by-ways of dermatological history.

Dermatitis venenata was defined as an eruption due to some chemical vegetable irritant coming in contact with the skin (Gardiner 1922); the term has since been more widely applied to contact dermatitis.

Many plants were used as topical therapeutic agants, and adverse reactions resulted from such medical use rather than by contact in the garden or industry. The ill-effects followed changing modes of treatment rather than fashions in horticulture.

Then, and now, Tincture of Arnica as a topical application caused often severe allergic contact dermatitis. Hebra in the 1880's advocated that if the remedy was for any topical use at all, which he disapproved, one drop of the tincture in a bucket of water was more than enough.

The North American weeds, poison-ivy oak (Toxicodendron), occasionally introduced into gardens elsewhere with disastrous results and an ornamental Primula introduced from China to households of North America and Europe with discomfitting results (or even murder, Brown 1906) have since 1609 and 1888 respectively, been prototypes for the investigation of allergic contact dermatitis.

Now the scourge of India, Parthenium hysterophorus (feverfew) introduced 20 years ago to Poona from America (Lonkar et al 1974) is producing epidemic contact dermatitis involving thousands of adult male patients.

These vast ecological and

biological natural experiments by interactions of afflicted people and quietly aggressive plants have perhaps subtly, but generously, benefitted clinical immunology.

A summary compilation of early reports of dermatitis from plants and plant products (to 1900 A. D.) is given in Table 1.

Table 1

Reports of adverse contact skin reactions to plants and plant products to 1900 A.D.

	Date	Author/Text	Plant/Plant Product	Reference
B.C.	Twenty-eight Century	Shennung Pentsao (Chinese text)	*Croton tiglium*, ?*Phytolacca* (Pokeberry)	Smith 1969
	Second millenium	Assyrian text (Thompson 1949)	*Brassica* (Mustard Plaster)	Woods 1962
	1400	Atharva Veda (Indian text)	*Psoralea corylifolia* (yields psoralen)	El Mofty 1968
	380-287	Theophrastus	*Euphorbia*, *Veratrum album* (white hellebore)	Woods 1962
	First Century	Lucretius	Exudations of trees	Lucretius (Rhys 1943)
A.D.	First Century	Petronius	*Ruta* (Rue)	Woods 1962
	First Century	Dioscorides	Numerous plant species	Dioscorides (Gunther 1959)
	23-79	Pliny	*Brassica* (mustard)	Woods 1962
	605-609	Ping-yuan-hon-lun (Chinese text)	*Rhus* vernicifera (Japanese lacquer tree)	Toyama 1918
	923-930	Wamyo-rui-ju-sho (Japanese text)	*Rhus vernicifera*	Toyama 1918
	Tenth Century	Ma Chi (Chinese text)	*Pinellia tubifera*	Smith 1969
	Thirteenth Century	Ibn El Bater (Egypt)	*Ammi majus* (yields psoralen)	El Mofty 1968
	Early Medieval	Al-Samarquandi (Arabian)	*Nigella sativa* (black cummin) *Euphorbia* (spurge)	Levey and Al-Khaledy 1967
	1492-1541	Paracelsus	Tincture of aloes and of hellebore	Kremers and Urdang 1940

A.D. 1535	Ovidio Y Valdes	*Comocladia*, *Metopium* (doctor gum) *Hippomane mancinella* (manchineel)	Pardo-Castello 1923
1594	Shakespeare	*Ruta* (rue)	Romeo and Juliet
1597	Gerard	Numerous	Gerard 1597
1609	Smith	*Toxicodendron*	McNair 1923
1615	Hernandez	*Hura crepitans* (sandbox tree)	Burkill 1935
1645	Digby	*Rosa* (rose)	Macalpine and Hunter 1956
1653	Culpeper	Numerous	Culpeper 1653
1673	Ligon	*Hura crepitans* (sandbox tree)	Woods and Calnan 1976
1674	Zacchia	*Thapsia*, *Clematis*, *Bryonia*, *Euphorbia*, *Taxus*, turpentine	Woods 1962
1678	Esquemeling	Palmae (palms)	Woods 1962
1690	Rumphius	Several	Burkill 1935
1693	Dale	*Humulus* (Hop)	O'Donovan 1924
1700	Ramazzini	Baker's itch, *Arum*, wood dust	Ramazzini 1713
1702	Dudley	*Toxicodendron*	Parish and Haviland 1974
1707	Sloane	*Mucuna pruriens* (cow-hage)	Shelley and Arthur 1955
1712	Kaempfer	Lacquer (*Rhus*)	Noojin 1954
1717	Montagu	Balm of Mecca (*Amyris opobalsamum*)	Woods and Calnan 1976
1719	DeAguilar	*Toxicodendron*	MaNair 1923
1720-21	Dudley	*Toxicodendron*	Rostenberg 1955
1748, 1750	Kalm	*Toxicodendron*	Rostenberg 1955, McNair 1923
1750	Rumphius	*Gluta renghas*	Sprague 1921
1755	Monti	*Toxicodendron*	McNair 1923
1760	de Sauvages	Indian varnish (*Rhus*)	Gray 1955
1763	dePréfontaine	*Anacardium occidentale*, *Simarouba*	dePréfontaine 1763
1774	Anon (Dictionary)	*Clematis vitalba*, *Ranunculus bulbosus* (Buttercup)	Piffard 1881

1777	Plenck	Indian varnish (Rhus)	Gray 1955
1777	Hunold, Gleditsch	Toxicodendron	McNair 1923
1780	Bulliard	Daphne mezereum, Anemone, Chelidonium majus (Celandine), Sedum acre (Stonecrop)	Bulliard 1780
1780	Ackerman	Dusty occupations	Ackerman 1780
1783	Pornai	Toxicodendron	McNair 1923
1784	Chamberlaine	Mucuna pruriens (Cow-hage)	Shelley & Arthur 1955
1786	Achard	Toxicodendron	McNair 1923
1787	Schoepf	Toxicodendron	Schoepf 1787
1787	Schoepf	Hippomane mancinella (manchineel)	Piffard 1881
1787	Fontana	Toxicodendron	White 1934
1788	Du Fresnoy	Toxicodendron	McNair 1923
1794	Barham	Lithraea brasiliensis, L. caustica, Hippomane mancinella (manchineel)	Barham 1794
1795	Fontana	Toxicodendron	McNair 1923
1797	Van Mons	Toxicodendron	McNair 1923
1798-1808	Willan, Bateman	Cashew nut oil (Anacardium) Indian varnish (Rhus) Valeriana, Sugar (Grocer's itch), spices	Adamson 1933 Bateman 1818
1798	Horsfield	Toxicodendron	McNair 1923, Rostenberg 1955
1801-4	Barton	Chimaphila umbellata, Rhus toxicodendron Ranunculus sceleratus, Nerium oleander	Piffard 1881
1801	Grant	Laportea gigas (a nettle)	Cleland 1914, 1925
1804	De Candolle	Ranunculus bulbosus (Buttercup) Daphne gnidium	Piffard 1881
1813-19	Gravmüller	Acontium neomontanum (aconite) Actaea spicata (bugbane) Anemone nemorosa, Bryonia alba (briony) Chelidonium majus (celandine) Ranunculus bulbosus (buttercup) R. acris, R. flammula, R. sceleratus	Piffard 1881

		Plumbago europaea *Anemone nemorosa*, *A. pulsatilla*, *Anemone* spp. *Lepidium sativum* (cress) *Drosera rotundifolia* (sundew) *Erysimum alliaria* *Delphinium staphisagria* *Clematis erecta*, *C. vitalpa* *Veratrum album* (white hellebore)	
1815	Chaumton	*Heracleum* (Cow parsnip)	White 1934
1817	Bigelow	*Phytolacca decandra*, *Rhus venenata*	White 1887, Piffard 1881
1818	Jahn	*Aconitum napellus*	Piffard 1881
1825	Boussingault & Rivero	*Hura crepitans*	Boussingault & Rivero 1825
1825	Jamison	*Laportea* (tree nettle)	Cleland 1925
1826	Frost	*Toxicodendron*	Frost 1826
1826	Zollickkoffer	*Asclepias tuberosa* (butterfly weed) *Bryonia alba*, *Euphorbia corollata*, *Sanguinaria canadensis* (blood root)	Piffard 1881
1828	Pointe	Tobacco	Fischer 1922
1832	Thackrah	Cake dough, sugar, tobacco	White 1934, Schwartz et al 1957
1834	Badham	*Humulus* (hop)	Smithies 1929
1834	Lindley	*Daphne mezereum*	Woods 1962
1834	Anon (Germany)	*Toxicodendron*	Pammel 1911
1835	Rayer	Mustard (*Sinapis*) Cherry laurel oil (*Prunus laurocerasus*)	Rayer 1835
1836	Le Soeuf	*Laportea gigas* (a nettle)	Cleland 1925
1836	Thompson	*Oenanthe crocata* (a fennel)	Piffard 1881
1837	Forcke	*Veratrum viride* (hellebore)	Forcke 1837
1837-8	Roques	*Cochlearia armoracia* (horseradish) *Urtica dioica* and *U. urens* (nettle)	Piffard 1881
1838	Batlett	*Toxicodendron*	McNair 1923

1839	Orfila	Toxicodendron	White 1934
1840	Trinquier	Arundo donax (fungus on reeds)	Fischer 1922
1841-42	Wibmer	Sedum acre (stonewort) Dioscorea alata (yam) Hippomane mancinella (manchineel) Plumbago europea, P. scandens (leadwort) Anemone nemorosa, Arnica montana Arum maculatum (spotted arum) Cereus grandiflora (cactus) Ruta graveolens (rue) Taxus baccata (yew) Urtica dioica and U. urens (nettle) Drosera rotundifolia (sundew)	Piffard 1881
1841	Dierbach	Sinapis alba and S. nigra (mustard) Aconitum (Aconitum napellus) Bryonia alba (briony) Capsicum annuum (Cayenne pepper) Euphorbia resinifera (spurge) Piper nigrum (pepper)	Piffard 1881
1842(?)	Dubreuil	Atropine (Atropa)	Dubreuil (1842?)
1842	Turnbull	Ipecacuanha (Cephaelis ipecacuanha)	Piffard 1881
1842	Hannay	Ipecacuanha (Cephaelis ipecacuanha)	Piffard 1881
1842	Cless	Baker's eczema	Teleky 1948
1844	Stickney	Anacardium occidentale topical application of oil	Stickney 1844
1844	Cazenave	Burgundy pitch (Pinus abies)	Piffard 1881
1845	Worcester	Spices, sugar, grocer's itch	Worcester 1845
1845	Miguel	Arundo donax (fungus on reeds)	Fischer 1922
1845	Leichhardt	Anacardium, Pandanus	Cleland 1925
1845-46	Hamilton	Hippomane mancinella (manchineel)	Hamilton 1845-46
1847	Brown	Grevillea (silky oak)	Leichhardt 1847
1848-55	Strumpf	Scilla maritima (squill), Iris florentina	Piffard 1881

1848	Lee	Maruta cotula (syn. Athemis cotula) Ranunculus bulbosus (buttercup)	Piffard 1881
1849	Popham	Brassica napus (mustard)	Piffard 1881
1851-52	Potton	Silkworm cocoons	Fischer 1922
1852	Thompson (Allen)	Anamirta cocculus	Piffard 1881
1852	Chevallier	Cinchona (quinine)	Fischer 1922
1852	Delioux	Ipecacuanha (Uragoga) (syn. Cephaelis)	Delioux 1852
1853	Duffors	Silkworm cocoons	Fischer 1922
1853	Türk	Arnica montana	Touton 1932
1855	Gerbaud	Fungi of reeds (Arundo)	Woods 1962
1856	Schroff	Juniperus sabina	Piffard 1881
1856	Oesterlen	Sanguinaria	White 1887
1856	Schroff	Scilla maritima (squill)	Piffard 1881
1857	Khittel	Toxicodendron	Broers 1926
1857	Buchheim	Euphorbia (spurge)	Touton 1932
1859	Maurin	Arundo donax (fungus on reeds)	Fischer 1922
1859	Lespian	Coal tar	Schwartz et al 1957
1861	Leon-Soubeiran	Ruta (rue)	Fischer 1922, Piffard 1881
1861	Imbert-Gourbeyre	Orange oil (Citrus)	Fischer 1922
1862	Beaugrand	Tanners' materials	Fischer 1922
1862	Guerard	Atropine (Atropa)	Guerard 1862
1862	Bazin	Classified the known agents of occupational dermatitis	Schwartz et al 1957 (Bazin 1862)
1862	Bentley	Podophyllum peltatum (may-apple)	Bentley 1862
1862	Walker	Aristida, Stipa	Cleland 1914
1863	Kleinhaus	Oil of Cade	Kleinhaus 1863
1864	Maish and Pfaff	Toxicodendron	White 1934
1866	Pereira	Mucuna pruriens (cow hage)	Piffard 1881
1868	Martin	Thapsia garganica (plaster resin)	Martin 1868

1868	Sanders	Toxicodendron	White 1934
1869	Baudot	Ipecacuanha (Uragoga syn. Cephaelis) Oil of cade (Juniperus oxycedrus)	Baudot 1869
1869	Hurlburt	Cypripedium (orchid)	McNair 1923
1870	Nothnagel	Ipecacuanha (Cephaelis), Juniperus communis, Pimpinella anisum (aniseed)	
1870-1887	Numerous authors	Cinchona,(quinine)	Morrow 1887
1871	Traube	Atropine (Atropa)	Traube 1871
1872	Yandell	Toxicodendron	White 1934
1872	Gray	Toxicodendron	McNair 1923
1873	Buchheim	Toxicodendron	White 1934
1874	Husemann	Pix liquida (Pinus palustris and Pinus spp.)	Piffard 1881
1874	Stillé	Croton oil (Croton tiglium) Daphne mezereum	Piffard 1881
1874	Husemann	Oil of Juniper (Juniperus communis)	Piffard 1881
1874	Purdon	Linum usitatissimum (flax)	Piffard 1881
1874	Tilbury Fox	Compound tincture of benzoin (Styrax) inhalation, Tincture of Arnica	Fox 1874
1874	Burness and Mavor	Turpentine	Piffard 1881
1874	Phillips	Conium maculatum, Burgundy pitch (Pinus abies), Anemone pulsatilla, Pimpinella anisum, Cochlearia armoracia, Arnica montana, Cinnamomum camphora, Capsicum annuum, Veratrum, Turpentine	Piffard 1881
1875	White	Tincture of Arnica	Morrow 1887
1875	Behier	Iris florentina	Piffard 1881
1875	Babcock	Cypripedium (an orchid)	White 1887
1875	Eulenburg	Veratrum	Eulenburg 1875
1875	Waring	Plumbago rosea (leadwort)	Piffard 1881
1876	Cantani	Turpentine (Pinus palustris) Thuja occidentalis	Piffard 1881

		(Arbor-vitae), *Anemone pulsatilla* and *Anemone* spp. *Lobelia inflata* (Indian tobacco), *Delphinium staphisagria*, *Euphorbia officinarum* (spurge)	
1876	Ringer	Ipecacuanha (*Cephaelis ipecacuanha*)	Piffard 1881
1876	Cazin	*Anemone nemorosa*, *Ranunculus bulbosus* (buttercup) *Arum maculatum*	Piffard 1881
1876	Guibout	Oil of Cade (*Juniperus oxycedrus*)	Piffard 1881
1876	Köhler	*Ferula galbaniflua* (gum galbanum), ipecacuanha (*Cephaelis ipecacuanha*), *Sinapsis alba* & *S. nigra* (mustard)	Piffard 1881
1876	Allen	*Capsicum* (pepper)	Allen 1876
1876	Köhler	*Scilla maritima* (Squill)	Piffard 1881
1876	Flückiger and Hanbury	*Sanguinaria canadensis* (blood root), *Chelidonium majus* (Celandine)	Piffard 1881
1876	Wood	Ipecacuanha (*Cephaelis ipecacuanha*)	Piffard 1881
1877	Putnam	Atropine (*Atropa*)	Putnam 1877
1877	Earle	*Arnica montana*	Piffard 1881
1878	Kaposi	Goa powder (*Andira*)	Morrow 1887
1878	Jarisch	Pyrogallic acid ointment	Jarisch 1878
1878	Duclaux	Zittwerblüten	Touton 1932
1878	Harnden	*Arnica montana*	Piffard 1881
1879	Poncet	Candied fruits	White 1934
1879	Farquharson	Chrysophanic acid ointment (*Andira*), coal tar	Farquharson 1879
1879	Tournadre	*Thapsia garganica* (plaster resin)	Tournadre 1879, Piffard 1881
1879	Farquharson	Tincture of *Arnica*	Morrow 1887
1879	Wilson	Tincture of *Arnica*	Morrow 1887
1879	Caesar	Atropine (*Atropa*)	Caesar 1879
1879	Phillips	*Capsicum* (cayenne pepper)	Phillips 1879
1879	Parsons	*Linum usitatissimum* (flax)	Piffard 1881

1879	Meyer	Japan wax (*Rhus*)	White 1934
1880	Trousseau	*Thapsia*, Burgundy pitch	Trousseau 1880
1880	Güntz	*Asparagus*	Güntz 1880
1880	Mögling	Peruvian balsam (*Myroxylon*)	Mögling 1880
1880	Blackwood	*Rhus* (poison ivy)	Blackwood 1880
1881	Morrow	*Thapsia garganica* (plaster resin)	Piffard 1881
1881	Porter	Oil of Tansy (*Tanacetum*) by ingestion	Porter 1881
1881	Dierbach	*Aconitum*	Dierbach 1881
?(1881)	Anon	*Caladium seguinum*	Piffard 1881
1881-82	Chislom	Atropine (*Atropa*)	Chislom 1881-82
1881	Piffard	*Viola tricolor*, *Arnica montana*	Piffard 1881
1881	Dierbach	Mustard (*Sinapis*)	Dierbach or Diehrbach 1881
1881(?)	Frost	*Stillingia sylvatica*	Piffard 1881
1882	Baltus	Fungi of reeds (*Arundo*)	Woods 1962
1881	Winterburn	*Podophyllum peltatum* (may-apple)	Winterburn 1882
1882	Lewin	*Anacardium occidentale* (bean used as necklace)	Lewin 1882
1882	Schwerin	*Anacardium occidentale* (bean inserted into ear canal)	Schwerin undated, cited by Morrow 1887, Lewin 1882
1882	Hikosaka	Japanese lacquer (*Rhus*)	Toyama 1918
1883	Kunze	*Toxicodendron*	McNair 1923
1883	Layet	*Vanilla*	Touton 1932
1883	Fialkouski	Atropine (*Atropa*)	Fialkouski 1883
1883	Vellebun	Candied fruits	White 1934
1883	Cundell-Juler, Leonard	*Toxicodendron*	McNair 1923
1884	Cartier	Tincture of *Arnica*	Morrow 1887
1884	Hendrix	Tincture of *Arnica*	Morrow 1887
1884	Cagny	Tincture of *Arnica* (in a horse)	Morrow 1887
1884	Cazenave	Burgundy pitch	Cazenave 1884

1885	Mackintosh	Belladonna (*Atropa*)	Mackintosh 1885
1885	Leloir	Flax (*Linum*)	Touton 1932
1886	de Molènes	Tincture of *Arnica*	Morrow 1887
1886	Allen	Pyrogallic acid ointment	Allen 1886
1886	Williamson	Tannic acid	Williamson 1886
1886	Abbott (Australia)	*Toxicodendron*	Cleland 1914
1886	Maisch, Barnes	*Toxicodendron*	McNair 1923
1886	Garland	Turpentine (*Pinus*) (administration)	Garland 1886
1886	Brocq	Chrysophanic acid ointment (*Andira*)	Brocq 1886
1887	Liebreich	Atropine (*Atropa*)	Leibreich undated, cited by Morrow 1887
1887	Cornevin	*Ailanthus altissima* (Tree of Heaven)	Woods & Calnan 1976
1887	White	100 plant species	White 1887
1887	Morrow	Turpentine (*Pinus*)	Morrow 1887
1887	Cornevin	*Bryonia dioica*, *Clematis vitalba* *Heracleum sphondylium*	Cornevin 1887
1887	Baldwin	*Toxicodendron*	McNair 1923
1887	Morrow	*Rhus toxicodendron*, *R. venenata*, *R. vernix*	Morrow 1887 cites numerous authors
1887	Morrow	Croton oil (*Croton*)	Morrow 1887 cites previous authors
1888	Collins	*Atropa* (atropine)	Collins 1887
1888	White	*Primula obconica*	White 1888, Touton 1932
1889	White	*Primula obconica*	Foerster 1910
1889	White	Boxwood (*Buxus*)	White 1889
1889	Albertin	Candied fruits	Albertin 1889
1889	Oldacres	*Primula obconica*	Oldacres 1889
1890	White	*Primula obconica*	Foerster 1910
1890	Lee	*Primula obconica*	Lee 1890
1890	Sym	*Primula obconica*	Sym 1890
1890	Clarke	*Primula obconica*	Clarke 1890

1890	Ferguson	*Primula obconica*	Ferguson 1890
1890	Rockstro	*Brya ebenus* (cocuswood)	Woods and Calnan 1976
1890	Sabra	Fungus spores on reed (*Arundo donax*)	Sabra 1890
1890	Paschikis	Henna (*Lawsonia*)	Touton 1932
1890	Mankowsky	*Bryonia alba* (Briony)	Touton 1932
1891	Stern	*Brya ebenus* (cocuswood)	Stern 1891
1891	Palm	*Ampelopsis hoggii* (Virginia creeper) in fact probably *Toxicodendron*	Palm 1891, Turton 1925
1891	Prichard (Britain)	*Toxicodendron*	Prichard 1891
1891	Swan	*Primula obconica*	Swan 1891
1891	Southern	*Primula obconica*	Southern 1891
1891	Anon	*Colocasia macrorrhiza*	Cleland 1914
1891	Cantrell	*Toxicodendron*	McNair 1923
1892	Blaschko	Candied fruits, turpentine	Blaschko 1892
1892	Samuel	Croton oil (*Croton*)	Touton 1932
1892	Hutchinson	*Vanilla*	Hutchinson 1892
1893	Ackland	*Primula obconica*	Ackland 1893
1893	Pooley	*Primula obconica*	Pooley 1893
1893	Jamieson	?*Primula*	Jamieson 1893
1893	Ehrhardt	*Narcissus*, *Leucojum*	Touton 1932
1894/95	MacDougal	*Cypripedium* (an orchid)	Touton 1932
1894	Bogue	*Toxicodendron*	McNair 1923
1895	Reihl	*Primula obconica*	White 1934
1895	Maiden	*Inula graveolens* (stinkwort)	Maiden 1895
1895	Grinden	*Ampelopsis quinquefolia* in fact probably *Toxicodendron*	Touton 1932
1896	Murrell	Japanese varnish (*Rhus*), *Primula*	Murrell 1896
1896	Gillett	*Primula obconica*	Gillett 1896
1896	Stott	*Primula obconica*	Stott 1896
1896	Hussmann	*Primula obconica*	White 1934

1896	Billet	Rhus vernicifera (Japanese varnish)	White 1934
1896	Maiden	Xanthium strumarium (cockle burr)	Maiden 1896
1896	Robinson	Atropine (Atropa), Belladonna plaster	Robinson 1896
1896	Müller'	Chrysarobin (Andira)	Touton 1932
1896	Anon	Teak (Tectona)	Lancet 1896
1897	Jamieson	Parsnip (Pastinaca)	Touton 1932
1897	Matignon	Atriplex littoralis	Touton 1932
1897	Arning	Vanilla	Arning 1897
1897	Pfaff, Hunt, Planchon	Toxicodendron	White 1934
1897	Woldo	Primula obconica	Woldo 1897
1898	Frank	Toxicodendron	White 1934
1898	Hudson	Toxicodendron	White 1934
1898	Chestnut	Toxicodendron	White 1934
1898	Dragendorff	Toxicodendron	Hurst 1942
1899	Nicholson (Britain)	Toxicodendron	Nicholson 1899
1899	Scott	Toxicodendron	White 1934
1899	Moebius	Rhus vernicifera	White 1934
1899	Hallopeau	Myroxylon (Peru Balsam)	Cummer 1927
1899	Kirk	Primula obconica	Kirk 1899
1899	Barton	Primula obconica	Barton 1899
1899	Brown	Toxicodendron	White 1934
1899	Lewin	Brassica (mustard)	Woods 1962
1899	Morrison	Phebalium argenteum	Cleland 1914
1899	Cooper	Primula obconica	Cooper 1899
1899	Noyes	Cassinia aculeata	Cleland 1914
1899	Burgenstein	Primula obconica	Burgenstein 1899
1899	Lewin	Mustard oil (Sinapis)	Touton 1932
1899	Pascal	Grain-dust (Gramineae)	Touton 1932
1899	Lewin	Achillea millefolium (milfoil)	Touton 1932

1900	Urban	Loasa (a nettle)	Touton 1932
1900	Urquhart	Croton oil (Croton)	Urquhart 1900
1900	Danlos	Hops (Humulus)	Danlos 1900
1900	Sabouraud	Croton oil (Croton), Thapsia garganica	Touton 1932
1900	Jarisch	Celery (Apium)	Touton 1932
1900-20	Nestler	Primula obconica	Nestler 1900-27
1900	Immerwahr	Toxicodendron	White 1934
1900	Shirasawa	Rhus vernicifera (Japanese varnish)	White 1934
1900	Kobert	Primula obconica	White 1934
1900	Peters	Primula obconica	White 1934
1900	Piza	Primula obconica	White 1934
1900	Munro	Hedera helix (ivy)	Munro 1900

REFERENCES

Ackermann, J.C.G. (1780) B. Ramazzinis Abhandlung von den Krankheiten der Künstler und Handwerker. New ed., revised and enlarged, Stendal.

Ackland, C.K. (1893) Poisoning by Primula obconica. Lancet 2, 289.

Adamson, H.G. (1933) The real position of Willan and Bateman's teaching in regard to eczema. Brit. J. Derm. Syph. 45, 493.

Albertin (1889) Note sur le mal des confiseurs. Gaz. Lebdom. 15 Marz cited by Touton 1932.

Allen (1876) Hughes' Manual of Pharmacodynamics. London p. 247, cited by Morrow, P. (1887) Drug eruptions, A clinical study of the irritant effects of drugs upon the skin. New York. Wm. Wood and Co.

Allen (1886) Journal of Cut. and Ven. Diseases. January cited by Morrow, J. (1887) Drug eruptions. A clinical study of the irritant effects of drugs upon the skin. New York. Wm. Wood and Co.

Arning, Ed. (1897) Dtsch. med. Wschr. 23, 435, cited by Touton 1932.

Barham, H. (1794) Hortus americanus, Kingston Jamaica.

Barton, E.A. (1899) On the effects of Primula obconica on the skin. Lancet 1, 1717.

Blackwood, W.R.D. (1880) Some thoughts on rhus poisoning. Philadelphia med. Tim. 19, 618, cited by Touton 1932.

Burgenstein (1899) Wien. illustr. Gartenbauztg. H.H. cited by Touton 1932

Blaschko (1892) Dermat. Wschr. 7 cited by Touton 1932.

Brown, W.H. (1906) Fatal blood poisoning following a wound by the Primula obconica. Lancet 1, 861.

Bateman, T. (1818) A Practical Synopsis of Cutaneous Diseases, first American edition from the fourth London Edition. Philadelphia. Collins and Croft.

Baudot (1869) Traité des Affect. de la Peau. Paris p. 155, cited by Morrow, P. (1887) Drug eruptions. A clinical study of the irritant effects of drugs upon the skin. New York. Wm. Wood and Co.

Bazin, P. (1862) Lecons Theo. et clinic. sur les affections Cutan. Artificielles. Paris.

Bentley (1862) Pharmaceutical Journ. and Trans. p. 462, cited by Morrow, P. (1887) Drug eruptions. A clinical study of the irritant effects of drugs upon the skin. New York. Wm. Wood and Co.

Bloch, B. (1924) Aetiologie und Pathogenese der Eczems. Arch. f. Derm. 154, 34.

Bloch, B. (1929) The role of idiosyncrasy and allergy in Dermatology. Archs. Derm. Syph. 19, 175.

Boussingault and Rivero (1825) Mémoire sur le lait vénéneus de l'hura crepitans. Annales de chimie et de physique 28, 430.

Brocq (1886) Jour. of Cutaneous and Venereal Diseases. January cited by Morrow, J. (1887) Drug eruptions. A Clinical study of the irritant effects of drugs upon the skin. New York. Wm. Wood and Co.

Bulliard, P. (1780) Histoire des Plantes Vénéneuses et Suspectes de la France. 2nd ed. Paris. A.J. Dugour.

Burkill, I.H. (1935) A Dictionary of the Economic Products of the Malay Peninsula. 2 Vols. London. Crown Agents for the Colonies.

Caesar, Julius (1879) Unusual effects of belladonna. Lancet 1, 431.

Cash, J.T. (1911) The dermatitis produced by East Indian Satinwood (Chloroxylon swietenia). Brit. Med. J. 2, 784.

Cazenave (1884) Annal. des Mal. de la Peau et Syph. p. 210, cited by Morrow, P. (1887) Drug eruptions. A clinical study of the irritant effects of drugs upon the skin. New York Wm. Wood and Co.

Chislom (1881-82) Maryland Med. Journal p. 375, cited by Morrow, J. (1887) Drug eruptions. A clinical study of the irritant effects of drugs upon the skin. New York. Wm. Wood and Co.

Chopra, R.N. and Chopra, I.C. (1955). A review of Work on Indian Medicinal Plants including Indigenous Drugs and Poisoning Plants. Indian Coun. Med. Res. Spec. Rep. Ser. No. 30, New Delhi.

Clarke F. H. (1890). Eczema caused by Primula obconica. Brit. Med. J. 2, 789.

Cleland, J.B. (1914). Plants, including fungi, poisonous or otherwise injurious to man in Australia Med. J. Australia 34, 554 and 570

Cleland, J.B. (1925) Plants including fungi, poisonous or otherwise injurious to man in Australia (Series II). Med. J. Australia 2, 443.

Collins E.T. (1888). Atropine irritation. Royal Ophth. Hosp. Rep. 12, 164.

Cooper, B. (1899) A case of poisoning by the Primula obconica. Brit. Med. J. 2, 1543.

Cornevin, C. (1887) Des Plantes Vénéneuses et des Empoisonments qu'elles déterminent. Paris. Firmin-Didot.

Culpeper, N. (1653) The Complete Herbal. Reprinted 1953, by Imperial Chemical (Pharmaceuticals) Ltd. Birmingham. The Kynoch Press.

Cummer, C.L. (1927) Dermatitis produced by Balsam of Peru. Archs Derm Syph 16, 44.

Dale, A.S. (1693) Pharmacologia Londini p. 133, cited by Touton 1932.

Danlos, M. (1900) Eczéma artificiel provoqué par le houblon. Ann. de Dermat. IV. s. 1, 392 cited by Touton 1932.

Dawson, W.R. (1929) The Origin of the Herbal. Aegyptus 10, 47.

Delioux (1852) Gazette Medicale de Paris. No. 6, cited by Morrow, P. (1887) Drug eruptions.

A clinical study of the irritant effects of drugs upon the skin. New York. Wm. Wood and Co.

Dierbach quoted by Piffard (1881) A treatise on the Materia Medica and Therapeutics of the skin. New York. Wm. Wood and Co.

Dioscorides, The Greek Herbal of: Englished by John Goodyer: A.D. 1655. Edited and first printed A.D. 1933 by R.T. Gunther 1959. New York Hafner Publishing Co.

Dubreuil (?1842) Journ. de Medicine p. 190 cited by Morrow, P. (1887) Drug eruptions, A clinical study of the irritant effects of drugs upon the skin. New York. Wm. Wood and Co.

Dulake, L. (1977) The Doctor's Tale 1662-1975. Published by the author. Redhill, Surrey.

Eulenburg (1875) Die Hypodermat. Injectionen. Berlin p. 278 cited by Morrow, P. (1887) Drug eruptions. A clinical study of the irritant effects of drugs upon the skin. New York. Wm. Wood and Co.

Farquharson, R. (1879) Various forms of skin irritations due to the administration of drugs. Brit. Med. J. 1, 223 and 266.

Ferguson, J. (1890) The Primula obconica. Brit. Med. J. 2, 954 (or 955).

Fialkouski (1883) Le Med. Practicien. Sept. p. 454 cited by Morrow, P. (1887) Drug eruptions. A clinical study of the irritant effects of drugs upon the skin. New York. Wm. Wood and Co.

Fischer, Joseph. History of the Occupational Dermatoses in Ullmann, Oppenheim, and Rille. "Injuries of the skin due to Professional and Industrial Work". Die Schädigungen der Haut durch Beruf und gewerbliche Arbeit. Leipzig 1922.

Foerster, O.H. (1910) Primula dermatitis. JAMA 55, 642

Forcke (1837) Physiol. u. Therapeut. Untersuch. über d. Veratrin. Hanover cited by Morrow, P. (1887) Drug eruptions. A clinical study of the irritant effects of drugs upon the skin. New York. Wm. Wood and Co.

Fox, T. (1874) Purpura urticans produced by inhalation of Friar's balsam. Lancet 1, 195.

Frost, J. (1826) Remarks on the erysipelatous inflammation produced by the juice of Rhus toxicodendron. London Medical and Physical Journal 55, 116.

Gardiner, F. (1922): Occupational dermatitis. Brit. J. Derm. Syph. 34: 297-320.

Garland (1886) Terebene rash. Lancet 1, 1005.

Gerard J. (1636) The Herball or Generall Historie of Plantes. The essence thereof distilled by M. Woodward (1927) from the edition of Th. Johnson 1630. London. Gerald Howe.

Gillett, J.F. (1896) The Poison of the Primula. Lancet 1, 1040.

Gray, A. (1955) The founders of modern Dermatology. Transactions and reports St. John's Hospital Dermatological Society. 35, 1

Grieve, M. (1970) A Modern Herbal. Darien, Conn. Hafner Publishing Co.

Guerard (1862) Des Erupt. Pathogénét. Thèse de Paris cited by Morrow, P. (1887) Drug eruptions. A clinical study of the irritant effects of drugs upon the skin. New York. Wm. Wood and Co.

Gunther, R.T. (1959) The Greek Herbal of Dioscorides. New York. Hafner.

Güntz, J.E. (1880) Miliaria - Ausschlag in Folge var Berührung mit roham Spargel (Asparagus officinalis) Vierteljahresschrift für dermatologie und Syphilis 7, 65.

Hall, A.J. (1921) The skin and its reactions. Lancet 1, 426.

Hamilton, W. (1845-46) On the properties of the Hippomane mancinella, or Manchineel Tree.

Pharmaceutical Journal 5, 408.

Hance, H.F. (1880) Stirpium duranum novarum e Primulacearum familia characteres. Journal of Botany 18, 234.

Hunt, E. (1931). A case of teakwood dermatitis. Lancet 1, 75.

Hurst, E. (1942) The Poison Plants of New South Wales. N.S.W. Poison Plants Committee; Sydney.

Hutchinson, J. (1892) An eruption caused by Vanilla. Arch. Surg. 4, 49.

Jadassohn, J. (1895) Zur Kenntniss der Medicamentösen Dermatosen. (Fifth German Dermatological Congress, Graz) Verh. Deutsch. Dermat. Ges. graz, cited by Rostenberg (1968).

Jadassohn, J. (1896) Zur Kenntniss der Medicamentösen Dermatosen, V. Deutscher Dermatologischen Kongress, Vienna. Wilhelm Braumueller.

Jadassohn, J. (1896) Zur Kenntniss der Arzweiexanthenei, Arch. Derm. u. Syph. 34, 103.

Jadassohn, J. (1904) Hautkrankheiten bei Stoffwechselanomalien. Fifth Internat. Dermat. Kong. Berlin 2, 231.

Jadassohn, J. (1923) Sensitization and desensitization in eczema. Klin. Wchnschr. 2, 1734.

Jamieson (1893) Brit. J. Derm. 5, 140 (untraced, not Brit. Med. J. nor Lancet).

Jarisch (1879) (Wiener. Med. Jahrbucher H. IV cited by Morrow, J. (1887) Drug eruptions. A clinical study of the irritant effects of drugs upon the skin. New York. Wm. Wood and Co.

Kaposi (1878) Wiener Med. Wochenschrift. No. 44 cited by Morrow, P. (1887) Drug eruptions. A clinical study of the irritant effects of drugs upon the skin. New York. Wm. Wood and Co.

Kesten, B. and Laszlo, E. (1931) Dermatitis due to sensitisation to contact substances. Dermatitis venenata, occupational dermatitis. Archs. Derm. Syph. 23, 221.

Kirk, R. (1899) On acute affections of the skin and mucous membrane of the mouth in an early stage of myxoedema. Primula obconica an alleged exciting cause in one case. Lancet 1, 579.

Kirk, R. (1899) On the effects of Primula obconica on the skin. Lancet 1, 1630.

Klaber, R. (1942) Phyto-photodermatitis. Brit. J. Dermat. 54, 193.

Kleinhaus (1863) Allg. Med. Cent. Zeit. No. 24, cited by Morrow, P. (1887) Drug eruptions. A clinical study of the irritant effects of drugs upon the skin. New York. Wm. Wood and Co.

Kremers, E. and Urdang, G. (1940) History of Pharmacy. Philadelphia Lippincott.

Lancaster, A.H. (1937) Clematis dermatitis. Southern Medical Journal 30, 207.

Lancet (1896) Letters 1, 1113, I, 1265.

Lane, J.E. (1933) Joseph Jacob Plenck 1738?-1807. Archs. Derm. Syph 28, 193.

Laszlo, H.G. de (1958) Library of Medicinal Plants Collected by Henry G. de Laszlo. Cambridge. W. Heffer and Sons. 56pp.

Lee, C.N. (1890) Eczema caused by Primula obconica. Brit. Med. J. 2, 790.

Leichardt, L. (1847) Journal of an overland expedition in Australia from Moreton Bay to Port Essington 1844-1845. London. Cited by Hurst (1942).

Levin, O.L. (1924) Dermatitis venenata from the lacquer on the boxes of Mah Jongg sets. JAMA 82, 465

Levin, O.L. (1933) Sawdust dermatitis. JAMA 100, 570

Levey, M. and Al-Khaledy, N., (1967) The Medical Formulary of Al-Samarqandi and the relation of early Arabic simples to those found in the indigenous medicine of the Near East and India. Philadelphia. University of Pennsylvania Press.

Lewin, L. (1882) The Incidental Effects of Drugs. New York., cited by Morrow, P. (1887) Drug eruptions. A clinical study of the irritant effects of drugs upon the skin. New York. Wm. Wood and Co.

Lonkar, A., Mitchell, J.C. and Calnan, C.D. (1974) Contact Dermatitis from Parthenium hysterophorus. The Transactions St. John's Hospital Dermatological Society. 60, 43.

Macalpine, I. and Hunter, R.A. (1956) A case of true allergy establshed by patch testing and reported by Sir Kenelme Digby in 1645. Brit. J. Derm. 68, 61

Mackintosh, M. (1885) Herpes after external use of belladonna and atropine. British Medical Journal 2, 739.

McNair, J.B. (1923) Rhus dermatitis from Rhus, Toxicodendron radicans and diversiloba (Poison Ivy). Its Pathology and chemotherapy. Chicago Univ. Chicago Press.

McNair, J.B. (1921) Pathology of Rhus dermatitis. Archives of Dermatology and Syphilogy 3, 383, cites many early references.

Maiden, J.H. (1895) Stink wort (Inula graveolens Desf.) Ag. Gaz. New South Wales 6, 667.

Maiden, J.H. (1896) The cockle burr (Xanthium strumarium L.) Ag. Gaz. New South Wales 7, 421.

Malten, K.E. (1972) The gap between clinical observation and scientific explanation. Nijmegen Dekker and Van de Vegt.

Markley, A.J. (1920) Anaphylactoid dermatitis due to direct contact with animal epidermal structures. Archs. Derm. Syph. 2, 723.

Martin (1868) Bull.Gen. de Therapeutique p. 170, cited by Morrow, P. (1887) Drug eruptions. A clinical study of the irritant effects of drugs upon the skin. New York. Wm. Wood and Co.

El Mofty, A.M. (1968) Vitiligo and Psoralens. Oxford. Pergamon Press. 234 pp.

Mögling (1880) Berlinger Klin. Wochenschrift. p. 557, cited by Morrow, P. (1887) Drug eruptions. A clinical study of the irritant effects of drugs upon the skin. New York. Wm. Wood and Co.

Morrow, Prince (1887) Drug eruptions. A clinical study of the irritant effects of drugs upon the skin. New York. Wm. Wood and Co.

Munro, W.J. (1900) A case of dermatitis venenata arising from a rare cause. Austr. Med. Gaz. 19, 25.

Munz, P.A. (1932) Dermatitis produced by Phacelia, (Hydrophyllaceae). Science 76, 194.

Murrell, W. (1896) The poison of the primula. Lancet 1, 1040.

Nestler, A. (1900) The irritant effect on the skin of Primula obconica Hance and Primula sinensis Lindl. Ber. d. Botan. Gesellsch 18, 189.

Nestler, A. (1904) Hautreizende Primeln. Gebr. Bornträger Verlag, Berlin.

Nestler, A. (1927) Zur Kenntnis der Primeldermatitis. Med. Klinik 23, 315.

Nicholson, F. (1899) A case of acute dermatitis caused by handling the Rhus toxicodendron. Brit. Med. J. 1, 530.

Nissen, C., (1958) Herbals of Five Centuries. Zurich. L'Art Ancien S.A. Antiquariat. Signawstrasse 6 Zurich 8. Switzerland.

Noojin, R.O. (1954) Brief history of Industrial Dermatology. Arch. Derm. Syph. 70, 723.

O'Donovan, W.J. (1924) Hop dermatitis. Lancet 2, 597.

Oldacres, C.E. (1889) Toxic symptoms produced by handling Primula obconica. Brit. Med. J. 2, 719 (Sept. 28). (refers to Gardener's Chronicle of Aug. 3 last).

Oppenheim, M. (1926) Discussion at the meeting of the Viennese Dermatological Society, (Oct. 20).

Orfila, M.J.B., (1814-15) Traité des Poisons tirés des Règnes minéral végétal et animal... 2 tom. Paris.

Palm, S. (1891) Eczema by Virginia creeper. Lancet 1, 142.

Pammell, L.H. (1911) A manual of Poisonous plants. Torch Press. Cedar Rapids, Iowa. Reprinted Univ. Microfilms Inc. Ann Arbor, Mich 1965.

Pardo-Castello, V. (1923) Skin Diseases in the New World. From Oviedo Y. Valdes, 1478-1557. Archs. Derm. Syph. 28, 22

Parish, L.C. and Haviland, T.N. (1974) The Saga of Poison Ivy. Trans. Stud. College Physicians, Philadelphia, 42, 88 (4th series)

Pepys, Samuel, The Diary of (1660-1669) 9 vol. ed. Latham, R. and Matthews, Wm. 1970-76. London, G. Bell and Sons.

Pfaff, F. (1897) On the active principle of Rhus toxicodendron and Rhus venenata. J. Exp. Med. 2, 181

Phillips (1879) Mat. Med. and Therapeutics New York p. 49, cited by Morrow, P. (1887) Drug eruptions A clinical study of the irritant effects of drugs upon the skin. New York. Wm. Wood and Co.

Piffard, H.G. (1881) A treatise on the Materia Medica and Therapeutics of the skin. New York. Wm. Wood and Co.

Pooley, E.B. (1893) Poisoning by Primula obconica. Lancet 2, 195.

Porter (1881) New York Medical Journal Oct. 15, cited by Morrow, P. (1887) Drug eruptions. A clinical study of the irritant effects of drugs upon the skin. New York Wm. Wood and Co.

Potton (1851-52) Mal de vers. Bull Acad. Med. 17, 803 cited by White 1887.

de Préfontaine (1763) Maison rustique, à l'usage de Cayenne. pp. 139, 152, 208-209. Paris, Bauche.

Prichard, A.W. (1891) Ivy dermatitis. Bristol Medico-Chirurgical Journal 9, 22.

Putnam (1877) Boston Med. and Surg. Journ. p. 142, cited by Morrow (1887) Drug eruptions. A clinical study of the irritant effects of drugs upon the skin. New York. Wm. Wood and Co.

Ramazzini, B., (1713) De Morbis Artificum. Bernardini Ramazzini (1633-1714). Diatriba. The Latin text of 1713, revised by Wright, W.C. 1940. The University of Chicago Press History of Medicine Series. No. 7. Library of the New York Academy of Medicine.

Rayer, (1835) Traité Théor. et Prat. des Mal. de la Peau. Paris p. 262, cited by Morrow, P. (1887) Drug eruptions. A clinical study of the irritant effects of drugs upon the skin. New York. Wm. Wood and Co.

Reihl (1895) On dermatitis from touching a Primula. Wien. Klin. Wochenschr p. 197 cited by White (1934)

Rhys, E. (1943) Lucretius 1st Cent. B.C. Of the Nature of Things. London. J.M. Dent. Bk. 6, 738.

Robinson, T. (1896) A case of cutaneous antipathy to atropine Lancet 2, 881

Rostenberg, A. Jr. (1955) An anecdotal biographical history of poison ivy. Archs. Derm. 72, 438.

Rostenberg, A. and Sulzberger, M.B. (1939). List of substances for patch testing and the concentration to be employed. J. Invest. Derm. 2, 93.

Rostenberg, A., Jr. and Solomon, L.M.

(1968). Jean Henri Fabre and the patch test. Archs. Derm. 98, 188.

Sabra (1890) Dermatite causata dalla spore di una ustilaginee, cited by Arch. f. Dermat. 22, 248, cited by Touton 1932

Schoepf Io. Davidis (1787) Materia medica americana potissimum regni vegetablis. Erlangae: sumtibus Joh. Jac. Palmii. Bulletin No. 6: Reproduction Series No. 3 by Lloyd J.U. and Lloyd C.G. (1903) Bulletin of the Lloyd Library of Botany, Pharmacy and Materia Medica. Cincinnati, Ohio.

Schwartz, L., Tulipan, L. and Birmingham, D.J. (1957) Occupational Diseases of the Skin. 3rd ed. Philadelphia. Lea and Febiger

Senear, F.E. (1933) Dermatitis due to woods. JAMA 101, 1527.

Sharpe, H.A. (1912) Primula dermatitis. Its occurrence in rural districts. JAMA 59, 2148.

Shaw, H.K.A. (1973) A Dictionary of the Flowering Plants and Ferns. (the late J.C. Willis) 8th. ed. Cambridge University Press.

Shelmire, B. (1939) Contact Dermatitis from Weeds; Patch Testing with Their Oleoresins. JAMA 113: 1085.

Shelmire, B. (1940) Contact Dermatitis from Vegetation; Patch Testing and Treatment with Plant Oleoresins. South. M. J. 33:337.

Shelley, W.B. and Arthur R.P. (1955) Studies on Cowhage (Mucuna pruriens) and its pruritogenic properties. Archs. Derm. 72, 399.

Simpson, C.A. (1917) Primrose dermatitis and its relation to anaphylaxis. JAMA 69, 95.

Smith, F.P. (1969) Chinese Materia Medica. Vegetable Kingdom 2nd ed. Rev. by Hei, P.D. Taipei, Taiwan. Ku T'ing Book House.

Smithies, B.M. (1929) The occupational diseases of hop-picking Lancet 2, 494.

Southern, G. (1891) Urticaria due to Primula obconica. Lancet 1, 112.

Sprague, T.A. (1921) Plant dermatitis. Journal of Botany 59, 308.

Stern, E. (1891) Über einige Hautkrankheiten der Musicker: ein Beitrag zu den professionellen Dermatosen. München. med. Wchnschr. 38, 739.

Stickney (1844) The Medical Examiner. Philadelphia p. 133, cited by Morrow, P. (1887) Drug eruptions. A clinical study of the irritant effects of drugs upon the skin. New York. Wm. Wood and Co.

Stott, F.W.A. (1896) The Poison of the Primula. Lancet 1, 1040.

Sulzberger, M.B. and Wise, F. (1931) Contact or patch test in Dermatology; its uses, advantages and limitations. Archs. Derm. Syph. 23, 519.

Swan, S.A.L. (1891) Poisonous properties of Primula obconica Lancet 1, 960.

Sym, A.C. (1890) Eczema caused by Primula obconica. Brit. Med. J. 2, 686.

Teleky, L. (1948) History of Factory and Mine Hygiene. New York Columbia University Press. pg. 342.

Tournadre (1879) Thèse de Paris No. 224, cited by Morrow, P. (1887) Drug eruptions. A clinical study of the irritant effects of drugs upon the skin. New York. Wm. Wood and Co.

Touton, K. (1932) Hauterkrankungen durch phanerogamische Pflanzen und ihre Produkte (Toxicodermia et Allergodermia phytogenes), in Barnewitz, J. et al Angeborene Anomalien, Lichtdermatosen, Pflanzengifte, Thermische Schädigungen, Einfluss Innerer Störungen auf die Haut. Berlin, Verlag von Julius Springer.

Toyama, I. (1918) Rhus dermatitis J. Cut. Dis. 36, 157.

Traube (1871) Beitr. zu Phys. u. Path. 2, 163, cited by Morrow, P. (1887) Drug eruptions. A clinical study of the irritant effects of drugs upon the skin. New York. Wm. Wood and Co.

Trousseau (1880) A Treatise on Therapeutics. New York. Vol. 1 p. 272 and 288, cited by Morrow, P. (1887) Drug eruptions. A clinical study of the irritant effects of drugs upon the skin. New York. Wm. Wood and Co.

Turton, P.H.J. (1925) Poisoning by ivy. British Medical Journal 2, 294.

Underwood, G.B. and Gaul, I.E. (1948) Overtreatment dermatitis in dermatitis venenata due to plants. JAMA 138, 570

Urquhart, A.R. (1900) Skin eruptions consequent on administration of croton oil. British Medical Journal 1, 633.

White, J.E. (1875) Ivy poisoning Boston Med. Surg. J. 93, 265-267

White, J.C. (1887) Dermatitis venenata. An account of external irritants upon the skin. Boston Cupples and Hurd.

White, J.E. (1888) Primula. Note in Garden and Forest 2, 94 (5 May).

White, J.C. (1889) Some unusual forms of dermatitis venenata. Boston medico-surgical Journal 121, 583

White, R.P. (1934) The Dermatergoses or Occupational affections of the skin 4th ed. London. H.K. Lewis and Co.

Williamson (1886) The Practitioner. July p. 37. cited by Morrow, J. (1887) Drug eruptions. A clinical study of the irritant effects of drugs upon the skin. New York Wm. Wood and Co.

Winterburn (1882) Louisville Med. News Apr. 21, cited by Morrow, P. (1887) Drug eruptions. A clinical study of the irritant effects of drugs upon the skin. New York. Wm. Wood and Co.

Woldo (1897) The poisoning by the Primula. Lancet 1, 1539, cited by Touton (1932) but not Lancet.

Woods, B. (1962) Irritant Plants. Transactions and reports St. John's Hospital Dermatological Society 48, 75.

Woods, B. and Calnan, C.D. (1976) Toxic Woods. Brit. J. Derm. 94, Suppl. 13, June.

Worcester, N. (1845) A Synopsis of the symptoms, diagnosis and treatment of the more common and important Diseases of the Skin. Philadelphia. Thomas Cowperthwirt Co.

Wren, R.W. (1968) Potter's New Cyclopaedia of Botanical Drugs and Preparations by Wren, R.C. Re-edit. by Wren, R.W., Potter and Clarke Ltd. Health Science Press. Rustington, Sussex.

The Doctrine of Signatures.

'Though Sin and Sathan have plunged mankinde into an Ocean of Infirmities, yet the mercy of God which is over all his workes, maketh Grasse to grow upon the Mountaines, and Herbes for the use of men, and hath not only stamped upon them a distincte forme, but also given them particular Signatures, whereby a man may reade, even in legible characters, the use of them' . (Coles 1687).

Coles, William, (1687).
The Art of Simpling.

It became doctrine that if a plant resembled a body organ (for example, Hepatics (Family Jubulaceae) and the liver), then the plant was helpful for treatment of diseases of that organ.

Adverse Reactions to Plants (Phytodermatitis)

The causes of adverse human skin reactions to plants can be summarized as follows:

1. Mechanical injury, e.g. from a spine.

2. Toxicological effects, e.g. alkaloidal poisoning from wood dust of Gonioma (family Apocynaceae).

3. Pharmacological effects, e.g. histamine, acetylcholine liberation by stinging hair of nettle, Urtica (family Urticaceae).

4. Contact dermatitis by irritancy. Chemical, e.g. from Euphorbia, (family Euphorbiaceae), or mechanical and chemical, e.g. granuloma from Opuntia (family Cactaceae).

5. Contact dermatitis by immunological effects. Immediate hypersensitivity (endogenous or contact urticaria), e.g. from Agave (family Agavaceae).

   Delayed hypersensitivity e.g. from Toxicodendron (family Anacardiaceae).

   (Epiphytodermatitis. Lichens and liverworts, Frullania (family Jubulaceae), can cause dermatitis which has incorrectly been attributed to trees such as oak, Quercus, family Fagaceae, and 'cedar', Thuja (family Cupressaceae), on which these epiphytic plants reside.)

6. Phytophotodermatitis. Evoked by linear furanocoumarins (psoralens) of some plants (Umbelliferae, Leguminosae, Rutaceae, etc.) and exposure of the skin to long-wave ultra-violet light (350 nm).

7. Pseudophytophotodermatitis. The skin lesions of phytophotodermatitis evoked by psoralen-containing plants can be mimicked by lesions produced by plant irritants with an added effect from sunburn (290-320 nm).

8. Pseudophytodermatitis. This term has been used for skin reactions such as those produced by the mite, Carpoglyphus on figs, Ficus (family Moraceae), by Schistoma infestation in growers of rice, Oryza (family Gramineae) and by contact with agricultural fungicides, pesticides, etc.

9. Parasitophytodermatitis, e.g. dermatitis produced by fungi parasitic on Arundo (family Gramineae).

10. Parasitophytophotodermatitis, e.g. the effects of the fungus Sclerotinia, parasitic on celery Apium (family Umbelliferae), which, in the parasitised state, yields psoralens which can evoke photodermatitis.

11. Heterophytodermatitis. This term might be suitable for the results of presently ill-defined biological phenomena such as the skin effects of chemical compounds, derived from plants, which become incorporated into other plants and render the recipient plants injurious to the skin.

12. Plant-animal dermatitis. Interactions of insects and plants can occur by which chemical compounds of plants, e.g. cucurtibacins and glucosinolates can act as insect 'hormones', and by which chemical compounds of insects influence the chemical constitution of plants. Such aspects of chemical ecology require investigation in respect to possible effects on humans.

"...the hony is too deare that is lickt from thorns",
(Gerard 1653).

MECHANICAL INJURY BY PLANTS

Some irritant, toxic, allergic and pharmacological effects of injury.

Mechanical injury by plants may be divided for convenience into the categories: trauma: injury with chemical irritation by plant juices: injury with allergic sensitization to plant juices or retained plant tissues: and injury with pharmacological effects from plant chemicals. A sharp distinction between these effects can not always be made.

Trauma and Micro-trauma

Trauma is the predominant cause of industrial illness amongst forest-workers who fall trees. In the sawmill, injury by slivers (splinters) of wood is an occupational hazard; bacterial infection can ensue. In the factory, sawdust can produce micro-trauma; irritation and sensitization can occur (Hanslian and Kadlec 1964, Zafiropoulo et al 1968).

Cuts

Cladium mariscus, (Razor Grass), and some other Sedges have long knife-like leaves armed with small sharp teeth. The stems of Tetracera affinis are covered with strong cutting hairs. In southern Africa, a spear or a thorn of Scolopia ecklonii var. engleri, to which has been applied the powdered root of a caper, Capparis tomentosa, is used to make incisions in the chest in ritual treatment of pneumonia (Watt and Breyer-Brandwijk 1962).

References

Hanslian, L. and Kadlec, K. (1964) Woods and wood dusts. Pracov. Lek 16, 276.

Watt, J.M. and Breyer-Brandwijk, M.G. (1962). The Medicinal and Poisonous Plants of Southern and Eastern Africa. Edinburgh. Livingstone

Zafiropoulo A, Audibert, A. and Charpin, J. (1968). Concerning accidents due to the handling of exotic woods. Rev. franc. Allerg. 8, 155.

Blunt Injury

Couroupita guianensis, (Cannon-Ball Tree) forms so large fruits as to prevent its use on roadsides (Corner 1952). The fruits of Treculia africana, (African Bread-fruit Tree) attain 45 cm. in diameter and up to 13 kg. in weight (Dalziel 1955). At Miami Beach, the coconuts are left upon the palm trees as a tourist attraction but, since a group of coconuts can weigh 6 or 7 kg., they are removed during a hurricane alert. In 1973, a two year old girl was killed and her 26 year old aunt was injured in a hail of 57 coconuts falling from a palm, 15 metres high, in Waikiki, Honolulu.

Durio zibethinus, (Durian) has a round or egg-shaped fruit, weighing up to 5 kg. and covered with stout, thickly set, sharp-pointed spines over one cm. long. These fruits, when they fall from the tree, are a hazard to passers-by; they give off a most disagreeable odour but have a delicious taste. Monodora myristica, (False Nutmeg) of the Annonaceae (Custard-Apple) family which grows to a height of 25 metres, produces very hard, woody, smooth, black globular fruits up to 30 cm. in diameter (Menninger 1967); the seeds are sometimes used as nutmegs (Myristica fragrans, Myristicaceae), (Shaw 1973). It is said to be dangerous to walk over the rotten taproot of Adansonia digitata, (Baobab), because one can drop down into the large cavity filled with decaying pulp (Irvine 1961). The juice of Saponaria vaccaria, a Soapwort of the Caryophyllaceae family, is slippery and when trod upon is apt to cause a fall; one of the Chinese princes forbade its being grown in the palace grounds (Smith 1969). The fruit skin of Musa (Banana) has a similar property. Sir Isaac Newton (1642-1727), was inspired to formulate the Law of Gravitation when he was struck on the head by a falling apple. Albizia falcata Batai tree) of the Pea family (Leguminosae) is one of the quickest growing trees in the world. The wood is soft, the root-system shallow and the crown large, consequently the full-grown tree is very apt to be blown down or damaged by wind. On this account it is not used as a roadside tree in Malaya (Corner 1952).

The dried seed of the edible Pea, Pisum sativum, is hygroscopic: attempts to syringe out a pea retained in the auditory canal give rise to severe pain owing to swelling of the plant tissue. In former times, an issue pea was placed in a surgical incision or artificial ulcer, known as an issue, to keep up irritation and so promote discharge (Treves 1923).

References

Corner, E.J.H. (1952) Wayside

Trees of Malaya. Singapore. Government Printer.

Dalziel, J.M. (1955) The useful plants of West Tropical Africa. London. Crown Agents for Oversea Governments and Administrations pg. 286.

Irvine, F.E. (1961) Woody plants of Ghana. London. Oxford University Press.

Menninger, E.A. (1967) Fantastic trees. New York. Viking Press pg. 69 and 84.

Shaw, H.K.A. (1973) A dictionary of the flowering plants and ferns. 8th ed. (The late J.C. Willis). Cambridge University Press. pg. 757.

Smith, F.P. (1969) Chinese Materia Medica. Vegetable Kingdom. 2nd. ed. Rev. by Hei, P.D. Taipei, Taiwan. Ku T'ing Book House.

Treves, F. (1923) The Elephant Man and other reminiscences. London, Cassell. pg. 55.

Occupational Marks

Certain occupations produce hallmarks or occupational stigmata.

Palm tree climbers in Nigeria develop fissured soles (Marshall 1964). 'Palm climbers' lumbar pads' are produced by the friction of knotted sappy cane as the climber hoists himself up the palm tree.

The friction of rattan rope over the outer surfaces of the arms produces hyperkeratosis known as 'Wine-tapper's arm'. The hyperkeratosis is usually accompanied by some hyperpigmentation and dermal fibrosis. Some forms of epidermal and dermal reaction to mechanical friction appear to be accelerated or intensified by tertiary yaws (Browne 1971).

The stripped stems of *Calamus* spp. (Palmae) named Rattan canes are used for making baskets; the hands of the workers develop painful longitudinal fissures of the palms; fungus infection of the canes was implicated (White 1934).

Workers who dehusk rice (*Oryza*, Gramineae) by rubbing it between their hands develop a characteristic type of callosity of the skin of the hypothenar eminence, over the first metacarpal bone and of the tips of the fingers (Diniz 1954).

Of 255 farmers examined, 58 displayed helioderma simplex of the left hand following continued use of a wood 'Glove' during harvesting (Despotov 1966). Infiltration of the subcutaneous tissue with cyanosis and atrophy of the skin of the forearms, more often the left, and of the buttocks from pressure contact with benches and hard stools were noted in 275 of 400 workers (Krasnopeeva and Tsukker 1962). Similar effects are seen from prolonged kneeling on hard surfaces in some persons and the disorder has been termed 'Nun's knees'. From sharpening millstones with a chipping hammer, millers can develop metal tattoos of the forearms, the 'Miller's sign' (Katzschmann 1965). 'Coal-miner's tattoo' is produced by particles of coal in the dermis. 'Colliers' stripes' were described by Bettley (1940). Plant potters show ulnar deviation of the proximal interphalangeal joints of the index fingers (Cohen 1947). 'Landscape gardeners' knuckles' are callosities caused by leaning on clenched fists in order to weed (Ronchese 1948).

'String-maker's thigh' is produced by the rolling of clay-moistened raffia (*Raphia* spp., Palmae) over the anterior surface of the thigh. 'Grass-cutters knee-elbow fibrosis', which is left-sided in the right-handed, is characterized by a long oval area of thickened skin just above the knee and a corresponding area over the elbow point (Browne 1971).

A Viola player developed pronounced callus formation on the tips of the fingers, from the string, on the thumb which guided the bow and on the skin of the chin and clavicular area on which the Viola rested (Leider and Golomb 1964). Acneform eruptions on the jawline (Ronchese 1947) and dermatitis from resin dust can occur in violinists (Beinhauer 1927).

Women working with apples (*Malus* sp.) and pears (*Pyrus* sp.) can develop painful swelling and immobility of the flexed fingers with hyperkeratosis and fissuring (Szego 1966).

'Crocodile hand' was a term used for the thickening of the skin which ultimately deformed the hands of labourers who sawed Chestnut wood, *Castanea* sp., Fagaceae; probably, tannins in the bark added to the mechanical effects, (Horand 1907).

In Hawaii, 'Carry Cane Ear' results from repeated injury to the pinna by bundles of Sugar cane, *Saccharum* sp., Gramineae. The disorder is unilateral according to the 'handedness' of the worker and resembles the 'Cauliflower Ear' of boxers (Ronchese 1947).

References

Beinhauer, L.G. (1927) Resin dermatitis. JAMA 81, 896

Bettley, F.R. (1940) Colliers' stripes - The coal-miners' dermatosis. Brit. J. Derm. 52, 159.

Browne, S.G. (1971) Skin diseases in the tropics in Modern Trends in Dermatology - 4. ed. Borrie P. London. Butterworths pg. 259-283.

Cohen, H. (1947) The hand of the plant potter: a stigma of the market gardener. Brit. J. Industr. Med. 4, 62

Despotov, B. (1966) Helioderma simplex in farmers. Dermatol. I. Venereol. 5, 124.

Diniz, O. (1954) Palmar keratosis in rice sorters. Arch. Argent. Derm. 4, 11.

Horand, R. (1907) Crocodile hand, an occupational dermatosis produced by chestnut wood. Gaz. Hop. 80, 255.

Katzschmann, R. (1965) 'The 'Miller's sign'. An occupational stigma that has become very rare. Z. Alternsforsch. 18, 244.

Krasnopeeva, L.F. and Tsukker, I.I. (1962) Occupational dermatoses in mica workers. Vestn. Derm. I. Vener. 5, 47.

Leider, M and Golomb, H. (1964) Occupational stigmata. Report of a case of pronounced formation of callus on finger tips, among other characteristic effects in a Viola player. Archs. Derm 89, 468.

Marshall, J. (1964) Skin diseases in Africa. Cape Town. Masken Miller

Ronchese, F. (1948) Occupational Marks. New York. Grune and Stratton pg. 22, 36, 109, 116.

Szego, L. (1966) Data on skin conditions caused by apples and pears in women working in canning factories. Borgyogy. Vener. Szle 42, 117

White, R.P. (1934) The Dermatergoses or Occupational Affections of the Skin. 4th. ed. London H.K. Lewis. pg. 182.

Thorns and Spines

A spine is a strong and sharp-pointed woody body mostly arising from the wood of the stem of a plant and is colloquially a thorn. A prickle is a small and weak spine-like body borne irregularly on the bark or epidermis of a plant.

The spines of *Cactus* spp., maintain a layer of still air close to the plant, retard transpiration, promote dew formation at their tips, protect from sunlight and from animals, and assist in vegetative propagation by animal dispersal.

In the deserts of southern Madagascar, East Africa and southwestern United States grow three botanically quite unrelated kinds of thorn trees - so-called because all of them have little or no foliage. Presumably because of the extremely dry climates where they grow, thorns have largely taken the place of leaves, as they allow less moisture to evaporate (Menninger 1967). However, *Fagara davyi*, (Horse's Teats) reaches 21 metres in height and grows in fairly moist dense forest. The thorns evidently do not serve the purpose of protecting the tree from grazing animals as is probably so in the instance of desert cactus-like plants (Menninger 1967).

Tribulus terrestris, (Caltrops) is a thorny creeping plant.

The mericarps have sharp rigid spines which can stick into the foot of an animal. If a spine enters the hoof of a horse, it completely rots the frog, thus crippling the animal. The plant was named Caltrops after the spiked instruments which ancient nations used to throw to maim horses on the field of battle.

Some spines are put to use. The Masai of southern Africa used the thorns of Balanites spp., to pierce the earlobes of children.

The thorny branches, with spines over 7 cm. long, of the Balanites aegyptica, (Desert Date), are used to fence cattle pens in Africa. Pithecellobium dulce, (Madras Thorn), makes an excellent hedge in Malaysia (Corner 1952). Acacia ataxacantha, which is widespread in tropical Africa, is a scrambling shrub with branchlets armed with recurved prickles and is used for an impenetrable barrier round villages. 'Wait a bit', a West African colloquial name for Capparis erythrocarpa, is probably used more generally for prickly climbing plants (Dalziel 1948). The thorns of the tree, Maytenus sp., are used by butcher birds, known as shrikes, for impaling their insect victims (Irvine 1961). The thorns of Acacia pennata, are used as fish hooks (Irvine 1961).

Opuntia dillenii, Cactaceae is a leafless succulent shrub with spines up to 6.0 cm. long, planted in Malawi to discourage lions (Williamson 1956). The correct variety must be chosen for this purpose since some varieties are spineless. In Africa, the 'leaves' of Opuntia spp. are placed outside houses as 'burglar alarms'. The fruit, shaped somewhat like a pear, is covered with short prickles (Irvine 1961).

For homicidal purposes the poisonous juice of Acokanthera venenata, (Bushman's Poison) is smeared on suitable prickly fruits e.g. Tribulus terrestris, and strewn on a path which is likely to be used by the victim (Watt and Breyer-Brandwijk 1962).

Scrapings of the canes of Calamus caesius,(Rattan) have glossy coats due to the presence of silica and have been used for criminal poisoning along with powdered glass (Burkhill 1935).

A Jujube Tree, Ziziphus spina-christi (Zizyphus) is said to have furnished the Crown of Thorns at the crucifixion of Jesus Christ. The names Paliurus spina-christi and Euphorbia splendens (E. milii), (Crown of Thorns) have this connotation.

The spiny leaf of Ilex aquifolia, Aquifoliaceae (Holly) is found in few other species of the genus Ilex and these appear to belong to the North temperate region. The tropical species have simply toothed or, in most cases, entire leaves (Corner 1952). At Christmas time in Malaysia, Streblus sp., Moraceae (Jungle Holly) which is thorny, is used as a substitute for Holly as a festive decoration. In Africa, thorny Drypetes spp., Euphorbiaceae which look somewhat like Ilex, are used for this purpose.

The sharp-pointed seeds of Themeda arguens, Gramineae are used for piercing ear-lobes. As they dry in the sun or are wetted with rain or dew, they twist and untwist by reason of their hygroscopic awn. By this method, they 'screw' themselves into the soil onto which they happen to fall (Burkill 1935).

The involucral bracts of Arctium spp., (Burdock), become hooked and woody after the flowers wither and by clinging to fur and clothing aid in dispersing the fruits (Shaw 1973). Parts of the burrs of Burdock, Lappa officinalis (Arctium), mixed with seeds are irritant and according to White (1887), workmen packing them always stood to windward.

The burr-plant Calotis cuneifolia, withers in the summer to a dust, leaving the almost invisible burrs on the ground. Travellers are irritated by this burr getting into their blankets. It also irritates the feet of dogs.

The sticky burr fruits of Pisonia aculeata (Parrot's Claws) adhere to birds' wings and impede their flying (Irvine 1961). On some Pacific Islands birds and even reptiles are ensnared and disabled and eventually killed by the masses of viscid anthocarps of Pisonia spp.

The spines of Maclura pomifera, (Osage Orange) can cause mechanical injury. The milky sap of the tree can cause dermatitis (Pammel 1911, Schur 1932).

Hura crepitans, (Monkey Dinner-Bell), is "quite a dangerous tree; it stabs, poisons and shoots" (Barrett 1956). The bark of the tree is thickly studded with prickles. The sticky sap is irritant and the pods, when ripe and dry, explode noisily and shower bystanders with seeds and sharp-pointed segments.

According to Shelley and Hurley (1958), granulomas in man can result from reaction to foreign bodies of plant origin viz. agar, cactus, camphorated oil, carboxymethyl cellulose, cotton fibres, grain, lipids, lycopodium, starch, vegetable matter and wood.

Injury by certain spines gives rise to distinctive reactions which suggest that the mechanical effects can be enhanced or modified by irritant or possibly allergenic agents as yet unidentified.

A male, aged 33 years, developed an itching, papular and nodular eruption on the dorsa of hands, forearms, arms, lower thighs and legs after he trimmed a barberry hedge. The eruption was persistent one month later. A biopsy of a nodule on the dorsum of the hand revealed a non-specific dermatitis (Schwartz 1938). A discussant of this case stated that he and his associates had seen several patients who presented a similar dermatitis after working around a barberry hedge. It was postulated that a foreign body reaction to such thorns or their chemical components could occur in a sensitized subject. In this report, the botanical name of the plant was not recorded; three natural (Fernald 1970) and twenty-one cultivated species (Bailey 1971) of Barberry, Berberis spp., Berberidaceae are listed as occurring in the United States. 'Barberry dermatitis' was mentioned in discussion of a case presented by Hollander (1927). Various species of Berberis yield alkaloids (Hegnauer 1964). Berberis vulgaris is the Common Barberry which is an alternate host for a rust Puccinia, parasite on wheat, Triticum, and other grasses, Gramineae (Shaw 1973). This shrub is also reported as a source of sporotrichosis (Foerster 1926, Blair and Yurian 1928). Further investigation of chemical irritation or sensitization from Berberis is required. Sporotrichosis has also been acquired from pit props used in mines where the organism is a saprophyte (Marshall 1964).

According to Giles (1889), the wood of Acacia aneura (Mulga) "used by the natives for spear-heads, contains a virulent poisonous property, and a spear or stake wound with it is very dangerous." Scratches from Acacia cyperophylla, (Red Mulga) were notable for festering (Cleland 1931). A sliver of this wood in the cheek of a patient caused a granuloma with foreign body giant cells (Cleland 1943). This author considered that this wood was not necessarily poisonous as was alleged in Australia and that the suppuration from Mulga spliners and other woods was facilitated by a deficiency of fresh foods and of vitamins in the interior of that country.

Slivers (splinters) of the wood of Gossweilerodendron balsamiferum, (Agba) are known in industry to be particularly prone to cause "festering" sores in the skin.

A particle of the shell of the Horse Chestnut, ?Aesculus sp., became embedded in the conjunctiva and caused necrosis and ulceration by a toxic effect (Grant 1962). The prickles of the Horse Chestnut are said to be relatively or completely innocuous to the eye (Duke-Elder and MacFaul 1972).

The thorns of Gleditschia chinensis (Gleditsia), are used in Chinese Medicine as needles in opening abscesses and as counter-irritants in tumours and growths (Smith 1969).

The large stout spines of Cudrania javanensis, (Cock's Spur) are regarded as poisonous (Hurst 1942).

Cuts from Buettneria aculeata (Byttneria), become considerably inflamed and seem to heal slowly (Allen 1943).

The thorns of Dichrostachys glomerata, (Marabou Thorn) are

considered poisonous in Tanganika (Irvine 1961). The spines of D. cinerea were reported to penetrate the skin and underlying structures causing great pain (Watt and Breyer-Brandwijk 1962).

Certain plant thorns, in or near bone, can cause a reaction in the tissues which may simulate a neoplasm or granuloma. The reaction can be osteolytic or osteoblastic or a combination of both. Reactions have been reported to thorns of Yucca sp., Rosa sp., (Rose) Phoenix (Date Palm) and to Cactus spines (Maylahn 1952, Costa 1943, Warthin and Davies 1924, Buhr 1960). Symptoms and sign also reported were burning, prickling, stinging, and redness, papulation or nodulation (Maylahn 1952).

A chronic subcutaneous nodule was found to be due to an unidentified plant spine (Gougerot and Eliascheff 1930).

The histopathological findings in five solitary intracutaneous nodules which occurred from retained wood and plant material were described by Mehregan and Faghri (1974). Like silica, wood particles are also best demonstrated by polarized light.

A Bathurst burr Xanthium spinosum, was inhaled by a five year old girl and caused a gross inflammatory reaction in the right bronchial tube (Cleland 1943).

An eruption confined to the skin of the limbs and resulting from the spines of cactus plants breaking off in the skin is comparatively common in the arid areas of the Western United States, most of those affected being gasoline truck drivers. Secondary infection and severe ulceration are common.

It is important to distinquish cactus-like Euphorbia species of the Spurge family, which characteristically have an irritant milky latex, from Cactus species which characteristically have a watery sap.

Sharp-tipped palm fronds lying beneath trees in places where children play can cause injuries, usually of the knee. No puncture wound may be discernible. In one case, one thorn was removed but persistent swelling resulted from other thorns which were not at first suspected to be present (Cozen and Fonda 1953).

Phoenix canariensis (Canary Date Palm) and Phoenix loureiri (Pigmy Date Palm) possess sharp thorns on the petioles. Punctures by the thorns are commonly experienced by nursery and landscape gardeners in Florida. The spines-tip may be broken off and serve as a foreign body but a chemical irritant may also be present in the thorns (Morton 1962).

The thorn from Prosopis chiliensis or P. glandulosa, (Mesquite) on penetrating the eye, causes an inflammation greater than expected from the degree of physical injury; the irritation has been attributed to a wax present in glands on the thorn and on its surface (Brunner and Bieberdorf 1950). Injection of cerotic acid, a component of the wax, is destructive to the eye (Duke-Elder and MacFaul 1972).

Ocular effects of alkaloids of Datura stramonium, (Thorn Apple) can occur from entry of seeds from the plant into the conjunctival sac; these effects occur accidentally in farmers at harvest time (Simmons 1957).

The hooked thorns of Uncaria rhynchophylla, (Gambir) are used as a drug in Japan; they contain a hypotensive alkaloid (Kariyone 1971).

Thorn injuries of the hands from Prunus spinosa, (Blackthorn or Sloe) which occurred in ten patients, required out-patient treatment nearly four times longer in duration than thorn injuries from Crataegus sp., (Hawthorn) and from Ribes sp., (Gooseberry), (Buhr 1960). William Withering (1741-1799), the pioneer of digitalis therapy, commented on countrymens' beliefs that Blackthorn injuries had some special poisonous effects. He wrote in 1801, "From some effects which I have repeatedly observed to follow the prick of the thorns, I have reason to believe there is something poisonous in them," (Buhr 1960).

The birds, known as shrikes, often impale their "kills" i.e. small birds or insects, on the thorns of the Blackthorn; it was suggested that the fly-infested putrefying bodies might be the source of an infection. It seems probable that the tip of the rough, long, brittle thorn of the Blackthorn snaps off more readily in the skin than the short sharp needle-sharp point of the Hawthorn; retention of Blackthorn plant tissues in the subcutaneous tissues is responsible for disability, (Buhr 1960).

Crataegus oxycantha (White Thorn) is particularly toxic to the eye and a corneal scratch can lead to blindness which occurred in 88 cases from 132 such accidents in Ireland (Smith 1940).

Salsola kali var. tenuifolia (S. pestifera), (Russian Thistle or Prickly Saltwort) has since about 1900 become a pest in North American agriculture (Shaw 1973). In New Mexico, U.S.A., a disorder known as 'Tumbleweed dermatitis' occurs from contact of this plant with the skin. Mechanical injury from sharp spines on the leaf tips appears to be responsible for the dermatitis (Smith 1972).

References

Allen, P.H. (1943) Poisonous and injurious plants of Panama. Am. J. Trop. Med. (Suppl.)23, 1.

Bailey, L. H. (1971) Manual of cultivated plants most commonly grown in the continental United States and Canada. New York Macmillan

Barrett, M.F. (1956) Common exotic trees of South Florida. Gainesville University of Florida Press

Blair, J. and Yurian, N.C. (1928) Two cases of sporotrichosis infection due to barberry. JAMA 91, 96.

Brunner, H. and Bieberdorf, F. (1950) The effects of the mesquite thorn on the human eye. Tr. Am. Acad. Ophth. 55, 595

Buhr, A.J. (1960) The thorn in the flesh. Lancet 1, 309.

Burkill, I. H. (1935) A dictionary of the economic products of the Malay peninsula. 2 vols. London Crown Agents for the Colonies

Cleland, J.B. (1931) Plants including fungi, poisonous or otherwise injurious to man in Australia. III. Med. J. Austr. 2, 775

Cleland, J.B. (1943) Plants, including fungi, poisonous or otherwise injurious to man in Australia. IV Med. J. Austr. 11, 161

Corner, E.J.H. (1952) Wayside trees of Malaya. Singapore. Government Printer

Costa, A.J. (1943) Cavernous lesion of the internal femoral condyle, produced by spine of cactus. Prensa Med. (La Paz) 3, 44.

Cozen, L. and Fonda, M. (1953) Palm thorn injuries. Difficulty in diagnosis of late sequelae. Calif. Med. 79, 40

Dalziel, J.M. (1948) The useful plants of West Tropical Africa. London. Crown Agents for Oversea Governments and Administrations pg. 20

Duke-Elder, S. and MacFaul P.A. (1972). System of Ophthalmology Vol. XIV. Injuries Part 1. Mechanical injuries. Extraocular foreign bodies. pg. 464-467 and Agricultural injuries pg. 32-34 London. Henry Kimpton

Fernald, M.L. (1970) Gray's Manual of Botany. 8th ed. New York. Van Nostrand Reinhold.

Foerster, H.R. (1926) Sporotrichosis and occupational dermatosis. Med. Jr. and Rec. 123, 530.

Giles, E. (1889) Australia Twice Traversed. London. 2 vols. Sampson, Low, Marston, Searle and Rivington Ltd. Facsimile ed 1964 London. Wm. Clowes.

Glass, E. (1927) Klinisch-experimenteller Beitrag zu den Verletzungen durch Kakteenstacheln Arch. Klin. Chir. 145, 658.

Gougerot, H. and Eliascheff, O. (1930) Chronic subcutaneous nodule from non-irritant foreign body (spine). Arch. Derm-syph. de Clin. L'Hopital Saint-Louis pg. 162

Grant, W.M. (1962) Toxicology of the eye. Springfield, Ill. Charles C. Thomas

Hegnauer, R. (1964) Chemotaxonomy of Plants. Vol. 3. Basel Birkhauser pg. 240.

Hollander (1927) Dermatitis venenata Archs. Derm. Syph. 15, 620

Hurst, E. (1942) The poison plants of New South Wales. Sydney. N.S.W. Poison Plants Committee

Irvine, F.R. (1961) Woody plants of Ghana. London. Oxford University Press

Kariyone, T. (1971) Atlas of Medicinal Plants. Osaka, Japan Takeda Chemical Industries

Kirsch, N. (1958) An unusual case of contact dermatitis. Connecticut Med. 22, 756.

MacPherson, J. (1932) Plants injurious to man in Australia. Med. J. Australia 1, 281.

Marshall, J. (1964) Skin diseases in Africa. Cape Town. Maskew Miller.

Maylahn, D.J. (1952) Thorn induced "Tumors" of bone. J. Bone Joint Surg. 34A, 386

Mehregan, A.H. and Faghri, B. (1974) Implantation Dermatoses. Acta. derm.-venereol 54, 61.

Menninger, E.A. (1967) Fantastic Trees. New York. Viking Press.

Morton, J.F. (1962) Ornamental plants with toxic and or irritant properties. II. Proc. Florida State Horticult. Soc. 75, 484

Pammel, L.H. (1911) A manual of poisonous plants. Torch Press Cedar Rapids, Iowa.

Schreiber, M.M., Shapiro, S.I. and Berry, C.Z. (1971) Cactus granulomas of the skin. Archs. Derm. 104, 347.

Schur, A. (1932) Dermatitis venenata Report of a case due to osage orange (Maclura pomifera) Archs. Derm. 26, 312.

Schwartz, W.F. (1938) Foreign body (Barberry) dermatitis. Archs. Derm. Syph. 37, 872.

Shanon, J. and Sagher, F. (1969) Sabra dermatitis. An occupational dermatitis simulating scabies due to the handling of prickly pears. In Essays on Tropical Dermatology ed. Simons R. and Marshall, J. Amsterdam. Excerpta Medica Foundation pg. 85-89

Shaw, H.K.A. (1973) A Dictionary of the Flowering Plants and Ferns. (the late J.C. Willis) 8th ed. Cambridge University Press.

Shelley, W.B. and Hurley (1958) The allergic origin of zirconium deodorant granulomas. Brit. J. Derm. 70, 75

Simmons, F.H. (1957) Jimson weed mydriasis in farmers. Am. J. Ophthal. 44, 109

Smith, F.P.E. (1940) Eye injuries in agriculture. Trans. Ophthal. Soc. U.K. 60, 252.

Smith, F.P. (1969) Chinese Materia Medica. Vegetable Kingdom. 2nd. ed. Rev. by Hei, P.D. Taipei, Taiwan. Ku T'ing Book House

Smith, E.B. (1972) University of New Mexico School of Medicine Personal communication.

Warthin, A.S. and Davies, J.E. (1924) Cactus-spine pseudotubercles. Ann. Clin. Med. 2, 248

Watt, J.M. and Breyer-Brandwijk, M.G. (1962) The Medicinal and Poisonous Plants of Southern and Eastern Africa. 2nd. ed. Edinburgh, Livingstone.

White, J.C. (1887) Dermatitis venenata. An account of the action of external irritants upon the skin. Boston. Cupples and Hurd.

Plant hairs

Plant hairs have been described as derived from perhaps five to six thousand species of plants. The various types of hairs were reviewed by Uphof and Hummeh (1962).

Plant hairs have been observed upon the skin surface and as laboratory contaminants (Pinkus 1969). Polemann (1960) reported that the bristles or trichomes of plants can cause an irritable eruption of the interdigital spaces simulating eczema or tinea.

In the cases of Primula obconica, Primulaceae: Toxicodendron spp. (Rhus), Anacardiaceae (Poison Ivy-Oak) and Parthenium hysterophorus, Compositae (Feverfew) disruption of the plant hairs results in the release of the respective allergens. Certain plant fibres and hairs have been found in the lungs, intestinal tract, blood and urine (Schreiber 1974).

The leaf hairs of Platanus orientalis, (Plane Tree) can produce conjunctival and respiratory irritation (Ross and Mitchell 1974). In that study, an allergic effect reported by Zaccharin (1933) could not be confirmed.

The Borage family (Boraginaceae) contains chiefly rough-hairy herbaceous plants (Fernald 1970). The coarse stiff hairs can cause mechanical irritation and so lead to difficulty in interpretation of patch test reactions (Woods 1962). Anchusa officinalis (Alkanet); Borago officinalis (Borage); Echium spp. (Viper's Bugloss); Lycopsis sp. Bugloss) and Lappula sp. (Eichinospermum) (Stickseed) can produce irritation by the mechanical action of their hairs. Pulmonaria officinalis (Lungwort) has rough hairs but is probably also allergenic (Woods 1962.

Opuntia basilaris (Beaver Tail) has irritant fine hair-like glochids (barbed bristles). If an attempt is made to suck out the glochid from the skin, it is likely to attach itself to the tongue. The best method for removal of glochids from the human skin is to spread adhesive plaster over the area affected and to rip it off quickly (Watt and Breyer-Brandwijk 1962). Melted wax has also been recommended (Shanon and Sagher 1969).

"Sore-mouth" in sheep, which are being fed Opuntia vulgaris (Prickly Pear), probably results from the glochids and possibly from the thorns (Watt and Breyer-Brandwijk 1962).

Macules and papules confined to the lateral and posterior surfaces of the left arm and to the antero-lateral and posterior aspect of the left thigh were observed in a female cactus fancier (Kirsch 1958). It was found that the forced warm air system of the woman's house blew detached 'spines' from Opuntia robusta, and these affixed themselves to her clothes; by movements of the body the 'spines' (probably glochids) were induced to penetrate the skin.

An occupational dermatitis from Opuntia ficus-indica, (Indian Fig. Cactus, Sabra) primarily affects the fingers but can affect any part of the skin and tends to simulate scabies. 'Sabra dermatitis' is an occupational disease of those engaged in the prickly pear trade and occurs when the fruit is in season which, in the Middle East, is from July to October. The hard palate and tongue are occasionally involved. The barbed glochids of the plant can be transferred to the workers' clothing and to other individuals. The prickly pear should be picked only when wetted and picking should be stopped when it is windy since the barbs can become airborne, (Shanon and Sagher 1969). Sagher (pers. comm. 1973) states that with improved economic conditions and disuse of the fruits of the plant for food, gathering of the plant seems to have ceased and the occupational disorder is no longer seen. However, the Indian Fig Cactus is widely naturalized in various parts of the world and 'Sabra dermatitis' has been seen in Mediterranean holiday makers.

Cactus glochids have been regarded as producing an irritative or toxic action in the skin (Glass 1927, Costa 1943). Alternatively, an allergic reaction was proposed because of the rarity of clinical lesions in contrast to the large number of cactus spine injuries suffered in Arizona (Schreiber et al 1971). These authors observed positive delayed skin test reactions in two-thirds of affected patients following intradermal injection of extracts of Cactus glochids.

Dogs, cats and grazing animals suffer irritation of the conjunctiva and of the nasal passages from dried awns of several kinds of grasses. Hooked seed pods adhere readily to clothing or blankets and once lodged they screw their way into cloth.

The awns of Avena fatua (Wild or Black Oat) can cause mechanical injury. The pointed calluses can injure the mouths of grazing cattle. The seeds may be found in the conjunctival sac, nasal cavity and external auditory meatus (MacPherson 1932).

The barbed hairs of the seeds of Arctium sp., (Common Burdock) can become embedded in the conjunctiva and cause opthalmia. The downy hairs of Cirsium spp. (Thistles) and the seed hairs of Helichrysum, (Everlasting Flowers) can produce small yellow conjunctival nodules.

The use of sticks for threshing Oryza spp. (Rice) can throw the grains up into the eyes. Resulting corneal abrasions usually show multiple spiky hairs projecting from the lesions, resembling nodose opthalmia caused by the hairs of caterpillars (Duke-Elder and MacFaul 1972).

Barley awns (Hordeum sp.) can cause an extensive papular dermatitis in farm workers and in others exposed to "barley dust", including children, in whom the cause is often unsuspected. The trichomes of the awns of some other cereals can produce papular urticaria in workers handling crops or straw. Whilst the majority of eruptions attributed to food grains appear to be caused by mechanical trauma, Immediate (Type I) amd delayed (Type IV) allergic sensitivity have been demonstrated (see Gramineae); mite infestation can also occur.

The fruit hairs of Crataegus (Hawthorn), can cause nodular conjunctivitis (Duke-Elder and MacFaul 1972).

The leaf of Cornus sanguinea, (Bloodtwig Dogwood) possesses T-shaped hairs which pierce the skin and produce erythema, or urtication, only when the leaf is rubbed on the skin in the direction of its long axis (Woods 1962). The leaves of Sparmannia africana were shown by Schulze (1940) to produce positive patch test reactions in 90 percent of controls as well as in patients with dermatitis from the plant. He concluded that the hairs were irritant; however, the plant may als be allergenic (Kuske and Bandi 1958)

'Hop Eye' is due, in part, t mechanical injury from spiny hairs o Humulus lupulus, Cannabidaceae (Adams 1893). Allergic kerato-conjunctivitis and dermatitis can also result from hop-picking.

The leaf hairs of Ulmus sp., (Elm) can produce irritation of the skin (Genner and Bonnevie 1938). A species of this family Celtis australis is known colloquially as the Nettle Tree. The Elm Family is taxonomically close, within the subclass Archichlamydeae, to the Nettle Family, Urticaceae and the Hop Famil Cannabidaceae which, respectively, contain species with urticant hairs and irritant prickles. However, suc taxonomic considerations are not of much relevance since stinging hairs are found in widely separated botanical families.

The stinging hairs of Tragia spp., Euphorbiaceae (Noseburn) cover the entire plant and possess sharp siliceous points which break off when touched and can penetrate the skin. Injury by the hairs results in sharp burning pain and inflammation. The colloquial name Pringamoza is used for this plant and also for Platygna pruriens, Euphorbiaceae and Urera baccifera, Urticaceae whic possess irritant hairs (Blohm 1962, Pardo-Castello 1923).

Stinging Spurges or Spurge Nettles, Cnidoscolus spp., Euphorbiaceae are perennial herbaceous plants or shrubs which are armed with stinging bristles (Fernald 1970). Contact with C. stimulosus (Tread Softly, Bull Nettle) can produce urtication. Some Dalechampi species, Euphorbiaceae, possess urticating hairs on all parts of the plant. The sepals of the female flowers of D. tiliaefolia are covere with stiff stinging hairs (Allen 1943). Sphaerostylis malaccensis (Climbing Croton) and Cnesmone spp. are other euphorbiaceous plants that possess stinging hairs.

The fallen fruits of the tree, Neesia sp., Bombacaceae in Malaya must be handled with the greatest care to prevent the bristles touching the skin; if their points once penetrate, it is impossible to get rid of them until the skin is naturally sloughed off. The bristles occur on the inner side of the woody fruit capsules (Corner 1952).

The capsule of Cnestis natalensis, Connaraceae is covered outside and inside with rigid brown hairs which easily penetrate the skin producing severe itching (Watt and Breyer-Brandwijk 1962).

Wigandia caracasana, (Ortiga), Hydrophyllaceae, is a large perennial herbaceous plant or undershrub grown in the garden for bold foliage effects (Bailey 1971): the leaves are covered with glistening stinging hairs (Allen 1943). Malpighia urens (Cow Itch Cherry), Malpighiaceae, has stinging hairs but some other members of the genus have toothed spines.

The epidermis of plants of the Loasa family bears hairs of various kinds: especially common are grapple-hairs (also called grapnel hairs) and stinging hairs. The rough barbed hairs of Mentzelia oliogosperma can irritate the skin (White 1887). The leaves of M. ornata possess hooked hairs (Pammel 1911). Gronovia scandens is armed with barbed stinging haris and Loasa spp. possess stinging hairs (Allen 1943). Loasa vulcanica, grown in Europe as a decorative half-hardy annual, has caused painful stinging in children (Rook, unpublished observations). Blumenbachia spp. (Sting Lily) and Caiophora spp. (Tingle Lily) have stinging hairs.

There is discussion in the literature concerning the presence or absence of irritant hairs on the leaves of Ficus spp., (Figs), Moraceae, and an allegation that the presence of stinging hairs on fig leaves is hardly in accord with their use as the primitive garment of Man. It appears that some species and kinds of Figs possess irritant hairs and others do not. The twigs, leaves and fruits of Ficus fulva (Stinging Fig) are set with short 'stinging' bristles (Corner 1952). A pruritogenic endopeptidase, ficin, is derived from Ficus (Arthur and Shelley 1955).

The hairs on the outside of the pods of Mucuna gigantea and M. pruriens, Leguminosae, are irritant to the skin and to the intestinal tract. They have been used for criminal poisoning, mixed in the case of M. gigantea with the slime of a slug to serve as a vehicle (Burkill 1935). The flowers and leaves of Laportea stimulans, Urticaceae, have been made up into cakes for vindictive poisoning (Gimlette 1929).

In Africa, the stinging hairs of Mucuna sloanei, (Horse-Eye Bean) are rubbed on the skin of small children to teach them to control urination (Irvine 1961). The hairs of Mucuna pruriens (Buffalo Bean, Cowhage) were formerly made into Unguentum urticans, an ointment of cowhage hairs 8 grains to one ounce of lard which, when rubbed on the skin, produced burning and urticaria. So much trouble was occasioned by handling Cowhage in the preparation of antihelmintics, that many in the trade refused to deal with it (White 1887). The stinging hairs of this (and other Mucuna spp.) are used by the Hausas in Africa in simulating leprosy, being applied first to the skin, which is then rubbed with the irritant latex of a cactiform Euphorbia. This procedure causes swelling and numbness likely to endure for several weeks (Dalziel 1948). Skin irritation of an urticarial type and conjunctivitis can occur from the hairs of Mucuna pruriens falling into the eyes (Dao 1967). The conjunctivitis occurs during the dry season when the hairs are shed from the plants. Dao (1967) observed 31 labourers with such skin irritation of the trunk and limbs; eight of them also had conjunctivitis. Keratitis can also occur. The hairs mixed in the soil irritate the feet of labourers who go bare-footed; for this reason irritation may occur from exposure to soil around a plant which has not yet produced its annual crop of stinging hairs.

The active pruritogenic principle is a proteolytic enzyme, mucunain (Arthur and Shelley 1955). The trichome also contains 0.015% of 5-hydroxytryptamine which is without pruritogenic properties. Mucunain is an endopeptidase with activity in the pH range of 7 to 8; when introduced into the skin, this chemical compound evoked pruritus without the appearance of any visible skin lesions. The endopeptidases, bromelin from plants of the Pineapple family, Bromeliaceae, papain from Carica papaya (Papaya) and ficin from Ficus sp., were also found to be active.

In the United Kingdom, Stinging Nettles are common weeds, the annual Urtica urens, Urticaceae: the perennial U. dioica: a third species U. pilulifera (Roman Nettle), which is the most virulent as regards its stings, is occasionally found (Chittenden 1974). Several other species occur in eastern North America (Fernald 1970).

The effects of contact with American and European species of Urtica, are trifling compared with those of species growing in the East Indies. The most venomous are U. urentissima, U. crenulata, U. stimulans and U. ferox (White 1887). A death was attributed to stinging by Urtica ferox (Onga Onga), (Cilles and Wright 1966). It is alleged that the application of a leaf of Rumex sp., (Dock) will allay nettlerash. It is possible that the time and attention devoted to finding such a Dock leaf may distract attention from the itching evoked by the nettle.

Members of the tribe Urticeae of the Urticaceae family which includes Urtica, Urera, and Laportea, possess stinging hairs. Members of five other tribes possess no stinging hairs (Shaw 1973). According to Allen (1943), Cecropia spp. Urticaceae (Pumpwood), possesses irritant hairs and a milky caustic sap; the hollow trunks and branches house stinging ants (Allen 1943). However, according to Shaw (1973), Cecropia spp. possess no stinging hairs. Acacia sphaerocephala forms spiny stipules which are hollow and become tenanted by ferocious ants (Corner 1952).

The tree nettles of New Guinea and Australia, Laportea spp., Urticaceae (Stinging Tree, Gympie) can produce severe stings. Acetylcholine, histamine and 5-hydroxytryptamine are present in the hairs together with a pain-producing substance (or substances) the chemical nature of which is unknown, (Cleland and Lee 1963, Macfarlane 1963). The chemical components of Urtica spp. (Emmelin and Feldberg 1947, Collier and Chesher 1956) and of Girardinia (Saxena et al 1964) are qualitatively similar but an unidentified active substance is present in the stinging fluid of Urtica dioica. The skin effects of U. urentissima (Devil's Leaf) are said to last for months and it is possible that retained siliceous hair tips contribute to the syndrome.

References

Adams, P.T. (1893) A special form of ophthalmia to which hop pickers are liable. Brit. Med. J. 1, 1000.

Allen, P. H. (1943) Poisonous and injurious plants of Panama. Am. J. Trop. Med. (Supp.) 23, 1.

Arthur, R.P. and Shelley, W.B. (1955) The role of proteolytic enzymes in the production of pruritus in man. J. Invest. Derm. 25, 341.

Bailey, L.H. (1971) Manual of Cultivated Plants. New York. Macmillan Co.

Blohm, H. (1962) Poisonous Plants of Venezuela, Cambridge, Mass. Harvard University Press.

Burkill, I.H. (1935) A Dictionary of the Economic Products of the Malay Peninsula. 2 vols. London, Crown Agents for the Colonies.

Cleland, J.B. and Lee, D.J. (1963) The Poisonous and Urticating Plants of Australia in Venomous and Poisonous Animals and Noxious Plants of the Pacific Region. ed. Keegan, H.L. and Macfarlane, W.V. Oxford Pergamon Press. pg.3-13.

Collier, H.O.J. and Chesher, G.B. (1956). Identification of 5-hydroxytryptamine in the sting of the nettle (Urtica dioica). Brit. J. Pharmacol. 11, 186.

Corner, E.J.H. (1952) Wayside Trees of Malaysia. Singapore, Government Printer

Dalziel, J.M. (1948) Useful Plants of West Tropical Africa. London. Crown Agents for the Colonies

Dao, L. (1967) Dermatitis from plants in the plains of Venezuela. Derm. Int. 6, 77.

Duke-Elder, S. and MacFaul, P.A. (1972) System of Opthalmology Vol. XIV. Injuries. Part 2,

Non-mechanical injuries. Irritant vegetable products pg. 1180-1196, and Self-inflicted injuries pg. 1016-1018. London Henry Kimpton

Emmelin, N. and Feldberg, W. (1947) The mechanism of the sting of the common nettle (Urtica urens) J. Physiol. 106, 440

Fernald, M.L. (1970) Gray's Manual of Botany. 8th ed. 1970. New York. Van Nostrand Reinhold Co.

Genner, V. and Bonnevie, P. (1938) Eczematous eruptions produced by leaves of trees and bushes. Archs. Derm. Syph. 37, 583.

Gilles, R.G. and Wright, A.S. (1966) Laportea, the Stinging Trees North Queensland Naturalist 33,2.

Gimlette, J.D. (1929) Malay Poisons and Charm Cures. London J. and A. Churchill.

Irvine, F.G. (1961) Woody Plants of Ghana. Oxford University Press London

Kuske, H. and Bandi, B. (1958) Dermatitis and eczema caused by an indoor linden. Dermatologica 116, 308.

Macfarlane, W.V. (1963) The pain-producing properties of the stinging tree, Laportea in Venomous and Poisonous Animals and Noxious Plants of the Pacific Region. ed. Keegan, H.L. and Macfarlane, W.V. Oxford. Pergamon Press. pg. 31-37

Pammell, L.H. (1911) A Manual of Poisonous Plants. Torch Press. Cedar Rapids, Iowa. Reprinted Univ. Microfilms Inc. Ann Arbor, Mich. 1965, pp.476

Pardo-Castello, V. (1923) Dermatitis venenata. A study of the tropical plants producing dermatitis. Archs. Derm. Syph. 7, 81.

Pinkus, H. (1969) Stellate plant hair contaminant in the laboratory. Archs. Derm. 100, 96.

Polemann, G. (1960) Durch Pflanzenhaare verursachte Pseudomykosontrichomatosen. Hautarzt 11, 181.

Ross, A.F. and Mitchell, J.C. (1974) Respiratory Irritation by Leaf Hair of the Tree Platanus. Ann Allergy 32, 94.

Saxena, P.R., Kishor, K., Pant, M.C. et al (1964) Pharmacologically active constituents of Girardinia heterophylla (Dcne,). J. Pharm. Pharmacol. 16, 361.

Schreiber, M.M, Shapiro, S.I. and Berry, C.Z. (1971) Cactus granulomas of the skin. Archs. Derm. 104, 374.

Schreiber, G. (1974) Ingested dyed cellulose in the blood and urine of man. Arch. Environ. Health 29, 39.

Schulze, W. (1940) Investigation of the irritative action of the leaves of African hemp. Arch. f. Derm. u. Syph. 181, 63.

Shaw, H.K.A. (1973) A Dictionary of the Flowering Plants and Ferns. (the late J.C. Willis) 8th ed. Cambridge University Press.

Uphof, J.C.T. and Hummeh, K. (1962) Plant hairs in Encyclopedia of Plant Anatomy. Vol. 4. Part V. Berlin-Nikolassen: Gebruden Borntraeger.

Watt, J.M. and Breyer-Brandwijk, M.G. (1962) The Medicinal and Poisonous Plants of Southern and Eastern Africa. 2nd. ed. Edinburgh, Livingstone.

White, J.C. (1887) Dermatitis venenata: An account of the action of external irritants upon the skin. Boston, Cupples and Hurd.

Woods, B. (1962) Irritant plants. Trans. St. John's Hosp. Derm. Soc. 48, 75.

Zacharin, D. (1933) Plane tree leaves a cause of seasonal asthma and hay fever. Med. J. Australia 1, 467.

DIAGNOSIS OF CONTACT DERMATITIS FROM PLANTS

Living plants and natural plant products such as balsams, turpentines and the aroma chemicals found in perfumes and in flavorings are among the commonest causes of contact dermatitis.

Plants are factories and store-houses of chemicals in great variety. Over 200 amino acids derived from plants are known, as compared with 30 from mammals. About 11,000 naturally occurring compounds are known from plants. About 12,000 of the half a million known plant species have been investigated in the laboratory. There are probably thousands of sensitizing chemicals in plants.

The quantity of a particular chemical produced by a plant depends not only on intrinsic factors such as genetic constitution, part of the plant, age and sometimes even sex, but also on extrinsic factors such as climate, moisture supply and soil fertility.

Toxicodendron (poison ivy-oak) in the United States and Primula obconica (primula) in Europe produce many cases of contact dermatitis and overshadow less well-known but significant plant irritants and allergens.

Our purpose is to outline a plan for the investigation of suspected plant dermatitis.

Clinical Patterns of Plant Dermatitis

There are 6 more or less distinct clinical types of eruption caused by contact with different types of vegetation, namely garden flowers, vegetables, weeds, sawdust of commercial woods, plant products and phototoxic plants. Sensitivity to flowers and shrubs of horticulture occurring in gardeners and florists usually is confined to the hands, forearms, face and neck; episodic acute vesicular reactions occur. Dermatitis in commercial flower growers usually does not come to the attention of dermatologists. Sensitivity to vegetables and fruits produces acute or chronic dermatitis and affects housewives, salad makers and truck gardeners.

Weed dermatitis affects primarily the exposed skin surfaces but may become disseminated. There is a remarkable resemblance to atopic dermatitis and photodermatitis (Lonkar et al 1947). In North America, dermatitis from ragweeds (Ambrosia) first occurs in the summer but may become perennial.

Sawdust dermatitis affects the eyelids, face, neck and moist skin folds such as the genital area where the wood dust lodges. Mild cases may resemble seborrhoeic dermatitis. Dermatitis from natural plant products such as turpentine, balsams and perfumes present additional clinical patterns.

Phytophotodermatitis

Phytophotodermatitis is evoked by exposure to sunlight, following exposure of the skin to the juice of a plant. The common denominator for the production of such phototoxicity is psoralens in the plants. Some other chemical compounds such as thiophenes (Chan et al 1975; Camm et al 1975) have so far been reported to induce phototoxicity only in microbial systems. Phytophotodermatitis can usually be diagnosed by the clinical history and characteristic skin lesions which follow exposure to psoralen-containing plants. The main features in differential diagnosis are listed in Table 1.

Botanical identification of the plant may confirm that it is one which yields psoralens, such as Heracleum (cow parsnip, wild rhubarb) (Camm et al 1976).

Exposure to Plants

In Europe, a patient may be lying in bed suffering from Primula dermatitis but denying any contact with or even possession of a plant when a specimen is present on the window sill. In considering the diagnosis, the most careful history is usually essential. Seasonal incidence is often suggestive but allergenic poison ivy (Toxicodendron) sap may be dried onto clothing or golf clubs. The patient's movements and activities before the last relapse may be informative. A spell in the greenhouse, a visit to a friend who has plants, a walk in the country may be remembered. A wide variety of potentially allergenic foreign plants are now grown increasingly in affluent societies, e.g. Humea elegans. A home visit is very worthwhile. Primula obconica has recently been offered for sale by California florists.

Dermatitis from plants is more common in hot climates than in cold climates. In hot climates, there is more skin exposure to plants as less

Table 1. Clinical Features of Poison Ivy-Oak (Toxicodendron) Dermatitis and of Phytophotodermatitis of Plants with Psoralens. (Sommer and Jillson 1967)

Disorder	Onset	Mechanism	Symptoms	Course	Residual effects
Poison-ivy dermatitis	First exposure can result in sensitization and dermatitis after 5 or more days; on re-exposure, dermatitis appears within 48 hours often within 12 hours	Contact allergic	Itching	Fresh disseminated lesions often appear during 1 week after re-exposure	None
Phytophotodermatitis	First exposure can result in redness and blistering of the skin which appears at about 48 hours; on re-exposure the reaction time is about 48 hours	Phototoxic	Burning pain	Reaction is confined to initial sites of contact	Hyperpigmentation often occurs and can persist for months

clothing is worn. In hot climates, horticultural plants require more pruning and trimming owing to their exuberant growth. Tropical plants seem to be storehouses of a wider variety of chemicals than are cold climate plants. In cold climates, however, hobby greenhouse gardening is providing an increasing source of exposure to exotic plants and thus, an interesting area for further study. Plants are common causes of occupational dermatitis (Gellin et al 1971).

Clinical and Botanical Investigation

When the dermatologist or his patient suspects that a plant is causing contact dermatitis, samples must be obtained of all the plants to which exposure may have occurred. Flowers and leaves of all the suspected plants should be brought in by the patient and stored temporarily in a refrigerator in the physician's office. The patient should be warned that he must be thorough and bring samples of all plants, including those which he would call "weeds" and therefore be inclined to overlook.

The plants selected for the first set of patch tests should be those recognized as causing dermatitis. If these first tests are negative, tests with the remaining plants should be carried out. In some instances, repeated search may be required before the offending plant is detected. An absolute necessity is botanical identification of the plants used for testing. Sources of information are listed in Table 2. It is fruitless and misleading to look up the common or colloquial name of the plant in any book. An expert identification of the suspected plants by a plant

Table 2. Sources for Botanical Identification of Plants Suspected of Causing Contact Dermatitis

Department of Botany at a University - Curator of Herbarium

Botanical gardens

Botanist (plant taxonomist if possible) at national, state or private herbarium or high school; county agricultural agents and soil conservation agents (U.S. Department of Agriculture)

taxonomist is essential.

Speed is essential in identifying a suspected plant. Wasted time leads to lack of interest by patient and physician and important information may be lost by delay. Each case is a minor or even a major research exercise. The suspected offending plant should promptly be divided into 3 approximately equal portions. One portion for botanical identification should be dried or stored in the freezer. The second and third portions should be stored in a freezer, one portion for patch test purposes and the other for possible later chemical studies.

An interested patient available for patch testing, the suspected plants reliably identified and the samples safely frozen in 3 portions provide the opportunity for a significant and rewarding investigation.

Armed with the names of the plants, one can turn to the literature.

It is useless to patch test with irritant plants; some plant families such as the Euphorbiaceae (Spurge) family contain mostly irritant plants. A knowledge of the botanical affinities of the plants derived from botanical treatises (Chittenden 1969; Fernald 1970; Bailey 1971) helps the physician avoid useless irritant patch tests. A partial list of irritant plant families appears in Table 3.

A suspected irritant plant may have known irritant relatives within the family and this information is helpful when starting patch-testing.

Some plant families contain plants whose main action on the skin is allergenic. Plants of about 22 genera of the family Anacardiaceae (poison ivy-oak family) have been reported to be allergenic. Any irritant effect of the juices of these plants is overshadowed by their strongly allergenic effect for sensitized persons.

Botanical taxonomy is not a static subject; nomenclature can change as new and old information is re-evaluated. According to Gillis (1975) the allergenic species of the genus Rhus of the Anacardiaceae family (poison ivy-oak family) are botanically sufficiently different to be separated off as the genus Toxicodendron of the Anacardiaceae (poison ivy-oak family).

It is still essential for meaningful scientific investigation of plant dermatitis that valid botanical names be used. An excursion into the complexities of botanical taxonomic nomenclature is necessary for a simplistic understanding of what is to be done with the safely stored and frozen 3 portions of plant specimens. Botanical terminology has much in common with dermatological terminology which is said to share a common origin from the writings of Jacob Plenck who was, among other activities, a botanist and a physician.

Plants are arranged by family tribe, genus and species as shown in Table 4 according to the system elaborated by Linnaeus, who also was a physician. A colloquial or common name has no scientific validity and is useless for scientific reports. Colloquial names for a plant species

Table 3. Botanical Families Which Contain Many Irritant Plants

Family	Genus
Euphorbiaceae (spurge)	Euphorbia (spurge)
Ranunculaceae (buttercup)	Ranunculus (buttercup) Clematis (pasque-flower) Anemone (wind flower)
Cruciferae (mustard)	Brassica (mustard)
Capparidaceae (caper)	Capparis (Cleopatra's needle)

Plants of the genera noted are often irritant.

Table 4. A Botanical Family, Tribe, Genus, Species and a Colloquial Name

Family:	Compositae (Chrysanthemum family)	Family:	The Smiths
Tribe:	Anthemidae	Tribe:	The New York-related Smiths
Genus:	Chrysanthemum	Genus:	Smith
Species:	Chrysanthemum maximum	Species:	Bill Smith
Colloquial name:	Shasta Daisy	Nickname:	Shorty

vary from one country to another, are misleading and numerous; for instance, Arum maculatum (spotted arum) has about 60 different colloquial names in the United Kingdom alone.

Botanical affinities allow the placing of a plant species in families. A tribe is a natural grouping of plants within a family. Allergenic plants may fall into certain tribes within a family, for instance, into the Anthemidae and Heliantheae tribes of the Compositae family (Chrysanthemum family) (Table 4) (Mitchell 1969). A genus is represented by an italicized noun, e.g. Chrysanthemum. A species is represented by an italicized adjective to form a binominal, e.g. Chrysanthemum maximum, similar in style to a dermatological name, e.g. acne vulgaris.

The authority for a name is shown in Table 5. The author who published a description of a plant is appended to the binominal, e.g. Toxicodendron radicans (Linnaeus) Kuntze. Linnaeus is often shortened to L. The author, Kuntze, revised the description of Linnaeus. As taxonomic research brings to light new information on authorities, the scientific name of a plant genus or species may be changed according to strictly established rules of nomenclature. For example, the familiar Vinca of chemotherapy is now named Catharanthus which leaves chemical names such as vincaleukoblastine in somewhat of a void.

In Table 6, examples are shown of a botanical variety, hybrid and cultivar which have scientific accuracy. Allergenicity may be confined to certain cultivars of a species. Some commercial flower growers sensitized to Chrysanthemum may be able to continue in their business, handling only cultivars of Chrysanthemum to which they react less or not at all. The word variety is used in horticulture for subtypes of a plant given common names; such names do not have scientific accuracy.

Table 5. Authority for a Botanical Species Name

Toxicodendron radicans (Linnaeus) Kuntze

Toxic epidermal necrolysis (Lyell)

Linnaeus (1707-1778) described the species.

Kuntze (1843-1907) revised the description

Table 6.

Botanical variety	Toxicodendron radicans var. littorale (East coast poison ivy)
Botanical hybrid	Chrysanthemum morifolium (C. sinense X C. indicum)
Horticultural cultivar	Chrysanthemum morifolium --Annie Curry

Table 7. Steps for Preserving Plants for Patch Testing

Recommended steps for patch testing with a plant:

1. Divide the plant into 3 parts. Air dry or freeze one part and keep for botanical identification (flowers needed). Label, date, source, geographic site obtained. Put 2 parts into freeze.
   a. For patch testing.
   b. For making extract dilutions and for chemical studies.
2. Patch test with leaf, flower-head, stalk, petal. Tests in control individuals are essential.

Patch Testing with Plants

The steps to be carried out are summarized in Table 7.

There is no point in patch testing with known irritant plants such as those shown in Table 3. If irritancy seems possible, it is necessary to patch test with caution (Kerner et al 1973). In all cases, patch tests to plants in a patient suspected to be allergic should be accompanied by control patch tests in at least 5, preferably 20, volunteer subjects. The literature abounds with invalid reports in which alleged allergenic plants have not received the simple but crucial tests for irritancy in controls. No plant can be considered proven allergenic unless tests are negative in a substantial number of controls.

The actual plants to which the patient was exposed should be used for patch-testing. Rarely is it possible to use dried herbarium specimens of identified species for this purpose.

Over 95% of all cases of patch-test proven plant dermatitis reported has been caused by plants in a small number of families (Table 8) (Hjorth 1966). Time can be wasted by repeated testing with innocuous plants but judgement is required if an infrequently allergenic plant is not to be missed, for example, Tolmiea (piggyback plant) yielded 4 positives and 89 negatives in 93 tests.

If there is a clinical suspicion of plant dermatitis but no clear lead is provided by the history, it may be useful to limit screening patch-testing to plants within these commonly offending families. Otherwise patch tests with innocuous but popular plants may continue to be performed.

One should wait until acute dermatitis has subsided before patch testing, in order to avoid the risk of provoking a focal or disseminated flare. The skin site selected for patch testing should be clear of dermatitis for at least 2 weeks and preferably for a month before such testing is carried out - hence the usefulness of freezing plants. An irritant plant, Ranunculus (buttercup), becomes more irritant after freezing; as the tissues are rewarmed, the cells burst and enzyme action releases an irritant compound, protoanemonin. Dried buttercups are hardly irritant at all since protoanemonin is converted into an innocuous polymer, anemonin. There is no firm evidence that plant allergens are made innocuous by freezing. False-positive reactions can result from testing during status eczematicus - the so-called angry back (Mitchell 1975). The back is more sensitive than are the

Table 8. Results of Aimed Patch-Tests with Plants in 6 Years. Hjorth, 1966

Species (number)	No. tests	Positive reactions No.	Positive reactions Percentage
23	595	58	9.7
227	1,513	0	0.0

Table 9. Steps Recommended for Patch Testing Workers Suspected of Allergy to Sawdust

Obtain botanical identification if possible from the wood (not the dust).
Place no reliance on trade (lumber) names.
Patch test with dry and then with damp sawdust. (Damp sawdust may release formic acid and other irritants).
It is best to patch test with freshly ground sawdust 10% in petrolatum and test controls.
Care must be taken not actively to sensitize workers by using allergens in too strong a concentration.

extremities. Confusion may occur from discoloration of the skin at the test site by the presence in a plant of a red dye which simulates an erythema. An irritant patch test reaction can never be reliably distinguished from an allergic patch test reaction.

Leaves and petals should be lightly crushed; stalks and thick leaves should be cut into thin slices.

Patch Testing with Sawdust

Colloquial, common and trade names of commercial woods can be completely misleading; for example, Canadian hemlock is often shipped as Alaska pine. A dictionary of commercial trees (Beckman 1964) lists the large number of trade names of commercial woods used in several languages. No reliance can be placed on the trade name of a wood as an indication of the botanical species of the tree from which the wood is derived. Expert identification by a department of botany or by a forest products laboratory is essential for meaningful tests in suspected contact allergy from sawdust. The steps recommended for patch testing workers who may be sensitized to commercial sawdusts are noted in Table 9.

Patch Testing with Bulbs

The bulbs of *Tulipa* (tulip), *Hyacinthus* (hyacinth) and *Narcissus* (daffodil) are important causes of contact dermatitis in the bulb-growing industry. The problem is well known to the growers but cases rarely are seen by a dermatologist. For patch testing, the thin dried outer scale of the bulb should be removed. The moist fleshy outer layers of the bulb which are actually leaves modified to storage, should be used for patch testing. Tests on control subjects are required to exclude irritancy.

Patch Testing with Hairy Plants

Patch testing with hairy plants can produce irritant patch test reactions. Some irritant hairy plants are listed in Table 10.

Table 10. Irritant Hairy Plants

Many plants of Borage family, *Borago*, etc.
Cortusa--relative of *Primula*
Bergonia rex and hybrids
Sparmannia (Indoor Linden) (This plant is also allergenic)
Ulmus (Elm)
Cornus sanguinea (Blood-twig dogwood)--T-shaped hairs
Nettles--*Urtica*

Table 11. Patch Testing with Irritant, Suspected Allergenic Plants

Patch testing with an irritant but suspected allergenic plant:

Make 10% aqueous extract. Allergen of Allium (garlic), is water soluble.
10% ethanol extract. Most plant allergens are soluble in organic solvents.

Patch test the patient and controls.

If negative, try 20% or greater to find a non-irritant, allergenic concentration. A variety of organic solvents can be tried.

Sparmannia (indoor linden) can produce irritant patch test reactions and is also probably allergenic, thus judicious patch testing with the plant and its extracts is required. The T-shaped hairs of Cornus sanguinea (blood-twig dogwood) produce urticarial reactions if the leaf is rubbed on the skin in the direction of its long axis.

Some other commonly grown hairy plants produce irritant patch test reactions from their leaves, e.g. Senecio (cineraria), Primula sinensis (primrose) and Ficus macrophylla (fig).

Photopatch testing

Phytophotodermatitis is caused by a photochemical reaction mediated by psoralens and possibly by other plant chemicals. No allergic mechanism is implicated and any individual exposed adequately to the plant juices and then to sunlight will react. Skin tests are meaningless if the suspected plant is known to contain psoralens but may be of interest if such information is lacking in the world literature and facilities for photochemical studies are not available. The tests can be carried out on any volunteer to avoid inconveniencing the patient, who is often a child.

Purification and Identification of Plant Allergens

Purification and identification of allergens of plants have been accomplished only in a few instances. The method used has been summarized by Benezra (1973). To carry an investigation this far is a major research exercise.

Some plants are irritant and allergenic. When such plants are suspect, it is necessary to use for patch testing plant extracts, diluted to a nonirritant level. This complex but not unimportant problem is summarized in Table 11.

Control Tests

Regarding controls, synthetic primin, the allergenic quinone of Primula obconica provides a useful example. Concentration 1 in 100 is always irritant: 1 in 1000 is often irritant: 1 in 10,000 produces active sensitization (sensitization by patch testing): 1 in 50,000 elicits positive reactions only in sensitized individuals. The allergen of Tulipa (tulip) (α-methylene - γ-butyrolactone) is irritant at a concentration 1 in 600 but produces positive patch test reactions in sensitized persons at 1 in 20,000. An overriding consideration is that the concentrations should not be great enough to cause active sensitization. 25-microliter pipettes may be used for applying the fluid extracts. The test response depends on the amount of allergen deposited per surface area and not on the total dose.

The patch test unit to be used requires consideration. The Al-test patches have a circular cellulose disc 1 cm. Plant chemicals in solution may be retained in the interstices of the cellulose disc. False-negative reactions can be thus produced. It is preferable to apply the solution to the skin, to await evaporation and then to occlude the site.

Patch Testing with Commerical Plant Extracts

Shelmire, (1939) the father of the ivestigation of "weed" dermatitis, used plant extracts for patch testing. His method forms the basis on which acetone extracts of plants are based. Such extracts which are usually in a concentration 10% w/v in acetone may be used for open tests.

Since false-negative test reactions can occur from open tests, closed tests are preferable. Closed tests, however, may produce severe reactions. For closed tests, the acetone solution is applied to the skin and allowed to evaporate. The site is then occluded by a patch test unit. The patient should be warned to remove the patch test unit if itching develops. In a severe reaction, this may occur as early as 6 hours after application of the patch. In such circumstances, occlusion for 48 hours may produce unnecessarily severe reactions which can be avoided by such a warning.

The commercial extracts have been dried in the dark and retain some plant pigments such as chlorophyll which stains the skin. Such stains are not difficult to distinguish from erythema. The use of added dyes in extracts, previously used to mark the sites of open tests, has been abandoned because of occasional contact sensitivity to the dye itself.

Evaporation of acetone from acetone extracts readily occurs from repeated opening of the container in which the extract is stored. Thus, old, frequently used acetone extracts may in time acquire an increased concentration and so produce irritant effects or even active sensitization by patch testing (spontaneous flare). Therefore, the extracts should be replaced by fresh extracts if such evaporation is suspected. The shelf life of such extracts is unknown. For office and clinic practice, replacement of the extracts every 6 or 12 months seems adequate.

Having established the allergenicity of a plant by suitable patch testing and by the use of controls, one can proceed to test more thoroughly with various parts of the plant -- root, stalk, leaf, flowerhead, parts of the flower. Controls are required for each part tested since the parts of a plant often vary in their chemical composition. Often, mature plants are more allergenic than immature plants. With age, secondary products of metabolism accumulate in plants since they have little or no excretory mechanisms. Therefore, mature plants should be used for patch testing. Some provisional evidence suggests that immature plants of _Asparagus_ (asparagus) and of _Chicorium_ (chicory) may be more allergenic than flowering specimens. If this is the case, these plants are exceptions to the rule noted previously. These plants are commonly used for commercial and culinary purposes when in a state of immaturity; therefore, maximum exposure occurs to immature rather than to mature plants. Until this aspect is clarified, it is probably best to use mature plants for patch testing.

Botanical Affinities and Phytochemical Investigation

To widen the scope of an investigation, patch tests may be carried out with related plants contained in the genus, tribe and family of a proven allergenic plant. Botanical affinities can thus suggest useful lines of investigation. More sophisticated information can be obtained from perusal of the phytochemical literature (Hegnauer 1962-73). In some instances, closely related chemicals are derived from botanically widely separated plants. Thus, sesquiterpene lactones are derived from _Frullania_ (liverwort) an evolutionarily lowly placed genus and from species of the Compositae (Chrysanthemum) family which are regarded as evolutionarily advanced. More closely related phytochemical affinities have been shown between _Tulipa_ (tulip) and _Alstroemeria_; cross-reactions occurring between these plant genera, which are of separate but related families, result from a common content of the allergen, alpha-methylene-gamma-butyrolactone which occurs both in _Tulipa_ and _Alstroemeria_.

Cross-sensitivity is important notably in dermatitis caused by species of the Compositae (Chrysanthemum) family.

A housecall to the patient's home and garden has proved most useful for supplementing the data. For instance, a patient who had _Chrysanthemum_ dermatitis did not recover in spite of avoidance of contact with

Chrysanthemum. A visit to the patient's garden revealed that he was pulling Tanacetum (tansy) weed which infested his flower beds. The dermatitis was perpetuated by exposure to tansy weed which is botanically and chemically related to chrysanthemum.

A patient who shows a positive patch reaction to ragweed (Ambrosia) may never have been exposed to this weed; he may actually have been sensitized to one of many other Compositate plants. Cross-reactions between Compositae are often observed owing to 600 cross-reacting allergenic sesquiterpene lactones distributed in this family. Cross-sensitivity also extends to Magnolia, Liriodendron (tulip tree), Frullania (liverwort), Laurel oil (Laurus), Champaca oil (Michelia), and Costus oil (Saussurea); these oils are used in perfumery. It is easy for the wrong plant to be incriminated.

Hyposensitization

Hyposensitization can be carried out for Toxicodendron (poison ivy) and for Ambrosia (ragweed) dermatitis. It is not safe to try hyposensitization with home-made extracts of other plants because of possible poisoning. Further efforts are needed to reduce the morbidity from various plant sources.

References

Bailey, L.H.: Manual of Cultivated Plants. New York, Macmillan, 1971

Beckmann, W.R.: Elsevier's Wood Dictionary in seven languages. Vol. 1. Amsterdam, Elsevier, 1964.

Benezra, C.: Allergenes vegetaux. Methodes chimiques d'isolement et d'identification. Rev. Franc. Allergol. 13:51, 1973.

Camm, E.L., Buck, H.W.L., and Mitchell, J.C.: Phytophotodermatitis from Heracleum mantegazzianum. Contact Derm. 2:68, 1976

Camm, E.L. , Towers, G.H.N. and Mitchell, J.C.: Ultraviolet-mediated antibiotic activity of some Compositae species. Phytochemistry 14: 2007, 1975.

Chan, G.F.Q., Towers, G.H.N., and Mitchell, J.C.: Ultraviolet-mediated antibiotic activity of thiophene compounds of Tagetes. Phytochemistry 14: 2295, 1975.

Chittenden, F.J.: The Royal Horticultural Society Dictionary of Gardening. 2nd. ed. Oxford, Clarenden Press, 1969.

Fernald, M.L.: Gray's Manual of Botany. 8th edition. New York, Van Nostrand Reinhold Co., 1970.

Gellin, G.A., Wolf, C.R., and Milby, T.H.: Poison ivy, poison oak and poison sumac. Common causes of occupational dermatitis. Arch. Environ. Health 22:280, 1971.

Gillis, W.T.: Poison-ivy and its kin. Arnoldia 34:93, 1975.

Hegnauer, R.: Chemotaxonomy of plants. 6 vols. Basel, Birkhauser, 1962-73.

Hjorth, N.: Contact sensitivity to plants and balsams. European Congress of Allergy 1965. Acta Derm. Venereol. page 65, 1966.

Kerner, J., Maibach, H.I., and Mitchell, J.C.: Irritant contact dermatitis from the plant Agave americana L. Arch. Derm. 108: 102, 1973.

Mitchell, J.C.: Allergic contact dermatitis from Compositae. Trans. St. John's Hosp. Derm. Soc. 55:174, 1969.

Mitchell, J.C.: The angry back syndrome. Contact Derm. 1:193, 1975.

Shelmire, B.: Contact dermatitis from weeds: Patch testing with their oleoresins. JAMA 113, 1085 1939.

Sommer, R.G., and Jillson, O.F.: Phytophotodermatitis (Solar dermatitis from plants). Gas Plant and Wild Parsnip. N. Engl. J. Med 276: 1484, 1967.

Alphabetical Listing of Plant Families and Genera.

ACANTHACEAE

Some 2,500 species in 250 genera are found mainly in the tropics, but some occur in the United States and the Mediterranean region. Some species are of horticultural value.

Chemistry is recorded by Hegnauer (1964).

Mechanical Injury

Anthacanthus spinosus (Catch and Keep) and Barleria lupulina are recorded as causing mechanical injuries (Oakes and Butcher 1962). Many other of the 230 species of Barleria are thorny.

References

Hegnauer, R. (1964) Chemotaxonomy of plants. Vol. 3. Basel, Birkhauser. pp.41

Oakes, A.J. and Butcher, J.O. (1962) Poisonous and Injurious Plants of the U.S. Virgin Islands. Misc. Publ. 82. U.S. Department of Agriculture, Washington, D.C.

ACERACEAE

About 200 species in three genera are found in northern temperate regions and on tropical mountains. The pollens of the anemophilous species, less commonly of the amphiphilous and entomophilous species are minor causes of hayfever (Wodehouse 1971).

Acer

About 200 species are found in northern temperate regions and on tropical mountains. Many species are found in China and Japan, a few in south-eastern Asia and one in western Malaysia. Acer saccharum and others of eastern North America yield maple sugar. Acer rubrum is used for an astringent effect for treating sore eyes by North American Indians (Wren 1968).

Acer spp. Maple

Inhalation of fungi of maple bark can produce maple bark disease, a form of allergic alveolitis (Morgan and Seaton 1975).

Maple was said to be a sensitizing wood by Weber (1953) repeated by McCord (1958). Airborne contact dermatitis was attributed to the tree-pollen oils of maple and box elder (Acer negundo) (Lovell et al 1955).

Acer spp. may be infested with aphides which drop from the tree and colonize the skin causing a form of pseudophytodermatitis (Mitchell 1975). Honeydew consists of the excretions of such insects.

Acer platanoides

The wood was listed as irritant (Hanslian and Kadlec 1966) probably from Weber (1953).

References

Hanslian, L. and Kadlec, K. (1966) Wood from the standpoint of hygiene VIII. Species with some or little biological effect. Drevo. 21, 229.

Lovell, R.G., Mathews, K.P. and Sheldon, J.M. (1955) Dermatitis venenata from tree pollen oils. J. Allergy 26, 408.

McCord, C.P. (1958) The toxic properties of some timber woods. Industr. Med. Surg. 27, 202.

Mitchell, J.C. (1975) Pseudophytodermatitis from honeydew and aphides. Derm. Int. 14, 761.

Morgan, W.K.C. and Seaton, A. (1975) Occupational Lung Diseases. Philadelphia, Saunders.

Weber, L.F. (1953) Dermatitis venenata from native woods. Arch. Derm. Syph. 67, 388.

Wodehouse, R.P. (1971) Hayfever Plants. 2nd. revised edition. New York, Hafner.

Wren, R.W. (1968) Potter's New Cyclopedia of Botanical Drugs and Preparations by Wren, R.C. Re-edit. by Wren, R.W. Potter and Clarke Ltd. Health Science Press. Rustington, Sussex.

AGAVACEAE

The topical and subtropical family contains about 670 species in 20 genera: they were formerly included in the Amaryllidaceae. Some species are cultivated as ornamental plants; Agave americana for spectacular display in favourable climates, and Sansevieria spp. as humble house plants. Human contact with many species is close and repeated, because of their economic value; several species of Agave yield strong fibres, e.g. A. sisalana, sisal and Phormium tenax, New Zealand Flax. The former is cultivated commercially in Malawi and elsewhere. The abundant sap of Agave americana, A. atrovirens and other species, is fermented to form the drink pulque, from which mescal is distilled.

Chemistry

Agave americana, A. vivipara, and A. fourcroydes, contain saponin and minute sharp crystals of calcium oxalate (Souder 1963), as do species of Furcraea, Phormium, Polianthes, Cordyline, Sansevieria and Yucca. Agave sisalana is said to contain a sensitizing agent (Schwartz et al 1957). An acrid volatile oil has been isolated from the leaf (Osol and Farrer 1955). Agave lechuguilla and Nolina texana contain a hepato-nephro-toxin, probably a saponin (Mathews 1938a) and a photodynamic substance with an action-spectrum similar to that of the photodynamic pigment of Fagopyrum (Mathews 1938b).

The chemistry is recorded by Hegnauer (1963).

Dermatitis

An irritant dermatitis and conjunctivitis has been attributed by many species, notably the widely grown Agave americana (Century Plant, American Aloe) (Schwartz et al 1957, Behl et al 1966, McCord 1962, Hardin and Arena 1969, Duke-Elder and MacFaul 1972). The skin of the leaf of A. americana has been shown to be irritant, and in parts of Africa is used as a rubefacient (Watt and Breyer-Brandwijk 1962). The sap has been noted to be intensely irritating (Maiden 1909). Other species, too, such as A. lechuguilla and A. sisalana (Sisal) have produced similar effects (Schwartz et al 1957). The sap of A. picta has been said to be particularly irritant, causing a burning rash (Morton 1971), and the sap of A. atrovirens has been described as caustic (Madinaveitia and Orozco 1940). An occupational dermatosis caused by mouldy sisal (Agave sisalana) was described by Faninger and Markovic-Brisk (1960). The use of a "cactus juice" shampoo derived from A. americana caused dermatitis (Kerner et al 1973): an open epicutaneous test produced contact urticaria followed by eczematous dermatitis.

Sanseverinia sp. (Mother-in-law's Tongue) may cause dermatitis (McCord 1962) which may be allergic (Hjorth 1968), although these plants are also irritant.

Furcraea spp (Figue), used for making coffee bags, has caused dermatitis in those who grow the plant, those who make the bags and those who put the coffee in the bags (Schwartz et al 1957).

Nolina texana (Bunch Grass) has caused an irritant dermatitis (Muenscher 1951).

The needle-sharp leaf-tips of many plants in this family may penetrate the skin (Oakes and Butcher 1962), and in or near bone may excite a reaction which may simulate a neoplasm (Maylan 1952).

Veterinary Aspects

Ingestion of Agave lechuguilla and Nolina texana have given rise in goats and sheep to photodermatitis accompanied by hepatic and renal damage (Mathews 1940).

Patch Testing

Preliminary open epicutaneous tests to the plants and their sap are recommended since closed patch tests may produce severe reactions (Kerner et al 1973).

References

Behl, P.N. Captain, R.M. Bedi, B.M.S. and Gupta, S. (1966) Skin-irritant and sensitising plants found in India. New Delhi. P.N. Behl.

Duke-Elder, S. and MacFaul, P.A. (1972) System of Opthalmology. Vol. XIV. Injuries Part. I. Mechanical Injuries. Extra-ocular foreign bodies. pp. 464-67 and Agricultural Injuries pp. 32-34. London. Henry Kimpton.

Faninger, A.A. and Markovic-Brisk, A. (1960) Occupational dermatosis caused by mouldy sisal. Srpski. Arkiv Celok Lek 88,303.

Hardin, J.W. and Arena, J.M. (1969) Human Poisoning from Native and Cultivated Plants, Durham, North Carolina, Duke University Press.

Hegnauer, R. (1963) Chemotaxonomy of plants. Vol. 2. Basel. Birkhauser. pp. 25-47.

Hjorth, N. (1968) at Finsen Institute. Personal communication.

Kerner, J., Mitchell, J.C. and Maibach, H.I. (1973) Irritant Contact Dermatitis from Agave americana. Archs. Derm. 108, 102.

McCord, C.P. (1962) The Occupational Toxicity of Cultivated Flowers. Ind. Med. Surg. 31, 365.

Madinaveitia, A. and F. and Orozco, D. (1940) Contribucion a la bioquimica del Agave. Anal. Inst. Biol. Mexico, 11, 373

Maiden, J.H. (1909) On some plants which cause inflammation or irritation of the skin. Agric. Gaz. New South Wales 20, 1073.

Mathews, F.P. (1938a) Lechuguilla (Agave lechequilla) poisoning in sheep and goats. J. Am. Vet. Med. Ass. 93, 168.

Mathews, F.P. (1938b) An experimental investigation of Lechuguilla poisoning. Arch. Path. 25, 661.

Mathews, F.P. (1940) Poisoning in sheep and goats by Sucahuiste (Nolina texana) buds and blooms. Texas Agr. Expt. Sta. Bull 585.

Maylahn, D.J. (1952) Thorn induced "Tumors" of bone. J. Bone Joint Surg. 34A, 386.

Morton, J.F. (1971) Plants Poisonous to People in Florida and Other Warm Areas. Miami, Florida. Hurricane House.

Muenscher, W.C. (1951) Poisonous Plants of the United States 2nd. ed. New York, Macmillan.

Oakes, A.J. and Butcher, J.O. (1962). Poisonous and Injurious Plants of the U.S. Virgin Islands. Misc. Publ. 882. U.S. Department of Agriculture, Washington, D.C.

Osol, A. and Farrer, G.E. (Ed.)(1955) Dispensatory of the U.S.A. Philadelphia J.B. Lippincott.

Schwartz, L., Tulipan, L. and Birmingham, D.J. (1957) Occupational Diseases of the Skin. 3rd. ed. Philadelphia, Lea and Febiger. pp. 637-672.

Souder, P. (1963) Poisonous Plants on Guam, in Venomous and Poisonous Animals and Noxious Plants of the Pacific Region. ed. Keegan, H.L. and Macfarlane, W.V. Oxford, Pergamon Press. pp.15-29.

Watt, J.M. and Breyer-Brandwijk, M.G. (1962) The Medicinal and Poisonous Plants of Southern and Eastern Africa. 2nd ed. Edinburgh. Livingstone.

AÏZOACEAE

The 1200 species in the 1?0 genera which make up this family are particularly strongly represented in South Africa, but some occur in tropical Africa, in Australia and in South and Central America and in California. Many species are decorative and are widely cultivated; some, notably Mesembryanthemum sp. (Ice plant), have become naturalised in many parts of Europe. Galenia africana is used in African indigenous medicine as a counter-irritant in the treatment of toothache (Watt and Breyer-Brandwijk 1962).

Chemistry is recorded by Hegnauer (1964).

Dermatitis

Mesembryanthemum sp. can apparently cause allergic dermatitis. One of 19 patients tested gave a positive reaction (Hjorth 1968).

When chewed Galenia africana may be vesicant for the oral mucous membrane (Watt and Breyer-Brandwijk 1962).

References

Hegnauer, R. (1964) Chemotaxonomy of Plants. Vol. 3. Basel. Birkhauser pp. 63.

Hjorth, N. (1968) at the Finsen Institute. Pers. comm.

Watt, J.M. and Breyer-Brandwijk, M.G. (1962) The Medicinal and Poisonous Plants of Southern and Eastern Africa. 2nd. ed. Edinburgh, E. and S. Livingstone, Ltd.

ALGAE

To the non-botanist the algae are a mystery. He may be aware that the seaweeds and the pond "blooms" are algae, but is unlikely to be aware of the almost universal distribution of these complex organisms in moist environments. The direct economic importance of the algae is considerable and is likely to increase rapidly, as the human population of the world expands faster than the conventional sources of protein foodstuffs. Some species, too, produce toxic secretions which are dangerous to domestic animals and to man himself.

It is certain that man's contact with algae will increase, and it is probable that the role of algae in human disease either as opportunistic pathogens (e.g. Protothecosis , Davies 1972) or as cutaneous irritants or sensitizers has been underestimated, because unsuspected.

Even to the botanist the algae present considerable problems. They are difficult to classify, and even to define, The outline which follows is based on the authoritative works by Prescott (1969) and by Chapman and Chapman (1973). Algae may be loosely defined as chlorophyll-bearing organisms (and their colourless relatives) which are thalloid - that is to say, have no true roots, stems or leaves. Some algae are commensually associated with fungi to form lichens.

Botanical classifications are based on morphology and are an indication of presumed evolutionary relationships. As has been shown in the account of many families of flowering plants, botanically closely related genera are more likely to show chemical similarities than are those less closely related, although there are notable exceptions to this generalization. There are a number of controversial features in any available classification of the algae, but the taxonomists agree about the grouping of algae into classes, though they differ concerning the grouping of the classes into phyla or divisions. Following Chapman and Chapman (1973) the following phyla or divisions may be listed. The genera so far proved to be of interest to the dermatologist are the only ones included.

Cyanophyta - Blue-green algae (not accepted as 'true' algae by all authorities)

Genera

Microcystis, *Anabaena* and *Lyngbya*.

Rhodophyta - Red algae
Chlorophyta - Green algae

Genera

Chlorella sp., *Prototheca*, *Scenedesmus*, *Ankistrodesmus*, *Chlorococcum*

Euglenophyta - Euglenoids
Chloromonadophyta - Chloromonads
Xanthophyta - Yellow-green algae
Bacillariophyta - Diatoms
Chrysophyta - Golden-brown algae

Genus

Fragillaria

Phaeophyta - Brown algae
Pyrrhophyta - Dinoflagellates
Cryptophyta - Cryptomonads

Chemistry

Phycocyanin in blue-green algae has been suspected of allergenicity on the basis of patch tests (Cohen and Reif 1953). A toxic principle which may play some part in causing dermatitis has been isolated (Chu 1969, Moikeha and Chu 1971, Moikeha et al. 1971).

A hepatotoxic and photosensitizing substance is present in *Microcystis* sp. and other water-blooms (Kingsbury 1964).

Dermatitis

Four clinical syndromes have been attributed to the effects of algae. An erythematous papulovesicular eruption on areas of skin not protected by a bathing costume was reported in a child who had swum in a lake with a 'bloom' of blue-green algae. Patch tests to

Anabaena were positive. Another blue-green alga, Lyngbya majuscula causes seabathers' dermatitis in Hawaii (Grauer and Arnold 1961). The dermatitis may affect only skin covered by a tight fitting costume (Grauer 1959). Blue-green algae of various genera produced toxic or allergic dermatitis in Czechoslovakia (Krauskopf 1973). Other cases in bathers were reviewed by Schwimmer and Schwimmer (1955) and Hardin (1961).

An eczematous eruption beginning on the hands, and sometimes becoming more extensive, has been shown (Fraser and Lyell 1963, Beer et al. 1968, Beer and Jones 1969) to be caused by the green alga Fragillaria striatulata, which becomes established in the summer months on the ropes of lobster-pots.

"Redfeed" dermatitis may ultimately be caused by certain coloured algae, perhaps Gymnodinium, which support the orange-red crustaceans, known as "Redfeed". Fish which have eaten this crustacean in any quantity do not keep well after being caught and fishermen and processers who handle them may develop irritation and ulceration of the skin of the hands. "Redfeed" dermatitis has been reported from the Baltic (Kersten and Zschunke 1955, Bowszyc 1966) and from the United States (Schwartz and Tabershaw 1945). The role of algae toxins is unproven.

An atopic sensitivity to algae has been reported. Heise (1949) found blue-green algae responsible for seasonal rhinitis, related to swimming in lakes. Many blue-green and green algae are airborne in significant numbers at certain seasons. This observation led McElhenney et al (1962) to skin test with algae children with respiratory allergic disorders; they obtained some positive reactions. Six strains of green algae commonly encountered in air, water and soil samples in the United States were used to skin-test 79 atopic patients; 47 gave positive results; species of Chlorella, Chlorococcum and Scenedesmus were chiefly involved (Bernstein and Safferman 1966). Further investigations (Bernstein and Safferman 1973) showed a high incidence of positive skin tests to a Chlorella species found in house dust, in patients with perennial rhinitis. Urticaria may accompany the rhinitis.

Sensitization to the algal component of lichens has also been reported.

Photosensitization has been reported in livestock drinking water containing heavy concentrations of blue-green algae (Wild 1961, Kingsbury 1965, Schwimmer and Schwimmer 1968). It accompanies blood in the faeces and icterus in those few cases of poisoning that are not rapidly fatal.

References

Beer, W.E., Jones, M. and Jones, W.E. (1968) Dermatoses in Lobster Fishermen. Br. med. J. 1, 807.

Beer, W.E. and Jones, W.E. (1969) Dermatoses in Lobster Fishermen. Brit. Med. J. 1, 572.

Bernstein, I.L. and Safferman, R.S. (1966) Sensitivity of Skin and Bronchial Mucosa to Green Algae. J. Allergy, 38, 166.

Bernstein, I.L. and Safferman, R.S. (1973) Clinical Sensitivity to Green Algae Demonstrated by Nasal Challenge and in Vitro Tests of Immediate Hypersensitivity. J. Allergy, 51, 22.

Bowszyc, J. (1966) Redfeed dermatitis. A professional disease of workers in the fishing industry caused by Baltic herring and mackerel. (Polish). Przegl. Derm. 53, 39.

Chapman, V.J. and Chapman, D.J. (1973) The Algae. London, Macmillan.

Chu, G.W. (1969) A unique toxic lipid from a Hawaiian dermatitis-producing marine alga. J. Formosan Med. Ass. 68, 570.

Cohen, S.G. and Reif, C.B. (1953) Cutaneous Sensitization to Blue-Green Algae. J. Allergy 24, 452.

Davies, R.R. (1972) Protothecosis and opportunist fungal infections. Trans. St. John's Hosp. Derm. Soc. 58, 38.

Fraser, J.H. and Lyell, A. (1963) Dogger Bank Itch. Lancet, i, 61.

Grauer, F.H. (1959) Dermatitis Escharotica Caused by a Marine Alga. Hawaii med. J. 19, 32.

Grauer, F.H. and Arnold, H.L. Jr. (1961) Seaweed Dermatitis. Archs. Derm. 84, 720.

Hardin, F.F. (1961) 'Seabathers eruption'. J. Med. Ass. Georgia 50, 450.

Heise, H.A. (1949) Symptoms of Hay Fever Caused by Algae. J. Allergy, 20, 383.

Kingsbury, J.M. (1964) Poisonous Plants of the United States and Canada. Englewood Cliffs, New Jersey.

Krauskopf, J. (1973) Phytodermatitis caused by Cyanophyta and Algae. Cs. Derm. 48, 195.

Kersten, E. and Zschunke, E. (1955) Redfeed dermatitis, a skin affection frequent in the fishing industries. Dtsch. Gesundhwes 10, 194.

McElhenney, T.R., Bold, H.C., Brown, R.M., Jr., and McGovern, J.P. (1962) Algae: a cause of inhalant allergy in children. Ann. Allergy 20, 739.

Moikeha, S.N. and Chu, G.W. (1971) Dermatitis-producing Alga *Lyngbya majuscula* Gomont in Hawaii II. Biological properties of the toxic factor. J. Phycol. 7, 8.

Moikeha, S.N., Chu, G.W. and Berger, L.R. (1971) Dermatitis-producing Alga *Lyngbya majuscula* Gomont in Hawaii I. Isolation and chemical characterization of the toxic factor. J. Phycol. 7, 4.

Prescott, G.W. (1969) The Algae: a Review. London, Nelson.

Schwartz, L. and Tabershaw, I.R. (1945) Dermatitis in the Fish Industry. J. Industr. Hyg. Toxicol. 27, 27.

Schwimmer, M. and Schwimmer, D. (1955) The role of algae and plankton in medicine. New York, Grune and Stratton.

Schwimmer, D. and Schwimmer, M. (1968) Medical aspects of Phycology, in Algae, Man and the Environment. Ed. D.F. Jackson. Syracuse University Press.

Wild, H. (1961) Harmful aquatic plants in Africa and Madagascar. Kirkia 2, 1.

ALTISMATACEAE

These cosmopolitan water or marsh plants comprise about 90 species in 13 genera and are related to Ranunculaceae.

Some species are cultivated for their edible rhizomes, e.g. *Alisma plantago-aquatica* (Water plantain) and others for their edible turions - winter buds - e.g. *Sagittaria sagittifolia* (Arrowhead).

Chemistry is recorded by Hegnauer (1963).

Dermatitis

The leaves of *Alisma* can irritate the skin (Dispensatory 1884). *Sagittaria* turions have caused dermatitis in those who handle them (Behl et al 1966).

References

Behl, P.N. et al (1966) Captain, R.M., Bedi, B.M.S. and Gupta, S. (1966) Skin irritant and Sensitizing Plants found in India, New Delhi. P.N. Behl, Irwin Hospital.

Dispensatory, The National (1884) Philadelphia, Stille and Maisch; cited by White, J.C. (1887).

Hegnauer, R. (1963) Chemotaxonomy of Plants. Vol. 2, Basel. Birkhauser. pp. 47.

White, J.C. (1887) Dermatitis Venenata: An Account of the Action of External Irritants Upon the Skin. Boston, Cupples and Hurd.

ALLIACEAE

This family of some 600 species in 30 genera is widely distributed throughout the world, with the exception of Australasia. The family is taxonomically intermediate between the Liliaceae and the Amaryllidaceae, and was formerly included in the Amaryllidaceae.

The most important genus numerically and economically is Allium, the 450 species of which are widely distributed in the Northern hemisphere. Some strongly flavoured species have been used since early times (Numbers) and garlic was an important food in the diet of the Egyptian slaves who built the Pyramids and among the legions of Ancient Rome (Collins 1964).

Many species of Allium have flowers which are sufficiently attractive to ensure their cultivation in gardens, despite their often disagreeable odour. The principal food species, Allium cepa (Onion), A. sativum (Garlic), A. schoenoprasum (Chives), A. ascalonicum (Shallot) and A. porrum (Leek) are very widely grown. In the wild, some species such as A. triquetrum have become abundant and troublesome weeds.

Species of Allium are used in folk medicine as such or as an ingredient of ointments (Burkill 1935).

The very beautiful South African genus of Agapanthus (5 species), notably A. orientalis, is cultivated wherever the winter climate is sufficiently mild or protection can be provided.

Chemistry

Sulphur-containing oils are present in many species of Allium, including A. sativum (garlic), A. cepa (onion), A. triquetrum (Triangle onion) and A. schoenoprasum (chives). They are pungent and irritant. Oil of garlic which contains allylpropyldisulphide and diallyldisulphide induces irritation or vesication of the skin (White 1887, Burkill 1935, Watt and Breyer-Brandwijk 1962). The concentration of oil in the bulb is 0.1 - 0.3% (Hurst 1942). Patch testing with the bulb is therefore not always a useful procedure since irritant reactions are obtained in most subjects (White 1887, Allen 1943, Edelstein 1950).

The fresh garlic bulb yields alliin, allicin and volatile and fatty oils. When the bulb is crushed the odourless alliin is converted by the enzyme alliinase to allicin, which has the characteristic smell (Merck 1968).

Although it has been assumed that the water soluble fraction of Allium species contains an allergenic substance (Burks 1954), this is by no means proven. The dermatitis attributable to Allium may be of irritant type. Four housewives with such a dermatitis related to handling A. cepa gave positive patch tests to alliin (Neves 1964). Allicin is certainly irritant to the skin (Merck 1968). The irritant properties of alliin appear not to have been studied. However the natural history of Allium dermatitis suggests that it usually has an allergic basis, and the fact that a substance is shown to be an irritant by no means excludes a capacity also to sensitize.

Many reports suggest that an identical or immunochemically related substance may be present in garlic and onion, but this assumption has often been based on patch tests of questionable reliability. However in the investigation of a male cook with eczema attributed to garlic, patch tests were positive to garlic but not to onion (Bleumink and Nater 1972). Ethanol and aqueous extracts of garlic were then used to patch test 125 persons; six reacted to the former and 10 to the latter; all these 10 subjects were women of average age 58, and all had been exposed to garlic in the course of food preparation. A latent subclinical allergic sensitivity was postulated. The relevance of cross-sensitivity with Tulipa is uncertain (Bleumink and Nater 1973).

In Mexico A. sativum appeared to cause photosensitization after it had been applied for the treatment of a variety of dermatoses, including lichen simplex and acne (Cueva and Duran 1955, Saul 1972). Lesions developed on non-exposed sites, including some to which the garlic had not been deliberately applied.

Although farmers and gardeners may frequently be exposed to Allium species, the most intimate and prolonged contact is liable to occur in cooks, housewives and other food handlers.

Eye irritation from the vapour of onions is attributed to allylpropyldisulphide (Feiner et al 1946), diallyldisulphide (Strong 1966) and propenylsulfinic acid (Virtanen 1961, Strong 1966).

Garlic as is and aqueous, ethanol and ether extracts of garlic produced positive patch test reactions. Some of the patients were also contact sensitive to chives (A. schoenprasum, onion (A. cepa), leek (A. porrum) and chicory (Cichorium).

These plants are probably marginal irritants by 2 day closed patch tests since they produce positive reactions in a few controls. One patient had a positive scratch test reaction indicating immediate hypersensitivity to garlic. Four patients who were contact sensitive to garlic showed positive patch test reactions to allyl disulphide 5% petrolatum which seems to be a common allergen of Allium spp. (Hjorth and Roed-Petersen 1976).

Dermatitis

The clinical syndrome most commonly reported has been a circumscribed, irritable, hyperkeratotic eczema of the tips of the fingers of one or both hands - usually the left hand which is used to grasp the bulb firmly, whilst a knife is held in the right hand (Borda and Bozzola 1961, Burks 1954, Burgess 1952). The sudden onset of eczema in this distribution has been observed in a male cook who had regularly handled garlic with impunity for over 20 years (Rook 1974).

Less distinctive patterns of eczema of hands or forearms have also been attributed to garlic, e.g. in a girl aged 12 (Sepulvedas 1933); in workers in a potato crisp factory (Inman 1965); in a meat-grinder (Edelstein 1950).

Handling dehydrated onions has been held responsible for an irritant dermatitis (Schwartz et al 1957).

A self-inflicted bullous eruption on the shins produced by garlic in a malingerer resembled pemphigus both histologically and cytologically (Pirogova and Katyukhina 1970).

The possible induction of photosensitivity by the medical use of Allium sativum has been mentioned above. A. schoenoprasum in an ointment has caused dermatitis in Japan.

A single case report (Black 1972) of facial oedema, coughing, sneezing and lacrimation one or two hours after handling A. triquetrum is difficult to evaluate. Subsequent consumption of onions was followed almost immediately by wheezing and a feeling of constriction in the throat. Tests for immediate type hypersensitivity were negative and patch tests were positive at 96 but not at 48 hours.

The major allergen of garlic and onion is allylsulphide, probably also of chives and leek (Hjorth and Roed-Petersen 1976).

Cross-sensitivity between garlic, onion and tulip (Tulipa) was described by Bleumink and Nater 1973).

References

Allen, P.H. (1943) Poisonous and injurious plants of Panama. Am. J. trop. Med. Suppl. 23, 1.

Black H. (1972) Contact Dermatitis from onion weed Plant. Personal Communication. Contact Dermatitis Newsletter 11, 282.

Bleumink E. and Nater, J.P. (1972) Garlic as possible cause of contact dermatitis. Personal Communication. Contact Dermatitis Newsletter 12, 310.

Bleumink, E. and Nater, J.P. (1973) Contact dermatitis to garlic: cross reactivity between garlic, onion and tulip. Arch. Dermatol. Forsch. 247, 117.

Borda, J.M. and Bozolla, C. (1961) Keratoses of the tips of the fingers due to contact with Liliaceae. Arch. argent. Derm 11, 293.

Burgess, J.F. (1952) Occupational dermatitis due to onion and garlic. Canad. med. Ass. J. 66, 275.

Burkill, I.H. (1935) A Dictionary of the Economic Products of the Malay Peninsula. 2 Vols. London, Crown Agents for the Colonies.

Burks, J.W. (1954) Classic Aspects of onion and garlic dermatitis in housewives. Ann. Allergy, 12, 592.

Collins, M. (1964) Spices of the World Cookbook by McCormick. New York. McGraw-Hill.

Cueva, J. and Duran, C.J. (1955) Dermatitis due to garlic. Rev. Med. Hosp. Gen. (Mex.) 18,29.

Edelstein, A.J. (1950) Dermatitis caused by garlic. Arch. Derm. Syph. 61, 111.

Feiner, B., Burke, W.J. and Baliff, J. (1946) An industrial hygiene survey of an onion dehydrating plant. J. Industr. Hyg. 28, 278.

Hjorth, N. and Roed-Petersen, J. (1976) Occupational protein contact dermatitis in food handlers. Contact dermatitis 2, 28.

Hurst, E. (1942) The Poison plants of New South Wales. Sydney. New South Wales Poison Plants Committee.

Inman, P.M. (1965) Dermatitis in a Crisp Factory. Acta derm. -vener. Stockh. 45, 295.

Merck Index (1968) ed. Stecher, P.G. 8th ed. Rahway, New Jersey, Merck.

Neves, R.G. (1946) Contact Dermatitis Caused by Liliaceous Bulbs. An. Brasil. Derm. 39, 23.

Pirogova, E.P. and Katyukhina, Z.D. (1970) Artificial dermatitis caused by garlic. Vest. Derm. Venereol 44, 53.

Rook, A.J. (1974) Unpublished observations.

Saul, A. (1972) Photosensitivity caused by garlic. Presentation to First Joint Dermatological Meeting, Mexico-Texas. Centro Dermatologico Pascua, Mexico City.

Schwartz, L, Tulipan, L. and Birmingham, D.J. (1957) Occupational Diseases of the Skin. Lea and Febiger

Sepulvedar, D. (1938) Un Caso de Dermatosis por Contacto con Aja. Rev. Chilena Pediat. 9, 339.

Strong, F.M. (1966) Naturally occurring toxic factors in plants and animals used as food. Canada Med. Ass. J. 94, 568.

Virtanen, A.I. (1961) Organic sulfur compounds in vegetables and their importance in human nutrition. Address before the Amer. Chem. Soc. Northeastern Sect. 12, Oct.

Watt, J.M. and Breyer-Brandwijk, M.G. (1962) The Medicinal and Poisonous Plants of Southern and Eastern Africa. 2nd. edit. Edinburgh, E. & S. Livingstone Ltd.

White, J.C. (1887) Dermatitis venenata: an Account of the Action of External Irritants upon the Skin. Boston, Cupples and Hurd.

ALSTROEMERIACEAE

There are about 200 species in the four genera of this family, which was formerly classified with the Amaryllidaceae. Although they are natives of Central and South America, some species of Alstroemeriaceae, notably *A. auriantiaca* and *A. ligtu*, are more or less hardy in temperate climates and are frequently cultivated in gardens and are increasingly popular in the cut-flower trade. Gardeners, florists and housewives are therefore at risk.

Chemistry

Alpha-methylene - gamma-butyrolactone, an allergenic lactone previously isolated from tulip bulbs, has been shown (Slob 1973) to be present in large amounts in the flowers and in moderate amounts in the leaves of *Alstroemeria auriantiaca* and of *A. ligtu*.

Dermatitis

Two cases of allergic contact dermatitis have been reported in florists (Rook 1970, Cronin 1972). Both patients were also allergic to tulips (*Tulipa*) Patch tests with *Alstroemeria* in normal subjects provoke no reaction (Rook 1970).

References

Cronin, E. (1972) Sensitivity to Tulip and Alstroemeria. Personal Communication. Contact Dermatitis Newsletter, 11, 286.

Rook, A.J. (1970) *Alstroemeria* Causing Contact Dermatitis in Florist also Allergic to Tulip.

Contact Dermatitis Newsletter, 7, 186.

Slob, A. (1973) Tulip Allergens in Alstroemeria and Some Other Liliiflorae. Phytochemistry 12, 811.

ALTINGIACEAE

This family, previously included in the related Hamamelidaceae consists of 10 species in 2 genera, native to Asia Minor, temperate and tropical South East Asia and North and Central America.

They are strongly resiniferous trees, some of which yield valuable timber and some of which are the sources of the various forms of storax (syn. styrax), a fragrant gum-resin with many pharmaceutical and industrial uses.

Sources of Storax:

Altingia excelsa Burmese storax

A. gracilipes Tonkin storax

Liquidambar formosanum Chinese storax

L. orientalis Levant storax (refined at Smyrna)

L. styraciflua American storax (produced mainly in Honduras)

Sources of Timber:

Many species provide useful timber but only one, L. styraciflua, is reported as causing dermatitis. The timber, known in the trade as Liquidambar or as Amberwood, is sometimes designated satin walnut, satinwood, American red gum, sweet gum, sap gum, hazel pine or bilsted.

Chemistry

Storax contains cinnamic acid and its esters, styrene and vanillin (Nayes and Mazuyer 1947, Merck 1968), and is known to be allergenic and to cross-react with Gum Benzoin derived from species of Styrax (Styracaceae); with Balsm of Peru derived from Toluifera (Myroxylon) (Leguminosae); with rosin from Pinaceae species; with vanilla, derived from Orchidaceae species; with orange peel (Rutaceae); with cinnamon (Lauraceae); with clove (Myrtaceae) and with other essential oils (Hjorth 1961, Hjorth 1965).

Dermatitis

Storax, rubbed on the skin, may cause irritation and wheals (Greenberg and Lester 1954). Medicaments containing storax may cause allergic dermatitis.

Satin walnut was said to be irritant Krais (1910) but Legge (1907) and Grossmann (1920) considered that the wood had been confused with irritant satinwoods e.g. Fagara . Nestler (1911) used an ether extract of American satin walnut (imported as "East Indian satinwood") to test his own skin; the extract induced painful bulla formation after five hours contact. The bulla healed very slowly and left a thickened scar. The sawdust had no effect. There are no recent reports of dermatitis from the wood which is a major timber in the United States but now not much imported to Europe (Hausen 1973).

References Liquidambar

Greenberg, I.A. and Lester, D. (1954) Handbook of Cosmetic Materials. New York. Interscience.

Grossmann, J. (1920) Gesundheitsschädliche Holzarten Der Holz-Käufer (Leipzig) 17, 529, 535, 540 and 545.

Hausen, B.M. (1973) Holzarten mit gesundheitsschädigenden inhaltsstoffen Stuttgart. DRW-Verlags-GmbH.

Hjorth, N. (1961) Eczematous allergy to Balsams, Allied Perfumes and Flavouring Agents. Copenhagen Munksgaard.

Hjorth, N. (1965) Contact sensitivity to plants and balsams. Europ. Congr. Alerg. 1965. Acta derm.-venereol. 65-79.

Krais, P. (1910) Gewerblishe Materialkunde. Vol. 1. Die Hölzer. Stuttgart, Krais.

Legge, T.M. (1907) Reports of the Chief Inspector of Factories and Workshops. p. 248. London.

Merck Index (1968) 8th ed. ed. Stecher, P.G. Rahway, New Jersey Merck & Co.

Naves, Y.R. and Mazuyer, G. (1947) National Perfume Materials. New York, Reinhold, p. 265.

Nestler, A. (1911) Die hautreizende Wirkung des Amberholzes. Ber dtsch. bot. Gesellschaft, 29, 672.

AMARANTHACEAE

This family consists of about 850 species in 65 genera, widely distributed over the temperate regions and tropics. Many are intimately associated with man as pot-herbs or as a source of edible seeds or as troublesome weeds of cultivated land.

Achryanthes

This tropical and subtropical genus may consist of only 3 to 5 very variable species, which have hitherto been considered to be up to 100 distinct species.

A. fauriei is a possible source of mechanical injury, by means of the hard spines at the bases of the utricles (Kariyone 1971).

Alternanthera

About 200 species are native to the tropics and substopics.

A. echinata

This plant, from Australia, is listed as irritant but no clinical details are given (Gardner and Bennetts 1956).

Alternanthera repens (syn. A. echinata)

Khaki-weed The plant was suspected of causing dermatitis in cattle (Webb 1948).

Amaranthus

The 60 species occur in tropical and temperate regions. Cattle and horses have been poisoned by eating these plants, probably by the high concentrations of potassium nitrate, which they may contain (Muenscher 1951, Kingsbury 1964). Photo-sensitivity seems not to be a feature of this syndrome.

A. blitoides Prostrate Amaranth, Spreading Pigweed

A. retroflexus Redroot Pigweed Careless Weed. These species produced positive patch test reactions in one of 50 patients who had 'weed dermatitis' (Shelmire 1939)

A. tamariscina (syn. Acnida) Western Water Hemp. The statement (Waldbott 1966) that contact sensitivity to this weed may occur in farmers, appears to lack confirmation (Shelmire 1939).

A. mangostenus
Ingestion of this plant is reported to cause photosensitivity in man (Cairns et al. 1968)

A. spinosus
Mechanical injury may be inflicted on man and stock (Pammel 1911, Watt and Breyer-Brandwijk 1962).

A. viridis is used as a sternutatory (Quisumbing 1951). The root of Deeringia amaranthoides of this family also causes violent sneezing (Burkill 1935).

References

Cairns, R.J., Champion, R.H. and Wilkinson, D.S. (1968) Cutaneous Reactions to Physical Agents in Textbook of Dermatology. Ed. Rook A.J., Wilkinson, D.S. and Ebling, E.J.G. 1st. Edit. Oxford, Blackwell, pp. 323-361.

Kariyone, T. (1971) Atlas of Medicinal Plants. Osaka, Japan, Takeda Chemical Industries.

Kingsbury, J.M. (1964) Poisonous Plants of the United States and Canada. Eaglewood Cliffs, New Jersey, Prentice Hall, Inc.

Muenscher, W.C. (1951) Poisonous Plants of the United States, 2nd. Edit. New York, The Macmillan Co.

Pammel, L.H. (1911) A Manual of Poisonous Plants. Cedar Rapids, Iowa, Torch Press. Reprinted Univ. Microfilms, Inc., Ann Arbor

Mich., 1965, pp. 476-7.

Shelmire, B. (1939) Contact dermatitis from Weeds: Patch testing with their oleoresins. JAMA 113, 1085 and unpublished table accompanying reprints.

Waldbott, G.L. (1953) Contact Dermatitis. Springfield, Ill., Charles C. Thomas.

Watt, J.M. and Breyer-Brandwijk, M.G. (1962) The Medicinal and Poisonous Plants of Southern and Eastern Africa. 2nd. Edit. Edinburgh, E.& S. Livingstone Ltd.

Burkill, I.H. (1935) A Dictionary of the Economic Products of the Malay Peninsula. 2 vols. London, Crown Agent for the Colonies.

Quisumbing, E. (1951) Medicinal Plants of the Philippines. Philipp. Dep. Agr. and Nat. Resources Tech. Bull. No. 16. Manila, Bureau of Printing.

Gardner, C.A. and Bennetts, H.N. (1958) The Toxic Plants of Western Australia. Perth West Australian Newspapers Ltd.

Webb, L.J. (1948) Guide to the medicinal and poisonous plants of Queensland. Bulletin No. 232. Council for Scientific and Industrial Research. Melbourne, Australia.

Centrostachya

The single species in this tropical genus is listed as causing mechanical injury (Oakes and Butcher 1962).

Reference

Oakes, A.J. and Butcher, J.O. (1962) Poisonous and Injurious Plants of the U.S. Virgin Islands. Misc. Publ. 882, U.S. Department of Agriculture, Washington, D.C.

Froelichia

About 20 species are distributed over the warmer parts of America and in the Galapagos.

F. floridana Cottonweed, Prairie Froelichia.

The species is listed by Shelmire (1940) as an infrequent sensitizer, but no clinical details are given.

Reference

Shelmire, B. (1940) Contact Dermatitis from Vegetation. Sth. med. J. 33, 338.

AMARYLLIDACEAE

This family of about 1,100 species, classified in 85 genera, is largely native to the tropics and subtropics, but some species occur naturally in temperate regions. The flowers of many species are of great beauty and are widely cultivated. The genus Narcissus (which includes the popular daffodil) is so extensively cultivated that the bulb and cut-flower industries bring many workers into frequent and prolonged contact with these plants, and this popularity ensures their contact also with amateur gardeners and housewives.

Some other genera such as Galanthus (snowdrop) are popular garden plants, but are innocent of any clinical consequences for the dermatologist. Others, less common, because more costly, may cause occasional problems for specialized gardeners or for those who chance to encounter them in the wild.

Chemistry: is recorded by Hegnauer (1963).

Hegnauer, R. (1963) Chemotaxonomy of Plants. Vol. 2. Basel Birkhauser. pp. 53-70.

Amaryllis. The single species A. belladonna (Belladonna Lily) is a native of Africa, but is cultivated widely in many cultivars.

It has been recorded as irritant (Gardner and Bennetts 1956).

Gardner, C.A. and Bennetts, H.W. (1956) The Toxic Plants of Western Australia. Perth, Western Australian Newspapers Ltd.

Boophone The five species in the genus are natives of Southern Africa. B. disticha is very poisonous. It is a skin irritant and, in Kenya, is popularly known as "sore-eye" (Kingsley 1967).

Kingsley, H.J. (1967) Personal Communication..

Crinum

There are over 100 species distributed over the warmer parts of the world, especially near sea coasts. Many species are cultivated for their beautiful flowers.

Dermatitis

At least some species are likely to be irritant. The bulbs of C. bulbispermum have been used as a rubefacient (Watt and Breyer-Brandwijk 1962), and those of C. zeylanicum for blistering cattle (Bailey 1906-7).

The bulb of C. latifolium is used as a rubefacient (Quisumbing 1951).

References

Bailey, F.M. (1906-7) Weeds and Suspected Poisonous Plants of Queensland. Brisbane. Quoted by Hurst, E. (1942).

Quisumbing, E. (1951) Medicinal Plants of the Phillipines. Phillip. Dep. Agr. and Nat. Resources Tech. Bull No. 16. Manila. Bureau of Printing.

Watt, J.M. and Breyer-Brandwijk, M.G. (1962) The Medicinal and Poisonous Plants of Southern and Eastern Africa. 2nd. ed. Edinburgh, E. & S. Livingstone Ltd.

Hurst, E. (1942) The Poison Plants of New South Wales. N.S.W. Poison Plants Committee; Sydney.

Haemanthus

Haemanthus. Over 50 species are natives of tropical and South Africa. Many species are cultivated for their decorative flowers.

Dermatitis

There is evidence that the juice of some species is irritant (Watt and Breyer-Brandwijk 1962)

Watt, J.M. and Breyer-Brandwijk, M.G. (1962) The Medicinal and Poisonous Plants of Southern and Eastern Africa. 2nd. Edit. Edinburgh, E. and S. Livingstone Ltd.

Hippeastrum

The 75 or more species in this genus are natives of tropical and subtropical America. Many are cultivated for their flowers.

Dermatitis

The positive patch test to the leaf of an unnamed cultivar is difficult to interpret (Agrup 1969). At least some species are irritant (Burkill 1935).

References

Agrup, G (1969) Hand Eczema and other Hand Dermatoses in South Sweden. Acta derm.-vener. Stockh. 49, Suppl. 61. p. 1-91.

Burkill, I.H. (1935) A Dictionary of the Economic Products of the Malay Peninsula. 2 vols. London, Crown Agents for the Colonies.

Hymenocallis

50 species are found in warm regions of America.

Hymenocallis declinata

The plant is very irritating to the skin (Altschul 1973).

Altschul, S. von R. (1973). Drugs and foods from little known plants. Cambridge, Mass. Harvard Univ. Press.

Leucojum

About 12 species occur in Southern Europe and Morocco. L. vernum (Snowflake) is often cultivated. It is said by Ehrhardt (1893) to cause dermatitis.

Reference

Ehrhardt (1893) Chemische Untersuchung der wesentlichen Bestandteile des Leucojum vernum und der Narcissus poeticus. Inaug.-Diss. Dorpat. Cited by Touton (1932).

Touton, K. (1932) Hauterkrankungen durch phanerogamische Pflanzen und ihre Produkte. In: Handbuch der Haut-und Geschlechtskrankheiten, ed. Jadassohn, J. Springer, Berlin.

Narcissus

Some 60 species are native to Europe, North Africa and West Africa, but many are amongst the most popular of plants and are widely cultivated wherever the climate is suitable. The narcissus industry is concerned with providing cut flowers for distribution to florists, and with the production of bulbs. Both sections of the industry have dermatitis problems, which have on occasions "caused serious dislocation" (Florist and Flower Grower 1933).

The vernacular nomenclature of the species is confusing. The term daffodil is commonly used for the trumpet narcissi, especially N. pseudo-narcissus, and the term narcissus for most of the remainder, but without consistency. The term jonquil is applied just as inconsistently, not only to N. jonquilla, but to a number of "wild daffodils", and to others thought to resemble them.

Narcissus species have been cultivated for over three hundred years, as have a number of naturally occurring hybrids. Deliberate hybridization was started in the nineteenth century by English gardeners and has since been carried out on such a large scale that the parentage of many popular cultivars is uncertain (Gorer 1970).

Chemistry

The bulbs of many species contain raphides of calcium oxalate. It is suggested (Walsh 1910) that these needle-like crystals account for their irritant properties. The stems and leaves also are mildly irritant.

These plants contain the alkaloid narcissin (Caldwell and Wallace 1955).

The nature of the allergen is unknown (Hjorth and Wilkinson 1968). It is present in the leaf, stem and petals (McCord 1962). The allergen is not soluble in ether, but is partially soluble in ethanol and sparingly in water (Report 1958). Nurserymen and pickers have repeatedly noted that some cultivars provoke dermatitis more readily than others; "Camparelle", "Ornatus", "Gloriosa" (Walsh 1910) and "Actaea" and "Princeps" (Rook 1961) have proved particularly troublesome. However the popularity of individual cultivars waxes and wanes, and new ones are constantly introduced. Only a large and experienced grower can advise on the relative sensitizing capacity of the cultivars in favour at a particular time and place.

Many authors refer loosely to "daffodils" or "narcissi", and little information is available concerning the sensitizing capacity of different species. However both N. poeticus and N. tazetta can sensitize (Agrup 1969) and so can N. jonquilla (Stryker 1936).

Dermatitis

Those who pick and pack the flowers are most heavily at risk; it has been estimated that up to 20% may be affected (Schwartz et al 1957). An expert picker may gather in a day up to 2,000 bunches, each of 12 blooms. The skin of the hands and forearms becomes macerated and abraded. If sensitization develops, eczematous dermatitis affects mainly the fingers, hands and forearms, but not uncommonly also affects the thighs and genitalia and may be generalized (Williams 1910, Palmer 1934). If warmer weather allows more scanty clothing to be worn, the principal sites affected may be the left forearm and the abdominal wall (Marshall 1967).

In florists, dermatitis from Narcissus is less common, and is often confined to the hands, but may involve the face.

Bulb handlers may develop dermatitis of the fingers (Van der Werff 1959), resembling tulip fingers, but usually less severe.

The flower and the leaf produced positive patch test reactions in a gardener who developed contact dermatitis of the hands from cutting and bunching daffodils (Bleumink and Nater 1974).

Dermatitis from Narcissus is probably always caused partly by irritant effects and partly by allergic mechanisms (Klaschka et al 1964). The clinical picture depends partly on the predominance of one or other mechanism and partly on the mode of exposure.

Patch testing

The leaf may be used for patch testing, although tests with stem and flower are often also positive (Heyl 1961). The authors have not seen irritant effects from patch tests with leaves, but it is a wise precaution always to test some normal controls, since the irritancy of some species and cultivars could be significant.

References

Agrup, G. (1969) Hand Eczema and Other Hand Dermatoses in South Sweden. Acta derm.-vener. Stockh. 49, Suppl. 61, pp 1-91.

Caldwell, J. and Wallace, T.J. (1955) Narcissus pseudonarcissus. J. Ecology, 43, 331.

Florist and Flower Grower (1933) March 25th; cited by Palmer 1934.

Gorer, R. (1970) The Development of Garden Flowers. London, Eyre and Spotiswoode, p. 132.

Heyl, T. (1961) Geneeskunde, 3, 296; by Personal Communication 1972.

Hjorth, N. and Wilkinson, D.S. (1968) Contact Dermatitis IV. Tulip Fingers, Hyacinth Itch and Lily Rash. Br. J. Derm. 80, 696.

Klaschka, F., Grimm, W. and Beiersdorff, H.U. (1964) Tulip Contact Eczema as Occupational Dermatosis. Hautarzt, 15, 317.

McCord, C.P. (1962) The Occupational Toxicity of Cultivated Flowers Ind. Med. Surg. 31, 365.

Marshall, J. (1967) Personal Communication.

Palmer, W.H. (1934) "Lily Rash": an Occupational Dermatitis. Lancet, ii, 755.

Report to College of General Practitioners (1958) Daffodil Dermatitis. J. Coll. Gen. Pract. 1, 78.

Rook, A.J. (1961) Plant Dermatitis. The Significance of Variety-specific Sensitisation. Br. J. Derm. 73, 283.

Schwartz, L., Tulipan, L. and Birmingham, D.J. (1957) Occupational Diseases of the skin. 3rd. Edit. Philadelphia, Lea and Febiger. Pp. 637-672.

Stryker, G.V. (1936) Contact Dermatitis Caused by the Jonquil (Narcissus jonquilla). J. industr. Hyg. Toxicol. 18, 462.

Walsh, D. (1910) Investigation of a Dermatitis amongst Flower-pickers in the Scilly Islands, the so-called "Lily rash". Br. med. J. ii, 854.

Bleumink, E. and Nater, J.P. (1974) Contact dermatitis in a gardener caused by daffodils. Berufsdermatosen 22, 123.

Pancratium

The 15 species are natives from the Mediterranean Region to tropical Asia and tropical Africa. Some species are cultivated for their flowers.

Dermatitis

The roots of *P. zeylanicum* and possibly of other species are irritant (Burkill 1935).

Reference

Burkill, I.H. (1935) A Dictionary of the Economic Products of the Malay Peninsula. 2 vols. London, Crown Agents for the Colonies.

ANACARDIACEAE

The 600 species in the 60 genera of this family include plants which probably cause more dermatitis than those in all other plant families combined. Most occur naturally in the tropics, and some of these species because of their economic importance have been widely cultivated beyond their limited area of origin. Some species occur in the Mediterranean region, in Eastern Asia and in America.

The resin-canals of the leaves do not open to the surface, and a leaf must therefore be injured to release the allergenic principles. The leaves of some species are covered with fine hairs; if these are broken the irritant sap exudes. The fruit of most species is a drupe with a resinous mesocarp. In some species containing irritant and sensitizing sap, the fruit at maturity may be eaten with safety (Merrill 1944).

Chemistry (reviewed by Whalley 1959)

The noxious substances in this family are mono- or dihydric phenols or monohydric phenolic acids, having an unbranched C_{15}-C_{17}-C_{19} partially unsaturated alkyl side chain (Wasserman and Dawson 1945).

The sap (latex) of each species contains in various proportions a mixture of phenols, some of which may be confined to a single or a few species, and others of which are widely distributed throughout the family. Moreover, chemically distinct substances may be immunochemically related, so that cross-reactions are frequent.

The following table, modified from Hausen (1970) shows the known distribution of most of the medically important phenols and phenolic acids.

Anacardium occidentale

Cardol

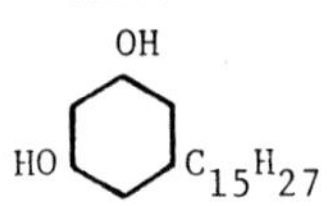

Anacardic Acid

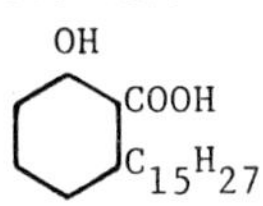

Semicarpus heterophylla

Renghol

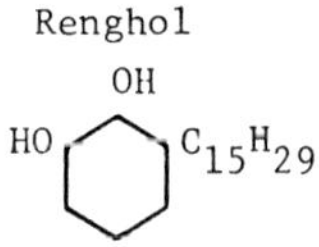

Semicarpus vernicifera

Semicarpus travancorica

Holigarna arnottiana

Rhus succedanea

Rhus orientalis

Laccol

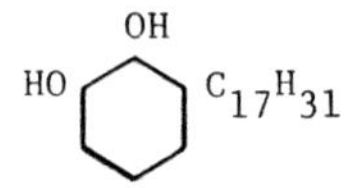

Gluta renghas

Glutarenghol

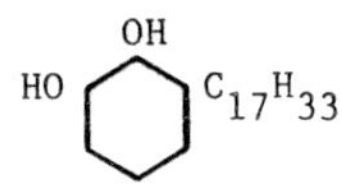

Rhus vernicifera

Rhus toxicodendron

Rhus radicans

Rhus vernix

Urushiol

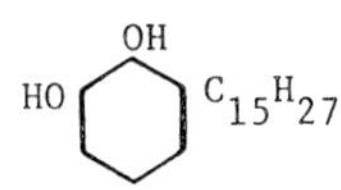

Experiments in guinea-pigs (Baer et al 1966) showed that the capacity of the catechols to induce delayed contact sensitivity depends on the nature of the ring substituents. Catechol and 3-n-alkylcatechols were equally effective in inducing sensitivity, but the degree of sensitivity as well as cross-reactivity depended upon the length of the side chain. Dermal toxicity was unrelated to sensitizing capacity (Baer et al 1967). Further studies (Baer et al 1968) emphasized the importance of the hydrocarbon side chain in determining antigenic specificity and non-reciprocal cross-reactivity. Cross-reactivity within this family was studied in guinea-pigs by Oliviera Lima (1953), who used the oleoresin of Lithraea molleoides as the primary sensitizer. The guinea-pigs were patch tested with the oleoresins of 12 species of Anacardiaceae in 7 genera. Only L. brasiliensis, L. caustica and Rhus radicans gave definite cross-reactions. A clinical study of patch tests in patients primarily sensitized by poison oak or poison ivy (Howell 1959) showed cross-sensitization to other Rhus species to be very frequent and cross-sensitization to other genera to be frequent, but inconstant. Further investigations are required. As a general practical principle cross-sensitization must be considered to be general within this family unless it has been positively excluded.

Dermatitis

The clinical features of the dermatitis they cause will be described in the individual accounts of the noxious genera of the Anacardiaceae. However the syndromes induced by the more potent sensitizers share certain distinctive characteristics.

In previously unsensitized individuals, exposure is followed by a latent period of about nine to fourteen days before dermatitis appears.

In sensitized individuals, symptoms develop from a few hours to several days after contact, with itching at the sites of contact, usually the fingers, hands, forearms and legs. Papules soon appear, often in linear pattern, and soon evolve into vesicles or bullae. In severe cases the eyelids, other parts of the face, the genitalia and the trunk may be affected. Except in regions well protected by hair, oedema may be considerable, and is particularly so in the eyelids and the male genitalia.

The allergen may be carried by the fingers from one site to another, but it is not present in the vesicle fluid. Carriage by the fingers obviously may extend the eventual distribution; it also accounts for the initial involvement of sites remote from those of greatest contact, as in lacquer dermatitis of the face in Mah Jongg players. The thicker horny layer on the fingers provides some protection.

In most noxious species the allergen is widely distributed throughout the plant. Digging the soil in which roots are growing may cause dermatitis. The pollen and flowers of Toxicodendron are not allergenic nor is smoke from the burning plant, unless the smoke contains incompletely burned plant material.

The evolution of the eruption occurs in crops, affecting first the sites where most allergen has been absorbed and then successively the less heavily contaminated sites. The dermatitis has commonly reached its full extent after 48 hours. Healing occurs within two weeks, without scars unless secondary infection has been introduced.

In dermatitis constitutional symptoms are usual, but if plant material is ingested there may be vomiting and diarrhoea and neurological symptoms simulating atropine poisoning - drowsiness or stupor, convulsions, delirium, fever, and pupillary dilation. Nephritis, too, may complicate poisoning, either by ingestion or after massive cutaneous vesication (Rytand 1948, Templeton et al 1947).

References

Baer, H., Watkins, R.C., Kurtz, A.P., Byck, J.S. and Dawson, C.R. (1967) Delayed Contact Sensitivity to Catechols. III. The Relationship of Side-Chain Length to Sensitizing Potency of Catechols Chemically Related to the Active Principles of Poison Ivy. Journal of Immunology 99, 370.

Baer, H., Dawson, C.R. and Kurtz, A.P. (1968) Delayed Contact Sensitivity to Catechols. IV Stereochemical Conformation of the Antigenic Determinant. Journal of Immunology 101, 1243.

Baer, H., Watkins, R.C. and Bowser, R.T. (1966) Delayed contact sensitivity to catechols and resorcinols. The relationship of structure and immunization procedure to sensitizing capacity. Immunochemistry 3, 479.

Hausen, B.M. (1970) Unteruchungen Über Gesundheitsschädigende. Holzer. Thesis. Hamburg.

Howell, J.B. (1959) Cross Sensitization in Diverse Poisonous Members of the Sumac Family (Anacardiaceae). Journal of Investigative Dermatology 32, 21.

Merrill, E.D. (1944) Dermatitis Caused by Representatives of Anacardiaceae in Tropical Countries. J. Amer. Med. Ass. 124, 222.

Oliviera Lima, A. (1953) Über das antigene Verhalten der Ölharze einiger Gattungen der Familie Anacardiaceae. Int. Arch. Allergy and Applied Immunology 4, 169.

Rytand, D.A. (1948) Fatal anuria, the adephrotic syndrome and glomerular nephritis as sequels of the dermatitis of poison oak. Am. J. Med. 5, 548.

Templeton, H.J., Lunsford, C.J. and Allington, H.V. (1947) Poison oak dermatitis: studies on haematologic, urinary and temperature changes. J. Invest. Derm. 8, 53.

Wasserman, D. and Dawson, C.R. (1545) Cashew Nutshell Liquid: Comparison of the Monophenol Isolated from Commercial Raw Cashew Nutshell Liquid and from Commercial Cardanol. Indust. Eng. Chem. 37, 396.

Whalley, W.B. (1959) The Toxicity of Plant Phenolics in the Pharmacology of Plant Phenolics. Ed. Fairburn, J.W. London, Academic Press. pp. 27-37

Anacardium

The fifteen species in this genus are natives of tropical America, but some are widely cultivated throughout the tropics.

Anacardium melanorrhoea

Rengas tree (This term is also applied to other trees in Malaya).

Contact dermatitis, said sometimes to have been fatal, has been attributed to this tree (Fasal 1945). Those cutting the tree have first anointed their bodies with sesame oil (Pedaliaceae) in an attempt to prevent dermatitis.

Anacardium occidentale

Cashew nut Tree. A. occidentale is a native of Brazil, but is cultivated in many parts of the tropics. Its timber, known as Acajou, is used for house and boat building in South America, but is not exported (Hausen 1973). The tree is however grown principally for its nuts, its oil, and its gum.

The distribution of irritants and sensitizers in the various tissues of this tree is such that many of those handling it, from the woodcutter to the consumer of cashew nuts, are exposed to some risk of dermatitis, though for the nut addict this risk is small indeed and can arise only in quite exceptional circumstances.

The bark of the tree contains a thick, resinous acrid sap, which blackens on exposure to air. The wood exudes a yellow gum, which can blister the skin. The yellow or red "cashew apple", technically a swollen peduncle, contains a juice which is astringent until the fruit is ripe, when it is acid but edible. This "apple" is the receptacle of the true fruit, the cashew nut, which is lightly attached to its apex, and which attains its full size before the receptacle enlarges to form the "apple", which is thus a false fruit. Between the smooth outer shell and the inner shell is a fibrous pulp containing a sticky brown oil, which is caustic and sensitizing. The kidney-shaped kernel is the cashew nut of commerce, and is innocuous unless contaminated with the shell oil, in which case it may be blackened.

The cashew apples with nuts attached fall from the trees when ripe. The nuts are dried in the sun and then roasted on an open fire, to dispel some of the caustic oil. The fumes from the fire are irritating to eyes, nose, throat and skin. The roasted nuts are split open and the edible kernels are removed (Morton 1961).

The oil is exported from India and other countries in drums, from which leakage is always possible.

The oil is used in indigenous medicine as a rubefacient and vesicant. It has also many industrial uses. It is used as a preservative for fishing lines and as an insect repellant in book bindings. A dilute extract has been used as a gloss on vanilla beans (Orchidaceae), and has been held responsible for 'vanilla itch' in workers handling the treated beans.

The sap of the tree and the oil are used for marking clothing and are less of a dermatitis hazard than marking-nut oil (Semecarpus). The gum is used as a varnish to protect books and woodcarvings from insects, and also as a substitute for gum arabic (Acacia, Leguminosae) in adhesives.

Chemistry (Backer and Haack 1941)

Cashew nut shell oil contains approximately 90% anacardic acid and 10% cardol, but the composition varies according to the method of extraction employed.

Anacardic Acic

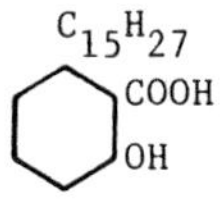

Cardol

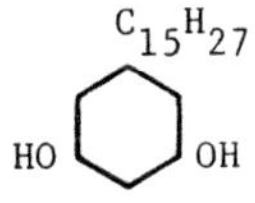

There are resorcinol derivatives which are a common molecular skeleton with the 3-pentadecyl phenols of poison ivy. Allergic cross-reactions are mentioned on page 64. The principal phenolic constituent of the Maidenhair tree (Ginkgo biloba) is closely related to anacardic acid (Furukawa 1934), since upon hydrogenation followed by decarboxylation it yields 3-pentadecyl phenol (Loev and Dawson 1958).

Cashew oil is applied ambiguously also to the innocuous oil extract from the kernel, which resembles almond oil.

Dermatitis (Neubauer 1926, Downing and Garney 1940)

Those falling the trees may suffer an irritant dermtitis (Hausen 1973). The sap caused a localised ulcerative lesion of the skin of a farmer's chest (Bedi 1971). Biting the unripe "apples" can cause dermatitis around the mouth (Bedi 1971). An additional hazard occurs when the tree is infested by caterpillars of Cricula, which have stinging hairs.

Exposure to the nuts in workers on Cashew nut farms may cause an acute dermatitis resembling that commonly observed in sensitized persons, but sometimes the only lesions are roughness, cracking and irritation of fingers and hands (Behl et al 1966, Bedi 1971, Cueva 1965). This chronic dermatitis afflicts particularly those employed in removing the kernels from the roasted nuts (Morton 1961).

Unprocessed nuts were responsible for dermatitis amongst dock workers who unloaded them, and in a secretary and a chemist who also handled them (Downing and Gurney 1940).

Roasted cashew nuts sold as ornaments or as the heads of "swizzle sticks" used for stirring drinks have caused dermatitis because they had been inadequately roasted and oil had seeped through the shell (Morton 1961).

Nine workmen developed dermatitis after dipping electrical equipment in a commercial varnish containing raw cashew nut oil (Lockey 1944). One of the nine developed exfoliative dermatitis and severe anaemia, haematuria and prostration.

Anacardium orientale

This East Indian tree is used locally as a timber and has caused dermatitis (Hausen 1973). A laboratory worker cutting sections of the fruit developed severe dermatitis (Fox 1921).

References

Backer, H.J. and Haack, N.H. (1941) Constituents of the Latex of Anacardium occidentale (French) Rev. Trav. Chim. 60, 661.

Bedi, B.M.S. (1971) Cashewnut Dermatitis (Report of two cases). Indian J. Derm. 16, 1

Cueva, L. (1965) A case of contact dermatitis caused by cashew nuts. J. Alergia (Mex). 12, 133.

Downing, J.G. and Gurney, S.W. (1940) Dermatitis from Cashew-Nut Shell Oil. J. indust. Hyg. 22, 169.

Fasal, P. (1945) Cutaneous Diseases in the Tropics. Arch. Derm. Syph. 51, 163.

Fox, H. (1921) Dermatitis Venenata from Oriental Cashew Nut. Arch. Derm. Syph. 3, 202.

Furukawa, S. (1934) Sci. Pap. Inst.

phys. chem. Res. (Tokyo) 24, 304 314, 320 (Cited by Watt and Breyer-Brandwijk 1962).

Hausen, B.M. (1973) Holzarten mit gesundheitsschädigenden inhaltsstoffen. Stuttgart, BMW-Verlags-GmbH.

Lockey, S.D. (1944) Cashew Nut Oil Dermatitis. Ann. Allergy 2, 22

Loev B. and Dawson, C.R. (1958) Cashew nut shell liquid. X. An investigation of the geometrical configuration of the olefinic components of cardinol and some observations concerning ginkgol. J. Am. chem. Soc. 80, 643.

Morton, J.F. (1961) The Cashew's Brighter Future. Econom. Bot. 15, 57.

Neubauer (1926) Akojounasse und Gefahren bei ihrer Vervundung Zentralbl. Gewerbehygiene 3, 188.

Watt, J.M. and Breyer-Brandwijk, M.G. (1962) The Medicinal and Poisonous Plants of Southern and Eastern Africa. 2nd. ed. Edinburgh, E. & S. Livingstone Ltd.

Astronium

The 15 species in this genus are native to Central and tropical South America and the West Indies.

Astronium fraxinifolium

The timber is used for construction work and for furniture, under the trade name Goncalo (Hausen 1973). The sawdust causes such intense skin irritation that the affected areas resemble second-degree burns (Freise 1932). Repeated contact is said to result in increased tolerance.

Astronium graveolens

The wood often resembles that of *Dalbergia* spp. and may be mixed with shipments of them (Record and Hess 1943).

References

Freise, F.W. (1932) Health Hazards from working with Toxic Woods. (German) Arch. Gewerbepath.-hyg. 3, 1.

Hausen, B.M. (1973) Timber Species with Constitutents Injurious to Health. (German) Stuttgart, D.R.W., p. 60.

Record, S.J. and Hess, R.W. (1943) Timbers of the New World. New Haven, Yale.

Buchanania

25 species are native to Indo Malaysia and tropical Australia.

Buchanania species

The black sap is said to be non-irritant (Burgess 1966) but the juice of *B. lucida* was noted by a plant collector to produce itching (Altschul 1973).

References

Altschul, S. von R. (1973) Drugs and foods from little-known plants. Cambridge, Mass. Harvard Univ. Press.

Burgess, P.F. (1966) Timbers of Sabah (Sabah Forest Records No. 6) Sabah, Malaysia, The Forest Department

Campnosperma

Some of the 15 species of this tropical genus are known in Malaya to produce dermatitis (Kochummen 1972).

Campnosperma auriculata is an evergreen tree the wood-sap of which causes dermatitis in some persons (Corner 1952, Burgess 1966). The plant yields a series of long-chain aklylquinols of which the nonadecyl homologue has been identified (Thomson 1971).

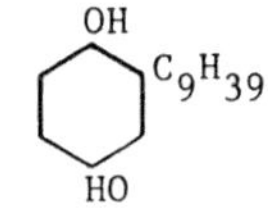

Campnosperma macrophylla and *C. minor* have similar effects on the skin (Corner 1952, Burgess 1966).

References

Burgess, P.F. (1966) Timbers of Sabah (Sabah Forest Records No. 6.) Sabah, Malaysia, The Forest Department.

Corner, E.J.H. (1952) Wayside trees of Malaysia. Singapore, Government Printer.

Thomson, R.H. (1971) Naturally Occuring Quinones. 2nd. ed. London Academic Press. p. 93.

Comocladia

The 20 species are natives of Central America and the West Indies. Oviedo reported (Standley 1927) that the Indian women of Santo Domingo used a vesicant paste made from the roots of Comocladia species, to soften and lighten the skin of their arms and faces. In 1845 Williams (1845-6) drew attention to a report by Otto in the Gardeners' Magazine of May 1842 of intensely severe oedema after minimal contact with the irritant sap of a Comocladia species. At least 17 of the 20 species are said to be capable of producing contact dermatitits (Pardo-Castello 1933).

Comocladia dentata

The timber known as Bastard Brazil is used locally for general purposes and can cause dermatitis (Standley 1927, Schwartz et al 1948). The dermatitis may be persistent as the resin contaminates clothing and tools (Pardo-Castello 1962).

Comocladia dodonaea
Christmas Bush

The spiny leaves can cause mechanical injury and the sap can produce severe dermatitis (Oakes and Butcher 1962).

Comocladia engleriana and C. mollifolia were noted as producing dermatitis (Altschul 1973)

References

Altschul, S. von R. (1973) Drugs and foods from little-known plants. Cambridge, Mass. Harvard Univ. Press.

Oakes, A.J. and Butcher, J.O. (1962) Poisonous and Injurious Plants of the U.S. Virgin Islands. Misc. Publ. 882. Washington,D.C., U.S. Department of Agriculture.

Pardo-Castello, V. (1933) Skin Diseases in the New World. From Oviedo Y. Valdes, 1478-1557. Arch. Derm. Syph. (Chicago), 28, 22.

Pardo-Castello, V. (1962) Common Dermatoses in Agricultural Workers in the Caribbean Area. Industr. Med. Surg. 31, 305.

Schwartz, L. Tulipan, L. and Peck, S.M. (1948) Occupational Diseases of the Skin. 2nd. ed Philadelphia, Lea and Febiger.

Standley, P.C. (1927) Poisonous Trees of Central America. Tropical Woods, 9, 3 (March) and 7, 8 (Sept.) 1926.

Cotinus (syn. Rhus)

One species is found in the south-eastern United States, one species from southern Europe to the Himalayas and China and one species in south-western China.

Cotinus coggygria
(syn. Rhus cotinus)
Wig tree, fustic wood, fisetholz

The wig tree which is native to regions from the Mediterranean to China is often cultivated in shrubberies. The wood yields the yellow dye 'young fustic'. The wood has caused dermatitis and general symptoms when cut for veneers (Hausen 1970).

Reference

Hausen, B.M. (1970) Untersuchungen über Gesundheitsschädigende Hölzer. Thesis, Hamburg.

Gluta

Of the 13 species in this genus, one is native to Madagascar and 12 to Indomalaysia. Many provide timber, and the sap of some species forms a good varnish. The heartwood of many species is blood red, sometimes with darker bands. It is excellent material for furniture and turning, and is used in Malaya for making "daching", Chinese weighing scales. It is hard, durable, and beautifully marked.

Rengas Trees

The name Rengas is given by Malays, sometimes wrongly, to several large jungle trees in five genera of the family Anacardiaceae which have black sap. In the timber trade the name Rengas or Renghas is reserved for the red heartwood of species of Gluta and of Melanorrhoea. Swintonia elmeri is believed to be a superfluous name for Melanorrhoea wallichii; its timber may be regarded as Rengas. The species of Gluta and Melanorrhoea have been inadequately collected because the irritant properties of the sap deter collectors. For the same reason the timber is obtainable only to very special order. The more 'poisonous' kinds, belonging to the genera Melanorrhoea and Melanochyla, are usually called in Malaya Kerbau Jalung, the Untamed Buffalo; it is unwise even to sit beneath these, for raindrops may carry down the poison from the leaves (Corner 1952). The wood of some species, even when thoroughly seasoned, remains irritant to sensitive skins. Furniture which had been in use for years has caused dermatitis (Hornsey 1914).

The various vernacular names: rengas (Malaya), hangus (Penang), rangus (Sakar), ruengas (Sudan), ingas (Indonesia), angas and ligas (Philippines), are applied to trees the sap of which produces sores on the skin. The species concerned are mainly in the genera Gluta and Melanorrhoea; their white irritant sap turns black on exposure to the air (Burkill 1935).

Rengas poisoning in the form of an acute dermatitis, with constitutional symptoms, is not uncommon in Malaya in estate labourers, gardeners and woodcutters (Gimlette 1929, Samuel 1935). Two companies of soldiers developed dermatitis after wading in a river the banks of which were covered with rengas trees which had contaminated the water with their fruits (Upwich 1894). The fruit juice can cause dermatitis (Noosten and Visser 1936).

Gluta benghas
(syn. Stagmaria verniciflua)

The species name is an old miswriting of rengas (Gimlette 1929). The sap is irritant (Gimlette 1929).

Gluta coarctata
Singapore Mahogany

The wood causes dermatitis and the fruit and leaves are also poisonous and have been used for criminal purposes (Ridley 1911, 1922).

Gluta elegans
Penang Rengas

The sap causes dermatitis (Burkill 1935, Corner 1952).

Gluta renghas
East Coast (Malaya) Rengas, Ape-nut

The timber of the large riverside tree is beautiful but its usefulness is limited by its sinister reputation amongst forestry workers (Foxworth 1927, Lewin 1928, Grevendtuk 1937). However it is used for building, for boats, for furniture and for inlay work, despite the fact that a chair made of this wood has caused dermatitis of the legs (Hausen 1973).

Chemistry

The vesicant sap of the fruit contains the monoethenoid alkyl catechol, glutarenghol (Whalley 1959). The chemical constituents of this species have been studied also by Backer and Haack (1941) and by Thiébault (1965).

Dermatitis

Those employed in felling the trees may develop an acute vesicular dermatitis (Ridley 1922).

Gluta tavoyana and Gluta turtur

The sap of both species is irritant (Thiébault 1965).

Gluta velutina
Water Rengas

The timber provokes skin reactions (Corner 1952) and the dried wood and sap retain their dermatitic properties (Burkill 1935).

Gluta virosa
Wild Buffalo Tree

This species can produce dermatitis (Gimlette 1929).

Gluta wrayi
Straits Mahogany

This species is said to be the most virulent of the rengas. (Ridley 1911, 1922, Burkill 1935)

The timber is beautifully marked.

References

Backer, N.J. and Haack, N.H. (1941) Le principe toxique de Gluta renghas.L.Rev. Trav. chim. Pays-Bas, 60, 856.

Burkill, I.H. (1935) A Dictionary of the Economic Products of the Malay Peninsula. 2 Vols. London, Crown Agents for the Colonies.

Corner, E.J.H. (1952) Wayside trees of Malaysia. Singapore, Government Printer.

Foxworth, P.W. (1927) Commercial Timber Trees of the Malay Peninsula. Malay. For. Rec. 3, 140.

Gimlette, J.D. (1929) Malay Poisons and Charm Cures. 3rd Ed. London J. & A. Churchill.

Grevendtuk, A. (1937) Vergiftungen durch Renghas. Samml. Vergift. 8A, 35.

Hausen, B.M. (1973) Holzarten mit gesundheitsschädigenden inhaltsstoffen. Stuttgart, DRW-Verlags-GmbH.

Hornsey, J.F. (1914) Rungus Dermatitis. Br. med. J. 1, 759.

Lewin, L. (1928) Gifte in Holzgewerbe. Beiträge zur Giftkunde. Heft 1. Berlin, Georg. Stilke Verlag.

Noosten, H.H. and Visser, J. (1936) Apropos the poisonous properties of rengas. (A clinical and experimental study of its blister forming constituent). Geneesk. tijdschr Nederl.-Indie.76, 1346.

Ridley, H.N. (1911) Rengas-poisoning. Malaya Med. J. 9 (pt. 2), 7-13 (April)

Ridley, H.N. (1922) Plant Dermatitis. J. trop. Med. Hyg. 25,225.

Samuel, J. (1935) Rengas Poisoning Malayan Med. J. 10, 14.

Senear, F.E. (1933) Dermatitis due to woods. J. Am. Med. Ass. 101, 1527.

Thiébault, A. (1965) Nomenclature Générale des Bois Tropicaux. L'Association Technique Internationale dés Bois Tropicaux, 45, bis Avenue de la Belle-Gabrielle, Nogent-sur-Marne, France.

Upwich, (1894) Geneesk. Tijdschr. v. Nederl-Indie 34,795, cited by Senear 1933.

Whalley, W.B. (1959) The Toxicity of Plant Phenolics in The Pharmacology of Plant Phenolics. Ed. Fairburn, J.W. London Academic Press, pp. 27-37.

Heeria

The single species H. argentea is a native of Southern Africa. It has been reported by Ross (1959) to have caused severe dermatitis in Pondoland. The Curator of the Pretoria Botanical Gardens had not seen reactions to the plant in visitors who had handled it.

References

Ross, C.M. (1959) Poison Ivy Dermatitis: the First South African Cases. S. Afr. med. J. 33, 657.

Holigarna

Eight species are native to Indo-Malaysia.

H. arnottiana contains a very acrid, black oleoresin, the powerfully vesicant properties of which are dreaded by local people (Behl et al 1966). Not all those in contact with the sap develop dermatitis (Chopra et al 1949), which suggests that sensitization rather than irritancy must be implicated.

H. grahamii and H. longifolia have similar properties. The latter yields a black varnish, which is caustic and vesicant. (Chopra et al 1949).

References

Behl, P.N., Captain, R.M., Bedi, B.M.S. and Gupta, S. (1966) Skin irritant and Sensitizing Plants Found in India. New Delhi, P.N. Behl, Irwin Hospital.

Chopra, R.N., Bhadwar, R.L. and Ghosh, S. (1949) Poisonous Plants of India. Sci. Monograph

No. 17. Delhi, The Indian Council of Agricultural Research.

Lannea

About 70 species are native to tropical Africa and one species to Indo-Malaysia. Some of the African species yield timber for local use, and others are employed for a variety of purposes in indigenous medicine (Watt and Breyer-Brandwijk 1962).

Lannea grandis, the East Indian member of the genus, is strongly irritant (Verbunt 1933).

References

Verbunt, J.A. (1933) Over een Huidaandoening door Geneeskrachtige Bladeren. Nederl. Tijdsch. v. Geneeskund. 77, 4436.

Watt, J.M. and Breyer-Brandwijk, M.G. (1962) The Medicinal and Poisonous Plants of Southern and Eastern Africa. 2nd Edit. Edinburgh, E. & S Livingstone Ltd.

Lithraea

The three species in this genus are natives of South America.

Lithraea brasiliensia. The timber, known in the trade as Aroeira or Pao bregre, is used for posts and fences, and sometimes for furniture. The sap is powerfully irritant (Mors and Rizzini 1961).

Lithraea caustica. The timber of this tree is also sold as Aroeira, but has the alternative name of Litre; it is used in Brazil and Chile, particularly for furniture (Hausen 1970).

Barham (1794) referred to swelling of the face and body from sleeping under the tree. The sap, and at certain times of the year, the exudate from the leaves are highly irritant (Sprague 1921).

The dried wood is said to be harmless (Webster 1911) but can cause dermatitis (Hausen 1970). Cross-sensitivity to Rhus, Maura and other Anacardiaceae was investigated by Lima (1953) and Hurtado (1968).

Feuillée, who visited South America in 1702-12, related that some of the seamen of his ship suffered severely as the result of cutting down some"Llithi" trees (Lithraea caustica) on the coast of Chile. By the following day their heads had swollen to an extraordinary size, and their features had become indistinguishable; and they might have been taken for monsters rather than men (Obs. ii. 33, t. 25, fig. dextra; 1725).

According to Molina (Hist., Engl. ed. 144; 1809), "the effluvium from this tree, especially in summer, produces painful pustules and swellings on the hands and faces of those who stop beneath its shade. This effect is various, however, with various persons: there are some who are very little, if at all, incommoded by it, while others, who merely pass by the tree, are severely affected; though never attended with fatal consequences, it is, nevertheless, very troublesome. Great precaution is requisite in cutting the tree, as its viscous juice is extremely caustic; but when dry, the wood loses all its injurious qualities." Molina, who has been described as "one of the most pernicious blunderers who have brought confusion into Natural History: (J. Ball, Notes Nat. S. Am. 175; 1887) is not very trustworthy; but, according to Gillies, "the statement made by Molina, relative to the poisonous nature of this tree, seems to be well founded; as I am informed, by several intelligent people, that individuals resting or sleeping under it at certain times of the year, are afterwards attacked with eruptions all over the body" (Hook. & Arn. Bot. Beechey's Voy. 16; 1832).

C. Gay (Fl. Chil. ii. 44; 1846) stated that the "Liti" or "Litre" tree (Lithraea caustica) is common on hills and sun-exposed plains in Central Chile, extending from Coquimbo to Arauco; and that the danger of remaining underneath it or of burning it is well known. It is mostly women, children, and persons of weak constitution who are affected (Sprague 1921).

References

Barham, H. (1794) Hortus americanus.

Kingston, Jamaica, cited by Woods and Calnan (1976).

Hausen, B.M. (1970) Untersuchungen über Gesundheitsschädigende Hölzer. Thesis, Hamburg.

Hurtado, I. de (1968) Studies on the biological activity of Rhus striata ('Manzanillo'). 2. Skin response to patch tests in humans. Int. Arch. Allerg. 33, 209.

Lima, A.O. (1953) Uber das antigene Verhalten der Olharze einiger Gattungen der Familie Anacardiaceae. Int. Arch. Allerg. Appl Immun. 4, 169.

Mors, W.B. and Rizzini, C.T. (1961) Die industriell verwertbaren Pflanzen Brasiliens. Sao Paulo. Deutsch-Brasilianische Ind. v. Handelskam.

Sprague, T.A. (1921) Plant Dermatitis. Journal of Botany 59, 308, cites references in text.

Webster (1911) New International Dictionary. Springfield, Mernam cited by Woods and Calnan (1976).

Woods, B. and Calnan, C.D. (1976) Toxic Woods. Brit. J. Derm. 94, Suppl. 13, June.

Loxopterygium

The five species are natives of tropical South America.

Loxopterygium huasango
Hualtaco Tree

Contact with the leaves can cause dermatitis but the wood does not seem to be irritant (Paulson 1942).

Loxopterygium lorentzii
(syn. Schinopsis lorentzii)

Reference

Paulson, G.A. (1942) Mango and Haultaco dermatitis (Dermatitis venenata produced by members of the Anacardiaceae family in northern Peru). Med. Bull. Standard Oil Co., New Jersey 5, 197.

Mangifera

The 40 species of Mango were originally natives of South East Asia and of Indo-Malaysia, but many species are now cultivated or have become naturalized in tropical regions throughout the world because of their importance as sources of food and timber.

Inconsistency in the use of trade names for timbers is particularly confusing in this genus. Asam is commonly applied to these timbers; the coloured heartwood present in some species is referred to as Figured Asam. Unfortunately the term Asam is applied also to timbers derived from the Burseraceae family (Canarium, Dacryodes, Santiria, Scutinanthe, Triomma).

Another trade name for the timber of M. indica is Aruba. Moreover there are a number of local names in current use: Machang (Malaya and Sarawak), Sepam (Malaya), Mango or Mangga (India and Pakistan), Thayet (Burma), Xoai (Vietnam) and Membatjang (Indonesia).

The identity of material from some Mangifera species is in doubt, as the genus awaits botanical revision (Burgess 1966). The following are commercial timber trees:

M. caesia, M. foetida, M. indica, M. macrocarpa, M. odorata, M. pajang, M. quadrifida.

Reference

Burgess, P. F. (1966) Timbers of Sabah (Sabah Forest Records No. 6). Sabah, Malaysia, The Forest Department.

Magifera caesia Binjai

This species is grown for its timber, and to some extent for its fruit, although the latter's foetid odour reduces its palatability (Corner 1952).

The sap of the fully grown tree is irritant and has been used for ciminal purposes. Raindrops contaminated by bruised foliage may irritate the skin.

The smoke from burning foliage or wood is unpleasantly acrid (Burkill 1935) and may cause dermatitis in those exposed to it (Simmons and Bolin 1921, Landor 1943).

Eating the fruit may cause dermatitis localized to the angles of the mouth (Simmons and Bolin 1921), or stomatitis (Fasal 1945).

References

Burkill, I.H. (1935) A Dictionary of the Economic Products of the Malay Peninsula. 2 Vols. London, Crown Agents for the Colonies.

Corner, E.J.H. (1952) Wayside trees of Malaysia. Singapore Government Printer.

Fasal, P. (1945) Cutaneous Diseases in the Tropics. Arch. Derm. Syph. 51, 163.

Landor, J.V. (1943) Dermatitis Venenata Caused by Smoke. Br. J. Derm. 55, 17.

Simmons, J.S. and Bolin, Z.E. (1921) Dermatitis Venenata Produced by an Irritant Present in the Stem Sap of the Mango (Mangifera indica, L.). Am. J. trop. Med. 1, 351.

Mangifera foetida Horse Mango

The sap of this unripe fruit, which often has a resinous smell, is particularly irritant (Corner 1952), and may cause dermatitis of the angles of the mouth (Simmons and Bolin 1921), or stomatitis (Fasal 1945).

Smoke from burning foliage may cause dermatitis (Fasal 1945).

References

Corner, E.J.H. Wayside trees of Malaysia. Singapore, Government Printer.

Fasal, P. (1945) Cutaneous Diseases in the Tropics. Arch. Derm. Syph. 51 163.

Simmons, J.S. and Bolin, Z.E. (1921) Dermatitis Venenata Produced by an Irritant Present in the Stem Sap of the Mango (Mangifera indica, L.). Am. J. trop. Med. 1, 351.

Mangifera indica Mango

The mango has been so extensively cultivated that there are large number of varieties, differing quantitatively in their chemical constituents, and hence in the quality of their fruit or timber. Varieties do not reliably reproduce their valuable qualities in their seedlings, and are therefore propagated vegetatively by grafting. Grafting may also confer other advantages. For example, in Malaysia M. indica is grafted on the locally vigorous M. foetida. The grafted trees grow less tall than the self-sown trees, so that the fruit is more easily picked, and the first fruits tend to be produced several years earlier. The fruit can be kept in storage for a month at a temperature of about 40°, and so can be despatched to distant markets. Chutneys are made from unripe mango fruits. Very young leaves, and flowers, may be eaten. The leaves are sometimes fed to cattle at times of scarcity.

The timber, sold under the trade name of Amba, is used locally for boat building and furniture, but is not exported (Hausen 1973).

Chemistry

The leaves, stems and timber and the pericarp of the fruit contain urushiol. (Keil et al 1946). Cross-sensitivity with 3-pentadecylcatechol was observed experimentally (Wechsler 1960).

Dermatitis

The growing plant itself and many of the commercial products derived from it are potential causes of dermatitis. Handling of the green fruits or breaking the branches may result in dermatitis, and contact with windblown pollen may also do so (Allen 1943). According to Lakhanpai and Nair (1953) the pollen is not anemophilous and Morton (1969, 1971) ascribed respiratory difficulty, in proximity to blooming trees in Florida, to emanations from the flowers.

Contact with the wood or its sawdust has caused dermatitis (Simmons and Bolin 1921). Dermatitis of irregular distribution may occur in children climbing the trees.

The most commonly observed clinical syndrome of mango dermatitis follows peeling and eating the fruit. The face, especially around the mouth, is most severely involved (Nasution et al. 1973), but the antigen may be carried by the fingers to the neck, and some dermatitis of the hands is not unusual (Kirby-Smith 1938). The linear vesicles of poison ivy dermatitis are not a feature. The antigen is found in stems, leaves and pericarp (peel) but not in the fruit juice, which may be drunk with impunity by sensitized subjects (Behl et al 1966). Zakon (1939) obtained a positive patch to the peel in one case of facial dermatitis. Goldberg (1954) reported two cases of facial dermatitis which followed peeling and eating mangoes, but patch tests were not carried out. In other cases (Brown and Brown 1941) patch tests were positive to an oil extracted from the peel, but not to the pulp of the fruit. The fruit can be eaten safely by sensitized subjects provided all contact with the peel or the stem can be avoided (Keil et al 1946). During harvesting of the fruit, stem sap may contaminate the peel which then shows patches which appear bleached, varnished or blackened. The sap may cause dermatitis localized to the angles of the mouth (Simmons and Bolin 1921), or stomatitis (Fasal 1945).

A reaction of a different type occurs more rarely. Contact with the peel may cause urticarial wealing (Behl et al 1966) and asthma (Kahn 1942). Urticaria alone or with shock has been reported after eating mangoes (Lindenbaum 1962, Rubin et al 1965, Dang and Bell 1937).

Incidence

Dermatitis from the mango occurs wherever this tree is grown. During its fruiting season in Hawaii it is the predominant cause of dermatitis from plants (Arnold 1972). It has been reported from the Philippine Islands (Gibson and Concepción 1914, Concepción 1914), from Argentina (Silva 1945), the Dutch West Indies (Tillema 1936) and Florida (Blank 1957), as well as from India, the East Indies and Japan (Asai 1939).

However mango appears to be a less powerful primary sensitizer than poison ivy. North Americans, already sensitized by poison ivy are more likely to develop mango dermatitis than are the inhabitants of the mango-growing regions (Blank 1957). Previous clinical or subclinical sensitivity to other anacardiaceous species will also influence the incidence of mango dermatitis. It seems probable, too, that varieties of mango differ in their allergenic potential (Blohm 1962).

The evidence for racial as distinct from environmental influences on the incidence of dermatitis is not conclusive.

References

Allen, P.N. (1943) Poisonous and Injurious Plants of Panama. Am. J. trop. Med. 23 (Suppl.) 3-76

Arnold, H.L., Jr. (1972) Honolulu, State of Hawaii. Personal communication.

Asai, T. (1939) Über Mango-Dermatitis. Jap. J. Derm. 46, 44.

Behl, P.N., Captain, R.M., Bedi, B.M.S. and Gupta, S. (1966) Skin irritant and Sensitizing Plants Found in India. New Delhi, P.N. Behl, Irwin Hospital.

Blank, H. (1957) Dermatitis from Anacardiaceae. Proc. Florida Mango Forum, Oct. 16th. 17th Annual meeting. Miami.

Blohm, H. (1962) Poisonous Plants of Venezuela. Cambridge, Mass., Harvard University Press.

Brown, A. and Brown, P.R. (1941) Mango Dermatitis. J. Allergy, 12, 310.

Concepción, I. (1914) Observation on Mango Rash. Philippines J. Sci. 9, 509.

Dang, R.W.M. and Bell, D.B. (1967) Anaphylactic Reaction to the Ingestion of Mango. Hawaii med. J. 27, 149.

Fasal, P. (1945) Cutaneous Diseases in the Tropics. Arch. Derm. Syph. 51, 163.

Gibson, R.B. and Concepción, I.

(1914) The Lymphagogic Action of the Philippine Mango, Mangi fera indica L. Philippines J. Sci. 9B:503

Goldberg, L.C. (1954) Mango dermatitis J. Am. med. Ass. 156, 954.

Hausen, B.M. (1973) Holzarten mit gesundheitsschädigenden inhaltsstoffen. Stuttgart, BMW-Verlags-GmbH.

Kahn, I.S. (1942) Fruit sensitivity. South. Med. J. 35, 858.

Keil, H. Wasserman, D. and Dawson, C. R, (1946) Mango Dermatitis and its Relationship to Poison Ivy Hypersensitiveness. Ann. Allergy, 4, 268.

Kirby-Smith, J.L. (1938) Mango Dermatitis. Am. J. trop. Med. 18, 373.

Lakhanpai, R.N. and Nair, P.K.K. (1958) Survey of the atmospheric pollen at Lucknow. J. Sci. Indust. Res. 17c, 80.

Lindenbaum, S. (1962) Allergic Reactions to Mangifera indica (Mango). Harefuah, 62, 422.

Morton, J.F. (1969) Some ornamental plants excreting respiratory irritants. Proc. Florida State Hort. Soc. 82, 415.

Morton, J.F. (1971) Plants poisonous to people in Florida and other warm areas. Miami, Fla. Hurricane House.

Nasution, D., Klokke, A.R. and Nater, J.P. (1973) A Survey of Occupational Dermatoses in Indonesia. Berufsdermatosen, 21, 215.

Rubin, J.M., Shapiro, J. Muehbauer, P. and Grolnick, M. (1965) Shock Reaction Following Ingestion of Mango. J. Am. med. Ass. 193, 397.

Silva, P. (1945) Dermatite de contacto causada pela manga (Mangifera indica L.) Hospital, Rio de Janeiro, 27, 231.

Simmons, J.S. and Bolin, Z.E. (1921) Dermatitis Venenata Produced by an Irritant Present in the Stem Sap of the Mango Mangifera indica L.) Am. J. trop. Med. I, 351.

Tillema, S. (1936) Huidaaveningen door manggifera-soorten. Geneesk Tijdschr. v. Nederland-Indie, 76, 2855.

Wechsler, H.L. (1960) Experimental contact dermatitis: effect of injections of 3-pentadecylcatechol (3-PDC) and mango feeding on cutaneous sensitivity to 3-PDC in guinea pigs. J. Invest. Derm. 34, 95.

Zakon, S.J. (1939) Contact Dermatitis due to Mango. J. Am. med. Ass. 113, 1808.

Mangifera kemanga

The resin is acrid and injurious to the skin of woodcutters (Senear 1933, Burkill 1935, Schwartz et al 1957).

References

Burkill, I.H. (1935) A Dictionary of the Economic Products of the Malay Peninsula. 2 vols. London, Crown Agents for the Colonies.

Schwartz, L. Tulipan, L. and Birmingham, D.J. (1957) Occupational Diseases of the Skin. 3rd. Edit. Philadelphia, Lea and Febiger, pp. 637-672

Senear, F.E. (1933) Dermatitis Due to Woods. J. Am. med. Ass. 101, 1527.

Mangifera lagenifera
Lanjut

The vapour of freshly bruised tissues, the smoke from a bonfire of their leaves or raindrops from the crown of the tree may affect the skin (Corner 1952).

Reference

Corner, E.J.H. (1952) Wayside trees of Malaysia. Singapore, Government Printer.

Mangifera odorata

The tree is extensively grown in Malaya although the fruit is inferior, because M. indica does not grow well in many parts of that country. The sap of the bark is irritant (Burkill 1935) but it is chiefly the sap of the unripe fruit which causes skin reactions (Corner 1952). The fruit has a strong turpentine-like smell but some varieties have a lesser smell.

Known as Sapian Mango in Guam, the plant is reported as causing dermatitis also by Souder (1963) and Ridley (1922).

References

Burkill, I.H. (1935) A Dictionary of the Economic Products of the Malay Peninsula. 2 Vols. London, Crown Agents for the Colonies.

Corner, E.J.H. (1952) Wayside trees of Malaysia. Singapore, Government Printer.

Ridley, H.N. (1922) Plant Dermatitis. J. trop. Med. Hyg. 25, 225.

Souder, P. (1963) Poisonous Plants on Guam In Venomous and Poisonous Animals and Noxious Plants of the Pacific Region. Ed. Keegan, H.L. and Macfarlane, W.V. Oxford, Pergamon Press, pp. 15-29.

Mauria

The twenty species are all natives of the Andes. M. birringo is said by the natives to be poisonous. The plant can cause dermatitis (Triana 1872). M. heterophylla produces skin eruptions in some persons (Altschul 1973). M. puberula is said to cause dermatitis (Hurtado 1968).

References

Altschul, S. von R. (1973) Drugs and foods from little known plants, Cambridge, Mass. Harvard University Press.

Hurtado, I. de (1968) Studies on the Biological Activity of Rhus striata ('Manzanillo') II. Skin Response to Patch Test in Humans. Int. Arch. Allergy, 33, 209.

Triana (1872) Ann. Sc. Nat. ser. 5. 14, 289, cited by Sprague (1921).

Sprague, T.A. (1921) Plant Dermatitis. Journal of Botany 59, 309.

Melanochyla

The 12 species are natives of Western Malaysia. They are often included with other genera, under the term rengas tree.

M. auriculata Swamp Rengas

This uncommon tree is not usually cut because of the irritant sap (Corner 1952, Burgess 1968) which is known to cause dermatitis (Senear 1933, Schwartz et al 1957).

M. beccanana and M. elmeri are also reported to cause skin reactions (Corner 1952)

References

Burgess, P.F. (1966) Timbers of Sabah (Sabah Forest Records No. 6). Sabah, Malaysia, The Forest Department.

Corner, E.J.H. (1952) Wayside trees of Malaysia. Singapore Government Printer.

Schwartz, L., Tulipan, L. and Birmingham, D.J. (1957) Occupational Diseases of the Skin. 3rd. Edit. Philadelphia, Lea and Febiger, pp. 637-672.

Senear, F. E. (1933) Dermatitis Due to Woods. J. Am. med. Ass. 101 1527.

Melanorrhoea

The 20 species are natives of South-East Asia, the Malay Peninsula and Borneo. They are among the trees known as Rengas in Malaya, and renowned collectively for the irritancy of their sap, though this varies from species to species (Burgess 1966). One unidentified species was so virulent that it was impossible to collect a specimen of its heartwood.

The timber of several species is hard and durable and has been sold as Singapore mahogany, but the irritancy of the sap limits its value and only two species (M. usitata and M. wallichii) are regularly distributed by the timber trade (Hausen 1973). Even thoroughly seasoned furniture may affect persons allergically sensitized to the poison. The black sap tends slowly to find its way through polish, but if a further application of a polish, particularly a modern polyurethane lacquer, is made after two or three years, further problems are likely to be avoided (Burgess 1966).

Some species yield a valuable black varnish.

The wood of several species contains silica and blunts saws.

M. aptera

M. beccarii

Both species have irritant sap (Burgess 1966).

M. curtisii

The sap causes dermatitis (Brown 1891, Mathes and Schreiber 1914, Senear 1933, Corner 1952). A scantily clad person who scrambles through the broken branches may suffer a widespread dermatitis, which may be complicated by fever and other constitutional symptoms and has occasionally proved fatal (Burkill 1935).

M. inappendiculata (Burgess 1966),
M. maingayi (Ridley 1911, Mathes and Schreiber 1914, Senear 1933, Schwartz et al 1957, Burgess 1966),
M. malayana (Corner 1952) and
M. speciosa (Burgess 1966) are all reported as irritant.
M. laccifera is a source of lacquer in Indo-China.
M. usitata is a source of lacquer in Burma.

The procedure for collecting the lacquer is essentially the same in both regions. The tree is tapped by making V-shaped cuts with a chisel. The bark above each cut is torn to form a cavity into which is inserted a shoot of bamboo, with an obliquely cut mouth, to form a spout.

The latex, which at first is yellowish-white, turns black, but remains fluid. It is stored in jars for distribution. It can be used as a varnish or, after mixing with sawdust, ashes or similar material, it can be moulded. For ornamental use it may be coloured by the addition of vermilion, or pigment, lampblack, indigo, gold leaf or silver leaf. The varnish has many uses. It is used on umbrellas, to give a surface to trays, drinking cups and similar articles and as the cement for Burmese glass mosaics (Watt 1906, Burkill 1935).

The timber of *M. usitata*, known in the trade as varnish tree or Mai Leek, is hard, durable and finely marked and is used for furniture and for inlay and similar work (Hausen 1973).

Chemistry

The main irritant and sensitizer of *M. usitata* is (Majima 1922, Backer and Haack 1941)

Thitsiol

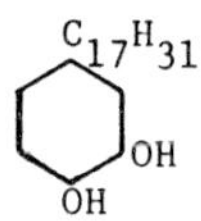

Cross reactions with other Anacardiaceae are recorded.

Dermatitis

The sap may splash the skin while the trees are being felled, and the sawdust of trees felled three or four years earlier, and even of old furniture, may cause dermatitis and irritation of mouth, nose and throat (Watt 1891, Schwartz et al 1957, Behl et al 1966).

M. wallichii

This beautifully coloured wood is used for furniture, and is one of the timbers known in the trade as Rengas. It has so far been imported to Europe only as samples (Hausen 1973). The irritant and sensitizer is moreakol, which is similar to, perhaps identical to thitsiol.

Felled trees are commonly left in the jungle for the sapwood to be destroyed by decay and by white ants, before they are dragged out.

The sap causes dermatitis (Ridley 1922, Lewin 1928, Thiébault 1965, Behl et al 1966).

M. Woodsiana

The sap causes dermatitis (Corner 1952, Burgess 1963).

References

Backer, H.J. and Haack, N.H. (1941) Le principe toxique de Gluta renghas L. Rev. Trav. chim. Pays-Bas, 60, 656.

Behl, P.N., Captain, R.M. Bedi, B.M.S. and Gupta, S. (1966) Skin-irritant and Sensitizing Plants Found in India. New Delhi, P.N. Behl, Irwin Hospital.

Brown, (1891) Journ. As. Soc. Straits 24, 83, cited by Sprague (1921).

Burgess, P.F. (1966) Timbers of Sabah (Sabah Forest Records No. 6). Sabah, Malaysia, The Forest Department.

Burkill, I.H. (1935) A Dictionary of the Economic Products of the Malay Peninsula. 2 vols. London, Crown Agents for the Colonies.

Corner, E.J.H. (1952) Wayside trees of Malaysia. Singapore, Government Printer.

Hausen, B.M. (1973) Holzarten mit Gesundheitsschädigenden Inhaltsstoffen. Stuttgart, DRW-Verlags-GmbH.

Lewin, L. (1928) Gifte in Holzgewerbe. Beiträge zur Giftkunde. Heft 1. Berlin, Georg Stilke Verlag.

Majima, R. (1922) Über den Haupbestandteil des Japanlacks. IX Chemische Untersuchung der verschiedenen natürlichen Lackarten, die dem Japanlack nahe verwandt sind. Ber. dtsch. chem. Ges. 55, 191.

Mathes, H. and Schreiber, E. (1914). Über hautreizende Hölzer. Ber. dtsch. pharm. Ges. 24, 385.

Ridley, H.N. (1911) Rengas-poisoning. Malaya Med. J. 9 (pt. 2), 7-13 (April).

Ridley, H.N. (1922) Plant Dermatitis. J. trop. Med. Hyg. 25, 225.

Schwartz, L., Tulipan, L. and Birmingham, D.J. (1957) Occupational Diseases of the Skin. 3rd Ed. Philadelphia, Lea and Febiger, pp. 637-672.

Senear, P.E. (1933) Dermatitis Due to Woods. J. Am. med. Ass. 101, 1527.

Sprague, T.A. (1921) Plant dermatitis. Journal of Botany 59, 309.

Thiébault, A. (1965) Nomenclature Générale des Bois Tropicaux. L'Association Technique Internationale des Bois Tropicaux, 45 bis Avenue de la Belle-Gabrielle, Nogent-sur-Marne, France.

Watt, G. (1891) Dict. Econ. Prod. India 5, 210, cited by Sprague (1921)

Watt, G. (1906) Kew Bulletin p. 137 cited by Burkill (1935).

Metopium

The three species are natives of the West Indies, Florida and Mexico.

Metopium brownei
(syn. Rhus metopium)

The timber, known as Black Poison Wood, is used locally for general purposes (Hausen 1973). The sap is irritant and can cause painful inflammation of the skin (Pardo-Castello 1923, Standley 1927, Baumer 1955).

Metopium toxiferum

Known as Poison Wood, this tree is widely distributed in Florida (Morton 1971), and the Caribbean region (Kingsbury 1964).

The sap of the plant and its fruit are irritant (Jackson 1946). When used in wreaths and bouquets the plant can cause dermatitis and it may do so also if overhanging branches brush against clothes hanging on a line (Morton 1971).

An outbreak of dermatitis occurred among Air Force personnel clearing undergrowth in the Bahamas, and in residents incautiously gathering trees for Christmas (Jackson 1946). In Florida, the trees often grow so close to pine trees that they escape destruction when land is cleared without removing the pines. The glossy leaves of young trees are attractive and inspire transplantation to gardens (Morton 1958).

The smoke from the burning wood is highly irritating (Dahlgren and Standley 1944).

Metopium venosum

Reports of dermatitis caused by this eastern Cuban species have not been traced, but its specific name suggests that it is, at the least, irritant.

References

Baumer, M. (1955) Que faut-il croire de la toxicité de certains bois tropicaux? Rev. Bois Forêts trop. 43, 27.

Dahlgren, B.E. and Standley, P.C. (1944) U.S. Bur. Med. Surg. Nav. Med. 127, quoted by Biology Data Book 1964.

Hausen, B.M. (1973) Holzarten mit Gesundheitsschädigenden Inhaltsstoffen. Stuttgart, DRW-Verlags-GmbH.

(Hausen, B.M. (1973) Timber species with Constituents Injurious to Health (German): Stuttgart DRW)

Jackson, W.P.U. (1946) Plant Dermatitis in the Bahamas. Br. med. J. 2, 298.

Kingsbury, J.M. (1964) Poisonous Plants of the United States and Canada. Englewood Cliffs, New Jersey, Prentice-Hall, Inc.

Morton, J.F. (1958) Ornamental plants with poisonous properties. Proc. Florida State Hort. Soc. 71, 372.

Morton, J.F. (1971) Plants Poisonous to People in Florida and Other Warm Areas. Miami, Florida, Hurricane House Publishers, Inc.

Pardo-Castello, V. (1923) Dermatitis Venenata. A Study of the Tropical Plants Producing Dermatitis. Archs. Derm. 7, 81.

Standley, P.C. (1927) Poisonous Trees of Central America. Tropical Woods, 9, 3-7 (March) and 7, 8 (Sept.), 1926.

Parishia

Twelve species are found in Burma and western Malaysia.

Parishia spp. Rengas

The wood used for fine furniture and ornamental work can cause dermatitis (Senear 1933).

Reference

Senear, F.E. (1933) Dermatitis due to woods. JAMA 101, 1527

Pentaspadon

The 5 species occur in Malaysia and the Solomon Islands.

Pentaspadon spp.

The sap in general is not dermatitic and indeed the oil from some species is used in Malaya for treating skin diseases (Corner 1952).

Pentaspadon officinalis

The oleo-resin is black and greatly irritant to the skin (Burkill 1935).

References

Burkill, I.H. (1935) A Dictionary of the Economic Products of the Malay Peninsula. 2 Vols. London, Crown Agents for the Colonies.

Corner, E.J.H. (1952) Wayside trees of Malaysia. Singapore, Government Printer.

Pseudosmodingium

The 7 species are natives of Mexico.

Pseudosmodingium perniciosum

This species can produce dermatitis (HBK 1825).

The plant was listed as irritant (Pammel 1911). The sap and wood are acrid, causing skin eruptions (Altschul 1973).

References

Altschul, S. von R. (1973) Drugs and foods from little-known plants. Cambridge, Mass. Harvard Univ.

Press.

HBK (1825) Nov. Gen. Sp. 7, 10. cited by Sprague (1921).

Pammel, L.H. (1911) A Manual of Poisonous Plants. Cedar Rapids, Iowa. Torch Press. Reprinted Univ. Microfilms Inc., Ann Arbor, Mich., 1965, pp. 476-7.

Sprague, T.A. (1921) Plant dermatitis. Journal of Botany 59, 309.

Rhus

There are over 200 species widely distributed over subtropical and warm temperate regions.

Rhus is closely related to Toxicodendron many species of which were formerly placed in the former genus. These include such plants as poison ivy.

Many Rhus species cause dermatitis. Some Indian villagers have an almost superstitious dread of all species; they believe that the smoke from the burning wood can cause swelling and vesication of the skin (Chopra et al 1949).

Reference

Chopra, R.N., Bhadwar, R.L. and Ghosh, S. (1949) Poisonous Plants of India. Sci. Monograph No. 17. The Indian Council of Agricultural Research, Delhi.

Rhus ambigua yields laccol (see R. succedanea) (Bertrand et al. 1939)

Reference

Bertrand, G., Backer, H.J. and Haack, N.W. (1939) Composition of Laccol. Bull. Soc. chem. (5), 6, 1670.

Rhus coriaria
Sumac (Southern Europe)

The finely ground leaves are used for tanning and dyeing. The plant has been suspected of causing dermatitis (Maiden 1909).

Reference

Maiden, J.H. (1909) On Some Plants which Cause Inflammation or Irritation of the Skin. Ag. Gaz. New South Wales, 20, 111.

Rhus cotinus
Smoke Tree, Venetian Sumac

The tree yields a yellow dye, (young fustic) (Schwartz et al 1957), and its leaf has a high tannin content and was formerly used for tanning (Hurst 1942). The timber is marketed as Fusticwood or Hungarian Yellow wood and is used for veneers. This plant is much cultivated in gardens. The sap can cause dermatitis (Maiden 1909, Behl et al 1966), attributable either to phenols or to hydroquinones (Hausen 1970). The plant is sometimes classified in a distinct mono-specific genus as Cotinus coggygria.

References

Behl, P.N., Captain, R.M., Bedi, B.M.S. and Gupta, S. (1966) Skin-irritant and Sensitizing Plants Found in India. New Delhi, P.N. Behl, Irwin Hospital.

Hausen, B.M. (1970) Untersuchungen über Gesundheitsschädigende Hölzer. Thesis. Hamburg.

Hurst, E. (1942) The Poison Plants of New South Wales. N.S.W. Poison Plants Committee, Sydney.

Maiden, J.H. (1909) On Some Plants which Cause Inflammation or Irritation of the Skin. Ag. Gaz. New South Wales, 20, 111.

Schwartz, L., Tulipan, L. and Birmingham, D.J. (1957) Occupational Diseases of the Skin. 3rd. Ed. Philadelphia, Lea and Febiger, pp. 637-672.

Rhus glabra Sumac

This species is said to cause dermatitis (Pardo-Castello 1923).

Reference

Pardo-Castello, V. (1923) Dermatitis Venenata. A Study of the Tropical plants Producing Dermatitis. Archs. Derm. 7, 81.

Rhus insignis

The leaves, fruit and bark can produce dermatitis; The sap is vesicant (Behl et al. 1966). The smoke from the burning wood has been reported to cause dermatitis (Watt and Breyer-Brandwijk 1962).

References

Behl, P.N., Captain, R.M., Bedi, B.M.S. and Gupta, S. (1966) Skin-irritant and Sensitizing Plants Found in India. New Delhi, P.N. Behl, Irwin Hospital.

Watt, J.M. and Breyer-Brandwijk, M.G. (1962) The Medicinal and Poisonous Plants of Southern and Eastern Africa. 2nd Edit. Edinburgh, E. and S. Livingstone Ltd.

Rhus juglandifolia
Hinchador

The plant is common in Costa Rica where its local name, Hinchador, meaning "the sweller", indicates that its toxic properties are well known. The shrub is of the right height to brush easily against face and hands (Standley 1927).

Reference

Standley, P.C. (1927) Poisonous Trees of Central America. Tropical Woods, 9, 3-7 (March) and 7, 8 (Sept.) 1926.

Rhus metopium
Coral Sumac, Mountain Machineel.

The sap is irritating (Weber 1937, Simons 1953). See also Metopium.

References

Simons, R.D.G. (1953) Jungle-Dermatitis (Dermatoses caused by tropical plants and woods) in Handbook of Tropical Dermatology and Medical Mycology. ed. Simons R.D.G. Vol. II. Amsterdam, Elsevier.

Weber, L.F. (1937) External Causes of Dermatitis. A List of Irritants. Arch. Derm. Syph. 35, 129.

Rhus punjabensis

The leaves, bark, fruit and sap can produce dermatitis (Behl et al 1966).

Reference

Behl, P.N., Captain, R.M., Bedi, B.M.S. and Gupta, S. (1966) Skin-irritant and Sensitizing Plants Found in India. New Delhi, P.N. Behl, Irwin Hospital.

Rhus pyroides

A scratch or prick from the sharp point of a twig (the plant has no thorns) is extremely painful and burns like fire, hence the specific name, pyroides (Watt and Breyer-Brandwijk 1962).

Reference

Watt, J.M. and Breyer-Brandwijk, M.G. (1962) The Medicinal and Poisonous Plants of Southern and Eastern Africa. 2nd Edit. Edinburgh, E. & S. Livingstone Ltd.

Rhus radicans
Poor Man's Liquid Amber

This plant caused allergic contact dermatitis in a woman in Australia (Turner 1972), see Toxicodendron.

Reference

Turner, T. (1972) Poison Ivy and Poor-man's Liquid Amber. Med. J. Austr. 2, 166.

Rhus semialata

This plant, which provides Chinese Nutgalls yields an irritant phenolic related to anacardic acid (Loev and Dawson 1958).

Reference

Loev, B. and Dawson, C.R. (1958) Cashew nutshell liquid. X. An investigation of the geometrical configuration of the olefinic components of cardinol and some observations concerning ginkgol. J. Am. Chem. Soc. 80, 643.

Rhus striata
Manzanillo (also applied to its timber)
(syn. Toxicodendron striatum)

This tree grows in Central America and northern South America. It has caused severe allergic contact dermatitis with blistering and oedema (Standley and Steyermark 1949, Hurtado 1965). In one case (Hurtado 1965) the dermatitis developed two days after sawing the wood, and persisted for two weeks.

The oleoresin shows haemolytic activity on human red cells (Hurtado et al 1965).

Cross reactions have been reported to *Toxicodendron radicans*, *Lithrea caustica*, *Mauria puberula* and *Rhus vernicifera* (Hurtado 1968).

The common name Manzanillo is applied also to the unrelated irritant plant *Hippomane* (Euphorbiaceae).

References

Hurtado, I. de (1965) Contact Dermatitis Caused by the "Manzanillo" (*Rhus striata*) Tree. Int. Arch. Allergy, 28, 321.

Hurtado, I. de (1968) Studies on the Biological Activity of *Rhus striata* ('Manzanillo'). II. Skin Response to Patch Test in Humans. Int. Arch. Allergy, 33, 209.

Hurtado, I. de, Burnell, R.H., Medina, J.D. et al (1965) Studies on the Biological Activity of *Rhus striata* ('Manzanillo'). I. Hemolytic Activity. Int. Arch. Allergy, 28, 261.

Standley, P.C. and Steyermark, J.A. (1949) Flora of Guatemala. Fieldiana Bot. 24, Part 6.

Rhus succedanea
Rhus Tree, Wax Tree

The exudate from incisions in this tree (as well as that from *R. vernicifera*) is collected for the manufacture of Japanese lacquer (Chopra et al 1949). The crushed berries yield wax.

Chemistry

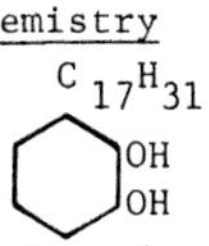

Laccol

The plant yields laccol.

Laccol, also present in *R. ambigua* and *Semecarpus vernicifera* is the diethenoid analogue of glutarenghol (from *Gluta renghas*), in which the exact positions of the double bonds have yet to be defined (Bertrand et al 1939).

Dermatitis

The leaves, fruit and bark can cause dermatitis (Guimaraes et al 1960, Behl et al 1966, Burry 1939). The sap is vesicant (Chopra et al 1949). The wax has caused dermatitis in workers handling fabrics waterproofed with it (Schwartz et al 1957).

References

Behl, P.N., Captain, R.M., Bedi, B.M.S. and Gupta, S. (1966) Skin-irritant and Sensitizing Plants Found in India. New Delhi, P.N. Behl, Irwin Hospital.

Bertrand, G., Backer, H.J. and Haack, N.H. (1939) Composition of Laccol. Bull. Soc. chem (5) 6, 1670.

Burry, J.N. (1969) The Value of Patch Testing: a Review of 363 Cases of Allergic Contact Dermatitis. Med. J. Aust. 1, 1226.

Chopra, R.N., Bhadwar, R.L. and Ghosh, S. (1949) Poisonous Plants of India. Sci. Monograph No. 17. The Indian Council of Agricultural Research, Delhi.

Guimaraes, O.P., Bento, D., Pickel, J. et al (1960) The toxico-allergic principle of the Anacardiaceae. The problem of *Rhus succedanea* in the city of Sao Paulo. Rev. Bras. Med. 17, 43.

Schwartz, L. Tulipan, L. and Birmingham, D.J. (1957) Occupational Diseases of the Skin. 3rd Edit. Philadelphia, Lea and Febiger, pp 637-672.

Rhus taitensis Lemayo

This native plant of Guam can produce dermatitis (Souder 1963).

Reference

Souder, P. (1963) Poisonous Plants on Guam, *in* Venomous and

Poisonous Animals and Noxious Plants of the Pacific Region. Ed. Keegan, H.L. and Macfarlane, W.V. Oxford, Pergamon Press pp. 15-29.

Rhus typhina

Staghorn Sumac, Antler Tree (Denmark)

This ornamental tree is a native of North America but is widely cultivated elsewhere. Its yellow soft and light timber is used for inlays (Hausen 1970). It is recorded as causing dermatitis (Grobmann 1910). The leaves are said to contain irritating sap (Lindemark 1971). However the plant produced no reactions in patch tests in normal subjects, but a positive reaction in one of ten subjects known to be sensitive to poison oak (*Toxicodendron*) (Maibach and Hjorth 1973). Ross (1974) observed a case of contact dermatitis from *R. typhina* in Newfoundland. It is possible that the species is not biochemically homogeneous and that some varieties, or cultivars, are allergenic.

References

Grobmann, J. (1910) Gesundheitsschad-liche Hölzer Bayr. Indust. Gewerbeblt. 96, 51.

Hausen, B.M. (1970) Untersuchungen Über Gesundheitsschädigende Hölzer. Thesis. Hamburg.

Lindemark, O. (1971) Vore giftige Blomsterplanter. Copenhagen, Gyldendal.

Maibach, H. and Hjorth, N. (1973) *Rhus typhina*, a Possible Cause of Contact Dermatitis. Personal Communication (Contact Dermatitis Newsletter), London, No. 13 (Jan.), p. 347.

Ross, J.B. (1974) Personal Communication.

Rhus vernicifera

Japanese Lacquer Tree

Rhus vernicifera, was distributed in Japan before 701 A.D. (White 1887). Every farmer in certain parts of Japan was obliged to establish plantations, and taxes were paid in lacquer. Lacquer was used in China as early as 2255 B.C. (Toyama 1926) and the art of lacquering was introduced to Japan in about 250 B.C. Lacquer dermatitis was described in China as early as 453 B.C.; a good description was given in Ping-yuan-hon-lun (605-609 A.D.) in China, and later in Wamyo-rui-ju-sho (923-930 A.D.) in Japan (Toyama 1918) and by Zan Yun Fang (c. 600 A.D.) (Toyama 1926). An early European account of lacquer dermatitis was published by Kaempfer (1712).

The lacquer is obtained by tapping the trees by incisions in the bark, just deep enough to reach the wood. Some lacquer is extracted from felled trees, under water. The latex flowing from the incised trees darkens on exposure to the air. As the quality is highest when the lacquer is light in colour, it is stored in bamboo tubes.

A volatile poisonous substance is associated with the fresh latex, and to eliminate it the latex is, in Japan, stirred for some hours in open vessels. The risk of dermatitis to tappers is reduced by the fact that they are a special class or caste of highly skilled workmen (Burkill 1935). The procedures followed in China and Burma differ in some particulars.

Chemistry
(Sunthankar and Dawson 1954)

The sensitizing substances are urushiol and its derivatives.

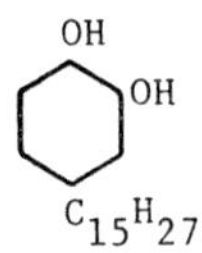

Urushiol

Their dermatitic properties depend on the two neighbouring hydroxyl groups and the degree to which the side chain is unsaturated (Majima 1922). Urushiol constitutes 35%-70% of Chinese lacquer and somewhat more of Japanese lacquer (Toyama 1923, 1926, Toyama and Usuba 1926).

Dermatitis

R. vernicifera and its lacquer can give rise to dermatitis at all stages from the initial collection of the latex to the final application of the lacquer, and even, it appears, a thousand years later; lacquer from a Chinese jar, which had been buried for about a millenium, caused dermatitis (Toyama 1918).

Contact dermatitis from handling the plant itself has been reported by Buraczynski (1903), by Bauer (1940) and by Rost (1914). A girl in North Vietnam developed dermatitis after wearing shoes made of the wood (Holcik 1959). Bullous occupational dermatitis, with systematic illness in workers was reported by Antonev et al (1964).

Contact dermatitis from the lacquer has been far more frequently reported because so many such cases have occurred in Western Europe or North America and because the sources of contact are sometimes exotic and unexpected. Men engaged in hanging embossed Japanese wallpaper are said to have been affected (White 1887). Some individuals become so sensitive that they cannot pass a furniture shop where articles are being varnished, without being affected. Others, less sensitive, react only on contact with freshly varnished furniture (Allen 1887).

When used for firewood the wood produces smoke with highly irritating particles (Holcik 1959).

In Hawaian pineapple factories, cans which were passed through a bath containing one part of lacquer to five parts of gasoline caused dermatitis in those handling the cans (Wayson 1923). A seller of toy canes used for flags developed dermatitis which was attributed to the lacquer on incomplete evidence (Pusey 1923). Lacquered lamp shades have also been incriminated, but inconclusively (Weber 1937). Lacquered bracelets and boxes have caused dermatitis in wood workers and others (Goldstein 1968). The lacquer on Japanese rifles caused dermatitis in American soldiers sensitive to poison ivy (Hinman 1946, Coomber 1947). Contact with a recently varnished bar in Japan caused dermatitis in 12 American officers; it is possible that some were previously sensitive to poison ivy (Etler 1951). In Scotland subjects sensitive to poison ivy developed dermatitis after contact with varnished boxes (Murrell 1896). Lacquer used as a spray has caused dermatitis (Queries and Minor Notes 1931). For 15 years a woman had suffered from recurrent dermatitis of fingers, palms and wrists; the cause was proved to be lacquered soup-bowls (Hollander and Shelton 1937).

The clinical features are almost infinitely variable, according to the mode and sites of contact and the degree of sensitivity. A study of affected workers in a factory (Riedel 1940) illustrated some of the problems. Repeated contact may lead to hyposensitization (Little 1924).

Cross-sensitivity to other anacardiaceous plants has been mentioned above. It has been investigated by Howell (1959); the range is wide but variable. Sturua (1963) found sensitivity to R. vernicifera to be specific with no cross-sensitivity to R. succedanea and Toxicodendron radicans (R. toxicodendron); tests were carried out with slices of twigs of the plant.

The experimental induction of sensitivity in guinea-pigs has been achieved in 44 of 63 exposed to an alcohol-ether extract of Rhus vernicifera (Toyama 1923).

References

Allen, H.N. (1887) Journal of Cutaneous and Genito-urinary Diseases, January. Cited by White, 1887.

Bauer, H. (1940) Über Sumachdermatitis. Med. Klin. 36, 48.

Buraczynski, A. (1903) Cited by Pusey, 1923.

Burkill, I.H. (1935) A Dictionary of the Economic Products of the Malay Peninsula. 2 Vols. London, Crown Agents for the Colonies.

Coomber, R.B. (1947) Dermatitis from Contact with Varnish of Japanese Rifles. Arch. Derm. Syph. 55, 110.

Etler, R.L. (1951) Dermatitis Caused by Japanese Lacquer. U.S. Armed Forces med. J. 2, 505.

Goldstein, N. (1908) The Ubiquitous Urushiols - Contact Dermatitis from Mango, Poison Ivy, and Other 'Poison'Plants. Cutis, 4, 679.

Antonev, A.F., Orlov V.M. and Raben, A.S. (1964) Occupational lesions of the skin caused by Far East (Chinese and Japanese) lacquer Vestn. Derm. Vener. 3, 26.

Hinman, F. Jr. (1946) Contact Dermatitis from Japanese Rifles. Ann. Allergy, 4, 384.

Holcik, L. (1959) Dermatitis from Rhus vernicifera (Czechoslovak). Csk. Derm. 34, 93.

Hollander, L. and Shelton, J.Z. (1937) Dermatitis due to Japanese Lacquer. Arch. Derm. Syph. 33, 1081.

Howell, J.B. (1959) Cross Sensitisation in Diverse Poisonous Members of the Sumac Family (Anacardiaceae). J. invest. Derm. 32, 21.

Kaempfer, (1712) Amoenitatum Exoticarum, cited by White, 1887.

Little, C. (1924) Dermatitis Produced by Chinese Lacquer. Br. med. J. 1, 1112.

Majima, R. (1922) Über den Hauptbestandeil des Japan Lacks. IX Chemische Untersuchung der verschiedenen natürlichen Lackarten, die dem Japan-Lack nahe verwandt sind. Ber. dtsch. chem. Ges. 55, 191.

Murrell, W. (1896) The Poison of the Primula. Lancet, 1, 1040.

Pusey, W.A. (1923) Lacquer Dermatitis. Arch. Derm. Syph. 7, 91.

Queries and Minor Notes (1931) Health Hazard of Lacquer Dyes Used as a Spray. J. Am. med. Ass. 96, 1894.

Riedel, H. (1940) Bemarkungen zur Entacabung der Lack-Krätze. Klin Wschr. 69, 159.

Rost, (1914) Wien med. Wchnschr. 27, 101. Cited by Pusey, 1923.

Sturua, G.A. (1963) The dermatitis caused by poisonous sumacs. Vestn. Derm. Vener. 2, 51.

Suthankar, S.V. and Dawson, C.R. (1954) The Structural Identification of the Olefinic Components of Japanese Lac. Urushiol. J. Am. chem. Soc. 76, 5070.

Toyama, I. (1918) Rhus dermatitis, J. Cutan. Dis. 36, 157.

Toyama, I. (1923) Further Observations on Lacquer Dermatitis. Far Eastern Assoc. trop. Med. Trans. Fifth. Bienniel Congress, Singapore, p. 824. Abstr., Trop Dis. Bull. (1925) 22, 231.

Toyama, I. (1926) Studies on Lacquer Dermatitis. III. Dermatitis Produced by Chinese Lacquer. Jap. J. Derm. Urol. 26, 927. Abstr. Bull. Hyg. (1927) 2, 808.

Toyama, I. and Usuba, T. (1926) Studies on Lacquer Dermatitis. IV. The Histopathology of Lacquer Dermatitis. Jap. J. Derm. & Urol. 26, 937. Abstr. Bull. Hyg. (1927) 2, 668.

Wayson, J.T. (1923) Lacquer Dermatitis or Dermatosis Industralis (Papulovesicular Lacquer). Arch. Derm. Syph. 8, 77.

Weber, L.F. (1937) External Causes of Dermatitis. A List of Iritants. Arch. Derm. Syph. 35 129.

White, J.C. (1887) Dermatitis Venenata: an Account of the Action of External Irritants upon the Skin. Boston, Cupples and Hurd.

Rhus wallichii

Japanese Wax Tree
Red Lac Sumac

This small tree is very closely allied to the Japanese lacquer tree and possesses similar properties (Behl et al. 1966).

Reference

Behl, P.N., Captain, R.M., Bedi, B.M.S. and Gupta, S. (1966) Skin-irritant and Sensitizing Plants Found in India. New Delhi, P.N. Behl, Irwin Hospital.

Schinopsis

The seven species in this genus are confined to South America.

Schinopsis lorentzii

Red Quebracho

(syn. Loxopterygium lorentzii)

This tree yields a timber useful for building constructional work (Hausen 1970) and is also a rich source of tannin.

The dermatitic agent in this species appears not to have been identified, but Lullo's (1934) suggestion that a substance similar to cardol is responsible seems probable. He showed that sensitization was involved since only a proportion of those exposed developed dermatitis, and this only after a latent period. It has been listed as an irritant wood (Schwartz et al 1957, Orsler 1973).

Contact with the branches or the leaves or the sawdust may provoke dermatitis in sensitive persons (Lullo 1928) and the condition is sufficiently common to have acquired the vernacular name of "Mal de quebracho".

The diagnosis may be confirmed (Lullo 1934) by patch testing with an alcoholic extract or with an aqueous distillate.

References

Hausen, B.M. (1970) Unteruchungen Über Gesundheitsschädigende Holzer. Thesis. Hamburg.

Di Lullo, O. (1928) Le "Paaj", dermite provoquée par le Quebrache rouge (Schinopsis lorentzii). Compte Rendu Soc. biol. 99, 1000.

Di Lullo, O. (1934) "El Paaj". Une Nouvelle Dermatite Vénéneuse. Rev. Sud. Amér. Med. Chir. 5, 513.

Orsler, R.J. (1973) Personal Communication from Forest Products Research Laboratory, Princes Risborough, Bucks, England.

Rendle, B.J. (1929) "Paaj" Dermatitis Produced by Red Quebracho. Tropical Woods, 17, 7. Review of di Lullo, O, "Paaj" dermatitis produced by red Quebracho. Comptes Rendus de Séances de la Société de Biologie et de ses Filiales, 99, 28, 1000, Paris, 1928.

Schwartz, L., Tulipan, L. and Birmingham, D.J. (1957) Occupational Diseases of the Skin. 3rd. Edit. Philadelphia, Lea and Febiger, pp. 637-672.

Schinus

The thirty species are native to northern and central South America, Central America and Mexico, but some are cultivated as ornamental or shade trees, wherever the climate is favourable.

Schinus sp. Aroeira

Von Bassewitz (1928) and Freise (1932) thought that aroeira was probably a species of Schinus but Astronium and Lithraea are also called aroeira.

The Aroeira Sickness was described by von Bassewitz (1928). This author established that up to 10% of the population of Southern Brazil has some degree of hypersensitivity to this wood. Those who were sensitive reacted not only to the tree itself but also to dry seasoned wood. Furniture which has been in use for long periods can provoke reactions.

References

Freise, F.W. (1932) Gesundheitsschädigungen durch Arbeiten mit giftigen Hölzern. Beobachtungen aus brasilianischen Gewerbebetrieben. Arch für Gewerbepathologie und Gewerbehygiene 3, 1.

von Bassewitz, E. (1928) Die südbrasilianische Aroeirakrankheit Arch. Schiffs. Tropenhyg 32,494.

Schinus molle

Brazilian Pepper Tree, Florida Holly Aroeira (timber)

The durable timber of this and probably of related species is used for bridge construction and for fencing (Hausen 1973). The fruit which is irritant to the throat (Aplin 1966) has been used as an adulterant of black pepper. The resin of the tree is a source of American mastic.

Chemistry

Phellandrene, carvacol and

pinene are derived from the fruit. The dermatitis is likely to be caused by a phenolic substance. (Hausen 1970).

Dermatitis

Dermatitis, resembling poison ivy dermatitis, occurs in those who become sensitized to the tree or its timber or sawdust.

Schinus terebinthifolius

Japanese Pepper, Florida 'Holly'

All parts of the tree contain a volatile resin, which produces dermatitis in susceptible subjects, especially when the tree is in full bloom, and in some people causes sneezing and asthma-like reactions (Aplin 1966, Hardin and Arena 1969, Morton 1971).

Respiratory symptoms can occur from proximity to the plant (Morton 1969).

References

Aplin, T.E.H. (1966) Poison Plants in the Garden. West Australian Dept. Agr. J. 7, 24.

Bassewitz, A. von (1928) The Aroeira Sickness of Southern Brazil (German) Arch. Schiffs. Tropen Hyg. 32, 494.

Hardin, J.W. and Arena, J.M. (1969) Human Poisoning from Native and Cultivated Plants. Durham, N. Carolina, Duke Univ. Press.

Hausen, B.M. (1973) Holzarten mit gesundheitsschädigenden inhaltsstoffen. Stuttgart, DRW-Verlags-GmbH.

Morton, J.F. (1969) Some ornamental plants excreting respiratory irritants. Proc. Florida State Hort. Soc. 82, 415.

Morton, J.F. (1971) Plants Poisonous to People in Florida and Other Warm Areas. Miami, Florida, Hurricane House Publishers, Inc.

Schinus velutinus

The foliage causes skin irritation (Altschul 1973).

Reference

Altschul, S. von R. (1973) Drugs and Foods from little-known plants. Cambridge, Mass. Harvard Univ. Press.

Sclerocarya

Five species are native to tropical and South Africa. The fruit is edible.

Sclerocarya caffra

Pammel (1911) noted that this species had an irritant effect.

Reference

Pammel, L.H. (1911) A Manual of Poisonous Plants. Torch Press. Cedar Rapids, Iowa. Reprinted Univ. Microfilms Inc., Ann Arbor, Mich. 1965. pp 476-7

Semecarpus

Some fifty species are native to Indo-Malaysia, Micronesia and the Solomon Islands. The young fruit of most, perhaps all species, yields an irritant resin, which can be used as a marking ink. Some of the species are rare and not well studied

Semecarpus anacardium

Indian Marking Nut Tree, Bhilawa

(Anacardium orientale, Semecarpus latefolius, Anacardium latefolium, Anacardium officinarum, King 1957)

The sap of this species, mixed with lime-water or alum, is used as marking ink in India and Malaya. Preparations of the nut were used in ancient medicine and still find a place in indigenous medicine. The ink is insoluble in water, but soluble in alcohol (Burkill 1935). The pedicel, which swells under the fruit, may be eaten. The pericarp and the ripe fruit contain bhilawa oil.

Trade in the bhilawa nut is very ancient, for this fruit was the "golden acorn" of Galen (A.D. 130-c.200) and Avicenna (d. 1037) (King 1957). It was estimated in 1946 that the crop consisted of about 50,000 tons of nuts containing 20% bhilawan oil (King 1957).

Chemistry

The dermatitic substance is bhilawanol (Mason 1945)

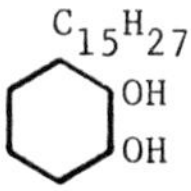

Dermatitis

Dermatitis occurs in those preparing the oil, or in those applying it to clothing in their capacity as laundrymen (called Dhobis in India) and in those wearing the marked clothing. The term "Dhobi itch" has been confusingly applied both to marking ink dermatitis and to tinea cruris (a ringworm infection of the groins).

There are two principal clinical patterns of dermatitis (Behl et al 1966). Those who use nut preparations medically or in treating sick animals may develop dermatitis of the hands and face. If they grind the nuts with the pestle in a mortar held between the knees, the feet and legs may also be affected.

The second clinical pattern involves those wearing the marked clothing. Fifty-two American soldiers serving in India were affected; about 14% of those exposed (Livingood et al 1943, Fitz-Hugh et al 1943). Indians appear to be less susceptible than Americans, but the difference is probably environmental and could be related to previous exposure of the latter to poison ivy or of the former to the relatively weaker sensitizing potential of *Mangifera* (Blank 1957). Since the Dhobi is accustomed to mark the inside of the shirt collar, brassiere, belt, vest and underpants, the site of the localised dermatitis tends to be the back of the neck or the lower back in men, and the mid or lower back in women. As the resin is not destroyed by boiling, the mark may continue to provoke dermatitis for the life of the garment (Fasal 1943). The mark must therefore be cut out or covered with adhesive plaster.

Extensive dermatitis occurred in a girl who accidentally contaminated her skin while marking her brother's clothing with pure Bhilawa juice (Behl et al 1966). The contamination of mail by a bottle of Bhilawol oil contained in the same sack caused dermatitis in 16 of 50 workers sorting the mail (Goldsmith 1943).

Cross sensitivity with other plants in the Anacardiaceae family has been studied (Howell 1959) but the lack of adequate phytochemical knowledge of some species makes any general conclusions premature.

References

Behl, P.N., Captain, R.M. Bedi, B.M.S. and Gupta, S. (1966) Skin-irritant and Sensitizing Plants Found in India. New Delhi, P.N. Behl, Irwin Hospital.

Blank, H. (1957) Dermatitis from Anacardiaceae. Proc. Florida Mango Forum. 17th Annual Meeting, Miami, Oct. 16th.

Burkill, I.H. (1935) A Dictionary of the Economic Products of the Malay Peninsula. 2 Vols. London Crown Agents for the Colonies.

Fasal, P. (1945) Cutaneous Diseases in the Tropics. Arch. Derm. Syph. 51, 163.

Fitz-Hugh, T. Jr., Livingood, C.S. and Rogers, A.M. (1943) Dhobie Mark Dermatitis. Bull. U.S. Army M. Dept. 69, 55.

Goldsmith, N.R. (1943) Dermatitis from Semecarpus anacardium (Bhilawanol or Marking Nut) Spread by Contaminated Mail. J. Am. med. Ass. 123, 27

Howell, J.B. (1959) Cross Sensitisation in Diverse Poisonous Members of the Sumac Family (Anacardiaceae). J. invest. Derm. 32, 21.

King, L.J. (1957) A Unique Reported Use for the Fruit of *Semecarpus anacardium* L.f. (Anacardiaceae) in Ancient Arabian and Indian Medicine. Econom. Bot. 11, 263.

Livingood, C.S., Rogers, A.M. and Fitz-Hugh, Jr., T. (1943) Dhobie Mark Dermatitis. J. Am. med. Ass. 123, 23.

Mason, H.S. (1945) The toxic principles of poison ivy. III. The structure of bhilawanol. J. Am. Chem. Soc. 67, 418.

Semecarpus atra

Contact with sap from the tree trunk caused dermatitis (Hitch 1944).

Hitch, J.M. (1944) Dermatitis venenata caused by Semecarpus atra. U.S. Nav. Med. Bull. 42, 1111.

Semecarpus australiensis

Tar tree

The black tarry sap causes severe dermatitis (Sulit 1940, Flecker 1945).

Flecker, H. (1945) Injuries produced by plants in tropical Queensland. Med. J. Australia 1, 636.

Sulit, M.D. (1940) Plants to be avoided or handled with care in the forest. Philipp. J. Forestry 3, 177.

Semecarpus cassuvium

The oil is used by the Amboinese as a varnish. The oily fruit has irritant properties (Burkill 1935).

Burkill. I.H. (1935) A Dictionary of the economic Products of the Malay Peninsula. 2 vols. London Crown Agents for the Colonies.

Semecarpus cuneiformis

The species was described as the most common of the contact poisons of the Phillipine Islands; rain dripping off the tree and the smoke of burning branches produced dermatitis (Burkill 1935). The oil of the pericarp is used as an escharotic and the sap produces violent dermatitis (Quisumbing 1951).

References

Burkill, I.H. (1935) A Dictionary of the economic products of the Malay Peninsula. 2 vols. London. Crown Agents for the Colonies.

Quisumbing, E. (1951) Medicinal Plants of the Philippines. Philipp. Dept. Agr. and Nat. Resources Tech. Bull. No. 16.

Semecarpus decipiens

The sap of the tree was found by a plant collector to be extremely irritant (Altschul 1973).

Altschul, S. von R. (1973) Drugs and foods from little-known plants. Cambridge, Mass. Harvard Univ. Press.

Semecarpus heterophylla

The resin of this Javanese plant, which turns black on exposure to air, produces severe dermatitis (Burkill 1935). The active principle is renghol (Backer and Haack 1938).

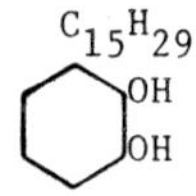

Renghol

References

Backer, H.J. and Haack, N.H. (1938). Le principe toxique des fruits de renghas Semecarpus heterophylla B.L. Rev. Trav. Chim. Pays-Bas 57, 225.

Burkill, I.H. (1935) A Dictionary of the Economic Products of the Malay Peninsula. 2 vols. London, Crown Agents for the Colonies.

Semecarpus laxiflora

This species causes dermatitis in Melanesia (Record 1945).

Reference

Record, M. (1945) A collection of woody plants from Melanesia. Tropical Woods 81 (Semecarpus pg. 11).

Semecarpus travancoricus

Marking nut tree, Bhilawa

The juice can cause dermatitis (Behl et al 1966).

Reference

Behl, P.N., Captain R.M., Bedi, B.M.S. and Gupta, S. (1966) Skin irritant and sensitizing plants found in India. New Delhi, P.N. Behl, Irwin Hospital.

Semecarpus venosa

This species was reported

to cause dermatitis by Iseki (1932).

Reference

Iseki, K. (1932) Fall von Dermatitis acuta durch "Aangot"-Baum (Semecarpus venosa Volk.) Acta. derm. (Kyoto) 19, 31.

Semecarpus vernicifera

This species provides Formosa lacquer (Hausen 1970).

Reference

Hausen, B.M.(1970) Untersuchungen Über Gesundheitsschädigende Hölzer. Thesis Hamburg.

Semecarpus vernicifera

The juice poisons the skin (Kumada 1940).

Reference

Kumada, T. (1940) Poisonous fishes and plants in the tropics. Trans. by K. Musya. U.S. Geological Survey. Pacific Geological Surveys. Military Geology Branch, U.S.G.S. Tokyo, Japan.

Semecarpus vitensis

Itchwood tree

This Pacific Island tree has an irritant milky juice (King 1957), suggested by its colloquial name.

Reference

King, L.J. (1957) A Unique reported use for the fruit of Semecarpus anacardium L.f. (Anacardiaceae) in ancient Arabian and Indian Medicine. Econom. Bot. 11, 263.

Smodingium argutum

Um-tovane, tovana

This monospecific genus is confined to South Africa. Although its poisonous properties were recognized by native tradition and by botanists it was not medically incriminated as a cause of contact dermatitis until recently (Findlay 1963).

Chemistry

The principal sensitizing agent appears to be a 17-carbon chain catechol (Findlay et al 1974).

Dermatitis

The sap is irritant in high concentration, but is also a potent sensitizer, causing severe contact dermatitis with oedema and bullae (Findlay 1963, Heyl 1972).

References

Findlay, G.H. (1963) Dermatitis of 'Poison Ivy' Type from an Indigenous South African Plant - Smodingium argutum E. Rey. (Anacardiaceae). S. Afr. Med. J. 37, 883.

Findlay, G.H., Whiting, D.A., Eggers, S.H. and Ellis, R.P. (1974) Smodingium (African "poison ivy") dermatitis, history, comparative plant chemistry and anatomy, clinical and histological features. Br. J. Dermatol. 90, 535.

Heyl, T. (1972) Personal Communication. Pretoria, Transvaal.

Spondias

There are 10-12 species native to Indo-Malaysia, south-east Asia and tropical America. The drupe of some species is edible. Four species are much cultivated throughout the tropics.

Spondias spp. Hog-Plum

The stone of the fruit is hard, round or ridged, generally prickly from woody fibres. All parts of the plants have a foetid turpentine-like smell when broken or bruised; the smell differs in each species and is characteristic. The fruits are edible (Corner 1952).

Spondias mombin

Mope, mombin, jobo

A sawyer who had dermatitis showed a strong positive patch test reaction to the sawdust of this species, and weak positive reactions to the sawdust of Pterygota macrocarpus and of Terminalia ivorensis. Control tests were not recorded (Woods and Calnan 1976).

Woods, B. and Calnan, C.D. (1976). Toxic Woods. Brit. J. Derm. 94, Suppl. 13, June.

Spondias pinnata   Hog Plum
(Spondias mangifera)

This tree is cultivated in India for its fleshy edible fruit, which is eaten raw or pickled. The bark of the tree is rubefacient, being used in indigenous medicine for rubbing on the skin over painful joints. The bark is irritant (Chopra et al 1958).

References

Chopra, R.N., Chopra, I.C., Handa, K.L. and Kapur, L.D. (1958) Chopra's Indigenous Drugs of India. 2nd. Edit. Calcutta, U.N. Dhur and Sons Ltd.

Corner, E.J.H. (1952) Wayside trees of Malaysia. Singapore, Government Printer.

Swintonia

There are 15 species in South-east Asia and West Malaysia.

Swintonia spp.

The plants were said to be as poisonous as Melanorrhoea (Foxworthy 1909), but according to Burgess (1966) the sap is apparently not irritating.

References

Burgess, P.F. (1966) Timbers of Sabah (Sabah Forest Records No. 6). Sabah, Malaysia, The Forest Department.

Foxworthy (1909) Philipp. J. Sci. Cited by Burkill, 1935.

Toxicodendron

The 15 species in this genus are native to East Asia and North and South America.

Changes of nomenclature, which are confusing to the non-botanist, are made only in accordance with strict internationally agreed taxonomic rules.

The most important cause of dermatitis in North America, Poison Ivy, has been known as Rhus toxicodendron and as Rhus radicans. It is correctly named Toxicodendron radicans (Kingsbury 1964, Gilles 1975).

The correct names for other important species in this genus are:

Western Poison Oak
Toxicodendron diversilobum

Eastern Poison Oak
Toxicodendron quercifolium

Poison Sumac
Toxicodendron vernix

Poison Ivy,
Toxicodendron radicans, occurs in a number of distinct forms of varieties (Kingsbury 1964), e.g.:

var. littorale	East Coast
var. radicans	Central states
var. verrucosum	Oklahoma, parts of Texas
var. eximium	Rio Grande basin
var. rydbergii	North West

Poison ivy occurs in all of the United States, east of the Cascade Mountains. It also occurs in Canada and in Mexico, Guatemala, and some Caribbean Islands. It has been introduced to Britain (Nicholson 1899, Nott 1910, Shadbolt 1916), Western Europe (Giuseppe 1928), South Africa (Ross 1959), Australia (Cleland 1914, Turner 1972), Bulgaria (Topalov 1957), Poland (Lukowska 1971) and Russia (Solomatin 1962).

Western Poison Oak, Toxicodendron diversiloba (which has been known as Rhus toxicodendron and Rhus diversiloba) is found in Western North America. It is closely related to Poison Ivy and hybrids occur between the species and Eastern Poison Oak, Toxicodendron quercifolium (which has been known as R. toxicodendron and R. diversiloba). It grows on sandy soils over a large part of central, eastern and southern North America. T. orientale (Khlebovich 1960) and poison sumacs (Lunin 1971) have been reported to cause dermatitis from Russia.

The dermatitic properties of these plants have long been recognized (McNair 1923, Rostenberg 1955).

The total incidence of sensitivity to these species is unknown, but may be in the region of 50% of the population of the United States (Kligman 1958). A larger proportion of positive reactors is obtained by patch testing with pure 3-n-pentadecyl-catechol: perhaps 10-15% are truly immune (Epstein 1973). There is no convincing evidence that children are less susceptible than adults and the incidence in all the younger age groups is a measure of exposure to the antigens (Strauss 1931, Epstein 1961). Sensitivity is most commonly acquired in childhood or early adult life and tends to decline in later life. There is no evidence for inborn immunity to sensitization or for familial predisposition to acquire sensitivity but atopic individuals may be less susceptible (Jones et al 1973). Immunity in Asiatics has been ascribed to exposure to Mangifera in early life (Epstein and Claiborne 1957). Dermatitis from the plants is an important problem (Epstein 1974).

References

Cleland, J.B. (1914) Plants, including fungi, poisonous or otherwise injurious to man in Australia. Australian Med. Gaz. 35, 569. idem. Tasmanian Ag. Gaz. 32, 361 and 401.

Epstein, E. and Claiborne, E.R. (1957) Racial and environmental factors in susceptibility to Rhus. Archs. Derm. 75, 197.

Epstein W.L. (1961) Contact-type delayed hypersensitivity in infants and children. Induction of Rhus sensitivity. Pediatrics. 27, 51.

Epstein, W.L. (1973) Personal communication.

Epstein, W.L. (1974) Poison Oak and poison ivy dermatitis as an occupational problem. Cutis 13, 544.

Gillis, W.T. (1975) Poison-ivy and its kin. Arnoldia 35, 93.

Giuseppe, A. (1928) The pathogenesis of Rhus toxicodendron dermatitis (Italian) Reforma Med. 44, 1344

Jones, H.E., Lewis, C.W. and McMarlin, S.L. (1973). Allergic contact sensitivity in atopic dermatitis. Archs. Derm. 107, 217.

Khlebovich, V.V. (1960) The 'Yperite-plant' of the Shikotan Island. Vestn. Derm. Vener. 34, 56.

Kingsbury, J.M. (1964) Poisonous Plants of the United States and Canada. New Jersey, Prentice-Hall.

Kligman, A.M. (1958) Poison ivy (Rhus) Dermatitis. Archs. Derm. 77, 149.

Lukowska, I. (1971) Allergic dermatitis due to occupational contact with Rhus toxicodendron. Przegl. Dermatol. 58, 481.

Lunin, M.M. (1971) Clinical form of affections by poison sumac. Vopr. Med. Khim. 17, 79.

McNair, J.B. (1923) Rhus dermatitis from Rhus Toxiçodendron Radicans and Diversiloba (Poison Ivy). Its Pathology and Chemotherapy. Chicago. Univ. Chicago Press.

Nicholson, F. (1899) A case of acute dermatitis caused by handling the Rhus Toxicodendron. Brit. Med. J. 1, 530.

Nott, H.W. (1910) A case of Rhus toxicodendron dermatitis. Brit. Med. J. 2, 545.

Ross, C.M. (1959) Poison-Ivy Dermatitis: the First South African Cases. S. Afr. med. J. 33, 657.

Rostenberg, A. Jr. (1955) An Anecdotal Biographical History of Poison Ivy. Archs. Derm. 72,438.

Shadbolt, L.P. (1916) Rhus toxicodendron poisoning. Brit. Med. 2, 480.

Solomatin, P. (1962) Rhus dermatitis. Vestn. Derm. I. Vener. 10, 38.

Strauss, H.W. (1931) Artificial Sensitization of Infants to Poison Ivy. J. Allergy 2, 137.

Topalov, Y.B. (1957) On a few cases of dermatitis caused by the plant Rhus toxicodendron. Savr. Med. 8,102.

Turner, T. (1972) Poison ivy and Poor-Man's Liquid Amber. Med. J. Australia 2, 166.

Chemistry

The elucidation of the chemical structure of the sensitizing agents of *Toxicodendron* has been largely the work of C.R. Dawson and his associates (Keil et al 1944, Dawson 1956, Kurtz and Dawson 1971) and of H. Baer and his associates (Baer et al 1967, 1968, Godfrey et al 1971, Johnson et al 1972). Poison Ivy contains four antigenic components; all are catechols with a 15-carbon atom side chain in the 3 position. By custom, the term urushiol is applied to this material.

Cross reactions occur with many other catechols in anacardiaceous plants and to some extent also with resorcinol, and to hydroquinone and to its monobenzyl ether (Kligman 1958).

Baer, H. et al (1967) Delayed contact sensitivity to catechols. III The relationship of side chain length to sensitising potency of catechols chemically related to the active principles of poison ivy. J. Immunology 99, 370.

Baer, H. et al (1968) Delayed contact sensitivity to catechols. IV Stereochemical configuration of the antigenic determinant. J. Immunology 101, 1243.

Dawson, C.R. (1956)The Chemistry of Poison Ivy. Trans. N.Y. Acad. Sci. 18, 427.

Godfrey, H.P., Baer, H. and Watkins, R.C. (1971) Delayed contact sensitivity to catechols. V Absorption and distribution of substances related to poison ivy extracts and their relation to the induction of sensitization and tolerance. J. Immunology 106, 91.

Johnson, R.A., Baer, H., Kirkpatrick, C.H. et al (1972). Comparison of the contact allergenicity of the four pentadecyl catechols derived from poison ivy urushiol in human subjects. J. Allergy Clin. Immunol 49, 27.

Keil, H., Wasserman, D. and Dawson, C.R. (1944). The Relation of Chemical Structures in Catechol Compounds and Derivatives to Poison Ivy Hypersensitiveness as Shown by the Patch Test. J. exp. Med. 80, 275.

Kligman, A.M. (1958) Poison Ivy (*Rhus*) Dermatitis. Archs. Derm. 77,149.

Kurtz, A.P. and Dawson, C.R. (1971) Synthesis of compounds structurally related to poison ivy urushiol 3. 3-n-pentadecylcatechol and 3-n-alkyl catechols of varying side-chain length. J. Med. Chem. 14, 729.

Kurtz, A.P. and Dawson, C.R. (1971) Synthesis of compounds structurally related to poison ivy urushiol 4. 3-(1-alkyl)alkyl catechols of varying side-chain shape and flexibility. J. Med. Chem. 14, 733.

Toxicodendron not *Rhus*

Four members of *Toxicodendron* which commonly produce dermatitis in the United States have recently received chemical study and taxonomic revision. (Gillis 1971, Gillis 1975, Gross et al 1975, Corbett and Billets 1975). Their current names are:

- *Toxicodendron radicans* (L.) Kuntze (*Rhus toxicodendron* L., *Rhus radicans* L.); Poison ivy, poison vine, markweed, three-leaved ivy, etc.
- *Toxicodendron toxicarium* (Salisb.) Gillis; Eastern poison oak, oakleaf ivy.
- *Toxicodendron diversilobum* (T. & G.) Greene; Western poison oak.
- *Toxicodendron vernix* (L.) Kuntze; Poison sumac, poison elder.

Allergenic catechols and derivatives of *Toxicodendron*

The allergenic catechols and their derivatives of 3 species are shown in the Figure. The minor antigenic component in poison ivy, saturated 3-pentadecylcatechol, has no double bonds in the side chain and therefore it is more stable and less reactive than the unsaturated catechols. Generally, the allergenic structure is an ortho catechol with a side chain at C3, 15 or 17 carbons long, with various degrees of unsaturation. The more unsaturated or the longer the side chain, the more

Figure: Chemical structures of the allergenic principles of <u>Toxicodendron</u> species

Compound	Poison ivy (<u>T. radicans</u>)	Poison oak (<u>T. diversilobum</u>)	Poison Sumac (<u>T. vernix</u>)
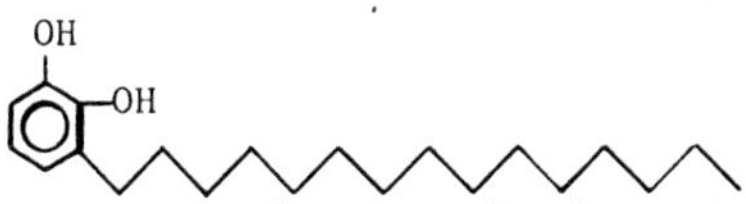 3-n-Pentadecylcatechol	0-7.6%	3.4-22.3%	15.3%
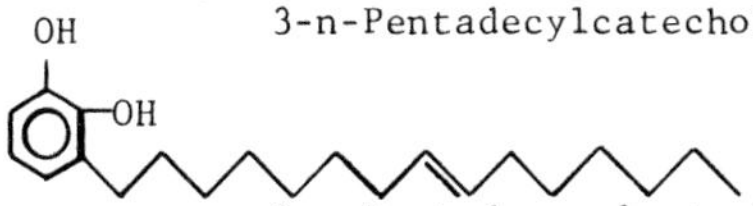 3-n-Pentadecenylcatechol	3.1-41.6%	1.4-8.4%	41.4%
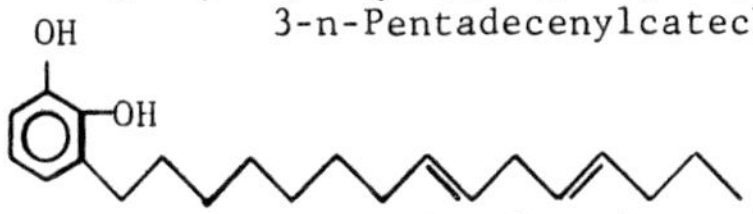 3-n-Pentadecadienylcatechol	17.9-83.1%	0.2-2.7%	32.7%
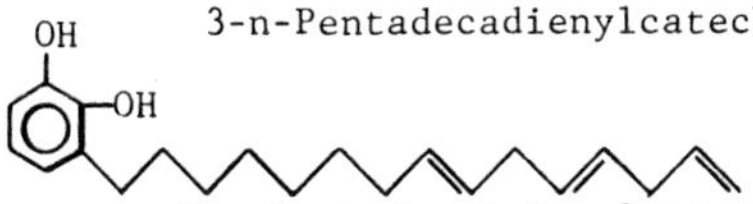 3-n-Pentadecatrienylcatechol	3.3-62.5%	0-0.6%	10.6%
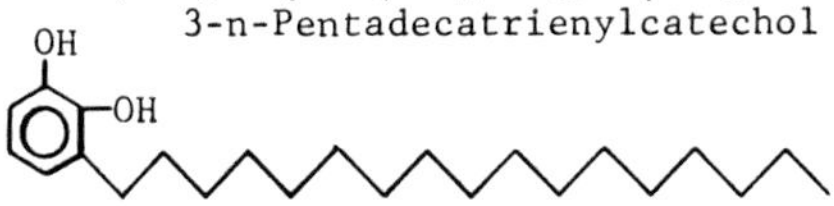 3-n-Heptadecylcatechol	0-0.2%	0-2.1%	0
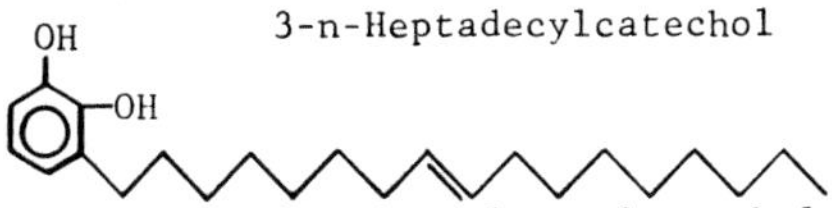 3-n-Heptadecenylcatechol	0-2.1%	5.7-10.7%	0
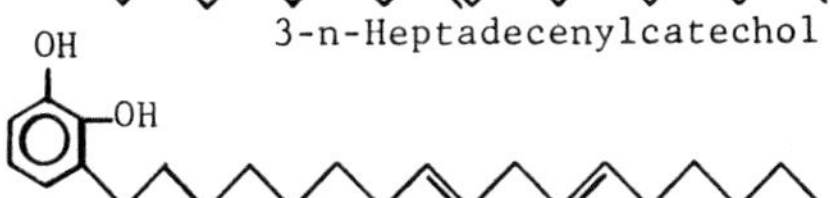 3-n-Heptadecadienylcatechol	0-22%	18.7-24.9%	0
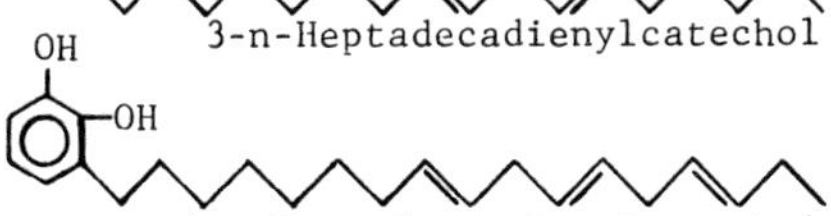 3-n-Heptadecatrienylcatechol	0-4.2%	35.1-62.5%	0
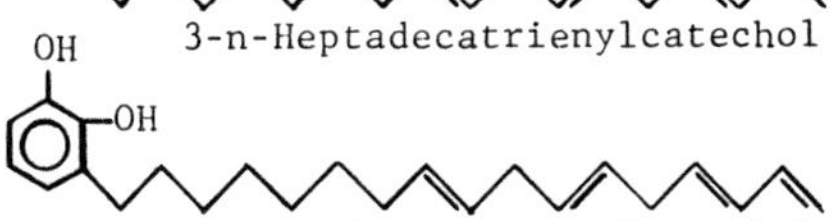 3-n-Heptadecatetraenylcatechol	0	0-1.3%	0

After Gross M, et al: Urushiols of poisonous Anacardiaceae: Phytochemistry 14:2263-2266; 1975 and Corbett M, Billets S: Characterization of poison oak urushiol. J. Pharm. Sci. 64:1715; 1975.

allergenically active it is. Thus 4-PDC is less reactive than 3-PDC. Western poison oak contains about 0.18 percent urushiol with a 17-carbon side chain which should be more allergenic than poison ivy urushiol which has a 15-carbon side chain. Western poison oak urushiol has unsaturated catechol congeners with 15- and 17-C side chains at C3 position and one to three double bonds in the side chain whereas poison-ivy urushiol has one $-CH_2CH_2-$ unit on the unbranched side chain (Corbett and Billets 1975). The allergenicity of PDC's derived from poison ivy urushiol were compared by Johnson et al (1972).

References

Corbett, M. and Billets, S. (1975) Characterization of poison oak urushiol. J. Pharm. Sci. 64, 1715.

Gillis, W.T. (1971) The systematics and ecology of poison-ivy and the poison oaks. Rhodora 73, 72 and 370 and 465.

Gillis, W.T. (1975) Poison-ivy and its kin. Arnoldia 35, 93.

Gross, M. et al (1975) Urushiols of poisonous anacardiaceae. Phytochemistry 14, 2263.

Johnson, R.A. et al (1972) Comparison of the contact allergenicity of the four pentadecylcatechols derived from poison ivy urushiol in humans. J. Allerg. Clin. Immunol 49, 27.

Dermatitis (reviewed by Gellin et al 1971).

Poison ivy and the two poison oaks are such an important source of the dermatitis so characteristic of the Anacardiaceae that its features have already been described in the general introduction to this family.

Early attempts to sensitize human volunteers (Biberstein 1929) soon established the basic sequence of events (Field and Sulzberger 1935). After the first effective contact the incubation period is usually 9 to 10 days. After subsequent exposures dermatitis develops in 24 - 72 hours; the interval may be shorter in highly sensitive subjects who are heavily exposed. Sensitive patients challenged with an oral extract developed degranulation of circulating basophils within an hour (Shelley and Resnik 1965).

Various methods of hyposensitization have been advocated, e.g. the application of gradually increasing doses to the skin (Maisel 1932) and graduated dosage orally of 10% cashew nut oil (Kligman 1958). A patient's attempt to desensitize himself by chewing poison ivy leaves caused stomatitis and dermatitis of the face and of the perianal skin (Silvers 1941). Oral hyposensitisation was demonstrated in some individuals (Kligman 1958) and confirmed in a study of larger groups (Epstein et al 1974). An adequate quantity of purified urushiol must be administered during a sufficiently long period of time and observation is required for cutaneous and systemic complications (Shelmire 1941, Shaffer et al 1951).

No propylactic applications are consistently effective (Howell 1943, Birmingham 1969). Urushiol is rapidly bound in the skin and washing with soap and water is only of value if carried out immediately after contact. Contaminated fomites, articles and animals may be sources of inadvertent re-exposure.

Prevention by controlling the offending plants was recommended as early as 1896 (Chesnut 1896) and later by Byram (1931) and Crooks and Klingman (1968), but this is practicable only in certain restricted areas. Some herbicides are listed by Maibach and Epstein (1964).

Biberstein, H. (1929) Skin reactions following the application of various species of Rhus. Klin Wschr. 8, 99.

Birmingham, D.J. (1969) Prevention of occupational skin disease. Cutis 5, 153.

Byram, A.T. (1931) Poison Ivy Control. Canadian Public Health Journal 22, 201.

Chesnut, V.K. (1896) Some common poisonous plants. Yearbook Department of Agriculture.p.137.

Crooks, D.M. and Klingman, D.L. (1968) Poison Ivy, Poison Oak, and Poison Sumac: Identification, precautions, eradication. Farmers' Bulletin 1972. U.S. Dept. Agriculture.

Epstein, W.L., Baer, H., Dawson, C.R. et al (1974) Poison oak hyposensitisation. Archs. Derm. 109, 356.

Field, H. and Sulzberger, M.B. (1935) Experiments in Poison Ivy Sensitivity. J. Allergy 7, 139.

Gellin, G.A., Wolf, C.R. and Milby, T.H. (1971) Poison ivy, poison oak, and poison sumac. Common causes of occupational dermatitis. Arch. Environ. Health 22, 280.

Howell, J.B. (1943) Poison ivy preventives prove ineffective. Archs. Derm. Syph. 48, 373.

Kligman, A.M. (1952) Cashew Nut Oil for Hyposensitization against *Rhus* dermatitis. Archs. Derm. 78, 359.

Kligman, A.M. (1958) Poison Ivy (*Rhus*) Dermatitis. Archs. Derm. 77, 149.

Maibach, H.I. and Epstein, W.L. (1964) Plant dermatitis: Fact and fancy. Postgrad. Med. 40, 571.

Maisel, F. (1932) Poison Ivy. A New Method of Immunization. J. Allergy 4, 35.

Shaffer, B., Burgoon, C.F. and Gosman, J.H. (1951) Acute glomerulonephritis following administration of *Rhus* toxin: report of a fatal and a near fatal case. JAMA 146, 1570.

Shelley, W.B. and Resnik, S.S. (1965) Basophil Degranulation Induced by Oral Poison Ivy Antigen. Archs. Derm. 92, 147.

Shelmire, B.S. (1941) Cutaneous and systemic reactions observed during oral poison ivy therapy. J. Allergy 12, 252.

Silvers, S.H. (1941) Stomatitis Venenata and dermatitis of the anal orifice from chewing poison ivy leaves. J. Am. med. Ass. 116, 2257.

ANNONACEAE Custard-Apple Family

About 2,100 species in 120 genera are mainly natives of the tropics; except for the genus *Annona*, they are especially of the Old World. Many yield edible fruit and some provide perfumes.

Chemistry is recorded by Hegnauer (1964).

Annona

120 species are found in warm regions, especially in America. Many contain insecticidal substances and also alkaloids of benzylisoquinoline type (Hausen 1973).

Annona cherimolia

Cherimoya

This Peruvian species, now widely established in the tropics, has edible fruit. The crushed seeds used in an alcoholic antiparasitic shampoo are said to have caused corneal ulcers (Romero 1947, Valdacasas 1947) and blindness (Allen 1943).

Annona chrysophylla

The sap of the trunk is said to be irritant (Watt and Breyer-Brandwijk 1962).

Annona glabra

This species contains a cytotoxic substance, liriodenin (Hausen 1973).

Annona muricata Sour Sop

The seeds contain 45% of an oil which in India and Mexico is applied to the hair to kill lice, though it is irritant to the eyes (Burkill 1935). The prickly fruit is edible.

Annona reticulata

Custard Apple, Bullock's Heart

The acrid sap is irritant and causes conjunctivitis (Watt and Breyer-Brandwijk 1962).

Annona squamosa

Sugar Apple, Sweet Sop

The powdered seed is irritant. It is applied as a pesticide and can cause conjunctivitis or even blindness (Burkill 1935, Morton 1958). A tincture of the seeds caused dermatitis of the face and eyelids (Barreto 1949).

References

Allen, P.H. (1943) Poisonous and Injurious Plants of Panama. Am. J. trop. Med. 23, Suppl., p. 3

Barretto, S.P. (1949) Dermatite et lésions conjonctivales et cornéennes consécutive à l'usage d'un insecticide populaire (estrait et teinture alcoolique de graines depinha). Arq. med. e. cirurgia de Pernambuco, 1, 99 (Abstr: Ann. ocul. 183, 720 1950).

Burkill, I.H. (1935) A Dictionary of the Economic Products of the Malay Peninsula. 2 Vols. London, Crown Agents for the Colonies.

Hausen, B.M. (1973) Holzarten mit gesundheitsschädigenden inhaltsstoffen. Stuttgart, DRW-Verlags. GmbH.

Hegnauer, R. (1964) Chemotaxonomy of plants. Vol. 3. Basel. Birkhauser, p. 116.

Morton, J.F. (1958) Ornamental plants with poisonous properties. Proc. Florida State Hort. Soc. 71, 372.

Valdecasas, P.G. (1947) Queratitis ocasionadas por le vapour del alcohol en el que semaceraron semillas de chirimoya. Arch. Soc. Oft. Hisp.-Amer. 7, 379.

Watt, J.M. and Breyer-Brandwijk, M.G. (1962) The Medicinal and Poisonous Plants of Southern and Eastern Africa. 2nd. Edit. Edinburgh, E. & S. Livingstone, Ltd.

Romero, E. (1947) Sobre la queratitis por vapor de alcohol. Arch. Soc. Oftal. Hipp.-Amer. 7, 912

Asimina

The genus consists of 8 species of eastern North American shrubs and trees.

Asimina triloba

Poor Man's Banana, Papaw (the tree Papaw is Carica papaya).

Some individuals develop dermatitis after handling the edible fruits (Muenscher 1951, Kingsbury 1964, Hardin and Arena 1969). Others who may not react to contact with the fruit may develop gastrointestinal symptoms after eating it (Barber 1905) perhaps because the bruised seeds are irritant and have emetic propensities (Grieve 1970).

References

Barber, M.A. (1905) Poisoning due to the Papaw (Asimina triloba) J. Am. med. Ass. 45, 2013.

Grieve, M. (1970) A Modern Herbal. 2 Vols. Darien, Connecticut, Hafner Publishing Co.

Hardin, J.W. and Arena, J.M. (1969) Human Poisoning from Native and Cultivated Plants. Durham, N. Carolina, Duke Univ. Press.

Kingsbury, J.M. (1964) Poisonous Plants of the United States and Canada. Eaglewood Cliffs, New Jersey, Prentice-Hall, Inc.

Muenscher, W.C. (1951) Poisonous Plants of the United States. 2nd. Edit. New York, The Macmillan Co.

Cananga

The two species are natives of tropical Asia south to Australia.

Cananga odorata

(syn. Canangium odoratum) Kenanga, Ylang-Ylang Tree

The Kenanga is a common village tree in Malaysia. Its fragrant flowers are worn for personal adornment and the oil distilled from them is known as Ylang-Ylang oil or Cananga oil. This oil, added to coconut oil and other ingredients, makes the Macassar oil (Corner 1952) so familiar to the well-groomed Victorian and Edwardian male. The flowers also yield a distillate used in perfumery (Burkill 1935, Arctander 1960). The term Macassar oil is also applied to a product of Schleichera, Sapindaceae.

Chemistry

Cananga oil is extracted from the flowers in Java by primitive machines and is said to contain fewer esters and more sesquiterpenes than Ylang-ylang oil which is grown on the Reunion, Madagascal and Comoro Islands (Nakayama et al 1974).

The constituents of Ylang-Ylang oil include (Greenberg and Lester 1954) geraniol and linalool esters of acetic and benzoic acids, p-cresol methyl ester, cadinene, a sesquiterpene and a phenol.

Perfumes colognes and toilet water containing essential oils of the plant can produce dermatitis in sensitized individuals (Greenberg and Lester 1954).

Ylang-Ylang oil has been accepted as an allergen and removed from certain cosmetics (Schieffelin 1973).

Cananga oil (15% in petrolatum) induced positive patch test reactions in 26 of 183 Japanese who had dermatitis from cosmetics. One of 40 control subjects showed a weak positive reaction. Ylang-Ylang oil (5% in petrolatum) induced positive patch test reactions in 25 of 183 such patients. There were no positive reactions in 40 control subjects (Nakayama et al 1974).

References

Arctander, S. (1960) Perfume and Flavor Materials of Natural Origin. Elizabeth, New Jersey. Publ. by the author.

Burkill, I.H. (1935) A Dictionary of the Economic Products of the Malay Peninsula. 2 Vols. London, Crown Agents for the Colonies.

Corner, E.J.H. (1952) Wayside Trees of Malaysia. Singapore, Government Printer.

Greenberg, L.A. and Lester D. (1954) Handbook of Cosmetic Materials. New York. Interscience.

Merck Index (1968) 8th ed. ed. Stecher, P.G. Rahway, New Jersey. Merck & Co.

Nakayama, H. (1973) Personal Communication.

Nakayama, H., Hanaoka, H. and Ohshiro, A. (1974) Allergen Controlled System (ACS). Tokyo. Kanehara Shuppan.

Schieffelin and Co. (1973) Almay Hypo-allergenic Cosmetics Product Formulary. 8th ed. Pharmaceutical Laboratories Division, 562 - 5th. Ave., New York, N.Y. 10036.

Enantia

Nine species are native to West Africa, one species to tropical East Africa.

Enantia polycarpa

African Yellow Wood

The bright yellow wood yields berberberine (Irvine 1961) which has elsewhere been found to produce distinctive cutaneous effects (Berberidaceae).

Reference

Irvine, F.R. (1961) Woody Plants of Ghana. London, Oxford University Press.

Monodora

20 species are native to tropical Africa and Madagascar.

Monodora myristica

Although the powdered seeds have been used as a pediculide, as in the case of other plants of this family, no ill-effects have been reported. A suggestion of irritancy comes from the use of the dried seeds as snuff and as a substitute for the spice, nutmeg (Myristica), (Irvine 1961).

Reference

Irvine, F.R. (1961) Woody Plants of Ghana. London, Oxford University Press.

Oxandra

About 22 species occur in Central and tropical South America and the West Indies. Several yield useful timber.

Oxandra lanceolata

Lancewood (The name is used for several strong elastic woods, Howes (1974).

The wood is used locally for spears, but is exported mainly for use in turnery and in the motor industry (Hausen 1973).

Since splinters of Australian lancewood, Acacia shirleyi were said to cause painful wounds (Maiden 1919), other lancewoods viz. O. lanceolata, Backhousia myrtifolia and Curtisia dentata have been included in lists of toxic woods (Howes 1951, McCord 1958) without any published evidence (Woods and Calnan 1976).

References

Hausen, B.M. (1973) Holzarten mit gesundheitsschädigenden inhaltsstoffen. Stuttgart, DRW-Verlags.-GmbH

Howes, F.N. (1951) Occupational dermatitis. Can. woodwork. 34 and 64.

Howes, F.N. (1974) A Dictionary of Useful and Everyday Plants and other Common Names. Cambridge University Press.

McCord, C.P. (1958) The Toxic Properties of Some Timber Woods. Industr. Med. Surg. 27, 202.

Maiden, J.H. (1919) Notes on Acacia, no.IV. J. Proc. Roy. Soc. New South Wales 53, 219-300 (whole paper 171-238 + plates).

Woods, B. and Calnan, C.D. (1976) Toxic Woods. Brit. J. Derm. 94, Suppl. 13, June.

Polyalthia

120 species are native to tropical regions especially Indo-Malaysia.

Polyalthia elongata

The plant, when chewed, produces itching (Altschul 1973).

Reference

Altschul, S. von R. (1973) Drugs and foods from little-known plants. Cambridge, Mass. Harvard Univ. Press.

Popowia

90 species are found from tropical Africa to tropical Australia.

Popowia diclina

The scented leaves provide a native perfume (Irvine 1961).

Reference

Irvine, F.R. (1961) Woody Plants of Ghana. London, Oxford University Press.

Steleocarpus

Five species are native to Thailand and Malaysia.

Steleocarpus burahol (Keppel)

Consumption of the edible fruit causes the sweat to smell like violets (Viola) and the trees were planted around Indonesian palace harems (Menninger 1967).

Reference

Menninger, E.A. (1967) Fantastic Trees. New York. The Viking Press.

Xylopia

100-150 species occur in the tropics, especially in Africa.

Xylopia aethiopica
Ethiopian Pepper

The fruits and seeds are used as a condiment, and as a rubefacient and counter-irritant in Africa. The seed oil is fragrant as is the bark (Irvine 1961).

Reference

Irvine, F.R. (1961) Woody Plants of Ghana. London, Oxford University Press.

APOCYNACEAE
Dogbane Family

This large family containing some 1500 species in 180 genera is of considerable economic and medical importance. Most of the species are tropical but a few are of common occurrence in temperate regions. The family yields many valuable timbers, pharmacologically active alkaloids, and decorative plants.

Chemistry

Of 200 alkaloids in the family, about 75 have been sufficiently studied to identify their chemical structure (Raffauf and Flagler 1960).

Acokanthera

The 15 species in this genus are natives of South Africa, tropical East Africa and Arabia.

Acokanthera ouabai
Ouabai, Wabai

In Abyssinia and Somalia the wood of this tree is the source of an extremely potent arrow poison. The poison, ouabain, is present also in such related species as A. longiflora and A. venenata (Hausen 1970).

Acokanthera spectabilis and A. venenata
Wintersweet, Bushman's Poison

These plants are cultivated for their decorative qualities. They are irritant to the skin, the eyes and the respiratory tract (Hurst 1942, Gardner and Bennetts 1956, Everist 1962).

References

Everist, S.L. (1962) A Review of the Poisonous Plants of Queensland. Proc. R. Soc. Queensland, 74, 1

Gardner, C.A. and Bennetts, H.W. (1956) The Toxic Plants of Western Australia. Perth, West Australian Newspapers Ltd.

Hausen, B.M. (1970) Untersuchungen über Gesundheitsschädigende. Hölzer. Thesis. Hamburg.

Hurst, E. (1942) The Poison Plants of New South Wales. N.S.W. Poison Plants Committee, Sydney.

Raffauf, R.F. and Flagler, M.B. (1960). Alkaloids of the Apocynaceae. Econ. Bot. 14, 37.

Allemanda (Syn. Allamanda)

There are 15 species native to tropical South America and the West Indies. Some have attractive flowers and are widely cultivated in appropriate climates. There are many cultivars of A. cathartica.

Allemanda cathartica
Yellow Allemanda

All parts of the plant may cause irritant dermatitis (Allen 1943, Morton 1971); that only susceptible individuals react, suggests that allergic sensitization also occurs. The sap may irritate the eyes and sucking the stems has caused swelling of the lips (Morton 1971, Blohm 1962, Hardin and Arena 1969).

References

Allen, P.H. (1943) Poisonous and Injurious Plants of Panama. Am. J. trop. Med. 23, Suppl., p. 3.

Blohm, H. (1962) Poisonous Plants of Venezuela. Cambridge, Mass., Harvard Univ. Press.

Hardin, J.W. and Arena, J.M. (1969) Human Poisoning from Native and Cultivated Plants. Durham, North Carolina, Duke University Press.

Morton, J.F. (1971) Plants poisonous to people in Florida, and other warm areas. Miami, Fla. Hurricane House.

Alstonia

50 species are found in Indomalaysia and Polynesia. The bark is used as a tonic.

Alstonia congensis Emien

Alstonia boonei

The wood is said in the trade to be irritant (Wendorff 1964). An alkaloid is present in a bark (Irvine 1961).

References

Irvine, F.R. (1961) Woody plants of Ghana. London. Oxford University Press.

Wendorff, G. von (1964) Pers. comm. to Woods and Calnan (1976).

Woods, B. and Calnan, C.D. (1976) Toxic Woods. Brit. J. Derm. 94,

Suppl. 13, June.

Aspidosperma

The 80 species are natives of tropical South America and the West Indies. Many species provide durable timber, resistant to weather and to fungus infection; these include (Hausen 1973):

Aspidosperma polyneuron
Peroba rosa

A. desmanthum Araracanga

A. inundatum Maparana

A. excelsum Carapanauba

A. macrocarpum Guatambu

A. eburnum Pequia marfim

A. gomesianum Peroba de campo

A. sessiflorum Peroba amarella

A. quebracho Quebracho

A. vargasii Amarillo, Pau marfum

A. peroba Peroba rosa

(The terms Peroba da campos and Peroba amarella are also applied to the somewhat similar, but botanically distinct, timber Paratecoma peroba).

Chemistry

The alkaloid macoubein has been isolated from all species investigated and is believed to be the cause of the dermatitis and other toxic effects. Other alkaloids are also present.

Dermatitis

The freshly cut wood and sap caused irritation of the eyes, nose and throat with general malaise. Contact of the sawdust with abrasions of the skin produced local burning and a vesicular eruption with general symptoms of muscular weakness and cramps, sweating, dryness of the mouth, drowsiness and faintness. Once the wood is thoroughly dry it loses its toxicity unless polishes or dyes in organic solvents are used on it (Freise 1932, 1937). Orsler (1973) received trade reports of irritation of the skin and respiratory tract in England from peroba rosa.

The bark and wood contain alkaloids (Hausen 1973).

References

Freise, F.W. (1932) Gesundheitsschädigungen durch Arbeiten mit giftigen Hölzern. Beobachtungen aus brasilianischen Gewerbebetriben. Archiv. fur Gewerbepathologie und Gewerbehygiene 3, 1.

Freise, F.W. (1937) Vergiftungen durch Brasilianische Werkhölzer I, II. Sammlung der Vergiftungsfällen, 8c, 13.

Hausen, B.M. (1973) Holzarten mit gesundheitsschädigenden inhaltsstoffen. Stuttgart, DRW-Verlags-GmbH.

Orsler, R.J. (1969) The effects of irritant timbers. Woodworking Industry. 26, 28.

Aspidosperma parvifolium

The wood dust caused dermatitis in sawyers (Peckolt 1909).

Reference

Peckolt, T. (1909) Heil-und Nutzpflanzen Brasiliens Berichte der deutschen pharmazeutischen Gesellschaft. 19, 529.

Cameraria

The four species are natives of Central America and the West Indies. The timber is used locally for general purposes (Hausen 1973).

Cameraria belizensis
White Poison wood, Savanna White Poison

C. latifolia
Bastard Manchineel

Both species are irritant and toxic (Standley 1927, Schwartz et al 1957, Hausen 1973).

Record and Hess (1943) refer to reputed burning and inflammation of th skin from contact with the sap of Cameraria latifolia (syn. C. belizensis) and C. angustifolia.

References

Hausen, B.M. (1973) Holzarten mit gesundheitsschädigenden Inhaltsstoffen. Stuttgart, DRW-Verlags-GmbH.

Record, S.J. and Hess, R.W. (1943) Timbers of the New World. New Haven, Yale.

Schwartz, L., Tulipan, L. and Birmingham, D.J. (1957). Occupational Diseases of the Skin. 3rd. Edit. Philadelphia, Lea and Febiger, pp. 637-672.

Standley, P.C. (1927) Poisonous Trees of Central America. Tropical Woods, 9, 3 (March) and 7, 8 (Sept. 1926).

Carissa

There are some 35 species in the warmer parts of Africa and Asia.

Carissa carandas

(Carissa spectabilis, Acokanthera spectabilis).

This thorny shrub has irritand latex (Burkill 1935).

Reference

Burkill, I.H. (1935) A Dictionary of the Economic Products of the Malay Peninsula. 2 Vols. London, Crown Agents for the Colonies.

Catharanthus

Five species are recorded from the tropics, notably from Madagascar. Catharanthus roseus, (syn. Vinca rosea), is a common weed throughout the tropics. Known as the Madagascar periwinkle it is familiar under its now obsolete scientific name as a source of the "Vinca" alkaloids.

Cerbera

Six species occur on tropical coasts of the Indian and West Pacific Oceans. Some former species have been reclassified as Thevetia.

The use of the colloquial name Buta Buta for both Excoecaria and some Cerbera species has led the latter to be falsely associated with intensely irritant and blinding properties (Corner 1952).

Cerbera manghas

The oil from the seed is rubefacient and the latex also may be so. (Corner 1952).

The white latex causes blindness if it gets to the eyes (Altschul 1973).

References

Altschul, S. von R. (1973) Drugs and foods form little-known plants. Cambridge, Mass. Harvard Univ. Press.

Corner, E.J.H. (1952) Wayside trees of Malaysia. Singapore, Government Printer.

Dyera

Two or three species are native to western Malaysia.

Dyera costulata Jelutong

Dyera lowii Jelutong

The sap and wood produced positive patch test reactions in six forest-workers; the leaf produced negative reactions (Siregar 1975).

Reference

Siregar, R.S. (1975) Occupational dermatoses among foresters. Contact Dermatitis 1, 33.

Geissospermum

Five species are found in tropical Brazil. The bark of G. laeve, cortex Pereirae, is officinal.

Geissospermum sericeum
Acari rana

The wood causes symptoms similar to those produced by Aspidosperma spp. (Freise 1937).

Reference

Freise, F.W. (1937) Vergiftungen durch Brasilianische Werkhölzer III. Samml. Vergift. 8c, 13.

Gonioma kamassi
South African Boxwood, Kynana Boxwood.

The solitary species in this genus is a native of South Africa. The hard timber has long been used as a substitute for true boxwood for shuttles, tool handles and similar objects (Hausen 1973).

Chemistry

The wood contains an alkaloid with curare-like effects (Watt and Breyer-Brandwijk 1962).

Dermatitis

Workers exposed to dust of African boxwood used for making shuttles developed irritation of the eyes and nose and general constitutional symptoms and some had asthma (Legge 1905, 1907, Hay 1907). The wood said to be Sarcocephalus sp. (Nauclea sp.) known as boxwood, was in fact Gonioma kamassi (Gibson 1906, Legge 1905). An alkaloid contained in the wood (Dixon 1911) was probably quebrachamine (Gellert and Witkop 1952). Only a few more cases were found (MacKenna and Horner 1954) and other woods have largely replaced this species in the trade.

References

Gellért, E. and Witkop, B. (1952) Die Identität der Alkaloids Kamassin mit Quebrachamin. Helv. Chim. Acta 35, 114.

Gibson, R.J.H. (1906) The physiological properties of 'West African Boxwood'. Biochem. J. 1, 39.

Hay, J. (1907) Special report on the condition of the workers employed in the manufacture of shuttles from African Boxwood. Report of the Chief Inspector of Factories and Workshops. London. pp. 266-268.

Legge, T.M. (1905, 1907) Reports of the Chief Inspector of Factories and Workshops. (1905), 380: (1907), 248.

MacKenna, R.M.B. and Horner, S. (1954) Occupational skin diseases. In: Industrial Medicine and Hygiene. ed. Merewether, E.R.A. London, Butterworth.

Watt, J.M. and Breyer-Brandwijk, M.G. (1962) The Medicinal and Poisonous Plants of Southern and Eastern Africa. 2nd. Edit. Edinburgh. E. and S. Livingstone Ltd.

Macoubea

The six species in this genus are natives of tropical America.

Macoubea guianensis
Molongo

The wood of this tree contains the cardiac glucoside macoubein, which has a curare-like action (Freise 1936, 1937). It is irritant and toxic.

References

Freise, F.W. (1936) Weiterer Beitrag zur Kenntnis des südamerikanischen Curare. Pharm. Ztg. 81, 818.

Freise, F.W. (1936) Vergiftungen durch brasilianische Werkhölzer I, II. Samml. Vergift. 7c, 1 and 61: (1937) III. 8c, 13

Nerium

The genus consists of three species and occurs naturally in the Mediterranean region to tropical Asia and Japan. N. indicum and N. oleander are widely cultivated; the latter species in particular has been introduced wherever the climate is suitable and is commonly used for roadside planting. In colder regions it has been cultivated under glass, or in tubs which can be taken under cover in winter.

Nerium indicum
(syn. N. odorum)

The sap is irritant, and circumstantial evidence suggests that it may contain an allergic sensitizer (Behl et al 1966).

Nerium oleander
Oleander

This shrub is too small for the timber to be of commercial value, but although its toxicity has long been known accidental poisoning from the use of the wood continues to occur. Pliny, Dioscorides and Galen were aware of the dangers. During the Peninsular wars some of Wellington's men were fatally poisoned by eating meat cooked on skewers of oleander (Francis and Southcott 1967) and children have been poisoned in the same manner (Hardin and Arena 1969). Smoke from a fire of oleander wood is toxic (Allen 1943, Hurst 1942, Steyn 1934), and meat cooked over such a fire may be poisonous (Burkill 1935). In some Florida communities the burning of oleander trimmings is prohibited (Morton 1958). Honey made from the nectar is toxic (Pammel 1911).

Chemistry

The plant contains oleandrine, a cardiac glucoside (Hausen 1973).

Dermatitis

In relation to the frequency with which exposure to Oleander occurs, rather few cases of dermatitis have been reported. In 1817 Bigelow said that oleander affected some persons like poison-ivy and Halstead (1889) reported similar effects. More recent reports (Dorsey 1962, Behl et al 1966) concern mainly children. The crushed leaves and stems are certainly irritant (Piffard 1881) but their allergenic properties have not been adequately studied. Hjorth (1968) obtained no positive patch tests in more than seven patients tested.

References

Allen, P.H. (1943) Poisonous and Injurious Plants of Panama. Am. J. trop. Med. 23, Suppl.p.3.

Behl, P.N., Captain, R.M., Bedi, B.M.S. and Gupta, S. (1966) Skin-irritant and Sensitizing Plants Found in India. New Delhi, P.N. Behl, Irwin Hospital.

Bigelow, (1817) American Medical Botany. Boston (1924), Florula Bostoniensis.

Burkill, I.H. (1935) A Dictionary of the Economic Products of the Malay Peninsula. 2 Vols. London, Crown Agents for the Colonies.

Dorsey, C.S. (1962) Plant dermatitis in California. Calif. Med. 96, 412.

Francis, D.F. and Southcott, R.V. (1967) Plants harmful to man in Australia. Misc. Bull. No. 1. Botanic Garden, Adelaide.

Halstead, B.C. (1889) Poisonous plants of New Jersey. New Jersey Ag. Expt. Stat. Bull. 135. quoted by Hurst 1942.

Hardin, J.W. and Arena, J.M. (1969) Human Poisoning from Native and Cultivated Plants. Durham, North Carolina, Duke University Press.

Hausen, B.M. (1973) Holzarten mit gesundheitsschädigenden Inhaltstoffen. Stuttgart, DRW-Verlags-GmbH.

Hjorth, N. (1968) At Finsen Institute. Personal Communication.

Hurst, E. (1942) The Poison Plants of New South Wales. N.S.W. Poison Plants Committee, Sydney.

Morton, J.F. (1958) Ornamental plants with poisonous properties Proc. Florida. State Hort. Soc. 71, 372.

Pammel, L.H. (1911) Manual of Poisonous Plants. Cedar Rapids, Iowa, Torch Press. Reprinted Univ. Microfilms, Inc., Ann Arbor, Mich., 1005, pp.476-7.

Piffard, H.G. (1881) A Treatise on the Materia Medica and Therapeutics of the Skin. New York. Wm. Wood and Co.

Steyn, D.G. (1934) The Toxicology of Plants in South Africa. Central News Agency Ltd. South Africa.

Plumeria

The seven species are natives of tropical America, but some are cultivated in other tropical regions, and, under glass, in temperate climates.

Plumeria sp.
Frangipani, Temple Tree

Unidentified species were reported as filled with copious latex, which is caustic and vesicant in "particularly susceptible" individuals (Allen 1943). Standley (1927) did not find the latex irritant on his own skin. The flowers of various species and hybrids are used for 'leis' (flower garlands) in Hawaii and cause no trouble except in very susceptible individuals (Arnold 1968).

Plumeria acuminata

The juice is rubefacient (Quisumbubg 1951).

Plumeria acutifolia

The latex is irritant (Allen 1943).

Plumeria alba
Pagoda Tree

The latex is rubefacient and irritant or corrosive (Allen 1943, Behl et al 1966). It has been used in the treatment of warts (Watt and Breyer-Brandwijk 1962).

Plumeria inodora

The latex is irritant (Allen 1943).

Plumeria rubra
Dogbane, Frangipani, Amapola

The latex is irritant (Allen 1943).

References

Allen, P.H. (1943) Poisonous and Injurious Plants of Panama. Am. J. trop. Med. 23, Suppl. p.3.

Arnold, H.L. (1968) Poisonous Plants of Hawaii. Rutland, Vermont, Charles E. Tuttle.

Behl, P.N., Captain, R.M., Bedi, B.M.S. and Gupta, S. (1966) Skin-irritant and Sensitizing Plants Found in India. New Delhi, P.N. Behl, Irwin Hospital.

Quisumbing, E. (1951) Medicinal Plants of the Philippines. Philipp. Dept. Agr. and Nat. Resources Tech. Bull. No. 16. Manila. Bureau of Printing.

Standley, P.C. (1927) Poisonous Trees of Central America. Tropical Woods, 9, 3 (March) and 7, 8 (Sept. 1926)

Watt, J.M. and Breyer-Brandwijk, M.G. (1962) The Medicinal and Poisonous Plants of Southern and Eastern Africa. 2nd. Edit. Edinburgh, E. & S. Livingstone Ltd.

Rauvolfia

About 100 species occur in the tropics and S. Africa. A few are cultivated elsewhere under glass.

Rauvolfia heterophylla

The latex is said to be irritant to "susceptible" subjects (Standley 1927).

Rauvolfia pentaphylla
Muirajussará rana

The wood causes symptoms similar to those produced by Aspidosperma (Freise 1937).

Reference

Freise, F.W. (1937) Vergiftungen durch Brasilianische Werkhölzer III. Samml. Vergift. 8c, 13.

Rauvolfia tetraphylla

The milky sap of the plant is irritant (Oakes and Butcher 1962).

References

Hanslian, L. and Kadlec, K. (1966) Drěvo z hlediska hygienickeho (VII) Biologicky silně agresívní drěviny. Drevo 21,157.

Standley, P.C. (1927) Poisonous Trees of Central America. Tropical Woods, 9, 3(March) and 7, 8 (Sept. 1926).

Oakes, A.J. and Butcher, J. (1962) Poisonous and injurious plants of the U.S. Virgin Islands. Misc. Publ. 882. U.S. Dept. Agriculture. Washington, D.C.

Rhabdadenia

There are four species known in Florida, Central and tropical South American and the West Indies.

Rhabdadenia paludosa

The copious latex is said to be vesicant in "susceptible" subjects (Allen 1943).

Reference

Allen, P.H. (1943) Poisonous and Injurious Plants of Panama. Am. J. trop. Med. 23, Suppl. p.3.

Tabernaemontana

There are about a hundred species, all confined to tropical regions.

Tabernaemontana crassa Ofuruma

The wood is used in West Africa; the latex is caustic (Irvine 1961).

Tabernaemontana citrifolia
Pegojo

The timber is used locally for general purposes in Central America (Hausen 1973). It contains an irritant glycoside. It has caused dermatitis (Pardo-Castello 1923) apparently with systemic toxicity.

Tabernaemontana macrophylla
Pequerete

The timber, which is used in Brazil for constructional work (Hausen 1973), contains a toxic glycoside said to be macoubein (Freise, 1937) and produces effects similar to those produced by Aspidosperma.

References

Freise, F.W. (1937) Vergiftungen durch brasilianische Werkhölzer III. Samml. vergift. 8c, 13.

Hausen, B.M. (1973) Holzarten mit gesundheitsschädigenden Inhaltsstoffen. Stuttgart, DRW-Verlags-GmbH.

Irvine, F.R. (1961) Woody plants of Ghana. London, Oxford University Press.

Pardo-Castello, V. (1923) Dermatitis venenata. Arch. Derm. Syph. 7,81.

Thevetia

Nine species are native to tropical America and the West Indies.

Thevetia nereifolia,
(syn. T. peruviana),
"Yellow Oleander".

Thevetia nitida

The latex of both species is reported to be irritant in some individuals (Allen 1943), and T. peruviana may cause dermatitis (Morton 1958).

References

Allen, P.H. (1943) Poisonous and Injurious Plants of Panama. Am. J. trop. Med. 23, Suppl. p. 3.

Morton, J.F. (1958) Ornamental plants with poisonous properties. Proc. Florida State Hort. Soc. 71, 372.

Vinca

The seven species retained in this genus are natives of Europe and Western Asia, but some are widely naturalized, notably V. major and V. minor, Some species formerly placed in this genus are now differentiated as Catharanthus.

Vinca sp. has been listed as a sensitizer (Shelmire 1940). Vinca major is very common in gardens in Britain and is used in Herbal medicine as an astringent but no proven case of dermatitis attributable to it has been reported.

Contact dermatitis occurred in 18/48 workers who prepared Vinca alkaloids. In 11 persons, sensitization to Vinca alkaloids was confirmed by patch tests; cross-sensitivity was demonstrated to alkaloids of Rauvolfia, reserpine and ajmalin, vegetable alkaloids of indolic structure (Valer 1965).

References

Shelmire, B. (1940) Contact Dermatitis from Vegetation. Sth. med. J. 33, 338.

Valer, M. (1965) Die bei der Erzeugung von Devincan auftretenden Hautläsionen. Berufsdermatosen 13, 96.

Zschokkea

The fifteen species are natives of tropical South America.

Zschokkea aculeata Tucujá

The wood produces symptoms similar to those produced by Aspidosperma and also asthmatic attacks (Freise 1937).

Reference

Freise, F.W. (1937) Vergiftungen

durch Brasilianische Werkhölzer III. Samml. Vergift. 8c, 13.

AQUIFOLIACEAE

400 species in two genera are found in tropical and temperate regions.

Ilex

400 species are of cosmopolitan distribution except in North America. *I. paraguariensis* provides Paraguay tea or maté, largely used in South America. The leaves contain caffeine.

Ilex sp.

The lichen *Parmelia caperata* growing on ilex trees and *Quercus* was implicated in 'wood-cutters' eczema (Ghillini 1954).

Reference

Ghillini, C.A. (1954) Un lichene causa di Allergosi cutanea. Rivista de Anatomia e Patologica. Oncologia 8, 755.

ARACEAE

This family contains about 2,000 species classified in 115 genera. Although some species are natives of temperate regions, 92% are tropical. They range in habit from small or large herbs to climbing shrubs and epiphytes and include marsh plants and one floating water plant. Many species are cultivated because they are decorative, and many of them are in particularly close contact with man because they are popular as "house plants". Man encounters some species because their starch-laden rhizomes are edible when suitably prepared by boiling or roasting.

The plants contain water insoluble calcium oxalate in bundles of fine, needle-like crystals packed in cells and surrounded by a mucilaginous liquid. Such bundles of crystals, called raphides, have the property of ejecting the individual needles on contact with water (Lampe and Fagerstrom 1968). It is suspected that these plants may contain other irritant compounds (Barnes and Fox 1955, Manno et al 1967).

Chemistry is recorded by Hegnauer (1963).

References

Barnes, B.A. and Fox, L.E. (1955) Poisoning with Dieffenbachia. J. Hist. Med. 10, 173.

Hegnauer, R. (1963) Chemotaxonomy of Plants. Vol. 2. Basel, Birkhauser pp. 73-98.

Lampe, K.F. and Fagerstrom, R. (1968) Plant Toxicity and Dermatitis. Baltimore, Williams and Wilkins.

Manno, J.E., Fochtman, R.W., Winek, C.L., et al (1967) Toxicity of plants of the genus *Dieffenbachia*. Tox. Appl. Pharmacol. 10, 405.

Acorus

The two species in this genus are widely distributed over Central and Eastern Europe, tropical and subtropical East Asia and North America.

Acorus calamus Sweet Flag

The sweet flag, not native to Britain, but naturalized many centuries ago, was used at least from the fifteenth century as a floor covering (Prime 1960).

The rhizome contains a pleasantly aromatic oil, the contents of which include asarone and eugenol (Merck 1968). The rhizome and its oil have been used in the indigenous medicine of many countries for millennia and were accepted in official medicine until recently (Flückiger and Hanbury 1874). The oil, known as Oil of Calamus, has been suspected of causing dermatitis (Klarmann 1958).

References

Flückiger, F.A. and Hanbury, D. (1874) Pharmacographia. A History of the Principal Drugs of Vegetable Origin, met with in Great Britain and British India. London, Macmillan & Co.

Klarmann, E.G. (1958) Perfume Dermatitis. Ann. Allergy, 16, 425.

Merck Index (1968) An Encyclopedia of Chemicals and Drugs. ed. Stecher, P.G. 8th ed. Rahway, N.J. Merck and Co. Inc.

Prime, C.T. (1960) Lords and Ladies. The New Naturalist. London,

Collins.

Aglaonema

Some 50 species have been recorded from Indo-Malaysia. The caustic effect of the leaves of some species, when used in folk medicine (Burkill 1935) suggests that, like some many other aroids, they contain irritants. The damaging effects on table tops of the exudation from the leaves of A. modestum (Western Garden Book 1961) provides further indirect evidence.

Aglaonema commutatum and A. modestum

These plants contain microscopic stinging crystals of calcium oxalate that are intensely irritating when brought in contact with the mucous membranes of mouth, nose and throat, or with tender skin; application of heat breaks down the crystals and thorough cooking makes the leaves edible (Souder 1963).

References

Burkill, I.H. (1935) A Dictionary of the Economic Products of the Malay Peninsula. 2 vols. London, Crown Agents for the Colonies.

Souder, P. (1963) Poisonous Plants on Guam, in Venomous and Poisonous Animals and Noxious Plants of the Pacific Region. Ed. Keegan, H.L. and Macfarlane, W.V. Oxford, Pergamon Press, pp. 15-29

Western Garden Book (1961) by the editors of Sunset Magazine and Sunset Books, Menlo Park, Calif. Lane Co.

Alocasia

The 70 or so species are natives of Indo-Malaysia. The taxonomy of the Araceae is complicated and several changes of nomenclature have proved necessary, e.g.:

Alocasia Neck = Dracunculus L. + Arisaema Mart.

Alocasia Schott (Rafin.) = Arisaema Mart.

All species seem to be irritant on account of their high content of needle-like crystals of calcium oxalate (Burkill 1935). Several species are cultivated under the collective popular name of Elephant's Ear.

The following species have been definitely recorded as irritant:

Alocasia cucullata (Burkill 1935)

Alocasia denudata (Burkill 1935, Uphof 1959)

Alocasia indica (Burkill 1935, Souder 1963)

Alocasia lowii (Burkill 1935)

Alocasia macrorrhiza
Cunjevoi (Australia), Ape (Hawaii)

This cultivated decorative plant contains an unknown poison as well as calcium oxalate crystals. Chewing any part of the plant causes swelling of the lips and tongue, and merely to touch the lips after handling the plant is painful (Cleland and Lee 1963).

To the eye the sap is powerfully and sometimes destructively irritant (Everist 1972, Souder 1963, Arnold 1968, Francis and Southcott 1967, Hurst 1942).

Alocasia sanderiana

Irritant (Souder 1963).

References

Arnold, H.L. (1968) Poisonous Plants of Hawaii. Rutland, Vermont, Charles E. Tuttle.

Burkill, I.H. (1935) A Dictionary of the Economic Products of the Malay Peninsula. 2 vols. London, Crown Agents for the Colonies.

Cleland, J.B. and Lee, D.J. (1963) The Poisonous and Urticating Plants of Australia in Venomous and Poisonous Animals and Noxious Plants of the Pacific Region. Ed. Keegan, H.L. and Macfarlane, W.V. Oxford, Pergamon Press. pp. 3-13.

Everist, S.L. (1972) Queensland Herbarium, Brisbane, Australia. Personal Communication Concerning Plants Recorded in Australia as Having Caused Dermatitis or Other Contact Injury to Man or Livestock.

Francis, D.R. and Southcott, R.V. (1967) Plants harmful to man in Australia. Misc. Bull. No.1 Botanic Garden, Adelaide, Australia.

Hurst, E. (1942) The Poison Plants of New South Wales. Sydney, N.S.W. Poison Plants Committee.

Souder, P. (1963) Poisonous Plants on Guam, in Venomous and Poisonous Animals and Noxious Plants of the Pacific Region. Ed. Keegan, H.L. and Macfarlane, W.V. Oxford, Pergamon Press, pp. 15-20.

Uphof, J.C. Th. (1959) Dictionary of Economic Plants. New York, Hafner Publ. Co.

Amorphophallus

There are about 100 species, native to the tropics of Africa and Asia.

Amorphophallus campanulatus
Zamindkand

The tubers contain abundant crystals of calcium oxalate, and are irritant. The edible tubers of the cultivated varieties are less irritant (Burkill 1935) but can cause pruritus, erythema and wealing in those who handle them. Chewing the tuber may cause a burning sensation, and urticaria may develop later.

The tubers and seeds are used as counter-irritants (Behl et al 1966).

Amorphophallus prainii

Amorphophallus variabilis

Both species are reported to irritate the oral cavity, when chewed (Burkill 1935).

Amorphophallus rivieri
(syn. Conophallus konjac)

The sap of the flower produces marked itching (Altschul 1973). The skin irritant effects of the root of the plant are used in Chinese Medicine (Smith 1969).

References

Altschul, S. von R. (1973) Drugs and foods from little-known plants. Cambridge, Mass. Harvard Univ. Press.

Behl, P.N., Captain, R.M., Bedi, B.M.S. and Gupta, S. (1966) Skin-irritant and sensitizing plants found in India, New Delhi, P.N. Behl, Irwin Hospital.

Burkill, I.H. (1935) A dictionary of the economic products of the Malay Peninsula. 2 vols. London, Crown Agents for the Colonies.

Smith, F.P. (1969) Chinese Materia Medica. Vegetable kingdom. 2nd ed. rev. by Hei, P.D. Taipei, Taiwan. Ku T'ing Book House.

Anthurium

Over 500 species are known from tropical America and the West Indies.

Anthurium andraenum
(Souder 1963)

Anthurium ferrierense
(Pammel 1911)

These two species are reported as irritant, and it is probably true that many others have similar properties. Some species are commonly cultivated.

References

Pammel, L.H. (1911) A Manual of Poisonous Plants. Cedar Rapids, Iowa, Torch Press. Reprinted Univ. Microfilms Inc., Ann Arbor, Mich., 1965, pp. 476-7.

Souder, P. (1963) Poisonous Plants on Guam, in Venomous and Poisonous Animals and Noxious Plants of the Pacific Region. Ed. Keegan, H.L. and Macfarlane, W.V. Oxford, Pergamon Press, pp. 15-29.

Arisaema

The genus contains about 150 species, mostly natives of tropical Asia, but some of East Africa and some of Atlantic North America to Mexico. Many species are cultivated for their horticultural merits, and some as food plants, but the starch-rich tubers contain abundant sharp crystals.

Arisaema atrorubens

Indian turnip, Jack-in-the-Pulpit

The leaves and tubers are irritant (McCord 1962, Kingsbury 1964).

Arisaema concinnum

Arisaema dracontium
Green Dragon

Both plants are irritant (Burkill 1935).

Arisaema japonicum

Arisaema ringeris

Arisaema thumbergii

These plants, too, are irritant, but their roots also have a numbing effect on the skin and were used as an ingredient of a local anaesthetic preparation applied in China to abscesses before these were opened surgically (Maxwell 1929).

Arisaema speciosum
Jack-in-the-Pulpit

The tuber is said to be violently irritant (Behl et al 1966)

Arisaema stewardsonii

The rhizomes are said to be particularly irritant (Kingsbury 1964).

Arisaema tortuosum

This species is described as violently irritant (Behl et al 1966).

Arisaema triphyllum
Indian turnip, Dragon-root, Jack-in-the-Pulpit, Pepper turnip, Bog-onion, Brown dragon, Starchwort.

Every part of this plant is acrid and irritant to the skin and mucous membranes (Muenscher 1951, Hardin and Arena 1969). Most careful preparation is needed to render the tuber edible.

Arisaema vulgare

The plant is listed as irritant (Pammel 1911).

References

Behl, P.N., Captain, R.M., Bedi, B.M.S. and Gupta, S. (1966) Skin-irritant and Sensitizing Plants Found in India. New Delhi, P.N. Behl, Irwin Hospital.

Burkill, I.H. (1935) A Dictionary of the Economic Products of the Malay Peninsula. 2 vols. London, Crown Agents for the Colonies.

Hardin, J.W. and Arena, J.M. (1909) Human Poisoning from Native and Cultivated Plants. Durham, North Carolina, Duke Univ. Press.

Kingsbury, J.M. (1964) Poisonous Plants of the United States and Canada. Englewood Cliffs, New Jersey, Prentice-Hall Inc.

McCord, C.P. (1962) The Occupational Toxicity of Cultivated Flowers. Ind. Med. Surg. 31, 365.

Maxwell, J.L. (1929) The Diseases of China including Formosa and Korea. Shanghai ABC Press.

Muenscher, W.C. (1951) Poisonous Plants of the United States, 2nd Edit. New York, Macmillan.

Pammel, L.H. (1911) A Manual of Poisonous Plants. Cedar Rapids, Iowa, Torch Press. Reprinted Univ. Microfilms Inc., Ann Arbor, Mich. 1965, pp. 476-7.

Arisarum

Three species are natives of the Mediterranean region. Prime (1960) considers it probable that the species referred to by Dioscorides in the first century A.D. and which has been interpreted as *Arum arisarum* was in fact *Arisarum vulgare*.

References

Dioscorides, The Greek Herbal of: Englished by John Goodyer: A.D. 1655. Edited and first printed A.D. 1933 by R.T. Gunther (1959) New York, Hafner Publishing Co. Book 2. pg. 198 (p.209) and Appendix p. 677.

Prime, C.T. (1960) Lords and Ladies. The New Naturalist. London, Collins.

Arum

The 15 species in this genus are found naturally in Europe and the Mediterranean region. The generic name Arum, or Arum Lily or Cunjevoi, has been used in some reports, and it is probable that all the species contain an acrid and irritant poison as well as calcium oxalate crystals (MacPherson 1929). The sap causes dermatitis (Lampe and Fagerström 1968).

Some species are cultivated for the beauty of their flowers, and others are in close contact with man as weeds of cultivated land.

Many plants previously named Arum are now placed in other genera, and many plants in other genera are popularly called arum, e.g. Lysichiton.

Arum arisarum
Arisaron, Cuckoo-pint.

The irritant effects of this plant have been known for many centuries. Ramazzini's (1713) account of genital dermatitis in an apothecary appears to have been plagiarized from Dioscorides (Mitchell 1974): (see Arisarum)

Arum cornutum
(syn. Sauromatum guttatum)
Voodoo Lily

This common houseplant in the United States is highly irritant.

Arum italicum

The sap contains crystals of calcium oxalate, and is intensely irritant to skin and mouth (Francis and Southcott 1967).

Arum maculatum
Cuckoo-pint, Wake-robin
Lords and Ladies.

The starch from the tubers was formerly used as food under such names as Portland arrowroot (Prime 1960). The poisonous principle is destroyed by cooking. The starch was used also to stiffen ruffs in the time of Queen Elizabeth I of England (Gerard 1597), but its use had to be abandoned because it irritated the hands of laundresses (Parkinson 1640, North 1967).

Gerard's (1597) stated that "it choppeth, blistereth and maketh the hands rough and rugged, and withall smarting".

Arum triphyllum
Wake Robin, Indian Turnip (N. America)

The fresh sap is vesicant (MacPherson 1929) and if the root is chewed it is burning and acrid (Wren 1968).

References

Francis, D.F. and Southcott, R.V. (1967) Plants harmful to man in Australia. Misc. Bull. No. 1 Botanic Garden, Adelaide, Australia.

Gerard, J. (1597) Leaves from Gerard's Herball. ed. Woodward, M. New York. Dover.

Lampe, K.F. and Fagerstrom, R. (1968) Plant Toxicity and Dermatitis. Baltimore, Williams and Wilkins.

MacPherson, J. (1929) The Toxicology of the Arum Lily and Cunjevoi Lily. Med. J. Australia 2,671.

Mitchell, J.C. (1974) Ramazzini and skin injury from the arum lily. Br. J. Derm. 91, 235.

North, P.M. (1967) Poisonous Plants and Fungi in Colour. London, Blandford Press Ltd.

Parkinson, J. (1640) Theatrum Botanicum, cited by Prime (1960).

Prime, C.T. (1960) Lords and Ladies. The New Naturalist. London, Collins.

Wren, R.W. (1968) Potter's New Cyclopaedia of Botanical Drugs and Preparations, by Wren, R.C. Re-edit. by Wren, R.W. Rustington, Sussex, Potter and Clarke Ltd. Health Science Press.

Caladium

There are 15 species which are natives of tropical South America, but many have very decorative foliage and are therefore widely cultivated as house-plants. They are often incorrectly called colocasias (Lampe and Fagerstrom 1968). Some species are cooked and eaten (Morton 1962, Souder 1963). All species contain irritant crystals of calcium oxalate, and can cause dermatitis.

Caladium bicolor

Caladium picturatum

Fancy-leaved caladium

These two species, in numerous named cultivars, are those most commonly cultivated.

Caladium sequinum

The juice of the leaves, when applied to the skin, produces intense itching and burning (Piffard 1881).

References

Lampe, K.F. and Fagerstrom, R. (1968) Plant Toxicity and Dermatitis. Baltimore, Williams and Wilkins.

Morton, J.F. (1962) Ornamental Plants with Poisonous Properties II. Proc. Florida Hort. Soc. 75, 484.

Piffard, H.G. (1881) A treatise on the Materia Medica and Therapeutics of the skin. New York. Wm. Wood and Co.

Souder, P. (1968) Poisonous Plants on Guam. In Venomous and Poisonous Animals and Noxious Plants of the Pacific Region. Ed. Keegan, H.L. and Macfarlane, W.V. Oxford, Pergamon Press, pp. 15-29.

Calla palustris

Wilk Calla,
Water Arum

The single species in this genus is a native of the north temperate and subarctic regions.

The plant is irritant, particularly its rhizome (Kingsbury 1964).

The Calla of gardeners is Zantedeschia.

Reference

Kingsbury, J.M. (1964) Poisonous Plants of the United States and Canada. Englewood Cliffs, New Jersey, Prentice-Hall Inc.

Colocasia

About 8 species are natives of Indo-Malaysia and Polynesia, but some have been extensively introduced into other tropical countries. The plants have a high content of calcium oxalate crystals, but these can be removed by careful cooking, and the tubers of several species are an important source of food.

Colocasia antiquorum

Cocco, Eddoes,
Elephant's Ears

Ingestion of any part of the plant in the raw state causes great pain and swelling of the lips, tongue and throat (Williamson 1956, Francis and Southcott 1967).

Colocasia esculenta

Taro, Cocco, Eddoes,
Elephant's Ears

The same irritant properties are shown by this species (Souder 1963, Francis and Southcott 1967, Arnold 1968).

Colocasia macrorrhiza

Cunjeboy, cunjevoi, Spoon Lily, Australian Cabbage.

The whole plant is irritant; the sap of leaves and petioles will blister the lips (MacPherson 1929). The young plant appears to be relatively innocuous, but the mature plant can cause severe dermatitis and conjunctivitis, intense enough to destroy vision. Eating a leaf caused death of a child from suffocation through swelling of the throat (Cleland 1914).

References

Arnold, H.L. (1968) Poisonous Plants of Hawaii. Rutland, Vermont, Charles E. Tuttle.

Cleland, J.B. (1914) Plants, including Fungi, Poisonous or Otherwise Injurious to Man in Australia. Australasian Med. Gazette, 35, 569. Idem, Tasmanian Agr. Gazette, 32, 361, and 401.

Francis, D.F. and Southcott, R.V. (1967) Plants harmful to man in

Australia, Misc. Bull. No. 1 Botanic Garden, Adelaide, Australia.

MacPherson, J. (1929) The Toxicology of the Arum Lily and Conjevoi Lily. Med. J. Australia, 2, 671.

Souder, P. (1963) Poisonous Plants on Guam, In Venomous and Poisonous Animals and Noxious Plants of the Pacific Region. Ed. Keegan, H.L. and Macfarlane, W.V. Oxford, Pergamon Press, pp. 15-29.

Williamson, J. (1956) Useful Plants of Malawi. Ed. Greenway, P.J. Zomba, Malawi, The Government Printer.

Culcasia

About 20 species are natives of tropical Africa.

Culcasia scandens

The sap of the stems irritates the skin (Williamson 1956).

Reference

Williamson, J. (1956) Useful Plants of Malawi. ed. Greenway, P.J. Zomba, Malawi, The Government Printer. Previously published as Useful Plants of Nyasaland.

Cyrtosperma

About 18 species are found in tropical countries, especially in New Guinea. The rhizome of Cyrtosperma edule is edible when cooked and is cultivated in Polynesia.

Cyrtosperma chamissonis
Giant Taro, Baba

The raw tuber is irritant to the mucous membrane of the mouth and to the skin (Souder 1963).

Reference

Souder, P. (1963) Poisonous Plants on Guam, In Venomous and Poisonous Animals and Noxious Plants of the Pacific Region. ed. Keegan, H.L. and Macfarlane, W.V. Oxford, Pergamon Press. pp.15-29.

Dieffenbachia

There are about 30 species, natives of tropical America and the West Indies. Some species are also cultivated elsewhere for their decorative foliage. They are commonly seen in hotel lobbies, waiting rooms and restaurants.

All species contain calcium oxalate crystals (Souder 1963), but their irritant effects on skin and mucous membranes are believed to be increased by the presence of other substances (Hardin and Arena 1969). It is possible that all species are irritant, but some species and cultivars are less so than others. The literature does not provide an unbiased assessment since species forming part of the environment of urban man are most likely to have their unpleasant propensities recorded in print.

Dieffenbachia aurantiaca

Dieffenbachia longispatha

Dieffenbachia oerstedii

Dieffenbachia pittieri

These species are all said to be irritant (Allen 1943).

Dieffenbachia picta
Dumb-cane

Dieffenbachia sequine

If the stem is bitten the resulting bullous stomatitis is of such severity that it renders the victim speechless (Francis and Southcott 1967). There may also be oedema of the skin around the mouth. Similar reactions have been reported to both species (Drach and Maloney 1963, Everist 1972, Behl et al 1966).

Patch tests on skin and lip were negative in this second case (Behl et al 1966) but it is not recorded whether the tests were carried out in the patient or in control subjects.

The species are very similar in appearance (Francis and Southcott 1967).

Contact with bruised plant tissues seems to be required for an irritant effect (Delph 1937, Occhioni and Rizzini 1958, Barnes and Fox 1955) since the plant sap of at least some species is not irritant (Arnold 1968). However, the plant juice itself, of Dieffenbachia picta has been described as highly irritating to the skin (Dahlgren and Standley 1944).

Tests on rabbits eyes have showed mild irritation from Dieffenbachia exotica and severe irritation from D. picta (Manno et al 1967, Fochtman et al 1969). The irritating component is probably a protein, probably not a saponin and certainly not calcium oxalate (Manno et al 1967, Pohl 1961, 1964, Fochtman et al 1969).

References

Allen, P.H. (1943) Poisonous and Injurious Plants of Panama. Am. J. trop. Med. Suppl. 23, 1.

Arnold, H.L. (1968) Poisonous plants of Hawaii. Rutland, Vermont. Charles E. Tuttle.

Barnes, B.A. and Fox, L.E. (1955) Poisoning with Dieffenbachia. J. Hist. Med. 10, 173.

Behl, P.N., Captain, R.M., Bedi, B.M.S. and Gupta, S. (1966) Skin-irritant and Sensitizing Plants found in India. New Delhi, P.N. Behl, Irwin Hospital.

Dahlgren, B.E. and Standley, P.C. (1944) Edible and poisonous plants of the Caribbean region. Bur. Med. Surg: Navy Dept. U.S. Gov't. Printing Office, Washington, D.C.

Delph, J.F. (1937) Chemical burns of oral cavity and oesophagus. Surg. Clin. North America 17, 585.

Drach, G. and Maloney, W.H. (1963) Toxicity of the Common Houseplant Dieffenbachia. Report of a Case. J. Amer. med. Ass. 184, 1047.

Everist, S.L. (1972) Queensland Herbarium, Brisbane, Australia. Personal Communication concerning Plants Recorded in Australia as Having caused Dermatitis or Other Contact Injury to Man or Livestock.

Fochtman, F.W., Manno, J.E., Winek, C.L. et al (1969) Toxicity of the genus Dieffenbachia. Tox. Appl. Pharmacol. 15, 38.

Francis, D.F. and Southcott, R.V. (1967) Plants harmful to man in Australia. Misc. Bull.No. 1. Botanic Garden, Adelaide, Australia.

Hardin, J.W. and Arena, J.M. (1969) Human Poisoning from Native and Cultivated Plants. Durham, North Carolina, Duke University Press.

Manno, J.E., Fochtman, F.W., Winek, C.L. et al (1967) Toxicity of plants of the genus Dieffenbachia Tox. Appl. Pharmacol. 12, 405.

Occhioni, P. and Rizzini, C.T. (1958) Toxic effect of Dieffenbachia spp. Rev. Brasil Med. 15, 10.

Pohl, R.W. (1961) Poisoning by Dieffenbachia. JAMA 177, 812.

Pohl, R.W. (1964) Dieffenbachia poisoning: a clarification. JAMA 187, 963.

Souder, P. (1963) Poisonous Plants on Guam, in Venomous and Poisonous Animals and Noxious Plants of the Pacific Region. Ed. Keegan, H.L. and Macfarlane, W.V. Oxford, Pergamon Press, pp. 15-29.

Dracunculus

The two species are natives of the Mediterranean region.

Dracunculus vulgaris

This is the Drakontium of Hippocrates. The root is irritant (Watt and Breyer-Brandwijk 1962).

Reference

Watt, J.M. and Breyer-Brandwijk, M.G. (1962) The Medicinal and Poisonous Plants of Southern and Eastern Africa. 2nd Ed. Edinburgh, E. and S. Livingstone Ltd.

Epipremnum

There are about 25 species in Indo-Malaysia.

Epipremnum gigantum
Rengut

This species is reported to be irritant (Gimlette 1929).

Reference

Gimlette, J.D. (1929) Malay Poisons and Charm Cures. 3rd Ed. London, J. & A. Churchill.

Homalomena

There are about 140 species in Asia and South America.

Homalomena spp.

Some species are irritant, probably H. purpurascens (Burkill 1935).

Reference

Burkill, I.H. (1935) A Dictionary of the Economic Products of the Malay Peninsula. 2 Vols. London, Crown Agents for the Colonies.

Monstera

About 50 species are native to tropical America and the West Indies.

Monstera spp. Ceriman

All species contain caustic and vesicant sap. The unripe fruit contains calcium oxalate crystals (Allen 1943).

Monstera deliciosa

Ceriman, Fruit-salad Plant.

This climbing plant is widely grown. The unripe fruit is acrid, and the ripe fruit may cause rapidly developing urticaria (MacPherson 1929, Francis and Southcott 1967). The spadix also is edible (Hurst 1942).

Young plants have been sold under the name of Philodendron pertusa (Prime 1960).

Monstera dilacerata

M. triedrichthalii

M. pertusa

M. schleichtleinii

These species are repoted to be irritant (Allen 1943, Souder 1963).

References

Allen, P.H. (1943) Poisonous and Injurious Plants of Panama. Am. J. trop. Med. Suppl. 23, 1.

Francis, D.F. and Southcott, R.V. (1967) Plants harmful to man in Australia. Misc. Bull. No. 1 Botanic Garden, Adelaide, Australia.

Hurst, E. (1942) The Poison Plants of New South Wales. N.S.W. Poison Plants Committee, Sydney.

MacPherson, J. (1929) The toxicology of the Arum lily and Cunjevoi lily. Med. J. Australia 2, 671.

Prime, C.T. (1900) Lords and Ladies. The New Naturalist. London Collins.

Souder, F. (1963) Poisonous Plants on Guam, in Venomous and Poisonous Animals and Noxious Plants of the Pacific Region. Ed. Keegan, H.L. and Macfarlane, W.V. Oxford, Pergamon Press, pp. 15-29.

Montrichardia
(syn. Pleurospa)

The two species in this genus are natives of tropical America.

Montrichardia arborescens
Rabano, Boroboro
(Venezuela)

The abundant sap of this plant has caused dermatitis in labourers cutting it with a machete. Erythema develops immediately on contact with the sap, and fades in 24-72 hours (Dao 1967).

Reference

Dao, L. (1967) Dermatitis por plantas en los llanos de Venezuela. Derm. Int. (Philadelphia) 6, 77.

Philodendron

About 275 species occur notably in tropical and subtropical America and in the West Indies. Several species are popular as house-plants in temperate regions, and the erratic specific nomenclature of the florists tends to be copied in medical reports. The species names, for example, have sometimes been used in meaningless isolation.

Philodendron sp.

Unnamed or incorrectly named species have caused dermatitis of face, neck, hands and arms in a florist (Dorsey 1958). A patch test to wet, crushed, stem and leaf was positive. Dermatitis was said to be not uncommon in nursery workers, but unusual in housewives who come into contact less often with the wet leaves. However Harris (1942) reported dermatitis of the eyelids in a housewife. Ayres and Ayres (1958) reported 12 cases of dermatitis. Conjunctivitis from contact and stomatitis from ingestion have also been noted (Everist 1972). Some species are irritant but possibly some can sensitize since Hjorth (1965) observed only one positive reaction in more than 50 patients tested. Dermatitis from Philodendron was reported by Zina and Bonu (1960); the patient also showed a positive patch test reaction to Primula.

Philodendron bipinnatifidum

This plant contains intensely irritating crystals of calcium oxalate (Souder 1963).

Philodendron consanguineum

Contact dermatitis is reported (Pardo-Castello 1923). A report of photodermatitis (Engel and Horn 1972) requires further evaluation since no plant in this family has been shown to contain a photosensitizing substance.

Philodendron cordatum

(P. oxycardium, P. scandens)

This species is particularly favoured as a house-plant. It has been reported to cause dermatitis (Ayres and Ayres 1958).

Philodendron hastatum

Philodendron var. Jaluit

Philodendron selloum

These species contain calcium oxalate crystals (Souder 1963). P. selloum is reported to cause dermatitis (Ayres and Ayres 1958).

Philodendron simsii

This species is reported as irritant (Pammel 1911).

Philodendron speciosum

Contact dermatitis is reported (Ayres and Ayres 1958).

References

Ayres, S. and Ayres, S. (1958) Philodendron as a Cause of Contact Dermatitis. Archs. Derm. 78, 330.

Dorsey, C.S. (1958) Philodendron Dermatitis. Calif. Med. 88, 329.

Engel, S. and Horn, K. (1972) Phytodermatosen durch Dictamnus alba, Sanicula europaea and Phyllodendron consanguineum. Derm.(Wschr. 158, 22.)

Everist, S.L. (1972) Queensland Herbarium, Brisbane, Australia. Personal Communication concerning Plants Recorded in Australia as Having Caused Dermatitis or Other Contact Injury to Man or Livestock.

Harris, H. (1942) Dermatitis of the Eyelids due to Philodendron (Scandens cardatum) Plants. Archs. Derm. 45, 1066.

Hjorth, N. (1965) Contact sensitivity to plants and balsams. Acta. derm.-venerol, Europ. Congr. Allerg. 65-79 and personal communication.

Pammel, L.H. (1911) A Manual of Poisonous Plants. Cedar Rapids, Iowa, Torch Press. Reprinted Univ. Microfilms Inc., Ann Arbor, Mich., 1965, pp. 476-7.

Pardo-Castello, V. (1923) Dermatitis venenata. Archs. Derm. 7, 80.

Souder, P. (1963) Poisonous Plants on Guam, in Venomous and Poisonous Animals and Noxious Plants of the Pacific Region. Ed. Keegan, H.L. and Macfarlane, W.V. Oxford, Pergamon Press, pp. 15-29.

Zina, G. and Bonu, G. (1960) Fitodermatosi di moda· eruzione allergica da contatto con Philodendron. Minerva Derm. 35, 157.

Pinellia

Seven species are natives of China, Japan.

Pinellia ternata

(P. tuberifera)

The fresh tuber contains a substance which is strongly irritating (Pammel 1911) and, when eaten, causes pharyngeal swelling which persists for several days (Kariyone 1971).

Pinellia tuberosa

The fresh tubers are bitter and acrid; for use in Chinese Medicine, they are soaked in warm water for seven days (Smith 1969).

References

Kariyone, T. (1971) Atlas of Medicinal Plants. Osaka, Japan, Takeda Chemical Industries.

Pammel, L.H. (1911) A Manual of Poisonous Plants. Cedar Rapids, Iowa, Torch Press. Reprinted Univ. Microfilms Inc., Ann Arbor, Mich. 1965, pp. 476-7.

Smith, F.P. (1969) Chinese Materia Medica. Vegetable Kingdom. 2nd Ed. Rev. by Hei, P.D. Taipei, Taiwan, Ku T'ing Book House.

Pothos

The 75 species are natives of Madagascar and Indo-Malaysia, but several are cultivated elsewhere in the tropics.

Pothos is used as a common name for some plants in other genera (e.g. Scindapsus and Anthurium) and reports of dermatitis unsupported by reliable botanical identification should be accepted with scepticism (Kelsey and Dayton 1942).

Pothos spp.

These plants are the commonest cause of plant dermatitis in Hawaii, except during the fruiting season of the mango, (Mangifera) when the latter predominates (Arnold 1972).

References

Arnold, H.L., Jr. (1972) Honolulu, State of Hawaii. Personal Communication.

Kelsey, H.P. and Dayton, W.A. (1942) Standardized Plant Names 2nd. ed. Harrisburg, Pa. J.F. McFarland.

Raphidophora

There are about 100 species in Indo-Malaysia and New Caledonia.

Rhaphidophora aurea
Hunter's Robe

Contact with the sap can cause dermatitis (Hardin and Arena 1969, Morton 1971).

Rhaphidophora gigantum
Rengut

The liquid contained in the spathe of flowers is very irritating. When the fruit decays bast cells and needle-shaped crystals are liberated. Malays are reluctant to touch the fruit as this irritant dust may cause blindness (Gimlette 1929).

References

Gimlette, J.D. (1929) Malay Poisons and Charm Cures. 3rd Ed. London, J. & A. Churchill.

Hardin, J.W. and Arena, J.M. (1969) Human Poisoning from Native and Cultivated Plants. Durham, North Carolina, Duke University Press.

Morton, J.F. (1971) Plants Poisonous to People in Florida and Other Warm Areas. Miami, Florida, Hurricane House Publishers, Inc.

Scindapsus

The 40 species are natives of South China, Southeast Asia and Indo-Malaysia, but some are cultivated elsewhere as ornamental plants.

Scindapsus aureus Engl.
(syn. Pothos aureus Lind.)
Hunter's Robe, Taro Vine

The juice is irritant and a frequent cause of dermatitis. Florida nurserymen who cut up stems for propogation commonly complain of "Pothos poisoning". Biting into the stem caused irritation of the mouth and tongue (Morton 1962, 1971). The plant contains stinging crystals of calcium oxalate that are intensely irritating (Souder 1963).

A case of allergic contact dermatitis from the plant was reported by Mobacken (1975). Patch tests were negative in 21 controls.

References

Mobacken, H. (1975) Alergic contact dermatitis from Scindapsus aureus. Contact dermatitis 1, 60.

Morton, J.F. (1962) Ornamental Plants with Poisonous Properties II. Proc. Florida hort. Soc. 75, 484.

Morton, J.F. (1971) Plants Poisonous to People in Florida and Other Warm Areas. Miami, Florida, Hurricane House Publishers, Inc.

Souder, P. (1963) Poisonous Plants on Guam, in Venomous and Poisonous Animals and Noxious Plants of the Pacific Region. Ed. Keegan, H.L. and Macfarlane, W.V. Oxford, Pergamon Press, pp. 15-29.

Spathiphyllum

There are 36 species in the Philippine Islands and in Central and tropical South America.

Spathiphyllum kochii var. clevelandii

The plant contains minute crystals of calcium oxalate that are intensely irritating (Souder 1963).

Reference

Souder, P. (1963) Poisonous Plants on Guam, in Venomous and Poisonous Animals and Noxious Plants of the Pacific Region. Ed. Keegan, H.L. and Macfarlane, W.V. Oxford, Pergamon Press, pp. 15-29.

Symplocarpus

The single species occurs in North East Asia, Japan and Atlantic North America.

Symplocarpus foetidus

Skunk Cabbage, Meadow Cabbage, Polecat Weed.

Bigelow (1817) stated that an acrid principle existed in the root, even when perfectly dry. Cheney informed White (1887) that the root produced intolerable itching and inflammation of the skin. The taste of the root is acrid and biting and the odour disagreeable (Wren 1968). The irritant properties particularly of the root are noted by Weber (1937), Lampe and Fagerstrom (1968) and Kingsbury (1964).

Lysichiton americanum is also known as Skunk Cabbage.

References

Bigelow, (1817) American Medical Botany. Boston (1824), Florula Bostoniensis. Cited by White, J.C. (1887). Dermatitis venenata: An account of the Action of External Irritants upon the skin. Boston, Cupples and Hurd.

Kingsbury, J.M. (1964) Poisonous Plants of the United States and Canada. Englewood Cliffs, New Jersey, Prentice-Hall Inc.

Lampe, K.F. and Fagerström, R. (1968) Plant Toxicity and Dermatitis. Baltimore, Williams and Wilkins.

Weber, L.F. (1937) External Causes of Dermatitis. A List of Irritants. Archs. Derm. 35, 129.

White, J.C. (1887) Dermatitis Venenata: an Account of the Action of External Irritants upon the Skin. Boston, Cupples and Hurd.

Wren, R.W. (1968) Potter's New Cyclopaedia of Botanical Drugs and Preparations, by Wren, R.C. Re-edit. by Wren, R.W. Rustington, Sussex, Potter and Clarke Ltd. Health Science Press.

Syngonium

The 20 species are found in Central and tropical South America and in the West Indies.

Syngonium podaphyllum

The plant contains irritating crystals of calcium oxalate (Souder 1963).

Reference

Souder, P. (1963) Poisonous Plants on Guam, in Venomous and Poisonous Animals and Noxious Plants of the Pacific Region. Ed. Keegan, H.L. and Macfarlane, W.V. Oxford, Pergamon Press, pp.15-29.

Typhonium

The 30 species are native of South East Asia and Indo-Malaysia.

Typhonium angustifolium Wanjallo

Typhonium brownii

The rhizomes are acrid (MacPherson 1929).

Typhonium cuspidatum
Pantake

The plant contains irritating crystals of calcium oxalate (Souder 1963).

Typhonium roxburghii

The tuber is very irritant (Burkill 1935).

References

Burkill, I.H. (1935) A Dictionary of the Economic Products of the Malay Peninsula. 2 Vols. London, Crown Agents for the Colonies.

MacPherson, J. (1929) The Toxicology of the Arum Lily and Cunjevoi Lily. Med. J. Australia, 2,671.

Souder, P. (1963) Poisonous Plants on Guam, in Venomous and Poisonous Animals and Noxious Plants of the Pacific Region. Ed. Keegan, H.I. and Macfarlane, W.V. Oxford, Pergamon Press, pp.15-29.

Typhonodorum

One species is found in tropical eastern Africa, Madagascar and the Mascarenes.

Typhonodorum lindleyanum

The roots are edible but poisonous unless repeatedly boiled and the water discarded (Wild 1961).

Reference

Wild, H. (1961) Harmful aquatic plants in Africa and Madagascar. Kirkia 2, 1.

Xanthosoma

Some 45 species are natives of tropical Central and South America and of the West Indies. Some have edible starchy tubers.

Xanthosoma brasiliense

The leaves are irritating unless scalded (Altschul 1973).

Xanthosoma sagittifolium
Yantia

Xanthosoma violaceum
Sunin Honolulu

Both species contain irritant crystals of calcium oxalate (Souder 1963).

Burkill (1935) noted that a cultivar or variety of Xanthosoma violaceum, withstreaked leaf-stalks, was particularly irritant to the mouth.

References

Altschul, S. von R. (1973) Drugs and foods from little-known plants. Cambridge, Mass. Harvard Univ. Press.

Burkill, I.H. (1935) A Dictionary of the Economic Products of the Malay Peninsula. 2 vols. London, Crown Agents for the Colonies.

Souder, P. (1963) Poisonous Plants on Guam, in Venomous and Poisonous Animals and Noxious Plants of the Pacific Region. ed. Keegan, H.L. and Macfarlane, W.V. Oxford, Pergamon Press, pp. 15-29.

Xenophya

Two species are found from the Molucca to the Bismarck islands.

Xenophya portei
(syn. Schizocasia)

The juice of a species of this genus, possibly Schizocasia portei, has irritant effects (Altschul 1973).

Altschul, S. von R. (1973). Drugs and foods from little-known plants. Cambridge, Mass. Harvard Univ. Press.

Zantedeschia

There are 8 or 9 species in tropical Africa.

Zantedeschia aethiopica
(syn. Richardia)
White Arum, Calla Lily

This plant, native of South Africa, is naturalized in parts of Australia and is widely cultivated elsewhere, including Europe and North America.

All parts of the plant contain calcium oxalate and an unknown toxic substance, which produces dermatitis. Attempts to utilize the starch in the tubers caused dermatitis in laundresses in Madeira (Johnson 1897).

Eating the plant causes swelling of lips, tongue and pharynx and gastrointestinal irritation (Everist 1962).

References

Everist, S.L. (1962) These plants can poison people. Queensland Agric. J. 88, 235.

Johnson, J.Y. (1897) Proc. Linn. Soc. 21st Jan., Quoted by Maiden, J.H. (1909) On some plants which cause inflammation or irritation of the skin. Agric. Gaz. of New South Wales 20, 1073.

ARALIACEAE

This family contains about 700 species in 55 genera. Most are natives of the tropics, particularly of Indomalaysia and America, but some species are natives of temperate regions and some have been widely distributed in horticulture.

The aromatic smell of crushed tissues results from the presence of oil glands (Corner 1952).

Chemistry is recorded by Hegnauer (1964).

References

Corner, E.J.H. (1952) Wayside trees of Malaysia. Singapore, Government Printer.

Henauer, R. (1964) Chemotaxonomy of Plants. Vol. 3. Basel, Birkhauser p. 173.

Aralia

There are some 35 species.

Aralia spinosa

Angelica Tree, Prickly Elder
Hercules' Club

The green bark irritates the hands of those collecting it (Cheney 1887, Massey 1941, Hardin and Arena 1969).

References

Cheney (1887) Personal communication to White (1887). Mr. Cheney was a wholesale dealer in medicinal vegetable drugs.

Hardin, J.W. and Arena, J.M. (1969) Human Poisoning from Native and Cultivated Plants. Durham, North Carolina, Duke University Press.

Massey, A.B. (1941) Plant Poisoning. Merck Reports 50, 24.

White, J.C. (1887) Dermatitis venenata: An account of the action of external irritants upon the skin. Boston. Cupples and Hurd.

Echinopanax

There are three species in North East Asia and North America.

Echinopanax horridum,
syn. Oplopanax David's Club

The prickles produce painful wounds (Muenscher 1951), but there is no evidence that they inflict more than mechanical injury.

References

Muenscher, W.C. (1951) Poisonous Plants of the United States. 2nd Edit. New York, Macmillan.

Hedera

The 15 species are natives of the temperate Old World countries, but many are naturalized elsewhere, and some species are widely cultivated in gardens or as house plants.

The ritual use of ivy as the archetypal evergreen, and its popularity as a decorative covering for walls and fences, bring it into unusually close contact with man.

The name "Ivy" is also applied to a variety of plants which are botanically unrelated to Hedera.

Hedera canariensis

Canary Island Ivy (U.K.),
Algerian Ivy (U.S.A.)

This ivy is tender in Britain, needing protection in winter, and is grown mainly as a house plant. In many parts of America and in Southern Europe it grows freely in the open, and is available in many named cultivars.

The substance causing dermatitis is water soluble (Dorsey 1957) and is probably an allergic sensitizer. The glucoside hederagenin may be the offending substance (Francis and Southcott 1967). It is released only when the leaves or stems are bruised. Dermatitis is commonly acquired in the process of cutting back the exuberant growth in the spring. In Europe, ivy on houses or walls is often clipped at this season.

Dermatitis is commonly confined to exposed skin, and may be diffusely eczematous or in linear, often vesicular, patterns (Rynes 1949, Dorsey, 1959).

Hedera helix

Common Ivy (U.K.),
English Ivy (U.S.A.)

This common European ivy has long been recognized as causing dermatitis (Zinsser 1909, Gutteling 1922, Roed-Petersen 1975). It contains hederagenin and patients allergic to H. cannariensis react also to H. helix. The clinical features of the dermatitis as described in case reports (Cleland 1925, Muenscher 1939) suggest that allergic sensitization may occur. Indeed the lesions may be linear and vesicular as in Toxicodendron dermatitis (Goldman et al 1956, Aplin 1966). Other similar cases have been reported by Thibierge (1969), and by Barry (1969).

An extract of the leaves, used as a corn-cure for the feet, caused dermatitis in a patient who later developed a recurrence after handling wet leaves (Munro 1900).

The evidence that H. helix is a sensitizer is largely circumstantial. In addition to the case reports already mentioned, Maiden (1909, 1911, 1921) and Allen (1943) state that it causes dermatitis only in some people. However, one of the authors (A.J.R.) has encountered four cases of dermatitis apparently attributable to this ivy; the clinical appearances were those of an irritant dermatitis; patch tests with fragments of bruised leaf were positive in only one patient, but also positive in 3 of 10 control subjects. Highman (1924) obtained a negative patch test with a leaf, but a positive reaction to an alcoholic extract of the leaves, which produced no reaction in two controls.

On present evidence it is reasonable to conclude that H. helix is an irritant plant, which may also, on occasions, induce sensitization. The morphological variability of the species is probably accompanied by an equivalent variation in chemical composition. A scarlatiniform eruption was produced by ingestion of ivy leaves (Turton 1925).

One of four patients who were contact sensitive to the plant was also contact sensitive to extracts of some Compositae species and to helenin (alantolactone) derived from Inula helenium (Roed-Petersen 1975).

A gardener in a cemetery developed eczema of the hands and forearms. A patch test to the leaf produced a positive reaction (Rothe 1968).

References

Allen, P.H. (1943) Poisonous and Injurious Plants of Panama. Am. J. trop. Med. 23, Suppl. 3.

Aplin, T.E.H. (1966) Poison Plants in the Garden. West Australian Dept. Agr. J. 7,24.

Burry, J.N. (1969) The value of patch testing: a review of 363 cases of allergic contact dermatitis. Med. J. Australia 1, 1226.

Cleland, J.B. (1925) Plants, including fungi, poisonous or otherwise injurious to man in Australia. Med. J. Aust. 2, 443.

Dorsey, C.S. (1957) Contact Dermatitis from Algerian ivy. Archs. Derm. 75, 671.

Dorsey, C.S. (1959) Algerian Ivy Dermatitis. A California Disease Calif. Med. 90, 155.

Francis, D.F. and Southcott, R.V. (1967) Plants harmful to man in Australia. Misc. Bull. No. 1 Botanic Garden, Adelaide, Australia.

Goldman, L., Preston, R.H. and Muegel, H.R. (1956) Dermatitis venenata from English Ivy (Hedera Helix). Archs Derm. 74, 811.

Gutteling (1922) Tijdschr. Geneesk. 3, 306, cited by Touton (1932).

Highman, W.J. (1924) The Pathogenesis of dermatitis, including eczema. A case of English Ivy poisoning. Archs Derm. Syph. 9, 344.

Maiden, J.H. (1909) On some plants which cause inflammation or irritation of the skin. Ag. Gaz. New South Wales, 20, 1073.

Maiden, J.H. (1911) Irritation of the skin by the common Ivy (Hedera helix) Ag. Gaz. New South Wales 22, 1069.

Maiden, J.H. (1921) Plants which cause inflammation or irritation of the skin. Ag. Gaz. New South Wales 32, 206, and 657.

Muenscher, W.C.L. (1939) Poisonous Plants of the United States. New York. The Macmillan Co.

Munro, W.J. (1900) A case of dermatitis venenata arising from a rare cause. Austr. med. Gaz. 19, 25.

Roed-Petersen, J. (1975) Allergic contact hypersensitivity to ivy (Hedera helix). Contact Dermatitis 1, 57.

Rothe, A. (1968) Berlin. Pers. Comm. 1975.

Rynes, S.E. (1949) House Ivy Dermatitis. Ann. Allergy 7, 62.

Schwartz, L., Tulipan, L. and Birmingham, D.J. (1957) Occupational Diseases of the Skin. 3rd. ed. Philadelphia, Lea and Febiger, pp. 637-672.

Thibierge, G. (1909) Eruption erythemato-ortiee a petites vesicules provoquee par le contact du lierre. Annales Derm. Syph. 10, 112.

Touton, K. (1932) Hauterkrankungen durch phanerogamische Pflanzen und ihre Produkte (Toxicodermia et Allergodermia phytogenes), in Barnewitz, J. et al angeborene Anomalien, Lichtdermatosen, Pflanzengifte, Thermische Schädigungen, Einfluss Innerer Störungen auf die Haut. Berlin, Verlag von Julius Springer.

Turton, P.H.J. (1925) Poisoning by ivy. Brit. Med. J. 2, 294.

Zinsser, F. (1909) Hautreizende Wirkung von Epheu. Munch. Med. Wschr. 56, 2706.

Polyscias (Syn. Nothopanax)

About 80 species are natives of the Old World tropics and of Australasia, but many are cultivated elsewhere.

Polyscias balfouriana (Syn. Aralia balfouriana) Balfour Polyscias

Generally referred to as "aralias" (Morton 1958).

Polyscias guilfoylei (Syn. A. guilfoylei) Guilfoyle Polyscias, "Aralias"

All parts contain saponin and the plants, commonly cultivated as hedges, are in south Florida, a frequent cause of dermatitis which may be provoked merely by brushing against the leaves. A more acute form may result from handling cuttings (Morton, 1971).

Polyscias species (known by their former name, Nothopanax) are popular as hedge plants in Hawaii. In 30 years of practice there Arnold (1972) has seen only 3 or 4 cases of dermatitis caused by them.

References

Arnold, H.L., Jr. (1972) Honolulu, State of Hawaii. Personal Communication.

Morton, J.F. (1971) Plants Poisonous to People in Florida and Other Warm Areas. Miami, Florida, Hurrican House Publishers, Inc.

Oplopanax (~ Echinopanax)

There are two species, natives of North-east Asia and Japan.

Oplopanax horridum
Devil's Club

The sharp spines on the stem are thought to be poisonous (Turner and Bell (1973).

Reference

Turner, N.C. and Bell, M.A.M. (1973) The Ethnobotany of the Southern Kwakiutl Indians of British Columbia. Economic Botany (in the press).

Schefflera

200 species are found in tropical and subtropical regions.

Schefflera actinophylla
Queensland umbrella tree, Octopus Tree

This species has on one occasion in Western Australia been suspected of causing an irritating rash to a person who handled it (Aplin 1976).

Reference

Aplin, T.E.H. (1976) Poisonous garden plants and other plants harmful to man in Australia. Western Australian Dept. of Agriculture Bull. 3964.

Tetrapanax papyriferum
(syn. Fatsia papyrifera), Chinese Rice Paper Plant.

The single species in this genus is a native of South China and Formosa, but is cultivated in the warmer parts of Europe and America.

The heavy yellow pollen is said to cause severe dermatitis (Dorsey 1962), but the report refers only to the common name of the plant and its identification is therefore not beyond question.

Reference

Dorsey, G.S. (1962) Plant Dermatitis in Californa. Calif. Med. 96, 412.

ARAUCARIACEAE

This family consists of some 38 species of trees, placed in the two genera Agathis and Araucaria, distributed over the Southern hemisphere, but not native to Africa.

Agathis

The 20 species are natives of the region extending from Indochina and West Malaysia to New Zealand. Several species furnish copals and dammars (Usher 1974), which are resins from which varnish is prepared. The highest quality copal is dug from the remains of trees long dead. Contact sensitivity to copal is noted under Trachylobium. Dammar used in adhesive plaster has caused dermatitis (White 1934). A variety of plants e.g. Canarium, Shorea furnish dammars (Usher 1974).

Araucaria

The natural distribution of this genus of 18 species is that of the family, but many species are widely cultivated elsewhere for their decorative virtues or for their timber.

Araucaria angustifolia
(syn. A. brasiliana)
Parana pine

This species, which originated in southern Brazil and northern Argentina, is known in the international timber trade as Parana or Perara Pine. The attractively coloured wood does not withstand the weather and is therefore used mainly for floor and staircases (Hausen 1973). This author refers to a febrile illness in a building worker handling the wood. Two alkaloids were isolated from the wood but their relevance could not be established as the patient was not available for tests. The tree was noted as a cause of dermatitis by Klauder and Gross (1951).

A carpenter showed positive patch tests to the wood and to Gonystylus, Tectona, epoxy resin, wood and coal tars (Woods and Calnan 1976).

Araucaria bidwilli

Bunya Bunya Pine (Queensland, Australia)

The leaves have sharp points. The nuts are said to have caused asthma (Cleland 1943).

Araucaria cunninghamii
Moreton Bay Pine, Hoop Pine, Queensland Pine

This tree has needle-like leaves, some with sharp bristle-like points (Corner 1952). The timber is listed as causing dermatitis (Commonwealth Department of Health 1926).

Araucaria excelsa
Norfolk Island Pine

Araucaria imbricata
(syn. A. araucana)
Monkey Puzzle Tree

These two species are popular with horticulturists. The latter species can cause unpleasant injuries in those foolish enough to climb it. Neither is listed as a cause of dermatitis, but they are included here because both are relatively common in many countries, and other related species are known to be dermatitic.

References

Cleland, J.B. (1943) Plants, including Fungi, Poisonous or Otherwise Injurious to Man in Australia. Med. J. Australia 11, 161.

Commonwealth Department of Health (1926) Division of Industrial Hygiene Bull. No. 4. Melbourne.

Corner, E.J.H. (1952) Wayside Trees of Malaysia. Singapore, Government Printer.

Hausen, B.M. (1973) Holzarten mit gesundheitsschädigenden inhaltsstoffen Stuttgart. DRW-Verlags.-GmbH.

Klauder, J.V. and Gross, B.A. (1951) Actual causes of certain occupational dermatoses. Archs. Derm. Syph. 63, 1.

Usher, G. (1974) A Dictionary of Plants used by Man. London. Constable.

White, R.P. (1934) The Dermatergoses or Occupational Affections of the Skin. 4th. ed. London. H.K. Lewis.

Woods, B. and Calnan, C.D. (1976) Toxic Woods. Brit. J. Derm. 94, Suppl. 13, June.

ARISTOLOCHIACEAE

This family contains about 400 species in 7 genera. Most species occur naturally in the tropics and subtropics, but a few are found in temperate regions.

Chemistry is recorded by Hegnauer (1964).

Aristolochia

This, the largest genus, contains about 350 species. Many are very decorative and are widely cultivated. The roots of some species have been used in folk medicine as abortifacients, as cures for snakebites, and for other purposes. Dermatitis appears not to have been reported, but the aromatic nature of the roots (Wren 1968) suggests that effects on the skin should be considered possible. Indeed A. clematitis has been reported as irritant (Perrot and Paris 1971).

Asarum

There are about 70 species. natives of north temperate regions. Many were cultivated for their alleged medicinal virtues: some are now cultivated for their horticultural interest.

Several species yield Oil of Asarum, which contains terpene (pinene), methyleugenol, borneol, linalool and geraniol (Merck 1968).

Asarum canadense
Wild Ginger

The leaves can cause dermatitis (Massey 1941).

Asarum arifolium

Asarum caudatum

Asarum europaeum Assarabacca

Asarum virginicum

These species are reported to be irritant (Pammel 1911).

Thottea

There are 9 species in Western Malaysia.

Thottea dependens

This species is reported as irritant (Pammel 1911).

References

Massey, A.B. (1941) Plant Poisoning. Merck Reports, 50, 24.

Merck Index (1968) ed. Stecher P.G. 8th. ed. Rahway, New Jersey, Merck & Co.

Pammel, L.H. (1911) A Manual of Poisonous Plants. Cedar Rapids, Iowa, Torch Press. Reprinted Univ. Microfilms, Inc., Ann Arbor, Mich., 1965, pp. 476-7.

Perrot, E. and Paris, R. (1971) Les plantes médicinales. 2 Vols. Paris, Presses Universitaires de France.

Wren, R.W. (1968) Potter's New Cyclopaedia of Botanical Drugs and Preparations, by Wren, R.C. Re-edit. by Wren, R.W. Rustington, Sussex, Potter and Clarke Ltd., Health Science Press.

Hegnauer, R. (1964) Chemotaxonomy of Plants. Vol. 3. Basel. Birkhauser p. 184.

ASCLEPIADACEAE

About 2,000 species in 130 genera are fairly widely distributed in the tropics and subtropics, but are rare as natives elsewhere, although some species are cultivated with artificial heat.

Chemistry is recorded by Hegnauer (1964).

Araujia

This small South American genus of twinning shrubs contains some species which are cultivated.

Araujia sericifera
"Cruel plant"

The latex of the species has been reported to be irritant to rabbit skin (Watt and Breyer-Brandwijk 1962), but the common name used at least in British horticulture, suggests that rabbits may not be its only victims.

Reference

Hegnauer, R. (1964) Chemotaxonomy of Plants. Vol. 3. Basel. Birkhauser p. 199.

Watt, J.M. and Breyer-Brandwijk, M.G. (1962) The Medicinal and Poisonous Plants of Southern and Eastern Africa. 2nd Edit. Edinburgh, R. & S. Livingstone Ltd.

Asclepias

There are about 120 species, most of which are natives of the Americas, particularly the United States. However many species are handsome border plants, hardy in the temperate regions, and are widely cultivated in Europe. Asclepias curassavica is the most popular species for greenhouse cultivation.

Asclepias curassavica

The plant's milky latex will produce dermatitis in "susceptible" individuals (Allen 1943, Blohm 1962).

Asclepias incarnata

A. syriaca

A. tuberosa

A. viridis

These species, which like others in this genus, are popularly known as "milkweeds", are listed as producing dermatitis (Shelmire 1940).

References

Allen, P.H. (1943) Poisonous and Injurious Plants of Panama. Am. J. trop. Med. 23 (Suppl.) 3.

Blohm, H. (1962) Poisonous Plants of Venezuela. Cambridge, Mass., Harvard Univ. Press.

Shelmire, B. (1940) Contact Dermatitis from Vegetation. Sth. med. J. 33, 338.

Calotropis

The six species in this genus are natives of tropical Africa and Asia. Some are of horticultural interest and are cultivated to a limited extent elsewhere.

Calotropics gigantea
Crown Flower, Madar, Giant Milkweed, Algodón de seda (Sp.)

The bark of this plant, the natural range of which is from Iran to China, yields a strong fibre, and the silky hairs from the seeds are woven into a fabric. (The Spanish name for the plant indicates its importance as a source of "silk".) The latex, which resembles gutta-percha, contains a proteolytic enzyme, and is irritant and caustic to the skin (Behl et al 1961, Morton 1962, Blohm 1962, Arnold 1968). It also causes keratoconjunctivitis (Muthayya 1948, Wong 1949, Crawford 1958, Sugiki 1966, Duke-Elder and MacFaul 1972).

This species, and C. procera, are the crown flowers of an Hawaiian "lei", and in this capacity can be violently irritant (Arnold 1968).

Calotropis procera
Sodom Apple, Swallow-wort

This plant too yields fibre and silky hairs, the latter being used to stuff mattresses. It is also used in indigenous medicine as a rubefacient (Irvine 1961) and a depilatory (Morton 1962).

The latex contains a proteolytic enzyme (Watt and Breyer-Brandwijk 1962).

The latex is caustic and irritant to the skin and dangerous to the eyes (Dalziel 1937, Willaimson 1956, Arnold 1968). Its medical use in India in the treatment of skin diseases may cause severe bullous dermatitis, leading sometimes to hypertrophic scars (Behl et al 1966).

References

Arnold, H.L. (1968) Poisonous Plants of Hawaii. Rutland, Vermont, Charles E. Tuttle.

Behl, P.N., Captain, R.M., Bedi, B.M.S. and Gupta, S. (1966) Skin-irritant and sensitizing plants found in India. New Delhi, P.N. Behl, Irwin Hospital.

Blohm, H. (1962) Poisonous Plants of Venezuela. Cambridge, Mass., Harvard Univ. Press.

Crawford, H.W. (1958) Crown flower keratoconjunctivitis. Hawaii Med. J. 17, 244.

Dalziel, J.M. (1937) The Useful Plants of West Tropical Africa. London, Crown Agents for the Colonies, P. 612.

Duke-Elder, S. and MacFaul, P.A. (1972) System of Ophthalmology. Vol. XIV. Injuries. Part 1. Mechanical Injuries, Extra-ocular Foreign Bodies pp.464-67, and Agricultural Injuries, pp.32-34. London, Henry Kimpton

Irvine, F.R. (1961) Woody Plants of Ghana. London, Oxford Univ. Press.

Muthayya, R.E.S. (1948) Madar Keratitis. Proc. All-India Opthal. Soc. 10, 44.

Sugiki, S. (1966) Crownflower or cornflower. Arch Ophth. 75, 736.

Watt, J.M. and Breyer-Brandwijk, M.G. (1962) The Medicinal and Poisonous Plants of Southern and Eastern Africa. 2nd. Edit. Edinburgh, E. & S. Livingstone Ltd.

Williamson, J. (1956) Useful Plants of Malawi. Ed. Greenway, P.J. Zoomba, Malawi, The Government printer. Previously published as Useful Plants of Nyasaland.

Wong, W.H. (1949) Crownflower Keratoconjunctivitis. Hawaii med. J., 8, 339.

Gymnema

25 species are palaeotropical, Southern Africa, Australia.

Gymnema sylvestre

The leaves contain gymnemin which obtunds taste for several hours for bitter or sweet, but not for sour, astringent or pungent substances (Webb 1948). The chemical responsible is gymnemic acid.

Reference

Webb, L.J. (1948) Guide to the medicinal and poisonous plants of Queensland. C.S.I.R. Bull. No. 232, cites Merck Index, 5th. ed. Merck & Co. Inc., Rahway, N.J.

Marsdenia

Between five and ten species are found in tropical regions. Some are ornamental and cultivated. M. tenacissima yields fibre used for bow strings.

Marsdenia erecta

The juice of this south-eastern European species blisters the skin (Howes 1974).

Reference

Howes, F.N. (1974) A dictionary of useful and everyday plants and their common names. Cambridge University Press.

Metaplexis

There are six species, natives of East Asia.

Metaplexis stauntonii

The crushed seeds are used in Chinese medicine as an astringent and haemostatic. They are thought to have escharotic properties if they are used frequently (Smith 1969).

Reference

Smith, F.P. (1969) Chinese Materia Medica. Vegetable Kingdom. 2nd Edit. Rev. by Hei, P.D. Taipei, Taiwan, Ku T'ing Book House.

Sarcostemna

There are 10 species in the tropics and subtropics of the Old World. Two species are cultivated, but to a limited extent.

Sarcostemna australe
Caustic Plant, Caustic Vine

This species has caustic sap (Hurst 1942, Webb 1948).

The plant contains a saponin, from the aglycone of which sarcostin, benzoic and cinnamic acids were obtained (Earl and Cornforth 1940). The latex blisters human skin (Everist 1972).

Sarcostemna viminale
(called *Euphorbia viminale* in the older literature)

The plant is said to produce urticaria on contact with the skin (Watt and Breyer-Brandwijk 1962).

References

Earl, J.C. and Cornforth, J.W. (1940) Sarcostin. Pt. 1. A Preliminary Study of its Behaviour with Reagents. J. chem. Soc. pp.1443-1447.

Everist, S.L. (1972) Queensland Herbarium, Brisbane, Australia. Personal Cummunication Concerning Plants Recorded in Australia as Having Caused Dermatitis or Other Contact Injury to Man or Livestock.

Hurst, E. (1942) The poisonous plants of New South Wales. Sydney, New South Wales Poisonous Plants Committee.

Watt, J.M. and Breyer-Brandwijk, M.G. (1962) The Medicinal and Poisonous Plants of Southern and Eastern Africa. 2nd. Edit. Edinburgh, E. and S. Livingstone Ltd.

Webb, L.J. (1948) Guide to the medicinal and poisonous plants of Queensland. Commonwealth Scientific and Industrial Research Bulletin. No. 232, Melbourne.

Sarcostemma australe

The milky juice was for corns and warts; it was also applied as a healing applicaton to wounds (MacPherson 1932).

Reference

MacPherson, J. (1932) Plants injurious to man in Australia. Med. J. Australia <u>1</u>, 281.

Tylophora

There are 50 species in palaeotropical regions and South Africa.

Tylophora spp.

Several species yield the skin-vesicant alkaloids tylophorine and tylocrebrine (related to cryptopleurine derived from *Cryptocarya*, Lauraceae (Donaldson *et al* 1968).

Reference

Donaldson, G.R., Atkinson, M.R. and Murray, A.W. (1968) Inhibition of Protein Synthesis by Tylophorine, Tylocrebrine and Cryptopleurine. Biochem. Biophys. Res. Comm., <u>31</u>, 104, and refs. therein.

AVICENNIACEAE

15 species are found on tropical coasts.

Avicennia

14 species are found as constituents of mangrove vegatation.

Avicennia tomentosa

The sap-wood is used in Java as a contraceptive (Quisumbing 1951) and the wood has been investigated as a source of paper pulp (Watt and Breyer-Brandwijk 1962). The heartwood yields lapachol, a sensitizer of Tectona.

References

Quisumbing, E. (1951) Medicinal Plants of the Philippines. Philipp. Dep. Agr. and Nat. Resources Tech. Bull. No. 16. Manila. Bureau of Printing 1234 pp.

Watt, J.M. and Breyer-Brandwijk, M.G. (1962) The Medicinal and Poisonous Plants of Southern Africa. 2nd. ed. Edinburgh. E. and S. Livingstone.

BALANITACEAE

25 species in one genus, found in tropical Africa and Asia, were formerly included in the family Zygophyllaceae.

Balanites

25 species are found from tropical Africa to Burma. The seeds yield oil.

Balanites spp.

Mechanical injury can result from these exceedingly spiny shrubs or trees of African bushland (Verdcourt and Trump 1969). The Masai of southern Africa used the thorns to pierce the earlobes of children (Watt and Breyer-Brandwijk 1962) and the thorny branches of B. aegyptica (Desert Date) are used as an obstacle to fence cattle pens (Irvine 1961).

References

Irvine, F.R. (1961) Woody plants of Ghana. Oxford University Press. London.

Verdcourt, B. and Trump, E.C. (1969) Common Poisonous Plants of East Africa. London. Collins.

Watt, J.M. and Breyer-Brandwijk, M.G. (1962) The Medicinal and poisonous plants of Southern Africa. 2nd. ed. Edinburgh. E. & S. Livingstone.

BALSAMINACEAE

600 species in four or five genera are found in Eurasia, Africa and North America.

Chemistry is recorded by Hegnauer (1964).

Reference

Hegnauer, R. (1964) Chemotaxonomy of plants. Vol. 3. Basel, Birkhauser p. 229.

Impatiens (syn. Balsamina)

Between five and six hundred species are found in tropical and temperate Eurasia and Africa and on mountains of India and Ceylon. About six species are found in North and Central America.

Impatiens sp.

Two of five patch tests to a species of the genus produced positive reactions suggesting irritancy (Hjorth 1968).

Impatiens biflora
Jewel Weed

This species which yields naphthaquinones (Hegnauer 1964) has been used in Herbal Medicine (Wren 1968, Lipton 1958) and to dye the fingernails (Smith 1969).

Impatiens nolitangera

This species has irritant properties (Pammel 1911).

References

Hegnauer, R. (1964) Chemotaxonomy of plants. Vol. 3. Basel, Birkhauser, p. 229.

Hjorth, N. (1968) at Finsen Institute. Pers. comm.

Lipton, R.A. (1958) The use of Impatiens biflora (Jewel Weed) in the treatment of rhus dermatitis. Ann. Allergy 16, 526.

Pammel, L.H. (1911) A Manual of Poisonous plants. Torch Press. Cedar Rapids, Iowa. Reprinted Univ. Microfilms Inc. Ann Arbor, Mich. 1965. pp. 476-7

Smith, F.P. (1969) Chinese Materia Medica. Vegetable kingdom. 2nd. ed. Rev. by Hei, P.D. Taipei, Taiwan. Ku T'ing Book House.

Wren, R.W. (1968) Potter's New Cyclopaedia of Botanical Drugs and Preparations by Wren, R.C. Re-edit. by Wren, R.W. Potter and Clarke Ltd. Health Science Press. Rustington, Sussex.

BARRINGTONIACEAE

53 species in five genera are found in palaeotropical regions.

Barringtonia

39 species are found in East Africa, Madagascar, Hainan, Formosa, north-eastern India, IndoMalaysia, Australia and the Pacific region.

Barringtonia racemosa

The powdered seed is irritant to the nasal cavity and produces sneezing. (Watt and Breyer-Brandwijk 1962).

Reference

Watt, J.M. and Breyer-Brandwijk, M.G. (1962) The Medicinal and poisonous plants of Southern Africa. 2nd ed. Edinburgh. E.& S. Livingstone.

BASELLACEAE

25 species in four genera are found in America, Africa and Asia.

Chemistry is recorded by Hegnauer (1964).

Reference

Hegnauer, R. (1964) Chemotaxonomy of Plants. Vol. 3. Basel, Birkhauser. p. 235.

Basella

Two species are found in tropical Africa, three species in Madagascar. One species, B. alba, of pantropical distribution is cultivated as spinach (Spinacia).

Basella rubra

This species is said to have rubefacient properties (Quisumbing 1951). The red juice of the berries is used for rouge and dyeing (Smith 1969).

References

Quisumbing, E. (1951) Medicinal Plants of the Philippines. Tech. Bull. 16. Manila, Philippine Islands. Manila Bureau of Printing. 1234 pp.

Smith, F.P. (1969) Chinese Materia Medica. Vegetable kingdom. 2nd ed. Rev. by Hei, P.D. Taipei, Taiwan. Ku T'ing Book House.

BEGONIACEAE

920 species in five genera are of tropical distribution.

Chemistry is recorded by Hegnauer (1964).

Reference

Hegnauer, R. (1964) Chemotaxonomy of Plants. Vol. 3. Basel, Birkhauser p. 237.

Begonia

900 species are found in tropical and subtropical regions especially in America. B. socotrana is the "tuberous" begonia. Many varieties and hybrids are cultivated.

Begonia sp.

Eight positive patch test reactions from 77 tests suggest irritancy from some species of the genus (Hjorth 1968).

A man who picked begonias and other plants developed allergic contact dermatitis from a mildew pesticide carbamate derivative (von Ketel 1976). Probably the pesticide was within the tissues of the plant as well as on the surface.

Reference

Van Ketel, W.G. (1976) Sensitivity to the pesticide benomyl. Contact Dermatitis 2, 290.

Begonia semperflorens
Fibrous-rooted begonia

Six positive patch test reactions from 101 tests suggest irritancy (Agrup 1969).

Begonia rex-cultorum
Rex begonia

One positive patch test reaction was observed from 33 tests (Agrup 1969).

References

Agrup, G. (1969) Hand Eczema and other hand dematoses in South Sweden. Acta derm.-venereol. 49. Suppl. 61. p. 1-91.

Hjorth, N. (1968) at Finsen Institute. Pers. comm.

BERBERIDACEAE

This family of some 575 species in 4 genera is of great horticultural importance. Natives of the north temperate region, of some mountainous areas in the tropics, and of South America, have been very widely introduced for use in landscape gardening and for ornamental hedges. Hundreds of named hybrids and cultivars are available.

Chemistry is recorded by Hegnauer (1964). Berberis vulgaris yields berberine (Schulz 1962). Local anaesthesic and hyperpigmentation can follow intracutaneous injection of berberine (Seery and Beiter 1940).

Berberis

The distribution of this large genus of 450 species is that of the family as a whole, and has been extended by cultivation to most climatically suitable areas.

The wood of Berberis vulgaris and of some other species has a limited use in turning and in-lay work. The wood contains a toxic alkaloid, and those who handle it may develop colic and diarrhoea (Hausen 1970). Many of the Asiatic species (often cultivated elsewhere) contain benzyl isoquinoline alkaloids (Tomita 1952). This species is an alternate host of a wheat rust, (Puccinia), and Berberis spp. are a source of infection with Sporotrichum schenckii (Foerster 1926). Ten of 14 employees in a tree nursery in Wisconsin, U.S.A. acquired this infection from this shrub. Two further cases acquired from the barberry were reported by Blair and Yarian (1928), and one of the authors (A.J.R.) has seen a student-gardener similarly infected.

The sharp brittle spines of some species can cause an irritable papular dermatitis in some individuals. Our experience confirms the evidence of scanty case reports (Schwartz 1938, Cole 1972), that those clipping or trimming barberry hedges are most at risk. The eruption consists of firm inflammatory papules and nodules at the sites of injury. They are histologically non-specific and they resolve in 7 to 10 days. It is not proven whether chemical irritation or a foreign body reaction is involved.

Since the wood of some species is irritant, the provocation of a similar dematitis as claimed by Miller in discussion of Hollander (1927) is possible, but not fully substantiated. Reactions to berberine are noted under Argemone.

References

Blair, J. and Yarian, N.C. (1928) Two Cases of Sporotrichosis Infection due to Barberry. J. Am. med. Ass., 91, 96.

Cole, H.N. (1938) In Discussion of Schwartz (1938).

Foerster, H.R. (1926) Sporotrichosis and Occupational Dermatosis. M.J. and Rec., 123, 530, and J. Am. med. Ass. 87, 1605.

Hausen, B.M. (1970) Untersuchungen über gesundheitsschädigende Hölzer. Thesis, Hamburg.

Hegnauer, R. (1964) Chemotaxonomy of Plants. Vol. 3 Basel. Birkhauser pg. 240.

Hollander, L. (1927) Dermatitis Venenata. Archs. Derm. Syph. 15, 620.

Schulz, E.R. (1962) Berberine in the common barberry (Berberis vulgaris) J. Am. Pharm. Ass. 15, 33.

Schwartz, W.F. (1938) Foreign Body (Barberry) Dermatitis. Archs. Derm. Syph. 37, 872.

Seery, T.M. and Bieter, R.N. (1940) A contribution to the pharmacology of berberine. J. Pharm. 69, 64.

Tomita, M. (1952) Die Alkaloide der Menispermaceae-Pflanzen in Zechmeister L. Fortschritte der Chemie organischer Naturstoffe. Wien. Springer Verlag. p. 175 and other papers cited by Hausen (1970).

BETULACEAE

This family consists of 95 species in 2 genera.

Chemistry is recorded by Hegnauer (1964).

Alnus

This genus of 35 species is widely distributed over the temperate regions of th Northern Hemisphere, and in America extends as far south as Peru.

The timber of some species is used for turnery, especially for tool handles, bobbins and clogs.

Alnus sp.

The name Alder is popularly applied not only to many different species of *Alnus*, but also to some botanically unrelated trees and shrubs.

An unspecified *Alnus* is said to have caused dermatitis in one man and three women who had been working with the wood for years (Brügel and Perutz 1927). Patch test findings suggested that a catechol was the sensitizer.

Alnus glutinosa

This species is common in Western and Central Europe. It has been listed as a wood causing dermatitis (Senear 1933, Genner and Bonnevie 1938, Weber 1953, Orsler 1973), but considering the fequency with which the wood is used, particularly in rural industries, the lack of detailed reports is surprising. Investigations by Dässler and Urzynicok (1958) led to the isolation of a tannin from the wood, but this provoked no reactions either in control subjects or in those suffering from alleged alder dermatitis.

References

Brügel, S. and Perutz, A. (1927) Clinical Features and Pathogenesis of Alderwood Dermatitis (German). Arch. Derm. u. Syph. 153, 661.

Dässler, H.G. and Urzynicok, H. (1958) The Tannin of the *Alnus glutinosa* (German). Holz. Rohwerkst. 16, 327.

Genner, V. and Bonnevie, P. (1938) Eczematous Eruptions Produced by Leaves of Trees and Bushes. Archs. Derm. Syph. 37, 583.

Orsler, R.J. (1973) Personal Communication from Forest Products Research Laboratory, Princes Risborough, Bucks, England.

Senear, F.E. (1933) Dermatitis due to Woods. J.Am. med. Ass. 101, 1527.

Weber, L.F. (1953) Dermatitis venenata due to Native Woods. Archs. Derm.

Hegnauer, R. (1964) Chemotaxonomy of Plants. Vol. 3. Basel, Birkhauser. p. 255.

Alnus

Apple (*Malus*), carrot (*Dauca*), parsnip (*Pastinaca*) and potato (*Solanum*) less often other vegetables produced immediate type hypersensitivity reactions in persons who were hypersensitive to birch pollen (*Alnus*) (Hannuksela and Lahti 1977).

Reference

Hannuksela, M. and Lahti, A. (1977) Immediate reactions to fruit and vegetables. Contact dermatitis 3, 79-84.

Betula

About 60 species occur, notably in the North Temperate regions, extending to the Arctic. The wood of some species is much used in turnery and especially for broom handles and similar purposes.

Betula alba

The bark of this species is used for tanning Russian Leather. Destructive distillation of the bark and wood yields birch tar oil, which contains phenol, cresol, xylenol and various terpenes (Merck 1968). Phototoxicity from birch juice (Espersen 1952) lacks substantiation.

The wood has been reported to cause dermatitis (Duke 1927, Howes 1951) with positive patch tests, but the nature of the allergen has not been established.

Betula lenta
Black Birch, Mountain Mahogany.

The bark yields methyl salicylate (oil of wintergreen), which is rubefacient.

Betula lutea

This species is listed as an irritant wood (Orsler 1973).

Betula papyrifera
Paper Birch

This species is used for making canoes. Dermatitis caused by this wood has been attributed to the fine powder beneath the bark, which causes folliculitis (Hardwood Record 1932).

Betula pendula

This species is listed as a wood causing dermatitis (Hanslian and Kadlec 1966).

References

Duke, W.W. (1927) Allergy, asthma, hay fever, urticaria and allied manifestations of reactions. 2nd. ed. London, Kimpton.

Espersen, E. (1952) Berlocque dermatitis. A survey and a case. Acta. Derm-Venereol. 32, 91. Suppl. 29.

Hanslian, L. and Kadlec, K. (1966) Drevo z hlediska hygienickehi VIII. Biologicky ucinne a malo ucinne dreviny. Drevo 21, 229.

Hardwood Record (1932) Sept.`10, p. 24, cited by Senear (1933).

Howes, H.C. (1951) Occupational dermatitis. Canad. Woodwork. 34 and 64.

Merck Index (1968) ed. Stecher P.G. 8th ed. Rahway, N.J. Merck and Co.

Orsler, R.J. (1973) Personal Communication from Forest Products Research Laboratory, Princes, Risborough, Bucks, England.

Senear, F.E. (1933) Dermatitis due to woods. JAMA 101, 1527.

BIGNONIACEAE

This predominantly tropical family consists mainly of trees and of shrubs, many of them climbers. There are some 650 species, placed in 120 genera. Many species yield valuable timber.

The family is rich in saponins, quinones and alkaloids (Hegnauer 1964, Thomson 1971). Among the most interesting is the naphthaquinone called lapachol (formerly known as Tecomin), which is 2-hydroxy-3-(3-methyl-2-butenyl)-1,4-naphthoquinone (Gibbs 1963). It is present in species of Tecoma, Paratecoma and Tabebuia, but whilst it is abundant in some species, it occurs only sparingly in others and is absent in others, apparently closely related such as Tabebuia pentaphylla. It is present however in Avicennia, now regarded as in a distinct family, but formerly classified with the Verbenaceae. It may well occur in other genera of Bignoniaceae, but its presense in other families is not proven.

Lapachol is an allergic sensitizer but a very much less potent one than deoxylapachol, which was first isolated from Tectona grandis (Verbenaceae) by Sandermann and Simatupang (1962, 1963). It was later isolated from Tabebuia species (Dietrichs 1964, Burnett and Thompson 1968) and may well be present in other Bignoniaceae (Hausen 1970).

Cross-sensitivity occurs between lapachol and deoxylapachol (Hausen 1970).

References

Burnett, A.R. and Thompson, R.H. (1968) Naturally occurring quinones. XII Extractives from Tabebuia chrysantha Nichols and

and other Bignoniaceae. J. chem. Soc. 850.

Dietrichs, H.H. (1964) Deoxylapachol in *Tabebuia* sp. Naturwiss. 17, 408.

Gibbs, R.C. (1963) History of Chemical Taxonomy in Chemical Plant Taxonomy. Ed. Swain, T. London, Academic Press.

Hausen, B.M. (1970) Untersuchungen über gesundheitsschädigenden Hölzer. Thesis Munich.

Hegnauer R. (1964) Chemotaxonomy of Plants. Vol. 3. Basel, Birkhauser P. 268.

Sandermann, W. and Simatupang, M.H. (1962) A Toxic Quinone from Teak Wood. Agnew. Chem.(Internat. Ed.) 1, 599.

Sandermann, W. and Simatupang, M.H. (1963) Über Inhaltsstoffe aus Teak (*Tectona grandis* L.) I. Isolierung und Konstitution eines toxischen Teakchinons. Chem. Ber. 96, 2182.

Thomson, R.H. (1971) Naturally Occurring Quinones, London. Academic Press.

Arrabidaea

70 species are found in tropical America.

Arrabidaea chica Chica

A red pigment from the leaves was used as a body paint by American Indians (Howes 1974).

Reference

Howes, F.N. (1974) A dictionary of useful and everyday plants and their common names. Cambridge. University Press.

Bignonia

Only one species *B. capreolata*, is now retained in this genus.

Bignonia brasiliana
one of many species known as Jacaranda

Under this name is listed a wood capable of causing dermatitis (Sandermann and Barghoorn 1956).
see *Jacaranda*

Reference

Sandermann, W. and Barghoorn, A.W. (1956a) Gesundheitsschädigende Nutzhölzer. Holz Roh-Werkst. 14, 37.

Sandermann, W. and Barghoorn, A.W. (1956b) Gesundheitsschädigende Hölzer. Holz Roh-Werkst. 14,87.

Campsis
Trumpet creeper

There are two species in this genus: *C. radicans* of the south east U.S.A., and *C. chinensis* of East Asia. Both are beautiful climbing plants which are extensively cultivated. *C. radicans* is hardy out of doors in the milder areas of Britain and Northern Europe.

The number of cases of dermatitis reported in those handling the flowers or leaves is likely to be a measure of their popularity rather than an indication of high sensitizing potential. All reports incriminate the commoner *C. radicans* but identification may not always have been reliable, since hybrids and cultivars are numerous (Pammel 1911, Muenscher 1951, Gardner and Bennetts 1956, McCord 1962, Hardin and Arena 1969).

References

Gardner, C.A. and Bennetts, H.W. (1956) The Toxic Plants of Western Australia. Perth, West Australian Newspapers Ltd.

Hardin, J.W. and Arena, J.M. (1969) Human Poisoning from Native and Cultivated Plants. Durham, North Carolina, Duke Univ. Press.

McCord, C.P. (1962) The Occupational Toxicity of Cultivated Flowers. Ind. Med. Surg. 31, 365.

Muenscher, W.C. (1951) Poisonous Plants of the United States. 2nd. Edit. New York, Macmillan.

Pammel, L.H. (1911) A Manual of Poisonous Plants. Cedar Rapids, Iowa, Torch Press. Reprinted Univ. Microfilms, Inc., Ann Arbor, Mich. 1965, pp. 476-7.

Catalpa

This genus contains 11 species of trees, natives of East Africa and of North and South America. Several species are extensively cultivated for their horticultural value, and some yield a useful timber.

Catalpa bignonioides
Indian Bean, Catalpa

This is the most popular species in cultivation for the beauty of its flowers. Its timber is durable.

The emanations of the fragrant flowers are said to be toxic and to irritate the skin and mucous membrane (White 1887, Pammel 1911, Weber 1937, Hurst 1943, Muenscher 1951), but the evidence seems inconclusive.

Catalpa speciosa
Western Catalpa

Handling the flowers has apparently caused dermatitis (Pammel 1911, Muenscher 1951). All listings appear to stem from anecdotal reports received by White (1887).

References

Hurst, E. (1942) The Poison Plants of New South Wales. N.S.W. Poison Plants Committee, Sydney.

Muenscher, W.C. (1951) Poisonous Plants of the United States. 2nd Ed. New York, The Macmillan Co.

Pammel, L.H. (1911) A Manual of Poisonous Plants. Cedar Rapids, Iowa, Torch Press. Reprinted Univ. Microfilms, Inc., Ann Arbor, Mich., 1965, pp. 476-7.

Weber, L.F. (1937) External Causes of Dermatitis. A List of Irritants. Archs. Derm. Syph. 35, 129.

White, J.C. (1887) Dermatitis venenata: an Account of the Action of External Irritants upon the Skin. Boston, Cupples and Hurd.

Jacaranda

There are about 50 species in Central and South America and the West Indies. Many of these trees and shrubs are very ornamental and are cultivated where conditions are suitable. The wood of J. chelonia is used in cabinet making.

Unfortunately the word Jacaranda is used as the common name for several trees in the Leguminosae family. It is therefore impossible to interpret many case reports of dermatitis, in which the responsible species has not been botanically identified. It is probable that in most such reports species of Dalbergia were responsible since some of them are potent sensitizers.

Jacaranda braziliensis

This species is said to contain lapachol (Schulz 1962, Krogh 1964).

It has been reported to cause dermatitis (Sandermann and Barghoorn 1956), probably referring to jacaranda (Dalbergia or Machaerium).

Jacaranda acutifolia

Jacaranda ovalifolia

These species are listed as irritant woods (Schwartz et al 1957).

Jacaranda
Boxwood substitutes (see Buxaceae)

Euxylophora and Jacaranda have been used as boxwood substitutes. Jacaranda as a genus name and jacaranda as a common name (e.g. for Dalbergia) and Machaerium have been confused. According to Woods and Calnan (1976), Sandermann and Barghoorn (1956) are not the only authors who have fallen into the trap of confusing Jacaranda, the scientific name of this genus of Bignoniaceae with jacaranda, the popular name in Brazil for several species of Dalbergia and Machaerium of the Leguminosae family.

References

Krogh, H.K. (1964) Contact Eczema Caused by True Teak (Tectona grandis). A Follow-up Study of a Previous Epidemiological Investigation, and a study into the Sensitizing Effect of Various Teak Extracts. Br. J. industr. Med. 21, 65.

Sandermann, W. and Barghoorn, A.W. (1956) Gesundheitsschädigende Nutzhölzer. Holz Roh-Werkst. 14, 37 and 87.

Schulz, K.H. (1962) Untersuchungen über die sensibilisierende Wirkung von Inhaltssoffen. Hölzer

Berufsdermatosen 10, 17

Schwartz, L., Tulipan, L. and Birmingham, D.J. (1957) Occupational Diseases of the Skin. 3rd. Edit. Philadelphia, Lea & Febiger, pp. 637-672.

Woods, B. and Calnan, C.D. (1976) Toxic Woods. Brit. J. Derm. 94, Suppl. 13, June.

Paratecoma peroba
(syn. Tecoma peroba)
Peroba da campos, White Peroba

In other languages the timber is known as "yellow peroba", e.g. peroba amarella, peroba jaune, etc.

The single species in this genus is a native of Brazil. The valuable timber is exported to Europe and elsewhere. Because the timber of Aspidosperma polyneuron is superficially similar, the latter is known as Peroba rosa, which introduces an additional hazard for the uninformed student of the literature of Peroba dermatitis. The wood has also been misnamed Illipe or Bassia.

Chemistry

Paratecoma was shown to contain lapachol, lapachonone and an alkaloid (De Jong et al 1951). In their patients with dermatitis patch tests incriminated lapachonone (lapachenole) as the sensitizer; lapachol was present only in small amounts, and the alkaloid provoked no reaction. Sandermann and Barghoorn (1955) showed that lapachonone is both irritant and sensitizing and they suggested that the wood also contained other compounds which might have effects on the skin. Sandermann et al (1968) subsequently isolated a new quinone. The complex chemistry of this species was reviewed by Thomson (1971) and Livingstone and Whiting (1955).

Dermatitis

This wood is among the six most commonly causing dermatitis in France (Zafiropoulo et al 1968). Early accounts of dermatitis from this species were that of Touraine et al 1932, Touraine and Golé (1934). Barnett (1948) described the extensive dermatitis caused by the sawdust, involving hands, face and neck, and sometimes axillae and groins. De Jong et al (1951) found 5 of 25 workers affected and with genital involvement in two of the cases. Patch tests with sawdust were positive in the patients but not in control subjects. The dermatitis relapsed when the patients entered the shed in which the timber was stored.

The sawdust can also cause asthma and conjunctivits (Orsler 1969, 1973, Zschunke 1963).

References

Barnett, (1948) Annual report of the Chief Inspector of factories and workshops. p. 93. London.

De Jong, J.C., Lenstra, J.B. and Vermeer, J.H. (1951) Eczema due to the Wood of Peroba da Campos: Isolation of the Allergen. Acta derm. -vener., Stockh. 31, 108.

Livingstone, R. and Whiting, M.C. (1955) The Structure of Lapachenole, a Hardwood Extractive. J. Chem. Soc. 138, 3631.

Orsler, R.J. (1969) The Effects of Irritant Timbers. Woodworking Industry, 26, 28.

Orsler, R.J. (1973) Personal Communication from Forest Products Research Laboratory, Princes Risborough, Bucks, England.

Sandermann, W. and Barghoorn, A.W. (1955) Über die Inhaltstoffe von Makoré und Peroba-Holz, sowie ihre gesundheitschädigende Wirkung. Holzforsch 9, 112.

Sandermann, W. Simatupang, M.H. and Wendeborn W. (1968) Neue Chinone aus dem Kernholz von Paratecoma peroba Kuhlm. Naturwiss 55, 38.

Thomson, R.H. (1971) Naturally Occurring Quinones. London. Academic Press.

Touraine, A. and Golé, L. (1934) Les dermatites par bois toxiques Paris méd. 91, 62.

Touraine, J.V., Hesse, J. and Golé (1932) Vingt cas de dermatite par bois satine ('Peroba grande amarella'). Bull. Soc. franc Derm. Syph. 39, 1392.

Zafiropoulo, A., Audibert, A. and Charpin, J. (1968) A propos des accidents due a la manipulation des bois exotiques. Rev. franc. Allerg., Vol. 8, 155.

Zschunke, E. (1963) Krankheiten durch den Umgang mit Holz Holztechn. 4, 51.

Pseudocalymma

There are four species, natives of tropical America and the West Indies.

Pseudocalymma alliaceum, Garlic Vine

Two workmen who trimmed this plant developed burning and swelling of the face (Golby 1971).

Reference

Golby, E. (1971) Personal Communication to Morton (1971).

Morton, J.F. (1971) Plants Poisonous to People in Florida and other warm areas. Miami, Fla. Hurricane House.

Tabebuia

About 100 species are distributed over an area ranging from Mexico to northern Argentina, including the West Indies.

Many species provide valuable timber, and many of them, perhaps all, can cause dermatitis in some individuals (Orsler 1973). Dogmatism is out of place, because the haphazard use of trade or popular names in many reports makes retrospective identification of the species uncertain.

Tabebuia avellanedae
Ipé prêto

The timber has many uses for internal and external constructional work and much is exported.

From 500 Gm of the heartwood, about 6 naphthaquinones and 9 anthraquinones and 9 mg of deoxylapachol have been isolated (Burnett and Thomson 1967).

Tabebuia lapacho Lapacho

The timber is used principally for furniture.

The wood contains lapachol, lapachonone and probably deoxylapachol (Hausen 1973).

Tabebuia pentaphylla Roble

Some of the timber is exported to Europe for use in furniture manufacture. At the turn of the century large quantities were used, especially in England, under the names of "Maracaibo boxwood" and "Zaputeau" (Hausen 1973).

The chemical composition is probably similar to that of the above species.

Tabebuia serratifolia
Ipé, Bethabara

The timber is harder and more durable than that of the other species of Tabebuia available in commerce.

The wood contains lapachol and deoxylapachol. Deoxylapachol is also derived from Tectona.

Tabebuia ipe
(syn. T. avellanedae)
Ipé, ipé tabaco, lapacho

Tabebuia serratifolia
(syn. Tecoma leucoxylon, Bignonia leucoxylon)
Bethabara, Surinam greenheart

Tabebuia guayacan
(syn. Tabebuia lapacho)
Guayacan

The sawdust of ipé tabaco irritates the nose, lungs and skin. Washing off the dust causes a change in colour of the skin from yellow-green to bright red (Woolston and Phillips 1955). 83 cases of dermatitis, respiratory and constitutional symptoms from sawdust of ipé were reported by Freise (1932, 1936). He reported three human deaths and expulsion of worms from swallowing the wood dust.

The woods of these species which were formerly often named Tecoma contain lapachol, lapachonone and small quantities of deoxylapachol. (Hausen et al 1971), (Hausen 1973), (Burnett and Thompson 1967). T. palmieri can cause dermatitis (Ortega 1926, Burnett and Thompson 1968).

The wood of Tabebuia spp. can cause dermatitis, conjunctivitis and respiratory symptoms (Weitbrecht 1967) and constitutional symptoms (Cordero and Lynch 1951).

References

Burnett, A.R. and Thompson, R.H. (1968) Extractives from Tabebuia chryantha Nichols. and other Bignoniaceae. J. Chem. Soc.(c) 850.

Freise, F.W. (1932) Gesundheitsschädigungen durch Arbeiten mit giftigen Hölzern. Beobachtungen aus brasilianischen Gewerbebetrieben. Archiv fur Gewerbepathologie und Gewbehygiene 3, 1

Freise, F.W. (1936) Vergiftungen durch Brasilianische Werkholzer I, II. Sammlung der Vergiftungsfällen 7C, 1 & 61.

Hausen, B.M., Simatupang, M.H. and Weitbrecht, U. (1971) Allergie gegen Bethabara-Holz. Berufsdermatosen 19, 324.

Hausen, B.M. (1973) Holzarten mit gesundheitsschädigenden inhaltsstoffen Stuttgart. DRW-Verlags-GmbH.

Burnett, A.R. and Thomson R.H. (1967) Naturally occurring quinones. X: The guinone constituents of Tabebuia avellanedae (Brynoniaceae) J. chem. Soc. 2100.

Cordero, A. and Lynch, H. (1951) Occupational Sensitization to Lapochowood Sawdust. Prensa méd. argent. 38, 838.

Orsler, R.J. (1973) Personal Communication from Forest Products Research Laboratory, Princes Risborough, Bucks, England.

Ortega (1926) quoted by Record, S.J. Tropical Woods 7, 37.

Weitbrecht, U. (1967) Allergy to Bethabara wood (German) Berufsderm. 15, 183.

Woolston, A. and Phillips, E.J. (1955) Utilization of some of the woods in Alto Paraguay. Tropical woods. 102, 23.

Tecoma

There are 16 species in the region between Florida and Argentina. Some produce a useful timber, others are used as a source of tecomin, a yellow dye, which turns red in alkaline solution.

Those species studied have been rich in quinones, which often include lapachol (Thomson 1971).

Several species, e.g. T. avellanaedae, T. pentaphylla and T. serratifolia are now transferred to the genus Tabebuia.

Tecoma impetiginosa
Ipé roxo

Tecoma insignis
Ipé tabacco

These species contain lapachol derivatives (Hausen 1973).

The Tecoma spp. reported by Freise in 1932 and 1936 to produce dermatitis, respiratory and constitutional symptoms have now been transferred to Tabebuia.

References

Hausen, B.M. (1973) Holzarten mit gesundheitsschädigenden inhaltstoffen Stuttgart, D.R.W.-Verlags.-GmbH.

Thomson, R.H. (1971) Naturally Occurring Quinones. London. Academic Press.

BIXACEAE

Four species in one genus are of tropical distribution.

Chemistry is recorded by Hegnauer (1964).

Reference

Hegnauer, R. (1964) Chemotaxonomy of Plants. Vol. 3. Basel, Birkhauser. p. 282.

Bixa

The species are native to tropical America and the West Indies.

Bixa orellana
Lipstick Tree

This species is cultivated for its seed which yields the food dye, annatto. Annatto was used as a red colouring for the body of South-American Indians (Corner 1952). The leaves and unripe fruits are said to have irritant properties.

Reference

Corner, E.J.H. (1952) Wayside Trees of Malaysia. Singapore, Government Printer.

BLEPHAROCARYACEAE

Two species in one genus found in northern and eastern Australia are tall trees. The family is closely related to Anacardiaceae.

Blepharocarya

The distribution is that of the family.

Blepharocarya involucrigera
Bolly Gum

North Queensland forest officers are unanimous in stating that the wood is poisonous if rubbed on the skin (Cleland 1943).

Reference

Cleland, J.B. (1943) Plants including fungi, poisonous or otherwise injurious to man in Australia. IV. Med. J. Australia. 11, 161.

BOMBACACEAE

180 species in 20 genera are found in tropical regions especially in America. Bombax malabaricum (syn. B. ceiba) furnishes Kapok.

Chemistry is recorded by Hegnauer (1964).

Reference

Hegnauer, R. (1964) Chemotaxonomy of Plants. Vol. 3. Basel, Birkhauser, p. 284.

Adansonia

Ten species are of palaeotropical distrubiton.

Adansonia digitata
Baobab

The seeds have a taste like ginger and the leaves and pounded bark are used as a condiment. The blossoms are extremely malodorous (Menninger 1967) and are pollinated by bats (Howes 1974). The tree burns with an irritating smoke. It can be dangerous to walk over the place where the rotten tap root of a Baobab is, because one can drop down into a large cavity filled with decaying pulp (Irvine 1961).

References

Howes, F.N. (1974) A Dictionary of Useful and Everyday Plants and their Common Names. Cambridge University Press. pp. 290.

Irvine, F.R. (1961) Woody plants of Ghana. Oxford University Press. London.

Menninger, E.A. (1967) Fantastic Trees. New York. The Viking Press.

Ceiba

Ten species are native to tropical America.

Ceiba pentandra
Silk Cotton Tree

This species, which is cultivated in West Africa, furnishes Kapok. The tree is not recommended for town planting since the floss of the seed-capsules is irritating to the eyes and nose. (Irvine 1961).

Reference

Irvine, F.R. (1961) Woody plants of Ghana. Oxford University Press. London

Durio

27 species are found in Burma and western Malaysia.

Durio zibethinus
Durian

The large spiny malodorous fruits are a hazard to passers-by as they fall from the tree (Menninger 1967). Eating the fruits can cause irritation especially in the angles of the mouth (Fasal 1945).

References

Fasal, P. (1945) Cutaneous Diseases

in the Tropics. Arch. Derm. syph. 51, 166.

Menninger, E.A. (1967) Fantastic Trees. New York. The Viking Press.

Neesia

Eight species are found in western Malaysia.

Neesia spp.

Bristles which are present on the inner side of the woody fruit capsules can produce mechanical injury to the skin (Burkill 1935, Corner 1952).

References

Burkill, I.H. (1935) A Dictionary of the Economic Products of the Malay Peninsula. 2 vols. London. Crown Agents for the Colonies.

Corner, E.J.H. (1952) Wayside Trees of Malaysia. Singapore, Government Printer.

Ochroma

One species is found from southern Mexico to Bolivia and in the West Indies.

Ochroma pyramidale Balsa
(syn. O. lagopus)

The wood is said to be irritant (Hanslian and Kadlec 1966).

Reference

Hanslian, L. and Kadlec, K. (1966) Wood from the standpoint of hygiene. VIII. Species with some or little biological effect. Drevo. 21, 229.

BORAGINACEAE

2000 species in 100 genera are found in tropical and temperate regions especially in the Mediterranean area. French women used Anchusa tinctoria to paint the face (Gerard 1639). Alkanna tinctoria yields the dye, alkannet. Lithospermum erythrorhizon is used to make a purple dye in Japan.

Chemistry is recorded by Hegnauer (1964).

References

Gerard, J. (1636) The Herball or Generall Historie of Plantes. The essence thereof distilled by M. Woodward (1927) from the edition of Th. Johnson 1630. London. Gerald Howe.

Hegnauer, R. (1964) Chemotaxonomy of Plants. Vol. 3. Basel, Birkhauser. p. 288.

Borago

Three species are found in the Mediterranean region, Europe and Asia.

Borago officinalis
Borage

Short bristly hairs on the leaves are irritant to the hands (Cheney cited by White 1887). This species is cultivated in gardens and as a bee-plant. It was formerly used in salads, but is now more commonly added to certain drinks, and is therefore handled by barmen.

Reference

White, J.C. (1887) Dermatitis venenata: An account of the Action of External irritants upon the Skin. Boston. Cupples and Hurd. Cheney was a dealer in medicinal plants.

Cynoglossum

Between 50 and 60 species are found in temperate and subtropical regions.

Cynoglossum officinale
Hound's Tongue

The fruits are covered with hooks. The plant is used in Herbal Medicine in an ointment for haemorrhoids (Wren 1968).

Reference

Wren, R.W. (1968) Potter's new Cyclopaedia of Botanical Drugs and Preparations by Wren, R.C. Re-edit. by Wren, R.W. Potter and Clarke Ltd. Health Science Press. Rustington, Sussex.

Echium

40 species are found in the

Canaries, Azores, northern and southern Africa, Europe and western Asia.

Echium plantagineum
Peterson's Curse

This species can cause a rash when handled by susceptible persons from the abrasive action of its stiff hairs and possibly from an allergenic property (Aplin 1966).

Echium vulgare
Viper's Bugloss

The hairs of the plant can cause dermatitis (Pammel 1911).

References

Aplin, T.E.H. (1966) Poison Plants in the Garden. West Australian Dept. Agr. J. 7, 24.

Pammel, L.H. (1911) A Manual of Poisonous plants. Torch Press. Cedar Rapids, Iowa. Reprinted Univ. Microfilms Inc. Ann Arbor, Mich. 1965. pp. 476-7.

Heliotropium

250 species are found in tropical and temperate regions.

Heliotropium sp.

A pharmaceutical worker developed dermatitis from contact with a species of this genus and from Duboisia (Trautner 1949).

Reference

Trautner, E.M. (1949) A contribution to the causation of atropine allergy. Med. J. Australia 2, 17.

Lappula

50 species are found in temperate Eurasia and Australia; five species are found in North America.

Lappula sp.
(syn. Echinospermum)

The wood of Echinospermum balthazarii (vinhatico) was reported to be injurious by Freise (1932).

Lappula myosotis

The fruits are armed with hooks.

Reference

Freise, F.W. (1932) Gesundheitsschädigungen durch Arbeiten mit giftigen Hölzern. Beobachtungen aus brasilianischen Gewerbebetrieben Arch. Gewerbepath. hyg. 3, 1.

Lycopsis

Three species are found in Europe and Asia.

Lycopsis arvensis Bugloss

The rough hairs of this species have irritant properties (Woods 1962).

Reference

Woods, B. (1962) Irritant Plants. Trans. St. John's Hosp. derm. Soc. 48, 75.

Myosotis

50 species are found in temperate Eurasia, on mountains of tropical Africa, in southern Africa, Australia and New Zealand.

Myosotis sp.
Forget-me-not

Species of this genus may produce irritant patch test reactions (Hjorth 1968).

Reference

Hjorth, N. (1968) at Finsen Institute. Pers. comm.

Pentaglottis
(syn. Anchusa)

One species is found in south-western Europe.

Pentaglottis sempervirens

The plant may have irritant properties from its rough hairs (Woods 1962).

Reference

Woods, B. (1962) Irritant Plants. Trans. St. John's Hosp. derm. Soc. 48, 75.

Pulmonaria

The 10 species are natives to Europe, but some are cultivated elsewhere.

Pulmonaria officinalis
Lungwort

One patient developed dermatitis after handling this plant in her garden. A patch test with a leaf provoked diffuse erythema and oedema: in 8 of 17 control subjects tested there was a mild punctate erythema; in the remainder there was no reaction (Woods 1962). It appears that there is individual variation in susceptibility to mechanical irritation by the hairs, and that allergic sensitization can also occur.

Reference

Woods, B. (1962) Irritant Plants. Trans. St. John's Hosp. derm. Soc., Lond. 48, 75.

Symphytum

25 species are found in Europe and from the Mediterranean region to the Caucasus. S. asperrimum is cultivated for fodder.

Symphytum officinale
Comfrey

The hairy or prickly leaves of this species have irritant properties (Woods 1962).

Reference

Woods, B. (1962) Irritant Plants. Trans. St. John's Hosp. derm. Soc. 48, 75.

Tournefortia

150 species are found in tropical and subtropical regions.

Tournefortia hirsutissima
Chiggernit

This hairy plant can produce mechanical injury (Oakes and Butcher 1962).

Reference

Oakes, A.J. and Butcher, J.O. (1962) Poisonous and injurious plants of the U.S. Virgin Islands. Misc. Publ. 882. U.S. Department of Agriculture, Washington, D.C.

BROMELLIACEAE

1400 species in 44 genera are found in tropical America and the West Indies.

Chemistry is recorded by Hegnauer (1962).

Reference

Hegnauer, R. (1962) Chemotaxonomy of Plants. Vol. 2. Basel, Birkhauser. p. 99.

Ananas

Five species are native to tropical America.

Ananas comosus
Pineapple Tree

"Pineapple estate pyosis", occurring in workers who gather the fruits, probably represents an acarus infestation with secondary bacterial infection (Simons 1952). The sharp spears on the pineapple and the high content of sugar which has a hygroscopic effect can cause injury to the hands (Schwartz et al 1957). The raw fruit, when eaten in large quantity, produces a burning sensation of the lips and mouth probably from the action of calcium oxalate crystals and the keratolytic enzyme bromelin (Watt and Breyer-Brandwijk 1962). Angular stomatitis can result from eating the fruit (Fasal 1945).

In workers employed in cutting up pineapples, pressure effects and the keratolytic effect of bromelin almost completely obliterated the finger prints by removal of the stratum corneum of the ridges. The nails were unaffected in contrast to the nail damage which occurs in workers exposed to proteolytic enzymes of animal origin. The variety named Mauritius pineapple seemed to be most injurious. Calcium oxalate crystals and citric acid were excluded as a cause of the skin changes. Moniliasis of the finger webs was occasionally observed in pineapple cutters (Polunin 1951). A positive patch test reaction to pineapple in a fruit handler (Morris 1954) cannot be interpreted in the absence of controls.

Ananas magdalenae

The strong sharp recurved hooks on the leaves can inflict mechanical injury (Allen 1943).

References

Allen, P.H. (1943) Poisonous and Injurious Plants of Panama. Am. J. Trop. Med. Suppl. 23, 1

Fasal, P. (1945) Cutaneous Diseases in the Tropics. Arch. Derm. Syph. 51, 166.

Morris, G.E. (1954) Dermatoses among Food Handlers. Industr. Med. Surg. 23, 343.

Polunin, I. (1951) Pineapple Dermatosis. Brit. J. Dermat. 63, 441.

Schwartz, L., Tulipan, L. and Birmingham, D.J. (1957) Occupational Diseases of the Skin. 3rd. ed. Philadelphia. Lea and Febiger. pp. 637-672.

Simons, R.D.G. (1952) Handbook of Tropical Dermatology. New York. Elsevier.

Watt, J.M. and Breyer-Brandwijk, M.G. (1962) The Medicinal and poisonous plants of Southern Africa. 2nd ed. Edinburgh. E. & S. Livingstone.

Ananas sativus

Ethyl acrylate, found in the fruits, produced sensitisation in 10 of 24 subjects by a maximisation test. The compound is used in soap, detergent, creams, lotions, perfumes and food (Opdyke 1974).

Reference

Opdyke, D.L.J. (1974) Monographs on fragrance raw materials. Ed. Cosmet. Toxicol. 12, 919.

Bromelia

40 species are found in tropical America and the West Indies. Some species provide edible fruit.

Bromelia pinguin

Recurved hooks on the leaf margins can produce mechanical injury (Allen 1943, Oakes and Butcher 1962). The fruit juice, when handled for a few hours, produces small painful ulcers on the fingertips. The juice contains the proteolytic enzyme, pinguinain (Asenjo et al 1944).

References

Allen, P.H. (1943) Poisonous and Injurious Plants of Panama. Am. J. Trop. Med. Suppl. 23, 1.

Asenjo, C.F., Guyco, J.A. and Fernandez, M. del C. (1944) Note on presence of calcium oxalate in maya fruit. J. Amer. Pharm. Ass. (Scient. Ed.) 33, 344.

Oakes, A.J. and Butcher, J.O. (1962) Poisonous and injurious plants of the U.S. Virgin Islands. Misc. Publ. 882. U.S. Department of Agriculture, Washington, D.C.

Karatas (syn. Bromelia)

Twenty species are found from Mexico to Argentina.

Karatas

The spines of the edible berries can produce mechanical injury (Burkill 1935).

Reference

Burkill, I.H. (1935) A Dictionary of the Economic Products of the Malay Peninsula. 2 vols. London. Crown Agents for the Colonies.

BRYOPHYTA

Within this natural group are mosses and hepatics. Sphagnum has been used as an absorbent for suppurating wounds (Answers 1917). Five species of moss were briefly reported to produce variable patch test reactions in workers sensitized to the hepatic Frullania (Mitchell et al 1969). Isothecium can grow in close proximity to Frullania. It seems likely that mosses are not in themselves allergenic but that they absorb and retain allergenic sesquiterpene lactones derived from neighbouring Frullania species. This hypothesis, which is based on the variability of patch test reactions to species of moss and on the known capacity of plants to absorb extraneous products (Towers 1969) requires further investigation.

The hepatics Porella and Marchantia have also been noted as

allergenic (Mitchell et al 1969).

References

Answers (1917) Sphagnum moss dressings. Brit.Med. J. 1,752.

Mitchell, J.C., Schofield, W.B., Singh, B. and Towers, G.H.N. (1969) Allergy to Frullania. Allergic contact dermatitis occurring in forest workers caused by exposure to Frullania nisquallensis. Archs. Derm. 100,46.

Towers, G.H.N. (1969) Pers. Comm.

Bryophyta Moss

Peat dust is irritant to the eye possibly from acid salts and silica spicules (Powell 1934).

Sphagnum moss was a source of sporotrichosis (D'Allessio et al 1965).

References

D'Alessio, D.J., Leavens, L.J., Strumpf, G.B. et al (1965). An outbreak of sporotrichosis in Vermont associated with sphagnum moss as a source of infection. New. Eng. J. Med. 272, 1054.

Powell, B.J. (1934) Uniocular conjunctivitis from peat dust. Am. J. Ophth. 17, 206.

BURSERACEAE

500 species in 16 genera are found in tropical regions. Many species provide resins.

Chemistry is recorded by Hegnauer (1964).

Reference

Hegnauer, R. (1964) Chemotaxonomy of Plants. Vol. 3, Basel, Birkhauser, p. 310.

Aucoumea

One species found in tropical West Africa yields a resin.

Aucoumea klaineana
Okumé, Gaboon Mahogany

A furniture maker developed dermatitis while working with okoumé. A patch test gave a positive reaction on a subject who had eczema, negative on a normal control; the furniture maker was not tested (Spitzer 1927). 'Okumen carcomido' produced conjunctivitis and nasal irritation in workers; few of them had skin irritation (Subiza 1958). A joiner who had dermatitis showed positive patch test reactions to gaboon and deal (?Pinus) (Woods and Calnan 1976).

The wood-dust can also produce respiratory symptoms (Gronemeyer and Fuchs 1967).

References

Gronomeyer, W. and Fuchs, E. (1967) Krankheiten durch inhalative Allergen-Invasion. in Hansen-Werner (1967) Lehrbuch der klinischen Allergie. Stuttgart. G. Thieme cited by Hausen(1973).

Hausen, B.M. (1973) Holzarten mit gesundheitsschädigenden Inhaltsstoffen. Stuttgart. DRW-Verlags-GmbH.

Spitzer, E. (1927) Gewerbedermatitis nach Okumé-holz. Zbl. Hat-Geschlkrkh. 22, 615.

Subiza, E. (1958) Pseudo allergia por maderas tropicales. Medicina y seguridad del trabajo 6, 74.

Woods, B. and Calnan, C.D. (1976) Toxic Woods. Brit. J. Derm. 94 Suppl. 13, June.

Boswellia

24 species are found in tropical Africa, Madagascar and tropical Asia. B. carteri and other species yield the resin frankincense or gum olibanum which was formerly officinal and is now used in incense. Other species e.g. B. dalzielii also yield fragrant resins.

Boswellia spp.

The use of olibanum in adhesive plasters (Greenberg and Lester 1954) and in perfumes (Schwartz et al 1957) has caused dermatitis in sensitive individuals. Sixteen patients contact sensitive to Balsam of Peru (Myroxylon) showed negative patch test reactions to olibanum (Hjorth 1961). Olibanum contains pinene, dipentene, etc. (Merck 1968); cross-sensitivity with turpentine (Pinus) requires investigation for apparently inexplicable contact sensitivity to turpentine which might result from exposure to incense and perfume.

References

Greenberg, L.A. and Lester, D. (1954) Handbook of Cosmetic Materials. New York. Interscience.

Hjorth, N. (1961) Eczematous Allergy to Balsams. Munksgaard, International Booksellers and Publishers Ltd. Copenhagen.

Merck Index (1968) An Encyclopedia of Chemicals and Drugs. ed. Stecher, P.G. 8th ed. Rahway, N.J. Merck and Co. Inc.

Schwartz, L., Tulipan, L. and Birmingham, D.J. (1957) Occupational Diseases of the Skin. 3rd. ed. Philadelphia. Lea and Febiger. pp. 637-672.

Bursera

80 species are found in tropical America. Bursera gummifera (Birch tree, Turpentine tree) furnishes the balsam resin known as American elemi.

Bursera spp.
especially B. delpechiana

These species yield Oil of Linaloe. Perfumes, colognes and toilet waters containing Oil of Linaloe may produce dermatitis in hypersensitive individuals (Tulipan 1938). The oil contains linalool, geraniol, etc. (Merck 1968). Linalool caused an outbreak of dermatitis among girls bottling perfume (Schwartz et al 1957). The sensitizing capacity of the oil is said to be due to a constituent, 1-linalool, (Klarmann 1958). One of 14 patients contact sensitive to Balsam of Peru (Myroxylon) showed a positive patch test reaction to elemi. Manila elemi is noted under Canarium.

References

Klarmann, E.G. (1958) Perfume dermatitis. Ann. Allergy. 16, 425.

Merck Index (1968) An Encyclopedia of Chemicals and Drugs. ed. Stecher, P.G. 8th ed. Rahway, N.J. Merck and Co. Inc.

Schwartz, L., Tulipan, L. and Birmingham, D.J. (1957) Occupational Diseases of the Skin. 3rd. ed. Philadelphia. Lea and Febiger. pp. 637-672.

Tulipan, L. (1938) Cosmetic irritants. Archs. Derm. Syph. 38, 906.

Canarium

75 species are found in tropical Africa, Asia, northern Australia and the Pacific region.

Canarium commune

The wood has produced dermatitis in wood-workers (Brezina 1912).

Canarium luzonicum

This species furnishes the resin Manila elemi and Oil of Elemi. Contact sensitivity to elemi is noted under Bursera. The oleoresin of the tree is used as a rubefacient (Quisumbing 1951).

Canarium muelleri
Scrub turpentine

The wood sap is reported to be poisonous when it enters a cut (Cleland 1943).

Canarium strictum

This and other species furnish some of the black dammar of commerce. Sensitivity to dammar is noted under Agathis.

References

Brezina, E. (1912) Internationale Übersicht über Gewerbekrankheiten in Teleky (1912 bis 1913) Wiener Arbeiten aus dem Gebiet der sozialen Medizin. Wien. A. Holder, cited by Hausen (1970).

Cleland, J.B. (1943) Plants including fungi, poisonous or otherwise injurious to man in Australia. IV. Med. J. Australia. 11, 161.

Hausen, B.M. (1970) Untersuchungen über Gesundheitsschädigende Hölzer. Thesis, Hamburg.

Quisumbing, E. (1951) Medicinal Plants of the Philippines. Tech. Bull. 16. Manila, Philippine Islands. Manila Bureau of Printing. 1234 pp.

Commiphora

185 species are found in warm regions of Africa, Madagascar and from Arabia to western India. C. opobalsamum is said to yield Balm of Gilead; other yield bdellium and other resins. A form of Balm of Gilead is derived from Abies balsamea.

Commiphora abyssinica

This and other species yield the gum resin myrrh. One of 13 patients contact sensitive to Balsam of Peru (Myroxylon) gives a positive patch test reaction to myrrh (Hjorth 1961).

Commiphora gileadense (syn. Balsamodendron)

Balsamodendron gileadense was suspected of producing allergic effects (Bardel 1935).

Commiphora pyracanthoides

This species produces a stinging burning sensation on the lips followed by swelling (Watt and Breyer-Brandwijk 1962).

References

Bardel, S. (1935) Les dermatoses par bois toxiques. These. Paris. 91 pp. cited by Hausen (1970).

Hausen, B.M. (1970) Untersuchungen über Gesundheitsschädigende Hölzer. Thesis, Hamburg.

Hjorth, N. (1961) Eczematous Allergy to Balsams. Munksgaard, International Booksellers and Publishers Ltd., Copenhagen.

Watt, J.M. and Breyer-Brandwijk, M.G. (1962) The Medicinal and poisonous plants of Southern Africa. 2nd. ed. Edinburgh, E. & S. Livingstone.

BUXACEAE

100 species in four genera are found in tropical and temperate regions.

Chemistry is recorded by Hegnauer (1964).

Reference

Hegnauer, R. (1964) Chemotaxonomy of Plants. Vol. 3. Basel, Birkhauser, p. 318.

Buxus

70 species are found in temperate Eurasia, tropical and southern Africa and Madagascar to the Malay Peninsula, Borneo, the Philippines and Lesser Sunda islands, North and Central America and the West Indies.

Buxus sempervirens Box

Acute dematitis of the face followed application of a decoction of the plant to the scalp for alopecia (White 1887, 1889). The juice of the plant can cause irritation and intense itching (Cheney cited by White 1887).

Some confusion may have arisen with Boxwood (Gonioma) which is indisputably irritant.

A watch maker who used box sawdust to clean gold developed asthma; a positive scratch to the dust was observed (Markin 1930). Contact dermatitis from the leaves was reported by Oppenheim (1913). Reports of dermatitis from the wood (Nestler 1929, Nordin 1947) are dubious.

Buxus macowani is known as East London or Cape Boxwood.

References

Hausen, B.M. (1973) Holzarten mit gesundheitsschädigenden Inhaltsstoffen. Stuttgart. DRW-Verlags-GmbH.

Markin, L.E. (1930) Boxwood sensitiveness. J. Allergy 1, 346.

Nestler, A. (1929) Hautreizende Pflanzen. Umschau 33, 611.

Nordin, J. (1947) Yrkessjukdomar (Industrial Diseases) 2, 605 Uppsala.

Oppenheim, M. (1913) Buchs. Baumdermatitis bei einem Gartner. Osterr. Sanitatsw 25, 1291.

White, J.C. (1887) Dermatitis venenata: An account of the Action of External irritants upon the Skin. Boston.

Cupples and Hurd. Cheney was a dealer in medicinal drugs.

White, J.C. (1889) Some unusual forms of dermatitis venenata. Boston med. Surg. J. 71, 583.

Boxwoods

Boxwoods are derived from several botanical species. Thus, the common names and botanical names of some boxwoods according to Woods and Calnan (1976) are as follows:

Abassian boxwood
Buxus sempervirens

African boxwood
Gonioma kamassi

Cape boxwood
Buxus macowani

East London boxwood
Buxus macowani

European boxwood
Buxus sempervirens

Iranian boxwood
Buxus sempervirens

Kamassi boxwood
Gonioma kamassi

Knysna boxwood
Gonioma kamassi

Maracaibo boxwood
Gossypiospermum praecox

Turkey boxwood
Buxus sempervirens

Venezuelan boxwood
Gossypiospermum praecox

West African boxwood
Nauclea trillesii (syn. *Sarcocephalus diderichii*)

West Indian boxwood
Gossypiospermum praecox

According to Woods and Calnan (1976) cocuswood (*Brya* syn. *Amerimnum*, *Inga*) replaced boxwood for some musical instruments.

Reference

Woods, B. and Calnan, C.D. (1976) Toxic woods. Brit. J. Derm. 94, Suppl. 13, June.

CACTACEAE

Perhaps 2,000 species in between 50 and 150 genera are chiefly found in the drier regions of tropical America.

Chemistry is recorded by Hegnauer (1964).

Reference

Hegnauer, R. (1964) Chemotaxonomy of plants. Vol. 3. Basel, Birkhauser, p. 324.

The members of this family are usually provided with spines which are sometimes barbed. *Opuntia* possesses, in additon to spines, tufts of short barbed hairs, named glochids, arising from cushion-like structures, named areoles. The sap of cacti is commonly watery or mucilaginous in contrast to the milky latex of cactiform *Euphorbia* spp.

Mechanical injury

The spines of the plants can cause mechanical injury. The Mexican Aztecs of about 1200-1600 A.D. ritually impaled victims on the tops of spiny cacti (Rowley 1960). Deep penetration of a cactus spine can produce a mass resembling sarcoma (Costa 1943) or pseudotuberculous lesions of bone (Warthin and Davies 1924, Buhr 1960).

The glochids of the plants can produce mechanical injury accompanied by local toxic and/or allergic effects which are described under *Cactus* and *Opuntia*.

References

Buhr, A.J. (1960) The thorn in the flesh. Lancet 1, 309.

Costa, A.J. (1943) Lesion cavernosa de condilo femoral interno, producida por espina de cactus Prensa Med (La Paz) 3, 44.

Rowley, G.C. (1960) A short history of succulent plants in A Handbook of Succulent Plants by Jacobsen, H. Vol. I. London. Blandford, p. 1.

Warthin, A.S. and Davies, J.E. (1924) Cactus-spine pseudotubercles. Ann. Clin. Med. 2,248.

The classification of the 2,000 or more species in this family is more than usually controversial. Some authorities recognise 50 genera, others three times as many. The Cactaceae are predominantly natives of the drier regions of tropical and subtropical America, but many species have been extensively naturalised in other countries with a suitable climate, notably the Mediterranean region, India, Africa and Australia. Moreover the greenhouse cultivation of "cacti" is a popular hobby in many parts of Europe.

Unfortunately the word "cactus" is applied very loosely by some authors to a wide range of succulent plants in other families and even to any spring plants having a superficial resemblance to a cactus. For example the "Candelabra Cactus" is *Euphorbia lactea*.

The genera and species reported as provoking skin reactions of various kinds are probably no more offensive than related species, which enjoy no such ill repute. The essential variable is the opportunity for human exposure to occur.

Many of the observations on the reactions to spines and glochids of *Opuntia* sp., are certainly applicable to other genera.

Acanthocereus

There are 8 species in this genus. *A.pentagonus* is listed as a cause of mechanical injury (Oakes and Butcher 1962), and doubtless other species share this property.

Reference

Oakes, A.J. and Butcher, J.O. (1962) Poisonous and Injurious Plants of the U.S. Virgin Islands. Misc. Publ. 882, U.S. Dept. of Agriculture, Washington, D.C.

Cactus

40 species are found in central and tropical South America and the West Indies.

Cactus spp.

Sutton (1918) described a disorder which was comparatively common in the arid regions of the western United States, most of those affected being gasoline tractor drivers. The eruption was confined to be skin of the limbs and resulted from the spines of cactus plants breaking off in the skin; secondary infection and severe ulceration were common. Local toxic effects from cactus spines were described by Hauffe (1926), Loewy (1926), Glass (1927) and Stein (1928). A pseudotuberculous lesion was described by Barney (1925). An unidentified spine produced a chronic subcutaneous nodule (Gougerot and Eliascheff 1930).

Glochids entering the skin can produce granulomatous reactions (Winer and Zeilenga 1955), which may be toxic or allergic. Since such reactions are uncommon compared to the large number of cactus injuries suffered in Arizona, an allergic mechanism was postulated by Schreiber et al (1971). They observed positive delayed skin test reactions in two-thirds of affected patients to intradermal injection of extracts of glochids.

Occasional case reports which use "cactus" as a common name are almost valueless, for it is not certain that the plants they refer to are even members of the Cactaceae.

References

Barney, R.E. (1925) Cactus Spine Pseudotubercle. Archs. Derm. 11, 331.

Glass, E. (1927) Klinisch-experimenteller Beitrag zu den Verletzungen durch Kakteenstacheln Arch. Klin. Chir. 145, 658.

Gougerot, H. and Eliascheff, O. (1930) Nodule chronique hypodermodermique par corps etranger non irritant (epine). Arch. Derm.-syph. de Clin. L'Hopital Saint-Louis. p. 162.

Hauffe (1926) Med. Klin. 22, 16, cited by Touton (1932).

Loewy, J. (1926) Uber eine lokale Toxikose nach Verletzung mit Kakteenstalcheln. Med. Klin. 22, 290.

Schreiber, M.M., Shapiro, S.I., Berry, C.A. (1971) Cactus Granulomas of the Skin. An Allergic Phenomenon. Arch. Dermatol. 104, 374.

Stein, R.O. (1928) Eigentümlich verlaufende Krankheitsbilder nach dem Eindringen von Cacteenstacheln in die Haut der Finger. Wien. Klin. Wschr. 2, 1729.

Sutton, R.L. (1918) in discussion of Lain, JAMA 71, 1116 (1918).

Touton, K. (1932) Hauterkrankungen durch phanerogamische Pflanzen und ihre Produkte (Toxicodermia et Allergodermia phytogenes), in Barnewitz, J. et al Angeborene Anomalien, Lichtdermatosen, Pflanzengifte, Thermische Schädigungen, Einfluss Innerer Störungen auf die Haut. Berlin, Verlag von Julius Springer.

Winer, L.H. and Zeilenga, R.H. (1955) Cactus granulomas of the skin: Report of a case. Arch. Derm. 72, 566.

Cereus

50 species are found in South America and the West Indies.

Cereus grandiflorus (syn. Cactus grandiflorus)

Application of the plant to the skin caused pruritus, pustules and excoriations (Piffard 1881).

Reference

Piffard, H.G. (1881) A treatise on the Materia Medica and Therapeutics of the Skin. New York.

Opuntia

250 species are native to America and the Galapagos islands. The fruits of O. vulgaris (Prickly Pear), O. ficus-indica (Indian Fig) and some other species are edible.

Opuntia spp.

Species of this genus are now widely naturalized in the Mediterranean region, Australia and South Africa.

The glochids can cause mechanical injury to the mouth of animals and human skin. If an attempt is made to suck out the glochid from the skin, it is likely to attach itself to the tongue. Glochids may be removed from the skin by application of adhesive plaster over the area of irritation; the plaster is then quickly ripped off (Watt and Breyer-Brandwijk 1962). Melted wax may also be used (Shanon and Sagher 1965). In Africa the plants are placed outside houses as 'burglar alarms' (Irvine 1961).

References

Irvine, F.R. (1961) Woody plants of Ghana. Oxford University Press. London.

Shanon, J. and Sagher, F. (1965) Sabra dermatitis. Occupational dermatitis caused by contact with the prickly pear. Derm. Int. 4, 125.

Watt, J.M. and Breyer-Brandwijk, M.G. (1962) The Medicinal and poisonous plants of Southern Africa. 2nd. ed. Edinburgh. E.& S. Livingstone.

Opuntia ficus-indica
Indian Fig Cactus, Sabra

Occupational dermatitis from gathering this species has long been recognized (Rossiter 1924, Cavallucci 1930). An outbreak in the Mediterranean region was described by Shanon and Sagher (1956, 1965, 1969). Glochids entering the skin of workers engaged in gathering the plant produced lesions of the skin between the fingers. Any part of the skin could be affected leading to a resemblance to scabies. The glochids were transferred to the workers' clothing and thence to other individuals. The hard palate and tongue were occasionally affected. The 'prickly pear' should be picked only when wetted and picking should be stopped when it is windy since the glochids can become air-borne. According to Behl et al (1966) the sap of the plant is irritant and can produce eczematous dermatitis. The epidemic of 'Sabra dermatitis' has ceased since with the increased prosperity, the prickly pear is no longer picked for food (Sagher 1973, pers. comm.).

Opuntia macrodasys
Bunny's Ears

This species is popular with green-house collectors. The glochids cause intense irritation (Behl et al 1966).

Opuntia robusta

The glochids produced an eruption on the left arm and left thigh. The forced warm air system of the house blew the glochids into the clothing covering these sites (Kirsch 1958).

One of us (A.J.R.) has seen extensive "Sabra dermatitis: of the back and thighs in a holiday maker who fell into a "prickly pear" in Majorca.

References

Behl, P.N., Captain, R.M., Bedi, B.M.S. and Gupta, S. (1966) Skin-irritant and sensitizing plants found in India, New Delhi. P.N. Behl, Irwin Hospital.

Cavallucci, U. (1930) Di una dermatite professionale da spine di fico d'India. Rinasc. med. 7, 90.

Kirsch, N. (1958) An unusual case of contact dermatitis. Connecticut Med. 22, 756.

Rossiter, C.B. (1924) Letters, Notes etc. Brit. Med. J. 2, 604.

Shanon, J. and Sagher, F. (1956) Sabra dermatitis. Harefuah 51, 271.

Shanon, J. and Sagher, F. (1956) Sabra dermatitis; occupational dermatitis due to prickly pear handling simulating scabies. Arch. Derm. 74, 269.

Shanon, J. and Sagher, F. (1965) Sabra dermatitis. Occupational dermatitis caused by contact with the prickly pear. Derm. Int. 4, 125.

Shanon, J. and Sagher, F. (1969) Sabra dermatitis. An occupational dermatitis simulating scabies due to the handling of prickly pears. In Essays on tropical Dermatiology. ed. Simons, R. and Marshall, J. Amsterdam. Excerpta Medica Foundation p. 85-89.

Opuntia microdasys

A description of keratoconjunctivitis in 2 cases caused by glochids was given by Whiting and Bristow (1975).

Reference

Whiting, D.A. and Bristow, J.H. (1975) Dermatitis and keratoconjunctivitis caused by a prickly pear (Opuntia microdasys). South Afr. Med. J. 49 1445.

CAMPANULACEAE

2000 species in 60 to 70 genera are found in temperate and subtropical regions and on tropical mountains. The plants often have an acrid milky juice (Bailey 1949).

Chemistry is recorded by Hegnauer (1964, 1966).

Campanula

300 species are found in north temperate regions especially the Mediterranean and on tropical mountains.

Campanula medium
(Canterbury Bell)

Contact dermatitis from Canterbury Bell was noted by Adamson (1952). He emphasized that high environmental temperature promoted the development of dermatitis.

Campanula isophylla

Sensitivity to this species was reported by Biberstein (1927).

Reference

Biberstein, H. (1927) Uberempfindlichkeit gegen Pflanzen (Sedum, Tradescantia, Campanula, Meerzwiebel, Myrthe, Alpenveilchen, Buntnessel) Zbl. Hautkrkh 22, 19, cited by Touton (1932).

Touton, K. (1932) Hauterkrankungen durch phanerogamische Pflanzen und ihre Produkte (Toxicodermia et Allergodermia phytogenes), in Barnewitz, J. et al Angeborene Anomalien, Lichtdermatosen, Pflanzengifte, Thermische Schädigungen, Einfluss Innerer Störungen auf die Haut. Berlin, Verlag von Julius Springer.

CAMPANULACEAE

Isotoma

Ten species are native to Australia, one species to central and South America and the West Indies.

Isotoma axillaris
(Australian Harebell)

The dried plant is irritating to the throat (Hurst 1942).

Isotoma longiflora
(syn. Hippobroma)
Star of Bethlehem

The juice of all parts of the plant can irritate the eyes and produce a burning sensation in the mouth and throat (Burkill 1935, Allen 1943). Souder (1963) noted that if a drop of the sap contacted the eye, blindness could result. The leaves are used as a counter-irritant (Burkill 1935). The plant has caused irritation in English gardeners (Phillips 1967).

Isotoma petraea
Cheeky Bugger

The dry dust or vapour from the plant is irritating to the eyes and throat (Higginson 1957, Cleland and Lee 1963).

References

Adamson, H.G. (1952) Sun heat and artificial heat in relation to skin eruptions due to local irritants. Brit. J. Derm. 64, 104.

Allen, P.H. (1943) Poisonous and injurious Plants of Panama. Am. J. Trop. med. 23 (suppl.) 3-76.

Bailey, L.H. (1949) Manual of Cultivated Plants: most commonly grown in the continental United States and Canada. Revised ed. New York. The Macmillan Co.

Burkill, I.H. (1935) A Dictionary of the Economic Products of the Malay Peninsula. 2 Vols. London. Crown Agents for the Colonies.

Cleland, J.B. and Lee, D.J. (1963) The Poisonous and Urticating Plants of Australia in Venomous and Poisonous Animals and Noxious Plants of the Pacific Region. Ed. Keegan, H.L. and Macfarlane, W.V. Oxford. Pergamon Press. pp. 3-13.

Hegnauer, R. (1964) Chemotaxonomy of plants. Vol. 3. Basel. Birkhauser 1964. p. 344.

Hegnauer, R. (1966) Chemotaxonomy of Plants. Vol. 4. Basel, Birkhauser. p. 404.

Higginson, A.R.R. (1957) Further notes on plants injurious to man. South. Aust. Nat. 32, 26.

Hurst, E. (1942) The Poison Plants of New South Wales. N.S.W. Poison Plants Committee; Sydney.

Phillips (1967) Pers. Comm. to A. Rook.

Souder, P. (1963) Poisonous plants on Guam. In Venomous and Poisonous Animals and Noxious Plants of the Pacific Region. ed. Keegan, H.L. and Macfarlane, W.V. Oxford. Pergamon Press. pp. 15-29.

Isotoma hypocrateriformis

The sap is very irritant to the eye (Aplin 1976).

Reference

Aplin, T.E.H. (1976) Poisonous garden plants and other plants harmful to man in Australia. Western Australian Dept. of Agriculture Bull. 3964.

Lobelia

200 to 300 species are cosmopolitan mostly in tropical and subtropical regions and especially America.

Lobelia spp.

The leaves, stems and fruits are said to be irritant and capable of producing dermatitis (Woods 1962, McCord 1962, Builliard 1780).

Lobelia excelsa

The leaves are smoked in India like tobacco. The acrid milky juice can produce irritant dermatitis. (Behl et al 1966).

Lobelia inflata
Indian Tobacco

Application of the plant to the skin can cause irritation (Piffard 1881); the taste is acrid and burning (Wren 1968).

Lobelia nicotinaefolia
Wild Tobacco

The milky juice can cause dermatitis and the dried plant irritates the nose like snuff (Behl et al 1966).

Lobelia philippinensis

The white milky juice is said to be capable of causing blindness (Altschul 1973).

References

Altschul, S. von R. (1973) Drugs and foods from little-known plants. Cambridge, Mass. Harvard Univ. Press.

Behl, P.N., Captain, R.M., Bedi, B.M.S. and Gupta, S. (1966) Skin-irritant and sensitizing plants found in India, New Delhi. P.N. Behl, Irwin Hospital.

McCord, C.P. (1962) The Occupational Toxicity of Cultivated Flowers. Ind. Med. Surg. 31, 365.

Piffard, H.G. (1881) A treatise on the Materia Medica and Therapeutics of the Skin. New York. Wm. Wood & Co.

Woods, B. (1962) Irritant Plants. Trans. St. John's Hosp. derm. Soc. 48, 75.

Wren, R.W. (1968) Potter's New Cyclopaedia of Botanical Drugs and Preparations by Wren, R.C. Re-edit. by Wren, R.W. Potter & Clarke, Ltd. Health Science Press. Rustington, Sussex.

Builliard (1780) Histoire des Plantes Veneneuses et Suspectes de la France. Paris, cited by Woods (1962).

Woods, B. (1962) Irritant Plants. Trans. St. John's Hosp. derm. Soc. 48, 75.

CANELLACEAE

16 species in five genera have a markedly discontinuous distribution in South America, the West Indies, eastern Africa and Madagascar.

Chemistry is recorded by Hegnauer (1964).

Reference

Hegnauer, R. (1964) Chemotaxonomy of Plants. Vol. 3. Basel, Birkhauser. p. 348.

Canella

Two species are found in southern Florida, the West Indies and tropical America.

Canella alba
(syn. C. winterana)
False Winter's Bark, White or Wild Cinnamon, Bahama White Wood

The plant is said to cause skin eruptions (Altschul 1973). The bark which is used as a spice and for flavouring tobacco yields, eugenol, etc. (Merck 1968). Winter's bark is derived from Drimys.

References

Altschul, S. von R. (1973) Drugs and foods from little-known plants. Cambridge, Mass. Harvard Univ. Press.

Merck Index (1968) An Encyclopedia of Chemicals and Drugs. ed. Stecher, P.G. 8th ed. Rahway, N.J. Merck and Co. Inc.

Cinnamodendron

Seven species are found in tropical South America and the West Indies.

Cinnamodendron corticosum
False Winter's Bark

The bark has astringent properties which are used in Herbal Medicine (Wren 1968).

Reference

Wren, R.W. (1968) Potter's New Cyclopaedia of Botanical Drugs and Preparations by Wren, R.C. Re-ed. by Wren, R.W. Potter and Clarke Ltd. Health Science Press. Rustington, Sussex.

Warburgia Three species are found in tropical East Africa.

Warburgia stuhlmannii

The inner bark and root bark have a pungent gingery or peppery taste. The wood yields a highly scented oil that is used in more pungent Oriental perfumes (Watt and Breyer-Brandwijk 1962).

Reference

Watt, J.M. and Breyer-Brandwijk, M.G. (1962) The Medicinal and poisonous plants of Southern Africa. 2nd ed. Edinburgh. E & S. Livingstone.

CANNABIDACEAE

Three species in two genera are found in north temperate regions.

Chemistry is recorded by Hegnauer (1964).

Reference

Hegnauer, R. (1964) Chemotaxonomy of Plants. Vol. 3. Basel, Birkhauser, p. 350.

Cannabis

One species, native to Central Asia, is cultivated.

Cannabis indica

A universal papular and vesicular eruption appeared in a man a few hours after he smoked an extract of the plant (Belyaev 1965). Oppenheim (1914) referred to a reaction to the plant.

Cannabis sativa
True Hemp, Indian Hemp.

A woman who worked in a hemp field developed dermatitis, blepharitis, conjunctivitis and keratitis; trichiasis resulted (Mieses-Reif 1936). Contact with the leaves or flowers can cause dermatitis in susceptible individuals (Behl et al 1966, Szego 1965).

The fibre, hemp, is derived from many botanical species (Howes 1974). Workers who process hemp fibre can develop maceration of the skin from standing in water in the retting basins, and irritation from the dust of the dried fibre. Secondary infection and reactions to oil used in the process can also occur (Slaviero 1915, Anon 1916, Schwartz et al 1957, Hegyi et al 1965). Dust containing silicious matter, a toxic alkaloid and sulphur which forms on the wetted fibre were implicated (Schwartz et al 1957). Porias (undated) refers to this topic.

References

Anon (1916) Disease among workers in hemp cultivation. Lancet 1, 580.

Behl, P.N., Captain, R.M., Bedi, B.M.S. and Gupta, S. (1966) Skin-irritant and sensitizing plants found in India, New Delhi. P.N. Behl, Irwin Hospital.

Belyaev, N.V. (1964) Universal Toxicoderma After Acute Cannabis Indica Poisoning. Vestn. Derm. Vener. 3, 77.

Hegyi, E., Jabojni, K.M., Korak, M., Hiavaty, P. et al (1965) Oil-induced skin damage. Cs. Derm. 40, 92.

Howes, F.N. (1974) A Dictionary of Useful and Everyday Plants and their Common Names. Cambridge University Press. pp. 290.

Mieses-Reif, M. (1936) A case of hemp hypersensitivity. Ztschr. f. Augenheilk. 98, 226.

Oppenheim, M. (undated) Zbl.Hautkrkh. 6, 500 and (1914) Wien. Klin. Wschr. 27, 63, cited by Touton (1932).

Porias (undated) Zbl. Hautkrkh. 6, 500, cited by Touton (1932).

Schwartz, L., Tulipan, L. and Birmingham, D.J. (1957) Occupational Diseases of the Skin. 3rd. ed. Philadelphia. Lea & Febiger. pp. 637-672.

Slaviro, G. (1915) Il Morgagni. Part 1. 30th Nov. abstr. (1916) Lancet 1, 380.

Szego, L. (1965) Sensitisation by Agricultural crops and crop-protection preparations I. Studies of plant (leaf) extracts. Acta Med. Acad. Sci. Hung. 21, 19 (Excerpta Medica XVII, 13,

3468).

Touton, K. (1932) Hauterkrankungen durch phanerogamische Pflanzen und ihre Produkte (Toxicodermia et Allergodermia phytogenes), in Barnewitz, J. et al Angeborene Anomalien, Lichtdermatosen, Pflanzengifte, Thermische Schadigungen, Einfluss Innerer Storungen auf die Haut. Berlin, Verlag von Julius Springer.

Humulus

Two species are found in north temperate regions south to IndoChina and the south-western United States.

Humulus lupulus Hop

The fruit is used in brewing beer. Dermatitis from hops has been long recognized (Dale 1693, Badham 1834, Adams 1893, Danlos 1900, Squire 1916, British Pharmaceutical Codex 1920, Lewith 1928). In addition to dermatitis of the hands and face, a purpuric eruption on the legs was attributed to hop-picking (Streich 1924).

The hands of hop-pickers are subject to irritation as the hop-cones are removed from their stalks; during wet or dewy weather the spines are made firmer and the skin is made soft by the moisture. Thus, mechanical abrasion by the rough hairs on the stems of the plants can occur (Maiden 1918). Hop-pickers can develop vesicular dermatitis of the exposed parts viz. hands, wrists, and face, and also of the genitals (Galbraith 1924, O'Donovan 1924, Jirasek and Trapl 1960). The eruption is often mistaken for sunburn, impetigo, erysipelas or urticaria (O'Donovan 1924). The true hop-rash is not difficult to distinguish from bites from 'hop-fleas', red spiders and harvest mites (Cookson and Lawton 1953, Van Thiel 1953).

The true incidence of 'hop rash' in pickers may be under-estimated since persons who are mildly affected leave the seasonal work. Although only one in 3000 hop-pickers received medical attention, about one in 30 were probably affected by dermatitis (Cookson and Lawton 1953). These authors obtained positive patch test reactions to fresh hop oil, humulone and lupulone. Fresh hop oil contains myrcene but this compound becomes oxidised and disappears from old hop oil. They concluded that myrcene of fresh hop oil was the responsible sensitizing agent. Irritant reactions were not excluded by their tests (Bettley 1953).

Hops in beer were alleged to cause dermatitis in a bar-tender (Hurst 1942). The disorder known as Hop Eye is probably due to mechanical injury of the conjunctiva from the spiny hairs found on the top bracts, leaves and bines of the plant; keratitis and hypopyon can result, (Adams 1893, Lewin and Guillery 1913). Hop Gout is a form of tenosynovitis in pickers (Smithies 1929).

Humulus japonicus

The wild hop of China and Japan is covered with fine prickles which chafe the skin when they come into contact with it (Smith 1969).

References

Adams, P.T. (1893) A special form of ophthalmia to which hop pickers are liable. Brit. Med. J. 1, 1000.

Badham, J. (1834) Exanthema and narcotism from the external application of hops. London. Med. Gaz. Oct. 25, cited by Smithies (1929).

Bettley, F.R. (1953) Hop dermatitis. Brit. Med. J. 2, 512.

British Pharmaceutical Codex (1920), pp. 636 and 849, cited by Broers (1926).

Broers, J.H. (1926) Occupationally acquired skin changes from materials chiefly vegetable in origin, in Injuries of the Skin, Oppenheim, Rille and Ullman. Leipzig. Vol. 2. pp. 509-549, cited by White 1934.

Cookson, J.S. and Lawton, A. (1953) Hop dermatitis in Herefordshire. Brit. Med. J. 2, 376.

Dale, A.S. (1693) Pharmacologia, Londoni p. 133, cited by Broers

(1926).

Danlos, M. (1900) Eczema artificiel provoqué par le houblon Ann. de. Dermat. IV. s. 1, 392, cited by Touton (1932).

Galbraith, S.N. (1924) Occupational diseases of hop-picking. Lancet 2, 885.

Hurst, E. (1942) The Poison Plants of New South Wales. N.S.W. Poison Plants Committee; Sydney Hurst cites Sydney Morning Herald (1939) Man's dermatitis. "Caused by hops in beer". March 24.

Jirasek, L. and Trapl. J. (1960) Dermatosis in hop-pickers with special reference to allergic hop-dermatitis. Acta. Univ. Carolinae. Ses. Med. Suppl. 10, 539.

Lewin, L. and Guillery, H. (1913) Die Wirkungen von Arzneimitteln und Giften auf das Auge. 2nd ed. 2 vols. Berlin. August Hirschwald.

Lewith, R. (1928) Uber Hopfender-matitis. Arch. f. Dermat. 154, 345, cited by Touton (1932).

O'Donovan, W.J. (1924) Hop dermatitis. Lancet 2, 597.

Smith, F.P. (1969) Chinese Materia Medica. Vegetable kingdom. 2nd ed. Rev. by Hei, P.D. Taipei, Taiwan. Ku T'ing Book House.

Smithies, B.M. (1929) The occupational diseases of hop-picking. Lancet 2, 494.

Squire (1916) Companion to the Pharmacopoeia. 19 Aufl, cited by Broers (1926).

Streich, C.J. (1924) Hop dermatitis. Lancet 2, 727.

Touton, K. (1932) Hauterkrankungen durch phanerogamische Pflanzen und ihre Produkte (Toxicodermia et Allergodermia phytogenes), in Barnewitz, J. et al Angeborene Anomalien, Lichtermatosen, Pflanzengifte, Thermische Schadigungen, Einfluss Innerer Storungen auf die Haut. Berlin, Verlag von Julius Springer.

Van Thiel, P.H. (1953) Arthropods and other animals in relation to Dermatology in Handbook of Tropical Dermatology and Medical Mycology, ed. Simons, R.D.G. Amsterdam. Elsevier Publ. Co. Vol. II, p. 908.

White, R.P. (1934) The Dermatergoses or Occupational Affections of the Skin. 4th. ed. London. H.K. Lewis.

CAPPARIDACEAE

650 species in 30 genera are found in tropical and warm temperate regions. The family is related to Cleomaceae and Cruciferae. All the species of the family which have so far been investigated contain thioglucosides from which 'mustard oils' are derived (Kjaer 1960, 1963). Mustard oils are considered under Cruciferae. Contact dermatitis from plants of this family was reviewed by Mitchell (1974).

Chemistry is recorded by Hegnauer (1964), Kjaer (1960, 1963) and Seidemann (1970). From the thioglucoside glucocapparin, the *iso*thiocyanate CH_3NCS is derived.

References

Hegnauer, R. (1964) Chemotaxonomy of plants. Vol. 3. Basel, Birkhauser p. 358.

Kjaer, A. (1960) Naturally derived *iso*Thiocyanates (Mustard Oils) and their parent glucosides in Progress in the Chemistry of Organic Natural Products. ed. Zechmeister, L. Vol. 18 Vienna. Springer-Verlag pp. 122.

Kjaer, A. (1963) The distribution of sulphur compounds in Chemical Plant Taxonomy. ed. Swain, T. London. Academic Press. p. 453.

Mitchell, J.C. (1974) Contact dermatitis from plants of the caper family, Capparidaceae. Brit. J. Derm. 91, 13.

Seidemann, J. (1970) Kapern (*Capparis spinosa* L.) Quart. J. Crude Drug Res. 10, 1516.

Boscia

37 species are found in tropical and southern Africa.

Boscia albitrunca

Boscia foetida

These species contain a pungent principle similar to that of Capparis (Watt and Breyer-Brandwijk 1962).

Reference

Watt, J.M. and Breyer-Brandwijk, M.G. The Medicinal and poisonous plants of Southern Africa. 2nd ed. Edinburgh. E. & S. Livingstone.

Buchholzia

Three species are found in tropical West Africa.

Buchholzia macrophylla
Abazzi

The wood of this species can cause dermatitis (Koelsch 1959).

Reference

Koelsch, F. (1959) Handbuch der Berufskrankheiten. 2 Aufl. Jena. Fischer

Capparis

250 species are found in warm climates. Many species climb by recurved thorns. The flowerbuds of C. spinosa are the capers used in flavouring; C. aphylla and C. mariana are also used.

Capparis arborea
(syn. Busbeckea)

This species is the caper-tree of New South Wales.

Capparis decidua
(syn. C. aphylla)

The shoots and young leaves contain a rubefacient and vesicant principle (Behl et al 1966).

Capparis erythrocarpa
Wait a Bit

The West African colloquial name is probably generally used for prickly climbing plants (Dalziel 1937).

Capparis micrantha
Cape-Thorn Melada

The Malay word, Melada, refers to the fact that the seeds are spicy and peppery. The same sharp cress - or mustard-like taste occurs also in the tissues of many other Capparis species (Corner 1952).

Capparis spinosa

Thioglucosides are present in the seeds and green parts of the plant (Kjaer 1960, 1963, Seidemann 1970).

Capparis tomentosa

The root is used as a counter-irritant in southern Africa (Watt and Breyer-Brandwijk 1962).

References

Behl, P.N., Captain, R.M., Bedi, B.M.S. and Gupta, S.(1966) Skin-irritant and sensitizing plants found in India, New Delhi. P.N. Behl, Irwin Hospital.

Corner, E.J.H. (1952) Wayside Trees of Malaysia. Singapore, Government Printer.

Dalziel, J.M. (1937) The Useful Plants of West Tropical Africa. London. Crown Agents.

Kjaer, A. (1960) Naturally derived isoThiocyanates (Mustard Oils) and their parent glucosides in Progress in the Chemistry of Organic Natural Products. ed. Zechmeister, L. Vol. 18. Vienna. Springer-Verlag. pp 122.

Kjaer, A. (1963) The distribution of sulphur compounds in Chemical Plant Taxonomy. ed. Swain, T. London. Academic Press. p. 453.

Seidemann, J. (1970) Kapern (Capparis spinosa L.) Quart. J. Crude Drug Res. 10, 1516.

Watt, J.M. and Breyer-Brandwijk, M.G. (1962) The Medicinal and poisonous plants of Southern Africa. 2nd ed. Edinburgh. E.& S. Livingstone.

Cleome

This genus is included in Cleomaceae.

Crateva
(syn. Crataeva)

Nine species are found in tropical regions excluding Australia and New Caledonia. Krateuas, physician to the Emperor Mithridates (131 - 63 B.C.) was renowned for his skill in poisoning.

Crateva nurvala Barna
(syn. C. religiosa)

The bark is biting and bitter in taste. The leaves have rubefacient and vesicant properties, (Burkill 1935). The root bark and young shoots are used as rubefacients (Behl et al 1966).

Crateva religiosa
(syn. C. adansonii)

The Yorubas and people in the Congo apply the leaf for counter-irritant purposes (Irvine 1961). The fresh leaves have rubefacient and vesicant properties (Quisumbing 1951).

Crateva roxburghii Dalur

Crateva lophosperma

The shoots and flowers are eaten in curries (Corner 1952).

Crateva tapia Toco

An irritant and vesicant principle is present in the roots. The wood when first cut has the odour of garlic (Allium). The sap is acrid and caustic and can produce dermatitis (Allen 1943, Blohm 1962). The roots are used to blister the skin (Usher 1974).

References

Allen, P.H. (1943) Poisonous and Injurious Plants of Panama. Am. J. Trop. Med. Suppl. 23, 1

Behl, P.N., Captain, R.M., Bedi, B.M.S. and Gupta, S. (1966) Skin-irritant and sensitizing plants found in India, New Delhi. P.N. Behl, Irwin Hospital.

Burkill, I.H. (1935) A Dictionary of the Economic Products of the Malay Peninsula. 2 vols. London. Crown Agents for the Colonies.

Blohm, H. (1962) Poisonous Plants of Venezuela. Cambridge, Mass. Harvard University Press.

Corner, E.J.H. (1952) Wayside Trees of Malaysia. Singapore, Government Press.

Irvine, F.R. (1961) Woody plants of Ghana. Oxford University Press. London.

Quisumbing, E. (1951) Medicinal Plants of the Philippines. Tech. Bull. 16. Manila, Philippine Islands. Manila Bureau of Printing. 1234 pp.

Usher, G. (1974) A Dictionary of plants used by man. London. Constable.

Maerua (syn. Courbonia)

100 species are found from tropical and southern Africa to India.

Maerua subcordata
(syn. Courbonia subcordata, C. tubulosa)

This species has rubefacient properties (Verdcourt and Trump 1969).

Reference

Verdcourt, B. and Trump, E.C. (1969) Common Poisonous Plants of East Africa. London. Collins.

CAPRIFOLIACEAE

450 species in 12 genera are mostly found in northern temperate regions and on tropical mountains. The family is closely related to Rubiaceae.

Chemistry is recorded by Hegnauer (1964).

Reference

Hegnauer, R. (1964) Chemotaxonomy of plants. Vol. 3. Basel. Birkhauser. p. 365.

Lonicera

200 species are found in North America (south to Mexico) and in Eurasia (south to North Africa, the Himalayas, the Philippines and south-western Malaysia).

Lonicera caprifolium
Honeysuckle

Dermatitis from this species was reported by Schoenfeld (1936).

Reference

Schoenfeld, W. (1936) Plant dermatitis, Med. Klin. 11, 1617.

Symphoricarpos

One species is found in central China, 17 species in North America.

Symphoricarpos racemosus

This species has irritant properties (Pammel 1911).

Reference

Pammel, L.H. (1911) A Manual of Poisonous plants. Torch Press. Cedar Rapids, Iowa. Reprinted Univ. Microfilms Inc. Ann Arbor, Mich. 1965. pp. 476-7.

Viburnum Snowball

200 species are found in temperate and tropical regions especially in Asia, North America; 16 species are found in Malaysia, excluding New Guinea. V. tinus is widely cultivated. V. opulus is the guelder-rose.

Viburnum sp.

McCord (1962) noted the availability of a commerical extract for patch-testing. There appear to be no reports of dermatitis from the plant.

Viburnum acerifolium
Arrow Wood

Viburnum dentatum

The young straight shoots of these species are used for arrows (Howes 1974).

References

Howes, F.N. (1974) A Dictionary of Useful and Everyday Plants and Their Common Names. Cambridge University Press. pp. 290.

McCord, C.P. (1962) The Occupational Toxicity of Cultivated Flowers. Ind. Med. Surg. 31, 365.

CARICACEAE

55 species in four genera are found in tropical regions of America and Africa.

Chemistry is recorded by Hegnauer (1964).

Reference

Hegnauer, R. (1964) Chemotaxonomy of Plants. Vol. 3. Basel, Birkhauser. p. 373.

Carica

45 species are found in America.

Carica papaya
Papaw, Papaya

This species is widely cultivated for its edible fruit. The leaves and unripe fruit contain a milky juice in which is present the proteolytic enzyme, papain. The concentration of papain in the unripe fruit reaches a maximum when the fruit is fully grown and decreases as the fruit ripens, apparently disappearing as full maturity is reached, (Watt and Breyer-Brandwijk 1962). The fresh roots have a rubefacient action (Quisumbing 1951). The milky sap of the plant is caustic; the juice of the ripe fruit is said not to be irritant (Arnold 1968), but Fasal (1945) states that eating the fruit can cause irritation especially in the angles of the mouth. The milky juice of the plant can produce conjunctivitis (Watt and Breyer-Brandwijk 1962), and dermatitis (Souder 1963) and is used to remove skin blemishes and warts (Gimlette 1929, Burkill 1935). Meat wrapped in the leaves and buried becomes tender through partial digestion of the fibres. Papain clots milk, unlike bromelin, an enzyme of Bromeliaceae and is not inactivated by human serum, unlike trypsin. Papain can produce allergic manifestations in workers in the pharmaceutical industry (Nava 1969, Osgood 1945) and burning itch when injected intradermally (Arthur and Shelley 1955). Papain is added to some cosmetic creams to smooth the skin (Kariyone 1971).

A powder of the pungent seeds is used to produce skin

irritation in Java (Burkill 1935). A thioglucoside glucotropaeolin, is present in the seeds and the enzyme, myrosinase, is present in the fruit pulp. The action of the enzyme is to release an irritant mustard oil as noted under Cruciferae (Kjaer 1960, 1963). Eating papaya caused a yellow colouration of the palms and soles similar to that produced by carotinemia (Okaya 1938).

References

Arnold, H.L. (1968) Poisonous Plants of Hawaii. Rutland, Vermont. Charles E. Tuttle.

Arthur, R.P. and Shelley, W.B. (1955) The role of proteolytic enzymes in the production of pruritus in man. J. Invest. Derm. 25, 341.

Burkill, I.H. (1935) A Dictionary of the Economic Products of the Malay Peninsula. 2 vols. London. Crown Agents for the Colonies.

Fasal, P. (1945) Cutaneous diseases in the tropics. Arch. Derm. 51, 163.

Gimlette, J.D. (1929) Malay Poisons and Charm Cures. 3rd. ed. London. J. and A. Churchill.

Kariyone, T. (1971) Atlas of Medicinal Plants. Osaka, Japan. Takeda Chemical Industries.

Kjaer, A. (1960) Naturally derived isoThiocyanates (Mustard Oils) and their parent glucosides in Progress in the Chemistry of Organic Natural Products. ed. Zechmeister, L. Vol. 18. Vienna. Springer-Verlag. pp. 122-176.

Kjaer, A. (1963) The distribution of sulphur compounds in Chemical Plant Taxonomy. ed. Swain, T. London. Academic Press. p. 453.

Nava, C. (1969) Allergic manifestations caused by papain in workers in the pharmaceutical industry. Med. Lavoro. 60, 732.

Okaya, N. (1938) A case of aurantiasis cutis caused by having taken much papaya. Mitt. d. ed. Gesellsch. z. u. Chiba, 16, H:2.

Osgood, H. (1945) Atopic sensitivity to caroid (papain). J. Allergy 16, 245.

Quisumbing, E. (1951) Medicinal Plants of the Philippines. Tech. Bull. 16. Manila, Philippine Islands. Manila Bureau of Printing 1234 pp.

Souder, P. (1963) Poisonous plants on Guam. In Venomous and Poisonous Animals and Noxious Plants of the Pacific Region. ed. Keegan, H.L. and Macfarlane, W.V. Oxford. Pergamon Press. pp. 15-29.

Watt, J.M. and Breyer-Brandwijk, M.G. (1962) The Medicinal and poisonous plants of Southern Africa. 2nd ed. Edinburgh. E. & S. Livingstone.

Jacaratia

Eight species are found in tropical regions of America and Africa.

Jacaratia digitata

The blossoms are extremely malodorous. The Indians of Peru fear to sleep beneath this tree lest they become afflicted with gangrenous sores which are attributed to the action of the sap (Menninger 1967).

Reference

Menninger, E.A. (1967) Fantastic Trees. New York. The Viking Press.

CARPINACEAE

47 species in three genera are found in north temperate regions.

Carpinus

35 species are found in north temperate regions chiefly in eastern Asia.

Carpinus betulus

The wood is said to have irritant effects (Hanslian and Kadlec 1966).

Reference

Hanslian, L. and Kadlec, K. (1966) Wood from the standpoint of hygiene VIII. Species with some or little biological effect.

Drevo. 21, 229.

Ostrya

Ten species are found in north temperate regions south to central America.

Ostrya virginiana
Lever-wood, Hop Horn Bean.

Stinging hairs at the base of the fruit can produce irritation of the hands (White 1896, 1903).

References

White, J.C. (1896) Hop Hornbean. J. Cutan. Dis. 14, 441.

White, J.C. (1903) Dermatitis Venenata. A Supplemental List. J. Cut. Dis. 21, 449.

CARYOPHYLLACEAE

1750 species in 70 genera are of cosmopolitan distribution.

Chemistry is recorded by Hegnauer (1964).

Reference

Hegnauer, R. (1964) Chemotaxonomy of plants. Vol. 3. Basel, Birkhauser. p. 378.

Agrostemma

Two species are found in Eurasia.

Agrostemma githago
Corn Cockle

The seeds have been placed in the conjunctival sac by patients with the intention of inducing kerato-conjunctivitis; to be effective for this purpose, the outer hull of the seeds must be removed or cut (Roberg 1950). The saponin, agrostemmin or githagin, has been shown to be irritating to the eye. The seeds of this plant and of Saponaria vaccaria can contaminate wheat (Triticum).

Reference

Roberg, M. (1950) Konjunktivitis durch Kornradesamen. Klin Mbl Augenheilk, 116, 426.

Dianthus

300 species are found in Europe, Asia and Africa especially in the Mediterranean region.

Dianthus caryophyllus
Carnation

A Malmaison carnation caused an erythematous eruption (Whitfield cited by White 1934). According to Shelmire (1940) acute dermatitis of the severity of a Toxicodendron or Primula eruption can be caused by carnations. Oil of carnation can cause dermatitis in dentists (Schwartz et al 1957).

References

Schwartz, L., Tulipan, L. and Birmingham, D.J. (1957) Occupational Diseases of the Skin. 3rd ed. Philadelphia. Lea & Febiger. pp. 637-672.

Shelmire, B. (1940) Contact dermatitis from vegetation. South Med. J. 33, 338.

White, R.P. (1934) The Dermatergoses or Occupational Affections of the Skin. 4th ed. London. H.K. Lewis.

Gypsophila

125 species are found in temperate Eurasia and Egypt, one species in Australia and New Zealand.

Gypsophila paniculata

An industrial antifoaming agent, 'Radix saponariae alba' derived from this plant caused dermatitis, rhinitis and asthma in 27 of 52 workmen exposed. Patch tests to the powder, aqueous 1 in 10, were positive in 23 cases. It was suggested that the strongly allergenic substance was of saponin type (Angelov and Minkov 1967).

Reference

Angelov, G. and Minkov, D. (1967) Occupational dermatitis caused by Gypsophila paniculata L. (Radix Saponariae Albae). Dermatol. Venereol. (Sofia) 6, 185.

Herniaria

35 species are found in Europe, from the Mediterranean region

to Afghanistan and in southern Africa.

Herniaria glabra

Herniaria hirsuta

The saponins of these plants were used for an irritant effect in the topical therapy of lupus vulgaris (Rock 1931).

Reference

Rock, H. (1931) Untersuchungen uber die Saponine der Herniaria glabra et hirsuta und ihre Wirkung bei Lupus vulgaris-Kranken. Arch. f. Dermat. 163, 187.

Lychnis

12 species are found in temperate Eurasia.

Lychnis githago
Corn Cockle

The poisonous constituent, a saponin, has a sharp burning taste and when inhaled causes violent sneezing (Hurst 1942). The flowers often contain a dark powder instead of pollen; this consists of the spores of the fungus Ustilago which are thus distributed from plant to plant, like pollen, by visiting insects (Shaw 1973).

References

Hurst, E. (1942) The Poison Plants of New South Wales. N.S.W. Poison Plants Committee; Sydney.

Shaw, H.K.A. (1973) A Dictionary of The Flowering Plants and Ferns. the late J.C. Willis. 8th ed. Cambridge University Press.

Saponaria

30 species are found in temperate Eurasia chiefly in the Mediterranean region.

Saponaria officinalis
Soapwort

The leaves form a lather if rubbed with water. The juice of the plant has an irritant action and, if inhaled, induces sneezing from a content of saponin (Perrot and Paris 1971, Watt and Breyer-Brandwijk 1962, Merck Index 1968). The taste of the leaves is bitter and acrid; the root is used for producing a head on beers (Wren 1968). According to Watt and Breyer-Brandwijk (1962) some of the literature concerning this plant actually refers to S. vaccaria.

Saponaria vaccaria

The plant is slippery and when trod upon is apt to cause a fall; one of the Chinese princes forbade its being allowed to grow in the palace grounds (Smith 1969).

References

Merck Index (1968) An Encyclopedia of Chemicals and Drugs. ed. Stecher, P.G. 8th ed. Rahway, N.J. Merck and Co. Inc.

Perrot, E. and Paris, R. (1971) Les plantes medicinales. 2 vols. Paris. Presses Universitaires de France. 245 (+ XXVI index) pp.

Smith, F.P. (1969) Chinese Materia Medica. Vegetable kingdom. 2nd ed. Rev. by Hei, P.D. Taipei, Taiwan. Ku T'ing Book House.

Watt, J.M. and Breyer-Brandwijk, M.G (1962) The Medicinal and poisonous plants of Southern Africa. 2nd. ed. Edinburgh. E. & S. Livingstone.

Wren, R.W. (1968) Potter's New Cyclopaedia of Botanical Drugs and Preparations by Wren, R.C. Re-edit. by Wren, R.W. Potter and Clarke Ltd. Health Science Press. Rustington, Sussex.

CASUARINACEAE

65 species in two genera are found in the Mascarenes, and from south-eastern Asia to north-eastern Australia and Polynesia.

Casuarina Australian oak

45 species are found in eastern Africa (query native), the Mascarenes, south-eastern Asia, Malaysia, Australia and Polynesia.

Casuarina spp.

The pollen is reported to cause hayfever in Florida (Wodehouse 1971).

Reference

Wodehouse, R.P. (1971) Hayfever Plants. 2nd rev. edition. New York, Hafner.

CELASTRACEAE

850 species in 55 genera are found in tropical and temperate regions. The root of Tripterygium wilfordi is used as an insecticide.

Chemistry is recorded by Hegnauer (1964).

Reference

Hegnauer, R. (1964) Chemotaxonomy of Plants. Vol. 3. Basel, Birkhauser. p. 395.

Elaeodendron

Sixteen or seventeen species are found in tropical and subtropical regions.

Elaeodendron australe
Olive-wood

Elaeodendron orientale
Olive plum

'Olive wood' noted as a cause of irritation by Legge (1907) was identified as this species by Smith (1920), possibly incorrectly. She listed the woods of the species as capable of causing irritation. She may imply sources as follows (Report 1907, Robinson 1907). According to Woods and Calnan (1976) the olive-wood referred to was more likely Olea.

References

Legge, T.M. (1907) Report of the Chief Inspector of Factories and Workshops. p. 248, London.

Smith, E.P. (1920) Plant dermatitis. J. Bot. 58, 130.

Report of the Departmental Commission on Compensation for Industrial Diseases (1907), p. 887.

Robinson (1907) Annual Report of H.H.C. Inspector of Factories.

Woods, B. and Calnan, C.D. (1976) Toxic Woods. Brit. J. Derm. 94, Suppl. 13, June.

Euonymus

176 species are subcosmopolitan in distribution with the greatest number of species in the Himalayas, China and Japan.

Euonymus europea
(syn. E. europaeus)

The wood which is used in turnery for spindles, etc. is reported to be injurious to wood-workers (Seidensticker 1886, Grobmann 1910).

The chemistry was investigated by Santavy and Reichstein (1948).

References

Grobmann, J. (1910) Gesundheitsschädliche Hölzer Bayr. Indust. Gewerbeblt. 96, 51. Cited by Hausen (1970).

Santavy, F. and Reichstein, T. (1948) Evonosid, ein kristallines, herzwirksames Glykosid aus Euonymus europea. Helo. Chim. Acta. 31, 655, cited by Hausen 1970.

Seidensticker A. (1886) Waldgeschichte der Alterthums Frankfurt/Oder. Bd. 1 u. 2. Trowitzsch and Sohn., cited by Hausen (1970).

Hausen, B.M. (1970) Untersuchungen über Gesundheitsschädigende Hölzer. Thesis, Hamburg.

Gymnosporia

100 species are found in tropical and subtropical regions especially in Africa. Many species have branches modified into thorns.

Gymnosporia buxifolia

The spines which are used as needles and for extracting the thorns of other plants from the skin of the feet are said to have an irritant and 'toxic' effect (Watt and Breyer-Brandwijk 1962).

Gymnosporia senegalensis
(syn. Maytenus senegalensis).

Thorns of this tree are used by butcher birds (shrikes) for impaling their insect victims (Irvine 1961).

References

Irvine, F.R. (1961) Woody plants of Ghana. Oxford University Press. London.

Watt, J.M. and Breyer-Brandwijk, M.G. (1962) The Medicinal and poisonous plants of Southern Africa. 2nd ed. Edinburgh. E.& S. Livingstone.

Hippocratea

120 species are found in tropical regions. This genus has been also described as a single American species.

Hippocratea indica
(syn. H. loesneriana)

The roots, chewed with hot oil, are blown on the skin as a counter-irritant (Harley 1941).

Reference

Harley, G.W. (1941) Native African Medicine. Cambridge Mass. Harvard University Press. pp. 294.

Kokoona

Five species are found in Ceylon, Burma and western Malaysia.

Kokoona zeylanica

The inner bark is used by jewellers for polishing (Howes 1974).

Reference

Howes, F.N. (1974) A Dictionary of Useful and Everyday Plants and their Common Names. Cambridge University Press. pp. 290.

Maytenus

225 species are found in tropical regions.

Maytenus thompsonii
Luluhut

This species can cause dermatitis (Souder 1963).

Reference

Souder, P. (1963) Poisonous plants on Guam. In venomous and poisonous animals and noxious plants of the Pacific Region. ed. Keegan, H.L. and Macfarlane, W.V. Oxford. Pergamon Press. pp. 15-29.

CERATOPHYLLACEAE

10 species in one genus are cosmopolitan rootless water plants.

Chemistry is recorded by Hegnauer (1964).

Reference

Hegnauer, R. (1964) Chemotaxonomy of plants. Vol. 3. Basel, Birkhauser, p. 408.

Ceratophyllum

The distribution of the genus is that of the family.

Ceratophyllum submersum

This species reported on circumstantial evidence to cause dermatitis in bathers (Touton 1928) as a form of Oppenheim's meadow dermatitis.

References

Touton, K. (1928) Eine Ursache beim Baden entstehender Hautausschlage. Dermat.Wschr. 87, 1931 cited by Touton (1932) and White (1934).

Touton, K. (1932) Hauterkrankungen durch phanerogamische Pflanzen und ihre produkte (Toxicodermia et Allergodermia phytogenes), in Barnewitz, J. et al Angeborene Anomalien, Lichtdermatosen, Pflanzengifte, Thermische Schadingungen, Einfluss Innerer Storungen auf die Haut. Berlin, Verlag von Julius Springer.

White, R.P. (1934) The Dermatergoses or Occupational Affections of the skin. 4th ed. London. H.K. Lewis.

CHENOPODIACEAE

1400 species in 102 genera are nearly all tolerant of salted earth in sea-shores and deserts, etc. Some are xerophytic and resemble Cactus. Salicornia fructicosa was used to provide the alkali for making soap in 2500 B.C.

Chemistry is recorded by

Hegnauer (1964).

Reference

Hegnauer, R. (1964) Chemotaxonomy of Plants. Vol. 3. Basel, Birkhauser, p. 409.

Atriplex

200 species are found in temperate and subtropical regions. Several species provide food for humans and animals.

A. canescens

A. halimus
Mediterranean Salt bush

A. hortensis
Garden Orach, Mountain Spinach

A. patula Orach

These species have been used as food by man (Usher 1974, Szczawinski and Hardy 1972).

References

Szczawinski, A.F. and Hardy, G.A. (1972) Guide to Common Edible Plants of British Columbia. Handbook No. 20. Dept. of Recreation and Conservation. Government of British Columbia, Victoria. B.C.

Usher, G. (1974) A dictionary of plants used by man. London. Constable.

Atriplex litoralis

The plant was reported to produce adverse effects by Matignon (1897, 1900).

Reference

Matignon (1897) Janus (Leyde) 2, 499 and 5, 250 (1900), cited by Touton (1932).

Touton, K. (1932) Hauterkrankungen durch phanerogamische Pflanzen und ihre Produkte (Toxicodermia et Allergodermia phytogenes), in Barnewitz, J. et al Angeborene Anomalien, Lichtdermatosen, Pflanzengifte, Thermische Schadigungen, Einfluss Innerer Storungen auf die Haut. Berlin, Verlag von Julius Springer.

Atriplex serrata
Noong Jang-ai

Women who ate the plant under famine conditions in China developed oedema and then a pruritic bullous eruption of the exposed skin surfaces. Men were rarely affected (Martin cited by Maxwell 1929). This disorder known as atriplicism has been interpreted as photosensitisation (Cairns et al 1958) and attributed to ingestion of A. serrata and Amaranthus mangostenus.

Species of these genera tend to grow on garbage dumps around human habitations (King 1966).

References

Cairns, R.J., Champion, R.H. and Wilkinson, D.S. (1968) Cutaneous reactions to physical agents in Textbook of Dermatology. Rook, A.J., Wilkinson, D.S. and Ebling, F.J.G. 1st ed. Oxford Blackwell. p. 323-361.

King, L.J. (1966) Weeds of the World. Biology and Control. London, Leonard Hill.

Martin, S.H. China Medical Journal 39, 808, cited by Maxwell(1929).

Maxwell, J.L. (1929) The Diseases of China including Formosa and Korea. Shanghai. ABC Press.

Bassia All.

Ten species are found from central Europe and the Mediterranean region to central Asia, 79 species in Australia.

Bassia paradoxa

The sharp-pointed fruits can produce mechanical injury (Cleland 1925).

Reference

Cleland, J.B. (1925) Plants, including fungi, poisonous or otherwise injurious to man in Australia. Med. J. Australia 2, 443.

Beta

Six species are found in Europe and the Mediterranean region.

From B. vulgaris (syn. B maritima), the Sea-beet are derived the garden beetroot, the sugar-beet and the mangold-wurzel. The sugar-beet is widely cultivated for its content of sugar. The leaves of the garden beet are sometimes eaten like spinach (Spinacia). B. vulgaris var. cicla (Swiss Chard) is eaten.

Beta spp.

Beet pollen can cause hayfever (Wodehouse 1971).

Beta vulgaris Beetroot

Dermatitis in the beet industry affected two-thirds of workers employed in the 'crystallizing department'. Sugar appears to be responsible for the dermatitis and secondary infection was common (White 1934).

A food handler who had contact dermatitis showed positive patch test reactions to beets and to Spinachia. Control tests were not recorded (Morris 1954).

A positive patch test reaction to beet pulp was observed in a dock worker who had allergic contact dermatitis from cattle fodder products including brans, maize (Zea) and barley (Hordeum) (Malten 1970).

References

Malten, K.E. (1970) Allergic contact dermatitis due to cattle fodder products. Contact Dermatitis Newsletter (London) 7, 158.

Morris, G.E. (1954) Dermatoses among Food Handlers. Industr. Med. Surg. 23, 343.

White, R.P. (1934) The Dermatergoses or Occupational Affections of the Skin. 4th ed. London. H.K. Lewis.

Wodehouse, R.P. (1971) Hayfever Plants. 2nd rev. edition. New York, Hafner.

Chenopodium

Between 100 and 150 species are found in temperate regions.

Some species are used as food or fodder.

Chenopodium alba
Lamb's Quarters

C. amaranticolor

C. ambrosiodes

C. bonus-henricus
(Syn. C. esculentus)
Good King Henry

C. canihua Canahua

C. capitum

C. foliosum

C. fremonti

C. leptophyllum

C. murale

C. nuttaliae

C. pallidicaule

C. quinoa

C. rhadinostachyum

C. rubrum

The above species have been used for food by man (Usher 1974).

Chenopodium spp.

A pellagra-like syndrome has occurred in starving persons who ate the plants (Gryzbowski 1948, Sebastynski 1960, Tyszukiewicz and Zelazowski 1964, Yu 1957, Lukacs 1958).

Contact with the plant has been reported to cause dermatitis (Becker and O'Brien 1959) and to evoke photodermatitis (Lubieniecki 1961). Poisoning in animals from ingestion of the plants and human poisoning from Oil of Wormseed, does not appear to produce features of photosensitivity (Kingsbury 1964). C. album is said to be useful in the treatment of vitiligo (Behl 1973). Keratitis from pigweed is noted under Amaranthus.

Chenopodium album
Lamb's Quarters,
White Goosefoot

This species produced a positive patch test reaction in one of 50 patients investigated for 'weed dermatitis' (Shelmire 1939).

Chenopodium botrys
Jerusalem Oak, Feather Geranium

This species produced negative patch test reactions in all of 50 patients investigated for 'weed dermatitis' (Shelmire 1939).

References

Becker, S.W. and O'Brien, M.P. (1959) Value of patch tests in Dermatology. Arch. Derm. 79, 569.

Behl, P.N. (1973) Personal Communication. Skin Institute 5-A, Jangpura, Mathura Road. New Delhi 14.

Gryzbowski, M. (1948) Peculiar, pellagra-like skin sensitization to light in starving persons. Brit. J. Derm. 60, 410.

Kingsbury, J.M. (1964) Poisonous Plants of the United States and Canada. Englewood Cliffs, New Jersey. Prentice-Hall Inc.

Lubieniecki, S. (1961) A case of photodermatitis after contact with Chenopodium. Pol. Tyg. Lek. 16, 105.

Lukacs, F.V. (1958) On a case of severe photodermatosis cured by means of hibernation. Ann. paediat 191, 183.

Sebastynski, T. (1960) Pellagroid due to consumption of Chenopodium. Pol. Tyg. Lek. 15, 688.

Shelmire, B. (1939) Contact Dermatitis from Weeds; Patch Testing with Their Oleoresins. JAMA 113, 1085.

Tyszukiewicz, D. and Zelazowski, K. (1964) Skin changes due to consumption of garden orach. Pol. Tyg. Lek. 19, 1166.

Yu, K.Y. (1957) Observations on Dermatitis solaris in China. Proc. XI th Int. Derm. Congress. 3, 538.

Chenopodium Goosefoot

The pollen of some species, especially C. album can cause hayfever (Wodehouse 1971).

Reference

Wodehouse, R.P. (1971) Hayfever Plants. 2nd rev. edition. New York, Hafner.

Cycloloma

One species is found in North America.

Cycloloma atriplicifolium
Winged pigweed

An extract of this species produced negative patch test reactions in all of 50 patients investigated for 'weed dermatitis' (Shelmire 1939).

Reference

Shelmire, B. (1939) Contact Dermatitis from Weeds; Patch Testing with Their Oleoresins. JAMA 113, 1085.

Kochia

90 species are found in central Europe, temperate Asia northern and southern Africa and Australia.

Kochia scoparia
Burning Bush

The pollen can cause hayfever (Wodehouse 1971).

Reference

Wodehouse, R.P. (1971) Hayfever Plants 2nd rev. edition. New York, Hafner

Salsola

150 species are cosmopolitan in maritime areas or on salt steppes.

Salsola kali Glasswort

The leaves end in spines.

Salsola kali var tenuifolia
(syn. S. pestifera)
Russian Thistle, Prickly Saltwort, Roly Poly

This species has become a pest of agriculture in North America since about 1900. The spines of the plant cause irritation to men and horses (Pammel 1911, Schwartz et al 1957). In New Mexico, U.S.A., a disorder known as 'tumbleweed dermatitis' occurs from contact of this plant with the skin; direct mechanical injury from the spines appears to be responsible; an extract of the plant produced negative patch test reactions in all of 50 patients investigated for 'weed dermatitis' (Shelmire 1939).

Reference

Pammel, L.H. (1911) A Manual of Poisonous plants. Torch Press, Cedar Rapids, Iowa. Reprinted Univ. Microfilms Inc. Ann Arbor, Mich. 1965. pp. 476-7.

Schwartz, L., Tulipan, L. and Birmingham, D.J. (1957) Occupational Diseases of the Skin. 3rd. ed. Philadelphia. Lea & Febiger. pp. 637-672.

Shelmire, B. (1939) Contact Dermatitis From Weeds; Patch Testing with Their Oleoresins. JAMA 113, 1085.

Salsola kali
Russian Thistle

Mechanical contact with plant branches as well as scratch, patch and photopatch tests with Russian thistle extract and scratch tests with 1.5% KNO_3, a plant constituent, were employed. These tests, along with transparent adhesive tape preparations and a skin biopsy, showed that in non-sensitive persons, dermatitits was due only to mechanical irritation of plant floral bracts. In sensitive individuals, Russian thistle floral bracts pierced the skin and stimulated an urticarial reaction, (Powell and Smith 1975).

Reference

Powell, R.F. and Smith, E.B. (1975) Unpublished Observations.

Salsola pestifer
Russian Thistle

The pollen can cause hayfever (Wodehouse 1971).

Reference

Wodehouse, R.P. (1971) Hayfever Plants. 2nd rev. edition. New York, Hafner.

Sarcobatus

One or two species are found in North America.

Sarcobatus vermiculatus
Greasewood

This plant which is poisonous to sheep probably from a content of oxalates is said to cause dermatitis (Dorsey 1962).

Reference

Dorsey, G.S. (1962) Plant Dermatitis in California. Calif. Med. 96, 412.

Spinacia

Three species are found from the eastern Mediterranean region to central Asia and Afghanistan.

Spinacia oleracea
Spinach

In the canning industry, workers employed in packing spinach are subject to a dermatitis resembling that produced by Toxicodendron (Schwartz et al 1957). Spinach can cause dermatitis in housewives (Shelmire 1940).

A food handler was contact sensitive to spinach and to Beta. A packer of spinach had oedema due to cold (Morris 1954). A vegetable dealer had dermatitis from contact with spinach and asthma from ingestion of spinach; he also had asthma from green peas (Pisum); a patch test to spinach produced a negative result (Zohn 1937).

References

Morris, G.E. (1954) Dermatoses among Food Handlers. Industr. Med. Surg. 23, 343.

Schwartz, L., Tulipan, L. and Birmingham, D.J. (1957) Occupational Diseases of the Skin. 3rd ed. Philadelphia. Lea & Febiger p. 637-672.

Shelmire, B. (1940) Contact dermatitis from vegetation. South Med. J. 33, 338.

Zohn, B. (1937) An unusual case of spinach hypersensitivity. J. Allergy 8, 381.

Tamarix

54 species are found in western Europe and from the Mediterranean region to India and northern China. T. mannifera produces the manna of the Bedouins.

Tamarix gallica Tamarisk

The pollen is reported to cause hayfever in Arizona (Wodehouse 1971).

Reference

Wodehouse, R.P. (1971) Hayfever Plants. 2nd rev. edition. New York, Hafner

Threlkeldia

Five species are found in Australia.

Threlkeldia proceriflorus

Ingestion of this species is reported to cause photosensitization in animals (Hurst 1942).

Reference

Hurst, E. (1942) The Poison Plants of New South Wales. N.S.W. Poison Plants Committee; Sydney.

CHRYSOBALANACEAE

400 species in 10 genera are found in tropical and subtropical regions. The fruit of C. icaco (Coco plum) is edible.

Parinari

Sixty species are found in tropical regions. Some species have edible seeds.

Parinari curatellaefolia

The trees are malodorous, smelling like an unwashed human body; only some individuals can detect an odour from the tree (Menninger 1967).

Parinari guianense (syns. Parinarium variegatum, Ferolia guyanensis)

Atlas wood, Guiana Satinwood, Antilles Satinwood.

The wood is said to be capable of causing dermatitis (Sandermann and Barghoorn 1956). Several botanical species are known as Satinwood. Brosimum and Fagara have been confused with species of this genus.

References

Menninger, E.A. (1967) Fantastic Trees. New York. The Viking Press.

Sandermann, W. and Barghoorn, A.W. (1956) Gesundheitsschädigende Nutzholzer. Holz Roh-Werkst 14, 37.

Ferolia (syn. Parinari)

A report of toxicity from the wood of bois de Féroles (Czimatis and Hagemann 1910) seems to refer to Brosimum parense and not to Ferolia spp. (Woods and Calnan 1976, citing Record and Hess 1943).

References

Czimatis and Hagemann (1910) Ueber Erkrankungen durch Holzstaub. Hygienische Rundschau 20, 761.

Record, S.J. and Hess, R.W. (1943) Timbers of the New World. New Haven, Yale.

Woods, B. and Calnan, C.D. (1976) Toxic Woods. Brit. J. Derm. 94. Suppl 13, June.

CLEOMACEAE

275 species in 12 genera are found in tropical and subtropical regions. The family is related to Capparidaceae and to Cruciferae.

Chemistry is recorded by Hegnauer (1964), (under Cleomoideae, a sub-family of Capparidaceae).

The seeds of species which have been examined contain the thioglucoside, glucocapparin, from which an irritant isothiocyanate, CH_3NCS, is derived. Isothiocyanates ('mustard oils') are noted under Cruciferae) (Kjaer 1960, 1963).

Dermatitis from plants of this family was reviewed by Mitchell (1974).

References

Hegnauer, R. (1964) Chemotaxonomy of Plants. Vol. 3. Basel, Birkhauser

p. 361.

Kjaer, A. (1960) Naturally derived isoThiocyanates (Mustard Oils) and their parent glucosides in Progress in the Chemistry of Organic Natural Products. ed. Zechmeister, L. Vol. 18. Vienna. Springer-Verlag. pp. 122-176.

Kjaer, A. (1963) The distribution of sulphur compounds in Chemical Plant Taxonomy. ed.Swain, T. London. Academic Press. p. 453.

Mitchell, J.C. (1974) Contact dermatitis from plants of the caper family, Capparidaceae. Brit. J. Derm. 91, 13.

Cleome

150 species are found in tropical and subtropical regions.

Chemistry

The seeds of nine species which have been examined contain glucocapparin (Kjaer 1960).

Cleome arabica

Cleome arborea

These species contain glucocapparin (Kjaer 1960).

Cleome felina Arivila

This species has irritant properties (Behl et al 1966).

Cleome graveolens

This species which has irritant properties (Pammel 1911) contains glucocapparin (Kjaer 1960).

Cleome gigantea

The species contains glucocapparin (Kjaer 1960).

Cleome icosandra (syn. *C. viscosa*) Wild Mustard

The brownish-black seeds are occasionally used for culinary purposes. Both the seeds and the leaves have rubefacient and vesicant properties (Behl et al 1966). This species is frequently confused with *Gynandropsis gynandra*; the plants may be found growing alongside each other (Behl et al 1966).

Cleome monophylla

This species contains glucocapparin (Kjaer 1960).

Cleome pentaphylla

This species is noted under *Gynandropsis gynandra*.

Cleome serrulata Stinking clover

This species is cultived (Wyman 1971).

Cleome speciosissima

This species contains glucocapparin (Kjaer 1960).

Cleome spinosa Spider Flower

This species is a half-hardy plant which is becoming increasingly popular in European gardens; one of us has seen a case of contact dermatitis from it. This species has also been known as *C. pungens* and *C. gigantea*. Its horticultural use is noted by Mitchell (1974) (Wyman 1971).

A gardener developed dermatitis of the hands from contact with the plant. Chromatography of chloroform and alcohol extracts revealed 10-12 coumarin-like substances. Patch tests with the extracts revealed an irritant effect which was enhanced by irradiation with a quartz lamp (Szego and Maacz 1968). The seeds of this species contain glucocapparin (Kjaer 1960).

Cleome trachysperma

This species contains glucocapparin (Kjaer 1960).

Cleome viscosa

The plant is used as a counter-irritant in West Africa (Dalziel 1937). The seeds contain glucocapparin (Kjaer 1960).

References

Behl, P.N., Captain, R.M., Bedi, B.M.S. and Gupta, S. (1966) Skin-irritant and sensitizing plants found in India, New Delhi. P.N. Behl, Irwin Hospital.

Dalziel, J.M. (1937) The Useful Plants of West Tropical Africa. London, Crown Agents.

Kjaer, A. (1960) Naturally derived isoThiocyanates (Mustard Oils) and their parent glucosides in Progress in the Chemistry of Organic Natural Products. ed. Zechmeister, L. Vol. 18. Vienna. Springer-Verlag.pp. 122-176.

Mitchell, J.C. (1974) Contact Dermatitis from Plants of the Caper Family, Capparidaceae. Brit. J. Derm. 91, 13.

Pammel, L.H. (1911) A Manual of Poisonous Plants. Torch Press, Cedar Rapids, Iowa. Reprinted Univ. Microfilms Inc. Ann Arbor, Mich. 1965.

Szego, L. und Maacz, J. (1968) Dermatitis als Berufskrankheit, hervorgerufen durch die "Kleopatra-Nadel" Cleome spinosa. Derm. Wochen. 154, 50

Wyman, D. (1971) Wyman's Gardening Encyclopedia. New York. Macmillan Co.

Gynandropsis (syn. Cleome)

One species, G. gynandra is recognized from tropical and subtropical regions.

Gynandropsis gynandra
Cat's Whiskers

The seeds are used like mustard (Brassica).

The bitter leaves are mildly irritant with a flavour like that of mustard oil (Brassica) (Burkill 1935). The seeds and bruised leaves have rubefacient and vesicant properties (Behl et al 1966, Oliver 1959, Quisumbing 1951). The plant has been confused with Cleome icosandra. According to Behl et al (1966) this species has been known as Cleome pentaphylla. The seeds contain glucocapparin (Kjaer 1960).

Gynandropsis pentaphylla

The plant is used as a counter-irritant in West Africa and is said to have acrid properties due to a content of an oil like that of garlic (Allium) or mustard (Brassica) (Dalziel 1937). The seeds and leaves have irritant properties (Watt and Breyer-Brandwijk 1962). The seeds of the plant contain an unidentified glucoside (Kjaer 1960). According to Landor (1940) the plant referred to as Gynandropsis gynandra or G. pentaphylla is known among Malays as maman puten, maman hantu, or kemaman, and among Tamils as valai or thair-velai. It is used by some as a vegetable; it is a common Malayan weed whose sap contains an irritant oil which is destroyed by cooking. The crushed fresh leaves are used as counter-irritant. The leaves were rubbed in the hands and applied to an axillary boil and a severe dermatitis soon followed. Patch tests to the crushed leaves produced strongly positive reactions; to the uncrushed leaf negative reactions (Landor 1940).

References

Behl, P.N., Captain, R.M., Bedi, B.M.S. and Gupta, S. (1966) Skin-irritant and sensitizing plants found in India, New Delhi. P.N. Behl, Irwin Hospital.

Burkill, I.H. (1935) A Dictionary of the Economic Products of the Malay Peninsula. 2 vols. London. Crown Agents for the Colonies.

Dalziel, J.M. (1937) The Useful plants of West Tropical Africa. London, Crown Agents.

Kjaer, A. (1960) Naturally derived isoThiocyanates (Mustard Oils) and their parent glucosides in Progress in the Chemistry of Organic Natural Products. ed. Zechmeister, L. Vol. 18. Vienna. Springer-Verlag. pp. 122-176.

Landor, J.V. (1940) Dermatitis venenata from a common Malayan plant. J. Malaya Branch Brit. Med. Ass. 3, 384.

Oliver, B. (1959) Nigeria's Useful Plants. Nigerian Field 24, 70.

Quisumbing, E. (1951) Medicinal Plants of the Philippines. Tech. Bull. 16. Manila, Philippine Islands. Manila Bureau of Printing. 1234pp.

Watt, J.M. and Breyer-Brandwijk, M.G. (1962) The Medicinal and poisonous plants of Southern Africa. 2nd ed. Edinburgh. E. & S. Livingstone.

Polanisia

Seven species are found in temperate North America.

Polanisia icosandra

According to Usher (1974) this species is named Cleome icosandra. The roots, leaves and seeds are used medicinally like mustard (Brassica). The whole plant, if bruised, is used as a counter-irritant and vesicant (Quisumbing 1951).

Polanisia uniglandulosa

The plant has rubefacient properties (Usher 1974).

References

Quisumbing, E. (1951) Medicinal Plants of the Philippines. Tech. Bull. 16. Manila, Philippine Islands. Manila Bureau of Printing. pp. 1234.

Usher, G. (1974) A Dictionary of Plants used by Man. London. Constable.

COCHLOSPERMACEAE

Between 20 and 25 species in two genera are of tropical distribution.

Chemistry is recorded by Hegnauer (1964).

Reference

Hegnauer, R. (1964) Chemotaxonomy of plants. Vol. 3. Basel. Birkhauser, p. 434.

Cochlospermum

Between 15 and 20 tropical species are mostly xerophytic.

Cochlospermum tinctorium

The rootstock yields a yellowish dye which is used to colour butter and to stain the mouth (Oliver 1961).

Reference

Oliver, B. (1958-61) Nigeria's Useful Plants. Nigerian Field Part V 26, 170.

COMBRETACEAE

600 species in 20 genera are found in tropical and subtropical regions.

Chemistry is recorded by Hegnauer (1964).

Reference

Hegnauer, R. (1964) Chemotaxonomy of plants. Vol. 3. Basel. Birkhauser. p. 437.

Combretum

250 species are found in tropical regions excluding Australia. C. butyrosum, of tropical Africa, yields a butter-like substance, chiquito, from the fruit.

Combretum sp.

The leaf, when used as an ophthalmic remedy stings the eyes (Watt and Breyer-Brandwijk 1962).

Combretum erythrophyllum
Hiccup nut

The tree is probably irritant (Watt and Breyer-Brandwijk 1962).

The fruit, when eaten, causes persistent hiccup (Greshoff 1909).

Combretum gueinzii

The leaf when pounded and soaked in water yields a red dye (Watt and Breyer-Brandwijk 1962).

Combretum krausii
Mdubu, Umbubu

The sawdust has been recorded as the cause of dermatitis of the hands of African forestry workers. A child who walked barefoot on the saw-dust developed blisters on the toes (Watt and Breyer-Brandwijk 1962). Hausen (1973) refers to reports of injurious effects of the wood.

Combretum platypetalum

Application of the powdered root to cuts in the skin produces pain (Watt and Breyer-Brandwijk 1962).

References

Greshoff, M. (1909) Lix.-Phytochemical investigations at Kew. Kew Bulletin (No. 10) p. 397.

Hausen, B.M. (1973) Holzarten mit gesundheitsschädigenden inhaltsstoffen Stuttgart. DRW-Verlags-GmbH.

Watt, J.M. and Breyer-Brandwijk, M.G. (1962) The Medicinal and poisonous plants of Southern Africa. 2nd ed. Edinburgh. E.& S. Livingstone.

Conocarpus

Two species are found in Florida, the West Indies, tropical America and north-eastern tropical Africa.

Conocarpus erectus
Button-wood, West Indian Alder

The latex is used as a styptic (Irvine 1961).

Reference

Irvine, F.R. (1961) Woody plants of Ghana. Oxford University Press. London.

Terminalia

250 species are found in tropical regions. The wood provides good timber and the bark provides tan.

Terminalia spp.
Framiré, Limba

Some species yield dyes (Irvine 1961). The wood can produce dermatitis and asthma (Zafiropoulo et al 1968). In one instance, a species of this genus and also Chlorophora and Triplochiton were implicated.

Terminalia alata
Indian Laurel

A veneer preparer who had dermatitis showed positive patch test reactions to this wood, to Tectona, Honduras mahogany, Jacaranda, Dalbergia, Primula and to dalbergiones (Woods and Calnan 1976).

Reference

Woods, B. and Calnan, C.D. (1976) Toxic Woods. Brit. J. Derm. 94, Suppl. 13, June.

Terminalia australis

The wood can produce dermatitis (Hanslian and Kadlec 1966).

Terminalia catappa

The fruit is edible (Country almond). The trunk is generally set with short woody spines.

Terminalia chebula
Myrobalans, Black Chebulic

The astringent fruits are used in Herbal Medicine (Wren 1968) and the black fruits are used for dyeing and tanning. This species was said to be toxic (Bernhard-Smith 1923).

Reference

Bernhard-Smith, A. (1923) Poisonous plants of all Countries. London. Baillière Tindall. 2nd. ed.

Terminalia glaucescens

The root-bark, when applied to wounds, produces a burning effect like iodine (Irvine 1961).

Terminalia ivorensis

The wood dust produces dermatitis and respiratory symptoms (Orsler 1973).

Terminalia melanocarpum
Stink tree

The offensive odour of the flowers account for the colloquial name (Menninger 1967).

Terminalia oblongata

Ingestion of the plant can cause photosensitisation in cattle (Everist 1962).

Terminalia subspathulata

This species is known to produce dermatitis in Malaya (Kochummen 1972).

Terminalia superba Limba

The wood can cause dermatitis and respiratory symptoms (Sandermann and Barghoorn 1956, Hausen 1973).

The splinters of limba produce prolonged infection. Vesicular dermatitis of the fingers was due apparently to limba sawdust (Nordin 1947). Hausen (1973) noted some brief reports of dermatitis from the wood. Asthma and contact urticaria from the wood were reported by Oehling (1963).

References

Everist, S.L. (1962) A review of the Poisonous Plants of Queensland. Proc. Roy. Soc. Queensland. 74, 1.

Hanslian, L. and Kadlec, K. (1966) Wood from the standpoint of hygiene VII Species with a highly aggressive biological effect. Drevo 21, 157.

Hausen, B.M. (1973) Holzarten mit gesundheitsschädigenden inhaltsstoffen Stuttgart. DRW-Verlags-GmbH.

Irvine, F.R. (1961) Woody plants of Ghana. Oxford University Press. London.

Kochummen, K.M. (1972) Forest Botanist. Forest Research Institute. Kepong, Selangor, Malaya. Personal communication.

Menninger, E.A. (1967) Fantastic Trees. New York. The Viking Press.

Nordin, J. (1947) Yrkessjukdomar (Industrial Diseases) 2, 605. Uppsala.

Oehling, A. (1963) Berufsallergie im Holzgewerbe Allergie u. Asthma. 9, 312.

Orsler, R.J. (1973) Personal communication from Forest Products Research Laboratory, Princess Risborough, Bucks. England.

Sandermann, W. and Barghoorn, A.W. (1956) Gesundheitsschadigende Nutzholzer. Holz Roh-Werkst. 14, (1), 37.

Wren, R.W. (1968) Potter's New Cyclopaedia of Botanical Drugs and Preparations by Wren, R.C. Re-edit. by Wren, R.W. Potter and Clarke Ltd. Health Science Press. Rustington, Sussex.

Zafiropoulo, A., Audibert, A. and Charpin, J. (1968) A propos des accidents dus a la manipulation des bois exotiques. Rev. Franc. Allerg. 8, 155.

COMMELINACEAE

500 species in 38 genera are mostly found in tropical and subtropical regions. Calcium oxalate is present in the tissues. Some species have edible rhizomes.

Chemistry is recorded by Hegnauer (1963).

Cyanotis

50 species are palaeotropical.

Cyanotis lanata

The plant is said to cause a sort of eczema of the muzzle of horses who browse amongst it (Dalziel 1937).

References

Dalziel, J.M. (1937) The useful plants of west tropical Africa. London. Crown Agents.

Hegnauer, R. (1963) Chemotaxonomy of plants. Vol. 2. Basel, Birkhauser p. 117.

Rhoeo

One species is native to Mexico, Central America and the West Indies.

Rhoeo spathacea
(syn. R. discolor)
Boat Lily

The plant can produce irritation of the hands, mouth, eye and respiratory tract. Handling, chewing and weeding amongst the plants can produce these effects. The juice is used to colour the cheeks, its irritant effect producing erythema (Morton 1962, 1971).

References

Morton, J.F. (1962) Ornamental Plants with Poisonous Properties II. Proc. Florida. Hort. Soc. 75, 484.

Morton, J.F. (1971) Plants Poisonous

to People in Florida and other warm areas. Miami, Florida. Hurricane House Publishers, Inc.

Setcreasea

Nine species are native to the southern United States and Mexico.

Setcreasea purpurea
Purple Queen

The juice of the plant can produce an instant stinging red rash in gardeners (Morton 1962, 1971). She noted that Florida gardeners who carry the plant while shirtless can show an eruption on the body.

References

Morton, J.F. (1962) Ornamental Plants with Poisonous Properties II. Proc. Florida Hort. Soc. 75, 484.

Morton, J.F. (1971) Plants Poisonous to People in Florida and other warm areas. Miami, Florida. Hurricane House Publishers, Inc.

Tradescantia

60 species are native to North America and tropical South America. Several species are popular houseplants, especially T. flumenensis and T. abiflora. T. virginiana (Common Spiderwort) is widely grown in gardens.

Tradescantia spp.

Biberstein (1927) referred to sensitivity to the plants. Dermatitis from handling the plant (Kirton 1974) which can affect the eyelids (Kaalung-Jorgenson 1951) may be allergic. Hjorth (1968) observed only one positive patch test reaction in more than 46 patients tested. An irritant effect, from calcium oxalate crystals, of some species, seems a possibility.

References

Biberstein, H. (1927) Überempfindlichkeit gegen Pflanzen. Zbl. Hautkrkh. 22, 19.

Hjorth, N. (1968) Pers. comm.

Kaalung-Jorgenson, O. (1951) Eczema perioculare (Dermatitis of the eyelids). Acta derm.-venereol 31, 83.

Kirton, V. (1974) Pers. comm.

COMPOSITAE

(syn. ASTERACEAE)

This family, consisting of 13,000 species in 900 genera, distributed over most of the world and living in almost every situation, is possibly the largest family of flowering plants, comprising more than ten percent of total species. The majority are herbaceous plants.

The Compositae family is divided into Asteroideae and Lactucoideae which show distinctive floral differences; the former contain oil canals and the latter contain latex. The Asteroideae are divided into twelve tribes (Hegnauer 1964). The tribes Anthemidae, Astereae and Heliantheae provide the largest number of plants reported to cause dermatitis. The major sensitizing agents of the family are sesquiterpene lactones and the distribution of these chemicals in the plants results in cross-sensitivity patterns between species. Consequently, a patient contact- sensitive to sesquiterpene lactones will frequently show positive patch test reactions to plants to which a history of exposure is lacking. Careful history taking is therefore essential in order to distinguish contact sensitivity resulting from relevant exposure to plants in the individual's environment from cross-sensitivity to immunochemically related plants. A yield of lactones also accounts for cross-sensitivity which has been observed to species of the Magnoliaceae family and to liverworts of the Jubulaceae family.

The principal immunochemical requisite of sesquiterpene lactones is an alpha-methylene group exocyclic to the gamma-lactone (Mitchell et al 1970).

The most important clinical pattern of Compositae dermatitis is 'weed dermatitis'. Adult males are most frequently affected by dermatitis, which is at first seasonal but may become perennial, and affects the exposed skin surfaces not ordinarily covered by clothing. Such allergic contact dermatitis is usually chronic and indurated or lichenified with marked chronicity although acute exacerbations are frequent. Vesicular or bullous dermatitis is rarely observed and the clinical picture of chronic cases of 'weed dermatitis' resembles atopic dermatits and photodermatitis (Mitchell 1969, Lonkar et al 1974). Patch test reactions to Compositae plants in sensitized individuals are frequently severe, vesicular or bullous, and persistent. Patients often react to other weeds of the Compositae family. It has been alleged that atopic individuals are particularly prone to weed dermatitis and that photosensitivity can develop. The data suggests that eczematous skin, whether atopic or not, is particularly prone to weed dermatitis and that sunlight induces photo-irritation of dermatitic skin (Lonkar et al 1974). The role of pollen is probably minimal; airborne dried plant material and contamination of fomites by weed 'oleoresins' can maintain or aggravate weed dermatitis (Lonkar et al 1974). The predeliction for middle-aged males, the rarity of affection of females and the sparing of children are unexplained.

Another clinical pattern of Compositae dermatitis is hand eczema from handling plants particularly Chrysanthemum and salad plants.

Although Compositae weed dermatitis has been previously regarded as a North American problem, European workers have recently reported unexpected cases, some previously diagnosed as photodermatitis (Roed-Petersen and Hjorth, Hjorth et al 1976).

References

Hegnauer, R. (1964) Chemotaxonomy of plants. Vol. 3 Basel. Birkhauser. pp. 449-554.

Hjorth, N. et al (1976) Airborne contact dermatitis from Compositae dermatitis simulating photodermatitis. Brit. J. Derm. 95, 613.

Lonkar, A., Mitchell, J.C. and Calnan, C.D. (1974). Comtact Dermatitis from Parthenium hysterophorus. Trans. St. John's Hosp. Derm. Soc. 60, 43.

Mitchell, J.C. (1969) Allergic Contact Dermatitis from Compositae. Trans. St. John's Hosp. Derm. Soc. 55, 174.

Mitchell, J.C., Fritig, B., Singh, B. and Towers, G.H.N. (1970). Allergic Contact Dermatitis from Frullania and Compositae. J. Invest. Derm. 54, 233.

Roed-Petersen, J. and Hjorth, N. (1976) Compositae sensitivity among patients with contact dermatitis. Contact Dermatitis 2, 271.

Hayfever from Compositae species.

The Compositae family is divided into fourteen tribes (Wodehouse 1971).

1 Heliantheae, Sunflower tribe

2 Ambrosieae, Ragweed tribe

3 Helenieae, Sneezeweed tribe

4 Arctotidae, African daisy tribe

5 Calenduleae, Calendula tribe

6 Inuleae, Inula tribe

7 Astereae, Aster tribe

8 Vernonieae, Ironweed tribe

9 Eupatorieae, Boneset tribe

10 Anthemideae, Chamomile tribe

11 Senecioneae, Groundsel tribe

12 Cynareae, Thistle tribe

13 Mutisieae, Mutisia tribe

14 Cichorieae, Chicory tribe

1. Heliantheae
Sunflower tribe

Sunflower (Helianthus), Dahlia, Cosmos, and black-eyed Susan (Rudbeckia) and others, both wild and cultivated, are known to cause hayfever when handled by susceptible individuals, and occasionally their pollen may even become atmospheric to a certain extent. Ragweed (Ambrosia) hayfever patients are invariably as sensitive to sunflower pollen as to that of ragweed, though resistant to the pollen of plants of other tribes. Feverfew (Parthenium hysterophorus) has been suspected of causing hayfever but is probably of only slight importance.

2. Ambrosieae

Classification of the Ambrosieae (Kahn 1924):

Iveneae

Oxytenia, Copperweeds

Chorisiva

Iva, Marshelders

Leuciva

Cyclachaena, Prairie ragweeds

Euphrosyne

Dicoria

Ambrosineae

Hymenoclea, Greasebushes

Ambrosia, Ragweeds

Franseria, False ragweeds

Xanthium, Cockleburs
Species of this tribe are important causes of hayfever.

Iva spp. Marshelders
Three of the eleven species of North America have been shown to cause hayfever, viz. I. oraria, I. ciliata and I. axillaris.

Cyclachaena spp. Prairie Ragweeds

C. xanthifolia can produce hayfever.

Dicoria spp.

D. canescens and D. brandegei have been suspected of causing hayfever.

Ambrosia spp. Ragweeds

Four species, short (A. eliator), tall (A. trifida), western (A. aptera) and southern ragweed (A. bidentata) are important causes of hayfever.

Franseria spp. False Ragweeds

Species of this genus, less common are less widely distributed than Ambrosia spp., can cause hayfever notably Bur ragweed (F. acanthicarpa), Slender ragweed (F. tenuifolia), Canyon Ragweed (F. deltiodea), Desert bur sage (F. dumosa) and Sonora-bur sage (F. ambroisoides).

Xanthium spp. The Cockleburs
Some species of this genus are minor contributing factors in hayfever.

Hymenoclea spp. Greasebushes.
Burro-weed (H. salsola) and H. monogyra can cause hayfever.

3. Helenieae Sneezeweeds

This tribe includes marigolds (Tagetes) and Gaillardia. Sneezeweed (Helenium) is suspected of causing hayfever.

4. Helenieae, Arctotidae, Calenduleae and Inuleae are almost entirely insect pollinated and of very little importance in hayfever.

7. Astereae

Aster, goldenrod (Solidago), cultivated asters (Callistephus), and English Daisy (Bellis) are mainly insect pollinated but occasional causes of hayfever. The plants are mainly insect pollinated but Solidago spp. can produce considerable amounts of airborne pollen. Baccharis spp. are local causes of hayfever.

8. Vernonieae spp. Ironweeds

Some species have been improbably suspected of causing hayfever (Wodehouse 1971).

9. Eupatorieae

Stevia (Piqueria trinervia) has been reported to cause hayfever.

10. Anthemideae

Most are insect pollinated. The insecticide Pyrethrum derived from C. cinerarieaefolium can cause hayfever and asthma.

Artemisia spp. Sagebrushes, Mugworts and Wormwoods

All species are wind pollinated and some are important causes of hayfever.

11. Senecioneae

Species of this tribe are insect-pollinated and of no importance

Principal Hayfever Species of Artemisia

Species	Group	Section
A. abrotanum		Abrotanum section
A. californica (Crossostephium californicum)		Abrotanum section
A. vulgaris (A. vulgaris typica)	A. vulgaris	Abrotanum section
A. heterophylla (A. vulgaris heterophylla)	A. vulgaris	Abrotanum section
A. ludoviciana (A. vulgaris ludoviciana)	A. vulgaris	Abrotanum section
A. gnaphalodes (A. vulgaris gnaphalodes)	A. vulgaris	Abrotanum section
A. serrata (A. vulgaris serrata)	A. vulgaris	Abrotanum section
A. wrightii (A. vulgaris wrightii)	A. vulgaris	Abrotanum section
A. biennis		Abrotanum section
A. annua		Abrotanum section
A. bigelovii		Abrotanum section
A. absinthium		Absinthium section
A. frigida		Absinthium section
A. dracunculoides (A. dracunculus glauca)		Dracunculus section
A. camporum (A. campestris pacifica)	A. campestris	Dracunculus section
A. caudata (A. campestris caudata)	A. campestris	Dracunculus section
A. canadensis (A. campestris borealis)	A. campestris	Dracunculus section
A. pycnocephala (A. campestris pycnocephala)	A. campestris	Dracunculus section
A. filifolia		Dracunculus section
A. spinescens		Dracunculus section
A. tridentata		Seriphidium section

in hayfever.

12. Cynareae

Some of the thistles (*Cirsium*) have been suspected of causing hayfever.

13. Mutisieae

Species of this tribe are not known to cause hayfever.

14. Cichorieae

The common dandelion (*Taraxacum officinale*) has been suspected of causing hayfever.

References

Kahn, I.S. (1924) The botany of south-west Texas with reference to hayfever and asthma. JAMA 82, 871.

Wodehouse, R.P. (1971) Hayfever Plants. 2nd rev. edition. New York, Hafner.

Many of eighty Compositae species tested were found to be phototoxic for *Candida albicans* (Camm et al 1975), notably *Tagetes*.

From phytochemical evidence of allergenic or potentially allergenic sesquiterpene lactones (Yoshioka et al 1973) and from cross-sensitivity studies, it seems likely that contact sensitivity to the plants listed in the Table results mainly from their lactone content. References to the molecular structures are from Yoshioka et al (1973) supplemented by some additional references noted.

Several sesquiterpene lactones have been shown to exhibit cytotoxic and anti-tumour activity (Kupchan 1970); the active group is the methylene group which can also determine antigenic activity.

Camm, E.L., Towers, G.H.N. and Mitchell, J.C. (1975). Ultra violet-mediated antibiotic activity of some Compositae species. Phytochemistry 14, 2007-2011.

Kupchan, S.M. (1970) Recent advances in the chemistry of tumor inhibitors of plant origin. Trans. N.Y. Acad. Sci. (Series II) 32, 85.

Mitchell, J.C., Fritig, B., Singh, B. and Towers, G.H.N. (1970). Allergic contact dermatitis from *Frullania* and Compositae. The role of sesquiterpene lactones. J. Invest. Derm. 54, 233.

Table

Arnica	Arnica	Yoshioka, H., Mabry, T.J. and Timmermann, B.N. (1973). Sesquiterpene Lactones. Chemistry, NMR and Plant Distribution. University of Tokyo Press.
Artichoke, Globe	Cynara	
Artichoke, Wild	Olearia	
Bitterweed	Helenium	
Boneset	Eupatorium	
Broomweed	Amphiachyris	
Burdock	Arctium	
Burrobrush	Hymenoclea	
Cape-weed	Cryptostemma	
Chamomile, German	Matricaria	
Chamomile, Roman	Anthemis	
Cocklebur	Xanthium	
Champaca of perfumery	Michelia (Magnoliaceae)	(Jalapatra et at 1973)
Chicory	Cichorium	
Chrysanthemum	Chrysanthemum	(Osawa et al 1973)
Cosmos	Cosmos	
Costus of perfumery	Saussurea	
Cottonthistle	Onopordon	
Encelia	Encelia	
Feverfew	Parthenium	
Fireweed	Gaillardia	
Fleabane	Erigeron	
Guayule	Parthenium	
Hempweed	Mikania	
Ironweed	Vernonia	
Laurel oil	Laurus (Lauraceae)	(Tada and Jakeda 1971)
Leafcup	Polymnia	
Lettuce	Lactuca	
Liverwort	Frullania	
Magnolia	Magnolia (Magnoliaceae)	(Wiedhopf et al 1973)
Marguerite	Chrysanthemum	
Marigold	Calendula	
Marshelder	Iva	
Oxeye	Telekia	
Pyrethrum	Chrysanthemum	
Ragweed	Ambrosia	
Sagebrush	Artemisia	
Sneezeweed	Helenium	
Sowthistle	Sonchus	
Starthistle	Centaurea	
Stinkwort	Inula	
Sunflower	Helianthus	
Tansy	Tanacetum	

Tulip-tree	Liriodendron	(Magnoliaceae)(Doskotch et al 1972,
Whitewood of commerce	Liriodendron	Doskotch and El-Feraly 1969)
Wormwood	Artemisia	
Yarrow	Achillea	

Chemistry

Recent advances

Potentially allergenic sesquiterpene lactones have been isolated from the following plants (Rodriguez, E., Pers. comm. 1975).

Liatris spp.

Herz, Z. et al (1975) Phytochemistry 14, 1561.
Kupchan, S.M. et al (1973) J. Org. Chem. 38, 1853.

Melampodium sp.

Neidle, S. and Rogers, D. (1972) Chem. Comm. 140.

Moquinia sp.

Tomassini, T.C.B. and Gilbert, B. (1972) Phytochemistry 11, 1177.

Montanoa sp.

Geissman, T.A. and Griffin, T.S. (1971) Rev. Latenoamer. Quim. 2, 811.

Polymnia sp.

Herz, W. and Bhat, S.V. (1973) Phytochemistry 12, 1737.

Pluchea sp.

Bohlmann, F. and Grenz, M. (1969) Tetrahedron Letters. 5111.

Vanillosmopsis sp.

Corbella, A. et al (1974) Phytochemistry 13, 459.

Bahia sp.

Herz, W. and Bhat, S.V. (1972) J. Org. Chem. 37, 906.
Wagner, H. et al (1972) Phytochemistry 11, 371.

Centaurea sp.

Gonzalez, A.G. et al (1973) Phytochemistry 12, 2997.
Harley-Mason, D.J. et al (1972) Chem. Comm. 460.

Cacalia

Hayashi, K. et al (1973) Phytochemistry 12, 2931.

Venegasia

Geissman, T.A. and Atala, S. (1971) Phytochemistry 10, 1075.

Eriophyllum, sp.

Geissman, T.A. and Atala, S. (1971) Phytochemistry 10, 1075

Chaenactis sp.

Geissman, T.A. and Atala, S. (1971) Phytochemistry 10, 1075.

Picridium sp.

Gonzalez, A.G. et al (1974) Phytochemistry 13, 611.

Pentzia sp.

Bohlmann, F. and Zdero, C. (1972) Tetrahedron Letters 621.

Lidbeckia sp.

Bohlmann, F. and Zdero, C. (1972) Tetrahedron Letters 621.

Jurinea sp.

Drozdz, B. et al (1973) Coll. Czech. Chem. Comm. 38, 727.

Iva spp.

Sundaraman, P. et al (1973) Tetrahedron Letters 3809.
Chikamatsu, H. and Herz, W. (1973 J. Org. Chem. 38, 585.
Herz, W. et al (1972) Phytochemistry 11, 1829.
Samek, Z. et al (1970) Coll. Czech. Chem. Comm. 35, 3818.

Inula graveolens

d.Alcontres, G.S. et al (1973) Gazz. Chim. Ital. 103, 239.

Hymenoxys sp.

Herz, W. et al (1970) J. Org. Chem. 35, 2611.

Eremanthus sp.

Vichneioski, W. and Gilbert (1972) Phytochemistry 11, 2563.

Eupatorium spp.

Kupchan, S.M. et al (1973) J. Org. Chem. 38, 2189.
Kupchan, S.M. et al (1973) J. Org. Chem. 38, 1260.

Enhydra sp.

Lartha, G. and Go, K.T. (1972) Chem. Comm. 1327.

Tribe: Heliantheae

Acanthospermum

Eight species are found mainly in the West Indies and South America.

Acanthospermum hispidum (Starr Burr)

Entry of a burr of the plant into the skin of the ankle caused a prolonged disability (Flecker 1945).

Flecker, H. (1945) Injuries produced by plants in tropical Queensland Med. J. Australia 1, 636.

Tribe: Anthemidae

Achillea

Two hundred species are found in north temperate areas.

Achillea lanulosa (Yarrow) and Achillea millefolium (Yarrow)

produced positive patch test reactions in 4 out of 21 patients who had weed dermatitis (Mackoff and Dahl 1951).

Desacetylmatricarin derived from A. lanulosa (Yoshioka et al 1973) produced positive patch test reactions in a sesquiterpene lactone sensitive patient (Mitchell 1973).

Mackoff, S. and Dahl, A.O. (1951) A botanical consideration of the weed oleoresin problem. Minn. Med. 34, 1169.

Yoshioka, H., Mabry, T.J. and Timmermann, B.N. (1973) Sesquiterpene Lactones. Chemistry, NMR and Plant Distribution. University of Tokyo Press.

Mitchell, J.C. (1973) Unpublished observations.

Tribe Anthemidae

Achillea millefolium (Milfoil, Yarrow)

Dermatitis from the plant was reported by Lewin in 1899. The powdered dry leaves are irritating to the nasal mucous membrane (Pammel 1911) and have long been used as a sternutatory. The plant caused dermatitis in bathers and, mixed with sheaves of barley, in a farmer (Low 1924). The plant was early suspected as a photosensitizer in Oppenheim's meadow dermatitis (Philadelphy 1828, Gans 1929, Créhange and Rosenthal 1933) but, under experimental conditions, extracts of the plant were found to show no photoxic activity (Van Dijk and Berrens 1964) and psoralens have not been reported from the plant. The plant applied as is by patch test is probably irritant (Gans 1929), but tests with extracts at non-irritant concentrations suggest that the plant is also a sensitizer (Shelmire 1939, Mackoff and Dahl 1951, Woods 1952). Drinking of Yarrow tea by a sensitized individual produced a generalized eruption (Gans 1929). The sesquiterpene lactones known from the plant (Yoshioka et al 1973) do not include a recognized sensitizer. Infraspecies differentiation in this plant (Ehrendorfer 1968) suggest the possibility of biochemical variation. Oil of Yarrow is produced from the plant (Merck 1968).

Achillea moschata yields an oil of flavouring and perfumery (Arctander 1960).

Arctander, S. (1960) Perfume and Flavor Materials of Natural Origin. Elizabeth, N.J., Published by the author.

Ehrendorfer, F. (1968) Geographical and ecological aspects of infraspecific differentiation. Chap. 17 in Modern Methods in Plant Taxonomy ed. Heywood, V.H. London Academic Press.

Gans, O. (1929) Ueber die Dermatitis durch Achillea millefolium. Ein Beitrag zur Aetiologie der beim Freibaden entstehenden Hautausschlage, Deutsche med. Wchnschr 55, 1213.

Low, R.C. (1924) Skin Sensitiveness to Non-Bacterial Proteins and Toxins. Brit. J. Derm. Syph. 31, 292.

Mackoff, S. and Dahl, A.O. (1951) A botanical consideration of the weed oleoresin problem. Minn. Med. 34, 1169.

Merck Index (1968) An Encyclopedia of Chemicals and Drugs. ed. Stecher, P.G. 8th ed. Rahway, N.J. Merck & Co. Inc.

Pammel, L.H. (1911) A Manual of Poisonous Plants. Torch Press. Cedar Rapids, Iowa. Reprinted Univ. Microfilms Inc. Ann Arbor, Mich. 1965. pp. 476-7.

Philadelphy, A. (1928) Eine bullose Hauterkrankung, hervorgerufen durch Achillea millefolium Wien. klin. Wchnschr. 41, 88.

Shelmire, B. (1939) Contact dermatitis from weeds: Patch testing with their oleoresins. JAMA 113, 1085 and unpublished table accompanying reprints.

Van Dijk, E. and Berrens, L. (1964) Plants as an etiological factor in phytophotodermatitis. Dermatologica (Basel) 129, 321.

Yoshioka, H., Mabry, T.J. and Timmermann, B.H. (1973) Sesquiterpene Lactones. Chemistry, NMR and Plant Distribution. University of Tokyo Press.

Créhange, J.L. and Rosenthal (no initial)(1933) Dermite bullense striée consecutive aux bains de soleil dans las prés. Bull Soc. franc. Derm. Syph. 40, 1261.

Achillea ptarmica (Sneezewort)

has been recognized as a sternutatory for centuries (Gerard 1636, Uphof 1959).

Gerard J. (1636) The Herball or Generall Historie of Plantes. The essence thereof distilled by M. Woodward (1927) from the edition of Th. Johnson 1630. London Gerald Howe.

Uphof, J.C.T. (1959) Dictionary of Economic Plants. New York. Hafner Publ. Co.

Tribe: Heliantheae (Ambrosieae)

Ambrosia (Ragweed)

35-40 species have been recognized.

Several different species are called Ragweed. Much confusion exists in the use both of the scientific and colloquial names of these species. Wagner (1959) recognized the following species:

Ambrosia artemisiifolia
(syn. A. eliator)
Common, Short, Low Ragweed

Ambrosia psilostachya
(syn. A. coronopilifolia)
Western, Perennial Ragweed.

Ambrosia trifida
(syn. A. Aptera)
Great, High, Tall Ragweed.

Fernald (1970) adds A. bidentata.

Wodehouse(1971) recognized some 21 species and recorded their distribution in North America with respect to pollinosis (Type I hypersensitivity).

Geographic distribution - North America

Ambrosia species are American in origin and are known ecologically as pioneer plants; that is to say they are well adapted to invade vacant soils, from which the customary vegetation has been removed. From a limited distribution, they have thrived with the coming of agriculture, disturbance of the land and interference with the ecology of the North American prairies and the south (Wodehouse 1971). The plants are still spreading and have invaded the Pacific North West (Perlman 1952). In Canada, Ragweeds are spreading northward and westward; each decade shows a westward spread; the West coast is still almost free (Bassett and Crompton 1966).

Geographic distribution - World

In Hawaii, Short Ragweed is reported to be present in a number of places. The presence of A. psilostachya in Australia was first reported in 1963 (Ford 1963). Ragweed was introduced from North America into Assam where it has now established itself as an escape (Behl et al 1966). The plants are limited in their distribution by length of day and temperature; they flower only under short day conditions of 12 hours or less sunlight. They are thus found in greater abundance between latitudes 45° and 30°. One noteworthy exception is they do not seem to naturalize generally in Japan (Wagner 1959). Ragweeds are scanty in the British Isles*(Queries and Minor notes 1948) but have colonized waste ground in some countries. Species are found in Germany, Belgium, France, Switzerland, Holland, Austria and other European countries (Lawalree 1947), in Sweden (Simmons 1928), Italy (Vignolo-Lutati 1939) and Argentina (Bozzola and Valentinetti 1955). Two introductions of local interest are along the railroad tracks of British Columbia and on the World War II invasion beaches of Normandy.

Bassett, I.J. and Crompton, C.W. (1966). Air-borne pollen surveys in British Columbia. Canada J. Plant. Sci. 47, 252.

Behl, P.N., Captain, R.M., Bedi, B.M.S. and Gupta, S. (1966) Skin irritant and sensitizing plants found in India, New Delhi. P.N. Behl, Irwin Hospital.

Bozzola, C.J. and Valentinetti, E. (1955) Contact dermatitis due to a fat-soluble portion of ragweed. Arch Argen. Dermat. 5, 181.

Fernald, M.L. (1970) Gray's Manual of Botany. 8th ed. 1970. New York. Van Nostrand Reinhold Co.

Ford, R.M. (1963) Ragweed pollenosis. Med. J. Australia. 1, 712.

Lawalree, A. (1947) Les Ambrosia adventices in Europe occidentale. Bull. Jard. Bot. Etat. Bruxelles 18, 305.

Perlman, F. (1952) Ragweed invasion of Oregon. J. Allergy 23, 452.

Queries and Minor Notes (1948) Ragweeds in Europe. JAMA 134, 1579.

Simmons, H.G. (1928) De i Sverige funna artenera Ambrosia L. (species of Ambrosia in Sweden). Sensk. Bot. Tidskr. 22, 437.

Vignolo-Lutati, F. (1939) Sulla sistematic di alcune Ambrosiae (Taxonomy of some ambrosias).

*"Ragweed" is the popular name in Britain for species of Jacobea.

Nuovo Gior. Bot. Ital. 46, 71.

Wagner, W.H. (1959) An annotated bibliography of Ragweed (Ambrosia). Rev. Allergy 13, 353.

Wodehouse, R.P. (1971) Hayfever Plants. 2nd Rev. ed. New York. Hafner Publ. Co. pg. 154.

Allergic contact dermatitis from Ambrosia species is the subject of an extensive literature dating at least from Hannah (1919) and Sutton (1919) and reviewed by Mitchell (1969). A distinction was made by Brown et al (1931) between contact dermatitis from the 'oleoresin' and Type I hypersensitivity from proteinaceous fractions of the pollen. The principal contact sensitizers are sesquiterpene lactones (Mitchell et al 1971). The precise biochemical nature of the atopens of the pollen has not yet been clarified. Cross-sensitivity between Ambrosia and other Compositae species was reported by Brunsting and Williams (1936) and elaborated by Shelmire (1939) and Mackoff and Dahl (1951). The biochemical basis of the cross-sensitivity is the presence of related sesquiterpene lactones in the plants (Mitchell and Dupuis 1971). Cross-sensitivity with pyrethrum (Chrysanthemum cinerariifolium) is probably based on lactone content but other terpenoids may also be involved. Persistence of Ragweed dermatitis may result from contact with fomites; grain and hay contaminated with ragweed oil or from exposure to other plants containing sesquiterpene lactones. Industrial feed and grain handlers can develop Ragweed dermatitis (Jordon et al 1942).

Ragweed pollen may be brought into a house with a Christmas tree (Wyse and Mallock 1970).

Brown, A., Milford, E.L. and Coca, A.F. (1931) Studies in contact dermatitis. I. The Nature and etiology of pollen dermatitis. J. Immunol. 20, 301.

Brunsting, L.A. and Williams, D.H. (1936) Ragweed (contact) dermatitis. Observations in 48 cases and report of unsuccessful attempts at desensitization by injection of specific oils. JAMA 106, 1533.

Hannah, L. (1919) Ragweed dermatitis

-a new treatment
report of a case. JAMA 22, 853.

Jordon, J.W., Campbell, P.C. and Osborne, E.D. (1942) Ragweed dermatitis among workers in the flour and grain industries. Arch. Derm. Syph. 46, 721.

Mackoff, S. and Dahl, A.O. (1951) A botanical consideration of the weed oleoresin problem. Minn. Med. 34, 1169.

Mitchell, J.C. (1969) Allergic Contact Dermatitis from Compositae. Trans. St. John's Hosp. Derm. Soc. 55, 174.

Mitchell, J.C. and Dupuis, G. (1971) Allergic Contact Dermatitis from sesquiterpenoids of the Compositae family of Plants. Brit. J. Derm. 8, 139.

Mitchell, J.C., Roy, A.E., Dupuis, G. and Towers, G.H.N. (1971) Allergic Contact Dermatitis from Ragweeds (Ambrosia Species). Arch.Derm. 104, 73.

Shelmire, B. (1939) Contact Dermatitis from weeds: Patch testing with their oleoresins. JAMA 113, 1085 and unpublished table accompanying reprints.

Sutton, R.L. (1919) Ragweed dermatitis. JAMA 73, 1433.

Wyse, D.M. and Mallock. D. (1970) Christmas tree allergy: mould and pollen studies. Canad. Med. Ass. J. 103, 1272.

A review of Ambrosia dermatitis has included the reports of Klauder (1929), Sulzberger and Wise (1930), Ramirez and Eller (1930), Milford (1930), Gay and Ketron (1932), Pascher and Sulzberger (1933), Frank (1935), Shelmire and Black (1937), Trunnell (1940), Sheldon and Blumenthal (1941), Case Presentation (1943), Slater et al (1946, 1947, 1948), Brachman and Roy (1954), Fisher (1957), Canizares and Trilla (1957), Trilla (1957), Fromer and Jenkins (1959), Cohen (1959), Strizler (1960), Spencer (1966). Other references are listed under individual species names.

Jillson et al (1959), Epstein (1960), Mitchell (1969) and Lonkar et al (1974) provide critical discussion.

Reports of specific hyposensitization by administration of Ambrosia extracts have rarely included evidence by quantitative patch testing. In such a study Fisher (1952) reported success by the oral route. Spontaneous desensitization was not observed. Some other references to Ambrosia dermatitis related to hyposensitisation were recorded by Mitchell (1969).

Brachman, E. and Roy, A.K. (1954) Oral hyposensitization by oleoresin extracts. Canad. Med. Assoc. J. 71, 4.

Canizares, O. and Trilla, E. (1957) Dermatitis venenata due to ragweed pollen. Discussion of two preceding cases. Arch. Derm. 75, 906.

Case Presentation (1943) Ragweed Dermatitis. Arch. Derm. Syph. 47, 714 and discussion.

Cohen, S.G. (1959) Seasonal ragweed dermatitis. Association of immediate and delayed types of pollen sensitivity. Arch. Derm. 79, 328.

Epstein, S. (1960) Role of dermal sensitivity in ragweed contact dermatitis. Arch. Derm. 82, 48.

Fisher, A.A. (1952) Some immunologic phenomena in treatment of and patch testing for ragweed oil dermatitis. J. Invest. Derm. 19 271.

Frank, L.J. (1935) Ragweed dermatitis J. Iowa M. Soc. 25, 283.

Fromer, J.L. and Jenkins, W.S. (1959) Ragweed oil dermatitis. Lahey Clinic Bull. 11, 75.

Gay, L.N. and Ketron, L.W. (1932) A case of ragweed dermatitis recurring over a period of 13 years. J. Allergy 3, 478.

Jillson, O.F., Curwen, W.L. and Alexander, B.R. (1959) Problems of contact dermatitis in the atopic individual: with reference to neomycin and ragweed oil sensitivity. Ann. Allergy 17, 215.

Klauder, J.V. (1929) Clinical aspects of allergy in Dermatology.

Arch.Derm. & Syph. 19, 198.

Lonkar, A., Mitchell, J.C. and Calnan, C.D. (1974) Contact Dermatitis from Parthenium hysterophorus. Trans. St. John's Hosp. Derm. Soc. 60, 43.

Milford, E.L. (1930) Studies in allergy. I. The specific activity of pollen oil. J. Allergy 1, 331.

Mitchell, J.C. (1969) Allergic contact dermatitis from Compositae. Trans. St. John's Hosp. Derm. Soc. 55, 174.

Pascher, F. and Sulzberger, M.B. (1933) Ragweed dermatitis. Report of two cases. Arch. Derm. & Syph. 28, 233.

Fisher, A.A. (1957) Dermatitis venenata due to ragweed pollen (disdussion of case) Arch. Derm. 75, 906.

Ramirez, M.A. and Eller, J.J. (1930) The patch test in 'Contact Dermatitis',(Dermatitis venenata) J. Allergy 1, 489.

Sheldon, J.N. and Blumenthal, F. (1941) Observations on the oral administration of ragweed oil. Amer. J. Med. Sci. 202, 98.

Shelmire, B. and Black, J.H. (1937) A method of patch testing with plant oil. JAMA 108, 719.

Slater, B.J., Norris, J.L. and Francis, N. (1946) Ragweed dermatitis. Occup. Med. 2, 298.

Slater, B.J., Norris, J.L. and Francis, N. (1947) Ragweed dermatitis (oral desensitization) N.Y. State J. Med. 47, 2322.

Slater, B.J., Norris, J.L. and Francis, N. (1948) Ragweed dermatitis, therapy by oral route. Ann. Allergy 6, 594.

Strizler, C. (1960) Ragweed dermatitis in a cemetery worker. Archs. Derm. 81, 1009.

Spencer, Mc(1966) Open versus closed patch testing with oleoresins. Archs. Derm. 93, 47.

Sulzberger, M.B. and Wise, F. (1930) Ragweed dermatitis with sensitization and desensitization phenomena. JAMA 94, 93.

Trilla, E. (1957) Dermatitis venenata due to ragweed pollen. Case report and discussion. Arch. Derm. 75, 905.

Trunnell, T.L. (1940) Weed dermatitis J. Iowa Med. Soc. 30, 390.

Tribe: Heliantheae

Ambrosia acanthicarpa
(see Franseria)

Ambrosia artemisiifolia
(syn. A. eliator) (Short ragweed) is found almost throughout the United States, extending in distribution from the Atlantic to the Pacific, throughout southern Canada and as far south as southern Florida, northern California and Cuba. Short ragweed is a complex and variable species consisting of a number of genotypes which, under natural environmental conditions, tend to segregate out (Wodehouse 1971). In various reports 14 of 18 (Brunsting and Anderson 1934), 37 of 40 (Brunsting and Anderson 1936), 23 of 50 patients (Shelmire 1939), and 23 of 25 patients (Mackoff and Dahl 1951) who had 'weed dermatitis' showed positive patch test reactions to this species.

Ambrosia bidentata
(Lance leaved Ragweed) was described as a plant of high-sensitizing capacity in the production of 'weed dermatitis' in the southern United States (Shelmire 1940).

Ambrosia psilostachya
(Western Ragweed)

"Weed dermatitis" from this plant was reported by Brunsting and Williams (1936) and Shelmire (1939, 1940). This species occurs in slightly different forms which are regarded by some taxonomists as different species (Wodehouse 1971). The plant displays an extremely variable morphology and different populations of the plants can yield different sesquiterpene lactones (Potter and Mabry 1971) which are proven or potentially allergenic (Mitchell and Dupuis 1971). The presence of delta-3-carene (Potter and Mabry 1971) may explain the cross-sensitivity between turpentine and Ragweed described by Fisher (1952).

Brunsting, L.A. and Anderson, C.R. (1934). Ragweed dermatitis. A report based on 18 cases. JAMA 103, 1285.

Brunsting, L.A. and Williams, D.H. (1936) Ragweed (contact) dermatitis. Observations in 48 cases and report of unsuccessful attempts at desensitization by injection of specific oils. JAMA 106, 1533.

Fisher, A.A. (1952) Some immunologic phenomena in treatment of and patch testing for ragweed oil dermatitis. J. Invest. Derm. 19, 271.

Mackoff, S. and Dahl, A.O. (1951) A botanical consideration of the weed oleoresin problem. Minn. Med. 34, 1169.

Mitchell, J.C. and Dupuis, G. (1971) Allergic Contact Dermatitis from Sesquiterpenoids of the Compositae family of Plants. Brit. J. Derm. 8, 139.

Potter, J.L. and Mabry, T.J. (1971) Origin of the Texas Gulf coast island populations of Ambrosia psilostachya: a numerical study using terpenoid data. Phytochemistry 11, 715.

Shelmire, B. (1939) Contact dermatitis from weeds: Patch testing with their oleoresins. JAMA 113, 1085 and unpublished table accompanying reprints.

Shelmire, B. (1940) Contact dermatitis from vegetation. South med. J. 33, 338.

Wodehouse, R.P. (1971) Hayfever Plants. 2nd Rev. ed. New York. Hafner Publ. Co. pg. 154.

Ambrosia trifida (Giant Ragweed) is of low sensitizing capacity (Brunsting and Williams 1936, Shelmire 1939) and rarely produces positive patch test reactions in Compositae sensitive patients.

Brunsting, L.A. and Williams, D.H. (1936) Ragweed (contact) dermatitis. Observations in 48 cases and report of unsuccessful attempts at desensitization by injection of specific oils. JAMA 106, 1533.

Shelmire, B. (1939) Contact dermatitis from weeds: Patch testing with their oleoresins. JAMA 113, 1085 and unpublished table accompanying reprints.

Tribe: Astereae

Amphiachyris

Two species are found in California.

Amphiachyris dracunculoides (Broom weed)

The plant produced positive patch test reactions in 6 of 50 patients with 'weed dermatitis' (Shelmire 1939).

Shelmire, B. (1939) Contact dermatitis from weeds: Patch testing with their oleoresins. JAMA 113, 1085 and unpublished table accompanying reprints.

Tribe: Anthemideae

Anacyclus

Twenty-five species are found in the Mediterranean region. Some species, notably A. depressus, are quite widely cultivated.

Anacyclus pyrethrum (Spanish Chamomile, Pellitory)

The root was used as a rubefacient and is a powerful irritant to the skin (Dispensatory 1884). The harvested flower-heads are dried in the sun and powdered between the thumb and fingers to yield a kind of Pyrethrum. Dermatitis can occur at these skin sites in workers who handle the plant (Chopra et al 1958).

Anacyclus pedunculatus was listed as an irritant by Pammel (1911).

Chopra, R.N., Chopra, I.C., Handa, K.L. and Kapur, L.D. (1958) Chopra's Indigenous Drugs of India. 2nd ed. Calcutta. U.N. Dhur & Sons Ltd.

Dispensatory, The National (1884). Philadelphia. Stille & Maisch.

Pammel, L.H. (1911) A Manual of Poisonous Plants. Torch Press. Cedar Rapids, Iowa. Reprinted

University Microfilms Inc., Ann Arbor, Mich. 1965. pg. 476-7.

Anthemis

200 species occur in Mediterranean areas of Europe extending to Iran.

Anthemis arvensis (Corn Chamomile)

Vesicular dermatitis occurred from picking the plant (Fivoli 1936). Patch tests were positive to the flowers and negative to the leaves. However in three cases Moslein (1963) obtained positive reactions to petals and leaves. Cross-sensitivity was observed with two other plants named Chamomile, Anthemis nobilis and Matricaria chamomilla.

Fivoli, C. (1936) Hypersensitivity to camomile: Dermatitis and general symptoms. Dermosifilografo 11, 614.

Moslein, P. (1963) Pflanzen als Kontakt-Allergene. Berufsdermatosen 11, 24.

Anthemis cotula (Stinking Mayweed, Dog Fennel, Dog Chamomile)

Several authors agree that the plant is a strong irritant (White 1887, Pammel 1911, Chopra and Badhwar 1940) and other reports suggest irritancy (Sequeira 1921, Rowe 1934, Underwood and Gaul 1948). Use of the plant in a shampoo caused dermatitis (Sternberg 1937).

Sixteen farm-workers developed a bullous eruption of the exposed parts (Grichener 1935); the hands and also the feet were affected in harvest workers who worked barefooted (Krantz 1938). Bullous dermatitis of the feet occurred in flax workers, barefooted in fields in which A. cotula was a common weed. (D'Agostino 1927). The plant is also probably allergenic since 5 of 25 patients who had 'weed dermatitis' showed positive patch test reactions to an extract of the plant (Mackoff and Dahl 1951). However, Shelmire (1940) observed urticarial patch test reactions lasting 12-14 hours and negative reactions at 24 hours.

Alleged phytophotodermatitis from the plant is incorrect. Sunlight is not necessary to produce the skin reactions and psoralens have not been reported from the plant (Woods 1962).

Chopra, R.N. and Badhwar, R.L. (1940) An account of the poisonous plants of India. Indian J. Agr. Sci. 20, 1.

Grichener, E. (1935) Dermatitis venenosa provocada por la manzanilla. Semana med. 2, 362.

Krantz, W. (1938) Bullous dermatitis in harvest workers. Munch. med. Wchnschr. 85, 1057.

Mackoff, S. and Dahl, A.O. (1951) A botanical consideration of the weed oleoresin problem. Minn. Med. 34, 1169.

Pammel, L.H. (1911) A Manual of Poisonous Plants. Torch Press. Cedar Rapids, Iowa. Reprinted Univ. Microfilms Inc. Ann Arbor, Mich. 1965. pg. 476-7.

Rowe, A.H. (1934) Camomile (Anthemis cotula) as a skin irritant. J. Allergy 5, 383.

Sequeira, J.H. (1921) A case of bullous eruption caused by May-weed. Lancet 2, 560.

Shelmire, B. (1940) Contact dermatitis from vegetation. South med. J. 33, 338.

Sternberg, L. (1937) Contact dermatitis. J. Allergy 8, 185.

Underwood, G.B. and Gaul, L.E. (1948) Overtreatment dermatitis in dermatitis venenata due to plants. JAMA 138, 570.

White, J.C. (1887) Dermatitis venenata: An account of the action of External irritants upon the skin. Boston. Cupples and Hurd.

Woods, B. (1962) Irritant Plants. Trans. St. John's Hosp. derm. Soc. 48, 75.

d'Agostino, M. (1927) Sobra una dermatitis eritematoampollosa observada en obreros occupados en la trilla del lino. Semana Medica 34, 641.

Anthemis nobilis is a strong-smelling perennial cultivated for ornamental purposes and for its fragrant herbage. The dried yellow flowers are used to make a medicinal tea and for wet compresses for the skin. Contact with the plant has caused dermatitis in farmers (D'Agostino 1935, Hissard 1946), in a plant collector (Babini 1949) and in pharmaceutical chemists (Schwartz et al 1957). Compresses of chamomile (Jadassohn and Zaruski 1927) and chamomile ointment (Beetz et al 1971) can cause dermatitis and drinking chamomile tea can exacerbate contact dermatitis (Babini 1949). An anaphylactoid reaction occurred from a tea (Benner and Lee 1973) and urticaria and asthma from an enema (Jaeggy 1931). The petals produced positive patch test reactions and cross-sensitivity was observed to *Anthemis arvensis* and *Matricaria chamomilla* (Moslein 1963). Cross sensitivity to *Chrysanthemum* has also been observed (Leipold 1938). Fivoli (1936) obtained positive patch test reactions with the blossoms, negative with the leaves. One of 290 (Meneghini et al 1971) and 3 of 200 patients in a skin clinic (Beetz et al 1971) showed positive patch test reactions to chamomile oil and chloroform extract of chamomile respectively.

The plant yields nobilin (Yoshioka et al 1973) a potentially allergenic sesquiterpene lactone.

In some reports the common name Chamomile may refer to *A. nobilis* (Roman Chamomile) or to *Matricaria chamomilla* (German Chamomile). *Anthemis nobilis* is now designated *Chamaemelum nobile*.

Babini, G. (1949) A not uncommon form of allergy to chamomile. Minerva Med. 2, 917.

Beetz, D., Cramer, H.J. and Mehlhorn, H. Ch. (1971). Zur haufigkeit der epidermalen allergie gegenuber Kamille in kamillenhaltigen arzneimitteln und kosmetica. Derm. Mschr. 157, 505.

Benner, M.H. and Lee, H.W. (1973) Anaphylactic reaction to Chamomile tea. J. Allerg. Clin. Immunol. 52, 307.

D'Agostino, M. (1935) Sobre la dermatitis venenosa provocada por la manzanilla. Semana med. 2, 510.

Fivoli, C. (1936) Hypersensitivity to camomile: Dermatitis and general symptoms. Dermosifilografo 11, 614.

Hissard, H. (1946) Dermatose bulleuse due à la camomille. Soc. franc. Derm. Syph. Séance. 11 July.

Jadassohn, W. and Zaruski, M. (1927) Idiosynkrasie gegen Kamillen Schweiz. med. Wochenschr 57, 868.

Jaeggy, E. (1931) Crises d'urticaire et d'asthma provoqueés par les lavements a la camomille. Schweiz. med. Wchnschr. 61, 572.

Leipold, H. (1938) Dermatitis der Hände und de Gesichts infolge Überempfindlichkeit gegen Chrysanthemem und Kamillen Zbl. Haut.-Geschlkrkh. 57, 248.

Meneghini, C.L., Rantuccio, F. and Lomuto, M. (1971) Additives, Vehicles and active drugs of topical medicaments as causes of delayed-type allergic dermatitis. Dermatologica 143, 137.

Moslein, P. (1963) Pflanzen als Kontakt-Allergene Berufsdermatosen 11, 24.

Schwartz, L., Tulipan, L. and Birmingham, D.J. (1957) Occupational Diseases of the Skin. 3rd. ed. Philadelphia. Lea & Febiger. pp. 637-672.

Yoshioka, H., Mabry, T.J.and Timmerman, B.N. (1973) Sesquiterpene Lactones. Chemistry, NMR and Plant Distribution. University Tokyo Press.

Tribe: Cynareae

Arctium

Five species are found in temperate regions. The burs cling to fur and aid in dispersing the fruits.

Arctium lappa
(syn. *Lappa vulgaris*) (Burdock)

The rough hairs can produce mechanical irritation of the skin (Sidi 1951) and of the cornea; the effects on the eye are both mechanical and toxic (Bruhn 1938, Havener et al 1955, Breed and Kuwabara 1966). The barbed needles attached to the seeds are responsible rather than the outer shafts that hook onto clothing (Duke-Elder and MacFaul 1972). A statement that the leaves can produce contact dermatitis (Massey 1941) requires confirmation.

Arctium officinalis
(syn. Lappa officinalis)

The rough leaves were used as a rubefacient; parts of the burrs mixed with seeds irritated workmen unless they stood to windward (White 1887).

Bruhn, A.M. (1938) Klinische und experimentelle Untersuchungen uber Augenschadigunger durch Klettenhaare. Klin. Monatsbl. Augengh. 101, 730.

Duke-Elder, S. amd MacFaul (1972a). System of Opthalmology. Vol. XIV. Injuries Part 1. Mechanical Injuries. Extra-ocular foreign bodies pp. 464-467 and Agricultural Injuries pp. 32-34. London Henry Kimpton.

Havener, W.H. et al (1955) Burdock bur opthalmia. Arch. opthalm. 53, 260.

Massey, A.B. (1941) Plant Poisoning. Merck Reports. 50, 24.

Sidi, E. (1951) Dermites par contact avec des plantes in Les Dermatoses Allergiques (Tzanck & Sidi) Paris Masson.

White, J.C. (1887) Dermatitis venenata: An account of the action of External irritants upon the skin. Boston. Cupples & Hurd.

Breed, F.B. and Kuwabara, T. (1966) Burdock ophthalmia. Arch. Ophthal 75, 16.

Arctotheca
(syn. Cryptostemma)

Four species occur in southern Africa, two in Australia.

Arctotheca calendulacea
(Capeweed)

The species is a native of South Africa, adventive to Australia (Hand 1944) and has also been known as Arctotis calendulacea in horticulture. Dermatitis occurred from contact with the plant (Farmer 1941, Hand 1944); the essential oil of the plant produced a positive patch test reaction when diluted 1 in 100 in one case and in a second, a generalized flare-up of dermatitis followed patch testing (Hand 1944). The fresh plant is irritant by closed patch test in almost every case tested (Burry 1973).

Burry et al (1973) observed positive patch test reactions from the plant in patients who had 'weed dermatitis' in Australia and cross-sensitivity with Chrysanthemum, Xanthium, Olearia and Inula species.

Burry, N. (1973) Personal communication.

Burry, J.N., Kuchel, R., Reid, J.G. and Kirk, J. (1973). Australian bush dermatitis: Compositae dermatitis in South Australia. Med. J. Australia. 1, 110.

Farmer, P.W., Jr. (1941) The patch test as a means of diagnosis in contact dermatitis. Med. J. Australia 1, 9.

Hand, E.A. (1944) Contact dermatitis due to capeweed. Archs. Derm. Syph. 49, 331.

Tribe: Sececioneae

Arnica

Thirty-two species occur in north temperate regions and in the Arctic.

Arnica montana
(Mountain Tobacco, Wolf's Bane)
provides officinal Tincture of Arnica which is made from all parts of the plant and which has been known to be capable of producing dermatitis since the 19th Century. According to White (1887), Hebra had seen many such cases and recommended, to those who advocated its use, that homeopathic amounts be made up, that is 'a drop of the tincture to a pail of water'. White (1887) also quoted Fox as stating in 1873, "Arnica may produce erythema and swelling of the part to which it is applied, or it may excite a real eczema"; the root was 'irritant' as well as the flowerhead.

The tincture made from the roots is liable to produce dermatitis in pharmacists and the plant has been responsible for dermatitis in gardeners. Cross-sensitivity between Arnica and Chrysanthemum has been observed (Paschoul 1956). Most of the reports of dermatitis from Arnica originate from Europe, where the plant has long been used in topical therapy (Muillot 1899, Biberstein 1927, Hausen and Schulz 1973). The plant yields an oil of perfumery (Arctander 1960). A sesquiterpene lactone (Zakharov et al 1971) which is potentially allergenic (Mitchell and Dupuis 1971) is derived from the plant.

Arctander, S. (1960) Perfume and flavor materials of natural origin. Elizabeth, New Jersey. Published by the author.

Biberstein, H. (1927) Zwei Fälle von Arnicadermatitis. Zbl. Haut. Geschl. Krkh 24, 586.

Hausen, B.M. and Schulz, K.H. (1973) Chrysanthemum-Allergie (1. Mitteilung). Berufsdermatosen 21, 199.

Muillot (1899). Arnica-Dermatitis. Derm. Centralbl. 3, 32.

Paschoud, J.M. (1956) Kontaktekxem durch Chrysanthemum. Gekreutze Uberempfindlichkeits-reaction mit Arnicatinctur. Hautarzt. 16, 229.

White, J.C. (1887) Dermatitis venenata: An account of the action of External irritants upon the skin. Boston. Cupples & Hurd.

Zakharov, P.I., Evstratova, R.I. and Rybalko, K.S. (1971) Mass-spectrometric study of arnifolin, a new sesquiterpene lactone from Arnica montana and A. foliosa. Chem. Nat. Comp. 7, 567.

Turk (1853) in France, Fox (1874) in England, White (1875) in America., Farquharson (1879), Wilson (1879) in England and Laissus (1883), Cartier (1884), Handrix (1884), Cagny (1884), de Molenes (1886) in France described vesicular dermatitis from applicaton of tincture of arnica.

Phillips (cited by Morrow 1887) asserts that the irritant effects of arnica never follow the use of an aqueous solution which contains none of the volatile oil. An insect in the flowers, Atherix maculatus, was implicated by Piffard (1881) who recommended that preparations of the root should be used for topical application.

References

White (1875) Boston Med. and Surg. Journal January.

Fox (1874) Treatise on Skin Diseases London.

Wilson (1879) Lectures on Eczema. London p. 338.

Farguharson (1879) Brit. Med. J. Feb. 15.

Laissus, M. (1887) L'Union Médicale Aug. 17.

Paule de Molenes (1886) Ann. derm. Syph. Feb.

Cartier (1884) Lyon Médical Apr. 13.

Hendrix (1884) St. Louis Méd. and Surg. Jour. June.

Cagny, P. (1884) Jour. de Med. et de Chirurg. Oct.

Piffard (1881) cited by Morrow (1887) Drug eruptions. A clinical study of the irritant effects of drugs upon the skin. New York. Wm. Wood and Co.

Touton, K. (1932) Hauterkrankungen durch phanerogamische Pflanzen und ihre Produkte (Toxicodermia et Allergodermia phytogenes), in Barnewitz, J. et al Angeborene Anomalien, Lichtdermatosen, Pflanzengifte, Thermische Schadidgungen, Einfluss Innerer Storungen auf die Haut. Berlin, Verlag von Julius Springer.

Turk (1853) Journ. des connaisances medico-chirurgicales cited by Touton (1932).

Tribe: Anthemidae

Artemisia (Sagebrush)

Four hundred species are found in north temperate regions and in southern Africa and South America. Species of this genus are common on arid soils of the Western United States and of the Russian steppes.

Artemisia dracunculus (Tarragon) is used for flavouring a vinegar and yields Oil of Tarragon which is used for flavouring and in perfumery (Merck Index 1968). The dried herb is frequently handled by cooks, for it is an essential ingredient of 'Sauce Béarnaise, of high gastronomic repute. A. judaica is said to be the bitter Wormwood of the Old Testament (Proverbs 5, 3). A. maritima yields Oil of Levant Woomseed which contains eucalyptol (cineol) (Merck 1968).

Some five Artemisia species yield oils of perfumery (Arctander 1960) (A. alba, A. annua, A. dracunculus, A. pallens and A. vulgaris).

Chemistry

About 35 species of this genus yield sesquiterpene lactones (Yoshioka et al 1973), many of which are proven or potentially allergenic (Mitchell et al 1970, Mitchell and Dupuis 1971). One such is A. tridentata, a Sagebrush of the southwest United States.

Arctander, S. (1960) Perfume and flavor materials of natural origin. Elizabeth, New Jersey. Published by the author.

Merck Index (1968) An Encyclopedia of Chemicals and Drugs. ed. Stecher, P.G. 8th ed. Rahway, N.J. Merck & Co. Inc.

Mitchell, J.C., Geissman, T.A., Dupuis, G. and Towers, G.H.N. (1970). Allergic contact dermatitis caused by Artemisia and Chrysanthemum species. J. Invest. Derm. 56, 98.

Mitchell, J.C. and Dupuis, G. (1971) Allergic Contact Dermatitis from sesquiterpenoids of the Compositae family of Plants. Brit. J. Derm. 8, 139.

Yoshioka, H., Mabry, T.J. and Timmerman, B.N. (1973) Sesquiterpene Lactones. Chemistry, N.M.R. and Plant Distribution. University Tokyo Press.

Artemisia absinthium (syn. Absinthium)

The flowers of this weed which is common in old gardens and road sides has caused a scarlatiniform eruption in sensitized persons working in its vicinity (Schwartz et al 1957). According to Behl et al (1966) the flowers have a greater sensitizing capacity than the leaves. Four patients, who had had plant dermatitis, showed positive patch test reactions to this plant which was a constituent of a proprietary remedy applied for dermatitis (Underwood and Gaul 1948). The plant is used for flavouring the beverage Absinthe and possibly also Vermouth and yields Oil of Wormwood.

Behl, P.N., Captin, R.M., Bedi, B.M.S. and Gupta, S. (1966) Skin irritant and sensitizing plants found in India, New Delhi. P.N. Behl, Irwin Hospital.

Schwartz, L., Tulipan, L. and Birmingham, D.J. (1957) Occupational Diseases of the Skin. 3rd ed. Philadelphia. Lea & Febiger pp. 637-672.

Underwood, G.B. and Gaul, L.E. (1948) Overtreatment dermatitis in dermatitis venenata due to plants. JAMA 138, 570.

Artemisia afra

This plant is one of the most widely used of herbal remedies in Southern Africa. Any irritant effects from it are probably due to camphor which is present in the volatile oil from the plant (Watt and Breyer-Brandwijk 1962).

Artemisia ludoviciana (Prairie Sage)

Contact sensitivity to Prairie Sage was reported by Brunsting and Anderson (1934) and has been observed by one of the authors (AJR) in a professional gardener. Seventeen of 25 patients who had 'weed dermatitis' showed positive patch test reactions to this plant with cross-sensitivity to other Compositae species (Mackoff and Dahl 1951). The plant yields sesquiterpene lactones (Yoshioka et al 1973), which are potentially allergenic (Mitchell and Dupuis 1971).

Artemisia mexicana (Mexican Mugwort)

None of 50 patients who had

weed dermatitis showed positive patch test reactions to an extract of this plant (Shelmire 1940). A sesquiterpene lactone derived from the plant (Yoshioka et al 1973) is potentially allergenic (Mitchell and Dupuis 1971).

Brunsting, L.A., and Anderson, C.R. (1934) Ragweed dermatitis. A report based on 18 cases. JAMA 103, 1285.

Mackoff, S. and Dahl, A.O. (1951) A botanical consideration of the weed oleoresin problem. Minn. med. 34, 1169.

Mitchell, J.C. and Dupuis, G. (1971) Allergic Contact Dermatitis from sesquiterpenoids of the Compositae family of Plants. Brit. J. Derm. 8, 139.

Shelmire, B. (1939) Contact dermatitis from weeds. Patch testing with their oleoresins. JAMA 113, 1085.

Watt, J.M. and Breyer-Brandwijk, M.G. (1962) The Medicinal and Poisonous Plants of Southern Africa. 2nd ed. Edinburgh. E & S Livingstone.

Yoshioka, H., Mabry, T.J. and Timmerman, B.N. (1973) Sesquiterpene Lactones. Chemistry, N.M.R. and Plant Distribution. University Tokyo Press.

Artemisia vulgaris (Common mugwort)

The ground leaves are used as a counter-irritant in Chinese Medicine (Smith 1969). This plant is listed as an agent of 'weed dermatitis' (Mackoff and Dahl 1951).

Mackoff, S. and Dahl, A.O. (1951) A botanical consideration of the weed oleoresin problem. Minn. Med. 34, 1169.

Smith, F.P. (1969) Chinese Materia Medica. Vegetable kingdom. 2nd ed. Rev. by Hei, P.D. Taipei, Taiwan. Ku T'ing Book House.

Tribe: Heliantheae

Aspilia

125 species are found in South America and in southern tropical Africa. *Aspilia latifolia* (Haemorrhage plant) is used as a haemostatic and is thought to have vaso-constrictor activity. (Oliver 1959).

Oliver, B. (1959) Nigeria's Useful Plants. Nigerian Field 24, 13.

Tribe: Astereae

Aster

500 species are found in Europe, Africa and America. *Aster* species are used in horticulture but the widely grown China Asters belong to the genus *Callistephus*. Therefore, reports of contact dermatitis in florists from colloquially named Asters (Dorsey 1962, Hjorth 1965) must be treated with caution. *Aster exilis* and *A. multiflorus* (Wild Asters) were implicated as infrequent sensitizers in 'weed dermatitis' (Shelmire 1940).

Dorsey, C.S. (1962) Plant Dermatitis in California. Calif. Med. 96, 412.

Hjorth, N. (1965) Contact sensitivity to plants and balsams. Europ. Congr. Allergy Acta derm-venereol. p. 65.

Shelmire, B. (1940) Contact dermatitis from vegetation. South Med. J. 33, 338.

Baccharis

400 species are found in America especially on the campos. Many are leafless xerophytes.

Baccharis spp.

Some species can cause hayfever (Wodehouse 1971).

Wodehouse, R.P. (1971) Hayfever Plants. 2nd rev. edition. New York. Hafner.

Bellis

15 species are found in Europe and the Mediterranean region.

Bellis sp.

Species of this genus e.g. *Bellis perennis* (English Daisy) are occasional causes of hayfever, (Wodehouse 1971).

Wodehouse, R.P. (1971) Hayfever Plants. 2nd rev. edition. New York. Hafner.

Tribe: Heliantheae

Bidens

230 species are cosmopolitan. Several species are known in horticulture as Bur-Marigold or Sticktights. Barbed bristles are present on the fruits and can cause mechanical injury (Muenscher 1951). The barbs of Bidens biternata (Beggar ticks) (Behl et al 1966), Bidens frondosa (White 1887), Bidens pilosa (Maiden 1895) can adhere to clothing or to the hair of animals and have caused dermatitis in South Africa (Scott 1967). Irritancy is ascribed to Bidens bipinnata (Pammel 1911) and Bidens frondosa (Coulter 1904, MacDougal 1894). Handling of Bidens frondosa causes itching (White 1887). In China, a black hair dye is made from Bidens tripartita (Smith 1969).

Reference

Behl, P.N., Captain, R.M., Bedi, B.M.S. and Gupta, S. (1966). Skin irritant and sensitizing plants found in India, New Delhi. P.N. Behl. Irwin Hospital.

Coulter, S. (1904) The poisonous plants of Indiana. Proc. Indiana Acad. Sci. 51-63.

MacDougal, D.T. (1894) Poisonous influences of various species of cyripedium. Minnesota Botan. Studies. pp. 32 and 450.

Maiden, J.H. (1895) The Weeds of New South Wales. Ag. Gaz. New South Wales. 6, 671.

Muenscher, W.C. (1951) Poisonous plants of the United States, 2nd ed. New York. The MacMillan Co.

Pammel, L.H. (1911) A Manual of Poisonous Plants. Torch Press. Cedar Rapids, Iowa. Reprinted Univ. Microfilms Inc. Ann Arbor, Mich. 1965. pp. 476-7.

Smith, F.P. (1969) Chinese Materia Medica. Vegetable kingdom. 2nd ed. Rev. by Hei, P.D. Taipei, Taiwan. Ku T'ing Book House.

White, J.C. (1887) Dermatitis venenata: An account of the Action of external irritants upon the skin. Boston. Cupples and Hurd.

Scott, F.P. (1967) Personal Communication.

Tribe: Inuleae

Blumea

50 species are distributed in tropical and southern Africa, India, eastern Asia and Australia.

Blumea balsamifera yields a camphor.

Blumea gariepina is reported to cause contact urticaria (Watt and Breyer-Brandwijk 1962).

Reference

Watt, J.M. and Breyer-Brandwijk, M.G. (1962) The medicinal and Poisonous Plants of Southern Africa. 2nd ed. Edinburgh. E. & S. Livingstone.

Tribe: Senecioneae

Brachyglottis

Two species are found in New Zealand.

Brachyglottis rapanda (Rangiora tree)

The wood is injurious to wood-workers from its alkaloid content (Aston 1923, Briggs 1946).

Reference

Aston, B.C. (1923) The poisonous, suspected and medicinal plants of New Zealand. New Zealand Agric. J. 78 and 149.

Briggs, L.H. (1946) Plant Products of New Zealand. J. Proc. Roy. Soc. N.S.W. 80, 151.

Poisonous honey is derived from this plant. The Maoris never take the wild honey when the rangiora is in blossom (Aston 1923).

Reference

Aston, B.C. (1923) The poisonous, suspected, and medicinal plants of New Zealand. New Zealand J. Argicult. 26, 78 and 149.

Tribe: Inuleae

Buphthalmum

Six species are found in Europe and Asia Minor.

Novak and Kolinsky (1960) reported dermatitis from a plant of this genus; they gave Telekia as a synonym for the plant. Shaw (1973) indicates a distinction between the genera.

Reference

Novak, J. and Kolinsky, J. (1960) Dermatitis phytogenes post. Telekiam Baumgartner (seu Buphthalmum) Cesk. Derm. 35, 113.

Shaw, H.K.Z. (1973) A Dictionary of the Flowering Plants and Ferns. (the late J.C. Willis) 8th ed. Cambridge University Press.

Tribe: Calenduleae

Calendula

Twenty or 30 species are found in the Mediterranean region east to Persia.

Calendula as a constituent of a proprietary remedy produced contact dermatitis in four individuals who had had plant dermatitis (Underwood and Gaul 1948). A plant of this genus is probably allergenic since Hjorth (1965) reported one positive patch test reaction from many tests.

Calendula officinalis

(Pot Marigold) is a common flower garden annual. Irritancy has been ascribed both to the plant itself and to a tincture made from it (Behl et al 1966). The plant yields an oil of perfumery (Arctander 1960).

A cultivar, Legion of Honour, of Calendula tagetes (Marigold) was reported as a cause of contact dermatitis by Harrison (1906).

References

Arctander, S. (1960) Perfume and flavor materials of natural origin. Elizabeth, New Jersey. Published by the author.

Behl, P.N., Captain, R.M., Bedi, B.M.S. and Gupta, S. (1966) Skin irritant and sensitizing plants, found in India, New Delhi. P.N. Behl, Irwin Hospital.

Harrison, A.J. (1906) Dermatitis from without and Dermatitis from within. Bristol. Med. Chir. J. 24, 325.

Hjorth, N. (1965) Contact sensitivity to plants and balsams. Europ. Congr. Allergy. Acta. Derm.-venereol. 65.

Underwood, G.B. and Gaul, L.E. (1948) Overtreatment dermatitis in dermatitis venenata due to plants. JAMA 138, 570.

Callistephus

One species is found in China and Japan.

Callistephus chinensis

The cultivated asters are occasional causes of hayfever (Wodehouse 1971).

Reference

Wodehouse, R.P. (1971) Hayfever Plants. 2nd rev. edition. New York. Hafner.

Tribe: Astereae

Calotis

Twenty species are found in Australia.

Calotis cuneifolia produces small 'almost invisible' burs which irritate the feet of dogs, and humans by getting into blankets (Maiden 1895).

Reference

Maiden, J.H. (1895) The Weeds of New South Wales. Ag. Gaz. New South Wales. 6, 671.

Tribe: Cynareae

Carduus (Thistle)

100 species are found in Europe, the mediterranean region and in Asia.

Carduus lanceolatus

(Black or Spear Thistle) can cause mechanical injury (Pammel 1911).

Reference

Pammel, L.H. (1911) A Manual of Poisonous Plants. Torch Press. Cedar Rapids, Iowa. Reprinted Univ. Microfilms Inc., Ann Arbor,

Mich. 1965. pp. 476-7.

Tribe: Astereae

Cassinia

Twenty-eight species are found in tropical and southern Africa, Australia and New Zealand.

Cassinia aculeata
(syn. Cassinia quinquefaris)
(Australian Dogwood)

Noyes (1899) described seven cases of eczema from this plant. Irritation occurred in skin folds where pollen or particles of bark accumulated. The disorder has been known as 'mountain itch' in Australia (Maiden 1909). According to Cleland (1943) the plant causes dermatitis of the exposed skin and probably also conjunctivitis. The workers employed in clearing the plant from the ground or working in Cassinia scrub developed dermatitis only after being exposed to it for a considerable time (Cleland 1943) suggesting an allergic effect. Bee farmers can develop itching from propolis derived from pollen of the plant (Rayment 1935).

References

Cleland, J.B. (1943) Plants including fungi, poisonous or otherwise injurious to man in Australia. IV. Med. J. Australia 11, 161.

Maiden, J.H. (1909) On some plants which cause inflammation or irritation of the skin. Ag. Gaz. New South Wales. 20, 111-117 & 1073-1082.

Noyes, A.W.F. (1899) Dermatitis produced by Cassinea aculeata. Intercol. Med. J. Aust. 4, 359.

Rayment, T. (1935) 'A Cluster of Bees'. pg. 398, cited by Cleland 1943.

Tribe: Vernonieae

Centaurea

600 species are found in Europe and North Africa to northern India and China, in temperate North and South America. One species occurs in Australia.

Centaurea species
(Knapweed, Star Thistle)

The spines can cause mechanical injury (Pammel 1911). Some species of the genus are probably allergenic since Hjorth (1965) recorded two positive patch test reactions among many tests.

Centaurea americana
(Sultana Star Thistle)

An extract of the plant produced positive patch test reactions in two of 50 patients who had 'weed dermatitis' in the southern United States (Shelmire 1940).

Centaurea calcitrapa

The plant is an irritant (Pammel 1911).

References

Hjorth, N. (1965) Contact sensitivity to plants and balsams. Europ. Congr. Allergy Acta. derm.-venereol 65 and personal communication.

Pammel, L.H. (1911) A Manual of Poisonous Plants. Torch Press. Cedar Rapids, Iowa. Reprinted Univ. Microfilms Inc., Ann Arbor, Mich. 1965 pp. 476-7.

Shelmire, B. (1940) Contact dermatitis from vegetation. South Med. J. 33, 338.

Tribe: Anthemidae

Centipeda

Six species are found in Madagascar, Afghanistan, eastern Asia, Indo-Malaysia, Australasia, Polynesia and Chile.

Centipeda cunninghamii
(Common Sneezeweed)

The powdered leaf is used as snuff. The plant was thought to cause swollen eyes and nostrils in sheep (Hurst 1942).

Centipeda minima

The plant is used as snuff in China. The leaves, when squeezed between the fingers, provoke sneezing (Smith 1969).

Centipeda minuta and
Centipeda orbicularis
(syn. Myriogyne) (Sneezewood)

The plants, when dry, cause irritation of the nasal mucous membrane (Maiden 1909).

References

Hurst, E. (1942) The Poison Plants of New South Wales. N.S.W. Poison Plants Committee; Sydney.

Maiden, J.H. (1909) On some plants which cause inflammation or irritation of the skin. Ag. Gaz. New South Wales. 20, 111-117 and 1073-1082.

Smith, F.P. (1969) Chinese Materia Medica. Vegetable kingdom. 2nd ed. Rev. by Hei, P.D. Taipai, Taiwan. Ku T'ing Book House.

Chrysanthemum

200 species are found in Europe and Asia. Some species are of commercial and horticultural importance. The insecticide, pyrethrum, is derived from Chrysanthemum cinerariifolium and also from C. coccineum and C. roseum. Dermatitis has been reported in field-workers, warehousemen, chemists and users of pyrethrum. C. morifolium (Chrysanthemum of florists) is probably the commonest cause of plant dermatitis in florists.

The horticultural Chrysanthemum C x hortorum was evolved largely from hybridisation of C. indicum and C. morifolium (Ackerson 1957). However, chromosome studies reveal inconsistencies which can be explained by apomixis, or more plausibly by polypoidy of one parent (Gorer 1970). Some more recent cultivars have a more mixed parentage, involving other species. The species names Chrysanthemum indicum (Hausen and Schulz 1973) and Chrysanthemum x morifolium (Rook 1960) have been used for Chrysanthemum of florists.

The following Chrysanthemum species have been reported to cause dermatitis:

Chrysanthemum species

(Dawson 1906, Waugh 1918, Goldstein 1931, McCormac 1932, Reyn 1933, Photinos 1934, Leipold 1938, Coste et al 1942, Fisher 1952, Olivier and Renken 1954, Blamoutier 1956, Paschould 1956, Hjorth 19675, and Hausen and Schulz 1973 (Review).

Chrysanthemum carinatum
(Robert 1951).

Chrysanthemum carneum
(McCord et al 1921).

Chrysanthemum cinerariifolium
(McCord et al 1921, Sequeira 1936, Martin and Kester 1941, Tonkin 1936, Editorial 1936) (See also Pyrethrum).

Pyrethrum (mainly Chrysanthemum cinerariifolium) (McCord et al 1921, Abramowitz 1927, Chevalier 1928, 1930, Marceron 1928, Sulzberger and Weinberg 1930, Hopkins 1930, Badham 1931, Feinburg 1934, Beinhauer and Perrin 1938, Epstein 1938, Anon 1942, Wilson and Ellis-Jones 1943, Keil 1944, Martin and Brightwell 1946, Lord and Johnson 1947, Zucker 1966, Rickett et al 1971, Griffin 1973).

(Kesten and Laszlo 1931, Brunsting and Anderson 1934, Sweitzer and Rusten 1938, Lord and Johnson 1947, Fisher 1957, Schwartz et al 1957, Key 1961, Rook 1961, McCord 1962, Watt and Breyer-Brandwijk 1962, Mitchell 1969, Mitchell et al 1971 and Burry et al 1973.)

Urticaria (Epstein 1938) and rhinitis and asthma have been reported from pyrethrum (Spratling 1893, Bigger 1923 and Ramirez 1930).

Sesquiterpene lactones of Chrysanthemum species.

The sesquiterpene lactones derived from species of the genus are listed by Yoshioka et al (1973). Many are reported allergenic or are potentially allergenic (Mitchell and Dupuis 1971, Mitchell, Dupuis and Geissman 1972). The principal allergen of pyrethrum is pyrethrosin (Mitchell et al 1972). Chrysanthemum indicum yields delta-3-carene (Demura 1961). A sesquiterpene lactone (Osawa et al 1973) which is potentially allergenic (Mitchell and Dupuis 1971) is derived from Chrysanthemum morifolium.

Alcohol extracts of pyrethrum flowers have been found to yield additional sesquiterpene lactones including beta-cyclopyrethrosin, chrysanolide and chrysanin (Doskotch and El-Feraly 1969, Doskotch et al 1971, Rickett and Tyszkiewicz 1974).

Chrysanthemum coccineum

(McCord et al 1921, Sequeira 1936, Rusten 1938 and Martin 1941).

Chrysanthemum indicum

(Hoffman 1904, Pilot 1932, Schlammadinger 1933, Bonnevie 1939 and Macharacek 1964).

Chrysanthemum leucanthemum

(Howe 1887, White 1887, Kren 1925, Oppenheim 1931, Bonnevie 1939, Ellerbroek 1952, Mackoff and Dahl 1951, Scarzella 1958 and Hjorth 1965).

Chrysanthemum maximum

(Nightingale 1931, Shelmire 1940, Gottron and Schonfeld 1959, Rook 1960 and Burry et al 1973).

Chrysanthemum morifolium

(Dawson 1906, Harrison 1906, Goldstein 1931, Leipold 1938, Osborne and Putnam 1932, MacCormac 1932, Mayers 1932, Reyn 1933, Photinos 1934, Davies 1939, Shelmire 1940, Coste et al 1942, Ellerbroek 1952, Fisher 1952, Olivier and Rankin 1954, Blamoutier 1956, Becker and O'Brien 1959, Rook 1960, Curtis 1960, Rook 1962, Macharacek 1964, Hjorth 1965, Paschoud 1965, Robertson and Mitchell 1967, Agrup 1969, Mitchell 1969 (Review), O'Quinn and Isbell 1969), Bleumink et al 1973, and Burry et al 1973).

Chrysanthemum parthenium

(Maiden 1909, Shelmire 1939, Robertson and Mitchell 1967, Tan and Mitchell 1968, Mitchell, Rook 1960 and O'Quinn and Isbell 1969).

Chrysanthemum roseum

(Editorial 1936 and McCord 1962).

Chrysanthemum vulgare
(Syn. Tanacetum vulgare)

(Greenhouse and Sulzberger 1933).

Chrysanthemum indicum

The biochemistry of the genus and the role of lactones in Chrysanthemum allergy were reviewed by Schulz et al (1975).

One of four sensitizing sesquiterpene lactones in C. indicum was found to be arteglasin-A which has previously been isolated from Artemisia douglasiana, (Hausen and Schulz 1975, 1976).

References

Hausen, B.M. and Schulz, K.H. (1975) A first allergenic sesquiterpene lactone from Chrysanthemum indicum L.: Arteglasin-A. Naturwissenschaften 62, 585.

Hausen, B.M. and Schulz, K.H. (1976) Chrysanthemum allergy III. Identification of the allergens. Arch. Derm. Res. 255, 111.

Schulz, K.H., Hausen, B.M. et al (1975) Chrysanthemum Allergy. Part 2. Arch. Derm. Forsch. 251, 235.

Doskotch, R.W. and El-Feraly, F.S. (1969) (+)-sesamin and betacyclopyrethrosin Can. J. Chem. 47, 1139 .

Doskotch, R.W., et al (1971) Sesquiterpene lactones from pyrethrum flowers. Can. J. Chem. 49, 2103.

Rickett, F.E. and Tyszkiewicz, K. (1974) Pyrethrum Dermatitis II. Pyrethrum Post. 12, 163.

Abromowitz, E.W. (1927) The systemic treatment of skin diseases. N.Y. State J. Med. 27, 877.

Ackerson, S. (1957) The complete Book of Chrysanthemum. New York. Doubleday.

Agrup, G. (1969) Hand Eczema and other hand dermatoses in South Sweden. Acta derm.-venereol 49. Suppl. 61 pp. 1-91

Anon (1942) Pyrethrum dermatitis. East African Med. J. 19, 137.

Becker, S.W. and O'Brien, M.P. (1959) Value of patch tests in dermatology. Archs. Derm. 79, 569.

Beinhauer, L.G. and Perrin, S.R. (1938) Pyrethrum dermatitis. Urol. Cut. Rev. 42, 910.

Badham, C. (1931) Report of the Director-General of Public Health, New South Wales, for year 1930:67.

Blamoutier, P. (1956) Un cas de sensibilization au chrysanthème. Sem. Hosp. Paris. 82, 2865.

Bleumink, E., Mitchell, J.C. and Nater, J.P. (1973) Contact dermatitis to Chrysanthemums. Archs. Derm. 108, 220.

Bonnevie, P. (1939) Atiologie und Pathogenese der Ekzemkrankheiten, Nord. Forl., Kopenhagen u. Verlag. J.A. Barth, Leipzig.

Brunsting, L.A. and Anderson, C.R. (1934) Ragweed dermatitis. A report based on 18 cases. JAMA. 103, 1285.

Burry, J.N., Kuchel, R., Reid, J.G. and Kirk, J. (1973). Australian bush dermatitis. Compositae dermatitis in South Australia. Med. J. Australia 1, 110 and Burry, J.N. (personal communication, 1973).

Chevalier, J. (1930) Le pyrèthre (chrysanthème insecticide) Activitié pharmacodynamique et therapeutique. Bull. Sci. Pharmacol. 37, 154.

Chevalier, J. (1928) Le pyrèthre nouvel anthelmintique vermicide. Bull. Acad. Med. Paris 109, 446.

Coste, F., Marceron, L. and Boyer, J. (1942). A propos d'un cas de dermosensibilisation aux chrysanthemes. Bull. Soc. franc. Derm. 259, 491.

Davies, J.H.T. (1939) Contact dermatitis. Practitioner 142, 636.

Dawson (1906) Chrysanthemum dermatitis. Brit. J. Derm. 18, 439.

Demura, Y. (1961) Fragrant components of a wild chrysanthemum-Chrysanthemum indicum L. Mem. Fac. Sci. Kyushu Univ. (C) 4, 145.

Editorial (1936) Pyrethrum dermatitis. Brit. Med. J. 1, 1262.

Editorial (1936) Pyrethrum dermatitis Lancet 114, 201.

Ellerbroek, U. (1952) Zur Beurteilung saisonbedingter Berufsdermatosen (Chrysanthemen-Krankheit). Derm. Gutacht. 1, 109.

Epstein, E. (1938) Urticaria due to an insecticide (pyrethrum). Urol. Rev. 42, 829.

Feinberg, S.M. (1934) Pyrethrum sensitization. Its importance and relation to pollen allergy. JAMA 102, 1557.

Fisher, A.A. (1952) Some immunologic phenomena in treatment of and patch testing for ragweed oil dermatitis. J. Invest. Derm. 19, 271.

Fisher, A.A. (1957) Dermatitis venenata due to ragweed pollen (in discussion of case). Archs. Derm. 75, 906.

Garrat, J.R. and Bigger, J.W. (1923) Asthma due to insect powder. Brit. Med. J. 2, 764.

Goldstein, M.B. (1931) Dermatitis venenata due to chrysanthemum leaves. JAMA 96, 1680.

Gorer, R. (1970) The Development of Garden Flowers. London, Eyre & Spottiswode p. 73.

Gottron, H.A. and Schonfeld, W. (1959) Dermatology and Venereology. Vol. 3. Stuttgart, Thieme.

Greenhouse, C.A. and Sulzberger, M.B. (1933) Common weed (Tanacetum vulgare) as a cause of eczematous dermatitis. J. Allergy 4, 523.

Griffen, C.S. (1973) Mammalian toxicology of pyrethrum. Pyrethrum Post. 12, 50.

Harrison, A.J. (1906) Dermatitis from without and Dermatitis from within. Bristol. Med. Chir. J. 24, 325.

Hausen, B.M. and Schulz, K.H. (1973) Chrysanthemum-Allergy. Berufsdermatosen 21, 199.

Hjorth, N. (1965) Contact sensitivity to plants and balsams. Europ. Congr. Allergy. Acta. derm.-venereol. 65.

Hoffmann, E. (1904) Uber die Primelkrankheit und andere durch Pflanzen verursachte Hautentzundungen. Munch. med. Wschr. 44, 1966.

Hopkins, M. (1930) Dermatitis venenata (insect powder). Archs. Derm. 21, 863.

Howe, J.S. (1887) Dermatitis caused by Leucanthemum vulgare. Boston Med. Surg. J. 116, 227.

Keil, H. (1944) The value of the patch test in poison ivy dermatitis with consideration of group reactions between Rhus extracts and turpentine, pyrethrum, ragweed oil and 3-geranyl catechol. J. Allergy 15, 259.

Kesten, B. and Laszlo, E. (1931) Dermatitis due to sensitization to contact substances. Dermatitis venenata, occupational dermatitis. Archs. Derm. Syph. 23, 211.

Key, M.M. (1961) Some unusual reactions in industry. Archs. Derm. 83, 3.

Kren, O. (1925) Ein Beitrag zur Pflanzendermatitis. Arch. f. Derm. Syph. 149, 96.

Leipold, H. (1938) Dermatitis der Hande und des Gesichts infolge Uberempfindlichkeit gegen Chrysanthemen und Kamillen. Zbl. Haut.-Geschlkrkh. 57, 248.

Lord, K.A. and Johnson, C.G. (1947) Production of dermatitits by pyrethrum and attempts to produce a nonirritant extract. Brit. J. Derm. 59, 367.

McCord, C.P., Kilker, C.H. and Minster, D.K. (1921) Pyrethrum dermatitis. JAMA 77, 448.

McCord, C.P. (1962) The occupational toxicity of cultivated flowers. Ind. Med. Surg. 31, 365.

MacCormac, H. (1932) Chrysanthemum dermatitis. Proc. Roy. Soc. Med. 25, 391.

Macharacek, V. (1964) Occupational eczema from Chrysanthemum. Cs. Derm. 39, 156.

Mackoff, S. and Dahl, A.O. (1951) A botanical consideration of the weed oleoresin problem. Minn. Med. 34, 1169.

Maiden, J.H. (1909) On some plants which cause inflammation or irritation of the skin. Agr.Gaz. New South Wales 20, 1073.

Malten, K.E. (1973) Chrysanthemum contact hypersensitivity. Contact Dermatitis Newsletter (London) 13, 357.

Marceron, M. (1928) Contact dermatitis provoked by a volatile insecticide. Bull. Soc. franc. Derm. 35, 829.

Martin, J.T. and Hester, K.H.C. (1941) Dermatitis caused by insecticidal pyrethrum flowers (Chrysanthemum cineriaefolium). Brit. J. Derm. 53, 127.

Martin, J.T. and Brightwell, S. (1946) Dermatitis caused by pyrethrum. J. Soc. Chem. Ind. 65, 379.

Mayers, M.R. (1932) Occupational dermatitis due to handling of plants, vegetables and fruits. Ind. Bull. 11, 342.

Mitchell, J.C. (1969) Allergic contact dermatitis from Compositae. Trans. St. John's Hosp. Derm. Soc. 55,174.

Mitchell, J.C., Geissman, T.A., Dupuis, G. and Towers, G.H.N. (1971). Allergic contact dermatitis caused by Artemisia and Chrysanthemum species. J. Invest. Derm. 56, 98.

Mitchell, J.C. and Dupuis,G. (1971) Allergic contact dermatitis from sesquiterpenoids of the Compositae family of plants. Brit. J. Derm. 84, 139.

Mitchell, J.C., Dupuis, G. and Geissman, T.A. (1972) Allergic contact dermatitis from sesquiterpenoids of plants. Additional allergenic sesquiterpene lactones. Brit. J. Derm. 87, 235.

Mitchell, J.C., Dupuis, G. and Towers G.H.N. (1972) Allergic contact dermatitis from pyrethrum. Brit. J. Derm. 86, 568.

Mitchell, J.C. (1974) Applied chemotaxonomy of plants I. A biological model. Contact Dermatitis Newsletter (London) 16, 494.

Nightingale, G.S. (1931) Chrysanthemum dermatitis. Lancet 1, 1132.

Olivier, J. and Renkin, A. (1954) Eczema par sensibilite a une seule variete de chrysanthemes. Arch. Belg. Derm. 10, 296.

Oppenheim, M. (1931) Uber empfindlichkeit gegen die Orakelblume Derm. Wschr. 93, 1706.

O'Quinn, S.E. and Isbell, K.H. (1969) Influence of oral prednisone on eczematous patch test reactions. Arch. Derm. 99, 380.

Osawa, T., Suzuki, A., Tamura, S. et al (1973) Structure of chlorochrymorin, a novel sesquiterpene lactone from Chrysanthemum morifolium (Ram.) Tetrahedron Lett. 52, 5135.

Osborne, E.D. and Putnam, E.D. (1932) Industrial dermatoses. JAMA 99, 972.

Paschoud, J.M. (1956) Kontaktekzem durch Chrysanthemen. Gekreuzte Uberempfindlichkeitsreaktion mit Arnikatinktur. Hautarzt 16, 229.

Photinos, P. (1934) Dermatitis durch Chrysanthemen. Zbl. Haut-Geschlkrkh. 48, 600.

Pilot, I. (1932) Dermatitis venenata due to chrysanthemums. J. Allergy 3, 404.

Ramirez, M.A. (1930) Pyrethrum, an etiologic factor in vasomotor rhinitis and asthma. J. Allergy 1, 148.

Reyn, A. (1933) Chrysanthemem dermatitis. Zbl. Haut-Geschlkrkh. 44, 14.

Rickett, F.E., Tyszkiewiczk and Brown, N.C. (1971) Pyrethrum dermatitis Part 1. The allergenic properties of various extracts of pyrethrum flowers. Pyrethrum.Part 11, 85.

Robert, P. (1951) Akutes Gesichtsekzem infolge Uberempfindlichkeit auf Chrysanthemum carnatum. Dermatologica 102, 318.

Robertson, W.D. and Mitchell, J.C. (1967) Allergic contact and photodermatitis. Canad. Med. Ass. J. 97, 380.

Rook A. (1960) Plant dermatitis. Brit. Med. J. 2, 1771.

Rook, A. (1961) Plant dermatis. Botanical aspects. Trans. St. John's Hosp. Derm. Soc. 46, 41.

Rook, A. (1961) Plant dermatitis. The significance of variety specific sensitisation. Brit. J. Derm. 73, 283.

Rusten, E.M. (1938) Seasonal contact dermatitis. Archs. Derm. Syph. 37, 727.

Szarzella, M. (1958) A case of contact dermatitis due to Leucanthemum vulgare. Minerva Pediat. 10, 34.

Schlammadinger, J. (1933) Phytogene Hauterkrankungen mit besonderer Rucksicht auf die Wiesendermatitis. Derm. Zschr. 67, 324.

Schulz, K.H., Hausen, B.M. et al (1975) Chrysanthemum allergy. Part 2. Arch. Derm. Forsch. 251, 235.

Schwartz, L., Tulipan, L. and Birmingham, D.J. (1957) Occupational Diseases of the Skin. 3rd ed. Philadelphia. Lea & Febiger.

Sequeira, J.H. (1936) Pyrethrum dermatitis. Brit. J. Derm. 48, 473.

Shelmire, B. (1939) Allergic reactions to plants. J. Allergy 11, 56.

Shelmire, B. (1940) Contact dermatitis from vegetation. South Med. J. 33, 338.

Spratling, W.P. (1893) Inflammation of upper air-passages and ears caused by inhalation of Persian insect powder. Med. Rec. 44, 584.

Sulzberger, M.B. and Weinberg, C.B. (1930) Dermatitis due to insect powder. JAMA 95, 111.

Sweitzer, S.E. and Rusten, E.M. (1938) Seasonal contact dermatitis. Archs. Derm. 37, 727.

Tan, K.S. and Mitchell, J.C. (1968) Patch and photopatch tests in contact dermatitis and photodermatitis. Canad. Med. Ass. J. 98, 252.

Tonking, H.D. (1936) Pyrethrum dermatitis in Kenya, East African Med. J. 13, 7.

Watt, J.M. and Breyer-Brandwijk, M.G. (1962) The Medicinal and Poisonous Plants of Southern and Eastern Africa. 2nd ed. Edinburgh Livingstone.

Waugh, E. (1918) Discussion of Lain, E.S. (1918) Dermatitis lycopersicum esculentum (Tomato plant) JAMA 71, 1116.

White, J.C. (1887) Dermatitis venenata: An account of the Action of External Irritants upon the skin. Boston Cupples and Hurd.

Wilson, H.T.H. and Ellis-Jones, D.W. (1943) Case of acute dermatitis occurring after handling pyrethrum powder with treatment. East Afr. Med. J. 20, 89.

Yoshioka, H., Mabry, T.J. and Timmermann, B.N. (1973) Sesquiterpene lactones. Chemistry, NMR and Plant distribution. University of Tokyo Press.

Zucker, A. (1966) Investigation of purified pyrethrum extracts. Ann Allergy 23, 335.

Tribe: Astereae

Chrysocoma

Fifty species are found in South America, tropical and southern Africa.

Chrysocoma tenuifolia

Photodermatitis occurred in kids and lambs whose mothers ate the plant during pregnancy (Watt and Breyer-Brandwijk 1962).

Watt, J.M. and Breyer-Brandwijk, M.G. (1962) The Medicinal and Poisonous Plants of Southern Africa. 2nd ed. Edinburgh, E. & S. Livingstone.

Tribe: Lactuceae (Cichorieae)

Cichorium

Nine species are found in Europe, the Mediterranean region and Abyssinia.

Cichorium endivia (Endive) is grown as a pot-herb and its blanched leaves are used for salad. A grocer who had recurrent contact dermatitis of the hands and forearms was found to be contact sensitive to this plant, to C. intybus (Chicory) and to Lactuca sativa var. longifolia (Romaine lettuce).

A patch test to a sesquiterpene lactone, alantolactone, was positive. Tests in controls were negative, (Vail and Mitchell 1973).

Chichorium intybus used as an additive to coffee caused dermatitis in workers (Bonnevie 1948). A grocer who handled vegetables was found to be contact sensitive to this plant and to C. intybus var. foliosum. Tests in controls were negative. (Friis and Hjorth 1973).

Bonnevie, P. (1948) Some experiences of war-time industrial dermatoses Acta derm.-venereol. 28, 231.

Friis, B. and Hjorth, N. (1973) Occupational dermatitis from Chicory salad (Cichorium intybus var foliosum). Contact Dermatitis Newsletter (London) 13, 349.

Vail, J.T., Jr. and Mitchel-, J.C. (1973) Occupational dermatitis from Cichorium intybus, C. endivia and Lactuca sativa var. longifolia. Contact Dermatitis Newsletter (London) 14, 413.

Tribe: Senecioneae

Cineraria

Fifty species are found in Africa. This genus has been placed within the genus Senecio which contains some irritant plants, (p. 216.)

Cineraria species The 'cineraria' of the florists is a popular houseplant. It is derived by selective breeding from Senecio cruentis, but has also been hybridized with other Senecio species. It is available in numerous named cultivars.

The leaf hair of C. maritima causes itching.

1.7 percent of 302 persons patch tested to the leaf showed positive reactions; Fregert and Hjorth (1968) concluded that some species are marginal irritants.

Reference

Fregert, S. and Hjorth, N. (1968) Results of Standard Patch tests with substances abandoned. Contact Dermatitis Newsletter (London) 5, 85.

Tribe: Cynareae

Cirsium

150 species are found in north temperate regions and are closely allied to Carduus.

Cirsium species (Thistle)

The spines of some species can cause mechanical injury. Transient papular urticaria can result from contact with a plant (Ross 1972), and the plant hairs can give rise to conjunctival nodules (Duke-Elder and MacFaul 1972).

Duke-Elder, S. and MacFaul (1972) System of Opthalmology Vol. XIV. Injuries Part I. Mechanical Injuries. Extra-ocular foreign bodies pp. 464-67 and Agricultural Injuries pp. 32-34. London Henry Kimpton.

Ross, J.B. (1972) Personal communication.

Tribe: Heliantheae

Cosmos

Twenty-five species are found in tropical and subtropical America and the West Indies. Several species, notably Cosmos bipinnatus, are cultivated in gardens.

Cosmos bipinnatus

Becker and O'Brien (1959) reported four positive patch test reactions to this plant; clinical details were not given.

Becker, S.W. and O'Brien, M.P. (1959). Value of patch tests in Dermatology. Arch. Derm. 79, 569.

The odour of Cosmos caused hayfever in a patient. Tagetes had a similar effect in this patient. (Biederman 1937).

Biederman, J.B. (1937) Sensitivity to flowers. Laryngoscope 47, 825.

Cyclachaena

Four species are found in North America. The genus has been included in Iva.

Cyclachaena xanthifolia
(Marshelder)

Contact dermatitis from this plant was reported by Huber and Harsh (1932).

Huber, H.L. and Harsh, G.F. (1932) Summer dermatitis caused by common weed. J. Allergy 3, 578.

Tribe: Cynareae

Cynara

Fourteen species are found in the Mediterranean region east to Kurdistan.

Cynara cardunculus
(Cardoon)

The leaves can be eaten as salad. Contact sensitivity to the leaf, flower-head and stem was observed in Australian bush workers who had weed dermatitis. Cross-sensitivity was observed to Arctotheca, Chrysanthemum, Inula, Olearia and Xanthium, (Burry et al 1973).

Cynara scolymus
(Artichoke)

Dermatitis from artichokes was reported by Davezac in 1908 (White 1934). Food-handlers, vegetable sellers and a housewife were affected by dermatitis of the hands, upper limbs and face from contact with the plant. Patch test reactions were found to be positive using the root and stem, negative using the leaf (Sidi et al 1950). Dermatitis was found to be common, affecting one fifth of workers who cleaned artichokes (Gougerot and Seringe 1936). A woman who picked artichokes while scantily dressed developed a widespread bullous linear dermatitis (Burry et al 1973). Artichokes produced contact dermatitis in market gardeners (Vallet 1964). Santori (1932) obtained positive patch test reactions with an ether extract.

The plant yields a sesquiterpene lactone (Yoshioka et al 1973) which is potentially allergenic.

References

Burry, J.N., Kuchel, R., Reid, J.G. and Kirk, J. (1973). Australian bush dermatitis. Compositae dermatitis in South Australia. Med. J. Australia 1, 110; and

Burry, J.N. (personal communication 1973).

Gougerot and Seringe (1936) Occupational eczema due to artichokes. Bull. Soc. franc. de dermat. et syph. 43, 1463.

Santori, G. (1932) Dermatite eczemada Cynara scolimus (carciofo); contributo allo studio dell'allergia cutanea. Policlinico (sez. med.) 39, 592.

Sidi, E., Morrill - Dobkevitch, S. and Godechot, R. (1950). Les dermites provoquees par les artichauts. Presse Med. 58, 328.

White, R.P. (1934) Occupational affections of the skin. 4th ed. H.K. Lewis and Co.

Yoshioka, H., Mabry, T.J. and Timmerman, B.N. (1973) Sesquiterpene Lactones. Chemistry, N.M.R. and Plant Distribution. University Tokyo Press.

Vallet, G. (1964) Allergy to certain market garden plants - artichokes, celery and parsley. Councours médical, Paris 86, 3603.

Artichokes contain a potentially allergenic sesquiterpene lactone, cynaropicrin (Schneider and Thiele 1974).

Reference

Schneider, von G. and Thiele, Kl. (1974) Eigenschaften und bestimmung des artischoken-bitterstoffen, cynaropicrin. Planta Medica 25, 149.

Tribe: Heliantheae

Dahlia

Twenty species originate from Central America.

Dahlia pinnata (McCord 1962) and three Dahlia species in Mexico (Cueva and Mingramm 1955) were briefly mentioned as plants capable of causing dermatitis.

A recurrent summer eruption in a woman was traced to a Dahlia species; the leaf was found to produce a positive patch test reaction in this patient, negative in controls (Calnan 1973).

A gardener's boy aged 15, who had worked for three years in a dahlia nursery, developed dermatitis of the face and hands. Patch tests with leaves and flowers were negative, but there was a strong reaction to the tuber (Vryman 1933).

References

Calnan, C.D. (1973) Dahlia Dermatits. Contact Dermatitis Newsletter (London) 13, 366.

Cueva, J.V. and Mingramm, C. (1955) Revista medica del hospital general (Mexico) Mayo 313-324.

McCord, C.P. (1962) The Occupational Toxicity of Cultivated Flowers. Ind. Med. Surg. 31, 365.

Vryman, L.H. (1933) Dahlia tuber Dermatitis (German) Arch. Derm. 168, 233.

Dicoria

5 species are found in the south-western United States and Mexico.

Dicoria spp.

Some species produce sesquiterpene lactones.

Tribe: Senecioneae

Doronicum

Thirty-five species are found in temperate Eurasia and northern Africa. Some are extensively cultivated.

Doronicum pardalianches (Leopard's Bane)

A woman developed acute eczema of the palms, wrists and face after handling the plant (Worsley 1898).

Reference

Worsley, R.C. (1898) Leopard's Bane. Brit. Med. J. 1, 1244.

Tribe: Heliantheae

Dyssodia

Fifty species are found in

the south western United States and Mexico.

Dysodia papposa (sic) was listed as an irritant plant (Pammel 1911).

Reference

Pammel, L.H. (1911) A Manual of Poisonous Plants. Torch Press. Cedar Rapids, Iowa. Reprinted Univ. Microfilms Inc. Ann Arbor, Mich. 1965. pg. 476-7.

Echinacea

Three species are found in Atlantic North America.

Echinacea

This plant, which was a constituent of a proprietary remedy, produced positive patch test reactions in four patients who had previously suffered plant dermatitis (Underwood and Gaul 1948).

Reference

Underwood, G.B. and Gaul, L.E. (1948) Overtreatment dermatitis in dermatitis venenata due to plants. JAMA 138, 579.

Tribe: Vernoniceae

Elephantopus

32 species are found in tropical regions.

Elephantopus scaber is an abundant and troublesome weed.

Elephantopus mollis

The hairs on the stem are irritating to the skin (Altschul 1973).

Reference

Altschul, S. von R. (1973) Drugs and foods from little-known plants. Cambridge, Mass. Harvard Univ. Press.

Tribe: Astereae

Erigeron

Over 200 species are cosmopolitan.

Erigeron canadensis (syn. Leptilon canadense) (Fleabane) has been reported as an irritant to the skin in persons who handle it (White 1887, Pammel 1911, Pope 1968). Oil of Fleabane derived from the plant is irritant to the skin and eyes. This plant together with Ambrosia was considered to be responsible for contact dermatitis (Lovell et al 1955) but the evidence is incomplete. In an investigation of 'weed dermatitis', one of 50 patients showed a positive patch test reaction to an extract of the plant (Shelmire 1939). The plant yields an oil of perfumery (Arctander 1960).

References

Arctander, S. (1960) Perfume and flavour materials of natural origin. Elizabeth, New Jersey. Published by the author.

Lovell, R.G., Mathews, K.P. and Sheldon, J.M. (1955) Dermatitis venenata from tree pollen oils. J. Allergy 26, 408.

Pammel, L.H. (1911) A Manual of Poisonous Plants. Torch Press. Cedar Rapids, Iowa. Reprinted Univ. Microfilms Inc. Ann Arbor, Mich. 1965.

Pope, W.T. (1968) Manual of Wayside Plants of Hawaii. Rutland, Vermont. Charles E. Tuttle Co.

Shelmire, B. (1939) Contact dermatitis from weeds: Patch testing with their oleoresins. JAMA 113, 1085 and unpublished table accompanying reprints.

White, J.C. (1887) Dermatitis venenata: An account of the action of external irritants upon the skin. Boston. Cupples & Hurd.

Erigeron linifolium was reported to cause dermatitis (Maiden 1909, Gardner and Bennetts 1956).

Erigeron philadelphicus

In an investigation of 'weed dermatitis', one of 50 patients showed a positive patch test reaction to an extract of the plant (Shelmire 1939).

Reference

Gardner, C.A. and Bennetts, H.W. (1956) The Toxic plants of Western Australia. Perth West. Australian Newspapers Ltd.

Maiden, J.H. (1909) On some plants which cause inflammation or irritation of the skin. Ag. Gaz. New South Wales 20, 111-117 and and 1073 and 1082.

Shelmire, B. (1939) Contact dermatitis from weeds: Patch testing with their oleoresins. JAMA 113, 1085 and unpublished table accompanying reprints.

Tribe: Eupatorieae

Eupatorium

1200 species are found, mostly in America, a few in Europe, Asia and Africa.

Eupatorium altissimum (Thoroughwort)

Recurrent seasonal dermatitis of the face and neck with a positive patch test reaction to an ether extract of the flowers was reported by Brier (1940).

Eupatorium serotinum

In an investigation of 'weed dermatitis', three of 50 patients showed positive patch test reactions to an extract of the plant (Shelmire 1939).

References

Brier, A.J. (1940) Contact dermatitis from the thurowort (Eupatorium altissimum) J. Allergy 11, 402.

Shelmire, B. (1939) Contact dermatitis from weeds. Patch testing with their oleoresins. JAMA 113, 1085 and unpublished table accompanying reprints.

Eupatorium capillifolium Dog Fennel

A female developed an itching rash on the neck and upper chest several hours after gathering up and packing the dried plants; the rash persisted for several days (Morton, J.F. 1975 Pers. Comm.)

Tribe: Heliantheae

Franseria (syn. Gaertneria)

Franseria species (False Ragweed) are similar and closely related to Ambrosia and to Xanthium forming a chain of connecting links between these two genera (Wodehouse 1971). According to Shaw (1973) Franseria = Ambrosia

Franseria acanthicarpa

In an investigation of weed dermatitis, this plant produced positive patch test reactions in 15 of 25 patients tested. Some of the patients were also contact-sensitive to Ambrosia, Iva, Xanthium, Parthenium and Helenium (Mackoff and Dahl 1951). Cross-sensitivity was also observed between this species and Chrysanthemum, Artemisia and Tanacetum (Mitchell 1972) Becker and O'Brien (1959) and Tan and Mitchell (1968) also observed contact sensitivity to the plant.

References

Becker, S.W. and O'Brien, M.P. (1959) Value of patch tests in Dermatology. Arch. Derm. 79, 569.

Mackoff, S. and Dahl, A.O. (1951) A botanical consideration of the weed oleoresin problem. Minn. Med. 34, 1169.

Mitchell, J.C. (1972) Plant dermatitis - note on inadequacy of some plant extracts. Contact Dermatitis Newsletter (London) 11, 271.

Shaw, H.K.A. (1973) A dictionary of the Flowering Plants and Ferns. (the late J.C. Willis). 8th ed. Cambridge University Press.

Tan, K.S. and Mitchell, J.C. (1968) Patch and photopatch tests in contact dermatitis and photodermatitis. Canad. Med. Ass. J. 98, 252.

Wodehouse, R.P. (1971) Hayfever Plants. 2nd Rev. ed. New York. Hafner. Publ. Co. pg. 154.

Tribe: Heliantheae

Gaillardia

Twenty-six species are found in North America, two species in temperate South America. 'Gaillardia' is a popular garden flower. The cultivars commonly grown are derived from G. aristata.

Gaillardia
(Firewheel, Blanket Flower)

Three cases of contact dermatitis from Gaillardia species were reported by Rostenburg and Good (1935); one of the three patients was also contact-sensitive to Ambrosia and pyrethrum (Chrysanthemum). Patients who were contact sensitive to Gaillardia also showed positive patch test reactions to Helenium, Parthenium and Tanacetum species (Mitchell 1972). Several species of the genus yield sesquiterpene lactones (Yoshioka et al 1973) which are potentially allergenic (Mitchell and Dupuis 1971).

Gaillardia pulchella,
including its variety G. picta

In an investigation of 'weed dermatitis', seven of 50 patients were found to be contact-sensitive to this species (Shelmire 1939).

A patch test to the pollen was positive in a flower-binder who had recurrent contact dermatitis from this plant (Zschunke 1955).

References

Mitchell, J.C. and Dupuis, G. (1971) Allergic Contact Dermatitis from sesquiterpenoids of the Compositae family of Plants. Brit. J. Derm. 8, 139.

Mitchell, J.C. (1972) Plant dermatitis - note on inadequacy of some plant extracts. Contact Dermatitis Newsletter (London) 11, 271.

Rostenburg, A., Jr. and Good, C.K. (1935) Gaillardia dermatitis: hitherto unreported plant cause of dermatitis venenata. JAMA 104, 1496.

Shelmire, B. (1939) Contact dermatitis from weeds: Patch testing with their oleoresins. JAMA 113, 1085 and unpublished table accompanying reprints.

Yoshioka, H., Mabry, T.J. and Timmerman, B.N. (1973) Sesquiterpene Lactones. Chemistry, N.M.R. and Plant distribution. University Tokyo Press.

Zschunke, E. (1955) Allergic dermatitis due to Gaillardia picta (Kokardenblume) Derm. Wschr. 132, 1321.

Tribe: Heliantheae

Galinsoja

Four species are found from Mexico to Argentina.

Galinsoja parviflora

This species has become a common weed in Europe (Shaw 1973). In cases of contact dermatitis from the plant, positive patch test reactions were observed, in one case, from the stem, leaf and petal; in a second case from application of the whole plant. In these cases patch test reactions to Anthemis species were negative (Moslein 1963).

References

Moslein, P. (1963) Pflanzen als. Kontakt-Allergene. Berufsdermatosen 11, 24.

Shaw, H.K.A. (1973) A Dictionary of the Flowering Plants and Ferns. (the late J.C. Willis) 8th ed. Cambridge University Press.

Gnephosis

15 species are found in temperate Australia.

Gnephosis sp.

Some Australian Compositae sensitive patients show positive patch test reactions to the plant (Kirk, J. 1977, pers. comm.).

Tribe: Astereae

Grindelia

Sixty species are found in the Americas especially in Central America.

Grindelia species

An unidentified species of Grindelia, which was a constituent of a proprietary remedy, produced positive patch test reactions in four patients who had previously suffered from plant dermatitis

(Underwood and Gaul 1948).

Reference

Underwood, G.B. and Gaul, L.E. (1948) Overtreatment dermatitis in dermatitis venenata due to plants. JAMA 138, 570.

Tribe: Calenduleae

Gynura

100 species are found in tropical Africa and eastern Asia.

Gynura pinnatifida
(Mountain varnish)

The root has the property of causing the edges of wounds to stick together (Smith 1969).

Smith, F.P. (1969) Chinese Materia Medica. Vegetable kingdom. 2nd ed Rev. by Hei, P.D. Taipei, Taiwan. Ku T'ing Book House.

Tribe: Heliantheae

Helenium

Forty species are found in western America.

Helenium autumnale
(Sneezeweed, False Sunflower)

The flowers have long been used as a sternutatory and the whole plant is acrid and pungent (Chesnut 1898, Hurst 1942). Balyeat et al (1932) reported contact dermatitis from this species.

In an investigation of 'weed dermatitis', 20 of 25 patients showed positive patch test reactions to an extract of the plant (Mackoff and Dahl 1951). These patients were also contact-sensitive to some other Compositae species. In three cases, cross-sensitivity was observed between this species and Chrysanthemum, Tanacetum and Ambrosia (Mitchell 1972).

References

Balyeat, R.M., Rinkel, H.J. and Stemen, T.R. (1932) Contact dermatitis (venenata). Distribution and importance of the Heleniums as a cause of contact dermatitis in the United States. Am. J. Med. Sc. 184, 547.

Chesnut, V.K. (1898) "Thirty Poisonous Plants of the United States." U.S. Dept. Agr. Farmers' Bull. 86.

Hurst, E. (1942) The Poison Plants of New South Wales. N.S.W. Poison Plants Committee; Sydney.

Mackoff, S. and Dahl, A.O. (1951) A botanical consideration of the weed oleoresin problem. Minn. Med. 34, 1169.

Mitchell, J.C. (1972) Plant dermatitis - note on inadequacy of some plant extracts. Contact Dermatitis Newsletter (London), 11, 271.

Helenium microcephalum
(Sneezeweed)

In an investigation of 'weed dermatitis', 29 of 50 patients showed positive patch test reactions to an extract of this species (Shelmire 1939).

Helenium tenuifolium
(Bitterweed)

In an investigation of 'weed dermatitis', 28 of 50 patients showed positive patch test reactions to an extract of this species (Shelmire 1939). This species causes allergic contact dermatitis in Arkansas, occurring from spring to frost, but handling of hay and silage during the winter may be responsible for perennial symptoms. Honeycutt (1972) observed 14 cases; 13 were male, average age 53 years and mostly farmers. The face, neck, dorsa of the hands, forearms, ankles and lower legs were affected with acute vesicular dermatitis proceeding to chronic lichenfied dermatitis with flexural involvement resembling atopic dermatitis. Patch tests to acetone extracts of the plant produced positive reactions. The clinical features thus closely resembled Ambrosia dermatitis but only one of the 14 cases also reacted to Ambrosia extract.

References

Honeycutt, W.M. (1972) Little Rock, Arkansas. Personal communication.

Shelmire, B. (1939) Contact dermatitis from weeds: Patch testing with their oleoresins. JAMA 113: 1085 and unpublished table accompanying reprints.

Helianthus

100 species are found in the Americas. The seeds of some species furnish oils. The tubers of Helianthus tuberosus (Jerusalem artichoke) are edible.

Dermatitis from Sunflower possibly of this genus was reported by Dreyer in 1906 (Touton 1932). A report of dermatitis in farmers from contact with sunflowers (Sneid 1955) is not well substantiated. Rajka (1948) reported an occupational dermatitis from sunflower seed with a positive patch test reaction to an aqueous extract of the seed: Greenberg and Lester (1954) briefly refer to dermatitis from picking sun-flower seeds.

Helianthus annuus (Sunflower)

Sunflower without botanical name usually means H. annuus.

This is an important crop-plant in many parts of the world.

In an investigation of 'weed dermatitis', one of 50 patients had a positive patch test reaction to an extract of the plant (Shelmire 1940). Noussitou and Cordero (1951) report two patients who, working with sunflower seeds, presented allergic dermatosis directly related to the pollen of the plant, demonstrated by scratch test and passive transfer. H. annuus may be a significant cause of dermatitis in countries where the plant is commonly grown. Of 1197 patch tests with the leaves in Hungary, 3.12% were positive. Positive reactions were most common in women land-workers (Ravnay and Garazsi 1955).

References

Dreyer (1906) Eine neue Pflanzendermatitis. Dermat. Zbl. Feb. cited by Touton (1932).

Greenberg, L.A. and Lester, D. (1954) Handbook of Cosmetic Materials. Their properties, uses and toxic dermatological actions with a bibliography of over 2500 titles. New York. Interscience Publishers Inc.

Noussitou, F.M. and Cordero, A.M. (1951) Dermatitis allergica por Girard. Prensa med. Argent. 38, 1052.

Rajka, O. (1948) Occupational dermatitis from Sunflower seed and linseed. Orvosok Lapja (Budapest) 4, 158.

Rávnay, T. and Garazsi, M. (1955) Investigation of occupational hypersensitivity to leaves of Helianthus annuus. (German) Z. Haut. -u. Geschlkrankh. 92, 320.

Shelmire, B. (1940) Contact dermatitis from vegetation. South med. J. 33, 338.

Sneid, P. (1955) Occupational health on the farm. Indust. Med. 24, 117.

Touton, K. (1932) Hauterkrankungen durch phanerogamische Pflanzen und ihre Produkte (Toxicodermia et. Allergodermia phytogenes), in Barnewitz, J. et al Angeborene Anomalien, Lichtdermatosen, Pflanzengifte, Thermische Schädigungen, Einfluss Innerer Storungen auf die Haut. Berlin, Verlag von Julius Springer.

Tribe: Inuleae

Helichrysum

500 species are distributed in Europe, Africa, Asia, India and Australia. The dried flower-heads of some species are used as 'everlasting flowers'. Since the dried flowers retain their colour, Helichrysum stoechas is used in potpourri (Wren 1968). Helichrysum angustifolium yields an oil of perfumery (Fenaroli 1971). The hairs on the seeds can produce small yellow conjunctival nodules (Duke-Elder and MacFaul 1972).

Helichrysum diosmifolium

Mair (1968) received a report of recurrent eczema from contact with the plant. The affected individual who tried eating the leaves in order to dispel the allergy, developed blistering of the mouth. An unaffected individual noted a sharp taste and stinging of the tongue from nibbling the plant.

References

Duke-Elder, S. and MacFaul (1972) System of Opthalmology. Vol. XIV Injuries Part 1. Mechanical Injuries. Extra-ocular foreign bodies. pp. 464-467 and Agricultural Injuries pp. 32-34. London. Henry Kimpton.

Fenaroli, G. (1971) Fenaroli's Handbook of Flavor Ingredients. ed. Furia, T.E. and Bellanca, N. Cleveland, Ohio. The Chemical Rubber Co.

Mair, K. (1968) Royal Botanic Gardens, Sydney. Personal communication.

Wren, R.W. (1968) Potter's New Cyclopaedia of Botanical Drugs and preparations by Wren, R.C. Re-edit. by Wren, R.W. Potter & Clarke Ltd. Health Science Press. Rustington, Sussex.

Helichrysum bractaetum

This plant displayed in a dried state as 'everlasting flowers' produced keratitis and a nodose type of conjunctivitis apparently from mechanical rather than toxic action. The lesion was not reproducible in rabbits (Karbe 1923).

Reference

Karbe, M. (1923) Ein Fall von Ophthalmia nodosa der Bindehaut bein einem Kind, hervorgerufen durch Spielen mit Strohblumen. Arch. Augenheilk 93, 160.

Helipterus

90 species are found in southern Africa and Australia. The dried flower-heads retain their colour and are sold as 'everlasting flowers'.

Helipterus charsleyae

Contact sensitivity to this plant was observed by Burry et al (1973).

Reference

Burry, J.N., Kuchel, R., Reid, J.G. and Kirk, J. (1973) Australian bush dermatitis. Compositae dermatitis in South Australia. Med. J. Australia 1, 110 and Burry, J.N. (personal communication 1973).

Tribe: Astereae

Heterotheca

Thirty species are found in the southern United States and Mecico

Heterotheca subaxillaris (Camphor Daisy)

In an investigation of 'weed dermatitis', two of 50 patients gave positive patch test reactions to an extract of this plant (Shelmire 1939).

Reference

Shelmire, B.(1939) Contact dermatitis from weeds: Patch testing with their oleoresins. JAMA 113, 1085 and unpublished table accompanying reprints.

Tribe: Lactuceae (Cichorieae)

Hieracium

Perhaps 5000 species are distributed in temperate regions, excluding Australasia, and on tropical mountains.

Hieracium auricula

This plant, used as rabbit food, caused recurrent springtime dermatitis of the face and forearms in a rabbit breeder (Bellonne 1948).

Reference

Bellonne, M.A. (1948) Dermite printaniere recidivante depuis onze and, provoquee par une herbe cueillie pour l'elevage des lapins. Bull. Soc. franc. Derm. Syph. 55, 290.

Hulsea

Eight species are found in the western United States.

Hulsea heterochroma

The juice, derived from the glands of the plant, is very irritant to the skin (Altschul 1973).

Reference

Altschul, S. von R. (1973) Drugs and foods from little-known plants.

Cambridge, Mass. Harvard University Press.

Tribe: Astereae

Humea

Seven species are found in Madagascar and South Australia. Resin canals are not known to be present in the leaves and stems (Metcalfe and Chalk 1950.

Humea elegans
(Crimson Shower)

The plant emits a scent when bruised. A woman who rubbed the leaves on her veil for their scent developed vesicular dermatitis of the nose and cheeks (Hearnden 1902). Reports of contact dermatitis caused by the plant in Australia (Maiden 1913, 1914) suggest allergenicity. Patch tests to the leaf were positive in two gardeners who developed dermatitis from contact with the plant (Cronin 1968, Rook 1970). According to Maiden (1913, 1914) the eyes might be affected by standing on the leeward side of a clump of plants when a breeze was blowing. Control tests with the plant to exclude irritancy, were carried out in four subjects by Rook (1970). There were no positive reactions. Absence of resin canals is unusual in allergenic Compositae species.

References

Cronin, E. (1968) Sensitivity to Humea elegans. Contact Dermatitis Newsletter (London) 3, 39.

Hearnden, W.C. (1902) A case of contact dermatitis caused by Humea elegans. Lancet 2, 216.

Maiden, J.H. (1913) Additional skin-irritating plants. Ag. Gaz. New South Wales 24, 778 and 916,917.

Maiden, J.H. (1914) On some plants which cause inflammation or irritation of the skin. Ag. Gaz. New South Wales. 25, 611.

Metcalf, C.R. and Chalk, L. (1950) Anatomy of the Dicotyledons Vol. 2. Oxford. Clarendon Press. p. 785.

Rook, A. (1970) Contact dermatitis from Humea elegans. Contact Dermatitis, Newsletter (London) 7, 164.

Tribe: Inuleae

Inula

200 species are found in Europe, Asia and Africa.

Inula brittanica

Exposure to hay which contained this plant caused dermatitis of the exposed skin surfaces. Patch test reactions were positive to this species and to Inula germanica, negative to four other Inula species (Hegyi 1967).

Inula graveolens
(Stinkwort)

The barbed pappuses can cause mechanical injury. Dermatitis occurred in workmen who pulled up this weed, only some of those exposed being affected (Maiden 1918). MacPherson (1932) reported dermatitis in a father and two sons. Other reports (Helms 1897, Seddon and Carne 1928, Wettenhall 1925, N.S.W. Dept. Agr. Rec. 1940, Hurst 1942, Scott 1967) suggest irritancy to man and animals. Burry et al (1973) reported contact sensitivity to the plant in three cases, positive patch test reactions to the leaf and cross-sensitivity with some other Compositae species. They found that the leaf, when dried, was not irritant by patch test. A fluorescent volatile oil is obtained from the plant (Watt and Breyer-Brandwijk 1962).

References

Burry, J.N., Kuchel, R., Reid, J.G. and Kirk, J. (1973) Australian bush dermatitis. Compositae dermatitis in South Australia. Med. J. Australia 1, 110 and Burry, J.N. (personal communication 1973).

Hegyi, E. (1967) Plant dermatitis (Inula brittanica L.) Contact Dermatitis Newsletter (London) 2, 18.

Helms, R. (1897) Stinkwort Jour. Ag. Western Australia. 4, 1311, quoted by Hurst (1942).

Hurst, E. (1942) The Poison Plants of New South Wales. N.S.W.

Poison Plants Committee; Sydney.

MacPherson, J. (1932) Plants injurious to man in Australia. Med. J. Australia. 1, 281.

Maiden, J.H. (1918) Plants which produce inflammation or irritation of the skin. Ag. Gaz. New South Wales 29, 344.

N.S.W. Dept. Ag. Rec. (1940) Unpublished files, etc.; quoted by Hurst (1942).

Scott, F.P. (1967) Personal communication.

Seddon, H.R. and Carne, H.R. (1928). Feeding tests with Mexican Poppy and Stinkwort. Ag. Gaz. New South Wales. 39, 527; quoted by Hurst (1942).

Watt, J.M. and Breyer-Brandwijk, M.G. (1962) The Medicinal and Poisonous Plants of Southern Africa. 2nd ed. Edinburgh. E and S. Livingstone.

Wettenhall, R.R. (1925) Dermatitis Venenata. Med. J. Australia. 2, 60.

Inula helenium (Elecampane)

Alantolactone has an inhibitory effect on seed germination and seedling growth of *Phaseolus mungo* (Dalvi et al 1971).

Reference

Dalvi, R.R., Singh, B. and Salunke, D.K. (1971) A study on phytotoxicity of alantolactone. Chem.-Biol. Interactions. 3, 13.

The root of the plant has been used medicinally since Roman times. The plant itself has not been reported to cause dermatitis but a sesquiterpene lactone, alantolactone, derived from it and formerly used as a vermifuge is an active sensitizer in a concentration 1 per cent in petrolatum (Hjorth 1970, Mitchell 1970). The lactone produced positive patch test reactions in some individuals who were contact sensitive to various Compositae. species and to *Frullania* (Liverwort), (Mitchell et al 1970). The plant is an occasional adulterant of Digitalis leaf (British Pharmaceutical Codex 1934).

Reference

British Pharmateutical Codex (1934) London. Pharmaceutical Society of Great Britain.

Hjorth, N. (1970) Active sensitization with alantolactone. Contact Dermatitis Newsletter (London) 8, 175 and 8, 180.

Mitchell, J.C., Fritig, B., Singh, B. and Towers, G.H.N. (1970). Allergic contact dermatitis from *Frullania* and Compositae. The role of sesquiterpene lactones. J. Invest. Derm. 54, 233.

Mitchell, J.C., Dupuis, G. and Geissman, T.A. (1972) Allergic contact dermatitis from sesquiterpenoids of plants. Additional allergic sesquiterpene lactones and immunological specificity of Compositae, liverworts and lichens. Brit. J. Derm. 87, 235.

Mitchell, J.C. (1970) Unpublished observations.

Piyankova and Nugmanova (1975) described cases of allergic contact dermatitis due to contact with elecampane. This medicinal herb is apparently widely used in the Soviet Union for self-treatment of skin ailments.

Alantolactone is toxic to cultured human lymphocytes (Dupuis and Brisson 1976); this activity does not seem to depend on the methylene group attached to the lactone.

References

Piyankova, Z.P. and Nugmanova, M.L. (1975) Dermatitis due to elecampane. Vestn. Derm. Vener. 51, 52. Dec.

Opdyke, D.L.J. (1976) Monographs on fragrance raw materials. Alantroot oil. Fd. Cosmet. Toxicol. 14, 307.

Dupuis, G. and Brisson, J. (1976) Toxic effect of alantolactone and dihydroalantolactone in *in vitro* cultures of lymphocytes. Chem.-Biol. Interactions 15, 205.

Tribe: Heliantheae

Iva Fifteen species occur in North and Central America and in the West Indies.

Iva angustifolia (Marshelder)

Smith et al (1942) reported dermatitis from this species. In an investigation of 'weed dermatitis' 18 of 50 patients showed positive patch test reactions to an extract of the plant (Shelmire 1939).

Iva ciliata (Marshelder)

Contact sensitivity to this plant was reported by O'Quinn and Isbell (1969). In Shelmire's (1939) series of 50 patients who had 'weed dermatitis', an extract of the plant produced negative patch test reactions.

Iva microcephala (Marshelder)

This species produced a positive patch test reaction in a patient who had'weed dermatitis', (Williams et al 1960).

Iva xanthifolia (Marshelder) (syn. Cyclachaena)

About two thirds of patients who had weed dermatitis showed positive patch test reactions to this species (Brunsting and Anderson 1934, Brunsting and Williams 1936 and Mackoff and Dahl 1951).

References

Brunsting, L.A. and Anderson, C.R. (1934) Ragweed dermatitis. A report based on 18 cases. JAMA 103, 1285.

Brunsting, L.A. and Williams, D.H. (1936) Ragweed (contact) dermatitis. Observations in 48 cases and report of unsuccessful attempts at desensitization by injection of specific oils. JAMA 106, 1533.

Mackoff, S. and Dahl, A.O. (1951) A botanical consideration of the weed oleoresin problem. Minn. Med. 34, 1169.

O'Quinn, S.E. and Isbell, K.H. (1969) Influence of oral prednisone on eczematous patch test reactions. Archs. Derm. 99, 380.

Smith, W.A., Prince, H.E. and Cole, M.L. (1942) Contact dermatitis from Narrow Leaf Marshelder (Iva angustifolia) J. Allergy 13, 371.

Shelmire, B. (1939) Contact dermatitis from weeds. Patch testing with their oleoresins. JAMA 113, 1085 and unpublished table accompanying reprints.

Williams, O., Speairs, R. and Boggs, H.W. (1960) Hypersensitivity to marshelder. Difficulties encountered in routine patch testing. J. Louisiana State Med. Soc. 112, 216.

Tribe: Lactuceae (Cichorieae)

Lactuca sativa (Lettuce)

Dermatitis from handling lettuce together with urticaria from ingestion were reported by Rinkel and Balyeat (1932). Morris (1954) reported a positive patch test reaction to the leaf. The milky sap which exudes from the cut stems caused occupational dermatitis and conjunctivitis; hydroxybutyraldehyde which was applied to the stems may have been responsible for these effects (Schwartz et al 1957). A gardener who had dermatitis from the mature plant showed positive patch test reactions to stem and leaf and to aqueous and ethanol extracts of fresh lettuce. Immature plants were innocuous (Krook 1973). The plant yields a sesquiterpene lactone (Yoshioka et al 1973) which is potentially allergenic. The dried juice of this species (and of Lactuca virosa) is known as Lactucarium formerly used medicinally; it contains some hyoscyamine and has been noted to induce mydriasis (Grant 1962).

Lactuca sativa var. longifolia (Romaine lettuce)

A grocer was contact-sensitive to this plant and to Cichorium (Vail and Mitchell 1973). A patch test to the leaf was positive, negative in one control.

Lactuca scariola

The cut stem exudes an irritant milky sap (Schwartz et al 1957).

References

Grant, W.M. (1962) Toxicology of the eye. Springfield, Ill. Charles C. Thomas.

Krook, G. (1973) Contact dermatitis due to lettuce, Lactuca sativa. Contact Dermatitis Newsletter 13, 346.

Morris, G.E. (1954) Dermatoses among food handlers. Indust. Med. Surg. 23, 343.

Rinkel, H.J. and Balyeat, R.M. (1932) Occupational dermatitis due to lettuce. JAMA 98, 137.

Schwartz, L., Tulipan, L. and Birmingham, D.J. (1957). Occupational Diseases of the Skin. 3rd ed. Philadelphia. Lea & Febiger.

Vail, J.T. and Mitchell, J.C. (1973) Occupational Dermatitis from C. intybus, C. endiva and Lactuca sativa. Contact Dermatitis Newsletter (London) 14; 413.

Yoshioka, H., Mabry, T.J. and Timmerman, B.N. (1973) Sesquiterpene Lactones. Chemistry, N.M.R. and Plant Distribution. University Tokyo Press.

Lactuca

Swelling of the oral mucous membrane and Eustachian tubes followed ingestion of lettuce (Closson 1974).

Salad makers were observed by Downing (1945) to develop dermatitis from contact with lettuce and from ingestion of lettuce.

Lactuca sativa and Cichorium produced immediate and delayed hypersensitivity (Krook 1977).

References

Closson, J.B. (1974) Oral allergy after lettuce ingestion. JAMA 230, 613.

Downing, J.G. (1945) in discussion of Templeton, H.J. (1945) Epidermal and dermal sensitisation (coexisting in the same individual) JAMA 127, 908.

Krook, G. (1977) Occupational dermatitis from Lactuca sativa and Cichorium (endive). Contact Dermatitis 3, 27.

Tribe: Anthemidae

Leucanthemum (syn. Chrysanthemum)

Twenty species are found in Europe, especially on the mountains of central Europe and in Northern Asia. Reports of dermatitis have been recorded under Chrysanthemum leucanthemum.

Matricaria

40 species are found in southern Europe and western Asia, 10 species in southern Africa and two species in western North America.

Matricaria chamomilla

The dried flowers are officinial. Some reports of dermatitis from Chamomile may refer to this plant known as German Chamomile or to Anthemis nobilis (Roman chamomile).

Two patients who developed dermatitis from the plant showed positive patch test reactions to the petals, negative reactions to the leaves (Moslein 1963). Cross-sensitivity was observed to Anthemis arvensis, and A. nobilis. The plant yields desacetyl matricarin which produced positive patch test reactions in a sesquiterpene-lactone sensitive patient (Mitchell 1973).

Matricaria inodora

Three farmers developed contact dermatitis from the plant. Patch test reactions were positive to M. inodora, negative to M. chamomilla (Kocsis 1961).

Reference

Kocsis, A. (1961) A case of hypersensitivity to Matricaria inodora. Borgyogy. Vener. Szemle 37, 232.

Mitchell, J.C. (1973) Unpublished observations.

Moslein, P. (1963) Pflanzen als Kontakt-Allergene. Berufsdermatosen 11, 24.

Tribe: Astereae

Microglossa

This genus contains Conyza:

sixty species in temperate and subtropical areas and Psiadia: sixty species mainly in tropical Africa.

Microglossa mespilifolia

The powdered plant is irritant to the eyes and respiratory tract (Watt and Breyer-Brandwijk 1962).

Microglossa pyrifolia (syn. M. volubilis)

The juice from crushed young roots is irritant to the eye (Irvine 1961, Watt and Breyer-Brandwijk 1962). A blistering necrotic action in wounds results from its use in an arrow poison (Kerharo and Bouquet 1950).

References

Irvine, F.R. (1961) Woody Plants of Ghana. Oxford University Press London.

Kerharo, J. and Bouquet, A. (1950) Plantes médicinales et toxiques de la Côte d'Ivoire - Haute - Volta. Ministère de la France d'outre Mer. office de la Recherche Scientifique Outre - Mer. Paris.

Watt, J.M. and Breyer-Brandwijk, M.G. (1962) The Medicinal and Poisonous Plants of Southern Africa. 2nd ed. Edinburgh. E. and S. Livingstone.

Tribe: Eupatorieae

Mikania

250 species are found in tropical America and the West Indies: two species in southern Africa.

Mikania capensis

The plant is caustic to the skin (Watt and Breyer-Brandwijk 1962).

Reference

Watt, J.M. and Breyer-Brandwijk, M.G. (1962) The Medicinal and Poisonous Plants of Southern Africa. 2nd ed. Edinburgh. E. and S. Livingstone.

Tribe: Astereae

Olearia

100 species are found in Australasia.

Olearia axillaris

Contact sensitivity to this plant and cross-sensitivity to other Compositae species was observed by Burry et al (1973).

Olearia decurrens

Maiden (1914) received a report of recurrent contact dermatitis from this species.

Olearia viscidula

Some persons who hand pull the weed suffer dermatitis (Maiden 1912, 1913, 1918).

References

Burry, J.N., Kuchel, R., Reid, J.C. and Kirk, J. (1973) Australian bush dermatitis. Compositae dermatitis in South Australia. Med. J. Australia. 1, 110 and Burry, J.N. (personal communication 1973).

Maiden, J.H. (1912) Additional skin-irritating plants. Ag. Gaz. New South Wales. 23, 604.

Maiden, J.H. (1913) Additional skin-irritating plants. Ag. Gaz. New South Wales. 24, 778, and 916-917.

Maiden, J.H. (1914) On some plants which cause inflammation or irritation of the skin. Ag. Gaz. New South Wales, 25, 611.

Maiden, J.H. (1918) Plants which produce inflammation or irritation of the skin. Ag. Gaz. New South Wales 29, 344.

Tribe: Cynareae

Onopordum (syn. Onopordon)

40 species are found in Europe, northern Africa and Western Asia.

Onoperdon acanthium (sic)
Cotton or Scotch Thistle

Topical use of the plant for cancerous affections of the skin

(Piffard 1881) suggests irritancy.

Piffard, H.G. (1881) A treatise on the Materia Medica and Therapeutics of the skin. New York. Wm. Wood and Co.

Tribe: Heliantheae

Oxytenia

One species is found in the southwestern United States.

A plant chemist developed dermatitis from this species. Patch tests to the plant and to an alcoholic extract were positive, negative to an ether extract (Schwartz and Warren 1940).

Reference

Schwartz, L. and Warren, L.H. (1940) Dermatitis caused by contact with copperweed (*Oxytenia acerosa*). J. Allergy 12, 63.

Parthenium

Fifteen species occur in America and the West Indies.

Parthenium argentatum
(Guayule)

Contact dermatitis from this species with a positive patch test was reported by Smith and Hughes (1938).

Parthenium hysterophorus, known in India as Congress Grass, Carrot Weed.

'Weed dermatitis' in the United States from this species was reported by French (1930), Kahn and Grothaus (1936) and Ogden (1957). Shelmire (1940) found that 27 of 50 patients showed positive patch test reactions to an extract of the plant. 19.0 grammes of oleoresinous material could be extracted from 0.45 kg. of dried plant. A sesquiterpene lactone, parthenin, derived from the plant produced positive patch test reactions in 27 of 50 Indian patients who had 'weed dermatitis' (Lonkar et al 1974). In this study and those of Shelmire (1939) and Mitchell et al (1971) the patients showed positive patch test reactions to some other Compositae species.

An extensive outbreak of 'weed dermatitis' involving perhaps 1000 patients with some deaths has been observed. The plant is believed to have been introduced to India about 1956. The outbreak has become a major health problem and also an agricultural problem owing to the aggressiveness and prolific growth of the plant (Ranade 1971, Lonkar et al 1974).

Parthenin is a major allergen of the species (Lonkar et al 1976).

Parthenium bipinnatifidum

This species has not been reported to cause dermatitis but yields a sesquiterpene lactone ambrosin, which produced positive patch test reactions in patients sensitized to *Parthenium hysterophorus* (Lonkar et al 1974).

References

French, S.W. (1930) A case of skin sensitivity to *Parthenium hysterophorus*. Mil. Surgeon 66, 673.

Kahn, I.S. and Grothaus, E.M. (1936) *Parthenium hysterophorus*. Antigenic properties, respiratory and cutaneous. Texas St. J. Med. 32, 284.

Lonkar, A., Mitchell, J.C. and Calnan, C.D. (1974). Contact dermatitis from *Parthenium hysterophorus*. Trans. St. John's Hosp. Derm. Soc. 60, 43.

Lonkar, A., Nagasampagi, B.Z., Naryyanan, C.R. et al (1976) An antigen from *Parthenium hysterophorus* L. Contact Dermatitis 2, 151.

Mitchell, J.C., Dupuis, G., Geissman T.A. and Towers, G.H.N. (1971) Allergic contact dermatitis caused by *Artemisia* and *Chrysanthemum* species. J. Invest. Dermat. 56. 98.

Ogden, H.D. (1957) Diagnosis and treatment of *Parthenium* dermatitis. J. Louisiana M. Soc. 109, 378.

Ranade, S.N. (1971) Generalized Eczematoid Dermatitis in Epidemic Form caused by *Parthenium hysterophorus* L. (Congress Grass). Maharashtra Medical Journal 17, 492.

Shelmire, B. (1939) Contact Dermatitis from weeds. Patch testing wiht their oleoresins. JAMA 113 1085 and unpublished table accompanying reprints.

Piqueria

20 species are found from Mexico to the Andes.

Piqueria trinervia
Stevia

This specis is used by florists in assembling bouquets and occasionally causes hayfever in florists and greenhouse workers (Langley and Sayer 1937).

Reference

Langley, W.D. and Sayer, M.D. (1937) Sensitivity to Piqueria pollen with a case report. J. Allergy 9, 60, 61.

Tribe: Anthemidae

Pyrethrum
(syn. Chrysanthemum)

100 species are found in temperate Eurasia. Reports have been listed under Chrysanthemum.

Tribe: Heliantheae

Rudbeckia

25 species are found in North America.

Rudbeckia hirta
(Black-eyed Susan)

Single instances of contact sensitivity to this species were reported by Lovell et al (1955), Shelmire (1939) and Mackoff and Dahl (1951).

References

Lovell, R.G., Mathews, K.P. and Sheldon, J.M. (1955) Dermatitis venenata from tree pollen oils. J. Allergy 26, 408.

Mackoff, S. and Dahl, A.O. (1951) A botanical consideration of the weed oleoresin problem. Minn. Med. 34, 1169.

Shelmire, B. (1939) Contact dermatitis from weeds. Patch testing with their oleoresins. JAMA 113, 1085 and unpublished table accompanying reprints.

Tribe: Inuleae

Rutidosis

Ten species are found in Australia.

Rutidosis helichrysoides

In an investigation of 'weed dermatitis', two patients were found to be contact-sensitive to this plant and to other Compositae species (Burry et al 1973).

Reference

Burry, J.N., Kuchel, R., Reid, J.G. and Kirk, J. (1973) Australian bush dermatitis. Compositae dermatitis in South Australia. Med. J. Australia 1, 110 and Burry J.N. (personal communication 1973).

Tribe: Cynareae

Saussurea

400 species are found in temperate Asia. Europe, Australia and western North America each provide one species.

Saussurea alpina of Europe has scented flowers, an unusual feature in Compositae species. The root of Saussurea auriculata of China is fragrant and used as incense and to darken the hair (Smith 1969).

Saussurea lappa

This species provides Costus Absolute and costus oil of perfumery (Arctander 1960). Costus Absolute is an active sensitizer. Individuals who were contact sensitive to the material showed positive patch test reactions to some other Compositae species (Mitchell and Epstein 1974).

References

Arctander, S. (1960) Perfume and Flavor Materials of Natural Origin Elizabeth, N.J. Published by the author.

Mitchell, J.C. and Epstein, W.L.

(1974) Contact hypersensitivity to a Perfume Material, Costus Absolute. The role of sesquiterpene lactones. Archs. Derm. 110, 871.

Smith, F.P. (1969) Chinese Materia Medica Vegetable kingdom. 2nd ed. Rev. by Hei, P.D. Taipei, Taiwan. Ku T'ing Book House.

Lactone free costus oil and hydrogenated costus oil lost their sensitizing capacity (Opdyke 1974).

Reference

Opdyke, D.L.J. (1974) Monographs on fragrance raw materials. Fd. Cosmet. Toxicol. 12, 867.

Tribe: Senecioneae

Senecio species, two to three thousand in number, are cosmopolitan. Cineraria has been placed in this genus. Cirrhosis is produced in animals by ingestion of some Senecio species (Hurst 1942).

Senecio cineraria

The hairy leaves can cause dermatitis (Schwartz et al 1957).

Senecio confusus

(Mexican Flame Vine) is a frequent source of dermatitis in persons who trim the plant (Morton 1958), all parts of the plant being incriminated (Hardin and Arena 1969).

Senecio hectori was reported to cause contact dermatitis in New Zealand (Maiden 1918).

Senecio jacobaea known in Britain as Ragweed was noted to cause dermatitis in some persons who handled it (Benson 1973) but has been used as a herbal remedy for inflamed eyes (Wren 1968). The plant is spreading in the United Kingdom owing to a decline in its natural controls, (North 1967).

References

Benson, R.L. (1973) Ragwort can be fatal. Oregon Farmer Stockman 96, 22.

Hardin J.W. and Arena, J.M. (1969) Human Poisoning from Native and cultivated plants. Durham, North Carolina. Duke University Press.

Hurst, E. (1942) The Poison Plants of New South Wales. N.S.W. Poison Plants Committee; Sydney.

Maiden, J.H. (1918) Plants which procue inflammation or irritation of the skin. Ag. Gaz. New South Wales. 29, 344.

Morton, J.F. (1958) Ornamental plants with poisonous properties. Proc. Florida State Hort. Soc. 71, 372.

North, P.M. (1967) Poisonous Plants and Fungi in Colour. London. Blandford Press Ltd.

Schwartz, L., Tulipan, L. and Birmingham, D.J. (1957). Occupational Diseases of the Skin. 3rd. ed. Philadelphia. Lea & Febiger. pp. 637-672.

Wren, R.W. (1968) Potter's New Cyclopaedia of Botanical Drugs and Preparations by Wren, R.C. Re-edit. by Wren, R.W. Potter & Clarke Ltd. Health Science Press. Rustington. Sussex.

Simsia

Forty species are found in tropical America and Jamaica.

Simsia annectens

The hairs on the stems have a slightly stinging property (Altschul 1973).

Reference

Altschul, S. von R. (1973) Drugs and foods from little-known plants. Cambridge, Mass. Harvard Univ. Press.

Tribe: Astereae

Solidago

100 species are found in America: one species, Solidago virgaaurea (Golden Rod) in Europe.

White (1887) observed several cases of dermatitis in persons who handled Solidago species but was unable to exclude inadvertent exposure to Toxicodendron. Two positive patch test reactions to Solidago species were recorded by Hjorth (1968).

Underwood and Gaul (1948) observed three cases of contact dermatitis from Goldenrod with strong positive patch test reactions.

Solidago odora

This plant has been used medicinally; the volatile oil derived from it is irritant and rubefacient (Dispensatory 1884). The plant yields an oil of perfumery (Arctander 1960).

Solidago serotina (Goldenrod)

In an investigation of 'weed dermatitis' 3 of 50 patients showed positive patch test reactions to an extract of this species (Shelmire 1939).

Solidago virgaaurea

The plant produced maculo-papular dermatitis with itching and a burning sensation of the skin of field-workers following three to twelve hours of work at hay making. The irritant is said to be carried by the pollen (Schwartz et al 1957). The flower heads tend to accumulate extraneous pollen from other plants.

References

Arctander, S. (1960) Perfume and Flavor materials of Natural Origin. Elizabeth, N.J. Published by the author.

Dispensatory, the National (1884) Philadelphia. Stille and Maisch cited by White (1887).

Hjorth, N. (1968) Finsen Institute. Personal Communication.

Schwartz, L., Tulipan, L. and Birmingham, D.J. (1957) Occupational Diseases of the Skin. 3rd. ed. Philadelphia. Lea & Febiger. pp. 637-672.

Shelmire, B. (1939) Contact dermatitis from weeds: Patch testing with their oleoresins. JAMA 113, 1085 and unpublished table accompanying reprints.

Underwood, G.B. and Gaul, L.E. (1948) Overtreatment dermatitis in dermatitis venenata due to plants. JAMA 138, 570.

White, J.C. (1887) Dermatitis venenata: An account of the action of external irritants upon the skin. Boston. Cupples and Hurd.

Stevia

150 species are found in tropical and subtropical America.

Stevia rebaudiana

The leaves of this Paraguay shrub have remarkable sweetening properties (Howes 1974).

Reference

Howes, F.N. (1974) A dictionary of useful and everyday plants and their common names. Cambridge. University Press.

Tribe: Calenduleae

Tagetes

Fifty species are found in warm regions of the Americas.

Tagetes species (Marigold)

Gerard (1636) cited Dodonaeus for the statement, "I did see a boy whose lippes and mouth, when hee began to chew the floures, did swell extreamely". Hjorth (1968) observed one positive patch test reaction in seven patients who were tested, suggesting potential irritancy.

Two intensely fluorescent compounds isolated from *Tagetes* root were found to be phototoxic for *Candida albicans* and identified as bithienyl and alpha-terthienyl (Chan et al 1975).

Tagetes erecta, African Marigold

According to Behl et al (1966) the leaves are irritant to some individuals. This species is widely cultivated in many named cultivars.

Alpha-terthienyl derived from the plant inhibits DNA repair in UV-irradiated cultured human fibroplasts (Stich et al 1975).

The odor of marigolds has been stated to cause hayfever symptoms even in the absence of pollen (Biederman 1937).

Tagetes glandulifera
(Stinking Roger)

Maiden (1895) received a report that the juice or seed irritated the eyes and bare arms of men working amongst the plant. The irritation was said to last for three or four days. The plant produced a strong scent which could be smelled at a distance. The plant yields an oil of perfumery (Arctander 1960). According to Chittenden (1974) Tagetes glandulifera is a synonym of Tagetes minuta.

Tagetes minuta
(Stinking Roger)

Maiden (1895) recorded that the juice of this species was irritant to the skin and eyes. The sharp seeds (Maiden 1895) and the stems (Watt and Breyer-Brandwijk 1962) can cause mechanical injury.

Scott (1967) and Findlay (1967) report this species to be a common cause of dermatitits in South Africa.

In three farmers, one female and two males, who had 'weed dermatitis', allergic contact dermatitis was demonstrated by patch testing with diluted extracts of the plant. The allergenic principle was found in the acetone soluble fraction of leaf and flower head. The fresh leaf and flower were irritant by patch test.

Patch tests to Tagetes erecta were negative. One of two patients who were tested showed a positive patch test reaction to pyrethrum (Chrysanthemum cinerariifolium). Two patients who were tested showed weak positive patch test reactions to the flower, negative to the leaf of Chrysanthemum morifolium. Positive patch test reactions were not augmented by exposure to ultraviolet light (Verhagen and Nyaga 1974). The leaf and stem were found to be phototoxic for Candida albicans (Camm et al 1975).

Tagetes patula
French Marigold

According to Behl et al (1966) the leaves of this commonly cultivated plant are irritant to some persons. The plant yields an oil of perfumery (Arctander 1960).

Tagetes

The odour of marigolds caused hayfever and asthma in two patients respectively. Cosmos had a similar effect in one of them.

Crown of Gold marigold which had odourless foliage, had no ill-effect (Biederman 1937).

References

Arctander, S. (1960) Perfume and Flavor Materials of Natural Origin. Elizabeth, N.J. Published by the author.

Behl, P.N., Captain, R.M., Bedi, B.M.S. and Gupta, S. (1966) Skin irritant and sensitizing plants found in India, New Delhi. P.N. Behl, Irwin Hospital.

Biederman, J.B. (1937) Sensitivity to flowers. Laryngoscope 47, 825.

Camm, E.L., Towers, G.H.N. and Mitchell, J.C. (1975) Ultraviolet-mediated antibiotic activity of some Compositae species. Lloydia 40, 487.

Chan, G.F., Towers, G.H.N. and Mitchell, J.C. (1977) Ultra violet-mediated antibiotic activity of thiophene compounds of Tagetes (Compositae) (in preparation)

Chittenden, F.J. (1974) The Royal Horticultural Society Dictionary of Gardening. 2nd ed. Oxford Clarendon Press.

Findlay, G.H. (1967) Personal Communication.

Gerard, J. (1636) The Herbal or Generall Historie of Plantes. The Essence thereof distilled by M. Woodward (1927) from the edition of Th. Johnson (1630) London. Gerald House.

Hjorth, N. (1968) Finsen Institute. Personal Communication

Maiden, J.H. (1895) The weeds of New South Wales. Ag. Gaz. New South Wales. 6, 671

Verhagen, A.R. and Nyaga, J.M. (1974) Contact dermatitis from Tagetes minuta. Archs. Derm. 110, 441.

Watt, J.M. and Breyer-Brandwijk, M.G. (1962) The Medicinal and Poisonous Plants of Southern Africa. 2nd ed. Edinburgh. E. & S. Livingstone.

Scott, F.P. (1967) Personal Communication.

Stich, H.F., Lam, P., Lo, L.W. et al (1975) The search for relevant short term bioassays for chemical carcinogens. Canad. J. Genet. Cytol. 17, 471.

Tribe: Anthemideae

Tanacetum (syn. Chrysanthemum)

Fifty to 60 species are found in north temperate regions.

Tanacetum vulgare (Tansy)

The plant is cultivated as a herbal remedy, for seasoning and for making a tea. The whole plant is strongly scented and has a bitter, acrid taste. Oil of Tansy has been used as a vermifuge since the Middle Ages. The plant yields an oil of perfumery (Arctander 1960).

Greenhouse and Sulzberger (1933) reported a case of contact dermatitis from the plant. Individuals who have contact dermatitis from Compositae species frequently show positive patch test reactions to acetone extracts of the plant (Robertsn and Mitchell 1967, Mitchell et al 1970, Mitchell 1972, Lonkar et al 1974). A gardener who had dermatitis from Chrysanthemum morifolium did not recover after discarding all his chrysanthemum plants. He continued to weed his flower beds and it was found, by a housecall, that the principal weed in his garden was Tanacetum vulgare to which he was also contact sensitive (Mitchell 1970).

This species yields the potentially allergenic sesquiterpene lactones, arbusculin-A and tanacetin (Rodriquez, E. pers. comm. 1975 cites Samek, Z. et al (1973) Coll. Czech. Chem. Comm. 38, 1971. Grabarczyk, H. et al (1973) Pol. J. Pharmacol. Pharm. 25, 95. Suchy, M. (1962) Coll. Czech. Chem. Comm. 27, 1958.)

References

Arctander, S. (1960) Perfume and Flavor materials of Natural Origin. Elizabeth, N.J. Published by the author.

Greenhouse, C.A. and Sulzberger, M.B. (1933) Common weed (Tanacetum vulgare) as a cause of eczematous dermatitis. J. Allergy 4, 523.

Lonkar, A., Mitchell, J.C., and Calnan, C.D. (1974) Allergic contact dermatitis from Parthenium hysterophorus. Trans. St. John's Hosp. Derm. Soc. 60, 43.

Mitchell, J.C. (1970) Unpublished observations.

Mitchell, J.C., Fritig, B., Singh, B. and Towers, G.H.N. (1970) Allergic contact dermatitis from Frullania and Compositae. The role of sesquiterpene lactones. J. Invest.Derm. 54, 233.

Mitchell, J.C. (1972) Plant dermatitis - note on inadequacy of some plant extracts. Contact Dermatitis Newsletter (London) 11, 271.

Robertson, W.D. and Mitchell, J.C. (1967) Allergic contact and photodermatitis. Canad. Med. Ass. J. 97, 380.

Tribe: Lactuceae (Cichorieae)

Taraxacum

Sixty species are found in north temperate regions, two species in temperate South America.

Taraxacum japonicum

This plant has not been reported to cause dermatitis but yields a sesquiterpene lactone, lactucopicrin (Kariyone 1971) which is potentially allergenic (Mitchell and Dupuis 1971).

Taraxacum officinale (Dandelion)

This species is almost cosmopolitan. The roasted roots are used as a coffee substitute (Wren 1968). Contact sensitivity to this species with cross-sensitivity to Anthemis nobilis and Apium graveolens was reported by Janke (1950).

Two patients who had 'weed dermatitis' showed positive patch test reactions to the plant; the patients were also contact sensitive to Chrysanthemum and Olearia and in one of the two cases to other Compositae species (Burry et al 1973).

References

Burry, J.N., Kuchel, R., Reid, J.D. and Kirk, J. (1973) Australian bush dermatitis. Compositae dermatitis in South Australia. Med. J. Australia 1, 110; and Burry, J.N. (personal communication 1973).

Janke, D. (1950) Durch Lowenzahn (Taraxacum officinale) verursachtes ekzem. Hautarzt 1, 177.

Kariyone, T. (1971) Atlas of Mecicinal Plants. Osaka, Japan. Takeda Chemical Industries.

Mitchell, J.C. and Dupuis, C. (1971) Allergic Contact Dermatitis from sesquiterpenoids of the Compositae family of Plants. Brit. J. Derm. 8, 139.

Wren, R.W. (1968) Potter's New Cyclopaedia of Botanical Drugs and Preparations by Wren, R.C. Reedit. by Wren, R.W. Potter and Clarke Ltd. Health Science Press. Rustington, Sussex.

Taraxacum officinale

Ingestion of a decoction of the plant produced itching and tingling erythema, papules and wheals, followed by desquamation (Smyth in The Lancet, cited by Piffard 1881).

Reference

Piffard, H.G. (1881) A treatise on the Materia Medica and Therapeutics of the skin. New York Wm. Wood & Co.

Tribe: Inuleae

Telekia

Two species are found in central Europe east to the Caucasus. A report of dermatitis from a species of this genus (Novak and Kolinsky 1960) is recorded under Buphthalmum.

Reference

Novak, J. and Kolinsky, J. (1960) Dermatitis phytogenes post. Telekiam Baumgartner (seu Buphthalmum). Cesk. Derm. 35, 113.

Tribe: Heliantheae

Tetradymia

Eight species are found in western North America.

Tetradymia canescens and T. glabrata (Horsebrush)

Ingestion of the plant may cause photodermatitis in sheep (Mathews 1937, Kingsbury 1964). Reported irritant effects of the plant for man (Muenscher 1951, Schwartz et al 1957) are not well-substantiated.

References

Kingsbury, J.M. (1964) Poisonous Plants of the United States and Canada. Englewood Cliffs, New Jersey. Prentice-Hall Inc.

Mathews, F.P.(1937) Photosensitisation and the photodynamic diseases of man and the lower animals. Arch. Path. 23, 399.

Muenscher, W.C. (1951) Poisonous plants of the United States, 2nd ed. New York. The MacMillan Co.

Schwartz, L., Tulipan, L. and Birmingham, D.J. (1957). Occupational Diseases of the Skin. 3rd. ed. Philadelphia. Lea & Febiger. pp. 637-672.

Thelesperma

Twelve species are found in warm regions of America.

Thelesperma gracilis (False Coreopsis)

The fruits have barbed bristles. McCord (1962) listed the plant as capable of producing dermatitis. Shelmire (1939) observed negative patch test reactions to an extract of the plant in 50 patients who had 'weed dermatitis'.

References

McCord, C.P. (1962) The Occupational Toxicity of Cultivated Flowers. Ind. Med. Surg. 31, 365.

Shelmire, B. (1939) Contact dermatitis from weeds: Patch testing with their oleoresins. JAMA 113, 1085; and unpublished table accompanying reprints.

Tragoceros

Five species are found in Mexico and Central America.

Tragoceros

Species of this genus have hooked fruits which attach themselves to animals (Howes 1974).

Reference

Howes, F.N. (1974) A Dictionary of useful and everyday plants and their common names. Cambridge University Press.

Tragopogon

50 species are found in temperate Eurasia, one species in southern Africa.

Tragopogon porrifolius
Salsify

This species is sometimes grown as a vegetable.

Tribe: Heliantheae

Verbesina

150 species are found in warm regions of America.

Verbesina enceloides
(Golden Crownbeard)

The achenes, when awned, can cause mechanical injury to animals (Hurst 1942). Shelmire (1940) observed contact urticaria from the plant.

References

Hurst, E. (1942) The Poison Plants of New South Wales. N.S.W. Poison Plants Committee; Sydney.

Shelmire, B. (1940) Contact dermatitis from vegetation. South Med. J. 33, 338.

Tribe: Vernonieae

Vernonia

About one thousand species are found in America, Africa, Asia and Australia.

Vernonia baldwinii
(Iron weed)

Contact sensitivity to this plant was observed in one of 50 patients who had 'weed dermatitis' (Shelmire 1939).

Reference

Shelmire, B. (1939) Contact dermatitis from weeds: Patch testing with their oleoresins. JAMA 113, 1085; and unpublished table accompanying reprints.

Vernonia anthelmintica

The fruits are used for skin diseases and for repelling moths from woollens (Howes 1974).

Reference

Howes, F.N. (1974) A dictionary of useful and everyday plants and their common names. Cambridge University Press.

Tribe: Heliantheae

Xanthium

Thirty species are cosmopolitan, having been unintentionally spread by animals and man.

Xanthium species

The hooked fruits become attached to animals and impair the value of sheeps' wool. The burs and the spines on the stems of some species can cause mechanical injury.

Fourteen of 25 patients who had 'weed dermatitis' showed positive patch test reactions to an extract of a species of this genus (Mackoff and Dahl 1951). Rook (1962) observed an individual who was contact sensitive to Xanthium, Chrysanthemum and other Compositae species.

Xanthium californicum

Four patients who had 'weed' dermatitis' were contact sensitive to this species and to some other Compositae species (Burry et al 1973). The cross-sensitivity pattern was not identical in the four cases.

Xanthium canadense

The plant was said to be a

skin irritant by MacDougal (1894). Brunsting and Anderson (1934) and Brunsting and Williams (1936) reported contact sensitivity to this plant and to other Compositae species in about one fifth of 32 patients who had 'weed dermatitis'.

Xanthium chinense

Dermatitis can be caused by handling the plant (Maiden 1918).

Xanthium occidentale

This species can cause mechanical injury to cattle and spoils sheeps' wool. The burs when ingested can cause intestinal obstruction. Ingestion of the immature plant, not the bur, can cause a fatal syndrome in cattle with fever, dermatitis and black faeces (Watt and Breyer-Brandwijk 1962).

Xanthium pungens

This species can cause mechanical injury to animals. Handling the plant was said to cause pruritus, erythema and urticaria (Watt and Breyer-Brandwijk 1962). Gardner and Bennetts (1956) list the plant as an agent of contact dermatitis without clinical details.

Xanthium speciosum

In an investigation of 'weed dermatitis', eleven of 50 patients showed positive patch test reactions to an extract of this plant (Shelmire 1939).

Xanthium spinosum

This species can cause mechanical injury to animals (Maiden 1895, Watt and Breyer-Brandwijk 1962). Rowe (1939) reported two cases of 'weed dermatitis' from the plant with positive patch test reactions to the leaves and, to a lesser degree, to the pollen. Four patients who had 'weed dermatitis' showed positive patch test reactions to this plant, to Xanthium californicum and to other Compositae species (Burry et al 1973).

Xanthium strumarium

The plant is rough to the touch and causes itching from the hairs or dust with which it is covered (Cheney 1887). The burs, if ingested, cause mechanical irritation of the mouth (Burkill 1935).

References

Brunsting, L.A. and Anderson, C.R. (1934) Ragweed dermatitis. A report based on 18 cases. JAMA 103, 1285.

Brunsting, L.A. and Williams, D.H. (1936) Ragweed (contact) dermatitis. Observations in 48 cases and report of unsuccessful attempts at desensitisation by injection of specific oils. JAMA 106, 1533.

Burkill, I.H. (1935) A Dictionary of the Economic Products of the Malay Peninsula. 2 Vols. London. Crown Agents for the Colonies.

Burry, J.N., Kuchel, R., Reid, J.G. and Kirk, J. (1973) Australian bush dermatitis. Compositae dermatitis in South Australia. Med. J. Australia 1, 110; and Burry, J.N. (personal communication 1973).

Cheney (1887) cited by White, J.C. (1887). Dermatitis venenata. An account of the action of external irritants upon the skin. Boston. Cupples and Hurd.

Gardner, C.A. and Bennetts, H.W. (1956) The Toxic plants of Western Australia. Perth West, Australian Newspapers Ltd.

MacDougal, D.T. (1894) Poisonous influences of various species of cypripedium. Minnesota Botan. Studies pp. 32 and 450.

Mackoff, S. and Dahl, A.O. (1951) A botanical consideration of the weed oleoresin problem. Minn. Med. 34, 1169.

Maiden, J.H. (1895) Plants which produce inflammation or irritation of the skin. Ag. Gaz. New South Wales. 29, 344.

Rook, A. (1962) Plant dermatitis in general practice. Practitioner 188, 627.

Rowe, A.H. (1939) Contact allergy to cocklebur (Xanthium spinosum) Archs. Derm. Syph. 39, 149.

Maiden, J.H. (1895) The weeds of New South Wales. Ag. Gaz. New South Wales. 6, 671.

Shelmire, B. (1939) Contact dermatitis from weeds. Patch testing with their oleoresins. JAMA 113, 1085.

Watt, J.M. and Breyer-Brandwijk, M. G. (1962). The Medicinal and poisonous plants of Southern Africa. 2nd ed. Edinburgh. E. & S. Livingstone.

White, J.C. (1887) Dermatitis venenata; an account of the Action of External irritants upon the skin. Boston. Cupples and Hurd.

Tibe: Heliantheae

Zinnia

Twenty species are found in the southern United States to Brazil and Chile. Many are cultivated in Europe, and are available in numerous named cultivars.

Zinnia species

Shelmire (1940) reported a species of this genus as a minor skin sensitizer without clinical details.

Zinnia elegans

This species was listed among plants which could cause contact dermatitis without clinical details (McCord 1962).

Zinnia pauciflora

The plant was suspected as a cause of photosensitisation by ingestion in animals (Hurst 1942).

References

Hurst, E. (1942) The Poison plants of New South Wales. N.S.W. Poison Plants Committee,

McCord, C.P. (1962) The Occupational Toxicity of Cultivated Flowers. Ind. med. Surg. 31, 365.

Shelmire, B. (1940) Contact dermatitis from vegetation. South Med. J. 33, 388.

CONNARACEAE

200 species in 25 genera are found in tropical regions.

Chemistry is recorded by Hegnauer (1964).

Cnestis

40 species are native to warm regions of Africa, Madagascar and Malaysia.

Cnestis corniculata

The bristles can produce mechanical injury (Watt and Breyer-Brandwijk 1962).

Cnestis natalensis

Penetration of the skin by rigid brown hairs, present on the inside and outside of the capsule, can produce severe itching (Watt and Breyer-Brandwijk 1962).

References

Hegnauer, R. (1964) Chemotaxonomy of plants. Vol. 3. Basel, Birkhauser. pg. 545.

Watt, J.M. and Breyer-Brandwijk, M.G. (1962) The Medicinal and Poisonous Plants of Southern Africa. 2nd ed. Edinburgh. E.& S. Livingstone.

CONVOLVULACEAE

1650 species in 55 genera are found in tropical and temperate regions. Some are thorny.

Chemistry is recorded by Hegnauer (1964).

Argyreia

90 species are native to IndoMalaysia, one species to Queensland.

Argyreia nervosa

The leaves have rubefacient and vesicant properties (Quisumbing 1951).

References

Hegnauer, R. (1964) Chemotaxonomy of plants. Vol. 3 Basel, Birkhauser. p. 547.

Quisumbing, E. (1951) Medicinal Plants of the Philippines. Philipp. Dep. Agr. and Nat. Resources Tech. Bull. No. 16. Manila. Bureau of Printing 1234 pp.

Convolvulus

250 species are cosmopolitan. The plants are subject to infection by a smut fungus, *Thecaphora seminisconvolvuli*. Some yield Rosewood oil.

Convolvulus arvensis
Bindweed

Striate bullous dermatitis occurring on the wrists and forearms and related to this plant on circumstantial evidence was considered to be an example of phytophotodermatitis (Klaber 1942). Under experimental conditions, extracts of the plant did not show any photosensitising activity (Van Dijk 1964). One can speculate that coumarins of plants may be changed to furanocourmarins by fungus infection as in *Apium*.

References

Klaber, R. (1942) Phyto-photo-dermatitis. Brit. J. Derm. Syph. 54, 193.

Van Dijk, E. and Berrens, L. (1964) Plants as an etiological factor in dermatitis venenata due to plants. Dermatologica 129, 321.

Convolvulus scoparius
(syn. *Rhodorhiza scoparia*)
Canary rosewood, lignum rhodii, bois de rose

An Oil of Rosewood used to be extracted from this shrub. It was replaced by a similar oil obtained from the wood of *Aniba rosaeodora* the source of which long remained uncertain (Record and Mell 1924). Grossman (1910, 1920) reported that men in his father's workshop could not work for long periods with 'rosewood' because of dermatitis and constitutional symptoms. He thought that the wood was *C. scoparius* but according to Woods and Calnan (1976) the wood was probably *Aniba*.

Reference

Grossman, J. (1910) Gesundheitsschädliche Hölzer Bayrische Industrielle Gewerbeblatt 96 (6), 51.

Grossmann, J. (1920) Gesundheitsschädliche Holzarten. Der Holzkäufer (Leipzig) 17, 529, 535, 540 and 545.

Record, S.J. and Mell, C.D. (1924) Timbers of Tropical America, New Haven, Yale.

Woods, B. and Calnan, C.D. (1976) Toxic Woods. Brit. J. Derm. 94, Suppl 13, June.

Dichondra

Four or five species are found in tropical and subtropical regions.

Dichrondra sp.

Dorsey (1962) received a report that a species of this genus was capable of producing dermatitis.

Reference

Dorsey, C.S. (1962) Plant Dermatitis in California. Calif. Med. 96, 412.

Ipomoea

500 species are found in tropical and warm temperate regions.

Ipomoea aculeatum
(syn. *Calonyction*)
Moonflower

Dermatitis can be produced in those who handle or trim the vine (Morton 1962).

Ipomoea batatas
(syn. *Batatas edulis*)
Sweet Potato

Parasitic infestation of the skin can be produced by *Trombiculum* (Batata Louse), (Simons 1952).

Ipomoea imperialis

The plant was listed as capable of producing dermatitis (Touton 1932).

Ipomoea pennata
(syn. *Quamoclit*)

The root has a sternutatory effect (Quisumbing 1951).

Ipomoea purga   Jalap

The root gives an acrid taste (Wren 1968).

References

Morton, J.F. (1962) Ornamental Plants with Poisonous Properties II. Proc. Florida Hort. Soc. 75, 474

Simons, R.D.G. (1952) Handbook of Tropical Dermatology. New York. Elsevier.

Touton, K. (1932) Hauterkrankungen durch phanerogamische Pflanzen und ihre Produkte (Toxicodermia et Allergodermia phytogenes), in Barnewitz J. et al Angeborene Anomalien, Lichtdermatosen, Pflanzengifte, Thermische Schadidgungen, Einfluss Innerer Storungen auf die Haut. Berlin. Verlag von Julius Springer.

Quisumbing, E. (1951) Medicinal Plants of the Philippines. Philipp. Dep. Agr. and Nat. Resources Tech. Bull. No. 16. Manila. Bureau of Printing. 1234 pp.

CORIARIACEAE

15 species in one genus are found in Eurasia, New Zealand and Central and South America. C. myrtifolia of the western Mediterranean yields tan, others a black dye.

Coriaria ruscifolia

Poisonous honey is derived from the plant; the toxic substance is mellitoxin, chemically related to tutin; the same substance was found in honey dew produced by an insect on the leaves. Tutin is an oxygenated lactone of the sesquiterpene series (Briggs 1946).

The chemistry is given by Hegnauer (1964).

References

Briggs, L.H. (1946) Plant products of New Zealand. J. Proc. Roy. Soc. New South Wales 80, 151.

Hegnauer, R. (1964) Chemotaxonomy of Plants. Vol. 3. Basel Birkhauser, p. 562.

CORNACEAE

100 species in 12 genera are found in northern and southern temperate regions and on tropical mountains.

Chemistry is recorded by Hegnauer (1964).

Reference

Hegnauer, R. (1964) Chemotaxonomy of Plants. Vol. 3. Basel. Birkhauser. p. 565.

Cornus

In a strict sense this genus consists of four species found from central and southern Europe to the Caucasus and eastern Asia and in California. The fruits of C. mas (Cornelian cherry) are used in preserves.

Cornus sanguinea

The leaf possesses T-shaped hairs which pierce the skin when rubbed on the skin in the direction of its long axis producing erythema or urticaria (Nestler 1913).

References

Nestler, A. (1913) Die hautreizende Wirkung des roten Hartriegels und der Kornelbirsche, Die Umschau 17, 860, cited by Woods and Calnan (1976).

Woods, B. and Calnan, C.D. (1976) Toxic Woods. Brit. J. Derm. 94 Suppl. 13, June.

CORYLACEAE

15 species in one genus are found in north temperate regions.

Corylus

The distribution of the genus is that of the family.

Corylus sp.   Hazel

Freshly cut hazel yields tannins which can produce painful fissures of the hands of woodworkers (Schwartz et al 1957).

Positive scratch tests to hazel nut were observed in two food handlers who had dermatitis (Hjorth and Roed-Petersen 1976).

Corylus sieboldiana

The bristles have an irritant inflammatory effect which can be counteracted by the leaves (Altschul 1973).

References

Altschul, S. von R. (1973) Drugs and foods from little-known plants. Cambridge, Mass. Harvard Univ. Press.

Schwartz, L., Tulipan, L. and Birmingham, D.J. (1957) Occupational Diseases of the Skin. 3rd ed. Philadelphia. Lea & Febiger. p. 637-672.

Hjorth, N. and Roed-Petersen, J. (1976) Occupational protein contact dermatitis in food handlers. Contact Dermatitis 2, 28.

CRASSULACEAE

1500 species in 35 genera are of cosmopolitan distribution but chiefly found in southern Africa Most species are xerophytic.

Chemistry is recorded by Hegnauer (1964),

Reference

Hegnauer, R. (1964) Chemotaxonomy of Plants. Vol. 3 Basel. Birkhauser. p 572.

Sedum

600 species are found in north temperate regions, one species in Peru. The plants are fleshy-leaved xerophytes.

Sedum acre
Mossy Stonecrop, Houseleek

Sedum alba

Sedum purpureum

The plants possess acrid properties and are irritant to the skin (Buillard 1780, Oesterlen 1856, Dispensatory 1884, Cheney 1887 cited by White 1887, Pammel 1911). Sensitivity to the plants was reported by Biberstein (1927). The acridity of the juice is said to be due to the presence of an alkaloid, sedine, which is related to piperine of pepper (Piper). An alkaloid, sedamine, was isolated by Kolsenikov and Shvattsman (1939).

Sedum roseum

The fleshy root stock, when cut or bruised, emits a fragrance like attar-of-roses.

References

Biberstein, H. (1927) Uberempfindlichkeit gegen Pflanzen (Sedum, Tradescantia, Campanula, Meerzwiebel, Myrthe, Alpenveilchen, Buntnessel). Zbl. Hautkrkh. 22, 19.

Builliard (1780) Histoire des Plantes Veneneuses et Suspectes de la France. Paris. cited by Woods (1962).

Dispensatory, the National (1884) Philadelphis. Stille and Maisch. cited by White (1887)

Kokesnikov and Shvattsman (1939) Alkaloids of Sedum acre L. J. Gen. Chem. U.S.S. Russia 9, 2156 (Chem. Abstr. 34, 4072.).

Oesterlen (1856) Handbuch der Heilmittellehre. Tubingern cited by White (1887).

Pammel, L.H. (1911) A Manual of Poisonous plants. Torch Press. Cedar Rapids, Iowa. Reprinted Univ. Microfilms Inc. Ann Arbor, Mich. 1965. pp. 476-7.

White, J.C. (1887) Dermatitis venenata: An account of the Action of External irritants upon the Skin. Boston. Cupples & Hurd.

Woods, B. (1962) Irritant Plants. Trans. St. John's Hosp. derm. Soc. 48, 75.

Kalanchoë

200 species are found from tropical and Southern Africa to China and Java; one species is found in tropical South America.

Kalanchoë blossfeldiana

This plant produced a positive patch test reaction in one patient (Agrup et al 1970).

Kalanchoë pinnata

The juice has been used for leg ulcers (Biberstein 1972).

References

Agrup, G. et al (1970) Value of History and Testing in Suspected Contact Dermatitis. Arch. Derm. 101, 212.

Bershtein, E.I. (1972) Use of *Kalanchoe pinnata* juice in the treatment of patients with trophic crural ulcers. Vestn. Khir. Im. I.I. Grekova 108, 116. BA: 56, 15910.

Sempervivum

25 species are found on the mountains of southern Europe to the Caucasus.

Sempervivum

The Ancient Greeks knew that a leaf tasted more acid in the morning than in the evening. Organic acids accumulate during the night and disperse during the day (Rowley 1960).

Sempervivum montanum
Hens and Chickens

The plant has irritant properties (Pammel 1911) and the leaves were said to cause dermatitis (McCord 1962).

Sempervivum tectorum
Houseleek

This species is planted on cottage roofs to keep slates in position. The juice is astringent and probably irritant (Wren 1968).

References

McCord, C.P. (1962) The Occupational Toxicity of Cultivated Flowers. Ind. Med. Surg. 31, 365.

Pammel, L.H. (1911) A Manual of Poisonous plants. Torch Press. Cedar Rapids, Iowa. Reprinted Univ.Microfilms Inc. Ann Arbor, Mich. 1965.

Bowley, G.C. (1960) A short history of succulent plants in A Handbook of Succulent Plants by Jacobsen, H. Vol. I. London. Blandford, p. 1.

Wren, R.W. (1968) Potter's New Cyclopaedia of Botanical Drugs and Preparations by Wren, R.C. Re-edit. by Wren, R.W. Potter and Clarke Ltd. Health Science Press. Rustington, Sussex.

CRUCIFERAE
(syn. BRASSICACEAE)

3200 species in 375 genera are of cosmopolitan distribution, chiefly in north temperate regions and especially in the Mediterranean area.

Chemistry is recorded by Hegnauer (1964), Kjaer (1960, 1963), Underhill and Wetter (1966), Ettlinger and Kjaer (1968).

This family is characterized by a yield of isothiocyanates ('mustard oils') which are derived from thioglucosides contained in the plant tissues and released by the action of the enzyme, myrosinase. The condiment, mustard (*Brassica*) provides a familiar example.

$$\text{Thioglycoside} \xrightarrow{\text{Myrosinase}} \textit{Iso}\text{thiocyanate}$$

*Iso*thiocyanates have irritant effects on the skin and can also be allergenic (Mitchell and Jordan 1974).

Brassica, *Sinapis* and *Eruca* have been suspected of evoking photosensitization in the causation of Oppenheim's meadow dermatitis but a combination of irritation from the plants and sunburn was probably responsible. Many plants of the family give rise to the tainting of milk or meat (Hurst 1942).

References

Ettlinger, M.G. and Kjaer, A. (1968) Sulphur compounds in plants. Chap. 3. in Recent Advances in Phytochemistry. Vol. I. ed. Mabry, T.J. New York Appleton-Century-Crofts. pp. 59-144.

Hegnauer, R. (1964) Chemotaxonomy of Plants. Vol. 3. Basel. Birkhauser p. 586.

Hurst, E. (1942) The Poison Plants of New South Wales. N.S.W. Poison Plants Committee; Sydney.

Kjaer, A. (1960) Naturally derived *iso*Thiocyanates (Mustard Oils) and their parent glucosides in Progress in the Chemistry of Organic Natural Products. ed. Zechmeister, L. Vol. 18. Vienna. Springer-Verlag pp. 122-176.

Kjaer, A. (1963) The distribution of sulphur compounds in Chemical Plant Taxonomy. ed. Swain, T. London. Academic Press. p. 453.

Mitchell, J.C. and Jordan, W.P. (1974) Allergic contact dermatitis from the radish, Raphanus sativus. Brit. J. Derm. 91, 183.

Underhill, E.W. and Wetter, L.R. (1966) Biosynthesis of mustard glucosides in Biosynthesis of Natural Compounds ed. Billek G. Oxford. Pergammon Press.

Thioglucosides

About 40 thioglucosides have been isolated from about 350 species of plants. Kjaer (1960, 1963) listed about 200 species studied. Apart from 10 species which are listed under the respective plant families Caricaceae, Euphorbiaceae, Limnanthaceae, Moringaceae, Phytolaccaceae, Plantaginaceae, Salvadoraceae and Tropaeolaceae, the plants which produce such thioglucosides and which may therefore be expected to be irritant for the skin are found in the families Cruciferae, Cleomaceae, Capparidaceae and Resedaceae. Of more than 200 species of Cruciferae so far studied, hardly any has been devoid of thioglucosides; it therefore seems safe to conclude that glucosides of this type are regular constituents of species of this family (Kjaer 1960, 1963). The large family Capparidaceae is an equally constant source of thioglucosides. Again, the limited number of Resedaceae that have been studied all contained thioglucosides of the same general type.

The side chains of sinigrin (Brassica) and of glucotropaeolin were identified in 1863 and 1899 respectively. The use of such plants as condiments, culinary herbs and herbal remedies is due to their containing isothiocyanate-producing glucosides.

In additon some of these plants contain non-protein sulphur amino acids, all derivatives of cysteine, which release sulphur containing compounds (Synge and Wood 1956). Thiophenol is allergenic (Gaul 1958).

References

Gaul, L.E. (1958) Sensitizing component in thiosalicylic acid. J. Invest. Derm. 31, 91.

Kjaer, A. (1960) Naturally derived isoThiocyanates (Mustard Oils) and Their parent glucosides in Progress in the Chemistry of Organic Natural Products. ed. Zechmeister, L. Vol. 18. Vienna. Springer-Verlag. pp. 122-176.

Kjaer, A. (1963) The distribution of sulphur compounds in Chemical Plant Taxonomy. ed. Swain, T. London. Academic Press. p. 453.

Synge, R.L.M. and Wood, J.C. (1956) (+)-(S-methyl-L-cysteine S-oxide) in cabbage. Biochem. J. 64, 252.

Distribution and quantitiy of thioglucosides in plant tissues of Cruciferae

The occurrence of more than one thioglucoside in a given plant species is the rule rather than the exception; as many as eight individual thioglucosides have been clearly distinguished in a single seed specimen. Within the thioglucoside-containing species, the compounds often seem to be distributed throughout the plant. The total and relative amounts of the individual thioglucosides in various parts of the plant vary during its growth cycle. The seeds seem to be particularly rich; considerable variations are observed in botanically identical seed specimens obtained from different sources. Hence it is imperative, here as in most provinces of natural product chemistry, to define the botanical source very carefully (Kjaer 1960, 1963). The amounts of thioglucoside in a plant vary from a trace to several per cent of the dry weight: in the case of fresh horse-radish (Armoracia), 3 kg. of fresh roots, containing 60-70% water, afforded 10.6 gm. of analytically pure sinigrin (Stoll and Seebeck 1948).

References

Kjaer, A. (1960) Naturally derived

isoThiocyanates (Mustard Oils) and Their patent glucosides in Progress in the Chemistry of Organic Natural Products. ed. Zechmeister, L. Vol. 18. Vienna. Springer-Verlag. pp. 122-176.

Kjaer, A. (1963) The distribution of sulphur compounds in Chemical Plant Taxonomy. ed. Swain, T. London. Academic Press. p. 453.

Stoll, A. and Seebeck, E. (1948) Die Isolierung von Sinigrin als genuine, kristalliserte Muttersubstanz des Meerrettichols. Helv. Chim. Acta. 31, 1432.

Irritancy of isothiocyanates

Those isothiocyanates which have been tested on human skin have been observed to produce irritant effects. A suitable patch test concentration to avoid irritant reactions to synthetic oil of mustard, CH_2=CH_2-CH-NCS, was found to be 0.1% in petrolatum (Gaul 1964). A concentration of 1% in alcohol was recommended by Rostenberg and Sulzberger (1939). Allyl-isothiocyanate 0.05% and benzyl isothiocyanate 0.1% in petrolatum were not irritant when tested in four males. Phenyl isothiocyanate 0.1% produced equivocal responses in two of the four individuals and may be a marginal irritant. There were no spontaneous flares (Maibach, H.I. pers. comm. 1973). Phenyl-mustard oils were shown to be more irritant for the skin and conjunctivae of dogs than were aliphatic mustard oils (Takahashi 1939).

Allergenicity of isothiocyanates

Mustard oil has been reported to produce allergic contact dermatitis in the guinea pig (Landsteiner and DiSomma 1938) and in man (Gaul 1964). Allyl- and benzyl isothiocyanate was not allergenic (Mitchell and Jordan 1974). These findings suggest that the presence of a methylene group is an immuno-chemical requisite. Mustard oil was found to be allergenic in 1 of 3,559 eczema patients (Desai et al 1965).

References

Desai, S.C., Dhurandhar, M:W. and Patnaik, R.N. (1965) The nature of allergic and eczematous dermatosis in a skin derpatment in Bombay. Ind. J. Dermat. and Venereal. 35, 98.

Gaul, L.E. (1964) Contact dermatitis from synthetic oil of mustard. Arch. Derm. 90, 158.

Landsteiner, K. and Di Somma, A.A. (1938) Studies on sensitization of animals with simple chemicals: sensitization to diazomethane and mustard oils. J. Exper. Med. 68, 505.

Mitchell, J.C. and Jordan, W.P. (1974) Allergic contact dermatitis from the radish, Raphanus sativus. Brit. J. Derm. 91, 183.

Rostenberg, A. and Sulzberger, M.B. (1939) List of substances for patch-testing and the concentration to be employed. Journal of Investigative Dermatology. 2, 93.

Takahashi, H. (1939) The irritative properties of mustard oils on the skin and mucous membranes. Mitteilungen der Medizinischen Gesellschaft zu Chiba 17, H2 (German summary p. 19).

Irritant clinical effects upon the skin.

White (1887) described the effects of a mustard plaster - (Brassica) as follows: "In a few minutes after applicaton, the skin begins to feel warm, and by the end of a half-hour, if the patient bears it so long, this sensation has increased to an intolerable burning. Within a few minutes redness appears, becomes intense, persists for a day or two and often leaves persistent dark brown pigmentation." On that account he warned against its use "upon the upper chest or other parts of a woman which the dress will not always conceal."

He noted that oil of mustard was a powerful irritant and caustic and that if the action of the mustard "be continued beyond its legitimate rubefacient effect, a period which varies greatly in persons, it may produce vesication, or even deep suppuration." Lepidium, Nasturtium, Sinapis, Sisymbrium and several other members of this family were typical rubefacients (White 1887).

Application of a mustard plaster produced a fatal result in a child (Fucci 1928).

Application of mustard oil, which was probably impure, produced acneiform lesions of the face of Indians (Bhutani et al 1970).

A vesicular eruption of the hands which occurred twice in a baker, was attributed to ground mustard, which was one of the various products handled by this man. No tests were carried out (Tara 1949).

Reports of cutaneous effects of mustard oils were provided by Lehner and Rajka (1925, 1927), Konrich and Mautsch (1931), Bacq (1946), Greenberg and Lester (1954), Grant (1962).

References

Bacq, Z.M. (1946) Substances thiolprives. Experientia 2, 349.

Bhutani, L.K., Malhotra, V.K. and Kandhari, K.C. (1970) Vegetable oil and acneiform lesions. Ind. J. Derm. Vener. 36, 120.

Fucci, A. (1928) Sopra un caso di grave cancrena cutanea con esito letali in una bambina per l' applicazioni di un cataplasma lievemente senapizzato Prat. pediatr. 6, 293, cited by Touton (1931).

Grant, W.M. (1962) Toxicology of the eye. Springfield, Ill. Charles C. Thomas.

Greenberg, L.A. and Lester, D. (1954) Handbook of Cosmetic Materials. New York. Interscience.

Konrich u Mautsch (1931) Zur biologischen Wirkung des Senfols. Klin Wschr. Nr. 25, cited by Touton (1932).

Lehner, E. and Rajka, E. (1925) Gelungener Ubertragungsversuch einer experimentele hervorgerufenden Senfoluberempfindlichkeit. Dtsch. med. Wschr. 51, 825.

Lehner, E. and Rajka, E. (1927) Ubertragung der Uberempfindlichkeit der menschlichen Haut auf das Kaninchenohr. Z. exper. Med. 53, 855.

Tara, M. (1949) Artificial dermatitis due to ground mustard. Le Medecin d'Usne, Paris 11, 286.

Touton, K. (1932) Hauterkrankungen durch phanerogamische Pflanzen und ihre Produkte (Toxicodermia et Allergodermia phytogenes), in Barnewitz, J. et al Angeborene Anomalien, Lichtdermatosen, Pflanzengifte, Thermische Schadigungen, Einfluss Innerer Storungen auf die Haut. Berlin, Verlag von Julius Springer.

White, J.C. (1887) Dermatitis venenata: An account of the Action of External irritants upon the Skin. Boston. Cupples and Hurd.

Genus:

Aethionema	Stone-Cress
Alliaria	Hedge garlic
Alyssum	Madwort
Arabis	Wall Rock Cress
Armoracia	Horse-radish
Aubrietia	Aubrietia
Barbarea	Winter Cress
Berteroa	
Biscutella	

Species of the above genera yield isothiocyanates (Kjaer 1960). Exposure risk for these plants was listed by Mitchell and Jordan (1974).

Armoracia rusticana (Horse radish) is a familiar irritant and lacyrymatory.

References

Kjaer, A. (1960) Naturally derived isoThiocyanates (Mustard Oils) and their parent glucosides in Progress in the Chemistry of Organic Natural Products. ed. Zechmeister, L. Vol. 18. Vienna, Springer-VErlag. pp. 122-176.

Mitchell, J.C. and Jordan, W.P. (1974) Allergic contact dermatitis from the radish, Raphanus sativus. Brit. J. Derm. 91, 183.

Brassica

This genus is native to Europe, the Mediterranean region and Asia. Many forms are cultivated (Nieuwhof 1969).

Brassica campestris
Turnip

The seeds are used as a counter-irritant in India (Behl et al 1966). Shelmire (1940) observed contact dermatitis of the hands in housewives from turnip greens and mustard greens.

Brassica integrifolia

The leaves, seeds and oil from the seeds are used as a counter-irritant (Quisumbing 1951).

Brassica napus
Rape

Mustard oils are derived from Brassica spp. (Kjaer 1960). Brassica spp. have been suspected of evoking photodermatitis (Pathak et al 1974, Ullmo 1932).

Colza oil derived from this species and used for polishing gold chains was reported to cause dermatitis (Weber 1937). Photosensitisation from ingestion was suspected in animals (Hansen 1924).

Brassica nigra
Mustard
(the seeds form the condiment)

The oil was employed as tear gas in World War I (Burkill 1935). The plant is irritant (Woods 1962). The condiment mustard is derived from the seeds.

During an Irish famine, peasants who ate large quantities of the plant developed blotches of deep red, resembling burns, on the backs of hands, dorsa of feet, nose and forehead sometimes followed by ulceration (Popham cited by Piffard 1881).

Punctate keratitis occurred in two workers with mustard (Bischler 1947).

Brassica oleracea
Cabbage

Races of this species provide cauliflower, broccoli, kale, brussel sprouts and kohlrabi. Sauerkraut is a form of cabbage.

Cabbage has been reported to cause occupational contact dermatitis (Leoni and Cogo 1964).

Brassica oleracea var botrytis
Cauliflower

Touton (1932) and Vaughan and Black (1954) refer to allergy to the plant. This species has been implicated in hand eczema (Agrup 1969).

A plant grower who had eczema of the hands was contact sensitive to B. oleracea var botrytis, tulip (Tulipa), tulipalin A. (alpha-methylene-gamma-lactone) derived from Tulipa, onion (Allium) and to the fungicide, tetramethylthiuramdisulfide. Aqueous and ethanol extracts of cauliflower, tulip and onion (10 gm. of fresh plant material with 100 ml. of water or thanol) produced positive patch test reactions in the patient, negative in ten controls (van Ketel W.G. 1975, pers. comm.)

References

Agrup, G. (1969) Hand Eczema and other hand dermatoses in South Sweden. Acta derm.-venereol. 49 Suppl. 61. pp.1-91.

Behl, P.N., Captain, R.M., Bedi, B.M.S. and Gupta, S. (1966) Skin-irritant and sensitizing plants found in India, New Delhi. P.N. Behl, Irwin Hospital.

Burkill, I.H. (1935) A Dictionary of the Economic Products of the Malay Peninsula. 2 vols. London Crown Agents for the Colonies.

Hansen, A.A. (1924) The Poison Plant situation in Indiana. J. Amer. Vet. Med. Ass. 66, 351.

Kjaer, A. (1960) Naturally derived isoThiocyanates (Mustard Oils) and their parent glucosides in Progress in the Chemistry of Organic Natural Products ed. Zechmesiter, L. Vol. 18. Vienna. Springer-Verlag. pp. 122-176.

Leoni, A. and Cogo, R. (1964) Occupational dermatitis caused by contact with cabbage. Minerva Derm. 39, 326.

Nieuwhof, M. (1969) Cole Crops. Cleveland, Ohio, CRC Press.

Pathak, M.A. (1974) Phytophotodermatitis. Chap. 32 in Sunlight and Man. ed. Pathak, M.A. et al. University of Tokyo Press. p. 495.

Piffard, H.G. (1881) A treatise on the Materia Medica and Therapeutics of the Skin. New York. Wm. Wood and Co.

Quisumbing, E. (1951) Medicinal Plants of the Philippines. Tech. Bull. 16. Manila, Philippine Islands. Manila Bureau of Printing. 1234 pp.

Shelmire, B. (1940) Contact dermatitis from vegetation. South Med. J. 33, 338.

Touton, K. (1932) Hauterkrankungen durch phanerogamische Pflanzen und ihre Produkte (Toxicodermia et Allergodermia phytogenes), in Barnewitz, J. et al Angeborene Anomalien, Lichtdermatosen Pflanzengifte, Thermische Schadigungen, Einfluss Innerer Storungen auf die Haut. Berlin, Verlag von Julius Springer.

Ullmo, A. (1932) Dermatitis bullose striata pratensis. Ann. Derm. Syph. 3, 31, cited by Klaber (1942).

Vaughan, W.T. and Black, H. (1945) Practice of Allergy. 3rd. ed. St. Louis. C.V. Mosby.

Weber, L.F. (1937) External causes of Dermatitis. A list of irritants. Arch. Derm. Syph. 35, 129.

Woods, B. (1962) Irritant plants. Trans. St. John's Hosp. derm. Soc. 48, 75.

Klaber, R. (1942) Phyto-photo-dermatitis. Brit. J. Derm. Syph. 54, 193.

Bischler (1947) Altérations oculaires professionnelles. Groupe opthalmologique du Léman 6-7.4. 1946. Opthalmologica 114, 56.

Bunias	
Cakile	Sea Rocket
Camelina	
Capsella	Shepherd's Purse
Cardamine	Cuckoo Flower
Cheiranthus	Wall-Flower
Cochlearia	Scurvy grass
Conringia	
Coronopus	
Crambe	
Dentaria (syn. Cardamine)	
Diplotaxis	
Draba	

Species of the above genera yield isothiocyanates (Kjaer 1960). Exposure risk for these plants was listed by Mitchell and Jordan (1974). *Cochlearia officinalis* is used as a rubefacient (Burkill 1935). The seeds of *Capsella bursa-pastoris* have rubefacient and vesicant properties (Behl et al 1966). *Diplotaxis erucoides* and *D. tenuifolia* have irritant properties (Pammel 1911).

References

Behl, P.N., Captain, R.M., Bedi, B.M.S. and Gupta, S. (1966) Skin-irritant and sensitizing plants found in India, New Delhi. P.N. Behl, Irwin Hospital.

Burkill, I.H. (1935) A Dictionary of the Economic Products of the Malay Peninsula. 2 vols. London. Crown Agents for the Colonies.

Kjaer, A. (1960) Naturally derived isoThiocyanates (Mustard Oils) and their parent glucosides in Progress in the Chemistry of Organic Natural Products. ed. Zechmeister, L. Vol. 18. Vienna. Springer-Verlag. pp. 122-176.

Mitchell, J.C. and Jordan, W.P. (1974) Allergic contact dermatitis from the radish, *Raphanus sativus*. Brit. J. Derm. 91, 183.

Pammel, L.H. (1911) A Manual of Poisonous plants. Torch Press. Cedar Rapids, Iowa. Reprinted Univ. Microfilms Inc. Ann Arbor, Mich. 1965 pp. 476-7.

Descurainia

55 species are found in cold and temperate regions of America, Eurasia and southern Africa.

Descurainia sophia
(syn. Sisymbrium sophia)

The plant which has a pungent odour and an acrid taste has been used externally to treat indolent ulcers (Unesco 1960).

Reference

Unesco (1960) Medicinal Plants of the Arid Zones. Arid Zone Research XIII. Paris. Place de Fontenoy.

Eruca

Six species are native to the Mediterranean region and north eastern Africa (Eritrea).

Eruca sativa
Rocket-salad, Taramira

The leaves are used for salad (Bailey's Manual 1971).

The seeds which are acrid and vesicant are used like mustard (Brassica). Taramira oil expressed from the seeds is used for culinary purposes. This oil when applied to the hair causes allergic dermatitis and photodermatitis of the scalp, neck and skin around the ears. Use of the oil by indigenous practitioners in India for vitiligo and other skin diseases can result in persistent melanosis (Behl et al 1966). The green parts of the plant and seeds yield 'mustard oil' (Kjaer 1960). The oil is used to adulterate mustard oil (Brassica).

References

Bailey, L.H. (1971) Manual of Cultivated Plants. New York. Macmillan Co.

Behl, P.N., Captain, R.M., Bedi, B.M.S. and Gupta, S. (1966). Skin-irritant and sensitizing plants found in India, New Delhi. P.N. Behl, Irwin Hospital.

Kjaer, A. (1960) Naturally derived isoThiocyanates (Mustard Oils) and their parent glucosides in Progress in the Chemistry of Organic Natural Products. ed. Zechmeister, L. Vol. 18. Vienna. Springer-Verlag. pp. 122-176.

Erucastrum

Erysimum — Blister Cress

Eutrema

Farsetia

Hesperis — Rocket

Hutchinsia

Iberis — Candy tuft

Isatis — Woad plant

Kernera (syn. Cochlearia)

Species of the above genera yield isothiocyanates (Kjaer 1960). Exposure risk for these plants was listed by Mitchell and Jordan (1974). Erysimum cheiranthoides has irritant properties (Pammel 1911). Application of E. alliaria to the skin produces vesication (Gravmuller 1813-1819 cited by Piffard 1881). The leaves of Isatis tinctoria were ground to a paste and fermented to provide the dye, woad, used by the Ancient Britons.

References

Kjaer, A. (1960) Naturally derived isoThiocyanates (Mustard Oils) and their parent glucosides in Progress in the Chemistry of Organic Natural Products. ed. Zechmeister, L. Vol. 18. Vienna. Springer-Verlag. pp. 122-176.

Mitchell, J.C. and Jordan, W.P. (1974) Allergic contact dermatitis from the radish, Raphanus sativus. Brit. J. Derm. 91, 183.

Pammel, L.H. (1911) A Manual of Poisonous plants. Torch Press. Cedar Rapids, Iowa. Reprinted Univ. Microfilms Inc. Ann Arbor, Mich. 1965. pp. 476-7.

Piffard, H.G. (1881) A treatise on the Materia Medica and Therapeutics of the skin. New York. Wm. Wood and Co.

Lepidium

150 species are of cosmopolitan distribution.

Lepidium campestre
Pepperwort, Cow Cress

This species, native to Great Britain, is found in dry pastures, on walls and banks, by waysides and in arable and waste land throughout England and Europe (Clapham et al 1962) and is found as a weed of waste places, roadsides and fields throughout eastern North America (Gray's Manual 1970). The seeds, green parts and seeds of the plant yield 'mustard oil' (Kjaer 1960).

Lepidium latifolium

The juice, when applied to the skin, excites redness, inflammation and purulent exudation (De Candolle 1804, cited by Piffard 1881).

Lepidium sativum
Garden Cress, Pepper Grass

The fresh leaves redden the skin (Piffard 1881). Irritant properties of the plant were known to Dioscorides (First Century A.D.) and are recorded by White (1887) and Weber (1937). The oil is vesicant akin to mustard oil (Brassica) and the plant is pounded and applied to the skin as a poultice; the plant has rubefacient properties (Burkill 1935). This species is both cultivated and found as a common winter weed in crop fields all over India. The seeds are mildly irritant, causing dermatitis in 'sensitive' individuals (Behl et al 1966).

The green parts and seeds of the plant yield 'mustard oil' (Kjaer 1960).

References

Behl, P.N., Captain, R.M., Bedi, B.M.S. and Gupta, S. (1966) Skin-irritant and sensitizing plants found in India, New Delhi. P.N. Behl, Irwin Hospital.

Burkill, I.H. (1935) A Dictionary of the Economic Products of the Malay Peninsula. 2 Vols. London. Crown Agents for the Colonies.

Clapham, A.R., Tutin, T.G. and Warburg, E.F. (1962) Flora of the British Isles. 2nd ed. Cambridge University Press.

Dioscorides, The Greek Herbal of: Englished by John Goodyer: A.D. 1655. Edited and first printed A.D. 1933 by R.T. Gunther 1959. New York. Hafner Publishing Co. 2, 206.

Gray's Manual of Botany (1970) 8th ed. by Fernald, M.L. New York. Van Nostrand Reinhold.

Kjaer, A. (1960) Naturally derived isoThiocyanates (Mustard Oils) and their parent glucosides in Progress in the Chemistry of Organic Natural Products. ed. Zechmeister, L. Vol. 18. Vienna. Springer-Verlag. pp. 122-176.

Piffard, H.G. (1881) A treatise on the Materia Medica and Therapeutics of the skin. New York. Wm. Wood and Co.

Weber, L.F. (1937) External causes of Dermatitis. A list of irritants. Arch. Derm. Syph. 35, 129.

White, J.C. (1887) Dermatitis venenata: An Account of the Action of External irritants upon the Skin. Boston. Cupples and Hurd.

Lunaria

Malcolmia — Virginian stocks

Matthiola — Stocks, Gilliflower

Nasturtium — Watercress

Neslia (syn. Vogelia)

Parrya

Species of the above genera yield isothiocyanates (Kjaer 1960). Exposure risk to the plants was listed by Mitchell and Jordan (1974). Gerard (1636) noted that Lunaria had a biting taste like mustard (Brassica). Matthiola spp. are used as a commercial crop by florists. Nasturtium officinale (watercress) caused contact dermatitis of the hands in housewives (Shelmire 1940).

References

Gerard, J. (1636) The Herball or Generall Historie of Plantes. The essence thereof distilled by M. Woodward (1927) from the edition of Th. Johnson 1630. London. Gerald Howe.

Kjaer, A. (1960) Naturally derived isoThiocyanates (Mustard Oils) and their parent glucosides in Progress in the Chemistry of Organic Natural Products. ed. Zechmeister, L. Vol. 18. Vienna. Springer-Verlag. pp. 122-176.

Mitchell, J.C. and Jordan, W.P. (1974) Allergic contact dermatitis from the radish, Raphanus sativus. Brit. J. Derm. 91, 183.

Shelmire, B. (1940) Contact dermatitis from vegetation. South Med. J. 33, 338.

Raphanus sativus
Radish

Dermatitis of the hands in housewives and in children playing with radish leaves was reported by Shelmire (1940), Waldbott and Shea (1948), Behl et al (1966). A waitress who chopped radishes developed dermatitis of the fingers. Patch tests revealed positive reactions to allyl- and benzyl isothiocyanate, negative to phenyl isothiocyanate; these findings suggest that a methylene group is an immunochemical requisite (Mitchell and Jordan 1974). The plant yields an isothiocyanate (Kjaer 1960).

References

Behl, P.N., Captain, R.M., Bedi, B.M.S. and Gupta, S. (1966) Skin-irritant and sensitizing plants found in India, New Delhi. P.N. Behl, Irwin Hospital.

Kjaer, A. (1960) Naturally derived isoThiocyanates (Mustard Oils) and thier patent glucosides in Progress in the Chemistry of Organic Natural Products. ed. Zechmeister, L. Vol. 18. Vienna. Springer-Verlag. pp. 122-176.

Mitchell, J.C. and Jordan, W.P. (1974) Allergic contact dermatitis from the radish, Raphanus sativus. Brit. J. Derm. 91, 183.

Shelmire, B. (1940) Contact dermatitis from vegetation. South Med. J. 33, 338.

Waldbott, G.L. and Shea, J.J. (1948) Causative diagnosis of contact dermatitis II. A classification of patterns on the hands. Archs. Derm. Syph. 57, 975.

Rapistrum

Schiverekia

These genera yield isothiocyanates (Kjaer 1960). Exposure risk to the plants was listed by Mitchell and Jordan (1974).

References

Kjaer, A. (1960) Naturally derived isoThiocyanates (Mustard Oils) and their parent glucosides in Progress in the Chemistry of Organic Natural Products. ed. Zechmeister, L. Vol. 18. Vienna. Springer-Verlag. p. 122-176.

Mitchell, J.C. and Jordan, W.P. (1974) Allergic contact dermatitis from the radish, Raphanus sativus. Brit. J. Derm. 91, 183.

Sinapis alba
White mustard

Irritation of the mouth occurs when animals eat cake containing the seeds, the plant with pods, or the stubble (North 1967).

Sinapis arvensis
Charlock, Wild Mustard

This species is common weed of cornfields. The plant was suspected of evoking photodermatitis (Spillman and Weiss 1931). Species of Sinapis yield isothiocyanates (Kjaer 1960).

References

Kjaer, A. (1960) Naturally derived isoThiocyanates (Mustard Oils) and their parent glucosides in Progress in the Chemistry of Organic Natural Products. ed. Zechmeister, L. Vol. 18. Vienna. Springer-Verlag p. 122-176.

North, P.M. (1967) Poisonous plants and fungi in colour. London. Blandford Press Ltd.

Spillman, L. and Weiss (1931) Dermites vésicantes d'origine végétale. Bull. Soc. fran Derm Syph. 38, 1095, cited by Klaber (1974).

Klaber, R. (1942) Phyto-photo-dermatitis. Brit. J. Derm. Syph. 54, 193.

Sisymbrium Hedge Mustard

Thlaspi Alpine Perny Cress

Vesicaria

The seeds of Sisymbrium irio (London Rocket) have a hot sharp taste and are rubefacient and vesicant for the skin (Behl et al 1966). Species of these genera yield isothiocyanates (Kjaer 1960). Exposure risk to the plants was listed by Mitchell and Jordan (1974).

References

Behl, P.N., Captain, R.M., Bedi, B.M.S. and Gupta, S. (1966) Skin-irritant and sensitizing plants found in India, New Delhi. P.N. Behl, Irwin Hospital.

Kjaer, A. (1960) Naturally derived isoThiocyanates (Mustard Oils) and their parent glucosides in Progress in the Chemistry of Organic Natural Products. ed. Zechmeister, L. Vol. 18. Vienna. Springer-Verlag. pp. 122-176.

Mitchell, J.C. and Jordan, W.P. (1974) Allergic contact dermatitis from the radish, Raphanus sativus. Brit. J. Derm. 91, 183.

Stanleya

Eight species are native to the western United States.

Stanleya pinnata

This species contains selenocystathionine which can cause hair loss by ingestion (see Lecythis ollaria) (Schoental 1965).

Reference

Schoental, R. (1965) Toxicology of natural products. Ed. Cosmet. Toxicol.

CRYPTERONIACEAE

Five species in two genera are found in tropical Asia.

Chemistry is recorded by Hegnauer (1964).

Reference

Hegnauer, R. (1964) Chemotaxonomy of Plants. Vol. 3. Basel. Birkhauser. p. 607.

Dactylocladus

One species is found in fresh water peat-swamps of Borneo.

Dactylocladus stenostachys
Jongkong, medang tabak

The wood is said to produce irritant effects in wood-workers (Orsler 1973).

According to Woods and Calnan (1976) the colloquial name 'tabak' which is used in Sarawak for the wood suggests that it is known there as a nasal irritant. They refer to the toxic wood, ipe tabaco (Tabebiua ipe) by analogy.

Reference

Orsler, R.J. (1973) Personal communication from Forest Products Research Laboratory, Princess Risborough, Bucks, England.

Woods, B. and Calnan, C.D. (1976) Toxic Woods. Brit. J. Derm. 94, Suppl. 13, June.

CUCURBITACEAE

640 species in 110 genera are most abundant in the tropics and wanting in the colder regions. Several have edible fruits, e.g. Cucurbita, Cucumis, Sechium, Lagenaria, etc.

Chemistry is recorded by Hegnauer (1964).

Bitterness of the plants is genetically determined and most, if not all, of the poisonous species are restricted to the sub-family Cucurbitae which includes Bryonia, Citrullus, Cucumis, etc.

Reference

Hegnauer, R. (1964) Chemotaxonomy of Plants. Vol. 3. Basel. Birkhauser. p. 608.

Bryonia

Four species are found in Europe, Asia, North Africa and the Canary Islands.

Bryonia sp.
Briony, Tetter-berry

The plant was used to cleanse tetters (pustular eruptions) (Culpeper 1653).

Bryonia alba
English Mandrake

The roots were sold as Mandrake (Podophyllum) (Wren 1968). The fresh plant when applied to the skin produces vesication and a pustular eruption (Dispensatory 1884, Dierbach 1841, Gravmuller 1813-1819 cited by Piffard 1881, Mankowsky 1890).

Bryonia dioica
Red Bryony, Devil's Turnip

The milky juice irritates the skin (North 1967) and mouth (Francis and Southcott 1967).

References

Culpeper, N. (1653) The Complete Herbal. Birmingham. Kynoch Press. (Imperial Chemical (Pharmaceuticals) Ltd.).

Dierbach, J.R. (1841) Synopsis Materiae Medicae. Heidelberg and Leipzig cited by Piffard (1881).

Dispensatory, The National (1834). Philadelphia. Stille and Maisch., cited by White (1887).

Francis, D.F. and Southcott, R.V. (1967) Plants harmful to man in Australia. Misc. Bull. No. 1. Botanic Garden, Adelaide, Australia.

North, P.M. (1967) Poisonous plants and fungi in colour. London. Blanford Press. Ltd.

Mankowsky (1890) Uber Bryonia alba. Histor. Studien aus derm.pharm. Institut. zu Dorpat, herausgegeben von. R. Kobert. 2, 143 Halle cited by Touton (1932).

Piffard, H.G. (1881) A treatise on the Materia Medica and Therapeutics of the skin. New York. Wm. Wood and Co.

Touton, K. (1932) Hauterkrankungen durch phanerogamische Pflanzen und ihre Produkte (Toxicodermia et Allergodermia phytogenes), in Barnewitz, J. et al Angeborene Anomalien, Lichtdermatosen, Pflanzengifte, Thermische Schadigungen, Einfluss Innerer Storungen auf die Haut. Berlin, Verlag. von Julius Springer.

White, J.C. (1887) Dermatitis venenata: An Account of the Action of External irritants upon the Skin. Boston. Cupples and Hurd.

Wren, R.W. (1968) Potter's New Cyclopaedia of Botanical Drugs and Preparations by Wren, R.C. Reedit. by Wren, R.W. Potter and Clarke Ltd. Health Science Press. Rustington, Sussex.

Citrullus

Three species are found in Africa, the Mediterranean region and tropical Asia. C. lanatus is the water-melon.

Citrullus colocynthis
(syn. Colocynthus vulgaris)

The juice is used to produce tissue irritation in an arrow-poison. The dried fruit pulp is irritating to the eye and nose (Watt and Breyer-Brandwijk 1962). The seed oil is used to blacken grey hair. Colocynth used as a denaturant in alcoholic hair tonics and brilliantines caused persistent eczema localized to the palm and finger web spaces of the left hand in three hair-dressers (Haxthausen 1930).

Reference

Haxthausen, H. (1930) Fall von Koloquinthekzem. Dermat. Wschr. 91, 1391.

Watt, J.M. and Breyer-Brandwijk, M.G. (1962) The Medicinal and poisonous plants of Southern Africa. 2nd ed. Edinburgh, E. & S. Livingstone.

Cucumis

25 species are mostly found in Africa, a few in Asia. C. melo (Melon) and C. sativus (Cucumber) have been cultivated from early times.

Cucumis sp.

An enema of the juice caused necrosis of the rectum and colon and death (Watt and Breyer-Brandwijk 1962).

Cucumis melo Melon

Sensitivity to melons is noted under Prunus persicaria.

Cucumis myriocarpus

Sheep developed sore lips from eating the plant (Hurst 1942). Ingestion of the plant has been suspected of evoking photosensitization in sheep (Watt and Breyer-Brandwijk 1962).

Cucumis sativus
Cucumber

This species occasionally produces stomatitis (Behl et al 1966).

References

Behl, P.N., Captain, R.M., Bedi, B.M.S. and Gupta, S. (1966) Skin-irritant and sensitizing plants found in India, New Delhi. P.N. Behl, Irwin Hospital.

Hurst, E. (1942) The Poison Plants of New South Wales. N.S.W. Poison Plants Committee; Sydney.

Watt, J.M. and Breyer-Brandwijk, M.G. (1962) The Medicinal and poisonous plants of Southern Africa. 2nd ed. Edinburgh. E. & S. Livingstone.

Cucurbita

15 species are found in America. C. pepo includes the vegetable marrow and some squashes.

Cucurbita moschata
Seminole Pumpkin

An individual who tied up the vine tips of this species to a fence developed skin irritation from the bristly hairs of the plant. Other persons have experienced a few hours of discomfort from handling the plant which is rough to the touch (Morton, J.F. 1965, pers. comm.).

Dendrosicyos

One species is found on the island of Socotra. The leaves are thorny. The milky white juice of the trunk and leaves produces severe pain if it enters the eye (Menninger 1967).

Reference

Menninger, E.A. (1967) Fantastic Trees. New York. The Viking Press

Ecballium

One species is found in the Mediterranean region.

Ecballium elaterium
Squirting Cucumber

The juice is irritant to the eye (Grant 1962).

Reference

Grant, W.M. (1962) Toxicology of the eye. Springfield, Ill. Charles C. Thomas.

Gurania

75 species are found in tropical America.

Gurania guaransenia

The plant has stinging hairs and harbours a butterfly larva having similar devices (Lewis & Elvin-Lewis 1977).

Reference

Lewis, W.H. and Elvin-Lewis, M.P.F. (1977) Medical Botany New York, John Wiley

Luffa

Six species are found in tropical regions. L. cylindrica (syn. L. aegyptica) furnishes the bath sponge known as loofah.

Luffa cylindrica var. lissa

The fruit has an intensely bitter taste and acrid properties (Watt and Breyer-Brandwijk, 1962).

Reference

Watt, J.M. and Breyer-Brandwijk, M.G. (1962) The Medicinal and poisonous plants of Southern Africa. 2nd ed. Edinburgh, E. and S. Livingstone.

Sechium

One species is found in tropical America.

Sechium edule
Chocho, Cohko

This plant is cultivated for its edible fruit. The juice of the skin of the fruit is said to have a paralysing effect upon the hands, if it comes into contact with them; possibly it has some sort of local anaesthetic action (Maiden 1918, Cleland 1915, Watt and Breyer-Brandwijk 1962).

References

Cleland, J.B. (1925) Plants including fungi, poisonous or otherwise injurious to man in Australia. (Series II). Med. J. Australia 2, 443.

Maiden, J.H. (1918) Note on the juice of the Choko (Sechium edule) Agr. Gaz. New South Wales 29, 531.

Watt, J.M. and Breyer-Brandwijk, M.G. (1962) The Medicinal and poisonous plants of Southern Africa. 2nd ed. Edinburgh. E. & S. Livingstone.

Kedrostis
(syn. Bryonopsis)

35 species are found in tropical and subtropical regions of Africa and Madagascar and in tropical regions of Asia and Malaysia.

Bryonopsis affinis

The sap is said to cause blindness (Altschul 1973).

Reference

Altschul, S. von R. (1973) Drugs and foods from little-known plants. Cambridge, Mass. Harvard Univ. Press.

Sicyos

15 species are found in Hawaii, Polynesia, Australia and tropical America.

Sicyos angulata
Bur Cucumber

The sap produces a burning sensation on contact with the skin. Penetration of the skin by a prickle of the plant produces an inflammatory reaction which may be of irritant or possibly of allergic nature (Pammel 1911, Gardner and Bennetts 1956, Watt and Breyer-Brandwijk 1962).

References

Gardner, C.A. and Bennetts, H.W. (1956) The Toxic Plants of Western Australia. Perth West. Australian Newspapers Ltd.

Pammel, L.H. (1911) A Manual of Poisonous plants. Torch Press. Cedar Rapids, Iowa. Reprinted Univ. Microfilms Inc. Ann Arbor, Mich. 1965. pp. 476-7.

Watt, J.M. and Breyer-Brandwijk, M.G. (1962) The Medicinal and poisonous plants of Southern Africa. 2nd ed. Edinburgh. E. & S. Livingstone.

Thladiantha

15 species native from eastern Asia to Malaysia are climbing herbs with root-tubers.

Thladiantha dubia

The plant caused severe contact dermatitis in a gardener (Hausen in press).

Reference

Hausen, B.M. (1978 in press) On the occurrence of the contact allergen primin and other quinoid compounds in species of the family Primulaceae. Archives of Dermatological Research.

CUNONIACEAE

25 species in 26 genera are chiefly found in regions between 13° and 35° S, a few in more northerly regions.

Chemistry is recorded by Hegnauer (1964).

Reference

Hegnauer, R. (1964) Chemotaxonomy of Plants. Vol. 3. Basel. Birkhauser p. 625.

Ceratopetalum

Five species of New Guinea and eastern Australia provide light timber.

Ceratopetalum apetalum

The wood of this tree can cause dermatitis in tradesmen (Mair 1968).

Reference

Mair, K. (1968) Director, Royal Botanical Gardens, Sydney, Australia, personal communication from records of the Herbarium.

Schizomeria

18 species are found in the Moluccas, New Guinea and Queensland.

Schizomeria ovata

The wood of this tree can cause dermatitis in tradesmen (Mair 1968).

Reference

Mair, K. (1968) Director, Royal Botanic Gardens, Sydney Australia, personal communication from Records of the Herbarium.

Davidsonia pruriens

This plant previously included in this family (Flecker 1945) is now represented in a monospecific family, Davidsoniaceae. The specific name indicates itching.

Reference

Flecker, H. (1945) Injuries produced by plants in tropical Queensland. Med. J. Australia 1, 636.

CUPRESSACEAE

130 species in 19 genera are of cosmopolitan distribution.

Chemistry is recorded by Hegnauer (1962).

Reference

Hegnauer, R. (1962) Chemotaxonomy of Plants. Vol. 1. Basel. Birkhauser. p. 342.

Callitris

16 species are found in Australia and New Caledonia.

Callitris spp.
Cypress Pine

The wood can produce dermatitis when cut in flower (Cleland 1925). The timber of commerce comes mainly from C. glauca (Boas 1947). C. articulata contains thymoquinone (Woods and Calnan 1976), a sensitizer of Calocedrus.

Reference

Boas, I.H. (1947) The Commercial timbers of Australia. Their Properties and Uses. Melbourne. Government Printer. Commonwealth of Australia. Council for Scientific and Industrial Research.

Cleland, J.B. (1925) Plants including fungi, poisonous or otherwise injurious to man in Australia. (series II) Med. J. Australia 2, 443.

Woods, B. and Calnan, C.D. (1976) Toxic Woods. Brit. J. Derm. 94, Suppl. 13, June.

Calocedrus

Three species are found in northern Burma, northeastern Siam, south-western China, Hainan; Formosa and Pacific North America.

Calocedrus decurrens
(syn. Libocedrus decurrens)
Californian white cedar,
Incense cedar

This species yields valuable timber.

Dermatitis occurred in a male carpenter and floor layer, affecting the groins, buttocks, thighs, legs and feet. From time to time he developed patches of an exudative dermatitis behind his ear which he attributed to holding a pencil there. The dermatitis on his feet followed a period of work sawing wood. Patch tests were positive to the wood of a pencil.

Dermatitis occurred in a female clerk aged 48 years affecting the right hand and the middle and ring fingers. Patch tests were positive to the wood of her pencil.

In the case of the carpenter, patch tests were positive to ether, water and ethanol extracts of the heartwood of L. decurrens. In both cases patch tests were positive to thymoquinone and hydrothymoquinone and in the case of the clerk to carvacrol; these compounds are known to occur in the steam volatile extract of the heartwood of L. decurrens (Anderson and Zavarin 1955). For possible cross-reactions of these compounds or possible multiple specific sensitivity, Calnan's (1972) paper should be consulted. Thymoquinone is very irritant in high concentrations and may be so at 1.0%; a concentration of 0.1% is recommended for patch testing (Calnan 1972).

Contact dermatitis from timbers is usually attributable to contamination of the skin from sawdust during machining. Handling of solid wood rarely induces dermatitis but Libocedrus and Dalbergia used for knife-handles, etc. and pencils may do so (Calnan 1972).

Calocedrus

Incense cedar and Virginian pencil cedar (probably Juniperus virginiana) are officially recognized causes of dermatitis in the German pencil industry (Koelsch 1931).

Reference

Koelsch (1931) Die Begutachtung der gewerblichen Dermatosen im Sinne der Verordnung vom 11 Februar 1929. Zentralblatt für Haut-ung Geschlechtskrankeiten 37, 1.

Anderson, A.B. and Zavarin, E. (1955) J. Instit. Wood. Sci. 15, 3, cited by Calnan (1972).

Calnan, C.D. (1972) Dermatitis from Cedar Wood Pencils. Trans. St. John's Hosp. derm. Soc. 58, 43.

Chamaecyparis (syn. Cupressus)

Seven species are found in North America, Japan and Formosa.

Chamaecyparis lawsoniana (syn. Cupressus lawsoniana) Port Orford cedar, Lawson's cypress

The foliage of this tree can produce dermatitis and the wood can cause asthma in wood-workers (Rasch 1923/24, Hausen 1970, Schonwald 1929, Stier 1929 and White 1934.)

The pollen causes hayfever (Wodehouse 1971).

White (1934) noted that splinter wounds from the wood were slow to heal.

The powerful resinous odour of the newly-cut wood was said to cause troublesome diuresis in saw-mill workers (Sargent 1896). Woods and Calnan (1976) found that none of Hausen's (1970) references for contact dermatitis was convincing on scrutiny. Unlike most Cupressaceae, this species contains very little beta-thujaplicin and no other tropolones (Zavarin et al 1959).

Chamaecyparis nootkatensis

This species yields carvacrol (Watt and Breyer-Brandwijk 1962), a sensitizer of Librocedrus.

References

Black, J.H. (1929) Cedar hayfever. J. Allergy 1, 87.

Hausen, B.N. (1970) Untersuchungen über Gesundheitsschädigende Hölzer. Thesis, Hamburg.

Wodehouse, R.P. (1971) Hayfever Plants. 2nd rev. edition. New York, Hafner.

Rasch, (1923/24) Cypresdermatitis. Verh. dan. dermat. Ges. 42 cited by Touton (1932).

Watt, J.M. and Breyer-Brandwijk, M.G. (1962) The Medicinal and poisonous plants of Southern Africa. 2nd ed. Edinburgh. E. & S. Livingstone.

White, R.P. (1934) The Dermatergoses or Occupational Affections of the Skin. 4th ed. London. H.K. Lewis.

Touton, K. (1932) Hauterkrankungen durch phanerogamische Pflanzen und ihre Produkte (Toxicodermia et Allergodermia phytogenes), in Barnewitz, J. et al Angeborene Anomalien, Lichtdermatosen, Pflangengifte, Thermische Schadigungen, Einfluss Innerer Storungen auf die Haut. Berlin, Verlag von Julius Springer.

Sargent, C.S. (1896) The Sylva of North America. Vol. 10, p. 120. Boston and New York, Houghton Mifflin, cited by Woods and

Calnan (1976).

Schonwald, P. (1929) in discussion of Black (1929) Journal of Allergy 1, 87.

Stier, R.F.E. (1929) in discussion of Black (1929) Journal of Allergy 1, 88.

White, R.P. (1934) The Dermatergoses of Occupational Affections of the Skin. 4th ed. London. H.K. Lewis.

Woods, B. and Calnan, C.D. (1976) Toxic Woods. Brit. J. Derm. 94, Suppl. 13, June.

Zavarin, E., Smith, R.M. and Anderson, A.B. (1959) Paper chromatography of the tropolones of Cupressaceae II. J. Org. Chem. 24, 1318.

Cupressus

15 - 20 species are found in the Mediterranean region, Sahara, Asia and North America. *C. macrocarpa* is the Monterey cypress largely planted for timber and shade in warm countries. Several species yield useful timber.

Cupressus spp.

The pollen of some species causes hayfever (Wodehouse 1971).

Cupressus sempervirens
Cypress

This species is the cypress of the Mediterranean region. The wood can cause dermatitis (Hausen 1970). The wood yields beta-thujaplicin which is a sensitizer of *Thuja* (Enzell and Erdtman 1957).

The pungent smell of cypress wood causes headaches in carpenters (Ramazzini 1713).

A man who was contact sensitive to *Dalbergia* showed transient erythema from a patch test with cypress wood (Lewith 1929).

References

Hausen, B.M. (1970) Untersuchungen uber Gesundheitsschadigende Holzer. Thesis, Hamburg.

Enzell, C. and Erdtman, H. (1957) The occurrence of Manool in *Cupressus sempervirens* L. Acta. Chem. Scand. 11, 902.

Lewith, R. (1929) Palisanderholzdermatitis Zentralblatt für Haut-und Geschlechtskrankheiten 30, 8.

Ramazzini, B. (1713) De Morbis Artificum. Bernardini Ramazzini (1633 1714). Diatriba. The Latin text of 1713, revised by Wright, W.C. 1940. The University of Chicago Press History of Medicine Series. No. 7. Library of the New York Academy of Medicine.

Wodehouse, R.P. (1971) Hayfever Plants. 2nd rev. edition. New York, Hafner.

Fitz-Roya

One species is found in Chile

Fitz-Roya cupressoides

The wood is irritant to the respiratory tract (Orsler 1973) and caused allergic contact dermatitis (Oleffe et al 1975).

References

Orsler, R.J. (1973) Personal communication from Forest Products Research Laboratory, Princess Risborough, Bucks., England.

Oleffe, J., Dedeken, H., Sporco, J., Hublet, P. (1975) Occupational skin allergy to Alerc. (*Fitzroya cupressoides*). Berufsdermatosen 23(6), 196.

Juniperus

60 species are found in the northern hemisphere. The wood of *J. virginiana* is the 'red cedar' used for making pencils.

Juniperus spp.

The sharp leaves of some species can cause punctate erythema or linear papules on the hands, wrists, forearms and ankles of person who weed or work amongst juniper shrubs. The reaction seems to be due to mechanical injury sometimes with an eczematous reaction from self-medication. Patch tests produced equivocal or negative results (Mitchell, J.C., unpublished observations).

Hjorth (1968) recorded a positive patch test reaction to juniper. Juniper wood can produce dermatitis and respiratory symptoms in wood-workers (Orsler 1973).

Juniperus communis

The fruit is used in making gin. The taste of the berries is aromatic, like turpentine (Pinus) (Wren 1968). Application of the plant to the skin produces burning and slight redness, sometimes vesicles (Nothnagel 1870, cited by Piffard 1881).

Juniperus oxycedrus

Irritant and probably allergic dermatitis can result from application of Oil of Cade derived from destructive distallation of the wood (White 1887, White 1889, Gougerot and Blamoutier 1922, Nelson 1932, Lord 1933, Grolnick 1938, Greenberg and Lester 1954). Acneiform eruptions can also result from use of Oil of Cade (White 1887).

Juniperus macropoda

This species can have irritant properties (Behl et al 1966).

Juniperus mexicana

The pollen is a common cause of hayfever in Texas. Some other Juniperus spp. can also cause hayfever (Wodehouse 1971).

Juniperus procera

The wood can cause dermatitis, conjunctivitis and rhinitis in wood-workers (Piorkowski 1944).

Juniperus sabina Savin

The plant was used as a counter-irritant (Merck 1968, Wren 1958). The twigs cause inflammation of the skin (Schroff 1856 cited by Piffard 1881).

Juniperus virginiana
Red Cedar, Savin

The leaves were used in an ointment for their irritant and rubefacient properties (White 1887). J. sabina yields podophyllotoxin (Merck Index 1968), an irritant of Podophyllum. The wood can cause dermatitis (Sandermann and Barghoorn 1956).

The use of toilet preparations containing cedarwood oils followed by exposure to various rays is sometimes the cause of dermatitis (Bray 1937, Greenbaum 1934, Tulipan 1938). Pigmentation may follow the topical application of cedarwood oil (del Vivo 1930, Sandler 1939). Phototoxicity from the oil could not be confirmed (Opdyke 1974). The oil is generally not irritant to the skin of animals although occlusion may produce irritation (Opdyke 1974). Oil of Juniper berries is reported to be not irritant (Lord 1933) and irritant to the skin and respiratory tract (Rothe et al 1973).

References

Behl, P.N., Captain, R.M., Bedi, B.M.S. and Gupta, S. (1966) Skin-irritant and sensitizing plants found in India, New Delhi, P.N. Behl, Irwin Hospital.

Bray, G.W. (1937) Recent Advances in Allergy. Blakiston, Philadelphia.

del Vivo, G. (1930) A proposito dell' azione di alcuni olii essenziali sulla pigmentazione. G. ital. Derm. Sif. 71, 467.

Wodehouse, R.P. (1971) Hayfever plants. 2nd ed. N.Y. Hafner.

Greenbaum, S.S. (1934) Cutaneous photopigmentation and cosmetics, with special reference to Berlock dermatitis. Penn. Med. J. 38, 28.

Greenberg, L.A. and Lester, D. (1954) Handbook of Cosmetic Materials. New York. Interscience.

Grolnick, M. (1938) Dermatitis due to haemorrhoidal ointment containing krameria and oil of cade. JAMA 110, 951.

Hjorth, N. (1968) at Finsen Institute. Pers. comm.

Lord, L.W. (1933) Oil of Cadeberry. A little known drug that is valuable in certain dermatoses. Arch. Derm. Syph. 28, 29.

Merck Index (1968) An Encyclopedia of Chemicals and Drugs. ed. Stecher, P.G. 8th ed. Rahway, N.J. Merck and Co. Inc.

Nelson, T. (1932) Contact dermatitis

to oil of cade. J. Allergy 3, 319.

Opdyke, D. (1974) Monographs on fragrance raw materials. Fd. Cosmet. Toxicol. 12, 807.

Orsler, R.J. (1973) Personal communication from Forest Products Research Laboratory, Princess Risborough, Bucks, England.

Piffard, H.G. (1881) A treatise on the Materia Medica and Therapeutics of the skin. New York. Wm. Wood and Co.

Piorkowski, F.O. (1944) Woodworkers' dermatitis in East Africa. East Afric. Med. J. 21, 60.

Rothe, A., Heine, A. and Rebohle, E. (1973) Oil from juniper berries as an occupational allergen for the skin and respiratory tract. Berufsdermatosen 21, 11.

Sandermann, W. and Barghoorn, A.W. (1956) Gesundheitsschadigende Nutzholzer. Holz. Roh-Werkst. 14, 37.

Sandler, I.L. (1939) Photosensitizing agents. A brief review of the literature. J. Am. med. Ass. 112, 2411.

Tulipan, L. (1938) Cosmetic irritants. Arch. Derm. And Syph. 38, 906.

White, J.C. (1887) Dermatitis venenata: An account of the Action of External irritants upon the Skin. Boston. Cupples and Hurd.

Gougerot and Blamoutier (1922) Intolérance anaphylactique aux applications médicamentenses externes ... huile de cade. Bulletin de la Société medicale des Hôspitaux de Paris 46, 733.

White, J.C. (1889) Some unusual forms of dermatitis venenata. Boston medico-surgical Journal 121, 583.

Wren, R.W. (1968) Potter's New Cyclopaedia of Botanical Drugs and Preparations by Wren, R.C. Re-edit. by Wren, R.W. Potter and Clarke Ltd. Health Science Press. Rustington, Sussex.

Libocedrus

Three species are found in New Caledonia, two species in New Zealand. *L. plumosa* yields valuable timber.

Libocedrus decurrens is now referred to *Calocedrus*.

Thuja

Five species are found in China, Japan and North America.

Thuja sp.

An irritant and possibly a sensitizer is present in the leaves (Sachs 1926, McCord 1962, Schwartz et al 1957).

Thuja douglasii

This species can cause eczema (Maiden 1904).

Thuja occidentalis
Arbor-Vitae

The plant or a decoction of it irritates and inflames the skin like *Juniperus sabina* (Cantani 1876 cited by Piffard 1881). The leaves have an irritant effect (Dispensatory 1884, Wren 1968). Oil of White Cedar was used as a rubefacient and in perfumes (Merck Index 1968).

Several men working with white cedar developed dermatitis of the hands; another man had pharyngitis and bronchitis but no dermatitis (Sachs 1920).

Thuja orientalis

The leaves and branches of this species and of *Th. occidentalis* can produce dermatitis in gardeners (Genner and Bonnevie 1938, Schwartz et al 1957). Contact dermatitis from a leaf of the tree was reported by Zubiri and Obras-Loscertales(1970).

Thuja japonica
Japanese Arbor Vitae

The wood can cause dermatitis and respiratory symptoms in woodworkers (Yasue 1973).

Thuja plicata
Western Red Cedar

The chemistry of the wood was reviewed by Barton and MacDonald (1971). A form of allergic contact dermatitis in forest-workers commonly known as 'cedar poisoning' results from exposure to lichens and liverworts (Frullania) which grow on the trees (Tan and Mitchell 1968, Mitchell et al 1972). Allergic contact dermatitis from the wood itself can occur in wood-workers; the sensitizing agents are tropolones (Bleumink et al 1973).

The wood-dust can produce allergic respiratory symptoms in wood-workers (Mitchell and Chan-Yeung 1974, Chan-Yeung et al 1973, Milne and Gandevia 1969, Doig 1949, Gandevia 1970, Gandevia and Milne 1970, Mitchell 1970, Mue et al 1973). The agent responsible is plicatic acid. Contact sensitivity to Thuja and to Libocedrus was reported by Calnan (1972).

76 cases of dermatitis from the sawdust were reported by Ishizaki et al (1973). Conjunctivitis, urticaria, rhinitis and asthma were also observed.

The main symptoms in 1,320 persons that appeared in connection with work with Western Red Cedar wood and the rate of occurrence per cent were asthma, 3.6%: nose inflammation 5.6%: urticaria 3.1%: skin infection, 3.0%: conjunctivitis 5.1%: total 21.1%. Only main symptoms were mentioned though several symptoms appeared simultaneously (Yasue 1973).

A number of persons living in houses built of Th. plicata after the 1923 Tokyo Earthquake developed 'beisugi asthma' (Hausen 1970). A joiner who had dermatitis showed positive patch test reactions to Th. plicata and Quercus, negative to some other woods (Woods and Calnan 1976).

References

Hausen, B.M. (1970) Untersuchungen über Gesundheitsschädigende Hölzer. Thesis, Hamburg.

Woods, B. and Calnan, C.D. (1976) Toxic Woods. Brit. J. Derm. 94, Suppl. 13, June.

Thuja standishii

The wood can cause dermatitis and respiratory symptoms in wood-workers (Ito 1963, Komatsu 1964). The contact sensitizing agent is beta-thujaplicin (Ito 1964).

References

Doig, A.T. (1949) Other lung diseases due to dust. Postgraduate Medical Journal 25, 639.

Gandevia, B. (1970) Ventilatory capacity during exposure to Western Red Cedar. Arch. Environ. Health 20, 59.

Gandevia, B. and Milne, J. (1970) Occupational asthma and rhinitis due to Western Red Cedar (Thuja plicata) with special reference to bronchial reactivity. Brit. J. Industr. Med. 27, 235.

Hausen, B.M. (1970) Untersuchungen über Gesundheitsschädigende Holzer. Thesis, Hamburg.

Ito, K. (1964) An antigenic substance beta-thujaplicin, in the steam-distillate of the sawdust of Thuja standishii Carr. Medical Journal of Shinshu University 9, 165.

Mitchell, C. (1970) Occupational asthma due to Western or Canadian red cedar (Thuja plicata) Med. J. Australia 57 (2), 233.

Mue, S., Ise, T., Ono, Y. et al (1975) A study of Western red cedar - induced asthma. Ann. Allerg. 34, 296.

Woods, B. and Calnan, C.D. (1976) Toxic Woods. Brit. J. Derm. 94, Suppl. 13, June.

Barton, G.M. and MacDonald, B.F. (1971) The chemistry, utilization of Western Red Cedar. Canadian Forestry Service Publ. No. 1023. Dept. of Fisheries and Forestry.

Bleumink, E., Mitchell, J.C. and Nater, J.P. (1973) Allergic contact dermatitis from cedar wood (Thuja plicata). Brit. J. Derm. 88, 499.

Calnan, C.D. (1972) Dermatitis from Cedar Wood Pencils. Trans. St. John's Hosp. derm. Soc. 58, 43.

Chang-Yeung, M., Barton, G.M., MacLean, L. et al (1973) Occupational asthma and rhinitis due to western red cedar (Thuja plicata). Amer. Rev. resp. Dis. 108, 1094.

Dispensatory, The National (1884) Philadelphia. Stille and Maisch., cited by White 1887.

Genner, V. and Bonnevie, P. (1938) Eczematous eruptions produced by leaves of trees and bushes. Arch. Derm. Syph. 37, 583.

Ishizaki, T., Shida, T., Miyamoto, T., Matsumara, Y., Mizuno, K. and Tomaru, M. (1973) Occupational asthma from Western Red Cedar dust (Thuja plicata) in furniture factory workers. J. Occup. Med. 15, 580.

Ito, K. (1963) Allergic disorders of upper respiratory tract by sawdust of Thuja standishii Carr. Rodo Kagaku 39, 27. 80, 501 and 568.

Ito, K. (1964) An antigenic substance, beta-thujaplicin, in the steam-destillate of the sawdust of Thuja standishii Carr. J. Jap. For. Soc. 35, 291.

Komatsu, F. (1964) Respiratory allergy in wood workers. Excerpta Medica. Int. Congr. Ser. 62, 1748.

McCord, C.P. (1962) The Occupational Toxicity of Cultivated Flowers. Ind. Med. Surg. 31, 365.

Maiden, J.H. (1904) Plants which induce eczema. Meeting of Therapeutical Society. Lancet 1, 1208.

Merck Index (1968) An Encyclopedia of Chemicals and Drugs. ed. Stecher, P.G. 8th ed. Rahway, N.J. Merck and Co. Inc.

Milne, J. and Gandevia, B. (1969) Occupational asthma and rhinitis due to Western Red Cedar (Thuja plicata). Med. J. Austr. 2, 741.

Mitchell, J.C., Dupuis, G., and Geissman, T.A. (1972) Allergic contact dermatitis from sesquiterpenoids of plants. Additional allergenic sesquiterpene lactones and immunological specificity of Compositae, liverworts and lichens. Brit. J. Derm. 87, 235.

Mitchell, J.C. and Chan-Yeung, M. (1974) Contact allergy from Frullania and respiratory allergy from Thuja. Canad. Med. Ass. J. 110, 653.

Piffard, H.G. (1881) A treatise on the Materia Medica and Therapeutics of the skin. New York. Wm. Wood and Co.

Sachs, O. (1926) Beitrag zur Frage der Uberempfindlichkeit der Haut. Wien. med. Wschr. 76, 933.

Tan, K.S. and Mitchell, J.C. (1968) Patch and Photopatch Tests in Contact Dermatitis and Photodermatitis. Canad. Med. Assoc. J. 98, 252.

Touton, K. (1932) Hauterkrankungen durch phanerogamische Pflanzen und ihre Produkte (Toxicodermia et Allergodermia phytogenes), in Barnewitz, J. et al Angeborene Anomalien, Lichtdermatosen, Pflanzengifte, Thermische Schädigungen, Einfluss Innerer Störungen auf die Haut. Berlin, Verlag von Julius Springer.

White, J.C. (1887) Dermatitis venenata: An account of the Action of External irritants upon the skin. Boston. Cupples and Hurd.

Wren, R.W. (1968) Potter's New Cyclopaedia of Botanical Drugs and Preparations by Wren, R.C. Reedit. by Wren, R.W. Potter and Clarke Ltd. Health Science Press. Rustington, Sussex.

Yasue, Y. (1973) Asthma due to Western Red Cedar. Mokuzai Kogyo (Wood Industry). 28, (No. 5), pp. 6-9.

Zubiri, A. and Obras-Loscertales, J.M. de las (1970) Caso curioso de dermatitis por contacto. Actas Dermosifilogr. 61, 277.

CURTISIACEAE

One species in one genus is found as a tree in southern Africa. The family was previously included in Cornaceae.

Curtisia

The distribution of the genus is that of the family.

Curtisia dentata

(syn. C. faginea)
Assegai-wood,
Cape Lancewood

Since splinters of Australian lancewood, Acacia shirleyi were said to cause painful wounds (Maiden 1919), other lancewoods, viz. C. dentata, Backhousia myrtifolia and Oxandra lanceolata have been included in lists of toxic timber (e.g. Schwartz et al 1957) without any published evidence (Woods and Calnan 1976).

The fruit pulp is bitter (Watt and Breyer-Brandwijk 1962).

References

Schwartz, L., Tulipan, L. and Birmingham, D.J. (1957) Occupational Diseases of the Skin. 3rd. ed. Philadelphia. Lea & Febiger. pp. 637-672.

Watt, J.M. and Breyer-Brandwijk, M.G. (1962) The Medicinal and poisonous plants of Southern Africa. 2nd ed. Edinburgh. E. & S. Livingstone.

Maiden, J.H. (1919) Notes on Acacia, no. IV. J. Proc. Roy. Soc. New South Wales. 53, 219 (whole paper 171-238 + plates).

Woods, B. and Calnan, C.D. (1976) Toxic Woods. Brit. J. Derm. 94, Suppl. 13, June.

CYCADACEAE

20 species in one genus are found in Madagascar, eastern Asia and IndoMalaysia.

Cycas

The distribution of the genus is that of the family.

Cycas circinalis

Cycas revoluta

These species are grown as ornamentals in Florida. The male 'cones' have acrid, repulsive odour which irritates the throat and respiratory passages (Morton 1969, 1971).

Aqueous emulsions of fresh cycad nuts have been used as dressings for skin ulcers. Systemic symptoms can result from absorption of cycasin (Schoental 1965).

Cycas rumphii

The pollen of the young cones has an unpleasant smell and causes sneezing (Benthall 1946).

References

Benthall, A.P. (1946) Trees of Calcutta and its neighbourhood. Calcutta. Thacker, Spink and Co. (1933) Ltd.

Morton, J.F. (1971) Plants poisonous to people in Florida and other warm areas. Miami, Florida. Hurricane House.

Schoental, R. (1965) Toxicology of Natural Products. Fd. Cosmet. Toxicol. 3, 609.

Morton, J.F. (1969) Some ornamental plants excreting respiratory irritants. Proc. Florida State Hort. Soc. 82, 415.

Toxic amblyopia may result from ingestion of cycad nuts and of cassava (Manihot) (Editorial 1972).

Reference

Editorial (1972) Food and cyanide. Brit. Med. J. 1, 481 (27 May).

CYPERACEAE

Carex

1500 - 2000 species are cosmopolitan especially found in temperate regions in marshes, etc.

New Zealand species of this genus are liable to cut the hands. (Howes 1974).

Reference

Howes, F.N. (1974) A Dictionary of Useful and Everyday Plants and their Common Names. Cambridge University Press. pp. 290.

About 4000 species in 90 genera are worldwide 'sedges'.

Cladium

Between 50 and 60 species

are found in tropical and temperate regions especially in Australia; one species is almost cosmopolitan.

Cladium mariscus
Razor Grass

This and related sedges have long knife-like leaves armed with small sharp teeth.

Carex

Between 1500 and 2000 species are cosmopolitan, especially found in temperate regions in marshes, etc.

Carex sp. Rush plant

The leaves which have fine sawing and cutting edges, made harder by the presence of silica in the superficial cells, can cause mechanical irritation of the hands of basket weavers and persons in allied occupations (Schwartz et al 1957).

Reference

Schwartz, L., Tulipan, L. and Birmingham, D.J. (1957) Occupational Diseases of the Skin. 3rd ed. Philadelphia. Lea & Febiger. pp. 637-672.

Cyperus

550 species are found in tropical and warm temperate regions.

Cyperus papyrus provided the well known papyrus of Egypt which afforded the Ancient Egyptians the compressed pith upon which they wrote their records. The stem was split into thin strips, which were pressed together while still wet (Burkill 1935).

Cyperus longus

The juice is irritant to the skin (Watt and Breyer-Brandwijk 1962).

Burkill, I.H. (1935) A Dictionary of the Economic Products of the Malay Peninsula. 2 vols. London. Crown Agents for the Colonies.

Watt, J.M. and Breyer-Brandwijk, M.G. (1962) The Medicinal and poisonous plants of Southern Africa. 2nd ed. Edinburgh. E. & S. Livingstone.

Gahnia

Forty species are native to China, IndoChina, Malaysia, Australia, New Zealand, Polynesia and Hawaii to the Marguesas.

Gahnia sp. Cutting Grass

A species of this genus, probably G. psittacorum, possesses leaf edges which can produce deep cuts in the skin (Cleland 1925).

Reference

Cleland, J.B. (1925) Plants, including fungi, poisonous or otherwise injurious to man in Australia. Med. J. Austr. 2, 444.

Scirpus

300 species are cosmopolitan.

Scirpus holoschaenus
Cultivated Bulrush

This species was incriminated in a case of Oppenheim's meadow dermatitis as evoking photosensitivity (Mariconda 1936).

Scirpus lacustris
Bulrush

The plant is used for chair-seats and mats. Dermatitis from reed matting derived from bulrushes was probably due to the reed bug Chilacis (Szego and Balogh 1965).

Scirpus paludosus
Bayonet Grass

The spiny leaves (Howes 1974) are capable of producing mechanical injury.

Howes, F.N. (1974) A Dictionary of Useful and Everyday Plants and their Common Names. Cambridge University Press. p. 290.

Mariconda, G. (1936) Observations and examinations in a sporadic case of "dermatitis bullose pratensis". Dermasifilografa 11, 117.

Szego, L. and Balogh, L. (1965) A form of occupational dermatitis due to the handling of reed matting. Borgyogy. vener. Szle. 41, 219.

Scleria

200 species are found in tropical and subtropical regions.

Scleria bracteata
Cut-grass

The rough edges of the leaves inflict painful cuts and scratches on any exposed surface of the skin (Allen 1943).

Scleria secans

The edges of the leaves, in common with the above species, may cut the skin like knives (Allen 1943).

Scleria oryzoides

The leaves are rough and used for polishing wood (Burkill 1935).

References

Allen, P.H. (1943) Poisonous and Injurious Plants of Panama. Am. J. Trop. Med. Suppl. 23, 1.

Burkill, I.H. (1935) A Dictionary of the Economic Products of the Malay Peninsula. 2 vols. London Crown Agents for the Colonies.

Scleria spp. Cut grass

The West Indian species of this genus are liable to cut the hands (Howes 1974).

Reference

Howes, F.N. (1974) A Dictionary of Useful and Everyday Plants and their Common Names. Cambridge University Press. pp. 290.

DAVIDSONIACEAE

One species in one genus found in North-east Australia is represented by a small slender tree (Shaw 1973).

Davidsonia

The tree bears irritant hairs.

Davidsonia pruriens
Davidsonian plum

This species, native to North Queensland produces a fruit which resembles a plum (Prunus). Eating the fruit produced a gastro-intestinal upset (Flecker 1945). He gives Cunoniaceae as the family of the plant. The affinities of the family are obscure (Shaw 1973).

References

Flecker, H. (1945) Injuries produced by plants in tropical Queensland. Med. J. Australia 1, 636.

Shaw, H.K.A. (1973) A Dictionary of the Flowering Plants and Ferns. (the late J.C. Willis) 8th ed. Cambridge University Press.

DENNSTAEDTIACEAE

The family consists of large much-divided ferns.

Pteridium

The genus contains one cosmopolitan species, P. aquilinum (Bracken).

Poisoning of animals from eating bracken produces symptoms which differ in various species. Blood dyscrasias with a bleeding tendency can produce petechiae and ecchymoses. Alterations in the hair have also been described (Kingsbury 1964, North 1967). The view that a photosensitising substance is found in the plants (Sampson and Malmsten 1935) has not been substantiated.

References

Kingsbury, J.M. (1964) Poisonous Plants of the United States and Canada. Englewood Cliffs, New Jersey. Prentice-Hall Inc.

North, P.M. (1967) Poisonous plants and fungi in colour. London. Blandford Press. Ltd.

Sampson, A.W. and Malmsten, H.E. (1935) Stock poisoning plants of California. Univ. California. Coll. Agr. Expt. Stat. Bull. 593.

DICHAPETALACEAE

200 species in five genera are of tropical distribution.

Chemistry is recorded by Hegnauer (1966).

Reference

Hegnauer, R. (1966) Chemotaxonomy of plants. Vol. 4. Basel Birkhauser. pg. 14.

Dichapetalum

150 to 200 species are found in tropical regions especially in Africa.

Dichapetalum spp.
Gifblaar (South Africa)

Fluoroacetate derived from this plant is poisonous; amongst the symptoms described resulting from contact with the powder were a tingling sensation around the corners of the mouth and in the nasal passages and numbness of the face (Grant 1962).

Dichapetalum cymosum

Handling the very young leaf causes a tingling and burning sensation of the skin, an effect not found with an old leaf (Watt and Breyer-Brandwijk 1962).

References

Grant, W.M. (1962) Toxicology of the eye. Springfield, Ill. Charles C. Thomas.

Watt, J.M. and Breyer-Brandwijk, M.G. (1962) The Medicinal and poisonous plants of Southern Africa. 2nd ed. Edinburgh. E. & S. Livingstone.

DIDIEREACEAE

Eleven species in four genera found in Madagascar are trees or shrubs with the habit of cacti or cactiform Euphorbia species.

Alluaudia

Six species in this genus found in Madagascar often have branches armed with thorns (Menninger 1967) which appear capable of producing mechanical injury.

Reference

Menninger, E.A. (1967) Fantastic Trees. New York. The Viking Press.

DILLENIACEAE

400 species in ten genera, found in tropical and subtropical regions, are well represented in the Australian scrub.

Chemistry is recorded by Hegnauer (1966).

Reference

Hegnauer, R. (1966) Chemotaxonomy of plants. Vol. 4 Basel, Birkhauser. p. 19.

Dillenia

Sixty species are found in the Mascarenes, south-eastern Asia, IndoMalaysia, northern Queensland and Fiji.

Dillenia indica
Elephant apple

This large tree has heavy fruits which make it unsuitable for planting on roadsides and it is seldom seen in gardens.

Tetracera

40 tropical species are recognized.

Tetracera sp. (syn. Delima)
Mempelas

The harsh leaves of this climbing plant are used for cleaning school boards (Corner 1952).

Tetracera affinis

The stems are covered with strong cutting hairs (Irvine 1961).

Tetracera rotundifolia

The young branches produce irritation on contact with the skin (Altschul 1973).

References

Altschul, S. von R. (1973) Drugs and foods from little-known plants. Cambridge, Mass. Harvard Univ. Press.

Corner, E.J.H. (1952) Wayside Trees of Malaysia. Singapore, Government Printer.

Irvine, F.R. (1961) Woody plants of Ghana. Oxford University Press. London.

DIOSCOREACEAE

750 species in five genera are found in tropical and warm temperate regions.

Chemistry is recorded by Hegnauer (1963).

Reference

Hegnauer, R. (1963) Chemotaxonomy of plants. Vol. 2. Basel, Birkhauser. p. 133.

Dioscorea

600 species are found in tropical and subtropical regions, three species in the Pyrenees, Balkan Peninsula and Caucasus. The tubers are known as yams.

Dioscorea spp.

The raw tubers are irritant to the skin. The skin of the fingers tingles slightly from continued contact (Burkill 1935). The tubers contain compounds which are used as a starting material for the manufacture of corticosteroid drugs (Oliver 1959).

Dioscorea alata White Yam

The raw tuber is irritant to the mucous membrane of the mouth (Burkill 1935). Application of the plant to the skin produces pruritus and desquamation (Piffard 1881).

Dioscorea dumetorum
syn. D. triphylla var. dumetorum)
(Verdcourt and Trump 1969)

Application of the tuber to the skin produces a burning sensation (Watt and Breyer-Brandwijk 1962). The plant yields a neurotoxic alkaloid (Verdcourt and Trump 1969).

Dioscorea hispida
Wild Yam

The tubers are edible after grating, boiling, repeated washing and soaking (Burkill 1935). Eating the raw tubers is a frequent cause of death in the Philippines (Quisumbing 1951). The toxic principle is dioscorine (Webb 1948).

Dioscorea transversa
Wild Hop Vine

Arrowroot, a starchy material also prepared from Arum, was prepared from the tubers in New South Wales. During washing of the pulp, workmen developed acute irritation of the hands and arms (Maiden 1914).

Dioscorea villosa
Wild Yam

The taste of the tuber is insipid, afterwards acrid (Wren 1968).

References

Burkill, I.H. (1955) A Dictionary of the Economic Products of the Malay Peninsula. 2 vols. London. Crown Agents for the Colonies.

Maiden, J.H. (1914) Dioscorea transversa R. Br. a yam, native of New South Wales and Queensland. Ag. Gaz. New South Wales 25, 612.

Oliver, B. (1959) Nigeria's Useful Plants. The Nigerian Field Part II (2) 24, 54.

Piffard, H.G. (1881) A treatise on the Materia Medica and Therapeutics of the skin. New York. Wm. Wood and Co.

Quisumbing, E. (1951) Medicinal Plants of the Philippines. Tech. Bull. 16. Manila, Philippine Islands. Manila Bureau of Printing. 1234 pp.

Verdcourt, B. and Trump, E.C. (1969) Common Poisonous Plants of East Africa. London. Collins.

Watt, J.M. and Breyer-Brandwijk, M.G. (1962) The Medicinal and poisonous plants of Southern Africa. 2nd ed. Edinburgh. E.& S. Livingstone.

Webb, L.H. (1948) Guide to the medicinal and poisonous plants of Queensland. C.S.I.R. Bull no. 232.

Wren, R.W. (1968) Potter's New Cyclopaedia of Botanical Drugs and Preparations by Wren, R.C. Reedit. by Wren, R.W. Potter and Clarke Ltd. Health Science Press. Rustington, Sussex.

Tamus

Five species are found in the Canaries, Madeira, Europe and the Mediterranean region.

Tamus communis
Black Bryony, Blackeye Root

The fresh root, when scraped, yields a slimy rubefacient paste (Wren 1968, Perrot and Paris 1971). Black eye root is a popular remedy for removing discoloration by bruises (Wren 1968). Bryony is also a common name for Bryonia.

References

Perrot, E. and Paris, R. (1971) Les plantes medicinales. 2 vols. Paris. Presses Universitaires de France. 245 (+XXVI index).

Wren, R.W. (1968) Potter's New Cyclopaedia of Botanical Drugs and Preparations by Wren, R.C. Re-edit. by Wren, R.W. Potter and Clarke Ltd. Health Science Press. Rustington, Sussex.

DIPSACACEAE

150 species in 8 genera are chiefly found in north temperate Eurasia and tropical and southern Africa.

Dipsacus

15 species are found in Eurasia, the Mediterranean region and tropical Africa. D. fullonum spp. sativus (fuller's teasel) has hooked bracts; the fruit heads are used for raising the nap upon cloth.

Dipsacus sylvestris

Use of the plant for warts (Piffard 1881) suggests an irritant effect.

Reference

Piffard, H.G. (1881) A treatise on the Materia Medica and Therapeutics of the skin. New York. Wm. Wood and Co.

DIPTEROCARPACEAE

580 species in 15 genera are of palaeotropical distribution and found chiefly in IndoMalaysia.

Chemistry is recorded by Hegnauer (1966).

Reference

Hegnauer, R. (1966) Chemotaxonomy of Plants. Vol. 4. Basel, Birkhauser. p. 31.

Dipterocarpus

76 species are found from Ceylon and India to Western Malaysia and Bali. Several yield wood-oil or gurjun balsam, a resin obtained by tapping, and used as a varnish.

Dipterocarpus alatus
Keruing, Gurjun

The wood dust has been reported to cause dermatitis in woodworkers (Wagenfuhr 1961, Hausen 1973, Orsler 1973). Balsam Gurjun (East Indian Copaiba) has not been reported to produce dermatitis (Greenberg and Lester 1954).

References

Greenberg, L.A. and Lester, D. (1954) Handbook of Cosmetic Materials. New York. Interscience.

Hausen, B.M. (1973) Holzarten mit gesundheitsschädigenden inhaltsstoffen Stuttgart. DRW-Verlags-GmbH.

Orsler, R.J. (1973) Personal communication from Forest Products Research Laboratory, Princess Risborough, Bucks, England.

Wagenführ, R. (1961) Gibt es giftige Hölzer Möbel und Wohnraum 4, 120.

Dryobalanops

Nine species are found in Sumatra, the Malay Peninsula and Borneo.

Dryobalanops aromatica

This and other species yield Borneo or Sumatra camphor, used chiefly in China. The camphor has rubefacient effects (Burkill 1935). Camphors are also obtained from Cinnamomum camphora and Blumea balsamifera. Borneol and isoborneol are used in perfumery and incense-making (Merck Index 1968).

References

Burkill, I.H. (1935) A Dictionary of the Economic Products of the Malay Peninsula. 2 vols. London. Crown Agents for the Colonies.

Merck Index (1968) An Encyclopedia of Chemicals and Drugs. ed. Stecher, P.G. 8th ed. Rahway, N.J. Merck & Co. Inc.

Shorea

180 species are found from Ceylon to southern China. western Malaysia, the Moluccas and the Lesser Sunda Islands. Some yield dammar (resin) used in varnishes. Shorea robusta known as Sal (India), Meranti, Luan or Seraya (Malay) and other species yield useful timber.

Shorea assamica   Meranti

Mucocutaneous reaction from this species in the wood working industry was reported by Hublet et al (1972).

Shorea meranti   Meranti

This Malaysian wood is irritant to the respiratory tract (Orsler 1973, Hausen 1973) possibly from a yield of terpenoids (Cocker 1964). Red Meranti is sometimes sold as western red cedar (Thuja).

References

Cocker, W. et al (1964) Extractives from woods. VI. Extractives from Shorea meranti. Perf. Essent. Oil. Rev. 55, 442.

Hausen, B.M. (1973) Holzarten mit gesundheitsschädigenden inhaltsstoffen Stuttgart. DRW-Verlags-GmbH.

Orsler, R.J. (1973) Personal communication from Forest Products Research Laboratory, Princess Risborough, Bucks, England.

Contact dermatitis from meranti wood (Shorea, Dipterocarpaceae) and jelutong wood (Dyera, Apocynaceae) was reported by Siregar (1975).

Reference

Siregar, R.S. (1975) Occupational dermatoses among foresters. Contact Dermatitis 1, 33.

Hublet, P., Sporcq, J., Oleffe, J. et al (1972) Etude sur les accidents cutanes et muqueux provoques par les bois tropicaus dans l'industrie due bois en Belgique. Arch. Belges. Med. Social. 30, 314.

Shorea spp.
Lauans, "Philippine mahogany"

The term "Philippine mahogany" is applied commercially in the United States to Philippine woods belonging to three genera: Shorea, Parashorea and Pentacme. The group is further sub-divided into types based on heartwood color as follows:

Dark red	
red lauan (Shorea negrosensis)	Dark reddish-brown to brick red
tanguile (Shorea polysperma)	Red to reddish-brown
Tianong (Shorea agsaboensis)	Light red to light reddish-brown
Light red	
Almon (Shorea almon)	Light red to pinkish
Bagtikan (Parashorea plicata)	Grayish-brown
Mayapis (Shorea squamata)	Light red to reddish-brown
White lauan (Pentacme contorta & P. mindanensis)	Grayish to very light red

The species within each group may be shipped interchangeably (Kukachka 1970).

Kukachka, B.F. (1970) Properties of imported tropical woods. USDA Forest Service Research Paper. FPL125 March. U.S. Dept. Agric. Forest Service. Forest Products Laboratory. Madison, Wis. U.S.A.

DROSERACEAE

105 species in four genera are recognized, mainly found in acid bogs. All are insectivorous. Aldrovanda is a submerged water plant.

Chemistry is recorded by Hegnauer (1966).

Reference

Hegnauer, R. (1966) Chemotaxonomy of plants. Vol. 4. Basel. Birkhauser. p. 40.

Drosera

100 species are found in tropical and temperate regions especially in Australia and New Zealand.

Drosera burmanni Sundew

Drosera indica

Drosera peltata
(syn. D. lunata)

The plants are insectivorous and contain a proteolytic enzyme of the pepsin type. The crushed leaves are acrid and vesicant (Behl et al 1966).

Drosera rotundifolia
Sundew

Application of the leaf to the skin will raise blisters (Culpeper 1653) and the juice of the plant was used to remove warts, corns, freckles and keratoses in eastern (Piffard 1881, White 1887) and western North America (Turner and Bell in press). Aldrovanda vesiculosa, Dionaea muscipula (Venus' Fly-trap), Drosophyllum lusitanicun and some Drosera spp. yield an irritant naphthaquinone, plumbagin (Thomson 1971) see Plumbago.

References

Behl, P.N., Captain, R.M., Bedi, B.M.S. and Gupta, S. (1966) Skin-irritant and sensitizing plants found in India, New Delhi, P.N. Behl, Irwin Hospital.

Culpeper, N. (1653) The Complete Herbal. Birminghams. Kynoch Press Imperial Chemical (Pharmaceuticals) Ltd.

Piffard, H.G. (1881) A treatise on the Materia Medica and Theraperutics of the skin. New York. Wm. Wood and Co.

Thomson, R.H. (1971) Naturally Occurring Quinones. 2nd ed. London. Academic Press.

Turner, N.C. and Bell, M.A.M. (in press) The ethnobotany of the southern Kwakiutl Indians of British Columbia. Economic Botany.

White, J.C. (1887) Dermatitis venenata: An account of the Action of External irritants upon the Skin. Boston. Cupples and Hurd.

EBENACEAE

500 species in three genera are found in tropical regions especially in IndoMalaysia.

Chemistry is recorded by Hegnauer, (1966).

Reference

Hegnauer, R. (1966) Chemotaxonomy of plants. Vol. 4. Basel, Birkhauser, p. 45.

Diospyros

500 species are found in warm regions. Many species yield the valuable wood, ebony. The sapwood is white and soft, the heartwood hard and black. Ebony refers to the heartwood of various species. The wood dust of some species is irritant to the respiratory tract (Orsler 1973). The wood of some species yields naphthaquinones including the irritant compound plumbagin (Thomson 1971), see Plumbago. An ebony bracelet produced dermatitis of the wrist (Nicolas and Pétouraud 1935). An ebony splinter wound produced dermatitis; no patch tests were recorded (Vonkennel 1929). Ebony sawdust added to snuff as a practical joke caused violent persistent irritation (Grossmann 1920).

References

Nicolas, J. and Pétouraud, C. (1935) Dermite eczématiforme due bras à la suite du port d'un bracelet d'ébène. Bull Soc. franc. derm. syph. 42, 27.

Orsler, R.J. (1973) Personal communication from Forest Products Research Laboratory, Princess Risborough, Bucks, England.

Thomson, R.H. (1971) Naturally Occurring Quinones. 2nd ed. London. Academic Press.

Grossmann, J. (1920) Gesundheitsschädliche Holzarten Der Holzkäufer (Leipzig) 17, 519, 535, 540 and 545.

Vonkennel (1929) Teakholzdermatitis. Zentr. Haut. Geschlechts. 30, 691.

Diospyros acris

This species has a vesicant action on the skin (White 1934).

Reference

White, R.P. (1934) The Dermatergoses or Occupational Affections of the Skin. 4th ed. London. H.K. Lewis.

Diospyros canaliculata
Flint Bark

A bark-extract blisters the skin (Irvine 1961).

Reference

Irvine, F.R. (1961) Woody plants of Ghana. Oxford University Press. London.

Diospyros celebica
Makassar, Coromandel

This species produced dermatitis (Buschke and Joseph 1927). Patch tests to the sawdust and an alcoholic extract produced negative results.

Reference

Buschke, A. and Joseph, A. (1927) Über Hautentzündung, hervorgerufen durch Makassarholz mit Berücksichtigung gewerbehygienischer Fragen. Deutsch. med. Wchnschr. 53, 1641.

Diospyros crassiflora
African Ebony

This species has been reported to cause dermatitis (Hausen 1973).

Reference

Hausen, B.M. (1973) Holzarten mit gesundheitsschädigenden inhaltsstoffen Stuttgart. DRW-Verlags-GmbH.

Diospyros discolor
Butter-fruit

The edible fruit has a dense covering of irritating silky hairs (Corner 1952).

Reference

Corner, E.J.H. (1952) Wayside Trees of Malaysia. Singapore, Government Printer.

Diospyros ebenaster

The bark and leaves are employed as a blistering plaster (Quisumbing 1951).

Reference

Quisumbing, E. (1951) Medicinal Plants of the Philippines. Tech. Bull. 16. Manila, Philippine Islands. Manila Bureau of Printing. 1234 pp.

Diospyros ebenum
(syn. Maba ebenus)
Ceylon ebony

This species has been reported to cause dermatitis (Hausen 1973, Herxheimer 1912).

References

Hausen, B.M. (1973) Holzarten mit gesundheitsschädigenden inhaltsstoffen Stuttgart. DRW-Verlags-GmbH.

Herxheimer,K. (1912) Über die gewerblichen Erkrankungen der Haut. Dtsch. med. Wschr. 1, 239.

Diospyros fischeri
(Syn. Royena)

Ulcerative stomatitis can result from using this plant to clean the teeth (Verdcourt and Trump 1969).

References

Verdcourt, B. and Trump, E.C. (1969) Common Poisonous Plants of East Africa. London. Collins.

Diospyros loureirana

Diospyros macrocalyx (syn. Royena)

These species are used in southern Africa to dye the teeth red (Watt and Breyer-Brandwijk 1962).

Reference

Watt, J.M. and Breyer-Brandwijk, M.G. (1962) The Medicinal and poisonous plants of southern Africa. 2nd ed. Edinburgh. E. & S. Livingstone.

Diospyros multiflora

The juice of the fruit is irritating to the skin; the bark and leaves are caustic (Quisumbing 1951).

Reference

Quisumbing, E. (1951) Medicinal plants of the Philippines. Tech. Bull. 16. Manila, Philippine Islands. Manila Bureau of Printing. 1234 pp.

Diospyros samoensis

The plant can cause dermatitis and the fruit juice can blister the skin (Uhe 1974).

Reference

Uhe, G. (1974) Medicinal plants of Samoa. Econ. Bot. 28, 1.

Diospyros villosa (syn. Royena)

The leaf and roots are vesicant for the skin (Watt and Breyer-Brandwijk 1962).

Reference

Watt, J.M. and Breyer-Brandwijk, M.G. (1962) The medicinal and poisonous plants of Southern Africa. 2nd ed. Edinburgh. E. & S. Livingstone.

Diospyros xanthochlamys (syn. D. canaliculata)

An extract of the bark has a strong vesicant action (Oliver 1959).

Reference

Oliver, B. (1959) Nigeria's Useful Plants. Part II (2). Nigerian Field 24, 54.

Euclea

20 species are found in Africa, the Comoro islands and Arabia.

Euclea daphnoides

The wood of this tree is never used as firewood by Zulus because this leads to quarrels and domestic unhappiness (Watt and Breyer-Brandwijk 1962).

Euclea fructuosa

This plant, when placed for medicinal purposes on cuts in the skin, is said to produce poisonous effects (Verdcourt and Trump 1969).

References

Verdcourt, B. and Trump, E.C. (1969) Common Poisonous Plants of East Africa. London. Collins.

Watt, J.M. and Breyer-Brandwijk, M.G. (1962) The Medicinal and poisonous plants of southern Africa. 2nd ed. Edinburgh. E. & S. Livingstone.

EHRETIACEAE

400 species in 13 genera are found in tropical and subtropical regions. The family is scarcely distinct from Boraginaceae in which it was formerly included.

Chemistry is recorded by Hegnauer (1964).

Reference

Hegnauer, R. (1964) Chemotaxonomy of plants. Vol. 3. Basel, Birkhauser, p. 288 (under Boraginaceae).

Coldenia

20 species are found in tropical and sub-tropical America; one species is palaeotropical.

Coldenia procumbens

The dried leaves, when pulverized, provoke sneezing (Quisumbing 1951).

Reference

Quisumbing, E. (1951) Medicinal plants of the Philippines. Tech. Bull. 16. Manila, Philippine Islands, Manila Bureau of Printing. 1234 pp.

Cordia

250 species are found in warm regions.

Cordia sp. Freijo

Guinea pigs were sensitized to ethanol/chloroform extracts of the wood. The species tested may have been C. goeldiana or C. millenii (Hausen 1974).

Cordia cylindrica

A woman had recurrent dermatitis of the hands from handling the leaves of this plant (Chan 1974).

References

Chan, M.K.C. (1974) Sabah, Malaysia Personal communication.

Hausen, B.M. (1974) Hamburg, Germany. Personal communication.

Cordia goeldiana
Brazilian walnut

Schwartz (1931) thought that Brazilian walnut which produced dermatitis might be Cordia goeldiana or Nectandra but the wood was Phoebe porosa (Record and Hess 1943).

References

Record, S.J. and Hess, R.W. (1943) Timbers of the New World. New Haven, Yale.

Schwartz, L. (1931) Dermatitis venenata due to contact with Brazilian walnut wood. Publ. Hlth. Rep. (Washington) 46, 1938.

ELAEOCARPACEAE

350 species in 12 genera are found in tropical and subtropical regions.

Sloanea

120 species are found in tropical Asia and America. The genus name Sloanea has also been applied to Apeiba of the Tiliaceae family.

Sloanea australis

The wood can cause dermatitis in tradesmen (Mair 1968). The family to which this species belongs has not yet been clarified.

Sloanea quadrivalvis Seem.

The seed capsules are densely covered with short, easily detachable bristles that are irritant to the skin and eyes (Allen 1943). He recorded this species as within Elaeocarpaceae.

References

Allen, P.H. (1943) Poisonous and injurious plants of Panama. Am. J. Trop. Med. Suppl. 23, 1.

Mair, K. (1968) Director, Royal Botanic Gardens, Sydney Australia. Personal communication.

Sloanea australis

"S australis is in the family Elaeocarpaceae in our view, although some authors regard the family Elaeocarpaceae as a group within the Tiliaceae" (Johnson 1976).

Reference

Johnson, L.A.S. (1976) Director, Royal Botanic Gardens and Natural Herbarium. Sydney, Australia. Per. Comm.

EPACRIDACEAE

400 species in 30 genera are found from IndoChina to New Zealand, Hawaii and South America but chiefly in Australia and Tasmania.

Chemistry is recorded by Hegnauer (1966).

Reference

Hegnauer, R. (1966) Chemotaxonomy of plants. Vol. 4. Basel, Birkhauser. p. 63.

Lissanthe

Four species are found in Australia.

Lissanthe strigosa

This species has been suspected as a cause of pustular dermatitis in sheep. (Hurst 1942).

Reference

Hurst, E. (1942) The Poison Plants of New South Wales. N.S.W. Poison Plants Committee; Sydney.

EPHEDRACEAE

40 species in one genus are found in northern and southern warm temperate regions.

Chemistry is recorded by Hegnauer, (1962).

Reference

Hegnauer, R. (1962) Chemotaxonomy of plants. Vol. 1. Basel, Birkhauser, p. 441.

Ephedra

The distribution of the genus is that of the family.

Ephedra equisetina
Ma Huang

Ephedra sinica

These species which are the main sources of natural ephedrine have been used in China since ancient times for treatment of hayfever and asthma. Contact dermatitis from ephedrine may occur soon after the start of applications or as long as two years after first usage. In some cases, a drug eruption accompanies the contact dermatitis (Abramovitz and Noun 1933). These authors reported the case of a woman who became contact sensitive to a spray used on her child. Most cases present dermatitis of the skin around the nose from the use of ephedride - containing nasal sprays (Scheer 1929, Ayres and Anderson 1931, Lewis 1944, Ramirez and Eller 1930). Localized contact sensitivity of the skin of the penis to ephedrine was reported by Hollander (1936). In a fixed drug eruption stereoisomeric specificity was observed (Brownstein 1968). Ephedrine can produce contact dermatitis of the skin of the eyelids from use in ophthalmic preparations. The two naturally occurring forms of ephedrine are l-ephedrine and d-pseudoephedrine. A chemically related compound derived from animal glands, epinephrine, can cause contact dermatits (Alani and Alani 1976) which can show isomeric specificity (Gibbs 1970).

References

Abramowitz, E.W. and Noun, M.H. (1933) Contact dermatitis from ephedrine. Brit. J. Derm. Syph. 45, 225.

Alani, S.D. and Alani, M.D. (1976) Allergic contact dermatitis and conjunctivitis frm epinephrine. Contact Dermatitis 2, 147.

Ayres, S. Jr. and Anderson, N.P. (1931) Dermatitis medicamentosa due to ephedrine and ephedrine inhalant. JAMA 97, 437.

Brownstein, M.H. (1968) Fixed eruptions due to an ephedrine isomer. Archs. Derm. 97, 115.

Gibbs, R.C. (1970) Allergic contact dermatitis to epinephrine. Arch. Derm. 101, 92.

Hollander, L. (1936) Dermatitis of the penis caused by ephedrin. JAMA 106, 706.

Lewis, G.M. (1944) Contact dermatitis-like lesions following intranasal application of ephedrine. Arch. Derm. Syph. 49, 379.

Ramirez, M.A. and Eller, J.J. (1930) The "Patch test" in "Contact Dermatitis" (Dermatitis venenata) J. Allergy 1, 489.

Scheer, M. (1929) A case of dermatitis venenata due to ephedrine. Arch. Derm. Syph. 20, 641.

EQUISETACEAE

This family consists of a single genus Equisetum containing 23 species which are cosmopolitan except in Australasia.

Chemistry is recorded by Hegnauer (1962).

Reference

Hegnauer, R. (1962) Chemotaxonomy of plants. Vol. 1. Basel, Birkhauser. p. 244 and 475.

The mechanical tissues of most species contain much silica and the stems of E. hyemale (Dutch rushes) and of other species are used for polishing (Shaw 1973, Wren 1968, Turner and Bell in press). E. limosum

(Schwartz et al 1957) and E. debile (Behl et al 1966) are said to be irritating to the skin. Equisetum spp. (Horsetails) contain a thiaminase; the effects of poisoning in animals from ingestion of the plants are similar to those of Vitamin B_1 deficiency (North 1967). An early report of a skin reaction attributed to the plants (Lohmann 1903/04 cited by Touton 1932, Kulp 1922) has not been obtained for review.

References

Behl, P.N., Captain, R.M., Bedi, B.M.S. and Gupta, S. (1966) Skin-irritant and sensitizing plants found in India, New Delhi, P.N. Behl, Irwin Hospital.

Kulp, (1922) Zur Atiologie und Pathologie toxischer Exantheme unter besonderer Berucksichtigung eines Falles von Erythema exsudativum multiforme toxicum nach Zinnkraut. Inaug. Diss. Munchen, cited by Touton (1932) and White (1934).

Lohmann 1903/04 cited by Touton (1932), Kulp (1922).

North, P.M. (1967) Poisonous plants and fungi in colour. London. Blandford Press Ltd.

Schwartz, L., Tulipan, L. and Birmingham, D.J. (1957) Occupational Diseases of the skin. 3rd ed. Philadelphia. Lea & Febiger. pp. 637-672.

Shaw, H.K.A. (1973) A Dictionary of the Flowering Plants and Ferns. (the late J.C. Willis) 8th ed. Cambridge University Press.

Touton, K. (1932) Hauterkrankungen durch phanerogamische Pflanzen und ihre Produkte (Toxicodermia et Allergodermia phytogenes), in Barnewitz, J. et al Angeborene Anomalien, Lichtdermatosen, Pflanzengifte, Thermische Schädigungen, Einfluss Innerer Störungen auf die Haut. Berlin, Verlag. von Julius Springer.

Turner, N.C. and Bell, M.A.M. (in press) The ethnobotany of the southern Kwakiutl Indians of British Columbia. Economic Botany.

White, R.P. (1934) The Dermatergoses or Occupational Affections of the Skin. 4th ed. London. H.K. Lewis.

Wren, R.W. (1968) Potter's New Cyclopaedia of Botanical Drugs and Preparations by Wren, R.C. Re-edit. by Wren, R.W. Potter and Clarke Ltd. Health Science Press. Rustington, Sussex.

ERICACEAE

1350 species in 50 genera are cosmopolitan except in deserts. The leaves of Ledum palustre are used as tea.

Andromeda arborea (Elkwood) (?syn. Oxydendrum)

One or two species are native to North temperate and cold regions.

White (1887) received a report that the tree is an acrid poison when handled.

Reference

White, J.C. (1887) Dermatitis venenata: An account of the Action of External irritants upon the Skin. Boston. Cupples & Hurd.

Erica

Over 500 species are native to Europe, Asia Minor and Africa.

Erica cinerea (Bell Heather)

Bell Heather briskly applied to skin produced a violent reaction. Ordinary heather (possibly E. tetralix) produced no reaction (Low 1924).

Reference

Low, R.C. (1924) Skin Sensitiveness to Non-Bacterial Proteins and Toxins. Brit. J. Derm. Syph. 31, 292

Gaultheria

200 species are native to regions around the Pacific Ocean. Two species are native to eastern North America and 8 species to Brazil.

Gaultheria procumbens (Tea Berry)

The fruit is edible. The leaves which yield methyl salicylate (Merck 1968) have been used as a counter-irritant (Hurst 1942). A possible hazard of exposure to the plant for aspirin-sensitive persons was noted by Shelley (1964).

Gaultheria shallon (Salal)

The berry is edible. The stiff leaves are a source of minor mechanical injury to bare ankles.

References

Hurst, E. (1942) The Poison Plants of New South Wales. N.S.W. Poison Plants Committee; Sydney.

Merck Index (1968) An encyclopedia of chemicals and drugs. ed. Stecher, P.G. 8th ed. Rahway, N.J. Merck & Co. Inc.

Shelley, W.B. (1964) Birch pollen and aspirin psoriasis: a study in salicylate hypersensitivity. JAMA 189, 985.

Kalmia

Eight species are native to North America and Cuba. Some species are cultivated.

Kalmia spp.
(Mountain Laurel)

The syndrome of poisoning from ingestion of the plant includes cutaneous effects - sweating and tingling sensations (Muenscher 1951). Some species yield poisonous honey (Morton 1964).

Oxydendrum

One species is native to eastern North America.

Oxydendrum arboreum
(Sorrel Tree)
(?syn. Andromeda)

The plant was listed as an irritant by Pammel (1911), Weber (1930).

References

Morton, J.F. (1964) Honeybee plants of South Florida. Proc. Florida State Horticult. Soc. 77, 415.

Muenscher, W.C. (1951) Poisonous plants of the United States, 2nd ed. New York. The MacMillan Co.

Pammel, L.H. (1911) A Manual of Poisonous plants. Torch Press. Cedar Rapids, Iowa. Reprinted Univ. Microfilms Inc. Ann Arbor, Mich. 1965. pp. 476-7.

Weber, L.F. (1937) External causes of dermatitis. Archs. Derm. Syph. 35, 129.

Rhododendron

Five to six hundred species are native to north temperate regions. Some yield poisonous honey (Morton 1964).

Rhododendron spp.

Cleland (1943) noted a report of dermatitis on the arms from cutting azaleas and rhododendrons. The leaf of Azalea (syn. Rhododendron) produced a positive patch test reaction in 1 of 87 patients tested (Fregert and Hjorth 1968). An apparently relevant report has not been obtained (Igumnov 1967).

Rhododendron indicum hybrid

A woman was contact-sensitive of this plant and to Streptocarpus, (Agrup and Fregert 1968).

Rhododendron simsii

Contact sensitivity to the leaf was observed in one patient (Agrup 1969).

Dermatitis from rhododendron was reported by Igumonov (1967).

References

Agrup, G. (1969) Hand eczema and other hand dermatoses in South Sweden. Acta. derm.-venereol 49 Suppl. 61. pp. 1-91.

Agrup, G. and Fregert, S. (1968) Patch test reactions to Streptocarpus. Contact Dermatitis Newsletter 4, 72.

Cleland, J.B. (1943) Plants including fungi, poisonous or otherwise injurious to man in Australia. IV. Med. J. Australia. 11, 161.

Fregert, S. and Hjorth, N. (1968) Results of standard patch tests with substances abandoned. Contact Dermatitis Newsletter 5, 85.

Igumnov, A.K. Rhododendron dermatitis in Transbaikalia. Vestn. Derm. Vener. 41, 70.

Morton, J.F. (1964) Honeybee plants of South Florida. Proc. Florida State Horticult. Soc. 77, 415.

ERYTHROXYLACEAE

250 species in two genera are found in tropical regions.

Chemistry is recorded by Hegnauer (1966).

Reference

Hegnauer, R. (1966) Chemotaxonomy of plants. Vol. 4. Basel, Birkhauser, p. 94.

Erythroxylum

About 250 species are found in tropical and subtropical regions chiefly in America and Madagascar.

Erythroxylum coca
Coca (Peru)

The leaves yield cocaine which can cause contact dermatitis of the eyelids and kerato-conjunctivitis (Duke-Elder 1965), and dermatitis of the fingers in dentists (Schwartz et al 1957).

References

Duke-Elder, S. (1965) System of Ophthalmology. Vol. VIII Diseases of the outer eye. Part 1. Allergic kerato-conjunctivitis. pp. 451. London. Henry Kimpton.

Schwartz, L., Tulipan, L. and Birmingham, D.J. (1957) Occupational Diseases of the Skin. 3rd. ed. Philadelphia. Lea & Febiger. pp. 637-672.

EUPHORBIACEAE

5000 species in 300 genera are of cosmopolitan distribution except in the Arctic. Few species have a very wide range; the most wide-ranging genus is Euphorbia.

Chemistry is recorded by Hegnauer (1966).

Reference

Hegnauer, R. (1966) Chemotaxonomy of plants. Vol. 4. Basel. Birkhauser. P. 103.

Euphorbiaceaous plants have been incriminated in Oppenheim's meadow dermatitis (Popoff and Zaharieff 1935) but probably a combination of irritant dermatitis and sunburn is actually responsible rather than phototoxicity.

Reference

Popoff, L. and Zaharieff, B. (1935) Ueber die Dermatitis bullosa, striata und pigmentosa (Feigenbaumdermatitis) und ihre klinischen und pathogenetischen Analogien mit der Dermatitis striata pratensis Oppenheim und der Dermatitis phytogenes, striata und pigmentosa durch Euphorbiaceae hervorgerufen, Jb. Univ. Sofia Med. Fak. 14, 153. (Abstracted in in Zentralbl. f. Haut-u. Geschlectskr. 54, 21, 1937)

Acalypha Copper Leaf

450 species are found in tropical and sub-tropical regions.

Acalypha hispida
Chenile, Redhot Cat-Tail

Acalypha indica
Hierba del cancer

Acalypha wilkesiana
Beef Steak Plant

Contact with the white latex of these species can cause acute dermatitis (Souder 1963).

Reference

Souder, P. (1963) Poisonous plants on Guam. In Venomous and Poisonous animals and Noxious plants of the Pacific Region. ed. Keegan, H.L. and Macfarlane, W.V. Oxford. Pergamon Press. pp 15-29.

Acidoton

Six species are found in the

West Indies, central America and northern tropical South America.

Acidoton microphyllus

Acidoton urens

These species can produce dermatitis (Pardo-Castello 1923). A. urens has stinging hairs (Altschul 1973). The word urens means burning or stinging.

References

Altschul, S. von R. (1973) Drugs and foods from little-known plants. Cambridge, Mass. Harvard Univ. Press.

Pardo-Castello, V. (1923) Dermatitis venenata. A study of the tropical plants producing dermatitis. Arch. Derm.Syph. 7, 81.

Agrostistachys

8 or 9 species are found from India and Ceylon to western Malaysia.

Agrostistachys spp.

Small black ants, which habitually make their nests on the stems among the bases of the leaves, fiercely resent interference with their abodes (Corner 1952).

Reference

Corner, E.J.H. (1952) Wayside Trees of Malaysia. Singapore, Government Printer.

Aleurites

Two species are found in tropical Asia, Malaysia and the Pacific region.

Chemistry is discussed by Emmel (1943), Kingsbury(1964).

References

Emmel, M.W. (1943) The toxic principle of Aleurites fordii Hemsl. J. Am. Vet. Med. Ass.103, 162.

Kingsbury, J.M. (1964) Poisonous Plants of the United States and Canada. Englewood Cliffs, New Jersey. Prentice-Hall.

Aleurites fordii

Tung Oil Tree,
China Wood-oil Tree

The liquid extruded by incision of the fruit exerts a local irritant effect on the skin (Carratala 1936).

The tree is cultivated for Tung oil contained in the seeds. The oil is used in varnishes, paints, etc. Contact with Tung oil can produce skin ulcers (Anon 1934), dermatitis of the groins and face or generalized dermatitis (Tupholme 1939). According to Swaney (1938) finished tung oil varnishes are innocuous but the vapour of heated Tung oil can produce allergic contact dermatitis. A small proportion of workers handling the oil, probably only heated oil, develop dermatitis (Watt and Breyer-Brandwijk 1962). Tung oil, which is the chief paint-oil of China, is often mixed with varnish derived from Rhus verniciflua. Chronic poisoning in animals from ingestion of the plant produces, as part of the syndrome, cracking of the skin of the muzzle (Oakes and Butcher 1962).

References

Anon (1934) Tung oil seed meal useless as stock food. Agric. Gaz. New South Wales 45, 102.

Carratala, R.E. (1936) Collective intoxication by the fruit of Aleurites fordii. Dia. Med. 8, 443 (Anales asoc. quim. Argentina 26, 138) Chem. Abstr. 32, 7134. 1938.

Oakes, A.J. and Butcher, J.O. (1962) Poisonous and injurious plants of the U.S. Virgin Islands. Misc. Publ. 882. U.S. Department of Agriculture, Wasington, D.C.

Swaney, M.W. (1938) Dermatitic Properties of tung oil. Industr. Engng. Chem. 30, 514.

Tupholme, C.H.S. (1939) Dermatitis from tung oil. Brit. J. Derm. 51, 138.

Watt, J.M. and Breyer-Brandwijk, M.G. (1962) The Medicinal and poisonous plants of southern Africa. 2nd ed. Edinburgh. E. & S. Livingstone.

Aleurites moluccana
Candle Nut Tree, Indian Walnut

The nut-oil is used as a rubefacient (Burkill 1935). Contact with the latex can cause acute dermatitis (Souder 1963).

Aleurites trisperma
Soft Lumbang

If the kernel of the nut is eaten, a burning sensation is experienced in the mouth and throat. The nut-oil is said to irritate the skin and cause eruptions but it certainly does not do so consistently (Burkill 1935). Souder (1963) notes dermatitis from the sap.

References

Burkill, I.H. (1935) A Dictionary of the Economic Products of the Malay Peninsula. 2 Vols. London. Crown Agents for the Colonies.

Souder, P. (1963) Poisonous plants on Guam. In Venomous and Poisonous Animals and Noxious Plants of the Pacific Region. ed. Keegan, H.L. and Macfarlane, W.V. Oxford. Pergamon Press. pp. 15-29.

Anthostema

Three species are found in tropical Africa and Madagascar.

Anthostema aubryanum

The latex is very caustic and can cause temporary blindness (Jones and Onochie quoted by Irvine 1961).

Anthostema senegalense

The latex is strongly caustic and dangerous to the eyes (Edwardson, S.L. pers. comm. to Irvine 1961).

Reference

Irvine, F.R. (1961) Woody plants of Ghana. Oxford University Press. London.

Antidesma is transferred to Stilaginaceae.

Baliospermum

Six species are found in India, south-eastern Asia, the Malay Peninsula, Java and Sumbawa.

Baliospermum montanum
(syn. B. axillare)
Jungle Jamalgota

The leaves and the oil from the seeds are irritant (Behl et al 1966).

Reference

Behl, P.N., Captain, R.M., Bedi, B.M.S. and Gupta, S. (1966) Skin-irritant and sensitizing plants found in India, New Delhi. P.N. Behl, Irwin Hospital.

Caperonia

60 species are found in tropical America and Africa.

Caperonia palustris

This species has stinging hairs (Altschul 1973).

Reference

Altschul, S. von R. (1973) Drugs and foods from little-known plants. Cambridge, Mass. Harvard University Press.

Chamaesyce (syn. Euphorbia)

250 species are of cosmopolitan distribution.

Chamaesyce hirta

From his personal experience, Arnold (1968), in Hawaii, states that the sap is not particularly irritating to the skin.

Reference

Arnold, H.L. (1968) Poisonous Plants of Hawaii. Rutland, Vermont. Charles E. Tuttle.

Chiropetalum
(syn. Argithamnia)

25 species are found from Mexico to South America.

Chiropetalum griseum

The plant has irritant effects on contact with the skin (Altschul 1973).

Reference

Altschul, S. von R. (1973) Drugs and

foods from little-known plants. Cambridge, Mass. Harvard University Press.

Claoxylon

80 species are found in palaeotropical regions.

Claoxylon marianum
Panao, Cator

Souder (1963) on Guam Island states that contact with the sap of this plant can produce acute dermatitis.

Reference

Souder, P. (1963) Poisonous plants on Guam. In Venomous and Poisonous Animals and Noxious Plants of the Pacific Region. ed. Keegan, H.L. and Macfarlane, W.V. Oxford. Pergamon Press. pp. 15-29.

Clutia

70 species are found in Africa and Arabia.

Clutia pulchella

The juice of the plant produces irritant effects (Watt and Breyer-Brandwijk 1962).

Reference

Watt, J.M. and Breyer-Brandwijk, M.G. (1962) The Medicinal and poisonous plants of Southern Africa. 2nd ed. Edinburgh. E. & S. Livingstone.

Cnesmone

10 species in Assam, southern China, south-eastern Asia and western Malaysia are climbing shrubs.

Cnesmone javanica

Cnesmone subpeltata

These climbing plants possess irritant hairs and are known to produce skin reactions in Malaya, (Kochummen 1972).

Reference

Kochummen, K.M. (1972) Forest Botanist. Forest Research Institute. Kepong, Selangor, Malaya. Personal communication.

Cnesmone spp.

Stinging hairs are known in species of this genus (Thurston and Lersten 1969).

Reference

Thurston, E.L. and Lersten, N.R. (1969) The morphology and toxicology of plant stinging hairs. Botan. Rev. 35, 393.

Cnidoscolus
Spurge Nettle

75 species are native to tropical America.

Cnidoscolus stimulosus
Tread-softly, Bull-nettle

This species, found in dry sandy woods, fields and sandhills from Florida to Texas and north to Virginia, has stinging bristles (Fernald 1970).

The word scolops means prickle or sting. Urticaria can arise from contact with the plant (Hardin and Arena 1969). Altschul (1973) notes stinging hairs of C. angustidens, C. multilobus, C. tubulosus, C. urens, C. cnicodendron, C. longipes, C. vitifolius and that the latex of some species is caustic.

References

Altschul, S. von R. (1973) Drugs and foods from little-known plants. Cambridge, Mass. Harvard Univ. Press.

Fernald, M.L. (1970) Gray's Manual of Botany. 8th ed. New York. Van Nostrand Reinhold.

Hardin, J.W. & Arena, J.M. (1960) Human Poisoning from Native and cultivated plants. Durham, North Carolina. Duke University Press.

Codiaeum

15 species are found in Malaysia, Polynesia and northern Australia.

Codiaeum variegatum
'Croton'

This species is cultivated for its coloured leaves. The plants, usually known as 'crotons', are also used as hedges. This genus is not to be confused with Croton. Different leaf forms and colour variations often appear on the same plant owing to genetic instability. The young leaves of certain of the yellow varieties are eaten as flavouring; old leaves irritate the mouth because their acridity increases with age (Brown 1960). The bark and roots are acrid and cause burning in the mouth if chewed. Although mature leaves may be irritant, the plant is rarely a cause of dermatitis despite much handling of foliage for decoration and of cuttings for propagation (Morton 1962). Souder (1963) refers to dermatitis from the plant and Allen (1943) stated that handling of, or even proximity to the plant in Panama, can produce dermatitis resembling erysipelas in many individuals. A positive patch test to the leaf was observed in one patient (Agrup 1969). A colourless liquid which bleeds from the broken leaf stem stains white cloth to a brownish colour which increases in darkness when the fabric is wetted; these markings have been mistaken for blood-stains (Brown 1960).

A flower grower who had hyperkeratotic eczema localized to the tips of the thumbs and index fingers showed positive patch test reactions to the leaf and stalk of the plant, negative in five controls. The sensitizer seemed to be soluble in water but not in alcohol (Tafelkruyer and van Ketel 1976).

References

Agrup, G. (1969) Hand eczema and other hand dermatoses in South Sweden. Acta derm.-venereol. 49 Suppl. 61. pp. 1-91.

Allen, P.H. (1943) Poisonous and Injurious Plants of Panama. Am. J. Trop. Med. Suppl. 23, 1.

Brown, B.F. (1960) Florida's Beautiful Crotons. American Codiaeum Society. Eau Gallie, Florida. Undersea Press.

Morton, J.F. (1962) Ornamental Plants with Poisonous Properties II. Proc. Florida Hort. Soc. 75, 484.

Souder, P. (1963) Poisonous plants on Guam. In Venomous and Poisonous Animals and Noxious Plants of the Pacific Region. ed. Keegan, H.L. and Macfarlane, W.V. Oxford. Pergamon Press. pp. 15-29.

Tafelkruyer, J. and van Ketel, W.G. (1976) Sensitivity to Codiaeum variegatum. Contact Dermatitis 2, 288.

The plant can produce allergic contact dermatitis (Schmidt and Olholm-Larsen 1977).

Reference

Schmidt, H. and Olholm-Larsen, P. (1977) Allergic contact dermatitis from croton (Codiaeum). Contact Dermatitis 3, 100.

Codiaeum

Soejarto et al (1977) pointed out confusion in the botanical nomenclature of Schmidt and Olholm-Larsen (1977) and suggested that Croton was implicated.

Reference

Soejarto, D.D., Kinghorn, A.D. and Farnsworth, N.R. (1977) Letter to editor. Contact Dermatitis 3, 276.

The plant was, in fact, Codiaeum (Schmidt and Larsen 1978).

Reference

Schmidt, H. and Larsen, P.O. (1978) Letter to the Editor. Contact Dermatitis 4, 113.

Codiaeum variegatum var pictum (syn. Croton variegatus)

The plant produced allergic contact dermatitis in a gardener (Hausen and Schulz 1977).

Reference

Hausen, B.M. and Schulz, K.H. (1977) Occupational contact dermatitis due to Croton (Codiaeum variegatum

(L.) A. Juss var. pictum (Lodd.) Muell. Arg.) Contact Dermatitis 3, 289.

Colliguaja

Five species are found in temperate South America.

Colliguaja odorifera

This species is said to be irritant (Schwartz et al 1957).

Reference

Schwartz, L., Tulipan, L. and Birmingham, D.J. (1957) Occupational Diseases of the Skin. 3rd. ed. Philadelphia. Lea & Febiger. pp. 637-672.

Croton

750 species are found in tropical and sub-tropical regions. C. cascarilla and C. eluteria yield cascarilla bark, used as a tonic and to scent tobacco (Nicotiana). C. laccifer yields a lac used in varnish-making. Several Brazilian species yield a dragon's-blood resin see Dracaena. Crotons of horticulture are of the genus Codiaeum.

Croton astroites
Maran

The plant possesses toxic properties similar to those reported for C. tiglium (Oakes and Butcher 1962). They stated that croton oils are concentrated in the seeds but also occur in the stems and leaves.

Croton capitatus
Hogwort

The plant can produce dermatitis (Shelmire 1940) and is described as an infrequent sensitizer. An extract of the plant produced a positive patch test reaction in one of 50 patients who had 'weed dermatitis' (Shelmire 1939).

Croton ciliato-glandulosa

The plant is said to irritate the eyes (Altschul 1973).

Croton cortesianus Pozual

The juice is caustic (Martinez 1969).

References

Altschul, S. von R. (1973) Drugs and foods from little-known plants. Cambridge, Mass. Harvard Univ. Press.

Martinez, M. (1969) The Medicinal Plants of Mexico. 5th ed. Mexico City. Andres Botas.

Oakes, J.J. and Butcher, J.O. (1962) Poisonous and injurious plants of the U.S. Virgin Islands. Misc. Publ. 882. U.S. Dept. of Agriculture. Washington, D.C.

Shelmire, B. (1939) Contact Dermatitis from Weeds; Patch testing with their oleoresins. JAMA 113, 1085.

Shelmire, B. (1940) Contact dermatitis from vegetation. South Med. J. 33, 338.

Croton gratissimus

The bark has irritant properties (Watt and Breyer-Brandwijk 1962).

Croton gubouga

A burning sensation in the mouth and throat is produced by chewing the seeds (Watt and Breyer-Brandwijk 1962).

Croton megalocarpus
Musine

The wood has been used for flooring in England. Its fresh wood has an objectionable smell and the sawdust irritates the nose and throat of some workmen (Anon 1951 cited by Woods and Calnan 1976). These authors may be referring to Anon (1957) since Anon (1951) is not listed in their references.

References

Anon (1957) Wood dust and the woodworker. Timber Technology 65, 205.

Woods, B. and Calnan, C.D. (1976) Toxic Woods. Brit. J. Derm. 94, Suppl. 13, June.

Croton monanthogynus

Shelmire (1940) stated that

the plant was an infrequent sensitizer. An extract of the plant produced negative patch test reactions in 50 patients who had 'weed dermatitis' (Shelmire 1939).

Croton sylvaticus

A burning sensation in the mouth and throat is produced by chewing the seeds (Watt and Breyer-Brandwijk 1962).

References

Shelmire, B. (1939) Contact dermatitis from weeds: Patch testing with their oleoresins. JAMA 113, 1085.

Shelmire, B. (1940) Contact dermatitis from vegetation. South Med. J. 33, 338.

Watt, J.M. and Breyer-Brandwijk, M.G. (1962) The Medicinal and poisonous plants of Southern Africa. 2nd ed. Edinburgh. E. & S. Livingstone.

Croton tiglium

The smoke from the burning wood irritates the eyes (Burkill 1935). The seeds have been employed for self-mutilation by malingerers (Duke-Elder and MacFaul 1972). The bark exudes a kino (astringent tannin). The plant seems to vary in toxicity in various districts. The oil becomes less irritating with aging by the action of a ferment within the seeds (Burkill 1935).

Croton oil

Oleum tiglii derived from the seeds was rubbed on a bald scalp as an irritant 'hair-producing' application (White 1887). The blistering effect of the oil is used in indigenous medicine (Quisumbing 1951).

Croton oil has been largely abandoned as a purgative in medical and veterinary practice as too violent in its action; it is employed to lubricate machinery. Its use as a counter-irritant by application and by pricking it into the skin for pulmonary disease, a process called "Baunscheitismus", fell into disuse (White 1887). Over 5000 pounds were imported into the United States in 1878 but, in 1883, only 300 pounds. The oil blisters the mucous membrane of the mouth; absorption of the irritant principle through the skin can produce a purgative action (Burkill 1935). Croton oil is used for illumination but only outdoors since the fumes of the burning oil are irritant to the eyes and intolerable (Burkill 1935).

Croton oil produces an erythematous or vesico-pustular reaction when applied to the skin depending on the amount applied and the duration of application (White 1887); folliculitis may also occur (Carvalho 1956). The action of croton oil was compared with that of some other irritants by Bjornberg (1968); 0.2% of croton oil in vaseline was found to produce erythema. A detailed histopathological study of the effects of croton oil on the skin was made by Bandmann (1960). Electron microscope studies of croton oil dermatitis were carried out by Metz (1972).

Phytochemistry

Although croton oil has been extensively used as an irritant and as a co-carcinogen (Berenblum 1941), its chemistry is not well-defined. According to Burkill (1935) a substance in the seeds, crotin, is a compound closely allied to ricin of castor oil (Ricinus) and to abrin of Abrus. The toxic principles are crotin, croton resin (Osol and Farrar 1955) and ricinine (Willaman and Schubert 1961). The fraction of the oil which is soluble in alcohol contains the skin irritant principle; the residue retains its purgative properties but is not vesicant (Anon 1965).

Croton oil has skin tumour-enhancing properties; identification of the active principles of croton oil has revealed two compounds (A and B) which together account for its toxic, inflammatory and co-carcinogenic properties. Compound A consists of a highly active compound (A_1) with a molecular formula $C_{36}H_{56}O_8$ which has been partially characterized as a non-aromatic compound with an α,β-unsaturated carbonyl group and three free and two esterified (acetate + myristate) hydroxyl groups, and an inactive compound (A_2). A partial structure for A_1 has been proposed.

Compound B consists of three components. Two of these (B_1 and B_2) are esters of the diterpenoid alcohol $C_{20}H_{28}O_6$; both B_1 and B_2 show high and comparable inflammatory activity compared with A_1.

Croton resin, the vesicant fraction of a croton seed extract, yielded a hydrogenation product with a proposed partial structure which is a fatty acid ester of a polyphenol containing 2-methylbutyric, capric and lauric acids.

This hydrogenation product may possibly be a mixture of the components B_1 and B_2. It is of interest that the partial structure proposed is similar to that of the long-chain olefinic catechols of Toxicodendron (Anon 1965).

References

Anon (1965) Probing deeper into croton oil. Food and Cosmetics Toxicol. 3, 339.

Bandmann, H.J. (1960) Contributions to the histopathology of allergic epicutaneous text reactions. Part 1. Allergic contact eczema and the epicutaneous patch test with previous research in the histopathology of reactions caused in the patch test. Hautarzt 11, 258, and 355.

Berenblum, I. (1941) The cocarcinogenic action of croton resin. Cancer. Res. 1, 44.

Björnberg, A. (1968) Skin reactions to primary irritants in patients with hand eczema. Goteborg. Oscar Isacson.

Burkill, I.H. (1935) A Dictionary of the Economic Products of the Malay Peninsula. 2 Vols. London. Crown Agents for the Colonies.

Carvalho de, L.P. (1956) Occupational contact allergens. Brasil-med. 70, 77.

Duke-Elder, S. and MacFaul, P.A. (1972) System of Opthalmology. Vol. XIV. Injuries Part. 1. Mechanical Injuries. Extra-ocular foreign bodies pp. 464-67 and agricultural injuries pp. 32-34. London. Henry Kimpton.

Metz, J. (1972) Electron microscopkal studies on allergic and toxic skin test reactions in humans. Arch. Derm. Forsch. 245, 125.

Osol, A. and Farrar, G.E. (1955) The Dispensatory of the United States of America. 25th ed. Philadelphia. Lippincott.

Quisumbing, E. (1951) Medicinal plants of the Philippines. Tech. Bull. 16. Manila. Philippine Islands. Manila Bureau of Printing. 1234 pp.

White, J.C. (1887) Dematitis venenata: An account of the action of external irritants upon the skin. Boston. Cupples and Hurd.

Willaman, J.J. and Schubert, B.G. (1961) Alkaloid-bearing plants and their contained alkaloids. U.S. Dep. of Agr. Tech. Bull. 1234.

Dalechampia

100 species are found in warm regions, especially in America.

Dalechampia dioscoreaefolia

Dalechampia ipomoeaefolia

Dalechampia panamensis

Dalachampia scandens

Dalechampia tiliaefolia

The plants possess stiff stinging hairs (Allen 1943, Altschul 1973).

References

Allen, P.H. (1943) Poisonous and injurious plants of Panama. Am. J. Trop. Med. Suppl. 23, 1.

Altschul, S. von R. (1973) Drugs and foods from little-known plants. Cambridge, Mass. Harvard Univ. Press.

Drypetes (syn. Putranjiva)

200 species are found in tropical regions, also in southern Africa and sub-tropical eastern Asia.

Drypetes pendula Sabre Leaf

Ants eat out the pith and live in the leaf twigs (Corner 1952).

Putranjiva roxburghii

The seeds contain thioglucosides from which irritant mustard oils are derived (see Cruciferae).

Reference

Corner, E.J.H. (1952) Wayside Trees of Malaysia. Singapore, Government Printer.

Elaeophorbia (syn. Euphorbia)

Five species are found in tropical and southern Africa.

Elaeophorbia drupifera

The latex, which causes considerable swelling if rubbed on the skin, is used to remove warts. It is dangerous to the eyes and can cause blindness (Oliver 1959, Irvine 1961).

Elaeophorbia grandifolia

This species contains caustic latex (Irvine 1961).

References

Irvine, F.R. (1961) Woody plants of Ghana. Oxford University Press. London.

Oliver, B. (1959) Nigeria's Useful Plants. Nigerian Field. Part II (2) 24, 54; 121.

Endospermum

12 or 13 species are found in south-eastern Asia, Malaysia and Fiji.

Endospermum moluccanum
Moon Tree

Contact with the sap causes acute dermatitis (Souder 1963).

Reference

Souder, P. (1963) Poisonous plants on Guam. In Venomous and Poisonous Animals and Noxious Plants of the Pacific Region. ed. Keegan, H.L. and Macfarlane, W.V. Oxford. Pergamon Press. pp. 15-29.

Euphorbia

2000 cosmopolitan species are chiefly found in subtropical and warm temperate regions. The genus is named for Euphorbus, physician of King Juba of Numidia. The culture of all the more interesting succulent plants has become an increasingly popular hobby in recent years.

Botanical descriptions of the succulent species of the genus are provided by Jacobsen (1960). Some are xerophytic and can produce mechanical injury by their spines (Oakes and Butcher 1962). The xerophytic species of Euphorbia resemble cacti but can be distinguished by their milky latex. Corner (1952) refers to cactus spines as being set in tufts whereas the spines of Euphorbia, when present, are in pairs.

Chamaesyce (syn. Euphorbia)

Elaeophorbia (syn. Euphorbia)

Tithymalus (syn. Euphorbia)

References

Corner, E.J.H. (1952) Wayside trees of Malaysia. Singapore, Government Printer.

Jacobsen, H. (1960) A Handbook of Succulent Plants. London. Blandford. p. 393.

Oakes, A.J. and Butcher, J.O. (1962) Poisonous and injurious plants of the U.S. Virgin Islands. Misc. Publ. 882. U.S. Dept. of Agriculture. Washington, D.C.

Euphorbia spp. Spurge

Theophrastus in the Fourth Century B.C. noted that the juice of the spurge could blind animals or even a man. Culpeper (1653) wrote of the irritant effect of spurges which "abound with a hot and acrid juice, which when applied outwardly, eats away warts and other excresences".

The milky latex is powerfully irritant to the skin and eyes and is used by Indian villagers to remove warts and as a rubefacient (Behl et al 1966). Application of juice, powder and extracts of the plant produces irritation, pustulation and even gangrene (Loudon 1855 and Van Hasselt 1882 cited by White 1887).

The irritant action of the

plants was reported by Lewis (1922), Mesa (1945), Williams (1949) Touton (1932), Brown (1954), Heyne (1950), Lipparoni(1951), North (1967), Morton (1958), Watt and Breyer-Brandwijk (1962). In Europe the plants are commonly called Wolf's milk (Wolfsmilch). Some 50 Euphorbia spp. said to have irritant properties were listed by Pammel (1911). Euphorbia juice is an ingredient of an arrow poison used by Bushmen in South Africa; it contains an irritant resin but it is probably used principally as a cement to fix onto the arrowhead other agents such as Acokanthera which are systemic poisons. E. lathyris is supposed to have been the active ingredient of the slow-acting poison employed by Catarina Sforza (1463-1509) (Raymond 1939).

Youngken (1948) and Connor and Adams (1951) refer to the chemistry of the irritant substances.

Noors honey is honey containing the nectar of Euphorbia spp. Such honey produces a hot, burning sensation in the mouth and throat which is increased rather than decreased by drinking water. The nectar of E. ingens, E. ledienii, E. triangularis, E. virosa and possibly E. cooperi, when incorporated into honey by bees, produces such irritant effects (Watt and Breyer-Brandwijk 1962). Morton (1964) discussed this topic also.

References

Behl, P.N., Captain, R.M., Bedi, B.M.S. and Gupta, S. (1966) Skin-irritant and sensitizing plants found in India, New Delhi. P.N. Behl, Irwin Hospital.

Biology Data Book (1964) ed. Altman, P.L. and Dittmer, D.S. Federation of American Societies for Experimental Biology. Washington, D.C.

Brown, W.H. (1954) Useful plants of the Phillipines. Tech. Bull. No. 10. Dept. of Agriculture and Natural Resources. Manila.

Corner, H.E. and Adams, N.M. (1951) New Zealand Dept. Sci. Ind. Res. Bull. 99, quoted by Biology Data Book (1964).

Culpeper, N. (1653) The Complete Herbal. Edition 1953. Birmingham, Kynoch Press.

Heyne, K. (1950) De nuttige Planten van Indonesie. ed. 3. N.V. Vitgeverijw, Wageningen, Netherlands:van Hoeve's Gravenhage Bandung.

Lewis, H. (1922) Some observations on South African toxicology. South. Afr. Med. Rec. 20, 350.

Loudon (1855) citedby White (1887).

Mesa, J.T. (1945) Plantes medicinales, aromaticas o venenosas de Cuba. Havana.

Morton, J.F. (1958) Ornamental plants with poisonous properties. Proc. Florida State Hort. Soc. 71,372.

Morton, J.F. (1964) Honeybee plants of South Florida. Proc. Florida State Hort. Soc. 77, 415.

Morton, J.F. (1972) Personal communication.

Lipparoni, E. (1951) Dermatitis due to ticks and vegetable substances. Arch. et al Sci. Med. Trop. 32, 913.

North, P.M. (1967) Poisonous plants and fungi in colour. London. Blandford Press.

Pammel, L.H. (1911) A manual of poisonous plants. Torch Press. Cedar Rapids, Iowa. Reprinted Univ. Microfilms Inc. Ann Arbor, Mich. 1965. pp. 476-7.

Raymond, W.D. (1939) Native poisons and native medicines of Tanganyika. J. Trop. Med. Hyg. 42, 295.

Touton, K. (1932) Hauterkrankungen durch phanerogamische Pflanzen und ihre Produkte (Toxicodermia et Allergodermia phytogenes), in Barnwitz, J. et al Angeborene Anomalien, Lichtdermatosen, Pflanzengifte, Thermische Schädidgungen, Einfluss Innerer Störungen auf die Haut. Berlin, Verlag von Julius Springer.

Van Hasselt (1882) cited by White (1887).

Watt, J.M. and Breyer-Brandwijk, M.G. (1962) The medicinal and poisonous plants of Southern Africa. 2nd ed. Edinburgh. E. &

S. Livingstone.

White, J.C. (1887) Dermatitis venenata: An account of the action of external irritants upon the skin. Boston. Cupples and Hurd.

Williams, R.O. (1949) Useful and Ornamental Plants in Zanzibar and Pemba, Zanzibar. Zanzibar Protectorate Gov't. Printer.

Youngken, H.W. (1948) Textbook of Pharmacognosy. Ed. b. Philadelphia. Blackiston.

Euphorbia abyssinica

The plant is used as a caustic on skin lesions (Watt and Breyer-Brandwijk 1962).

Reference

Watt, J.M. and Breyer-Brandwijk, M.G. (1962) The medicinal and poisonous plants of Southern Africa. 2nd ed. Edinburgh. E. & S. Livingstone.

Euphorbia acaulis
(syn. *E. fusiformis*)

The plant is irritant (Behl et al 1966) and the latex has been used in the treatment of chronic eczema for a mild irritant action (Agrawal et al 1971).

References

Agrawal, D.K. et al (1971) Clinical studies of *Euphorbia acaulis* Roxb. in cases of eczema. Indian. J. Derm. 16, 57.

Behl, P.N., Captain, R.M., Bedi, B.M.S. and Gupta, S. (1966). Skin-irritant and sensitizing plants found in India, New Delhi. P.N. Behl, Irwin Hospital.

Watt, J.M. and Breyer-Brandwijk, M.G. (1962) The medicinal and Poisonous plants of Southern Africa. 2nd ed. Edinburgh. E. & S. Livingstone.

Euphorbia antiquorum

In Malaya, this species forms a spiny cactus-like shrub or tree up to 4.5 m. in height (Corner 1952). The latex is irritant to the skin (Burkill 1935, Behl et al 1966) and blindness is reported from its contact with the eyes (Souder 1963).

References

Behl, P.N., Captain, R.M., Bedi, B.M.S. and Gupta, S. (1966). Skin-irritant and sensitizing plants found in India, New Delhi. P.N. Behl. Irwin Hospital.

Burkill, I.H. (1935) A dictionary of the economic products of the Malay Peninsula. 2 vols. London. Crown Agents for the Colonies.

Corner, E.J.H. (1952) Wayside trees of Malaysia. Singapore. Government Printer.

Souder, P. (1963) Poisonous plants on Guam. In venomous and poisonous animals and noxious plants of the Pacific Region. ed. Keegan, H.L. and Macfarlane, W.V. Oxford. Pergamon Press. pp. 15-29.

Euphorbia antisyphilitica

This species is irritant (Schwartz et al 1957).

Reference

Schwartz, L., Tulipan, L. and Birmingham, D.J. (1957) Occupational diseases of the skin. 3rd ed. Philadelphia. Lea and Febiger. pp. 637-672.

Euphorbia balsamifera
Balsam Spurge

The latex is corrosive (Aubréville 1936, 1950).

References

Aubréville, A. (1936) La Flore Forestière de la Côte d'Ivoire. 3 vols. Paris.

Aubréville, A. (1950) Flore forestière soudano-guineene. Afrique occidentale francaise (A.O.F.) Cameroun-Afrique équatoriale francaise (A.E.F.) Paris cited by Irvine (1961).

Irvine, F.R. (1961) Woody plants of Ghana. Oxford University Press. London.

Euphorbia calyculata

The juice produces swelling and itching of the skin (Martinez

1969).

Reference

Martinez, M. (1969) The medicinal plants of Mexico. 5th ed. Mexico City. Andres Botas.

Euphorbia candelabrum

The wood produced dermatitis in workers who used in to make caskets in Somalia (Lipparoni 1951).

Reference

Lipparoni, E. (1951) Dermatiti da zecche e dermatiti da sostange vegetali. Archivio italiano di Scienze Mediche Tropicali 32, 913.

Euphorbia caput-medusae

The latex is said to be highly acrid and irritant (Watt and Breyer-Brandwijk 1962).

Reference

Watt, J.M. and Breyer-Brandwijk, M.G. (1962) The medicinal and poisonous plants of Southern Africa. 2nd ed. Edinburgh. E. & S. Livingstone.

Euphorbia cattimando
(syn. E. trigona)

This species is irritant (Behl et al 1966).

Reference

Behl, P.N., Captain, R.M., Bedi, B.M.S. and Gupta, S. (1966) Skin-irritant and sensitizing plants found in India, New Delhi. P.N. Behl, Irwin Hospital.

Euphorbia chamissonis
Beach Spurge

This species is irritant (Souder 1963).

Reference

Souder, P. (1963) Poisonous Plants on Guam. In venomous and poisonous animals and noxious plants of the Pacific Region. ed. Keegan, H.L. and Macfarlane, W.V. Oxford. Pergamon Press. pp.15-29

Euphorbia cooperi

This species is a tree-like succulent grown as a garden plant in Australia and often called a cactus but with copious milky sap and no spines. The latex is irritant to the skin and eyes; washing with water will not remove the irritant latex (Everist 1962). The latex is so irritant that a slight smear on the face or tender skin produces a blister within a short time. The latex is also irritant to the eyes and can produce blindness. If a person stands in close proximity to a bleeding plant, inhalation of the air from the neighbourhood produces a burning sensation in the throat (Watt and Breyer-Brandwijk 1962).

References

Everist, S.L. (1962) These plants can poison people. Queensland Agric. J. 88, 235.

Watt, J.M. and Breyer-Brandwijk, M.G. (1962) The medicinal and poisonous plants of Southern Africa. 2nd ed. Edinburgh. E. & S. Livingstone.

Euphorbia corollata
Snakemilk

The juice produces vesication (Gray 1870 cited by White in 1887). Coulter (1906) carried out an irritancy test for human skin with a positive result.

References

Coulter, S. (1904) Poisonous Plants of Indiana. Proc. Indiana Acad. Sci. 51-63.

Gray (1870) cited by White (1887)

White, J.C. (1887) Dermatitis venenata: An account of the action of external irritants upon the skin. Boston. Cupples and Hurd.

Euphorbia cotinifolia
Red Spurge

This central American species is condemned as poisonous but is extensively planted for hedges in Guatemala city (Standley 1927). The foliage causes blisters in animals who eat it, except in goats (Blohm 1962). The sap produces inflammation and blistering of the skin (Blohm 1962). Because of its attractive dark-red foliage, this shrub was introduced into the nursery trade in Florida but somr who planted it as a hedge had it removed because it was a prime contact poison. Simply touching the leaves can produce an overall rash in 'sensitive' individuals. The milky sap is highly irritant, commonly producing inflammation and blistering and, in the eye, at least temporary blindness (Morton 1962).

References

Blohm, H. (1962) Poisonous plants of Venezuela. Cambridge, Mass. Harvard University Press.

Morton, J.F. (1962) Ornamental plants with poisonous properties II. Proc. Florida Hort. Soc. 75, 484.

Standley, P.C. (1927) Poisonous trees of Central America. Tropical Woods 9, 3.

Euphorbia cyathophora
Dwarf Poinsettia

This species is irritant to the mucous surfaces (Everist 1972) and to the skin (Souder 1963). Arnold (1968) stated that this plant and also P. geniculata had varying degrees of the toxicity of the well-known E. pulcherrima.

References

Arnold, H.L. (1968) Poisonous plants of Hawaii. Rutland, Vermont. Charles E. Tuttle.

Everist, S.L. (1972) Queensland Herbarium, Brisbane, Australia. Personal communication concerning plants recorded in Australia as having caused dermatitis or other contact injury to man or livestock.

Souder, P. (1963) Poisonous plants on Guam. In venomous and poisonous animals and noxious plants of the Pacific Region. ed. Keegan, H.L. and Macfarlane, W.V. Oxford. Pergamon Press. pp. 15-29.

Euphorbia deightonii
(syn. E. kamerunica)

This thorny plant which grows to 6 m in height has caustic latex (Dalziel 1937, Irvine 1961).

References

Dalziel, J.M. (1937) The useful plants of west tropical Africa. London. Crown Agents.

Irvine, F.R. (1961) Woody plants of Ghana. Oxford University Press. London.

Euphorbia drummondii
Caustic weed, Milk weed

There is conflicting data concerning the effects of this plant. Apparently the fresh milky sap is considered by Australian bushmen to possess great healing qualities for they make constant use of it (Hurst 1942). She stated that the head of a sheep, which has eaten the plant, swells to an enormous extent and becomes so heavy that the animal cannot support it. Eating the flesh of pigeons which have fed on the fruit of the plant causes sickness in man (Cleland 1914). Orchard (1954) states that the plant was irritant to human skin but Stanley (1896) found that the latex had no caustic or even irritant action on the eye of the sheep or dog.

References

Cleland, J.B. (1914) Plants, including fungi, poisonous or otherwise injurious to man in Australia. Australian Med. Gaz. 35, 569. idem. Tasmanian Ag. Gaz. 32, 361 and 401.

Hurst, E. (1942) The Poison Plants of New South Wales. N.S.W. Poison Plants Committee, Sydney.

Orchard, H.E. (1954) Snow-on-the-Mountain (Euphorbia marginata Pursh.) J. Agric. South Australia 57, 337.

Stanley, E. (1896) Euphorbia drummondii. Agr. Gaz. New South Wales. 7, 619

Euphorbia esculenta

This plant and also E. hamata are used as animal fodder suggesting that they are not strongly irritant (Jacobsen 1960).

Reference

Jacobsen, H. (1960) A Handbook of Succulent Plants. Vol. I. London.

Blandford. p. 394.

Euphorbia esula
Wolf's Milk

The word esula is from the Celtic, esu, and refers to the acrid milky juice (Fernald 1970).

Reference

Fernald, M.L. (1970) Gray's Manual of Botany. 8th ed. New York. Van Nostrand Reinhold Co.

Euphorbia exigua
Dwarf Spurge

This species is irritant (North 1967).

Reference

North, P.M. (1967) Poisonous plants and fungi in colour. London. Blandford Press. Ltd.

Euphorbia fulgens

Two cases of dermatitis occurred from contact with this plant (Hausen, B.M. 1974, pers. comm.).

Inhalation of the pollen can cause occupational allergy (Hausen et al 1976).

Reference

Hausen, B.M. et al (1976) Berufsbedingte Inhalations - allergie durch pollen von Euphorbia fulgens Karw. Deutsch. med. Wochen. 101, 567.
See also E. pulcherrima.

Euphorbia genistoides

This species is irritant to the skin of sheep (Watt and Breyer-Brandwijk 1962).

Reference

Watt, J.M. and Breyer-Brandwijk, M.G. (1962) The Medicinal and poisonous plants of Southern Africa. 2nd ed. Edinburgh. E. & S. Livingstone.

Euphorbia gomerifera

Contact with the latex produces acute dermatitis (Souder 1963).

Reference

Souder, P. (1963) Poisonous plants on Guam. In venomous and poisonous animals and noxious plants of the Pacific Region. ed. Keegan, H.L. and Macfarlane, W.V. Oxford. Pergamon Press. pp. 15-29

Euphorbia gorgonis

The latex is used as a styptic (Watt and Breyer-Brandwijk 1962).

Reference

Watt, J.M. and Breyer-Brandwijk, M.G. (1972) The Medicinal and poisonous plants of Southern Africa. 2nd ed. Edinburgh. E. & S. Livingstone.

Euphorbia grandidens

This species is thought to be capable of producing irritation of the skin and blindness (Watt and Breyer-Brandwijk 1962).

Reference

Watt, J.M. and Breyer-Brandwijk, M.G. (1962) The medicinal and poisonous plants of Southern Africa. 2nd ed. Edinburgh. E. & S. Livingstone.

Euphorbia grantii
(syn. Synadenium grantii)

The plant is irritant to the skin and eyes (Raymond 1939).

Reference

Raymond, W.D. (1939) Native poisons and native medicines of Tanganyika. J. Trop. Med. Hyg. 42, 295.

Euphorbia guadichaudii

Contact with the latex produces acute dermatitis (Souder 1963).

Reference

Souder, P. (1963) Poisonous plants on Guam. In venomous and poisonous animals and noxious plants of the Pacific Region. ed. Keegan, H.L. and Macfarlane, W.V. Oxford. Pergamon Press. pp.15-29.

Euphorbia helioscopia
Sun Spurge, Wolf's Milk, Wartweed

Severe kerato-conjunctivitis can result in man from exposure of the eye to this plant but, experimentally, rabbits were not susceptible (Guggenheim 1926). Cleland (1931) received a report that this species caused dermatitis when handled. Varca (1937) reported two cases of a diffuse itching eruption on the face, neck and forearms after contact with the plant. The plant was suspected of causing acute dermatitis in cows (Hurst 1942). Watt and Breyer-Brandwijk (1962) cite various authors who stated that the plant is irritant and vesicant to the hands and face and that severe ulceration of the skin has followed application of a poultice of the bruised plant. Some children who played with the plant in New South Wales developed blisters followed by permanent scars on their faces (Mair 1968). Formerly the juice was used for treating warts on the fingers; blistering of the lips and tongue occurred if the fingers were subsequently sucked (North 1967).

References

Cleland, J.B. (1931) Plants including fungi, poisonous or otherwise injurious to man in Australia III. Med. J. Australia 2, 775.

Guggenheim, I. (1926) Bindehaut-und Hornhautentzundung durch Sart der Euphorbia helioscopa (Wolfmilch). Klin. Mbl. Augenheilk 77, 521.

Hurst, E. (1942) The poison plants of New South Wales. N.S.W. Poison Plants Committee; Sydney.

Mair, K. (1968) cited personal communication to himself from F.C. Morris, District Agronomist, Mudgee, N.S.W.

North, P.M. (1967) Poisonous plants and fungi in colour. London. Blandford Press. Ltd.

Varca, C. (1937) Dermatitis due to euphorbia. Boll. occ. region Soc. ital. dermat. 1, 29.

Euphorbia heterophylla
(syn. Poinsettia heterophylla)
Painted Leaf, Wild Poinsettia, Mexican Fire plant.

This plant, a common native weed of Florida, has an abundant milky sap which is irritant (Morton 1962) and can produce dermatitis (Allen 1943, Orchard 1954, Pope 1968). The latex of the plant is used as an antidote for the irritation produced by other species of Euphorbia; since the leaf and the acrid latex is poisonous, it is difficult to know why such therapy sould be efficacious (Watt and Breyer-Brandwijk 1962).

References

Allen, P.H. (1943) Poisonous and injurious plants of Panama. Am. J. Trop. Med. Suppl. 23, 1

Morton, J.F. (1962) Ornamental plants with poisonous properties II. Proc. Florida Hort. Soc. 75, 484.

Orchard, H.E. (1954) Snow-on-the-Mountain (Euphorbia marginata Pursh.). J. Agric. South Australia. 57, 337.

Pope, W.T. (1968) Manual of wayside plants of Hawaii. Rutland, Vermont. Chales E. Tuttle Co.

Watt, J.M. and Breyer-Brandwijk, M.G. (1962) The Medicinal and poisonous plants of Southern Africa. 2nd ed. Edinburgh. E. & S. Livingstone.

Euphorbia hirta
(syn. E. pilulifera)
Asthma plant, Hairy Spurge

The first common name is derived from the use of a tea made from the dried plant for the relief of asthma (Wren 1968). The sap can cause dermatitis (Pammel 1911, Watt and Breyer-Brandwijk 1962, Souder 1963, Behl et al 1966). This species is a common lawn weed in Florida and gardeners who pull it can develop dermatitis of the hands, particularly of the sides of the fingers (Morton 1972).

References

Behl, P.N., Captain, R.M., Bedi, B.M.S. and Gupta, S. (1966) Skin-irritant and sensitizing plants found in India, New Delhi. P.N. Behl, Irwin Hospital.

Morton, J.F. (1972) Personal communication.

Pammel, L.H. (1911) A Manual of Poisonous plants. Torch Press.

Cedar Rapids, Iowa. Reprinted University Microfilms Inc. Ann Arbor, Mich. 1965. pp. 476-7.

Souder, P. (1963) Poisonous plants on Guam. In venomous and poisonous animals and noxious plants of the Pacific Regions. ed. Keegan, H.L. and Macfarlane, W.V. Oxford. Pergamon Press. pp. 15-29.

Watt, J.M. and Breyer-Brandwijk, M.G. (1962) The medicinal and poisonous plants of Southern Africa. 2nd ed. Edinburgh. E. & S. Livingstone.

Wren, R.W. (1968) Potter's New Cyclopaedia of Botanical Drugs and Preparations by Wren, R.C. Reedit. by Wren, R.W. Potter and Clarke Ltd. Health Science Press. Rustington, Sussex.

Euphorbia hoffmanniana

This species is abundant in central Costa Rica, especially in fence rows, and was said to cause swelling and inflammation but Standley (1927) observed that poeple seemed to pay little attention to the shrub and he did not believe it to be very noxious.

Reference

Standley, P.C. (1927) Poisonous trees of Central America. Tropical Woods 9, 3.

Euphorbia hypericifolia

The juice is used as a caustic on skin lesion (Watt and Breyer-Brandwijk 1962).

Reference

Watt, J.M. and Breyer-Brandwijk, M.G. (1962) The Medicinal and poisonous plants of Southern Africa. 2nd ed. Edinburgh. E. & S. Livingstone.

Euphorbia ipecacuanha

The plants are irritant to those who collect and handle them (Cheney 1887 cited by White 1887).

References

Cheney was a dealer in medicinal plants.

White, J.C. (1887) Dermatitis venenata: An account of the action of external irritants upon the skin. Boston. Cupples and Hurd.

Euphorbia ingens

Contact with this plant produced an acute bullous dermatitis (H.J. Kingsley, pers. comm. to Arthur Rook).

Euphorbia jolkini

This species yields an irritant substance, ingenol (Uemura and Hirata 1973).

Reference

Uemura, D. and Hirata, Y. (1973) Isolation and structures of irritant substances obtained from Euphorbia species (Euphorbiaceae). Tetrahedron Lett. 11, 881.

Euphorbia lactea
Candelabra Cactus, Cardon

The plant forms a spiny shrub which is widely planted in tropical America and, as an adventive to India, is now completely naturalized and found all over the country especially near habitation, (Bailey 1949 , Behl et al 1966). The cristate form of the plant is grown in India as an ornamental succulent (Behl et al 1966). They refer to an irritant and vesicant action of the plant.

This species, and also E. tirucalli, are often planted in foundation boxes in Florida. Since they outgrow such locations and have to be cut back, the trimmer is exposed to the free-flowing sap which can cause a rash and blisters, intense burning and temporary blindness (Morton 1958). Contact with the plant can produce severe oedematous and oozing dermatitis and also conjunctivitis; the face, scrotum and hands are most commonly affected as is the case from exposure to Hura crepitans and Hippomane mancinella (Pardo-Castello 1923, 1962). The sap forms a rubbery clot about one minute after collection. Crowder and Sexton (1964) observed eight cases of keratoconjunctivitis from this plant or from E. tirucalli during a three year period in Florida. They exposed the eyes of dogs to the plant juice and observed corneal opacities which appeared after 24-36 hours and cleared in one to three weeks.

References

Bailey, L.H. (1949) Manual of Cultivated Plants: most commonly grown in the continental United States and Canada. Revised ed. New York. MacMillan Co.

Behl, P.N., Captain, R.M., Bedi, B.M.S. and Gupta, S. (1966) Skin-irritant and sensitizing plants found in India, New Delhi. P.N. Behl, Irwin Hospital.

Crowder, J.I. and Sexton, R.R. (1964) Keratoconjunctivitis resulting from the sap of Candelabra Cactus and the Pencil Tree. Arch. Opthal. 72, 476.

Morton, J.F. (1958) Ornamental plants with poisonous properties. Proc. Florida State Hort. Soc. 71, 372.

Pardo-Castello, V. (1923) Dermatitis venenata. Arch. Derm. Syph. 7, 81.

Pardo-Castello, V. (1962) Common dermatoses in agricultural workers in the Caribbean area. Industr. Med. Surg. 31, 305.

Euphorbia lancifolia Ixbut

It seems that the plant is not strongly irritant since, in Guatemala, the leaves or stems are drunk in a herbal tea as a galactagogue in a dose of five leaves per cup, five cups per day (Time 1949). Blohm (1962) refers to the purgative effects of an overdose.

References

Blohm, H. (1962) Poisonous plants of Venezuela. Cambridge, Mass. Harvard University Press.

Time (1949). Ixbut 54, 38.

Euphorbia laterifolia

The juice is corrosive to flesh, acting as an escharotic, and has been used to produce white patches on the skin in order to simulate leprosy (Irvine 1961).

Reference

Irvine, F.R. (1961) Woody plants of Ghana. Oxford University Press. London.

Euphorbia lathyris
Caper Spurge, Mole Plant

This European species which grown as an annual to 0.9m in height is naturalized in the eastern United States and California and is sometimes planted to drive away moles or gophers. The first common name refers to a resemblance of the fruits to capers (*Capparis*). The plant does not lose its toxicity on drying or storage (North 1967). Persons who eat the fruits develop a severe burning sensation in the mouth and throat (Anon 1893). The juice is irritant and, when applied to the skin, causes redness, itching, pimples and sometimes gangrene (Bazin cited by White 1887, Chesnut 1898, Lander 1926, Atkinson 1926, Raymond 1939). Kerato-conjunctivitis can result from exposure to the sap (Geidel 1962). Experimentally, guinea pigs, but not rabbits, were susceptible (Lewin and Guillery 1913). The seeds contain 50 percent and the kernels 70 percent of a toxic oil; a crystalline substance separates in the oil and when this is removed the oil loses its toxicity. A steroid, $C_{29}H_{36}O_7$ known as euphorbiosteroid, is considered to be responsible for the toxic action (Dublyanskaya 1937, 1939).

References

Anon (1893) Caper Spurge - a poisonous plant. Agr. Gaz. New South Wales 4, 215.

Atkinson, E. (1926) Weeds and their identification. Caper Spurge (*Euphorbia lathyrus*) New Zealand Jour. Agr. 32, 404.

Chesnut, V.K. (1898) "Thirty Poisonous Plants of the United States." U.S. Dept Agr. Farmers' Bull. 86.

Crowder, J.I. and Sexton, R.R. (1964) Keratoconjunctivitis resulting from the sap of Candelabra Cactus and the Pencil Tree. Arch. Opthal. 72, 476.

Dublyanskaya, N.F. (1937) Biokhimiya 2, 521. (abstr. in Chem. Zeutr. (1938) 3926).

Dublyanskaya, N.F. (1939) The biological effect of the fractions responsible for the toxicity of Euphorbia lathyris oil. Farmatsiya i Farmakol No. 11-12, 50-56 (Abstr. in Chem. Zeutr. (1939) 1977).

Geidel, K. (1962) Clinical observations and animal experimental studies on effect of sap of Euphorbia lathyris on eye. Klin. Mbl. Augenheilk. 141, 374.

Hurst, E. (1942) The Poison Plants of New South Wales. N.S.W. Poison Plants Committee, Sydney.

Lander, G.D. (1926) Veterinary Toxicology. 2nd ed. London, cited by Hurst (1942).

Lewin and Guillery (1913) Die Wirkungen von Arzneimitteln und Giften auf das Auge. S699 cited by Crowder and Sexton (1964).

North, P.M. (1967) Poisonous plants and fungi in colour. London. Blandford Press. Ltd.

Raymond, W.D. (1939) Native poisons and native medicines of Tanganyika. J. Trop. Med. Hyg. 42, 295.

White, J.C. (1887) Dermatitis venenata: An account of the action of external irritants upon the skin. Boston. Cupples and Hurd.

Euphorbia maculata
Spotted Spurge, Eyebane

This native plant of the eastern and mid-western United States occurs as an occasional weed in the Pacific States and has irritant latex (Hardin and Arena 1969).

Reference

Hardin, J.W. and Arena, J.M. (1969) Human Poisoning from native and cultivated plants. Durham, North Carolina. Duke University Press.

Euphorbia marginata
Snow-on-the-Mountain

In parts of Texas, the plant was formerly used for branding cattle, the juice having a caustic, blistering action on the animals' skin. The plant is dangerous to handle since contact with the copious milky juice causes swelling and an eruption (Orchard 1954). The plant was grown for its ornamental foliage in Australia but has been declared a noxious weed. The latex is irritant to the skin and eyes (Aplin 1966, Francis and Southcott 1967, Everist 1972, Mair 1968). When the juice of the plant is placed on the skin the area becomes erythematous almost immediately and there is a slight sensation of stinging at the contact site. The erythema disappears rapidly but is followed after a latent period by a constant, follicular, papulo-pustular irritative reaction (Shelmire 1940). Honey derived from the plant is poisonous (Morton 1964).

References

Aplin, T.E.H. (1966) Poison Plants in the garden. West Australia Dept. Agr. J. 7, 24.

Everist, S.L. (1972) Queensland Herbarium, Brisbane, Australia, Personal communication concerning plants recorded in Australia as having caused dermatitis or other contact injury to man or livestock.

Francis. D.F. and Southcott, R.V. (1967) Plants harmful to man in Australia. Misc. Bull. No. 1 Botanic Garden, Adelaide, Australia.

Mair, K. (1968) Information in the Records of the Herbarium of the Royal Botanic Gardens, Sydney.

Morton, J.F. (1964) Honeybee plants of South Florida. Proc. Florida State Hort. Soc. 77, 415.

Orchard, H.E. (1954) Snow-on-the-Mountain (Euphorbia marginata Pursh). J. Agric. South Australia 57, 337.

Shelmire, B. (1940) Contact dermatitis from vegetation. South Med. J 33, 338.

Euphorbia milii
(syn. E. splendens)
Crown-of-thorns

This plant is grown as a garden subject in western Australia. The stems are armed with sharp spikes and the sap is corrosive and caustic to the skin and eyes causing temporary blindness (Morton 1962, Aplin 1966). The plant yields an irritant substance, milliamine Uemura and Hirata 1973). Patch tests were carried out with a young flowering greenhouse specimen identified as Euphorbia milii Ch. des Moulins (syn. E. splendens Hook) by Camm and Mitchell (1974 unpublished observations). Fresh milky sap, crushed flowers and bruised leaves were applied by 48 hours closed patch tests to the forearm flexures of three healthy white volunteers. No irritant effect was observed.

References

Aplin, T.E.H. (1966) Poison plants in the garden. West Australia Dept. Agr. J. 7, 24.

Morton, J.F. (1962) Ornamental plants with poisonous properties II. Proc. Florida Hort. Soc. 75,484.

Uemura, D. and Hirata, Y. (1973) Isolation and structures of irritant substances obtained from Euphorbia species (Euphorbiaceae). Tetrahedron Lett. 11, 881.

Euphorbia myrsinites

Rasch cited by Touton (1932) referred to dermatitis from the plant. The sap is irritant (Sierputowska and Sliwinska 1968).

References

Sierputowska, M. and Sliwinska, M. (1968) Dermatitis toxica bullosa phytogenes wywolane przez Euphorbia myrsinites. Przegl. Derm. 55, 787.

Touton, K. (1932) Hauterkrankungen durch phanerogamische Pflanzen und ihre Produkte (Toxicodermia et Allergodermia phytogenes), in Barnewitz, J. et al. Angeborene Anomalien, Lichtdermatosen, Pflanzengifte, Thermische Schädidgungen, Einfluss Innerer Sterungen auf die Haut. Berlin, Verlag von Julius Springer.

Euphorbia neglecta

The plant is irritant to the skin and eyes (Raymond 1939).

Reference

Raymond, W.D. (1939) Native poisons and native medicines of Tanganyika. J. Trop. Med. Hyg. 42, 295.

Euphorbia neriifolia

The spiny plant is used as a hedge plant in India. The milky juice is irritant to skin and throat (Burkill 1935, Corner 1952, Souder 1963, Watt and Breyer-Brandwijk 1962, Behl et al 1966).

References

Behl, P.N., Captain, R.M., Bedi, B.M.S. and Gupta, S. (1966) Skin-irritant and sensitizing plants found in India, New Delhi. P.N. Behl, Irwin Hospital.

Burkill, I.H. (1935) A Dictionary of the Economic Products of the Malay Peninsula. 2 vols. London. Crown Agents for the Colonies.

Corner, E.J.H. (1952) Wayside trees of Malaysia. Singapore, Government Printer.

Souder, P. (1963) Poisonous plants on Guam. In venomous and poisonous animals and noxious plants of the Pacific Region. ed. Keegan, H.L. and Macfarlane, W.V. Oxford. Pergamon Press. pp. 15-29.

Watt, J.M. and Breyer-Brandwijk, M.G. (1962) The medicinal and poisonous plants of Southern Africa. 2nd ed. Edinburgh. E. & S. Livingstone.

Euphorbia nivulia

The latex is irritant (Behl et al 1966).

Reference

Behl, P.N., Captain, R.M., Bedi, B.M.S. and Gupta, S. (1966) Skin-irritant and sensitizing plants found in India, New Delhi. P.N. Behl, Irwin Hospital.

Euphorbia obliqua

The sap is used in conjunction with charcoal for tatooing to produce blue marks (Altschul 1973).

Reference

Altschul, S. von R. (1973) Drugs and foods from little-known plants. Cambridge, Mass. Harvard Univ. Press.

Euphorbia officinarum

The sap is irritant to wounds and to the eye (Rowley 1960).

Reference

Rowley, G.D. (1960) A short history of succulent plants in A Handbook of Succulent Plants by Jacobsen, H. Vol. 1. London. Blandford. p. 1.

Euphorbia orabensis

The sap is irritant to wounds and to the eye (Rowley 1960).

Reference

Rowley, G.D. (1960) A short history of succulent plants in A Handbook of Succulent Plants by Jacobsen, H. Vol. 1. London. Blandford.p.1.

Euphorbia paralias? Sea Spurge

Gerard (1636) wrote about a sea-shore plant, "I tooke but one drop of it (the sap) into my mouth; which neverthelesse did so inflame and swell in my throte that I hardly escaped with my life". His companion was similarly affected.

Reference

Gerard, J. (1636) The Herball or Generall Historie of Plantes. The essence thereof distilled by M. Woodward (1927) from the edition of Th. Johnson 1630. London. Gerald Howe.

Euphorbia pekinensis (syn. E. lasiocaula)

The root has a bitter acrid taste, causing a scratching sensation in the throat (Smith 1939).

Reference

Smith, F.P. (1969) Chinese Materia Medica. Vegetable kingdom. 2nd ed. Rev. by Hei, P.D. Taipei, Taiwan. Ku T'ing Book House.

Euphorbia peplus

This plant is a cosmopolitan weed and one of the commonest weeds in gardens of Australia. Handling of the plant when weeding is a common source of irritation of the skin, particularly of the face, and of the eyes and lips (Francis and Southcott 1967). The juice has been employed for destroying rodent ulcers by its irritant action (Maiden 1917) and produces buccal irritation in animals who eat the plant (Hurst 1942). The latex is irritant (Bernhard-Smith 1923, Behl et al 1966, North 1967, Everist 1972). Volatile emanations of the plant were observed to affect photographic plates (Chapman and Petrie 1912). Calnan (1975) reported dermatitis from the plant and positive patch test reactions in all of six controls. Uveitis resulted in a man from accidental instillation of the sap into the eye (Hartmann 1940). The milky sap is effective for treating solar keratoses (Wilkinson, D.S. 1974, pers. comm.).

References

Behl, P.N., Captain, R.M., Bedi, B.M.S. and Gupta, S. (1966) Skin-irritant and sensitizing plants found in India, New Delhi. P.N. Behl, Irwin Hospital.

Bernhard-Smith, A. (1923) The Poison Plants of all countries. 2nd ed. London. Bailliere, Tindall & Cox.

Calnan, C.D. (1975) Spurge dermatitis. Contact Dermatitis 1, 128.

Chapman, H.C. and Petrie, J.M. (1912) Action of the latex of Euphorbia peplus on the photographic plate. Rep. Australasian Assoc. Adv. Sci. 13, 30.

Everist, S.L. (1972) Queensland Herbarium, Brisbane, Australia. Personal communication concerning plants recorded in Australia as having caused dermatitis or other contact injury to man or livestock.

Francis, D.F. and Southcott, R.V. (1967) Plants harmful to man in Australia. Misc. Bull. No. 1. Botanic Garden, Adelaide, Australia.

Hartmann, K. (1940) Augenschadigung durch den Saft der Euphorbia peplus. Klin. Mbl. Augenheilk 104, 324.

Hurst, E. (1942) The poison plants of New South Wales. N.S.W. Poison Plants Committee; Sydney.

Maiden, J.H. (1917) On some plants which cause inflammation or irritation of the skin. Ag. Gaz. New South Wales 28, 400

North, P.M. (1967) Poisonous plants and fungi in colour. London. Blandford Press Ltd.

Euphorbia preslii
Pasture Spurge, Spotted Spurge, Eye-bright

Application of the juice to the eyes causes severe irritation with smarting, burning, lachrymation and momentary blindness (True quoted by Pammel 1911).

Reference

Pammel, L.H. (1911) A manual of poisonous plants Torch Press. Cedar Rapids, Iowa. Reprinted Univ. Microfilms Inc. Ann Arbor, Mich. 1965.

Euphorbia procumbens

The juice is used as a caustic on skin lesions (Watt and Breyer-Brandwijk 1962).

Reference

Watt, J.M. and Breyer-Brandwijk, M.G. (1962) The medicinal and poisonous plants of Southern Africa. 2nd ed. Edinburgh. E. & S. Livingstone.

Euphorbia prostrata
(syn. Chamaesyce prostrata)

The plant occurs as a weed in the Sydney district of Australia and is common in townships in Queensland (Blakely 1923). The milky sap is sometimes applied to sores on the skin and is not known to be irritant (White 1927). Souder (1963) on Guam Island refers to irritation by this species. Martinez (1969) noted a report of an irritant action in a Materia Medica and applied the juice to the eyes of animals but did not see the irritant action which he expected.

References

Blakely, W.F. (1923) Weeds of New South Wales. Prostrate Spurge (Chamaesyce prostrata (Ait.) Small.) Ag. Gaz. New South Wales 34, 286.

Martinez, M. (1969) The medicinal plants of Mexico. 5th ed. Mexico City. Andres Botas.

Souder, P. (1963) Poisonous plants on Guam. In venomous and poisonous animals and noxious plants of the Pacific Region. ed. Keegan, H.L. and Macfarlane, W.V. Oxford. Pergamon Press. pp. 15-29.

White, C.T. (1927) Answers to correspondents. Queensland Agr. J. 27, 481. ditto (1929) 31, 313.

Euphorbia pubescens

The plant is said to be irritant in Europe (Watt and Breyer-Brandwijk 1962).

Reference

Watt, J.M. and Breyer-Brandwijk, M.G. (1962) The medicinal and poisonous plants of Southern Africa. 2nd ed. Edinburgh. E. & S. Livingstone.

Euphorbia pulcherrima
(syn. Poinsettia pulcherimma)
Poinsettia

The plant is named for Joel Poinsett who studied Medicine at Edinburgh and was first United States Minister to Mexico (MD of Canada 1972). The plant is grown as a garden subject in Australia and Africa and is cultivated for the Christmas trade as a houseplant in colder regions. The plant has small, inconspicuous flowers but white, pink or red bracts (specialized leaves). The latex is irritant to the skin and eye (Rock 1920, Allen 1943, Morton 1958, Blohm 1962, Aplin 1966, Francis and Southcott 1967). In a case reported by D'Arcy (1974) the eruption appeared about 24 hours after contact; allergy was suggested but patch tests were not recorded.

Patch tests were carried out with a young flowering greenhouse specimen (red bracts) identified as Euphorbia pulcherrima Willd. by Camm and Mitchell (1974 unpublished observations). Fresh milky sap, crushed flowers and bruised leaves were applied by 48 hour closed patch tests to the forearm flexures of three healthy white volunteers. No irritant effect was observed.

The saps of this species and of E. fulgens have given evidence of sensitising capacity (Hausen and Schulz 1977).

Reference

Hausen, B.M. and Schulz, K.H. (1977) Occupational contact dermatitis due to Croton (Codiaeum variegatum (L.) A. Juss var. pictum (Lodd.) Muell. Arg.) Contact Dermatitis 3, 289.

Allen, P.H. (1943) Poisonous and injurious plants of Panama. Am. J. Trop. Med. Suppl. 23, 1.

Aplin, T.E.H. (1966) Poison plants in the garden. West Australia Dept. Agr. J. 7, 24.

Blohm, H. (1962) Poisonous plants of Venezuela. Cambridge, Mass. Harvard University Press.

D'Arcy, W.G. (1974) Severe contact dermatitis from Poinsettia. Archs. Derm. 109, 909.

Everist, S.L. (1962) These plants can poison people. Queensland Agric. J. 88, 235.

Francis, D.F. and Southcott, R.V. (1967) Plants harmful to man in Australia. Misc. Bull. No. 1. Botanic Garden, Adelaide, Australia.

MD of Canada (1972) Flower of Fire. December pp. 76

Morton, J.F. (1958) Ornamental plants with poisonous properties. Proc. Florida State Hort. Soc. 71, 372.

Souder, P. (1963) Poisonous plants on Guam. In venomous and poisonous animals and noxious plants of the Pacific Region. ed. Keegan, H.L. and Macfarlane, W.V. Oxford. Pergamon Press. pp. 15-29.

Watt, J.M. and Breyer-Brandwijk, M.G. (1962) The medicinal and poisonous plants of Southern Africa. 2nd ed. Edinburgh. E. & S. Livingstone.

West, E. (1957) Poisonous plants around the home. Fla. Agr. Expt. Sta. Circ. S-100.

Euphorbia ramosissima

The latex is irritant (Souder 1963).

Reference

Souder, P. (1963) Poisonous plants on Guam. In venomous and poisonous animals and noxious plants of the Pacific Region. ed. Keegan, H.I. and Macfarlane, W.V. Oxford. Pergamon Press. pp. 15-29.

Euphorbia resinifera

This species is the source of officinal Gum Euphorbium. The latex is collected by making incisions in the stem and is then dried. The taste is extremely acrid and persistent and the dust excites violent sneezing (Burkill 1935, Wren 1968, Blacow 1972). The juice was used to destroy warts (Bigelow 1818) and as an ingredient of a rubefacient plaster (White 1934). Dioscorides and Pliny described the method of collecting the juice so as to prevent irritation of the hands and face (Dispensatory 1884). The men who collect the exuded dried latex muffle their faces to prevent the dust getting into their mouths and nostrils. The action upon man is first to cause sneezing, then irritation of the skin and mucous membrane, vomiting, diarrhoea and death (Burkill 1935). The drug is no longer used medicinally but serves to make an anti-fouling paint for ships' bottoms. The plant is used to make a vesicant ointment in veterinary Medicine (Perrot and Paris 1971).

References

Bigelow (1818) cited by White (1887).

Blacow, N.W. (1972) Martindale. The Extra Pharmacopoeia. London. The Pharmaceutical Press.

Burkill, I.H. (1935) A Dictionary of the Economic Products of the Malay Peninsula. 2 Vols. London. Crown Agents for the Colonies.

Dispensatory, United States (1884) cited by White (1887).

Perrot, E. and Paris, R. (1971) Les

plantes medicinales. 2 vols. Paris. Presses Universitaires de France. pp. 245 (+XXVI (index)).

White, J.C. (1887) Dermatitis venenata: an Account of the action of external irritants upon the skin. Boston. Cupples & Hurd.

Wren, R.W. (1968) Potter's New Cyclopaedia of Botanical Drugs and Preparations by Wren, R.C. Re-edit. by Wren, R.W. Potter and Clarke Ltd. Health Science Press. Rustington, Sussex.

Euphorbia rigida

This species caused dermatitis (Smirnov and Efrenov 1970).

Reference

Smirnov, L.D. and Efremov, A.I. (1970) Dermatitis due to Euphor bia rigida. Vestn. Derm. Vener. 44, 67.

Euphorbia rothiana

Euphorbia royleana

These species have irritant properties (Behl et al 1966, Sofat et al 1972, Sood et al 1971).

Reference

Behl, P.N., Captina, R.M., Bedi, B.M.S. and Gupta, S. (1966) Skin-irritant and sensitizing plants found in India, New Delhi. P.N. Behl, Irwin Hospital.

Sofat, B.K. et al (1972) Euphorbia royleana latex dermatitis. Amer. J. Ophth. 74, 634.

Sood, et al (1971) Injury of the eye by the sap of Euphorbia royleana. Brit. J. Ophth. 55, 856.

Euphorbia serrulata

This species is irritant (Souder 1963).

Reference

Souder, P. (1963) Poisonous plants on Guam. In venomous and poisonous animals and noxious plants of the Pacific Region. ed. Keegan, H.L. and Macfarlane, W.V. Oxford. Pergamon Press. pp. 15-29.

Euphorbia splendens
(syn. E. milii)
Crown-of-Thorns

The taxonomy of this plant is discussed by Jacobsen (1960). E. milii var. splendens appears to be the correct name. The prickly plant has irritant latex (Orchard 1954, Souder 1963, Behl et al 1966).

Arnold (1968) in Hawaii, stated that from personal experience the sap of E. splendens was not particularly irritating to his own skin whereas that of E. tirucalli was extremely irritating.

References

Arnold, H.L. (1968) Poisonous plants of Hawaii. Rutland, Vermont. Charles E. Tuttle.

Behl, P.N., Captain, R.M., Bedi, B.M.S. and Gupta, S. (1966) Skin-irritant and sensitizing plants found in India, New Delhi. P.N. Behl, Irwin Hospital.

Jacobsen, H. (1960) A Handbook of Succulent plants. Vol. 1. London. Blandford. p. 452.

Orchard, H.E. (1954) Snow-on-the-Mountain (Euphorbia marginata Pursh). J. Agric. South Australia. 57, 337.

Souder, P. (1963) Poisonous plants on Guam. In venomous and poisonous animals and noxious plants of the Pacific Regions. ed. Keegan, H.L. and Macfarlane, W.V. Oxford. Pergamon Press. pp. 15-29.

Euphorbia striata

Handling of the fresh plant can produce dermatitis (Steyn 1928 cited by Watt and Breyer-Brandwijk 1962).

Reference

Watt, J.M. and Breyer-Brandwijk, M.G. (1962) The medicinal and poisonous plants of Southern Africa. 2nd ed. Edinburgh. E. & S. Livingstone.

Euphorbia terracina
False Caper

The milky sap of this plant, which has a repulsive smell, causes inflammation of the eyes and of the softer portions of the human body when the plants are pulled by hand and the workers are heated (J. Agric. South Australia 1947). Orchard (1954) refers to irritation by the plant. The plant is also said to have no odour or only a very faint odour (South Australian Naturalist 1952).

The latex was reported to cause severe corneal ulcerations in a man (Aplin 1976).

Reference

Aplin, T.E.H. (1976) Poisonous garden plants and other plants harmful to man in Australia. Western Australian Dept. of Agriculture Bull. 3964.

Orchard, H.E. (1954) Snow-on-the-Mountain (Euphorbia marginata Pursh).

Euphorbia tetragona

The plant is irritant and vesicant to the skin and produces severe irritation or even blindness when accidentally applied to the eyeball (Watt and Breyer-Brandwijk 1962).

Reference

Watt, J.M. and Breyer-Brandwijk, M.G. (1962) The medicinal and poisonous plants of Southern Africa. 2nd ed. Edinburgh. E. & S. Livingstone.

Euphorbia thomsoniana

This species is irritant (Behl et al 1966).

Reference

Behl, P.N., Captain, R.M., Bedi, B.M.S. and Gupta, S. (1966) Skin-irritant and sensitizing plants found in India, New Delhi. P.N. Behl, Irwin Hospital.

Euphorbia thymifolia
Thyme-leaved Spurge

The plant is irritant (Pammel 1911, Souder 1963) and the milky juice is vesicant for the skin of 'many individuals' (Allen 1943).

References

Allen, P.H. (1943) Poisonous and injurious plants of Panama. Am. J. Trop. Med. Suppl. 23, 1.

Pammel, L.H. (1911) A manual of poisonous plants. Torch Press. Cedar Rapids, Iowa. Reprinted Univ. Microfilms Inc. Ann Arbor, Mich. 1965.

Souder, P. (1963) Poisonous plants on Guam. In venomous and poisonous animals and noxious plants of the Pacific Region. ed. Keegan, H.L. and Macfarlane, W.V. Oxford. Pergamon Press. pp.15-29.

Euphorbia tirucalli
Naked Lady, Pencil Tree, Indian Tree Spurge, Milk Bush.

This plant and also E. lactea are often planted in foundation boxes in Florida. They outgrow such locations and have to be cut back exposing the trimmer to the free-flowing sap which can cause skin eruptions and blisters, intense burning and temporary blindness (Morton 1958). Keratoconjunctivitis from the plant (Crowder and Sexton 1964) is noted under E. lactea. The plant is grown as a garden subject in Western Australia, as the common 'rubber hedge' of Southern Rhodesia planted around African kraals as a deterrent to marauders, as a live hedge plant and on graves in Malawi where it discourages browsing animals. Planted in India as a cattle fence, it used to be a formidable obstacle to cavalry. From India it has been reported to be used by criminals to destroy the eyes of domestic animals; it is established there as a common road-side tree. The latex is violently irritant to the skin and eye (Aplin 1966, Francis and Southcott 1967, Raymond 1939, Watt and Breyer-Brandwijk 1962, Behl et al 1966, Williamson 1956, Burkill 1935, Everist 1962, Corner 1952, Arnold 1972, Oliver 1959). Washing with water will not remove the irritant latex which forms a rubbery clot after one minute's exposure to the air (Crowder and Sexton 1964, Everist 1962). Roe and Field (1965) tested the latex of nine Euphorbia species and found E. tirucalli to be the most irritant and tumorigenic for mouse skin. The latex contains triterpene alcohols (Warren and Watling 1958).

References

Aplin, T.E.H. (1966) Poison plants in the garden. West Australia Dept. Agr. J. 7, 24.

Arnold, H.L. (1972) Honolulu, State of Hawaii. Personal Communication.

Behl, P.N., Captain, R.M., Bedi, B.M.S. and Gupta, S. (1966) Skin-irritant and sensitizing plants found in India, New Delhi. P.N. Behl, Irwin Hospital.

Burkill, I.H. (1935) A dictionary of the economic products of the Malay Peninsula. 2 vols. London. Crown Agents for the Colonies.

Corner, E.J.H. (1952) Wayside trees of Malaysia. Singapore, Government Printer.

Crowder, J.I. and Sexton, R.R. (1964) Keratoconjunctivitis resulting from the sap of Candelabra Cactus and the Pencil Tree. Arch. Opthal 72, 476.

Everist, S.L. (1962) These plants can poison people. Queensland Agric. j. 88, 235.

Francis, D.F. and Southcott, R.V. (1967) Plants harmful to man in Australia. Misc. Bull. No. 1 Botanic Garden, Adelaide, Australia.

Morton, J.F. (1958) Ornamental plants with poisonous properties. Proc. Florida State Hort. Soc. 71, 372.

Oliver, B. (1959) Nigeria's Useful Plants. Nigerian Field 24, 70.

Raymond, W.D. (1939) Native poisons and native medicines of Tanganyika. J. Trop. Med. Hyg. 42, 295.

Roe, F.J.C. and Field, W.E.H. (1965) Chronic toxicity of essential oils and certain other products of natural origin. Food, Cosmet. Toxicol. 3, 311.

Warren, F.L. and Watling, K.H. (1958) The euphorbia resins. Part X: The structural differences between euphol and tirucallol. J. Chem. Soc. 179.

Watt, J.M. and Breyer-Brandwijk, M.G. (1962) The medicinal and poisonous plants of Southern Africa. 2nd ed. Edinburgh. E. & S. Livingstone.

Euphorbia triangularis

Honey containing the nectar of this plant is said to be irritant but the latex has been used for making rubber and chewing gum and does not appear to be irritant (Watt and Breyer-Brandwijk 1962).

Reference

Watt, J.M. and Breyer-Brandwijk, M.G. (1962) The medicinal and poisonous plants of Southern Africa. 2nd ed. Edinburgh. E. & S. Livingstone.

Euphorbia trigona (syn. E. neriifolia)

The latex of this Indian shrub is irritant but less so that that of its close relatives (Burkill 1935).

Reference

Burkill, I.H. (1935) A dictionary of the economic products of the Malay Peninsula. 2 vols. London. Crown Agents for the Colonies.

Euphorbia variegata
Japanese edelweiss

A man aged 50 years and a female aged 18 years developed marked swelling, erythema and vesiculation a few hours after gathering and binding this plant. Application of the milky sap and of an ether extract of the sap to the skin of the patients and of control subjects produced erythema and papules (Musger 1935).

Reference

Musger (1935) Two cases of toxicoderma phytogenes. Oesterreichische dermatologische Gesellschaft. Wien. Oct. 17.

Samokhval, G.T. and Krivchak, G.G. (1974) Dermatitis caused by a decorative plant, Euphorbia variegata. Vestn. Dermatol. Venerol 48, 85..

Euphorbia venenata

Chewing the plant produces stomatitis (Watt and Breyer-Brandwijk 1962).

Euphorbia virosa

Honey containing the nectar of this plant is irritant and the latex is said to be irritant (Watt and Breyer-Brandwijk 1962).

Reference

Watt, J.M. and Breyer-Brandwijk, M.G. (1962) The medicinal and poisonous plants of Southern Africa. 2nd ed. Edinburgh. E. & S. Livingstone.

Excoecaria

40 species are found in tropical Africa and Asia.

Excoecaria sp.

The milky juice of a species of this genus was noted to produce severe inflammation of the conjunctiva and even temporary blindness (Spencer and Gillen cited by Cleland 1914).

Excoecaria agallocha
Milky Mangrove, River Poison Tree, Aloewood, Geor.
Blind-your-eyes (Australia), Buta-buta (Malaysia)

The milky juice in the bark is strongly irritant and an axe-blow may bespatter the wood-cutter with it causing blisters on the bare skin and irritation of the eyes. Experienced wood-cutters remove the bark before felling a tree so that no harm results (Burkill 1935). Because of its irritancy, the tree is rarely cut in Sabah (Burgess 1966). The smoke from the burning wood is very irritating so the wood is little used for firewood and workmen making charcoal from it are said to suffer (Burkill 1935, Souder 1963).

Diseased wood is fragrant and aromatic and is sold as Bastard Aloeswood; it burns with a scent which is stronger than benzoin. The wood loses its fragrance in a few years (Burkill 1935). Burgess (1966) also refers to its use as an incense wood and notes that in areas where other wood is in short supply, E. agallocha is used for making packing cases, clogs, matches, toys and furniture.

The wood is said to irritate the skin and eyes even when dry (Lewin 1928).

The sap is known to be irritant in Australia (Banfield cited by Cleland 1914, Logan 1925, Maiden 1904, 1909, Gardner and Bennetts 1956, Hurst 1942, Cleland and Lee 1963, Francis and Southcott 1967), in India (Behl et al 1966) and on Guam island (Souder 1963). Volatile emanations from the tree are also said to be irritant. A single drop of the sap getting into the eye can produce severe irritation and temporary blindness.

The sap is used as a caustic application for chronic ulcers in Malaysia (Burkill 1935) and in India where it is known as Tiger's Milk (Behl et al 1966).

Children have used the sap of this species for chewing gum in mistake for the sap of a fig (Ficus macrophylla) with fatal results (Logan 1925, Cleland and Lee 1963, Francis and Southcott 1967).

Excoecaria dallachyana
Bush Poison Tree

The milky sap is irritant to the skin and erosive to the cornea (Burkill 1935, Hurst 1942, Everist 1972).

Excoecaria grahami

This species is irritant (Burkill 1935).

Excoecaria macrophylla

This species is dreaded by natives of the Phillipine Islands because it is strongly irritant to the skin (Burkill 1935).

Excoecaria oppositifolia

This tree of upper Burma is probably irritant (Burkill 1935).

Excoecaria parvifolia
Gutta Percha tree

The sap is acrid and drastically irritant to the human skin and eye and to mouths of humans and of sheep, (Maiden 1909, Logan 1925, Cleland 1914, Hurst 1942, Cleland and Lee 1963). Maiden (1909) says the juice is more or less volatile.

References

Behl, P.N., Captain, R.M., Bedi, B.M.S. and Gupta, S. (1966) Skin-irritant and sensitizing plants found in India, New Delhi. P.N. Behl, Irwin Hospital.

Burgess, P.F. (1966) Timbers of Sabah, (Sabah Forest Records No. 6). Sabah, Malaysia. The Forest Department.

Burkill, I.H. (1935) A dictionary of the economic products of the Malay Peninsula. 2 vols. London. Crown Agents for the Colonies.

Cleland, J.B. (1914) Plants, including fungi, poisonous or otherwise injurious to man in Australia. Australasian Med. Gaz. 35, 569. idem. Tasmanian Ag. Gaz. 32, 361 and 401

Cleland, J.B. and Lee, D.J. (1963) The Poisonous and Urticating Plants of Australia in venomous and poisonous animals and noxious plants of the Pacific Region. ed. Keegan, H.L. and Macfarlane, W.V. Oxford. Pergamon Press. pp. 3-13.

Everist, S.L. (1972) Queensland Herbarium, Brisbane, Australia. Personal communication concerning plants recorded in Australia as having caused dermatitis or other contact injury to man or livestock.

Francis, D.F. and Southcott, R.V. (1967) Plants harmful to man in Australia. Misc. Bull. No. 1. Botanic Garden, Adelaide, Australia.

Gardner, C.A. and Bennetts, H.W. (1956) The toxic plants of Western Australia. Perth West. Australian Newspapers Ltd.

Hurst, E. (1942) The poison plants of New South Wales. N.S.W. Poison Plants Committee, Sydney.

Logan, D.A. (1925) Gutta Percha tree (Excoecaria parviflora) and its effect on sheep. Queensland Agr. J. 24, 232.

Maiden, J.H. (1909) On some plants which cause inflammation or irritation of the skin. Ag. Gaz. New South Wales. 20, 111, 1073.

Maiden, J.H. (1904) Plants which induce eczema. Meeting of Therapeutical Society. Lancet 1, 1208.

Lewin, L. (1928) Gifte im Holzgewerbe. Berlin, Stilke.

Souder, P. (1963) Poisonous plants on Guam. In venomous and poisonous animals and noxious plants of the Pacific Region. ed. Keegan, H.L. and Macfarlane, W.V. Oxford. Pergamon Press. pp. 15-29.

Glochidion

300 species are found in Madagascar, from tropical Asia to Queensland and Polynesia and in tropical America. Some species are widely used in Asia and Malaysia as timber and for tanning (Burkill 1935).

Glochidion marianum
Chosgo

This species can cause contact dermatitis (Souder 1963).

References

Burkill, I.H. (1935) A dictionary of the economic products of the Malay Peninsula. 2 Vols. London. Crown Agents for the Colonies.

Souder, P. (1963) Poisonous plants on Guam. In venomous and poisonous animals and noxious plants of the Pacific Region. ed. Keegan, H.L. and Macfarlane, W.V. Oxford. Pergamon Press. pp. 15-29.

Hevea

12 species are native to tropical America.

Hevea brasiliensis
Pará rubber

This tree is the source of the best natural rubber which is the coagulated milky latex. Contact with the latex of the tree can cause dermatitis (Souder 1963). Seeberg cited by Pirila (1947) presented a case in which there was simultaneous sensitivity to caoutchouc (rubber), Swedish turpentine and cymene. Isoprene, the parent molecule of natural rubber, is a polymer of both Vitamin A and squalene.

Ingestion of Vitamin A and squalene, inhalation of the vapour of synthetic neoprene rubber and topical application of neoprene compounds have been reported to produce alopecia (Sulzberger and Lazar 1951, Flesch and Goldstone 1952, Wilson et al 1953). A systemic rather than a local action is responsible for the effect.

References

Flesch, P. and Goldstone, S.B. (1952) Local depilatory action of unsaturated compounds. J. Invest. Derm. 18, 267.

Pirila, V. (1947) On occupational diseases of the skin among paint factory workers, painters, polishers and varnishers in Finland. Acta. Derm-venereol. 17: Suppl. 16, 163.

Souder, P. (1963) Poisonous plants on Guam. In venomous and poisonous animals and noxious plants of the Pacific Region. ed. Keegan, H.L. and Macfarlane, W.V. Oxford. Pergamon Press. pp. 15-29.

Sulzberger, M.B. and Lazar, M.P. (1951) Hypervitaminosis A. Report of a case in an adult. JAMA 146, 788.

Wilson, J.W. et al (1953) Temporary depilation of the scalp resulting from the use of a new 'antifugal chemical'. J. Invest. Derm. 21, 131.

Hippomane

Five species are found in Mexico and the West Indies.

Hippomane mancinella
Manchineel, beach apple, arvore da morte.

This tree, perhaps the most notorious of all irritant trees, has acquired an extensive mythology (Bodeau 1936).

The species name is derived from the Latin American name manzanillo - "little apple". The early Spanish explorers discovered that the fruits were poisonous (Standley 1927). He stated that this tree is the most poisonous of all the euphorbiaceous trees but happily it never grows outside a narrow belt fringing the seashore. The tree has been largely eliminated in southern Florida except from the Everglades National Park; persons wishing to fish in certain parts of that area are permitted to do so after proving to Park authorities that they can recognize the manchineel tree and so avoid poisoning (Morton 1958). The tree grows to about 6 m. in height and spreads about 6 m. It is sought by the unwary for shelter and even rain falling from the tree can cause skin irritation. Woodcutters char the bark before cutting the tree down (Barham 1794, Allen 1943). The wood is used locally for turnery and cabinet-work, but the sawdust causes rhinitis and cough and some men refuse to work with it (Earle 1938).

All parts of the plant contain a caustic milky juice which produces severe burning and swelling on contact with the skin and temporary blindness if rubbed into the eyes. The smoke of the wood, if used for fuel, is intensely irritating to the eyes (Allen 1943). The wood, if thoroughly dried, is said to lose its irritant properties and it is used for utensils (Standley 1926).

Biting into the fruit causes large blisters on the cheeks and lips which become extremely swollen. Grana (1946) reported 13 cases of acute conjunctivitis and dermatitis due to contact with the tree on beaches. The sap was used by exiled prisoners in French Guiana to provoke dermatitis and conjunctivitis (Allen 1943) and by persons to the skin of their backs to simulate the effects of a beating (White 1887). According to Pardo-Castello (1962) dermatitis from contact with the plant effects principally the face, scrotum and hands. Satulsky (1943), Satulsky and Wirts (1943), Earle (1938), provided a clinical description. Soldiers training in the West Indies during World War II developed bullous dermatitis and conjunctivitis after accidental contact with the sap.

Workers who cut down the tree were affected by blistering of the skin; a white cedar (*Bignonia*) which grew in close proximity to the tree was said to be an effective antidote (Hamilton 1845-46).

The tree is said to be more toxic in summer than in winter. An alkaloid and a sapogenin are said to be the irritant principles (Lauter and Foote 1955, Schaeffer et al 1954, Carroll et al 1957). Rao (1974) reviewed the chemistry.

The irritant can be effectively removed from the skin within 30 minutes by soap and water, or more traditionally by plain seawater as the tree is usually found on or near beaches (Snow and Harley 1944).

Dermatitis from the tree is known in the Barbados and in Cuba (Sheard 1974).

References

Sheard, C. (1974) Manchineel dermattitis. Cutis 14, 751.

Rao, K.V. (1974) Toxic principles of Hippomane mancinella. Planta Med. 25, 166.

Allen, P.H. (1943) Poisonous and injurious plants of Panama. Am. J. Trop. Med. Suppl. 23, 1.

Carroll, M.N., Fox, L.E. and Ariail, W.T. (1957) Investigation of the toxic principles of Hippomane mancinella L. III. Toxic actions of extracts of Hippomane mancinella L. J. Am. Pharm. Assoc. 46, 93.

Grana, P.C. (1946) Conjunctivitis and dermatitis due to "Beach Apple". Report of 13 cases. Arch. Opthal. 35, 421.

Hamilton, W. (1845-46) On the properties of the Hippomane mancinella, or Manchineel Tree. Pharm. J. 5, 408.

Lauter, W.M. and Foote, P.A. (1955) Investigation of the toxic principles of Hippomane mancinella L. II. Preliminary isolation of a toxic principle of the fruit. J. Am. Pharm. Ass. Sci. Ed. 44, 361.

Morton, J.F. (1958) Ornamental plants with poisonous properties. Proc. Florida State Hort. Soc. 71, 372.

Pardo-Castello, V. (1962) Common dermatoses in agricultural workers in the Caribbean area. Industr. Med. Surg. 31, 305.

Satulsky, E.M. (1943) Dermatitis venenata caused by the Manzanillo tree. Arch. Derm. Syph. 47, 36.

Schaeffer, H.J., Lauter, W.M. and Foote, P.A. (1954) A preliminary phytochemical study of Hippomane mancinella L. J. Am. Pharm. Ass. 43, 43.

Standley, P.C. (1926) Trees and shrubs of Mexico. Part 5. Contr. U.S. Nat. Herb. 23.

Standley, P.C. (1927) Poisonous Trees of Central America. Tropical Woods. 9, 3 and 7, 8 (1926).

White, J.C. (1887) Dermatitis venenata: An account of the action of external irritants upon the skin. Boston. Cupples and Hurd.

Barham, H. (1794) Hortus americanus. Kingston, Jamaica.

Bodeau (1936) Apropos de quelques accidents dus au mancenillier. Archives de Medécine et Pharmacie Navales 126, 122.

Earle, K.V. (1938) Toxic effects of Hippomane mancinella. Trans. Roy. Soc. Trop. Med. Hyg. 32,363.

Satulsky, E.M. and Wirts, C.A. (1943) Dermatitis caused by the Manzanillo tree. Archs. Derm. Syph. 47, 797.

Snow, U.S. and Harley, R.D. (1944) Dermatitis venenata and keratoconjunctivitis caused by the manzanillo tree. Archs. Derm. Syph. 49, 236.

Homolanthus

35 species are found in Indo-Malaysia and Polynesia. *H. populifolius* yields a black dye.

Homolanthus spp.

Some species of this genus have irritant properties (Burkill 1935).

Homolanthus acuminatus

The wood dust is irritating to the nose and throat (Uhe 1974).

Homolanthus nutans

The plant is irritant (Uhe 1974).

References

Burkill, I.H. (1935) A dictionary of the economic products of the Malay Peninsula. 2 Vols. London. Crown Agents for the Colonies.

Uhe, G. (1974) Medicinal plants of Samoa. Econ. Bot. 28, 1.

Hura

Two species are found from Mexico to tropical South America and in the West Indies.

Hura brasiliensis

This plant has properties similar to those of *H. crepitans* (White 1887).

Hura crepitans
Hura, assacú, sandbox, possentrie, possumwood, javillo, sablier, ceiba blanca

The common names possen- and possum tree are corruptions of poison tree (Record and Mell 1924).

'The fellers, as they cut them down, are very careful of their eyes; and those that have Cipers (kerchiefs), put it over their faces; for if any of the sap fly into their eyes, they become blind for a month'. (Ligon 1673).

The bark of the young tree is studded with stout prickles. The fruits explode violently when ripe and the noise, which they make, gives rise to the West Indian name, Monkey's Dinner Bell. The noisy explosion of the ripe dry pods showers by-standers with seeds and sharp-pointed segments sometimes to a distance of 60 m. The tree thus "stabs, poisons and shoots" (Barrett 1956). The seed-pod was filled with sand to provide a sand-box for goose quills which were formerly used for writing (Menninger 1967).

Men engaged in felling the tree developed swelling of the face and hands from contact with the acrid sap (Allen 1943). The sap from broken leaves, branches and from the bark is vesicant for the skin and the saw-dust is irritant to carpenters (White 1887, Pardo-Castello 1923, Standley 1927, Allen 1943, Kerharo and Bouquet 1950, Blohm 1962 Arnold (1968), in Honolulu, did not find the plant noticeably irritant to his own skin. The sap is said to be milky (White 1887, Standley 1927) but Morton (1972 pers. comm.) in Florida found it to be clear and sticky but not milky.

The segments of the woody fruits can cause dermatitis when they are used in bracelets and necklaces (Morton 1958).

Chemistry

It was one of the first toxic woods to be chemically investigated. Boussingault and Rivero (1825), working in Bogota, found a vesicant essential oil in the latex, the vapour from which inflamed their faces severely while it was being boiled down. Richet (1909, 1910) studied anaphylaxis provoked in animals by an albuminoid extract of the latex which he called crepitine, but this was not the irritant principle.

The plant contains a toxalbumin, hurin, related to ricin or *Ricinus* and crotin of *Croton* and tetracyclic triterpenes (Ponsinet and Ourisson 1965, 1968). The wood exported to Europe has caused dermatitis (Hausen 1970).

References

Allen, P.H. (1943) Poisonous and injurious plants of Panama. Am. J. Trop. Med. Suppl. 23, 1.

Arnold, H.L. (1968) Poisonous plants of Hawaii. Rutland, Vermont. Charles E. Tuttle.

Barrett, M.F. (1956) Common exotic trees of South Florida. Gainesville. University of Florida Press.

Blohm, H. (1962) Poisonous plants of Venezuela. Cambridge, Mass. Harvard University Press.

Kerhargo, J. and Bouquet, A. (1950) Plantes medicinales et toxiques de la Côte d'Ivoire-Haute-Volta. Ministère de la France d'outre mer. office de la Recherche Scientifique Outre-Mer. Paris p. 291.

Menninger, E.A. (1967) Fantastic trees. New York. The Viking Press.

Morton, J.F. (1958) Ornamental plants with poisonous properties. Proc. Florida State Hort. Soc. 71, 372.

Ponsinet, G. and Ourisson G. (1965, 1968) Etudes chimiotaxohomique dans la famille des Euphorbiacées II Triterpenes de Hura crepitans L. Phyto-chem. 4, 813: 7, 89.

White, J.C. (1887) Dermatitis venenata: An account of the Action of external irritants upon the skin. Boston. Cupples and Hurd.

Boussingault and Rivero (1825) Mémoire sur le lait vénéneux de l'hura crepitans. Annales de chimie et de physique 28, 430.

Hausen, B.M. (1970) Untersuchungen über Gesundheitsschädigende Hölzer Thesis, Hamburg.

Ligon, R. (1673)A True and Exact History of the Island of Barbados. London, Parker.

Ponsinet, G. and Ourisson, G. (1965, 1968) Etudes chimo-taxonomiques dan la famille des Euphorbiacees. Phytochemistry 4, 813: 7, 89.

Record, S.J. and Mell, C.D. (1924) Timbers of Tropical America. New Haven, Yale.

Richet, C. (1909. 1910) Etudes sur la crépitine (toxine de Hura crepitans) Annales de l' Institut Pasteur, Paris 23, 745: 24, 609.

Pardo-Castello, V. (1923) Dermatitis venenata; a study of the tropical plants producing dermatitis. Archs. Derm. Syph. 7, 81.

Hyaenanche Lamb.
(syn. Toxicodendrum Thunb.)

One species is found in southern Africa.

Hyenanche globosa

Hausen (1970) cites Anon (1940) and Briggs (1946) for an injurious effect of the wood and Henry (1920) for chemical aspects.

References

Anon, (1940) Giftige en voor de gezondheid nadeelige houtsoorten. Hout 20, 184.

Briggs, L.H. (1946) Plant Products of New Zealand. J. Proc. Roy. Soc. N.S.W. 80, 151.

Hausen, B.M. (1970) Untersuchungen über Gesundheitsschädigende Hölzer. Thesis. Hamburg.

Henry, T.A. (1920) Hyenanchin and other constituents of Hyenanche globosa Lamb. J. Chem. Soc. 117, 1619.

Jatropha

175 species are principally found in tropical and subtropical regions but also in North America and southern Aprica. Tapioca is prepared from the root of J. manihot.

Jatropha curcas Physic Nut

The tree is used for hedges and planted in graveyards (Barrett 1956, Irvine 1961). The sap of the tree turns brown and brittle when dried, stains linen and can be used as a marking ink (Oliver 1961). The seeds are poisonous, producing burning in the throat. Toxicity varies from tree to tree, some bearing apparently harmless seeds, others violently purgative (Morton 1958). Burkill (1935) refers to two races in Malaysia, one with dark seeds and one with pale seeds. Frequent eating of roasted seeds, even from an apparently harmless tree, can produce sores in the mouth (Morton 1958). The greenish viscid juice and pounded leaves are rubefacient and styptic and can cause inflammation of the eyes (Irvine 1961). The sap can cause dermatitis (Hurst 1942, Morton 1958, Watt and Breyer-Brandwijk 1962) but is used by children in Malaysia and in Africa for blowing bubbles. (Burkill 1935, Irvine 1961).

A poultice of the seed or the seed-oil when applied to the skin causes erythema then a pustular eruption (Burkill 1935). The seed oil known as Hell oil is used for soap and illumination and is known as Chinese Castor Oil. Penetration of the skin by the stiff hairs of the fruit causes great pain for 24 hours or longer, accompanied by fever. (Watt and Breyer-Brandwijk 1962). The husks of the seeds contains a toxalbumin, curcin, related to ricin of Ricinus and crotin of Croton (Webb 1948).

Jatropha gossypiifolia

A yellowish-brown substance in the pith of old stems is used to provoke sneezing (Quisumbing 1951, Irvine 1961). Contact with the sap can produce dermatitis (Souder 1963). The seeds are toxic but less so than those of J. curcas, (Oakes and Butcher 1962).

Jatropha janipha

The powdered root is used to remove pock-marks, stains and pigmentary deposits from the face (Smith 1969).

Jatropha multifida
Coral plant

The oil from the seeds, named Pinhoen oil, has properties similar to that of J. curcas (Burkill 1935) and the plant is poisonous (Oakes and Butcher 1962). Contact with the sap can cause dermatitis (Souder 1963). The latex contains a thioglucoside which yields irritant mustard oil (Cruciferae) (Kjaer 1960, 1963).

Jatropha podagarica
Gout stick

Contact with the sap can cause dermatitis (Souder 1963).

Jatropha urens
Pringamoza, Ortiga

The whole plant is covered with stiff white stinging hairs which produce intense pain and inflammation if they enter the skin; ulceration can result (Pardo-Castello 1923, Allen 1943). Entry of about ten hairs into the skin resulted in severe local and disseminated urticaria followed by severe constitutional symptoms and coma (Lutz 1914 cited by Blohm 1962). Cattle are also affected by the stinging hairs and ordinarily do not eat the plant; if they do so, swelling of the lips results. When the plant dries, the hairs are shed and can enter the eye causing conjunctivitis and can irritate the skin producing an urticarial eruption (Dao 1967).

Jatropha urens var. stimulosa
(syn. Cnidoscolus stimulosus)

This species which has stinging hairs (Standley and Steyermark 1949) is noted under Cnidoscolus.

References

Allen, P.H. (1943) Poisonous and injurious plants of Panama. Am. J. Trop. Med. Suppl. 23, 1.

Barrett, M.F. (1956) Common exotic trees of South Florida. Gainesville University of Florida Press.

Blohm, H. (1962) Poisonous plants of Venezuela. Cambridge, Mass. Harvard University Press.

Burkill, I.H. (1935) A dictionary of the economic products of the Malay Peninsula. 2 vols. London. Crown Agents for the Colonies.

Dao, L. (1967) Dermatitis from plants in the plains of Venezuela. Derm. Internat. 6, 77.

Hurst, E. (1942) The poison plants of New South Wales. N.S.W. Poison Plants Committee; Sydney.

Irvine, F.R. (1961) Woody plants of Ghana. Oxford University Press. London.

Kjaer, A. (1960) Naturally derived isoThiocyanates (Mustard Oils) and their parent glucosides in Progress in the Chemistry of Organic Natural Products. ed. Zechmeister, L. Vol. 18. Vienna. Springer-Verlag. pp. 122-176.

Kjaer, A. (1963) The distribution of sulphur compounds in Chemical Plant Taxonomy. ed. Swain T. London Academic Press. p. 453.

Lutz, O. (1914) The poisonous nature of the stinging hairs of Jatropha urens. Am. J. Pharm. 86, 527, cited by Blohm (1962).

Morton, J.F. (1971) Ornamental plants with poisonous properties. Proc. Florida State Hort. Soc. 71,372.

Morton, J.F. (1971) Plants poisonous to people in Florida and other warm areas. Miami, Florida. Hurricane House Publishers Ltd.

Oliver, B. (1958-61) Nigeria's Useful Plants. Nigerian Field Part V 26, 170.

Pardo-Castello, V. (1923) Dermatitis venenata. Arch. Derm. Syph. 7, 81.

Quisumbing, E. (1951) Medicinal plants of the Phillipines. Tech. Bull. 16. Manila, Phillipine Islands. Manila Bureau of Printing 1234 pp.

Smith, F.P. (1969) Chinese Materia Medica. Vegetable kingdom. 2nd ed. Rev. by Hei, P.D. Taipei, Taiwan. Ku T'ing Book House.

Souder, P. (1963) Poisonous plants on Guam. In venomous and poisonous animals and noxious plants of the Pacific Region. ed. Keegan, H.L. and Macfarlane, W.V. Oxford. Pergamon Press. pp. 15-29.

Stanley, P.C. and Steyermark, J.A. (1949) Flora of Guatemala. Fieldiana Bot. Vol. 24. Pt. 6. quoted by Morton (1971).

Watt, J.M. and Breyer-Brandwijk, M.G (1962) The medicinal and poisonous plants of Southern Africa. 2nd ed. Edinburgh. E. & S. Livingstone.

Webb, L.J. (1948) Guide to the medicinal and poisonous plants of Queensland. C.S.I.R. Bull. No. 232.

Oakes, A.J. and Butcher, J.O. (1962) Poisonous and injurious plants of the U.S. Virgin Islands. Misc. Publ. 882. U.S. Department of Agriculture, Washington, D.C.

Macaranga

280 species are found in tropical Africa, Madagascar, IndoMalaysia, Australia and the Pacific region. Some have hollow stems inhabited by stinging ants (Corner 1952). Some yield kino gum.

Macaranga hispida

This species has brittle irritating hairs (Altschul 1973).

Macaranga thomsonii
Pengua

Contact with the sap can cause dermatitis (Souder 1963).

References

Altschul, S. von R. (1973) Drugs and foods from little-known plants. Cambridge, Mass. Harvard Univ. Press.

Corner, E.J.H. (1952) Wayside Trees of Malaysia. Singapore, Government Press.

Souder, P. (1963) Poisonous plants on Guam. In venomous and poisonous animals and noxious plants of the Pacific Region. ed. Keegan, H.L. and Macfarlane, W.V. Oxford. Pergamon Press. pp. 15-29.

Mallotus

Two species are found in tropical Africa and Madagascar. 140 species are found in eastern and south-eastern Asia and from IndoMalaysia to New Caledonia and Figi, northern and eastern Australia. M. philippensis yields Kamala dye.

Mallotus oppositifolius

The fresh leaves are applied as a styptic (Salziel 1937).

Mallotus subulatus

The seeds are beaten and used for marking the faces of young persons (Irvine 1961).

References

Dalziel, J.M. (1937) The useful plants of west tropical Africa. London. Crown Agents.

Irvine, F.R. (1961) Woody plants of Ghana. Oxford University Press. London.

Manihot

170 species are found from the south-western United States to tropical South America. Several species yield rubber.

Manihot esculentus
Cassava

Sweet and bitter cultivars are known (Robers 1963).

This species is cultivated

for manioc or cassava meal (Brazilian arrowroot) and tapioca. The poisonous juice is processed to yield an antiseptic, cassareep, used in preserving meat. Contact with the sap of this and also of M. glaziovii can cause dermatitis (Souder 1963).

References

Rogers, D.J. (1963) Studies of Manihot esculenta Crantz and related species. Bull. torr. Bot. Club. 90, 43.

Souder, P. (1963) Poisonous plants on Guam. In venomous and poisonous animals and noxious plants of the Pacific Region. ed. Keegan, H.L. and Macfarlane, W.V. Oxford. Pergamon Press. pp.15-29.

Mareya

Three species are found in tropical West Africa.

Mareya micrantha
(syn. M. spicata)
Executioner

The plant is said to have local anaesthetic properties. The common name is derived from its use as an abortefacient (Irvine 1961).

Reference

Irvine, F.R. (1961) Woody plants of Ghana. Oxford. University Press. London.

Melanolepis

One or two species are found in Formosa, IndoChina, Malaysia and the Pacific region.

Melanolepis multiglandulosa
var. glabrata
Alom

Contact with the sap can cause dermatitis (Souder 1963).

Reference

Souder, P. (1963) Poisonous plants on Guam. In venomous and poisonous animals and noxious plants of the Pacific REgion. ed. Keegan, H.L. and Macfarlane, W.V. Oxford. Pergamon Press. pp. 15-29.

Mercurialis

Eight species are found from the Mediterranean region and temperate Eurasia to northern Siam.

Mercurialis perennis

This species has irritant properties (Pammel 1911).

References

Pammel, L.H. (1911) A Manual of Poisonous Plants. Torch Press. Cedar Rapids, Iowa. Reprinted Univ. Microfilms Inc. Ann Arbor. Mich. 1965.

Pachystylidium

One species is found in peninsular India, Siam, Indochina, the Phillipines and Java.

Pachystylidium spp.

These species possess stinging hairs (Thurston and Lersten 1969).

Reference

Thurston, E.L. and Lersten, N.R. (1969) The morphology and toxicology of plant stinging hairs. Botan. Rev. 35, 393.

Pedilanthus

14 species are found from Florida and Mexico to tropical South America and in the West Indies.

Pedilanthus latifolius
Christmas Candle

The stems, leaves and roots possess a very caustic milky juice which can produce severe irritation of the skin (Mesa 1953 cited by Oakes and Butcher 1962).

Pedilanthus tithymaloides
Red-Bird Cactus, Slipper Bush
Christmas Candle, Candedilla

The milky sap is caustic and can cause irritation and vesication of the skin and conjunctivitis (Allen 1943, Morton 1958, Blohm 1962, Martinez 1969). Some horticultural varieties of the plant have irritant properties (Behl et al 1966).

References

Allen, P.H. (1943) Poisonous and

injurious plants of Panama. Am. J. Trop. Med. Suppl. 23, 1.

Behl, P.N., Captain, R.M., Bedi, B.M.S. and Gupta, S. (1966) Skin-irritant and sensitizing plants found in India. New Delhi. P.N. Behl, Irwin Hospital.

Blohm, H. (1962) Poisonous plants of Venezuela. Cambridge, Mass. Harvard University Press.

Martinez, M. (1969) The Medicinal Plants of Mexico. 5th ed. Mexico City. Andres Botas.

Mesa Roig, Y.T.J. (1953) Diccionario Botanico de los nombres vulgares cubanos. Ed. 2. Vol.1-2. La Habana cited by Oakes and Butcher (1962).

Morton, J.F. (1958) Ornamental plants with poisonous properties. Proc. Florida State Hort. Soc. 71, 372.

Oakes, A.J. and Butcher, J.O. (1962) Poisonous and injurious plants of the U.S. Virgin Islands. Misc. Publ. 882. U.S. Dept. of Agriculture, Washington, D.C.

Pera

40 species are found from Mexico to tropical South America and in the West Indies. The genus has been placed in a family Peraceae.

Pera ferruginea

The root bark yields a napthaquinone, plumbagin, which has vesican properties (Thomson 1971). The action of the chemical is noted under *Plumbago*.

References

Thomson, R.H. (1971) Naturally Occurring Quinones. 2nd. ed. London. Academic Press.

Piscaria (syn. *Eremocarpus*)

Two species are found in the north western United States.

Piscaria (syn. *Eremocarpus*) *setigerus*
Turkey-Mullein, Dove-Weed

This hairy plant causes mechanical injury to the gut of animals (Muenscher 1951).

References

Muenscher, W.C. (1951) Poisonous plants of the United States. 2nd ed. New York. The MacMillan Co.

Phyllanthus

600 species are found in tropical and subtropical regions except in Europe and northern Asia. The fruits of *P. emblica* (Emblic, Myrobalan) are made into jam.

Many species are used medicinally (Watt and Breyer-Brandwijk 1962) and some have irritant properties (Souder 1963).

References

Souder, P. (1963) Poisonous plants on Guam. In Venomous and Poisonous Animals and Noxious Plants of the Pacific Region. ed. Keegan, H.L. and Macfarlane, W.V. Oxford. Pergamon Press. pp.15-29.

Watt, J.M. and Breyer-Brandwijk, M.G. (1962) The Medicinal and Poisonous Plants of Southern Africa. 2nd ed. Edinburgh. E. & S. Livingstone.

Platygyna

Five species are found in Cuba.

Platygyna hexandra

The plant has stinging hairs (Altschul 1973).

Platygyna pruriens
Pringamoza
(syn. *P. urens*)

The plant has irritant hairs (Pardo-Castello 1923).

References

Altschul, S. von R. (1973) Drugs and foods from little-known plants. Cambridge, Mass. Harvard University Press.

Pardo-Castello, V. (1923) Dermatitis venenata. A study of the tropical plants producing dermatitis. Arch. Derm. Syph. 7, 81.

Ricinus

One species is found in tropical Africa and Asia. Varieties are known in cultivation.

Ricinus communis
Castor Oil Plant

The castor bean yields an oil; the residual meal or pomace which is left after extraction of the oil is used as a fertilizer. The pomace contains ricin, a highly toxic protein and a water-soluble, carbohydrate-free allergenic protein substance. There is great variation in toxicity from plant to plant. The pomace, used in a dry dusty state, can produce asthma and urticaria (Brugsch 1960, Wolfromm et al 1967). He reviewed the literature concerning Type I hypersensitivity reactions to the pomace. Anaphylaxis resulted from biting into a bean (Arnold 1968) and contact urticaria resulted from wearing a necklace of beans (Lockey 1968). Family members at home can develop Type I hypersensitivity reactions from dust carried on workers' clothing (Zerbst 1944). Panzani (1962) reported cross-sensitivity between bean dust and a mould Spondylocladium. Dermatological effects apart from urticaria and conjunctivitis appear to be rare (Key 1961). Dermatitis can occur from contact with the plant and its seeds (beans) (Behl et al 1966, Watt and Breyer-Brandwijk 1962, Souder 1963). In a patch test study of hospitalized patients from an agricultural region, Szego (1965) observed positive patch test reaction to the leaf. The pomace was found to be a contact allergen (Klauder 1962).

Castor oil is said to produce contact dermatitis (Karabow 1927, Coca et al 1931). Contact dermatitis from castor oil and Vitamin B was attributed to pyridine derivatives (Kadlec and Hanslian 1965). Sulphonated castor oil used as a fabric finish for stockings had irritant effects (Schwartz 1934). Methyl heptine carbonate, a semi-synthetic chemical derived from the beans and used for the production of artificial violet and jasmine odours can produce contact dermatitis (Rattner 1934, Tulipan 1938, Klarmann 1962).

References

Arnold, H. (1968) Poisonous Plants of Hawaii. Rutland, Vermont. Charles E. Tuttle.

Behl, P.N., Captain, R.M., Bedi, B.M.S. and Gupta, S. (1966) Skin-irritant and sensitizing plants found in India. New Delhi. P.N. Behl, Irwin Hospital.

Brugsch, H.G. (1960) Toxic Hazards. The Castor Bean. New Eng. J. Med. 262, 1039.

Coca, A.F., Walzer, M. and Thommen, A.A. (1931) Asthma and hayfever in Theory and Practice. Springfield, Ill. Charles C. Thomas.

Kadlec, K. and Hanslian, L. (1965) Gruppenallergie gegen Pyridinderivate. Berufsdermatosen, 13, 283.

Karabow, A.S. (1927) An occupational affection of the skin in workers preparing Castor Oil. Mosk. med. j. 7, 47.

Key, M.M. (1961) Some unusual reactions in industry. Arch. Derm. 83, 3.

Klauder, J.V. (1962) Actual causes of certain occupational dermatoses. Arch. Derm. 85, 451.

Klarmann, E.G. (1962) Cosmetic Chemistry for Dermatologists. Springfield, Ill. Charles C. Thomas.

Lockey, S.D. (1968) Anaphylaxis from an Indian necklace. JAMA 206, 2900.

Panzani, R. (1962) Study of cross-sensitivity between castor oil bean dust and Spondylocladium. Int. Arch. Allergy 21, 288.

Rattner, H. (1934) Dermatitis of eyelids. JAMA 103, 180.

Schwartz, L. (1934) Actual causes of dermatitis attributed to socks. Pub. Health Rep. 49, 1176.

Souder, P. (1963) Poisonous plants on Guam. In Venomous and Poisonous Animals and Noxious Plants of the Pacific Region. ed. Keegan, H.L. and Macfarlane, W.V. Oxford. Pergamon Press. pp.15-29

Szego, L. (1965) Sensitisation by agricultural crops and crop-protection preparations I. Stuties of plant (leaf) extracts. Acta. Med. Acad. Sci. Hung. 21, 19. (Excerpta Medica XVII, 13, 3468).

Tulipan, L. (1938) Cosmetic irritants. Archs. Derm. Syph. 38, 906.

Watt, J.M. and Breyer-Brandwijk, M.G. (1962) The Medicinal and Poisonous Plants of Southern Africa. 2nd ed. Edinburgh. E. & S. Livingstone.

Zerbst. G.H. (1944) Unusual hazard in a fertilizer factory. Industr. Med. 13, 552.

Wolfromm, R. et al (1967) Epidemic of ricin allergy in Dieppe (1963-1965) Presse Med. 75, 2157.

Sapium

120 species are found in tropical and subtropical regions and in America south to Patagonia.

Sapium spp.
Palo de la flecha, Arrow-wood

Evidence concerning trees of this genus is contradictory. In Mexico, the milky sap is reputed harmful and it is reported on good authority that the Indians utilized it for poisoning their arrows. In Salvador, the sap is claimed to be poisonous and blistering in effect if in contact with the skin for which reason the trees are often left standing when land is cleared. A colloquial name in Salvador is 'chile', the common hot pepper, a name used also to express the idea of burning or smarting. In Costa Rica, where the Sapiums are called 'Yos', they are not reported poisonous and the same is true in Panama where the name 'olivo' is usually applied to the trees. It seems probable that the species of Sapium differ in their properties and that while some may be harmful, others are innocuous (Standley 1927).

Reference

Standley, P.C. (1927) Poisonous Trees of Central America Tropical Woods 9, 3 and 7, 8 (1926).

Sapium aubletianum

The latex is irritant and the skin of the hands may be made painful and swollen by grasping the fresh leaves (Burkill 1935).

Reference

Burkill, I.H. (1935) A Dictionary of the Economic Products of the Malay Peninsula. 2 Vols. London. Crown Agents for the Colonies.

Sapium biloculare
Hierbe de flecha

North-American Indians of southern California claimed that this, their arrow tree, was dangerous and warned travellers that if they fell asleep under it they would wake up blind (Menninger 1967).

Reference

Menninger, E.A. (1967) Fantastic Trees. New York. The Viking Press.

Sapium ellipticum
Tomi

The wood is used locally but is not of commercial importance.

Sapium glandulosum

The white latex is caustic (Altschul 1973).

Reference

Altschul, S. von R. (1973) Drugs and foods from little-known plants. Cambridge, Mass. Harvard University Press.

Sapium grahamii

The latex of the root has vesicant and escharotic properties (Dalziel 1937); when ground with a little water, it produces red or black marks on the face, causing swelling and ultimately tattoo-like marks. When applied to fresh tribal markings it ensures scarification. The juice from the crushed leaves is less irritant but is used by small boys to raise blisters (Irvine 1961).

References

Dalziel, J.M. (1937) The Useful Plants of West Tropical Africa. London. Crown Agents.

Irvine, F.R. (1961) Woody Plants of Ghana. London. Oxford University Press.

Sapium indicum

The latex blisters the skin. The fruits are used by Malay children to play 'marbles'. The seeds can be eaten when quite ripe but care should be taken to put nothing more than the seed into the mouth, as the latex, which is in the fruit-wall, is caustic (Burkill 1935, Irvine 1961).

References

Burkill, I.H. (1935) A Dictionary of the Economic Products of the Malay Peninsula. 2 Vols. London Crown Agents for the Colonies.

Irvine, F.R. (1961) Woody Plants of Ghana. London. Oxford University Press.

Sapium insigne

The tree yields an acrid, vesicant milky juice (Behl et al 1966). Pammel (1911) referred to its irritant properties.

References

Behl, P.N., Captain, R.M., Bedi, B.M.S. and Gupta, S. (1966) Skin-irritant and sensitizing plants found in India. New Delhi. P.N. Behl, Irwin Hospital.

Pammel, L.H. (1911) A Manual of Poisonous Plants. Torch Press. Cedar Rapids, Iowa. Reprinted Univ. Microfilms Inc. Ann Arbor, Mich. 1965, pp. 467-7.

Sapium macrocarpum

The plant is reported to be very poisonous to the skin (Altschul 1973).

Reference

Altschul, S. von R. (1973) Drugs and foods from little-known plants. Cambridge, Mass. Harvard University Press.

Sapium malagascariense

The milky juice of the plant is vesicant for the skin and smoke from the burning of leaves can produce blindness (Watt and Breyer-Branwijk 1962).

Reference

Watt, J.M. and Breyer-Brandwijk, M.G. (1962) The Medicinal and Poisonous Plants of Southern Africa. 2nd ed. Edinburgh. E. and S. Livingstone.

Sapium reticulation

The seed with a living grub in it, which is known as 'jumping bean, hops about when warmed, a result of the activities of the grub (Burkill 1935).

Reference

Burkill, I.H. (1935) A Dictionary of the Economic Products of the Malay Peninsula. 2 Vols. London. Crown Agents for the Colonies.

Sapium sebiferum
Tallow tree

The native Tallow tree of southern China is now naturalized in many parts of the world. The plant has a waxy covering yielding a tallow-like substance which is used for making candles. The tree yields an acrid vesicant milky juice (Behl et al 1966). Pennington (1958) refers to its effects.

References

Behl, P.N., Captain, R.M., Bedi, B.M.S. and Gupta, S. (1966) Skin-irritant and sensitizing plants found in India. New Delhi. P.N. Behl, Irwin Hospital.

Hausen, B.M. (1970) Untersuchungen über Gesundheitsschädigende Hölzer. Thesis. Hamburg.

Pennington, C.W. (1958) Tarahumar fish stupefaction plants. Econ. Bot. 12, 95, cited by Hausen (1970).

Sebastiana

95 species are found in tropical America and the Atlantic United States. One species is found in tropical West Africa and from India to southern China and Australia. Three species are found in western Malaysia.

Sebastiana lucida
West Indian Poison tree

The wood is listed as injurious by Hausen (1970) citing Bernard-Smith (1923) and Pennington

(1958).

Sebastiana

In Belize, Honduras the plants are known to cause dermatitis (Towers, G.H.N., pers. comm.).

References

Bernhard-Smith, A. (1923) The Poisonous Plants of all Countries. 2nd ed. London. Bailliere, Tindall & Cox.

Hausen, B.M. (1970) Untersuchungen über Gesundheitsschädigende Hölzer. Thesis. Hamburg.

Pennington, C.W. (1958) Tarahumar fish stupefaction plants. Econ. Bot. 12, 95, cited by Hausen (1970).

Sphaerostylis

8 species are found in tropical East Africa, Madagascar and western Malaysia.

Sphaerostylis malaccensis
Climbing Croton

This climbing stinging plant (Burkill 1935) possesses irritant hairs and is known to produce skin reactions in Malaysia (Kochummen 1972).

References

Burkill, I.H. (1935) A Dictionary of the Economic Products of the Malay Peninsula. 2 Vols. London. Crown Agents for the Colonies.

Kochummen, K.N. (1972) Forest Botanist. Forest Research Institute. Kepong, Selangor, Malaya. Personal communication.

Sphaerostylis
(syn. Tragiella)

Eight species are found in tropical East Africa, Madagascar and western Malaysia.

Sphaerostylis spp.

Stinging hairs are known in species of this genus (Thurston and Lersten 1969).

Reference

Thurston, E.L. and Lersten, N.R. (1969) The morphology and toxicology of plant stinging hairs. Botan. Rev. 35, 393.

Spirostachys

Three or four species are found in eastern tropical and southern Africa.

Spirostachys africanus
(syn. Excoecaria africana)
African sandalwood, Tambooti, sandalo africano, tomboti, tambootie

The sap of the tree is irritant to the skin and conjunctivitis results from exposure to the sawdust. (Codd 1951, Pardy, 1954). It is exported from East Africa as a substitute for sandalwood in making furniture. The wood is unsuitable for ox-yokes since it produces a 'burning' effect on the animals' necks (Davy 1929). Necklaces, however, are made of it (Watt and Breyer-Brandwijk 1962).

References

Watt, J.M. and Breyer-Brandwijk, M.G. (1962) The Medicinal and Poisonous Plants of Southern Africa. 2nd ed. Edinburgh. E. & S. Livingstone.

Codd, L.E.W. (1951) Trees and shrubs of the Kruger National Park. Pretoria. Department of Agriculture.

Davy, J.B. (1920) African 'Sandaleen' wood. Tropical Woods. 17, 15.

Pardy, A.A. (1954) Notes on indigenous trees and shrubs of Southern Rhodesia. Rhodesia agricultural Journal 51, 489.

Stillingia

One or two species are found in the Mascarene Islands, one in eastern Malaysia and Fiji, 30 in warm America.

Stillingia sylvatica
Queen's Root, Queen's Delight, Yaw Root

The juice of the green root is acrid; it inflames and swells the hands (Dispensatory 1884, Cheney 1887) producing smarting and irritation (Frost cited by Piffard 1881).

Stillingia texana

The milky sap is said to produce blisters on the skin (Altschul 1973).

References

Altschul, S. von R. (1973) Drugs and foods from little-known plants. Cambridge, Mass. Harvard University Press.

Cheney (1887) Personal communications to White (1887).

Dispensatory, The National (1884) Philadelphia. Stille and Maisch, cited by White (1887).

Piffard, H.G. (1881) A Treatise on the Materia Medica and Therapeutics of the Skin. New York. Wm. Wood and Co.

White, J.C. (1887) Dermatitis venenata: An account of the action of external irritants upon the skin. Boston. Cupples and Hurd.

Synadenium

15 species are found in warm regions of Africa, Madagascar and the Mascarene Islands.

Synadenium cupulare

The plant is irritant and vesicant, producing dermatitis and conjunctivitis which may lead to blindness. The latex gives off an irritant vapour which produces the same effects if held at arm's-length. Tests have shown that the latex is quite as irritant as that of Euphorbia ingens.

Synadenium grantii
African Milk Bush

The plant is widely grown as an ornamental plant in the tropics and under glass in colder regions. The latex is extremely irritant (Watt and Breyer-Brandwijk 1962, Everist 1972) and was used by the Masai people of South Africa as a blistering remedy for East Coast fever, the applicaton being made over the swollen glands (Mettam 1932). Injection of the latex into guinea pigs produced necrosis and sloughing in the area of injection (Thorold 1953).

A report of dermatitis from the plant (Raymond 1939) is noted under Euphorbia grantii.

A gardener noted that the latex dripped from the cut stems onto the arms and forearms. She experienced no immediate discomfort but four hours later a burning sensation was felt and eight hours after exposure, streaky erythema and blisters appeared. Applicaton of a drop of latex to the forearm of a volunteer was followed, after six hours, by intense irritation then by blistering (Rook 1965).

Synadenium kirkii

The latex is apparently irritant (Watt and Breyer-Brandwijk 1962).

References

Everist, S.L. (1972) Queensland Herbarium, Brisbane, Australia. Personal communication concerning plants recorded in Australia as having caused dermatitis or other contact injury to man or livestock.

Mettam, R.W.M. (1932) Poisonous plants of East Africa. Uganda. Gov't Press.

Raymond, W.D. (1939) Native Poisons and Native Medicines of Tanganyika. J. Trop. Med. Hyg. 42,295.

Rook, A.J. (1965) An unrecorded plant irritant, Synadenium grantii. Brit. J. Derm. 77, 284.

Thornold, P.W. (1953) Suspected malicious poisoning. J. South Afr. Vet. Med. Ass. 24, 215.

Watt, J.M. and Breyer-Brandwijk, M.G. (1962) The Medicinal and Poisonous Plants of Southern Africa. 2nd ed. Edinburgh. E. and S. Livingstone.

Tithymalus

200 species are found in north temperate reigons and in the Andes. The genus is closely related to Euphorbia.

Tithymalus cyparissias

The sap of this plant has given rise to violent iridocylitis with hypopyon (Duke-Elder and MacFaul 1972).

Tithymalus esula

The sap is irritant to the eye (Duke-Elder and MacFaul 1972).

References

Duke-Elder, S. and MacFaul, P.A. (1972) System of Opthalmology Vol. XIV Injuries Part 1. Mechanical Injuries. Extra-ocular foreign bodies, pp. 464-67 and Agricultural Injuries pp. 32-34. London. Henry Kimpton.

Tragia

100 species are found in tropical and subtropical regions.

Tragia adenanthera

The plant is irritant to the skin (Watt and Breyer-Brandwijk 1962).

Tragia bicolor
Noseburn

The stinging hairs which cover the entire plant have sharp siliceous points which break off when touched and penetrate the skin. In addition to mechanical injury, sharp burning pain and inflammation occur like the effects produced by nettles (Urtica) (Behl et al 1966).

Tragia cannabina

This plant has effects similar to those of T. bicolor (Behl et al 1966).

Tragia cordifolia

The plant has a vesicant effect (Pammel 1911).

Tragia hispida

The plant has stinging hairs (Altschul 1973). The effects are similar to those of T. bicolor (Behl et al 1966).

Tragia hirsuta

The plant is irritant to the skin (Altschul 1973).

Tragia involucrata

The plant has a vesicant effect (Pammel 1911). The effects are similar to those of T. bicolor (Behl et al 1966).

Tragia laevis

This climbing plant of Malaya possesses irritant hairs and is known to produce skin reactions (Kochummen 1972). Burkill (1935) noted that the plant stings, but not badly.

References

Allen, P.H. (1943) Poisonous and Injurious Plants of Panama. Am. J. Trop. Med. Suppl., 23, 1.

Altschul, S. von R. (1973) Drugs and foods from little-known plants. Cambridge, Mass. Harvard University Press.

Behl, P.N., Captain, R.M., Bedi, B.M.S. and Gupta, S. (1966) Skin-irritant and sensitizing plants found in India. New Delhi. P.N. Behl, Irwin Hospital.

Burkill, I.H. (1935) A Dictionary of the Economic Products of the Malay Peninsula. 2 Vols. London. Crown Agents for the Colonies.

Fernald, M.L. (1970) Gray's Manual of Botany. 8th ed. 1970. New York. Van Nostrand Reinhold Co.

Kochummen, K.M. (1972) Forest Botanist. Forest Research Institute. Kepong, Selangor, Malaya. Personal communication.

Oakes, A.J. and Butcher, J.O. (1962) Poisonous and injurious plants of the U.S. Virgin Islands. Misc. Publ. 882. U.S. Dept. of Agriculture, Washington, D.C.

Pammel, L.H. (1911) A Manual of Poisonous Plants. Torch Press. Cedar Rapids, Iowa. Reprinted Univ. Microfilms Inc. Ann Arbor, Mich. 1965. pp. 476-7.

Pardo-Castello, V. (1923) Dermatitis venenata. A study of the tropical plants producing dermatitis. Arch. Derm. Syph. 7, 81.

Watt, J.M. and Breyer-Brandwijk, M.G.

(1962) The Medicinal and Poisonous Plants of Southern Africa. 2nd ed. Edinburgh. E. and S. Livingstone.

FAGACEAE

Between 800 and 900 species are of cosmopolitan distribution excluding tropical South America and tropical and southern Africa.

Chemistry is recorded by Hegnauer (1966).

Reference

Hegnauer, R. (1966) Chemotaxonomy of Plants. Vol. 4. Basel. Birkhauser p. 141.

Castanea

Twelve species are found in north temperate regions.

Castanea mollissima
Chinese Chestnut Tree.

The wood is said to be irritant (Schwartz et al 1957).

Reference

Schwartz, L., Tulipan, L. and Birmingham, D.J. (1957) Occupational Diseases of the Skin. 3rd. ed. Philadelphia. Lea & Febiger. pp. 637-672.

Castanea sativa
(syn. C. vulgaris)
Sweet Chestnut, Spanish Chestnut

The wood is useful and the bark is used in tanning. Basket makers working with chestnut wood were said to develop herpes labialis (Weber 1953). Workers in tanneries develop characteristic sub-ungual hyperkeratoses (Silva and Cozzolino 1952, Silva 1957). Labourers who sawed chestnut wood developed erythema and remarkable thickening of the skin which ultimately deformed the hand; this condition was called 'crocodile hand' (Horand 1907) and attributed mainly to tannin. Contact sensitivity to the wood was reported by Navarro Martin and Ordax (1932).

References

Horand, R. (1907) Mains de crocodile, dermatose professionnelle produite par le bois de chataignier. Gaz. Hôp. 80, 255.

Navarro Martin, A. and Ordax, J.T. (1932) Estudio de la alergia en un caso de eczema de los lenadores. Acta dermosifiliograf. 25, 41.

Silva, Ramos E.J. (1957) Dermatoses professionnelles au Bresil. Brazil Med. 71, 286.

Silva, Ramos E.J. and Cozzolino, D. (1952) Algunas observaciones de una dermatosis profesional sui-generis: tilosis sub-ungueal. Arch. Argent. Derm. 2, 93.

Weber, L.F. (1953) Dermatitis venenata from native woods. Arch. Derm. Syph. 67, 388.

Castanea vesca

The wood is listed as irritant (Hanslian and Kadlec 1966).

Reference

Hanslian, L. and Kadlec, K. (166) Wood from the standpoint of hygiene VIII Species with some or little biological effect. Drevo. 21, 229.

Fagus

Ten species are found in north temperate regions and in Mexico.

Fagus sylvatica
Beech

Dermatitis attributed to contact with beech trees (Longin 1929, 1930) may actually be caused by lichens and liverworts (Jubulaceae) present on the bark of the trees (Spillman 1921, LeCoulant and Lopes 1960). Dermatitis (Howes 1951, Jones 1946) and asthma (Hausen 1973) have been reported in wood-workers. Oleum Fagi and Oleum Betulae (Betula) (of each 5%) produced positive patch test reactions in 3% of patients with stasis dermatitis (Rudzki and Baranowska 1974).

Woodworkers in the High Wycombe area of England have a higher incidence of adenocarcinoma of the paranasal sinuses than the general population (Acheson et al 1968). It is not known which sawdust, if any, might be responsible but beech is the most largely used wood.

References

Acheson, E.D., Cowdell, R.H., Hadfield, E. et al (1968) Nasal cancer in wood-workers in the furniture industry. Brit. med. J. 2, 587.

Rudzki, E. and Baranowska, E. (1974) Contact sensitivity in stasis dermatitis. Dermatologica 148, 352.

Howes, H.C. (1951) Occupational dermatitis. Can. Woodwork. 34 and 64.

Jones, I. (1946) Dermatitis, causes and prevention. Furniture Development Council Inform. Serv. Inf. rep. (London) 6, 2.

LeCoulant, P. and Lopes, G. (1960) Rôle pathogène des muscinées-hépatiques dans les industries du bois. Arch. mal. prof. 21, 374.

Longin, L.A. (1929) Une tirade éruptive provoquée par les essences forestières. Ann. Dermat. 10, 178: (1930) Bull. Soc. franc. Derm. 37, 741.

Spillman, L. (1921) Dermite artificielle due à l'action du chêne. Bull Soc. franc. Derm. 6, 33.

Hausen, B.M. (1973) Holzarten mit gesundheitsschädigenden inhaltsstoffen. Stuttgart. DRW-Verlags-GmbH.

Quercus

450 species are found from North America to western tropical South America, in temperate and subtropical Eurasia and northern Africa. Q. tinctoria yields a yellow dye from the bark. The bark of several species is used for tanning.

Quercus robur (syn. Q. pedunculata) Oak

Spillman (1921) described dermatitis on the ear and right side of the neck in a man who had carried freshly-cut oak logs on his shoulder and suggested that fungi on the bark might be responsible. Oak was implicated in 'wood-cutters' eczema (Schulman and Detouillon 1932) now known to be caused by lichens and liverworts (Frullania) (LeCoulant and Lopes 1960). Woods and Calnan (1976) reported three patients who had positive patch test reactions to oak. The results were of doubtful clinical relevance. One of the patients was sensitized to Calocedrus. One of the patients also showed a positive patch test reaction to Tectona.

A joiner who had dermatitis showed positive patch test reactions to Thuja plicata and to oak (Woods and Calnan 1976).

The wood is said to be more irritant when moist than when dry (Schulman and Detouillon 1932). Wood workers can develop asthma from oak wood dust (Scheven et al 1963, Sosman et al 1969).

The oak processionary caterpillar can cause dermatitis (Gougerot and Carteaud 1952, Touraine et al 1947).

References

Gougerot, H. and Carteaud, A. (1952) Les Dermatoses Professionelles. Paris, Libraine Maloine.

Touraine, A., Thomas, J. and Caldera, R. (1947) Presse méd. 55, 654.

Woods, B. and Calnan, C.D. (1976) Toxic Woods. Brit. J. Derm. 94, Suppl. 13, June.

LeCoulant, P. and Lopes, G. (1960) Rôle pathogène des muscinées-hépatiques dans les industries du bois. Arch. mal. prof. 21, 374.

Schulman, E. and Détouillon, P. (1932) L'eczéma du bois et la sensibilisation sylvestre. Paris. Med. 1, 55.

Spillman, L. (1921) Artificial dermatitis due to the action with oak. Bull. Sco. franc. Derm. Syph. 6, 33.

Scheven, H. et al (1963) Zum Antigenkatalog gewerblicher Inhalationsallergien. Allerg. Asthma 9, 286.

Sosman, A.J., Schlueter, D.P., Fink, J.N. and Barboriak, J.J. (1969) Hypersensitivity to wood dust.

New Eng. J. Med. 281, 977.

Spillman, L. (1931) Deux cas de dermite artificielle dues vraisemblent à l'action de substances végétales chez des bûcherons. Bull. Soc. franc Derm. 38, 339.

Quercus suber
Cork oak

In Spain and Portugal exposure to the bark is reported to produce a respiratory disorder, suberosis. The disorder starts with rhinitis, cough and dyspnoea and proceeds to chronic bronchitic changes or extrinsic allergic alveolitis (Avila 1972). The cork contains much silica (Schepers 1964, Cancella 1955, 1963).

References

Avila, R. (1972) Some aspects of suberosis. Les Bronches (Paris) 22, 121.

Cancella, L. de C. (1955) On a special kind of pneumoconiosis: the suberosis. A Medicina contemporânae (Lisbon) 73, 235.

Canella, L. de C. (1963) Suberosis: a pneumoconiosis due to cork dust - the present stage of the problem. Ind. Med. Surg. 32, 435.

Schepers, G.W.H. (1964) Suberosis in Sensitivity Chest Diseases. ed. Harris, M.C. and Shure, N. Philadelphia, Davis.

Tannins

Tannic acid occurs in the bark and fruit of many plants notably in the bark of the oak (Quercus spp.), sumac (Rhus semialata, Anacardiaceae) and myrobalan (Terminalia, Combretaceae). It is produced from nutgalls which are excrescences from the young twigs of Quercus infectoria and other allied species of Quercus; the constituents of nutgall include 50-60% tannic acid, 2-4% gallic acid (Merck 1968). Tannic acid is used medicinally as a mild astringent and allergic sensitivity appears to be rare; an authentic case seems to be that reported by Lewis (1944); clinical dermatitis from application of tannic acid compresses was confirmed by positive patch tests to an aqueous solution 0.25 per cent; positive patch tests were also observed to ink (in the preparation of which, tannic acid may be used), and to pyrogallol. Cross-sensitivity between pyrogallol and resorcin and related compounds has been observed (Caron and Calnan 1962, Keil 1962). The chemistry of the tannins is complex and non-uniform (Merck 1968). Gallates (propyl-, octyl-, and lauryl-) used as antioxidants in margarine have been observed to cause allergic contact dermatitis (Brun 1964, 1970: Burckhardt and Fierz 1964: Roed-Petersen, and Hjorth, 1976) and the same compounds may be present in vegetable oils, chocolate (Theobroma cacao, Sterculiaceae), fruit juices, rice oil, therapeutic creams and natural essences such as anise, orange and bergamot. The shells of the seeds of Theobroma cacao are used in the manufacture of caffeine and theobromine and the handling of them occasionally caused allergic contact dermatitis (Merck 1968). Tanning agents of plant origin are responsible for some cases of shoewear dermatitis; in Britain, lining leathers are almost all vegetable tanned but the real causes of tanned shoe leather sensitivity are difficult to find or are unknown (Calnan and Sarkany 1959). The chemical compound responsible for dermatitis from Indian tanned buffalo-hide sandals has not been found (Lynch and Rudolph 1969, Cronin 1966, Rothenborg and Hjorth 1971, Pilgram et al 1970, Minkin et al 1971). Tanning agents can cause contact dermatitis (Hailey and Burks 1960). Laborie and Laborie (1958) discussed cross-sensitivity between tannins, terpenes and flavones, all of which contain benzene rings with OH radicals that can be easily oxidised.

Propyl gallate, when used in sun screens in high concentration, has sensitizing properties (Kahn 1972). Contact sensitivity to tannic acid oleate (digalloyl trioleate) was observed by Sams (1956).

References

Brun, R. (1964) Kontaktekzem auf Laurylgallat und p-Hydroxybenzoesäureester. Berufsdermatosen 12, 281.

Brun, R. (1970) Contact eczema from an antioxidant of margarine (Gallate) and change of occupation. Dermatologica 140, 390.

Burckhardt, W. and Fierz, U. (1964) Antioxydation in der Margarine als Ursache von Gewerbeekzemen. Dermatologica 129, 431.

Calnan, C.D. and Sarkany, I. (1959) Studies in Contact Dermatitis. IX Shoe dermatitis. Trans. St. John's Hosp. Derm. Soc. 43, 8.

Caron, G.A. and Calnan, C.D. (1962) Studies in contact dermatitis XIV Resorcin. Trans. St. John's Hosp. Derm. Soc. 48, 149.

Cronin, E. (1966) Shoe dermatitis. Brit. J. Derm. 78, 617.

Hailey, C. and Burks, J.W. (1960) Contact dermatitis from currently popular tanning agents. JAMA 174, 2072.

Kahn, G. (1972) Report to the Pacific Dermatologic Association. Dermatology News. Vol. 4. No. 2 pg. 2, Oct-Nov 1972 (Syntex Labs. Ltd.).

Keil, H. (1962) Group reactions in contact dermatitis due to resorcinol. Arch. Derm. 86, 212.

Laborie, F. and Laborie, R. (1958) Intolerance to certain chemical groups in cutaneous allergy. J. Med. Bordeaux 135, 43.

Lewis, G.M. (1944) Dermatitis venenata due to tannins. Archs. Derm. Syph. 50, 138.

Lynch, P.J. and Rudolph, A.J. (1969) Indian sandal strap dermatitis. JAMA 209, 1906.

Merck Index (1968) An Encyclopedia of Chemicals and Drugs. ed. Stecher, P.G. 8th ed. Rahway, N.J. Merck and Co. Inc.

Minkin, W., Cohen, H.J. and Frank, S.B. (1971) Contact dermatitis to East Indian leather. Archs. Derm. 103, 522.

Pilgram, R.E. et al (1970) Indian sandal strap dermatitis. JAMA 211, 1378.

Roed-Petersen, J. and Hjorth, N. (1976) Contact dermatitis from antioxidants. Brit. J. Derm. 94, 233.

Rothenborg, H.W. and Hjorth, N. (1971) Indian Sandal dermatitis. Ugeskr. Laeg. 133, 802.

Sams, W.M. (1956) Contact photodermatitis. Arch. Derm. 73, 142.

FLACOURTIACEAE

1000 species in 93 genera are found in tropical and subtropical regions as trees and shrubs. The fruits of Oncoba spinosa are used as snuff-boxes (Irvine 1961).

Chemistry is recorded by Hegnauer (1966).

References

Hegnauer, R. (1966) Chemotaxonomy of plants. Vol. 4 Basel, Birkhauser, p. 155.

Irvine, F.R. (1961) Woody plants of Ghana. Oxford University Press. London.

Carpotroche

Fifteen species are found in tropical America.

Carpotroche amazonica

The bark is used as a caustic (Altschul 1973).

Reference

Altschul, S. von R. (1973) Drugs and food from little-known plants. Cambridge, Mass. Harvard Univ. Press.

Doryalis
(syn. Dovyalis)

30 species are found in Africa and Ceylon. Some have edible fruit.

Doryalis caffra

This species (Williamson 1956) and others (Burkill 1935) are used as live fences because of their spiny branches.

Doryalis hebecarpa
(syn. Dovyalis)

Fine hairs upon the fruit are irritant to the mouth

and the fruit is almost too acid to eat raw but is used in jams (Burkill 1935).

References

Burkill, I.H. (1935) A Dictionary of the Economic Products of the Malay Peninsula 2 vols. London. Crown Agents for the Colonies.

Williamson, J. (1956) Useful Plants of Malawi. ed. Greenway, P.J. Zomba, Malawi. The Government Printer. Previously published as Useful Plants of Nyasaland.

Flacourtia

Fifteen species are found in tropical and southern Africa, south-eastern Asia, Malaysia and Fiji. F. remontchi (Madagascar plum) and others have edible drupes. Many have spiny trunks and F. flavescens (Niger plum) has stout thorns on the stem and makes a good hedge (Irvine 1961).

Flacourtia rukam
Indian Prune

The ripe fruit is acid and astringent but rubbing it between the hands bruises the flesh of the fruit and causes a chemical change to take place which renders it sweet and palatable (Corner 1952).

References

Corner, E.J.H. (1952) Wayside Trees of Malaysia. Singapore, Government Printer.

Irvine, F.R. (1961) Woody plants of Ghana. Oxford University Press. London.

Gossypiospermum

Two species are found in Cuba and tropical South America.

Gossypiospermum praecox
West Indian Box-wood

The wood is said to be irritant (Schwartz et al 1957, Orsler 1973).

Gossypiospermum praecox (syn. Casearia praecox)
Maracaibo boxwood

Maracaibo boxwood from this species is widely used and has not been reported to cause ill-effects in wood-workers. According to Woods and Calnan (1976), the Maracaibo boxwood which was reported by Dr. T.F. Young at a medical meeting in 1902 to cause irritation of the throat and eyes may have been Gonioma These authors state that Dr. Young's Maracaibo boxwood was incorrectly identified as Tabebuia pentaphylla by Oliver (1908). For this information, they cite Record and Mell (1924).

References

Orsler, R.J. (1973) Personal communication from Forest Products Research Laboratory, Princess Risborough, Bucks, England.

Schwartz, L., Tulipan, L. and Birmingham, D.J. (1957) Occupational Diseases of the Skin. 3rd ed. Philadelphia. Lea & Febiger. pp. 637-672.

Oliver, T. (1908) Diseases of Occupation. London, Methuen.

Record, S.J. and Mell, C.D. (1924) Timbers of Tropical America. New Haven, Yale.

Woods, B. and Calnan, C.D. (1976) Toxic Woods. Brit. J. Derm. 94, Suppl. 13, June.

Ryania

Eight species are found in northern tropical South America and Trinidad.

Ryania mansoana
Mata collado, Silent Killer

The fumes of the burning plant are lethal, if inhaled (Smith 1971).

Reference

Smith, A. (1971) Mato Grosso. Last virgin land. New York. E.P. Dutton and Co.

FLAGELLARIACEAE

Three species in one genus found in tropical Africa, Asia and the Pacific region are high-climbing lianes.

Flagellaria

The distribution of the genus is that of the family.

Flagellaria guineensis

A poultice of mashed berries is irritant to the skin (Watt and Breyer-Brandwijk, 1962).

Reference

Watt, J.M. and Breyer-Brandwijk, M.G. (1962) The Medicinal and Poisonous Plants of Southern Africa. 2nd ed. Edinburgh. E. & S. Livingstone.

FLINDERSIACEAE

17 species in two genera found in southern India, Ceylon, eastern Malaysia, eastern Australia and New Caledonia are trees or shrubs often with hard, bright yellow wood.

Chloroxylon

One species is found in south-western India and Ceylon.

Chloroxylon swietenia
Satinwood, East Indian Satinwood

The timber is very lasting and is largely used in veneering. The tree also yields a gum.

Two outbreaks of dermatitis occurred in cabinet-makers working with East Indian satinwood in Glasgow ship-building yards; not all the men exposed were affected. The latent period became shorter in successive attacks (Jones 1904). Legge (1907) wrote: 'there can be no doubt that East Indian satinwood possesses much more irritant properties than the West Indian variety'. West Indian satinwood is a name for Fagara flava. Bidie (1905) proposed exactly the opposite view. According to Woods and Calnan (1976) both types of satinwood had been imported into England since about 1780; they cite Sheraton (1803). Genuine satinwoods were increasingly replaced by substitutes. The identity of the wood is therefore uncertain but Auld (1909) investigated the wood of C. swietenia and found, among other substances, an alkaloid chloroxylonine. The skin effects of this compound were investigated by Cash (1911) on his own person and volunteers. He observed what has since come to be known as allergic sensitization by a spontaneous flare phenomenon (active sensitization by patch testing); 0.0000165 gm. of the compound produce positive patch test reactions. He distinguished the wood of C. swietenia from West Indian Satinwood (Fagara flava); the latter was not allergenic but slightly irritant by patch test. Hausen (1970) suggests that substitutions for satinwoods may have produced fluctuations in toxicity and that photosensitisation by chemical compounds of Fagara flava may have played a role. According to Woods and Calnan (1976) C. swietenia also contains photosensitizers. They cite the finding of xanthyletin in the plant by King et al (1954). Wilkinson (1971, pers. comm.) cited by Woods and Calnan (1976) has seen a case of clinical photosensitivity to C. swietenia but the findings could not be confirmed experimentally. Gardiner (1908) also referred to satinwood dermatitis. According to McCord (1958) exposure to the wood can cause gastrointestinal disturbances and headache.

References

Auld, S.J.M. (1909) An examination of irritant woods. I. Chloroxylonine from East Indian satinwood. J. Chem. Soc. 95, 964.

Bidie, G. (1905) Satinwoods and dermatitis. Brit. med. J. 1, 74.

Cash, J.T. (1911) The dermatitis produced by E. Indian satinwood (Chloroxylon swietenia). Brit. med. J. 2, 784.

Gardiner, F. (1908) Satinwood-dermatitis. Brit. med. J. 1, 1231.

Hausen, B.M. (1970) Untersuchungen über Gesundheitsschädigende Hölzer. Thesis, Hamburg.

Jones, H.E. (1904) Acute dermatitis produced by satinwood irritation. Brit. med. J. 1, 1484.

King, F.E., Housley, J.R. and King, T.J. (1954) Coumarin constituents of Fagara macrophylla, Zanthoxylum flavum and Chloroxylon swietenia. J. Chem. Soc.1392.

Legge, T.M. (1907) Report of the

Chief Inspector of Factories and Workshops, 248, London.

McCord, C.P. (1958) The toxic properties of some timber woods. Industr. Med. Surg. 27, 202.

Sheraton, T. (1803) The cabinet dictionary, London.

Woods, B. and Calnan, C.E. (1976) Toxic Woods. Brit. J. Derm. 94, Suppl. 13, June.

Flindersia

Sixteen species are found in the Moluccas, New Guinea, eastern Australia and New Caledonia.

Chemistry is reported by Brown et al. (1954). Alkaloids are derived from the wood.

Reference

Brown, R.F.C. et al (1954) The chemical constituents of Australian Flindersia species. VI. Aust. J. Chem. 7, 348.

Flindersia australis
Moah, Crow's ash, Australian teak

Early reports of dermatitis from the wood were reviewed by Hausen (1973). Mill-hands noted reactions to the wood (Cleland 1943).

The Australian moah wood, reported by Pflanz (1908) to produce dermatitis of the face, hands and arms in wood-workers has been considered by some authors to be Madhuca sp., but according to Woods and Calnan (1976) Flindersia was also named Australian moah at that time. Pflanz (1908) could not reproduce the eruption which occurred in his woodworker patients with the sawdust or extracts of the wood, either on the patients or himself. African moah is a name for Madhuca sp. The chemistry of Flindersia spp. was investigated by Ritchie (1964).

Flindersia brayleyana

A factory worker developed a severe skin eruption from handling the wood (Cleland 1943).

Flindersia chatawaiana
Queensland Maple

A cabinet maker developed dermatitis of the hands, forearms, neck and face after working with this wood for over 20 years. Respiratory symptoms occurred in other workers (MacPherson 1925).

Flindersia pimenteliana

A factory worker developed a severe skin eruption from handling the wood (Cleland 1943).

References

Cleland, J.B. (1943) Plants including fungi, poisonous or otherwise injurious to man in Australia IV. Med. J. Australia. 11, 161.

Pflanz, V. (1908) Interessante Fälle von 'Dermatitis venenata'. Med. Klin. 4, 832.

Ritchie, E. (1964) Chemistry of Flindersia species. Review of pure and applied Chemistry. 14, 47.

Woods, B. and Calnan, C.D. (1976) Toxic Woods. Brit. J. Derm. 94, Suppl. 13, June.

Hausen, B.M. (1973) Holzarten mit gesundheitsschädigenden inhaltsstoffen Stuttgart. DRW-Verlags.-GmbH.

MacPherson, J. (1925) Dermatitis caused by Queensland maple. Med. J. Australia. 2, 542.

FUMARIACEAE

450 species in 16 genera are found in north (especially warm) temperate regions, a few on mountains of eastern and southern Africa.

Fumaria (Fumitory) was mentioned as a remedy for ingrowing eyelashes by Dioscorides in the First Century A.D. (Gerard 1636).

Reference

Gerard, J. (1636) The Herball of Generall Historie of Plantes. The essence thereof distilled by M. Woodward (1927) from the edition of Th. Johnson 1630. London. Gerald Howe.

Dicentra

20 species are found from the

western Himalayas to eastern Siberia, Japan and western China and in North America.

Dicentra spectabilis
Bleeding Heart

A male greenhouse worker, aged 19 years, developed dermatitis of the hands, forearms and neck. A second attack followed re-exposure to this plant. Patch tests with the pulverized leaves were positive: negative with the pulverized leaves of primrose, chrysanthemum, begonia, geranium and asters. Patch tests with an alcoholic solution of an ether extract of the plant were also positive. Control tests were not recorded (Harville 1933).

Reference

Harville, C.H. (1933) Contact dermatitis due to a common plant. J. Allergy 4, 527.

FUNGI

Fungi

Allergic reactions to moulds were reviewed by Finegold (1976).

Reference

Finegold, I. (1976) Allergic reactions to moulds. Cutis 17, 1080.

Unidentified and various fungi

Smuts and rusts have been suspected of producing skin irritation, stomatitis and inflammation of mucous membranes (Hurst 1942).

Workers who make baskets from rattan (Calamus) develop an eruption on the palms attributed to a fungus on the rattan (Schwartz et al 1957).

White (1934) observed two adult males who suddenly developed an erythematous eruption on the face and exposed parts of the hands and arms following sweeping out a cellar containing a quantitiy of dry decaying wood. The eruptions subsided in 36 hours. He stated that the "dry rot" fungus was the probable irritant.

Dry fruit packers developed palmar dermatitis; a fungus was isolated from the skin (Myers 1927).

A black powdery mould coats the macerated dry stalks of sugar canes (Saccharum) and produces dermatitis in some of the workmen who handle it (Schwartz et al 1957).

Inhalation of fungi from various sources can produce allergic alveolitis (McCombs 1972, Morgan and Seaton 1975).

Brewery workers who scrape off masses of yeasts adhering to fermentation casks with their fingernails develop crusted excrescences beneath the nails and destruction of the nail-plates (White 1934).

Powdery moulds on dry bales of cotton may have been the cause of dermatitis of one hand in workers who picked handfuls of the cotton (Gossypium) (White 1934); however, he speculated that a poisonous weed may have been present.

Various moulds have been suspected as causes of dermatitis viz. Mucor mucedo, Rhizopus nigricans, Aspergillus glaucus and Penicillium glaucum (White 1934).

McCord (1958) refers to Towey's disease which results from exposure to fungi of various trees or logs.

Pammel (1911) referred to an irritant effect of various fungi.

References

Hurst, E. (1942) The Poison Plants of New South Wales. N.S.W. Poison Plants Committee; Sydney.

McCord, C.P. (1958) The toxic properties of some timber woods. Industr. Med. Surg. 27, 202.

McCombs, R.P. (1972) Diseases due to immunologic reactions in the lungs. New Eng. J. Med. 286, 1186 and 1245.

Morgan, W.K.C. and Seaton, A. (1975) Occupational Lung Diseases. Philadelphia. Saunders.

Myers, H.B. (1927) An unappreciated fungicidal action of certain volatile oils. JAMA 89, 1834.

Pammel, L.H. (1911) A Manual of

Poisonous Plants. Torch Press. Cedar Rapids, Iowa. Reprinted Univ. Microfilms Inc. Ann Arbor, Mich. 1965. pp. 476-67.

Schwartz, L., Tulipan, L. and Birmingham, D.J. (1957) Occupational Diseases of the Skin. 3rd ed. Philadelphia. Lea and Febiger. pp. 637-672.

White, R.P. (1934) The Dermatergoses or Occupational Affections of the Skin. 4th. ed. London. H.K. Lewis.

Agaricus

Mushrooms (Agaricus campestris) were reported to be the cause of contact dermatitis of the hands and face in a male mushroom-grower. Patch tests implicated the mushroom rather than the insecticide used (Hopkins 1952).

Inhalation of fungi of mushroom compost can produce mushroom worker's lung, a form of allergic alveolitis (Morgan and Seaton 1975).

Workers in canneries who prepare mushrooms are subject to keratitis, lachrymation and other ocular affections accompanied by such constitutional symptoms as vomiting and jaundice. Helvellic acid which becomes vaporized in the air when the mushrooms are washed in cold water is believed to be the cause (Schwartz et al 1957).

References

Hopkins, H.H. (1952) Mushroom dermatitis. Maryland State Med. J. 1, 504.

Morgan, W.K.C.and Seaton, A. (1975) Occupational Lung Diseases. Philadelphia, Saunders.

Schwartz, L., Tulipan, L. and Birmingham, D.J. (1957) Occupational Diseases of the Skin. 3rd. ed. Philadelphia. Lea and Febiger. pp. 637-672.

Alternaria

Eczematous dermatitis has been attributed to contact with and inhalation of Alternaria, Aspergillus and Penicillium (Fujisawa et al 1966, Feinberg 1940, Tuft et al 1950, Prince et al 1960, Rajka 1963, Jillson and Adami 1955, Jillson 1957, Ofuji et al 1961, Strauss and Kligman 1957, Ofuji et al 1961, Gomez-Orbanaja and Quinones-Caravia 1954, Watanabe and Fujisawa 1965, Bocobo et al 1954, Albert and Walzer 1940, Storck 1955). Crude extracts of moulds produced eczematous changes by patch test and also by inhalation. Type I hypersensitivity reactions can occur from inhalation of fungi (Bruce 1963). Baer et al (1964) reported sensitivity to moulds.

References

Albert, M. and Walzer, M. (1940) Contact Reactions in Atopy: II. The Incidence of contact reactions with various allergens. J. Invest Derm 3, 119.

Baer, R.L. et al (1964) Changing patterns of sensitivity to common mould antigens. Archs. Derm 89, 3.

Bocobo, F.C., Curtis, A.C. and Stubbart, J. (1954) Studies on fungi encountered in the atmosphere II. Production of dermatitis in guinea pigs by crude ether-soluble extracts of Alternaria, Hormodendrum, Penicillium and Aspergillus. J. Invest Derm 23, 489.

Bruce, R.A. (1963) Bronchial and skin sensitivity in asthma. Int. Arch. Allergy 22, 294.

Feinberg, S.M. (1940) Seasonal atopic dermatitis. Archs Derm 40, 200.

Fujisawa, S. et al (1966) Eczematous dermatitis produced by air-borne moulds. Archs. Derm. 94, 413.

Gomez-Orbanaja, J. and Quinones-Caravia, P.A. (1954) La alergia a inhalantes (hongos) en el eczema de las manos. Acta Dermosifiliogr 44, 610, 1953; Z Haut Geschlechtskr 89, 289,1954.

Jillson, O.F. and Adami, M. (1955) Allergic dermatitis produced by inhalant moulds. Archs. Derm 72, 411.

Jillson, O.F. (1957) Allergic dermatitis produced by pathogenic and saprophytic fungi. Ann Allerg. 15, 14.

Ofuji, S. et al (1961) Studies on the role of airborne fungi in several skin diseases. Acta. Derm. 56, 205.

Prince, H.E., Kaplan, M.A. and Halpin, L.J. (1960) The Importance of Inhalant Mold Sensitivity in Atopic Dermatitis. Ann Allerg 18, 186.

Rajka, S. (1963) Studies in Hypersensitivity to Molds and Staphylococci in Prurigo Besnier. Acta Dermatovener 43 (supp 54),1.

Storck, H. (1955) Ekzem Durch Inhalation. Schweis Med Wschr 85, 608.

Strauss, J.S. and Kligman, A.M. (1957) The Relationship of atopic allergy and dermatitis. Archs Derm 75, 806.

Tuft, L., Tuft, H.S. and Heck, V.M. (1950) Atopic dermatitis I. An experimental clinical study of the role of inhalant allergens. J. Allerg 21, 181.

Watanabe, S. and Fujisawa, S. (1965) Eczematous hypersensitivity to molds. Jap. J. Med. Mycol 6, 276.

Aspergillus

See Unidentified Fungi and Alternaria.

Autoerythrocyte sensitisation, which apparently resulted from mould antigen absorption onto the red cell, was found responsible for recurrent urticaria (Shelley and Florence 1961). The patient was sensitive to trichophytin with a cross-sensitivity to mould-derived antibiotics and the common saprophytes such as Aspergillus and Alternaria.

Reference

Shelley, W.B. and Florence, R. (1961) Chronic urticaria due to mold hypersensitivity. A study in cross-sensitisation and autoerythrocyte sensitisation. Archs Derm 83, 549.

Boletus

Two cases of cutaneous sensitization to edible mushrooms (Boletus edulis, Boletus luteus, Lactarius deliciosus and Clavaria flava) were reported. In one case hypersensitivity was also demonstrated after eating the mushrooms in question, fried. Boiling seems to destroy the antigenic effect of mushrooms. From a practical point of view, it is important to be familiar with the cases, as for example in differentiating between similar eruptions caused by sunlight or hypersensitivity to autumn flowers. (Hellerstrom 1941).

Reference

Hellerstrom, S. (1941) Sensitization to edible mushrooms. Acta. Dermato-Venereologica 22, 331.

Candida

Candida allergy produced skin and systemic disease (Joseph et al 1965). Oidomycin, an extract of Candida, produces positive delayed intracutaneous test reactions in sensitized persons.

Reference

Joseph, R., Vialatte, J., Job, J.C. et al (1965) A report of two cases of allergy from Candida albicans in the child, in which respiratory, digestive and skin disorders were combined with articular manifestations. Rev. franc. Allerg. 5, 37.

Cereosporella

An eruption of the wrists of women sorting and packing dried fruits from the Orient was attributed to a mould Cereosporella. The wrists rubbed against the sacking on the tables containing the fruit (Russ 1923).

Reference

Russ, C. (1923) A skin eruption due to a mould. Lancet 1, 77.

Clavaria

See Boletus.

Claviceps

Ingestion of Claviceps on various graminaceous plants can cause ergotism (Sollman 1957).

Reference

Sollman, T.H. (1957) A manual of pharmacology. 8th ed. Philadelphia. W.B. Saunders Co.

Coleosporium

A species of this genus has irritant effects (Pammel 1911).

Reference

Pammel, L.H. (1911) A Manual of Poisonous Plants. Torch Press. Cedar Rapids, Iowa. Reprinted Univ. Microfilms Inc. Ann Arbor, Mich. 1965.

Coprinus atramentarius
Ink Cap

Poisoning occurs only when the fungus is consumed with alcohol. The onset of symptoms varies from 20 minutes to 2 hours. The symptoms are reddening of face, spreading over body with sensation of heat and increase in pulse rate. These last a short time but return if further alcohol is consumed (North 1967).

Reference

North, P.M. (1967) Poisonous plants and fungi in colour. London. Blandford Press. Ltd.

Gyromitra esculenta
Lorchel

The skin and the eyes may be irritated by handling the fungus (North 1967).

Reference

North, P.M. (1967) Poisonous plants and fungi in colour. London. Blandford Press Ltd.

Hebeloma crustuliniforme
Poison Pie

This fungus smells of radish (Raphanus) (North 1967).

Reference

North, P.M. (1967) Poisonous plants and fungi in colour. London. Blandford Press Ltd.

Lactarius

See Boletus.

Lycoperdon

Lycoperdon bovista (Puff Ball) is used in Herbal Medicine as a haemostatic (Wren 1968).

Inhalation of the spores of the puffball (Lycoperdon) can possibly produce allergic alveolitis (Morgan and Seaton 1975).

References

Morgan, W.K.C. and Seaton, A. (1975) Occupational Lung Diseases. Philadelphia, Saunders.

Wren, R.W. (1968) Potter's New Cyclopaedia of Botanical Drugs and Preparations by Wren, R.C. Re-edit. by Wren, R.W. Potter and Clarke Ltd. Health Science Press. Rustington, Sussex.

Morchella

Industrial workers preserving an edible fungus, Morchella (Morel) developed keratoconjunctivitis and respiratory irritation (Pick 1927, Grant 1962).

References

Grant, W.M. (1962) Toxicology of the eye. Springfield, Ill. Charles C. Thomas.

Pick, L. (1927) Augen- und Schleimhauterkrankungen durch Morchelausdunstungen (gewerbliche Massenerkrankung). Zbl. Augenheilk, 61, 325.

Mucor

See Unidentified fungi.

Parietaria officinalis

This species can cause contact dermatitis (Noferi 1970).

Reference

Noferi, A. (1970) Difficulties and limitations of specific hyposensitization in patients sensitized to Parietaria officinalis. Folia Allergol (Roma) 17, 256.

Pencillium

See Unidentified Fungi and Alternaria.

Pithomyces

See Sporidesmium.

Puccinia

The wheat (Triticum) rust (Puccinia) has been reported to cause dermatitis (Schwartz et al 1957).

Puccinia coronata can cause contact dermatitis (Leonardi 1954).

Reference

Leonardi, G. (1954) Spore di lichene boschivo (Palmeria caperata) causa di allergosi cutanea. Folia Allerg. 1, 219.

Schwartz, L., Tulipan, L. and Birmingham, D.J. (1957) Occupational Diseases of the Skin. 3rd ed. Philadelphia. Lea and Febiger. pp. 637-672.

Rhizopus

See Unidentified Fungi.

Saccharomyces

Saccharomyces cerevisiae, a yeast used in baking has been reported to cause dermatitis.

Scopulariopsis

Binders and vendors of hay, straw and rushes, those engaged in putting matting around bottles and in seating cane-bottomed chairs may be affected by fungi. White (1934) speculated that Scopulariopsis koninjii might be responsible; the fungus occurs in litter, straw and manure.

Reference

White, R.P. (1934) The Dermatergoses or Occupational Affections of the Skin. 4th ed. London. H.K. Lewis.

Spondylocladium

Cross-sensitivity was observed between castor oil bean dust (Ricinus) and a mould, Spondylocladium (Panzani 1962).

Reference

Panzani, R. (1962) Study of cross sensitivity between castor oil bean dust and Spondylocladium. Int. Arch. Allergy 21, 288.

Sporidesmium

Cattle who ingest Sporidesmium, Pithomyces can develop eczema and liver disease (Leach and Tulloch 1971, Russell 1960).

References

Leach, C.M. and Tulloch, M. (1971) Pithomyces chartarium, a mycotoxin-producing fungus, isolated from seed and fruit in Oregon. Mycologia 63, 1086.

Russell, D.W. (1960) Sporidesmolide I, a metabolic product of Sporidesmium bakeri Syd. Biochim. Biophys. Acta. 45, 411.

Sporotrichum

The reeds of Provence (Arundo), used to make sieves, trellises and ceilings when piled in heaps carry a dry white mould (Sporotrichum) which produces dermatitis in workers who strip the stalks (Schwartz et al 1957).

Ustilago hypodites was incriminated and positive epicutaneous tests to the fungus were observed in rabbits (Gerbaud 1885 Ann. de Derm. et Syph. November cited by White 1887). This represents an early use of the epicutaneous test. For Ustilago, see p. 314.

References

Schwartz, L., Tulipan, L. and Birmingham, D.J. (1957) Occupational Diseases of the Skin. 3rd ed. Philadelphia. Lea & Febiger. pp. 637-672.

White, J.C. (1887) Dermatitis venenata: An account of the Action of External irritants upon the skin. Boston. Cupples and Hurd.

Tilletia

Some species of this genus including T. foetens have irritant effects (Pammel 1911).

Reference

Pammel, L.H. (1911) A Manual of Poisonous plants. Torch Press. Cedar Rapids, Iowa. Reprinted Univ. Microfilms Inc. Ann Arbor, Mich.

1965. pp. 476-7.

Trichophytum

See Aspergillus.

Trichophytin, an extract of the fungus, produces positive delayed intracutaneous test reactions in sensitized persons.

Ustilago

A species of this genus was incriminated in dermatitis from reeds as noted under Sporotrichum.

Ustilago bromivora

This smut frequently affects the prairie grass Bromus catharcticus (usually called Bromus unioloides) (Cleland 1943). It was reported to him by a Mr. Goldsack that this smut causes severe hay fever and raises wheals on any part of my body that may be scratched. One smut body in a glass of water gave a solution which gave rise to large wheals when applied to skin that had been broken.

Ustilago has been reported to produce dermatitis (Barjaktarovic and Bogdanovic 1933).

A disorder resembling acrodynia occurs from ingestion of the corn smut Ustilago (Watt and Breyer-Brandwijk, 1962). See also p. 312.

References

Barjaktarovic, S.S. and Bogdanovic, S.B. (1933) Untersuchungen uber die Wirkung des Maisbrandes (Ustilago maidis). Arch f exper Path in Pharmakol 173, 381.

Cleland, J.B. (1943) Plants including fungi, poisonous or otherwise injurious to man in Australia. IV. Med. J. Australia. 11, 161.

Watt, J.M. and Breyer-Brandwijk, M.G. (1962) The Medicinal and poisonous plants of Southern Africa. 2nd ed. Edinburgh. E. & S. Livingstone.

Ustilago avenae, U. hordei, U. neglecta, U. nuda, U. tritica and U. utriculosa have irritant properties (Pammel 1911).

Reference

Pammel, L.H. (1911) A Manual of Poisonous plants. Torch Press. Cedar Rapids, Iowa. Reprinted Univ. Microfilms Inc. Ann Arbor, Mich. 1965. pp. 476-7.

GERANIACEAE

750 species in five genera are cosmopolitan.

Erodium

90 species are found in Europe, the Mediterranean area to central Asia, temperate Australia and southern tropical South America. The mericarp has a sharp point with backward-pointing hairs.

Erodium cicutarium (Common Crowfoot)

The sharp pointed fruits can injure the skin, especially of sheep (Hurst 1942). Alleged photodermatitis from ingestion of the plant is probably incorrect (Watt and Breyer-Brandwijk 1962).

Erodium moschatum

The pointed seeds can produce mechanical injury (Watt and Breyer-Brandwijk 1962).

References

Hurst, E. (1942) The Poison Plants of New South Wales. N.S.W. Poison Plants Committee; Sydney.

Watt, J.M. and Breyer-Branwijk, M.G. (1962) The Medicinal apd Poisonous Plants of Southern Africa. 2nd ed. Edinburgh. E. & S. Livingstone.

Geranium

400 species are cosmopolitan, especially found in temperate regions.

Geranium dissectum (Cranesbill Herb) and G. maculatum (American Cranesbill)

The roots of these plants have astringent and styptic properties (Wren 1968) from a content of tannin (Kariyone 1971).

References

Kariyone, T. (1971) Atlas of Medicinal Plants. Osaka, Japan.

Takeda Chemical Industries.

Wren, R.W. (1968) Potter's New Cyclopaedia of Botanical Drugs and Preparations by Wren, R.C. Re-edit. by Wren, R.W. Potter & Clarke, Ltd. Health Science Press. Rustington, Sussex.

Pelargonium

250 species are native to tropical regions especially South Africa. Geraniums of florists belong to this genus. Some are fragrant especially when bruised.

Pelargonium species

Patch testing with the leaf can cause irritant reactions and reactions registered as allergic should be accepted with caution (Agrup 1969). Four of 52 patients tested showed a positive reaction (Hjorth 1968). However in another study none of 400 persons tested showed a positive reaction (Fregert and Hjorth 1968). The reports of dermatitis from species of this genus are lacking in sufficient detail to confirm an allergenic effect (Schwartz et al 1957, McCord 1962, Anderson 1923, Kaalund-Jorgenson 1951, Freundenthal 1924, Imschenetzky 1928, Williams 1924, Becker and O'Brien 1959).

Pelargonium odoratissimum

Oil of Geranium is derived from this and allied species (Arctander 1960). The constituents include esters of geraniol, citronellol and linalool (Merck 1968). The composition of the oil can vary according to the source (Algerian, French, Bourbon). Oil of Geranium has been reported to cause contact dermatitis and cheilitis (Klarmann 1958). Geraniol was reported to have sensitizing properties by Keil (1947). Oil of Geranium - East Indian is derived from Andropogon, Gramineae.

Agrup, G. (1969) Hand Eczema and other hand dermatoses in South Sweden. Acta derm.-venereol. 49 Suppl. 61.

Anderson, J.W. (1923) Geranium Dermatitis. Archs. Derm. Syph. 7, 510.

Arctander, S. (1960) Perfume and Flavor Materials of Natural Origin. Elizabeth, N.J. Published by the author.

Becker, S.W. and O'Brien, M.P. (1959) Value of patch tests in dermatology. Archs. Derm. 79, 569.

Fregert, S. and Hjorth, N. (1968) Results of Standard Patch tests with substances abandoned. Contact Dermatitis Newsletter 5, 85.

Freundenthal, W. (1924) Primula and Pelargonium dermatitis. Zbl. Hautkrkh. 13, 240.

Hjorth, N. (1968) Personal communication.

Imschenetzky, A. (1928) Dermatitis from Heracleum and Geranium. Russk. Vestn. Dermat. 6, 3.

Kaalund-Jorgenson, O. (1951) Eczema perioculare (Dermatitis of the eyelids). Acta. derm.-venereol. 31, 83.

Keil, H. (1947) Contact dermatitis due to oil of citronella. Report of 3 cases with experimental studies on ingredients and related substances. J. Invest. Derm. 8, 327.

Klarmann, E.G. (1958) Perfume dermatitis. Ann. Allergy 16, 425.

McCord, C.P. (1962) The Occupational toxicity of cultivated flowers. Ind. Med. Surg. 31, 365.

Merck Index (1968) An encyclopedia of chemicals and drugs. ed. Stecher, P.G. 8th ed. Rahway, N.J. Merck & Co. Inc.

Schwartz, L., Tulipan, L., and Birmingham, D.J. (1957) Occupational Diseases of the Skin. 3rd ed. Philadelphia. Lea & Febiger pp. 637-672.

Williams, C.M. (1924) in discussion of Highman, W.J. (1924) The pathogenesis of dermatitis including eczema. Archs. Derm. Syph. 9, 344.

GESNERIACEAE

2000 species in 120 genera are mainly distributed in tropical and subtropical regions.

Chemistry is recorded by Hegnauer (1966).

Reference

Hegnauer, R. (1966) Chemotaxonomy of plants. Vol. 4. Basel, Birkhauser. p. 202.

Columnea

200 species are native to tropical America.

Columnea pilossisima

Two patients who had contact dermatitis from Streptocarpus showed positive patch test reactions to the leaf, negative to the petal of this plant (Van Ketel 1973).

Reference

Van Ketel, W.G. (1973) Allergic contact eczema from the leaves of Streptocarpus. Trans. St. John's Hosp. Derm. Soc. 59, 73.

Saintpaulia

12 species are native to tropical East Africa.

Saintpaulia spp.
African Violet

Plants of this genus, commonly cultived indoors, are some of the more popular house-plants of North America. Positive patch test reactions to the hairy leaf may indicate irritancy (Hjorth 1968); therefore, anecdotal reports of dermatitis from the plants must be treated with caution.

Saintpaulia ionantha
African Violet

Several varieties and many cultivars are known. The flower produced positive patch test reactions in three patients and the leaf in two of 154 patients tested (Agrup 1969). Heyl (1972) briefly noted two cases of contact dermatitis from the plant. No fully documented case has been found.

References

Agrup, G. (1969) Hand Eczema and other hand dermatoses in South Sweden. Acta. derm.-venereol. 49 Suppl. 61.

Heyl, T. (1972) Pretoria, Transvaal. Personal communication.

Hjorth, N. (1968) at the Finsen Institute. Personal communication.

Sinningia

20 species are native to Brazil.

Sinningia speciosa
Gloxinia

The hairy leaves can produce irritant patch test reactions (Rook 1968, Hjorth 1968). Such reactions (Agrup 1969, Heyl 1972) may not be significant.

References

Agrup, G. (1969) Hand Eczema and other hand dermatoses in South Sweden. Acta. derm.-venereol. 49 Suppl. 61.

Hayl, T. (1972) Pretoria, Transvaal. Personal communication.

Hjorth, N. (1968) at the Finsen Institute. Personal communication.

Rook, A. (1968) Contact dermatitis caused by Streptocarpus, a popular greenhouse plant. Contact Dermatitis Newsletter 3, 52

Streptocarpus

100 species are native to tropical and South Africa and to Madagascar.

Streotocarpus sp.
Trumpet Flower

Three women developed striate dermatitis of the arms, neck and face. Patch test reactions to the leaf and flower were positive, negative in 17 of 18 controls. Additional contact sensitivity was found in two of the cases; in the first to Primula obconica, Rhododendron indicum, Cyclamen persicum, and Fuchsia; in the second, to Browallia, (Agrup and Fregert 1968). Two women had dermatitis of the hands and forearms resembling nummular eczema. Patch tests to the leaf produced positive reactions, negative to the petal; tests in ten controls were negative. The patients showed positive patch test reactions to Columnea pilossisima, Balsam of Peru (Myroxylon), cinnamic and caffeic acids: negative to *Saintpaulia*, *Gloxinia* and *Episcia* (Van Ketel 1973). Of 21 patients tested one showed a positive patch test reaction to the leaf and one to the flower (Agrup 1969).

Streptocarpus rexii
Cape Primrose

Two female horticulturalists developed acute vesicular striate dermatitis of the hands resembling *Primula* dermatitis. Patch tests to the leaf produced positive reactions, negative in seven controls (Rook 1968).

References

Agrup, G. (1969) Hand Eczema and other hand dermatoses in South Sweden. Acta. derm.-venereol. 49 Suppl. 61.

Agrup, G. and Fregert, S. (1968) Patch test reactions to *Streptocarpus*. Contact Dermatitis Newsletter 4, 72.

Rook A. (1968) Contact dermatitis caused by *Streptocarpus*, a popular greenhouse plant. Contact Dermatitis Newsletter 3, 52.

Van Ketel, W.G. (1973) Allergic contact eczema from the leaves of *Streptocarpus*. Trans. St. John's Hosp. Derm. Soc. 59, 73.

GIGARTINACEAE

Chondrus crispus
Irish Moss

Gigartina mammillosa

Subcutaneous injection into rats of carragenin derived from these species induces sensitivity to cold. Necrotizing lesions occur in the nose, paws and tail (Selye 1965). Carragenin is said to stimulate collagen production in wounds (Grant 1962). Injection of carragenin into the cornea of guinea pigs causes granuloma formation (Burns and Beighle 1960).

References

Burns, R.P. and Beighle, R. (1960) Experimental carragenin granuloma of the cornea. Arch. ophth. 64, 712.

Grant, W.M. (1962) Toxicology of the eye. Springfield, Ill. Charles C. Thomas.

Selye, H. (1965) Induced hypersensitivity to cold. Science 149, 201

GINKGOACEAE

Maiden-Hair Family

Fossil species are known but one existing species of the one genus is found in eastern Asia. The plant is widely cultivated as an ornamental but since the fruits are malodorous, male trees are preferred for gardens. Historical aspects were discussed by Franklin (1959).

Chemistry

Ginkgol, hydroginkgol, bilobol and hydrobilobol were isolated from the fruit pulp by Furakawa (1934, 1935).

Ginkgolic acid is the major phenolic, vesicant constituent of the fruit and is closely related to anacardic acid since upon hydrogenation followed by decarboxylation, it yields 3-pentadecyl phenol (Walley 1959). Bilobol is chemically related to cardol. The formulae of the four chemical derivatives of the fruit are given by Sowers et al (1965).

Ginkgolic acid (Sowers et al 1965 from Furakawa (1934)).

OH

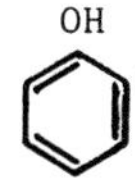

COOH

$(CH_2)_7$-CH=CH-$(CH_2)_5$-CH_3

Ginkgo biloba
Maiden-Hair, Ginkgo Tree

The plant is cultivated and perhaps found wild in eastern China. Since ancient times, in Japan, the leaves have been inserted between the pages of books as a preservative. The green seed-kernel is edible (Watt and Breyer-Brandwijk 1962). An early report of the noxious effects of the fruits was provided by Starr (1913). Saito (1929, 1930) observed dermatitic effects of the fruit juice for humans and rabbits.

Contact with the fruit caused partially generalized dermatitis; patch testing with the fruit pulp produced an irritant reaction (Bolus 1939). The shell and kernel also produced positive patch test reactions (Vollmer and Halter 1939). An epidemic of linear vesicular dermatitis principally on the legs occurred in 35 North American schoolgirls who walked through the crushed fruits under a tree(Sowers et al 1965). These authors confirmed that undiluted fruit pulp was irritant but acetone extracts of the pulp diluted to non-irritant concentration produced positive patch test reactions in the patients and in other individuals who had had dermatitis from Toxicodendron. Additional evidence of cross-sensitivity with Anacardiaceae was provided by the finding that Ginkgo sensitive patients showed positive patch test reactions to pentadecylcatechol (Sowers et al 1965). Handling the intact fruit is said not to cause dermatitis. Patch tests with the leaves have apparently not been performed. Ingestion of the fruit caused stomatitis and pruritus ani (Becker and Skipworth 1975). Their patient had a history of Toxicodendron dermatitis.

Washing old fruits of the previous year produced dermatitis (Watt and Breyer-Brandwijk 1962). The significance of patch tests (Minaki 1969) and of open tests (Becker and Skipworth 1975) is doubtful because of probable irritancy of the fruit pulp.

References

Becker, L.E. and Skipworth, G.B. (1975) Ginkgo-tree dermatitis, stomatitis and proctitis. JAMA 231, 1162.

Bolus, M. (1939) Dermatitis venenata due to Ginkgo berries. Archs. Derm. Syph. 39, 530.

Franklin, A.H. (1959) Ginkgo biloba L.: Historical summary and bibliography. Va. J. Sci. 10, 131.

Furakawa, S. (1934) Constituents of Ginkgo biloba L. fruits: I and II. Sci. Papers Inst. Phys. Chem. Res. 24, 304, cited by Sowers et al (1965) who provide the other references.

Minaki, S. (1969) Rinsho to Kenkyu 46, 145, cited by Ito, K. (1972) Pers. comm.

Saito, J. (1929) Research about skin burning from ginkgo meat. Jap. J. Derm. Urol. 129, 105. cited by Becker and Skipworth (1975) and Watt and Breyer-Brandwijk (1962).

Saito, J. (1930) Tohuku J. exp. Med. 16, 413, cited by Watt and Breyer-Brandwijk 1962.

Saito, J. (1930) Tohuku J. exp. Med. 16, 385, cited by Watt and Breyer-Brandwijk (1962).

Sowers, W.F., Weary, P.E., Collins, O.D. et al (1965) Ginkgo-Tree Dermatitis. Archs. Derm. 91,452.

Starr, A.M. (1913) Poisoning by Ginkgo. Bot. Gaz. Chicago 55, 251.

Vollmer, H. and Halter, K. (1939) Dermatitis due to the fruit of Ginkgo biloba. Zentbl. Haut. Geschlechtskr. 62, 208.

Watt, J.M. and Breyer-Brandwijk, M.G. (1962) The Medicinal and Poisonous Plants of Southern Africa. 2nd ed. Edinburgh. E. & S. Livingstone.

Whalley, W.B. (1959) The Toxicity of Plant Phenolics in The Pharmacology of Plant Phenolics. ed. Fairburn, J.W. London. Academic Press Ltd.

GOODENIACEAE

300 species in 14 genera are chiefly Australian (especially in the southwest) a few in New Zealand, Polynesia and tropical coasts.

Scaevola

80 to 100 species are found in tropical and subtropical regions especially in Australia and Polynesia. S. taccada and S. plumieri widely distributed in tropical beach jungle furnish a kind of rice paper.

Scaevola spinescens
Maroon bush

The plants which bear spines or barbs can cause injuries to humans and livestock (Aplin 1976).

Reference

Aplin, T.E.H. (1976) Poisonous garden plants and other plants harmful to man in Australia. Bull. 3964 Western Australian Department of Agriculture. W.C. Brown. Gov't Printer, Western Australia.

GRAMINEAE (POACEAE)

Grass family

10,000 species in about 620 genera are found in all regions where plants can survive. From this family are derived the majority of the food grains: Avena (Oats): Hordeum (Barley): Oryza (Rice): Panicum, Pennisetum, Sorghum (Millets): Secale (Rye): Triticum (Wheat) and Zea (Corn, Maize). The name Corn is used for various cereal grains - Zea in the United States: Triticum in England: Avena in Scotland.

Chemistry is recorded by Hegnauer (1963).

Coumarin is responsible for the odour of new-mown hay (Whalley 1959). Anthoxanthum odoratum (Sweed Vernal Grass) and Hierochloe odorata have a marked odour of coumarin.

References

Hegnauer, R. (1963) Chemotaxonomy of plants. Vol. 2. Basel, Birkhauser. p. 156.

Whalley, W.B. (1959) The Toxicity of Plant Phenolics in The Pharmacology of Plant Phenolics. ed. Fairburn, J.W. London Academic Press Ltd.

Irritant and allergic contact dermatitis and contact urticaria

Microtrauma, irritant dermatitis and Types IV and I hypersensitivity reactions can result from exposure to plants of this family. A distinction between these effects is not readily made.

A papular urticarial type of dermatitis can result from contact sensitivity to straw and cereal chaff (Michelson 1921). Moor-Millett used for making brooms (Fiocco 1936), grass (Robinson 1937) and Zea (Maize) (Goldshtein and Speransky 1962). have been reported to cause contact dermatitis. Poultry feed workers developed dermatitis of the exposed skin surface and of the intertriginous areas from the dust of Hordeum (Barley) and of Avena (Oats), (Weekly Bulletin 1942). Contact with hay produced urticaria and rhinitis (Bonnevie 1935).

Urticaria (Marcussen 1935) and eczema (Marcussen 1937) resulted from contact with straw. Positive patch test reactions were observed, in one case, to Secale (Rye), Triticum (wheat) Hordeum, (barley), Avena (Oats), Cock's-foot (?Dactylis glomerata) and Phleum (Timothy Grass) (Marcussen 1937).

A cattle fodder worker who had contact-type dematitis showed positive patch test reactions to brans, to Zea (Maize), Hordeum (Barley) and to Beta (Malten 1970); an intracutaneous test to grass pollen produced a negative result. Pesticides and additives used for the plant products can cause dermatitis.

References

Bonnevie, P. (1935) Urticaria following contact with hay. Vereinigung Duesseldorfer Dermatologen Nov. 18.

Fiocco, G.B. (1936) Dermatoses evoked by moor grass (Millet); the industrial dermatoses of broom makers. Boll. sez. region Soc. ital. dermat. 1, 42.

Goldshtein, L.M. and Speranski, W.N. (1962) Maize contact dermatitis Sborn. Nauch. Rab Po Leprol. I Dermatol. 16, 160.

Malten, K.E. (1970) Allergic contact dermatitis due to cattle fodder products. Contact Dermatitis Newsletter 7, 158.

Marcussen, P.V. (1935) Contact urticaria from straw. Vereinigung Duesseldorfer Dermatologen Nov. 18.

Marcussen, P.V. (1937) Combined eczematous and urticarial hypersensitivity to hay and straw. Acta Derm.-Venereol. 18, 186.

Michelson, H.E. (1921) Grain dust dermatoses. Acta derm.-venereol. 2, 262.

Robinson, S.S. (1937) Grass dermatitis. Calif. and West. Med. 47,252.

Weekly Bulletin (1942) Dermatitis due to grain dust. California State Dept. of Health 20, 51, 104.

Parasitophytodermatitis

Parasites of grain were suspected as a cause of skin irritation from grain dust by Ramazzini (1713). 'Straw-itch', 'grain-itch' and itching from contact with cereals can be caused by *Pyemotes ventricosus* (*Pediculoides*). Flour can be infested with the mites *Tyroglyphus farinae*, *T. siro*, *T. longior* and *Glyciphagus domesticus* which are causes of 'baker's itch' (van Thiel 1953).

Dermatitis of the exposed skin surfaces due to tyroglyphid mites in straw can be indistinguishable from contact dermatitis but *Pediculoides* infestation from grain produces a clinical picture more suggestive of bites (Saunders 1944) affecting the covered parts of the body (Fine and Scott 1965). The mite *Pyemotes ventricosus* is parasitic on the larvae of many insects. Such insects, accompanied by their mite, can infest straw, grain, hay, bromegrass seed (*Bromus*), termite infested wood (Fine and Scott 1965), cereals and cotton (*Gossypium*) (van Thiel 1953). Outbreaks of mite bites followed fumigation of houses for termites; termite carcasses are a ready source of food for newly arriving mites (Arnold and Haramoto 1962).

'Harvester's itch' can be caused by a mite *Leptus autumnalis* (Von Mallinckrodt-Haupt 1930, Oppenheim 1942). 'Grass itch' can be caused by *Trombicula deliensis* and by *Acomatacarus australiense* (Belisario 1948).

Packing straw (Legge 1921, Fidanza 1936) and straw bags (palliasses) (O'Donnell 1949) can be infested with mites. Dermatitis in *Sorghum* cutters was probably caused by mites (Hoffer 1918). A zoological classification of these animal parasites in relation to Dermatology was provided by Rook (1972).

References

Arnold, H.L., Jr. and Haramoto, F.H. (1962) 'Grain itch' following fumigation for termites. Derm. Trop. 1, 1.

Belisario, J.C. (1948) Some aspects of occupational dermatitis in Australia. Proc. Brit. Med. Ass. Excerpta Medica Sect. 13 (1948) 3 Abstr. 2808 pp. 590.

Fidanza (1936) Papulovesicular dermatitis due to straw from Guinea. Rev. argent. dermatosif. 20, 403.

Fine, R.M. and Scott, H.G. (1965) Straw itch mite dermatitis caused by *Pyemotes ventricosus*. South. Med. J. 58, 416.

Hoffer, G. (1918) Dermatitis in Sorghum harvesters. Policlinico. Rome. 25(15), 341. abstr. JAMA. 70, 1801, 1918.

Legge, R.T. (1921) Occupational diseases of the skin and hands in California industry. Calif. State. J. Med. 19, 461.

O'Donnell, J.M. (1949) A brief review of industrial dermatoses in Western Australia. Med. J. Australia 2, 200.

Oppenheim, M. (1942) Dermatitis striata pratensis bullosa (Grass or Meadow dermatitis). Arch. Derm. Syph. 46, 541.

Ramazzini, B. (1713) De Morbis Artificum. Bernardini Ramazzini (1633-1714). Diatriba. The Latin Text of 1713, revised by Wright, W.C. (1940). The University of Chicago Press History of Medicine Series No. 7. Library of the New York Academy of Medicine.

Rook, A. (1972) Skin diseases caused by anthropods and other venomous or noxious animals in Textbook of Dermatology. ed. Rook, A., Wilkinson, D.S. and Ebling, F.J.G. 2nd ed. Oxford. Blackwell. p. 845.

Saunders, T.S. (1944) Dermatitis from Tyroglyphidae in handlers of straw. Arch. Derm. Syph. 50, 245.

van Thiel, P.H. (1953) Arthropods and other animals in relation to Dermatology in Handbook of Tropical Dermatology and Medicine-Mycology. Vol II ed. Simons, R.D.G. Amsterdam. Elsevier.

Von Mallinckrodt-Haupt, A. (1930) The harvest itch in Europe. Urol. Cut. Rev. 34, 744.

Mechanical Injury

Many grasses can traumatize the skin by their prickly spikes or by laceration (Behl et al 1966).

Conjunctival reactions can be caused by vegetable matter such as a piece of chaff, straw or a grain of corn, barley (Hordeum), flax-seed (Linum) or cotton (Gossypium) in the eye (Duke-Elder and MacFaul 1972).

Abscesses in the soft palate and lung have been caused by grass seeds (Cleland 1931).

References

Behl, P.N., Captain, R.M., Bedi, B.M.S. and Gupta, S. (1966). Skin-irritant and sensitizing plants found in India, New Delhi. P.N. Behl, Irwin Hospital.

Cleland, J.B. (1931) Plants including fungi, poisonous or otherwise injurious to man in Australia III. Med. J. Australia 2, 775.

Duke-Elder, S. and MacFaul (1972) System of Opthalmology. Vol. XIV. Injuries Part 1. Mechanical Injuries. Extra-ocular foreign bodies. pp. 464-67 and Agricultural Injuries p. 32-34. London. Henry Kimpton.

Fungi

An early report concerning Arundo is that of Sarra (1890)

Smuts and rusts on cereal grains can produce contact sensitivity in wheat-harvesters (Prisco 1952) and respiratory allergy in grain elevator and flour mill workers (Wittich and Stakman 1936-37).

Fungi of Saccharum can produce dermatitis and fungi of Arundo can produce dermatitis and respiratory disease. Claviceps infection of grain can cause ergotism.

References

di Prisco, L. (1952) Dermatite da ruggini del grano nei contadini Folia med. 35, 377.

Sarra (1890) Dermatite causata dalla spore di una ustilaginee. Ref. Arch. f. Dermat 22, 248. Cited by Touton 1932.

Wittich, F.W. and Stakman, E.C. (1936) Case of respiratory allergy due to inhalation of grain smuts. J. Allergy. 8, 189.

Microtrauma

Grain dust (Michelson 1921) and straw dust (Szego et al 1962) can cause mechanical irritation of the skin. Dirt, extraneous vegetable matter of protein nature and prior irritation of the skin were also implicated (Queries and Minor Notes 1928). The irritating properties of Hordeum (Barley) and other cereal dusts are due to sharp trichomes from the awns. Millets (e.g. Pennisetum), Oryza (Rice) and Bambusa (Bamboo) have similar spicules which can produce urticarial papules in workers handling crops or litter straw (Faninger 1960, 1961). Dermatitis has been reported in Europe and America from dehusking Oryza (Rice), Millets (e.g. Pennisetum), and Hordeum (Barley)(Schwartz et al 1957, Woods 1962) but Behl et al (1966) in India saw few cases where dermatitis could be definitely attributed to working with these grains.

References

Behl, P.N., Captain, R.M., Bedi, B.M.S. and Gupta, S.(1966) Skin-irritant and sensitizing plants found in India, New Delhi, P.N. Behl, Irwin Hospital.

Faninger, A. (1960) Berufsdermatosen durch Trichome von Cereallen. Berufsdermatosen 8, 313.

Faninger, A. (1961) Beitrag zur Kenntnis von Berufsdermatosen durch trichome. Berufsdermatosen 9, 130.

Michelson, H.E. (1921) Grain dust dermatoses. Acta derm.-venereol 2, 262.

Queries and Minor Notes (1928) Skin irritations among workers in grain elevators. JAMA 91,1129.

Schwartz, L., Tulipan, L. and

Birmingham, D.J. (1957) Occupational Diseases of the Skin. 3rd ed. Philadelphia. Lea & Febiger. pp. 637-672.

Szego, L., Szabo, P., Cservenka, I. and Lengyel, B. (1962) Dermatitis of the genital regions. An occupational disease of farmers stacking straw. Borgyogy. Vener. Szle. 38, 206.

Woods, B. (1962) Irritant Plants. Trans. St. John's Hosp. derm. Soc. 48, 75.

Heterophytodermatitis

A variety of weeds can occur as satellite plants of food crops (King 1966).

Compositae species especially Ambrosia (Ragweed) can cause dermatitis in workers exposed to graminaceous plants. Nine workers in the flour and cattle feed industries had dermatitis of the exposed skin surfaces from Ambrosia (Ragweed) and other Compositae species which contaminated grain and grain dust. The dermatitis occurred at all times of the year but was most common and severe in hot weather when perspiration caused dust particles to adhere to the skin (Jordan et al 1942). Avena (Oats) and hay contaminated by Ambrosia can cause Ambrosia contact dermatitis or can be responsible for persistence into the winter of previously seasonal dermatitis originally caused by Ambrosia itself (Case Presentation 1943). Threshing of cereal plants, silo-filling and grinding of Avena (Oats) can cause dermatitits actually due to Ambrosia and other weeds (Epstein 1961).

References

Case Presentation (1943) Ragweed dermatitis. Arch. Derm. Syph. 47, 714 and discussion.

Epstein, S. (1961) Occupational dermatitis among farmers. Postgrad. Med. 30, 1.

Jordon, J.W., Campbell, P.C. and Osborne, E.D. (1942) Ragweed dermatitis among workers in the flour and grain industries. Arch. Derm. Syph. 46, 721.

King, L.J. (1966) Weeds of the World. Biology and Control. New York. Interscience.

Pollen

Allergic contact dermatitis form Phleum (Timothy Grass), Artemisia (Pasture Sage) and Plantago (Plantain) with positive patch tests to the oils of the pollens was reported by Michelson (1936). Positive patch test reactions to the pollen of Zea (Corn), of some other grasses and of Ambrosia (Ragweed) in a farmer's daughter were reported by Curtis (1960). In a screening study, none of 533 persons patch tested to a grass-pollen oleoresin, one percent in vaseline, showed positive reactions (Fregert and Hjorth 1968). In Type I hypersensitivity from pollen, in-vitro Type IV reactions have been described (Maini et al 1971). Combined sensitivity has been described (see Phleum).

References

Curtis, G.H. (1960) Plant dermatitis. Virgin. Med. Month 87, 301.

Fregert, S. and Hjorth, N. (1968) Results of standard patch tests with substances abandoned. Contact Dermatitis Newsletter 5, 85.

Maini, R.N., Dumonde, D.C., Faux, J.A. et al (1971) The production of lymphocyte mitogenic factor and migration-inhibition factor by antigen-stimulated lymphocytes of subjects with grass pollen allergy. Clin. Exp. Immunol. 9, 449.

Michelson, H.E. (1936) Dermatitis due to pollen. Archs. Derm. Syph. 33, 897.

Agricultural chemicals

Hjorth and Wilkinson (1968) found that dermatitis from pesticides is regarded as rare. Impurities cause more trouble than the active pesticides; thus contaminants of DDT, Malathion and Lindane were responsible for contact dermatitis. Patch testing with pesticides diluted to an non-irritant concentration can produce false negative patch test results. Selection of an appropriate concentration requires caution since systemic toxicity from absorption can occur. The true incidence of sensitivity will not be known until pure substances are available in proper vehicles and concentrations for patch testing.

The following chemicals have been reported to cause dermatitis: thiurams: Zineb and Maneb, respectively zinc and manganese ethylene bis-dithiocarbamate, DDT, 1,1,1-trichloro-2,2-bis(p-chlorophenyl)ethane: Lindane, gamma-hexachlorocyclohexane: Malathion, S-(1,2-dicarbethoxyethyl)O,O-dimethyldithiophosphate: Parathion, diethyl-p-nitrophenylthiophosphate: Captan or Orthocide, N-(trichloromethylthio)-4-cyclohexane-1,2-dicarboxiimide: (Hjorth and Wilkinson 1968). Germisan, a mordant containing mercury can produce bullous dermatitis and systemic toxicity (Szego 1963). Insecticides (Janson 1951) and plant protective chemicals (Szego 1965) caused dermatitis.

References

Hjorth, N. and Wilkinson, D.S. (1968) Contact Dermatitis II. Sensitisation to pesticides. Brit. J. Derm. 80, 272.

Janson, P. (1951) Skin lesions: in F drug intoxication. Z. Haut.-u. GesehlKr. 11, 507.

Szego, L. (1963) Dermatitis bullosa caused by Germisan, a mordant powder, occurring during wheat-sowing with a machine. Borgyogy. Vener. Szle. 39, 282.

Szego, L. (1965) Experiments with agricultural plant extracts and plant protective substances. Borgyogy. Vener. Szle. 41, 78.

Molinari, R. (1957) Professional papulo-necrotic dermatitis. Riv. Infort. Mal. Prof. 44:556.

Animal feed additives

An extensive list of animal feed additives was provided by Burrows (1975) who reported contact dermatitis from ethoxyquin. Furazolidone (Scharfenberg 1967) cobalt (Bruecker and Hofs 1966), calcium cyanamide (Downing 1935), the antibiotic, tylosin (Neldner 1972), fertilizers and agricultural chemicals (Tamas 1962, Laborie and Laborie 1965) and quinoxaline dioxide (Dawson and Scott 1972) have been reported to cause dermatitis.

References

Breucker, G. and Hofs, W. (1966) Fodder containing cobalt for ruminants as an occupational eczematogen. Derm. Wschr. 152, 528.

Burrows, D. (1975) Contact dermatitis in animal feed mill workers. Brit. J. Derm. 92, 167.

Dawson, T.A.J. and Scott, K.W. (1972) Contact eczema in agricultural workers. Brit. Med. M. 2, 469.

Downing, J.G. (1925) Industrial dermatoses: treatment and legal aspects: review of recent literature. J. Indust. Hyg. Toxicol. 22, 169.

Laborie, F. and Laborie, R. (1965) Pathogenesis of allergic diseases in an agricultural environment. Statistics and ways of prophylaxis. Concours Med. 87, 4783.

Neldner, K.H. (1972) Contact dermatitis from animal feed additives. Archs. Derm. 106, 722.

Scharfenberg, B. (1967) Chicken feed containing nitrofuran as the cause of occupational eczema. Derm. Wschr. 153, 60.

Tamas, R. (1962) Occupational dermatoses of agricultural workers. Borgyogy. Never. Szle. 38, 49.

Gluten

Ingestion of gluten derived from cereals can cause eczema associated with malabsorption (Friedman and Hare 1965).

Reference

Friedman, M. and Hare, P.J. (1965) Gluten-sensitive enteropathy and eczema. Lancet 1, 521.

Starch

Starch is derived from Triticum (Wheat), Solanum (Potato) Oryza (Rice), Zea (Corn), etc. (Merck 1968). Starch (Morris 1954) and a mixture of starches and dextrin (Forstall 1926, Downing 1935) were reported to cause dermatitis. Starch used as a sizing for cloth was incriminated in weaver's asthma

(Murray et al 1957). Wheat and rice starch are considered to be known allergens, and are removed from certain cosmetics (Schieffelin 1973). Starch used for surgical gloves can provoke granulomatous peritonitis (Coder and Olander 1972, Ignatius and Hartman 1972). Alcalase and amylase protease, used as enzyme detergents, produced dermatitis (Bernstein 1972).

Starch

Two cases of dermatitis were reported from dextrin in glue on stamps and labels (Walters and Stern 1941).

References

Walters, J.C. and Stern, E.C. (1941) Dermatitis due to dextrins used as an adhesive on tax stamps. JAMA. 116, 1518.

Bernstein, I.L. (1972) Enzyme allergy in populations exposed to long term, low level concentrations of household laundry products. J. Allerg. Clin. Immunol. 49, 219.

Coder, D.M. and Olander, G.A. (1972) Granulomatous peritonitis caused by starch glove powder. Arch. Surg. 105, 83.

Downing, J.G. (1935) Industrial dermatoses: Treatment and legal aspects: review of recent literature. J. Industr. Hyg. 17, 138.

Forstall, W.C. (1926) Industrial dermatitis. JAMA. 86, 1996.

Ignatius, J.A. and Hartman, W.H. (1972) The glove starch peritonitis syndrome. Ann. Surg. 175, 338.

Merck Index (1968) An encyclopedia of chemicals and drugs. ed. Stecher, P.G. Rahway, New Jersey. Merck Co.

Morris, G.E. (1954) Dermatoses among food handlers. Industr. Med. Surg. 23, 343.

Murray, R., Dingwall-Fordyce, I. and Lane, R.E. (1957) An outbreak of weaver's cough associated with tamarind seed powder. Brit. J. Industr. Med. 14, 105.

Schieffelin and Co. (1973) Almay Hypo-allergenic cosmetics product formulary. 8th ed. Pharmaceutical Laboratories Division 562, 5th. Avenue. New York, N.Y. 10036.

Glycopeptides

Plant material notably glycopeptides was considered to be a significant material in atopic allergens of house dust (Morris et al 1965, Berrens et al 1965).

References

Berrens, L., Morris, J.H. and Versie, R. (1965) The complexity of house dust, with special reference to the presence of human dandruff allergen. Int. Arch. Allergy 27, 129.

Morris, J.H., Berrens, L. and Young, E. (1965) The carbohydrate moiety of house dust allergen. Clin. Chim. Acta. 12, 407.

Flour

Flour is derived from various plants, especially in the East from *Oryza* and in the West from *Triticum*.

Bakers' eczema was described by Bateman (1817). Early reports (Tankard 1923, DeJong 1923, Parsons 1924, White 1925, Walker 1925, Mummery 1925, Schmitt 1927, Starobinski 1927, Stern 1927, Vonno 1930, 1931, Hansman 1931, Queries and Minor Notes 1931, Rothmann 1931 and Wise 1931) were summarized by Zitzke (1932), Downing and Welch (1932), White (1934). The exposed parts were exposed to low grade mechanical irritation from flour particularly dough. Sources of dermatitis were considered to be flour itself, calcium sulfate in confectioner's flour, potassium bicarbonate, salt, sugar, bran, acarids, wetness, sensitisation to wheat protein, yeasts, fungi and the flour improvers potassium and ammonium persulphate. DeJong (1923) found that dermatitis was more common in bakers than in flour mill workers although the latter were more exposed to flour dust.

Tankard (1923) appears to have been the first to report the effects of potassium persulphate which has subsequently been found to be the major cause of bakers' eczema. Reports are scanty from France where the improvers have been little used and legislative banning of persulphates has been followed by a reduction in the number of cases in some other countries (Young 1974). Increase of mechanical rather than hand mixing of the dough has also led to a decline in the number of cases (Kilpinen 1947).

Atopic respiratory symptoms from inhalation of flour (Baker's asthma) were described by Baagöe (1933) and Salen and Juhlin-Dannfelt (1935).

Some bakers show positive skin tests for Type I hypersensitivity to flour extracts (Van Nonno et al 1934, Kilpinen 1947, Subiza 1951, Grianti and Bartalini 1953). Ammonium persulphate acts as a histamine liberator in some persons (Molesworth 1930, Calnan and Shuster 1963). According to van Dishoeck and Roux (1940) dermatitis from flour results from inhalation and is more common in atopic persons who are sensitive to grass pollen. Contact urticaria from flour was observed by Urbach and Wiethe (1931).

Flour and starch derived from various plants have been incriminated in weaver's asthma (Murray et al 1957).

Wüthrich (1970) found that intracutaneous tests with flour extracts were not only specific for flour as such but also for each kind of flour.

Some contaminants of flour in mill dust were considered to be allergenic viz. Penicillium, Aspergillus, rusts and smuts, mites namely Glyciphagus and Tryroglyphus and some insects (Jimenez-Diaz et al 1947).

Benzoic acid, 6% in petrolatum, produced a positive patch test reaction in a baker who had dermatitis (Baird 1945).

Benzoyl peroxide was found to be a significant sensitizer for bakers by Grosfeld (1951). A material used to raise bread, named 'lockerine or diafarine' caused dermatitis in a baker (Chanial and Joseph 1965).

The use of chemicals which are added to flour varies between different countries. For Holland, Young (1974) recommended the following for screening patch testing: Ammonium persulphate 1% aqueous: benzoyl peroxide 1% petrolatum: Potassium bromate 5% aqueous: cinnamic oil 0.5% Petrolatum: limonene 5% olive oil: Balsam of Peru 25% petrolatum: para-amino azobenzene 0.25% petrolatum. Limonene was used as a component of Citrus. Aimed patch testing should include the flour used by a patient and other individual items. Flour extracts should be used for Type I hypersensitivity tests. Flour free of improvers e.g. persulphates should be used for such tests. Heyl and Reinert-Dilthey (1968) and Young (1964, 1974) consider that inhaled flour can act as an atopen and so produce atopic dermatitis and dyshidrotic eczema.

Flour accumulating in the conjunctival sac of bakers in the humid atmospheres of flour-mills can produce a chronic occupational keratoconjunctivitis (Duke-Elder and MacFaul 1972).

Baker's psoriasis is a name for palmar keratoderma of bakers (Wüthrich 1970). Historical aspects of bakers' eczema were discussed by Fisher (1919).

Dermatitis from contact with flour and recurrence of dermatitis following ingestion of flour was reported by Templeton (1945).

References

Baagöe, K.H. (1933) Flour allergy as a cause of vasomotor rhinitis and asthma. Acta med. Scandinav. 80, 310.

Baird, K.A. (1945) Allergy to chemicals in flour: A case of dermatitis due to benzoic acid. J. Allergy 16, 195.

Calnan, C.D. and Shuster, S. (1963) Reactions to ammonium persulphate. Archs. Derm. 88, 812.

Chanial, G. and Joseph, J.-Y. (1965) Allergy to a product of breadmaking in a young baker. Bull. Soc Derm. franc Syph. 72, 99.

DeJong, O. (1923) Etiology of

dermatitis in bakers. Lancet 1, 894.

Dishoeck, H.A.E. v. and Roux, D.J. (1939) Sensitization to flour and flour illnesses amongst flour workers. J. Hyg. 39, 674.

Downing, J.G. and Welch, C.E. (1932) Industrial Dermatoses and their treatment. Review of 10 year's literature. New Eng. J. Med. 206, 666.

Duke-Elder, S. and MacFaul (1972) Systme of Opthalmology. Vol. XIV. Injuries Part 1. Mechanical injuries. Extra-ocular foreign bodies. pp. 464-67 and Agricultural Injuries pp. 32-34. London. Henry Kimpton.

Fischer, J. (1919) History of the professional dermatoses. Urol. Cut. Rev. (Jan) 35-43 cited by White (1934).

Grianti, V. and Bartalini, E. (1953) Allergy in workmen in mills. Rass. Med. Industr. 22, 257.

Grosfeld, J.C.M. (1951) Onderzoekingen over het ontstaan van eczeem bij bakkers. Thesis, Amsterdam; cited by Young (1974).

Hansman, F.S. (1931) Ammonium persulphate in "yeast foods" as a cause of allergic dermatitis in bakers. Med. J. Australia. 2, 94.

Heyl, U. und Reinert-Dilthey, I. (1968) Neue Gesichtspunkte bei der Beurteilung des 'Backerekzems'. Berufsdermatosen 16, 204.

Jimenez-Diaz, C., Lahoz, C. and Canto, G. (1947) The allergens of mill dust. Ann. Allergy 5, 519.

Kilpinen, O. (1947) On bakers' eczema in Finland. Acta derm.-venereol 27, 216.

Kilpinen, O. (1947) Bakers' eczema in Finland. Duodecim 63, 158.

Legge, R.T. (1921) Occupational diseases of the skin ahd hands in California industry. Calif. State J. Med. 19, 461.

Molesworth, E.H. (1930) Allergy as applied to Dermatology. Urol. Cut. Rev. 34, 647.

Parsons, A.C. (1924) Bakers' dermatitis. Brit. J. Derm. 36, 193.

Queries and Minor Notes (1931) Bakers' dermatitis. JAMA 97, 1170.

Rothmann (1931) Bäckerekzem. Dermat. Wschr: 93, No. 50; cited by Touton (1932).

Salen, E.B. and Juhlin-Dannfelt, C. (1935) On the development of so-called latent allergy. Acta med. Scandinav. 86, 505.

Schmitt, P.W. (1927) Allergische Hautproben beim Bäckerekzem. Munch. med. Wschr. 74, Nov. 29, 1957. Arch. f. Dermat. 156, 247; cited by Touton (1932).

Stern, C. (1927) Untersuchung zur Entstehung des Bäckerekzems, zugleich Beitrag zur Frage der Funktionsprüfung der Haut. Arch. f. Dermat. 153, H_2. 286; cited by Touton (1932).

Subiza, E. (1951) Eczema and asthma caused by the combination of flour and ammonium persulphate. Alergologia (Madr.) 1, 343.

Tankard, A.R. (1923) Note on "bakers' excema". Lancet 2, 279.

Templeton, H.J. (1945) Epidermal and dermal sensitisation (Co existing in the same individual) JAMA 127, 908.

Touton, K. (1932) Hauterkrankungen durch phanerogamksche Pflanzen und ihre Produkte (Toxicodermia et Allergodermia phytogenes), in Barnewitz, J. et al Angeborene Anomalien, Lichtdermatosen, Pflanzengifte, Thermische Schädidgungen, Einfluss Innerer Störungen auf die Haut. Berlin, Verlag von Julius Springer.

Urbach, E. and Wiethe, C. (1931) Experimentelle Untersuchungen beieinem nasal gegen verschiedene Mehlarten überempfindlichen Bäcker. Münch. med. Wchnschr. 78, 1470.

Van Dishoeck, H.A.E. and Roux, D.J. (1939) Sensitization to flour and flour illnesses among flour workers. J. Hyg. 39, 665.

Van Dishoeck, H.A.E. and Roux, D.J. (1940) The pathogenesis of flour and persulphate hypersensitivity in flour workers. Ned. T. Geneesk 84, 2320.

Van Dishoeck, H.A.E. and Roux, D.J. (1940) Pathogenesis of hypersensitivity to flour and persulfate in workers handling flour. Arch. f. Dermat. u. Syph. 181, 34.

van Vonno, N.C. (1930) Ekzem der Bäcker. Ned. T. Geneesk. 2, 4388; cited by Touton (1932).

van Vonno, N.C. (1931) Contribution to the knowledge of "Bakers' Eczema" ("Bakers' Itch)". Acta. derm.-venereol. 12, 1; cited by Touton (1932).

van Vonno, N.C., Struycken, J. and Bonnevie, P. (1934) Baker's eczema. Acta derm.-venereol. 15, 343.

Walker, J.T.A. (1925) Baker's itch and workmen's compensation. Lancet 1, 1163 and 1, 1205.

White, R.P. (1925) Eczemas of bread bakers and confectioners. Brit. J. Derm. Syph. 37, 163.

White, R.P. (1934) The Dermatergoses or Occupational Affections of the Skin. 4th ed. London. H.K. Lewis.

Wüthrich, B. (1970) Zur Genese des Bäckerekzems. Hautarzt 21, 214.

Young, E. (1964) Dysidrotic (endogen) eczema. Dermatologica, Basel 129, 306.

Young, E. (1974) Allergic reactions among bakers. Dermatologica 148, 39.

Zitzke, E. (1932) Allergic nature of baker's eczema. Derm. Wchnschr. 95, 1009; abstr. JAMA. 92, 1210.

Zitzke, E. (1934) Value of suitability tests for bakers in the field of industrial direction. Derm. Wchnschr. 99, 878.

Onychia and paronychia

Blackish discoloration of the finger nails probably of bacterial origin was observed in confectioners (Clermont-Ferrand 1950). Infection by yeasts or fungi of flour in bakers was postulated by Mummery (1925), Starobinski (1927).

References

Clermont-Ferrand, C.J. (1950) Onychia and paronychia as an occupational disease of confectioners. Arch. Mal. Prof. 11, 151.

Mummery, H.H. (1925) Baker's dermatitis. Lancet 2, 647.

Starobinski, A. (1927) La dermite des boulangers. Rev. franc. Derm. venereol. 3, 618.

Stigma of bakers

Ramazzini (1713) observed that bakers had thickened hands.

Reference

Ramazzini, B. (1713) De Morbis Artificum. Bernardini Ramazzini (1633-1714). Diatriba. The Latin text of 1713, revised by Wright, W.C. 1940. The University of Chicago Press History of Medicine Series. No. 7. Library of the New York Academy of Medicine.

Grocer's itch and sugar itch

Sugar is derived from various plants e.g. *Saccharum*, *Beta*. Refined and double-refined white sugar was more likely to be one of the causes of grocer's itch than brown sugar. Sugars often contained an abundance of mites (White 1887). The literature was reviewed by White (1934); maceration of the hands in syrups to make candied fruits was responsible for paronychia and skin ulceration. Diacetyl-2,3-butanedione used as a flavoring was found to be the agent of contact dermatitis in 7 of 8 confectionery workers (Hegyi 1971).

Carcinoma

Carcinoma of the skin of the thumb of a baker resulted from friction of hot metal (O'Donovan 1922).

References

Hegyi, E. (1971) Contact sensitivity to flavourings. Contact

Dermatitis Newsletter, London, 9. 206.

O'Donovan, W.J. (1922) Industrial dermatitis. Lancet 2, 570.

White, J.C. (1887) Dermaitis venenata: an account of the Action of External irritants upon the Skin. Boston. Cupples and Hurd.

White, R.P. (1934) The Dermatergoses or Occupational Affections of the Skin. 4th ed. London. H.K. Lewis.

Photosensitization

Reports of phytophotodermatitis from grasses and reeds (Klaber 1942) lack substantiation and psoralens are not known from plants of this family. Oppenheim's meadow dermatitis is produced by Pastinaca and other plants containing psoralens.

Reference

Klaber, R. (1942) Phyto-photo-dermatitis. Brit. J. Derm. Syph. 54, 193.

Andropogon

113 species are native to tropical and subtropical regions.

Andropogon aciculatus

The seeds stick on touch to clothing and animal skin (Das).

Andropogon nardus

Varieties of this plant yield lemon Grass Oil (see Cymbopogon), (Fenaroli 1971).

Andropogon rufus

This species has stinging hairs but many cases of supposed 'grass dermatitis' result from chigger bites (Simons 1952).

References

Das, S.K. (undated) Medicinal, Economic and Useful Plants of India.

Fenaroli, G. (1971) Fenaroli's Handbook of Flavor Ingredients ed. Furia, T.E. and Bellanca, N. Cleveland, Ohio. The Chemical Rubber Co.

Simons, R.D.G. (1952) Handbook of Tropical Dermatology. New York. Elsevier.

Agropyron

100-150 species are found in temperate regions.

Agropyron spp.
Wheatgrass, twitch-grass
couchgrass

The pollens of A. repens and A. smithii are contributing factors in hayfever (Wodehouse 1971). A. repens (twitch - grass, couch-grass) is a troublesome weed.

Reference

Wodehouse, R.P. (1971) Hayfever Plants. 2nd rev. edition. New York, Hafner.

Agrostis

150 and 200 species are cosmopolitan but chiefly north temperate.

Agrostis alba and
Agrostis spp.

Redtop or Herd's grass

The pollen can cause hayfever (Wodehouse 1971).

Reference

Wodehouse, R.P. (1971) Hayfever Plants. 2nd rev. edition. New York, Hafner.

Alopecurus

50 species are found in temperate Eurasia and temperate South America.

Alopecurus pratensis
Meadow foxtail

The pollen can cause hayfever (Wodehouse 1971). The plant is cultivated for pasture.

Reference

Wodehouse, R.P. (1971) Hayfever Plants. 2nd rev. edition. New York, Hafner.

Anthoxanthum

20 species are found in north temperate regions and on tropical mountains of Africa.

Anthroxanthum odoratum
Sweet vernal grass

The pollen is an important cause of hayfever (Wodehouse 1971). The stems contain large quantities of coumarin to which the smell characteristic of new mown hay is due; it may be recognized by chewing a stalk.

Reference

Wodehouse, R.P. (1971) Hayfever Plants. 2nd rev. edition. New York, Hafner.

Avena

70 species are native to temperate regions and tropical mountains. A. sativa, the cultivated Oat is perhaps derived from A. fatua (Wild or Black Oat).

Avena fatua

The awns can cause mechanical injury (Muenscher 1951) and the pointed callus of the fruits can injure the mouths of cattle (Watt and Breyer-Brandwijk 1962). The seeds may be found in the conjunctival sac, nasal cavity and external auditory meatus (MacPherson 1932), and can cause conjunctival reactions (Duke-Elder and MacFaul 1972).

Avena sativa

Excessive consumption of the grain as groats or oatmeal has been thought to cause skin eruptions in man (Newsom et al 1937) and dermatitis from oats has been described in animals (Suppel and Brunside 1954). 'Oat epithelioma' of the tongue of rats may be due to mechanical irritation (Stahr 1921). Ambrosia (ragweed) contaminating oats can cause contact dermatitis (Epstein 1961).

References

Duke-Elder, S. and MacFaul (1972) System of Opthalmology. Vol. XIV. Injuries Part 1. Mechanical Injuries. Extra-ocular foreign bodies. pp. 464-67 and Agricultural Injuries p. 32-34. London, Henry Kimpton.

Epstein, S. (1961) Occupational dermatitis among farmers. Postgrad. Med. 30, 1.

MacPherson, J. (1932) Plants injurious to man in Australia. Med. J. Australia. 1, 281.

Muenscher, W.C. (1951) Poisonous plants of the United States, 2nd ed. New York. The Macmillan Co.

Newson, I.E., Stout, E.N., Thorp, F. et al (1937) Oat hay poisoning J. Am. Vet. Med. Ass. 90, 66.

Sippel, W.L. and Burnside, J.E. (1954) Oat Dermatitis. Georgia Vet. 6(2), 3.

Stahr (1921) Deutsch. med. Wchnschr. 47, 1452 cited by White, R.P. (1934).

Watt, J.M. and Breyer-Brandwijk, M.G. (1962) The Medicinal and Poisonous Plants of Southern Africa. 2nd ed. Edinburgh. E. & S. Livingstone.

Arundo

12 species are found in tropical and temperate regions.

Arundo donax

The stems of the plant are used as lathes and fishing rods. 'Mal des cannes de Provence' was first described by Chaptal in 1750. Stacked reeds become covered with a white powdery fungus which can produce dermatitis, conjunctivitis and respiratory symptoms in workmen who strip the canes. White (1928) reviewed an extensive French literature.

Wetting the canes to prevent dissemination of the fungus provides relief. The fungus is Ustilago (Timpano 1921) or Sporotrichum dermatodes (White 1928) or Alternaria (Gate et al 1952).

Reeds are derived from various botanical species e.g. Arundo, Phragmites; reed grass is a common name for Calamagrostis, (Kelsey and Dayton 1942).

Unspecified reeds have been reported to cause cheilitis and

dermatitis (Fellner 1930, Lerner 1941, Jansen 1973). A report of phytophotodermaitis from reeds (Siemens 1927) lacks substantiation. Dermatitis from reed matting derived from bulrushes (?Scirpus) was probably due to the reed bug Chilacis (Szego and Balogh 1965).

References

Fellner, M. (1930) Die desensibilisierende Wirkung der Höhensonne als Heilfaktor bei einem Berufsekzem (Saxophondermatitis). Derm. Wchnschr. 90, 480.

Gate, J., Coudert, J. and Therre, P. (1952) A new aspect of the disease of the 'canne de Provence' due to its use in the building industry. Ann. Derm. et. Syph. 79, 398.

Jansen, G.T. (1973) Quoted by Arnold, H.L. and Rees, R.B. (1973). Report of Congress. American Academy of Dermatology. Dec.4-9, 1971. Int. J. Derm. 12, 209.

Kelsey, H.P. and Dayton, W.A. (1942) Standardized Plant Names. 2nd ed. Harrisburg, Pa. J.H. McFarland.

Lerne, C. (1941) Cheilitis (with dermatitis) caused by Italian reed. Urol. and Cutan. Rev. 45, 195.

Siemens, H.W. (1927) Systematized bullous dermatitis probably caused by contact with reeds. Derm. Wchnschr. 85, 1577.

Szego, L. and Balogh, L. (1965) A form of occupational dermatitis due to the handling of reed matting. Borgyogy. vener. Szle. 41, 219.

Timpano, P. (1921) Dermatite da canna. Il. Policlinico 28, 6.

White, R.P. (1928) The Dermatergoses or Occupational Affections of the Skin. 3rd. ed. London. H.K. Lewis & Co. Ltd.

Arundinaria

150 species are found in warm regions.

Arundinaria alpina
Bamboo

Dermatitis attributed to this species (Schiff 1951, Bencel 1951) is said to be due to varnish applied to the bamboo or to insects (Simons 1952).

References

Bencel (1951) cited by Simons, R.D.G. (1952).

Schiff, B.L (1951) Contact dermatitis caused by bamboo. Arch. Derm. Syph. 64, 66.

Simons, R.D.G. (1952) Handbook of Tropical Dermatology. New York. Elsevier.

Aristida

330 species are found in temperate and subtropical regions.

Aristida spp.
Spear Grass

The awns can produce mechanical injury to the skin of sheep and humans (Cleland 1914). A. adscensionis (Oakes and Butcher 1962), A. dichotoma, A. longiseta and A. oligantha (Muenscher 1951) have this property. The sharp callus of the fruits of A. congesta can cause a 'traumatic purulent dermatitis' in sheep(Watt and Breyer-Brandwijk 1962).

References

Cleland, J.B. (1914) Plants, including fungi, poisonous or otherwise injurious to man in Australia. Australasian Med. Gaz. 35, 569. idem. Tasmanian Ag. Gaz. 32, 361 and 401

Muenscher, W.C. (1951) Poisonous plants of the United States. 2nd ed. New York. The Macmillan Co.

Oakes, A.J. and Butcher, J.O. (1962) Poisonous and injurious plants of the U.S. Virgin Islands. Misc. Publ. 882. U.S. Dept. of Agriculture, Washington, D.C.

Watt, J.M. and Breyer-Brandwijk, M.G. (1962) The Medicinal and poisonous plants of southern Africa. 2nd ed. Edinburgh. E. & S. Livingstone.

Bambusa

70 species native to tropical and subtropical regions of Asia, Africa and America are the typical genus of bamboos.

Bambusa spp.

Tawny or red hairs on the sheaths of bamboo shoots can cause mechanical injury to the skin and gastrointestinal tract; they have been used for criminal poisoning (Burkill 1935).

Schiff (1951) investigated dermatitis in a factory when tennis-rackets were made of bamboo; the exposed skin surfaces were affected and hyperpigmentation ensued. The workers were sanding bamboo stems from which the bark and hairs had been removed. Patch tests with bamboo shavings produced positive reactions; control tests were not recorded.

An affliction of the Orient is bites from insects which live between the canes of bamboo chairs, affecting some persons who sit on the chairs. Eating of the shoots of B. spinosa is said to cause alopecia (Smith 1969).

Dermatitis can be produced not by the bamboo itself but by saprophytic fungi or varnish applied to the surface.

References

Burkill, I.H. (1935) A Dictionary of the Economic Products of the Malay Peninsula. 2 Vols. London. Crown Agents for the Colonies.

Schiff, B.L. (1951) Contact dermatitis caused by bamboo. Arch. Derm. Syph. 64, 66.

Smith, F.P. (1969) Chinese Materia Medica. Vegetable kingdom 2nd ed. Rev. by Hei, P.D. Taipei, Taiwan. Ku T'ing Book House.

Bouteloua

40 species are found from Canada to South America, especially in the south-western United States.

Bouteloua spp.
Grama

The pollen of some species is a minor cause of hayfever (Wodehouse 1971).

Reference

Wodehouse, R.P. (1971). Hayfever Plants. 2nd rev. edition. New York, Hafner.

Brachiaria

50 species are found in warm climates.

Brachiaria brizantha

Ingestion of the plant is said to produce hepatic photosensitisation in sheep (Hurst 1942).

Brachiaria nigropedata

The juice is irritant to the skin (Watt and Breyer-Brandwijk 1962).

References

Hurst, E. (1942) The Poison Plants of New South Wales. N.S.W. Poison Plant Committee; Sydney.

Watt, J.M. and Breyer-Brandwijk, M.G. (1962) The Medicinal and Poisonous Plants of Southern Africa. 2nd ed. Edinburgh. E. & S. Livingstone.

Bromus

50 species are found in temperate regions and on tropical mountains.

Bromus spp. Brome Grass

The plants can cause mechanical injury to the skin (Behl et al 1966). Brome grass seed can be infested by the biting mite, Pyemotes ventricosus (Fine and Scott 1965). A smut which infects the plants is said to produce contact urticaria.

The barbed fruits work into the eyes, nostrils and mouth of stock causing serious injury. The pollen of some species especially B. rigidans, can cause hayfever (Wodehouse 1971).

Bromus tectorum
Downy Brome Grass

The awns can cause mechanical injury to the skin (Muenscher 1951).

References

Behl, P.N., Captain, R.M., Bedi, B.M.S. and Gupta, S. (1966) Skin-irritant and sensitizing plants found in India, New Delhi. P. N. Behl, Irwin Hospital.

Fine, R.M. and Scott, H.G. (1965) Straw itch mite dermatitis caused by Pyemotes ventricosus. South Med. J. 58, 416.

Muenscher, W.C. (1951) Poisonous plants of the United States. 2nd ed. New York. The Macmillan Co.

Wodehouse, R.P. (1971) Hayfever Plants. 2nd rev. edition. New York, Hafner.

Cenchrus

25 species are found in tropical and warm temperate regions.

Cenchrus spp.

Species of this genus have hooked fruits which attach themselves to animals (Howes 1974).

Cenchrus biflorus (Bhandari 1974), Cenchrus echinatus (Burgrass) (Oakes and Butcher 1962) and C. pauciflorus (Muenscher 1951) can cause mechanical injury to the skin by their spiny burs.

Cenchrus tribuloides

The spikelets surrounding the fruits become hard and prickly acting as a means of distribution by animals and their entanglement in wood can be injurious to sheep.

References

Bhandari, M.M. (1974) Famine foods in the Rajasthan desert. Lloydia 28, 73.

Muenscher, W.C. (1951) Poisonous plants of the United States. 2nd ed. New York. The Macmillan Co.

Oakes, A.J. and Butcher, J.O. (1962) Poisonous and injurious plants of the U.S. Virgin Islands. Misc. Publ. 882. U.S. Dept. of Agriculture, Washington, D.C.

Howes, F.N. (1974) A Dictionary of Useful and Everyday Plants and their Common Names. Cambridge University Press. pp. 290.

Chloris

40 species are found in tropical and warm temperate regions. Several species are useful pasture grasses.

Chloris truncata
Windmill Grass

Ingestion of this plant is said to produce photosensitisation in animals (Hurst 1942). A report from Australia of dermatitis from the plant (Gardner and Bennetts 1956) may refer to the above statement.

References

Gardner, C.A. and Bennetts, H.W. (1956) The Toxic plants of Western Australia. Perth West. Australian Newspapers Ltd.

Hurst, E. (1942) The Poison Plants of New South Wales.N.S.W. Poison Plants Committee; Sydney.

Cortaderia

Fifteen species are found in New Zealand and South America.

Cortaderia selloana
Pampas grass

The plant can cause cuts and itchiness in humans (Aplin 1976).

Reference

Aplin, T.E.H. (1976) Poisonous garden plants and other plants harmful to man in Australia. Bull. 3964. Western Australia Department of Agriculture. W.C. Brown, Gov't. Printer, Western Australia

Cymbopogon

60 species are native to tropical and subtropical regions of Africa and Asia. Several species yield aromatic essential oils used

in soaps and perfumery.

Chemistry of some of the essential oils from species of this genus is given by Fenaroli (1971).

Cymbopogon citratus and C. flexuosus

These plants in Ceylon and Southern India yield Lemon-Grass Oil which has rubefacient properties (Behl et al 1966). Vesicular dermatitis of the face, forearms and ankles appeared in eight workers who were exposed to a ship's cargo of Lemon Grass Oil (Mendelsohn 1944). Undiluted oil is irritant by patch test; sensitization to the oil can probably occur (Mendelsohn 1946). the oil from this plant contains 72 to 81% citral (Merck 1968). Citral is considered a sensitizer of perfumery (Greenberg and Lester 1954). Lemon Grass Oil may be used to adulterate Lemon Oil (Citrus).

Cymbopogon nardus

Contact sensitivity to Oil of citronella resulted from two isomers of citronellol and geraniol of the oil. Cross-sensitivity was observed with Palmarosa oil (Cymbopogon martini) and some other chemicals (Paschoud 1963).

Reference

Paschoud, J.M. (1963) Qulques cas d'eczema de contact avec sensibilisation de groupe. Dermatologica. 127, 349.

Cymbopogon martini

The plant in India yields Palmarosa (East Indian geranium) Oil (Fenaroli 1971). The oil can produce dermatitis in hypersensitive individuals (Greenberg and Lester 1954).

Cymbopogon winterianus (syn. Andropogon nardus) and C. nardus (Andropogon nardus)

These plants yield Java and Ceylon Citronella oils respectively (Fenaroli 1971). Follicular contact dermatitis from Citronella oil was observed by Lane (1922). In two cases of contact dermatitis from the oil positive patch test reactions were observed to citronellal; weaker positive reactions were observed to citronellol, hydroxycitronellal, citral and geranylacetate and in one of the two cases to geraniol (Keil 1944, 1947).

For the precise botanical sources of oils from Cymbopogon and Andropogon Fenaroli (1971) and Arctander (1960) and Hegnauer (1963) may be consulted.

References

Arctander, S. (1960) Perfume and Flavor Materials of Natural Origin. Elizabeth, N.J. Published by the author.

Fenaroli, G. (1971) Fenaroli's Handbook of Flavor Ingredients ed. Furia, T.E. and Bellanca, N. Cleveland, Ohio. The Chemical Rubber Co.

Hegnauer, R. (1963) Chemotaxonomy of plants. Vol. 2 Basel, Birkhauser p. 185.

Keil, H. (1944) The value of the patch test in Poison Ivy dermatitis, with consideration of group reactions between Rhus extracts and Turpentine, Pyrethrum, Ragweed oil and 3-geranyl catechol. J. Allergy 15, 259.

Keil, H. (1947) Contact dermatitis due to oil of citronella. Report of 3 cases with experimental studies on ingredients and related substances. J. Invest. Derm. 8, 327.

Lane, C.G. (1922) Dermatitis caused by Oil of Citronella. Archs. Derm. 5, 589.

Greenberg, L.A. and Lester, D. (1954) Handbook of Cosmetic Materials New York. Interscience.

Behl, P.N., Captain, R.M., Bedi, B.M.S. and Gupta, S. (1966) Skin-irritant and sensitizing plants found in India, New Delhi. P.N. Behl. Irwin Hospital.

Fenaroli, G. (1971) Fenaroli's Handbook of Flavor Ingredients ed. Furia, T.E. and Bellanca, N. Cleveland, Ohio. The Chemical Rubber Co.

Greenberg, L.A. and Lester, D. (1954) Handbook of Cosmetic Materials.

New York. Interscience Publishers, Inc.

Mendelsohn, H.V. (1944) Dermatitis from Lemon Grass Oil (Cymbopogon citratus or Andropogon citratus). Arch. Derm. Syph. 50, 34.

Mendelsohn, H.V. (1946) Lemon Grass Oil; a primary irritant. Arch. Derm. Syph. 53, 94.

Merck Index (1968) An Encyclopedia of Chemicals and Drugs. ed. Stecher, P.G. Rahway, New Jersey. Merck Co.

Cynodon

10 species are found in tropical and subtropical regions. C. dactylon is cosmopolitan.

Cynodon dactylon
Bermuda Grass

In an investigation of 'weed dermatitis', Shelmire (1939) observed positive patch test reactions to an extract of this plant in 7 of 50 patients tested.

Reference

Shelmire, B. (1939) Contact Dermatitis from Weeds; patch testing with their oleoresins. JAMA 113, 1085.

The pollen is an important cause of hayfever. No cross-reaction has been noted with other grasses (Wodehouse 1971).

Reference

Wodehouse, R.P. (1971) Hayfever Plants. 2nd rev. edition. New York, Hafner.

Dendrocalamus

20 species are native to China and IndoMalaysia.

Dendrocalamus giganteus
and D. strictus

Minute brown bristles on the 'collars' at the joints of the poles are irritant to the skin and eye (Allen 1943).

Dactylis

Five species are native to temperate Eurasia.

Dactylis glomerata
Cock's-foot

This pasture grass is widely naturalized or cultivated in North America and South Africa. For reactions to the grass see Phleum. The pollen can cause hayfever (Wodehouse 1971).

References

Allen, P.H. (1943) Poisonous and injurious plants of Panama. Am. J. Trop. Med. (Suppl.) 23, 1.

Wodehouse, R.P. (1971) Hayfever Plants. 2nd rev. edition. New York, Hafner.

Digitaria

380 species are found in warm regions.

Digitaria spp. Crab Grass
(syn. Syntherisma)

Contact dermatitis from Crab Grass was reported by Underwood and Gaul (1948), of 20 patients, 12 were children. The plant produced positive patch test reactions only at certain stages of its growth. Control tests were not recorded. In an investigation of 'weed dermatitis', Shelmire (1939) observed positive patch test reactions to an extract of Syntherisma sanguinalis (Crab Grass) in 5 of 50 patients tested.

References

Shelmire, B. (1939) Contact dermatitis from weeds; patch testing with their oleoresins. JAMA. 113, 1085.

Underwood, G.B. and Gaul, L.E. (1948) Overtreatment dermatitis in dermatitis venenata due to plants JAMA 138, 570.

Echinochloa

30 species are found in warm regions.

Echinochloa crus-galli
(syn. Panicum) Panic Grass

The plant can cause mechanical injury (Behl et al 1966).

Refernece

Behl, P.N., Captain, R.M., Bedi, B.M.S. and Gupta, S. (1966) Skin-irritant and sensitizing plants found in India, New Delhi. P.N. Behl, Irwin Hospital.

Eragrostis

300 species are cosmopolitan, mostly tropical.

Eragrostis sp.
Tumble Grass

The juice is irritant to the skin (Watt and Breyer-Brandwijk 1962). Tumble Grass was said to cause contact dermatitis by Underwood and Gaul (1948). They obtained strong positive patch test reactions in three cases but controls were not recorded.

References

Underwood, G.B. and Gaul, L.E. (1948) Overtreatment dermatitis in dermatitis venenata due to plants. JAMA 138, 570.

Watt, J.M. and Breyer-Brandwijk, M.G. (1962) The Medicinal and poisonous plants of Southern Africa. 2nd ed. Edinburgh. E. & S. Livingstone.

Erianthus

30 species are found in a disjunct distribution in America, southeastern Europe, etc.

Erianthus ravennae
Plume Grass

The rough sharp edges of the leaves can cause mechanical injury (Behl et al 1966).

References

Behl, P.N., Captain, R.M., Bedi, B.M.S. and Gupta, S. (1966) Skin-irritant and sensitizing plants found in India, New Delhi. P.N. Behl. Irwin Hospital.

Festuca

80 species are cosmopolitan. Many are good pasture grasses.

Festuca spp. Fescues

The pollen of some species can cause hayfever (Wodehouse 1971).

Reference

Wodehouse, R.P. (1971) Hayfever Plants. 2nd rev. edition. New York, Hafner.

Guadua

30 species are found in tropical America.

Guadea aculeata,
G. angustifolia and G. latifolia

Minute brown bristles on the 'collars' at the joints of the poles are irritant to the skin and eye (Allen 1943).

Reference

Allen, P.H. (1943) Poisonous and injurious plants of Panama. Am. J. Trop. Med. (Suppl) 23, 1.

Heteropogon

120 species are found in tropical regions.

Heteropogon contortus

The sharp callus of the fruits can puncture the skin, mouth and gut of animals (Burkill 1935, Watt and Breyer-Brandwijk 1962).

References

Burkill, I.H. (1935) A Dictionary of the Economic Products of the Malay Peninsula. 2 Vols. London. Crown Agents for the Colonies.

Watt, J.M. and Breyer-Brandwijk, M.G. (1962) The Medicinal and Poisonous Plants of Southern Africa. 2nd ed. Edinburgh. E. & S. Livingstone,

Holcus

Eight species are found in the Canary islands, northern Africa, Europe to Asia Minor and the Caucasus, one species in Southern Africa.

Holcus lanatus
Velvet grass

The pollen can cause hayfever

(Wodehouse 1971).

Reference

Wodehouse, R.P. (1971) Hayfever Plants. 2nd edition.New York, Hafner.

Hordeum

20 species are found in temperate regions.

Hordeum vulgare (syn. H. sativum) Cultivated Barley

The awns of Hordeum can produce microtrauma and irritation of the skin (Thompson 1925). 'Barley itch' in dock-workers was attributed to Mucuna pruriens among the barley (White 1934); in barley-sifters to an acarus Sphaerogyna cerealella which was parasitic on moth larvae among the barley (Pascal 1900). 'Maltster's itch' was attributed to malt dust (Spillman 1924). Fermented barley caused generalized dermatitis in seven members of a family (Marinoso 1947). Urbach and Steiner (1927) reported contact sensitivity to barley dust. Barley grains can cause conjunctival reactions (Duke-Elder and MacFaul 1972). Some other effects attributed to barley will be found in the introduction to this family.

References

Marinoso, J. (1947) Cereals itch in a family. Acta Dermo-Sifiliograficas 38, 523.

Pascal (1900) A generalized desquamating scarlatiniform erythema of parasitic origin. Ann. Derm. Syph. Aug.-Sept; p. 947. abstr. Brit. J. Derm. 13, 37. 1901.

Thompson, A.G.G. (1925) Barley Itch. Brit. Med. J. 1, 71.

Spillman, M.L. (1924) Maltster's itch. Bull. Soc. Franc. Derm. Syph. May. p. 17 cited by White 1937.

Urbach, E. and Steiner, M. (1927) Barley-dust idiosyncrasy: A contribution to physical allergy of the skin. Arch. f. Derm. u. Syph. 153, 772.

White, R.P. (1934) The Dermatergoses or Occupational Affections of the Skin. 4th ed. London. H.K. Lewis.

Imperata

10 species are found in tropical and subtropical regions.

Imperata cylindrica Cotton Grass

This species can produce mechanical injury (Behl et al 1966).

Reference

Behl, P.N., Captain, R.M., Bedi, B.M.S. and Gupta, S. (1966) Skin-irritant and sensitizing plants found in India, New Delhi. P.N. Behl, Irwin Hospital.

Koeleria

60 macrospecies (100 microspecies) are found in north and south temperate regions.

Koeleria spp. Western June grass

The pollen can cause hayfever (Wodehouse 1971).

Reference

Wodehouse, R.P. (1971) Hayfever Plants. 2nd rev. edition. New York, Hafner.

Lagurus

One species is native to the Mediterranean region.

Lagurus ovatus

This species was reported to cause occupational dermatitis (Benini et al 1970).

Reference

Benini, F. et al (1970) A case of occupational phytodermatitis caused by Lagurus ovatus and Antriscus cerefolium. Arcisp. S. Anna Ferrara. 23, 427.

Leersia

15 species are found in tropical and warm temperate regions.

Leersia spp. Cut grass

North American species of the genus are liable to cut the hands (Howes 1974).

Leersia oryzoides Cut grass

This European and British species has a similar property.

Reference

Howes, F.N. (1974) A Dictionary of Useful and Everyday Plants and their Common Names. Cambridge University Press. pp. 290.

Lolium

12 species are native to temperate Eurasia.

Lolium spp. Ryegrass

The pollen of some species can cause hayfever (Wodehouse 1971).

Lolium perenne
Darne, Ryegrass

Facial eczema occurring in animals which ingest the plant may result from photosensitivity (Hurst 1942).

References

Hurst, E. (1942) The Poison Plants of New South Wales. N.S.W. Poison Plants Committee; Sydney

Wodehouse, R.P. (1971) Hayfever Plants. 2nd rev. edition. New York, Hafner.

Melinis

One species is native to tropical South American and the West Indies, 17 species to tropical and South Africa.

Melinis minutiflora
Molasses grass

This fodder grass has stinging hairs. Many cases of 'grass dermatitis' are caused by chigger bites (Simons 1952). The seeds of Melinis can cause mechanical injury by their prickles (Wimmer).

The pollen has been suspected of causing hayfever (Wodehouse 1971).

References

Simons, R.D.G. (1952) Handbook of Tropical Dermatology. New York. Elsevier.

Wimmer cited by White, R.P. (1934) The Dermatergoses of Occupational Affections of the Skin. London. H.K. Lewis.

Wodehouse, R.P. (1971) Hayfever Plants. 2nd rev. edition. New York, Hafner.

Miscanthidium

Seven species are found in tropical and South Africa.

Miscanthidium sorghum

The leaf is irritant to the skin (Watt and Breyer-Brandwijk 1962).

Reference

Watt, J.M. and Breyer-Brandwijk, M.G. (1962) The Medicinal and Poisonous Plants of Southern Africa. 2nd ed. Edinburgh. E. & S. Livingstone.

Oryza

25 species are found in tropical regions.

Oryza Rice

The plant is cultivated in shallow water till nearly ripe when the water is drained off. The stagnant water contains putrescent matter, uprooted weeds and the remains of fish and molluscs. Maceration of the feet and hands, trauma and infection can produce skin disease in rice-field workers (Schwartz et al 1957, White 1934). Water plants such as Najas which have toothed leaves can cause mechanical injury to the legs. A nonspecific papulo-pustular eruption can affect the immersed skin, (Gianotti and Luvoni 1958, Pardo-Castello 1962). A major cause of disability is cercarial dermatitis which has been reported from many countries (Gianotti and Luvoni 1958, Rácz and Lengyel 1966, Bearup and Langsford 1966, Yang et al 1965, Kaijima 1958, Landman et al 1961, Pardo-Castello 1962, Malheiro 1960).

Szego (1965) observed positive patch test reactions to the leaf of the plant in some agricultural workers. Mechanical irritation by rice dust and allergy to rice protein are noted by Nasution et al (1973). Workers who dehusk rice by rubbing it between their hands develop a characteristic type of callosity (Diniz 1954).

Spiky hairs of the plant can cause a type of nodose opthalmia and blasticidin powder used on the plants has been reported to inflame the eye (Duke-Elder and MacFaul 1972). Rice starch is considered to be a known allergen and removed from certain cosmetics, (Schieffelin 1973).

References

Bearup, A.J. and Langsford, W.A. (1966) Schistosome dermatitis in association with rice-growing in the Northern Territories of Australia. Med. J. Australia 53, 521.

Diniz, O. (1954) Queratosis palmar de los classificadores de arroz. Arch. Argent. Derm. 4 11.

Duke-Elder, S. and MacFaul (1972) System of Opthalmology. Vol. XIV Injuries Part 1. Mechanical Injuries. Extra-ocular foreign bodies. pp. 464-67 and Agricultural Injuries pp. 32-34 London. Kenry Kimpton.

Gainotti, F. and Luvoni, R. (1957) Cutaneous Pathology of Persons weeding Rice Fields and Transplanting Rice. G. Ital. Derm. 99, 377.

Kaijima, H. (1958) Paddy field dermatitis in Nagano Prefecture. Shinshu Med. J. 7, 603.

Landman, H., Thai, D.D., Ngoan, T.V. and Nga, V.B. (1961) Cercaria-dermatitis in Vietnamese rice-planters. Zbl. Bakt. I. Abt. Orig. 182, 410.

Malheiro, L. (1960) Dermatitis of Rice Weeders. J. Soc. Cienc. Med. Lisbon 124, 673.

Nasution, D., Klokke, A.H. and Nater, J.P. (1973) A survey of occupational dermatoses in Indonesia. Berufsdermatosen 21, 215.

Pardo-Castello, V. (1962) Common dermatoses in Agricultural Workers in the Caribbean Area. Industr. Med. Surg. 31, 305.

Racz, I. and Lengyel, B. (1966) Occupational dermatitis of rice-field workers. Borgyogy Vener. Szle. 42, 208.

Schieffelin and Co. (1973) Almay Hypo-allergenic cosmetics product formulary. 8th ed. Pharmaceutical Laboratories Division. 562 - 5th Avenue, New York, N.Y. 10036.

Schwartz, L., Tulipan, L. and Birmingham, D.J. (1957) Occupational Diseases of the Skin. 3rd. ed. Philadelphia. Lea & Febiger, pp. 637-672.

Szego, L. (1965) Sensitisation by agricultural crops and crop-protection preparations. I. Studies of plant (leaf) extracts. Acta. Med. Acad. Sci. Hung. 21, 19 (Excerpta Medica XVII, 13, 3468).

White, R.P. (1934) The Dermatergoses or Occupational Affections of the Skin. 4th ed. London. H.K. Lewis.

Yang, K-L., Tschou, T-K., T'ang, C-C. Ho, T-K. and Luo, H-C (1965) A study on dermatitis in rice farmers. Chin. Med. J. 84, 143.

Oxytenanthera

20 species are found in tropical Africa, eastern Asia and IndoMalaysia.

Oxytenanthera sp.

The brown hairs on the leaf-sheaths are an irritant poison (Burkill 1935).

Reference

Burkill, I.H. (1935) A Dictionary of the Economic Products of the Malay Peninsula. 2 Vols. London. Crown Agents for the Colonies.

Panicum

500 species are found in tropical and warm temperate regions.

Panicum effusum Millet

In certain stages of growth the plant is said to be photosensitising for guinea pigs and sheep (Hurst 1942).

Panicum maximum

Photodermatitis ('dikoor') clinically similar to tribulosis (Tribulus) is reported from ingestion. It is possible that a smut infeciton (Ustilago sp.) is involved (Watt and Breyer-Brandwijk 1962).

Panicum pyramidale
Sett or Sadd

This water-grass causes dermatitis in Egypt named Sett or Sadd dermatitis (Simons 1952).

References

Hurst, E. (1942) The Poison Plants of New South Wales. N.S.W. Poison Plants Committee; Sydney.

Simons, R.D.G. (1952) Handbook of Tropical Dermatology. New York. Elsevier.

Watt, J.M. and Breyer-Brandwijk, M.G. (1962) The Medicinal and Poisonous Plants of Southern Africa. 2nd ed. Edinburgh. E. & S. Livingstone.

Paspalum

250 species are found in warm lands. In temperate America they form a large proportion of the pasture of the campos, pampas, etc.

Paspalum spp. Bull grass

The pollen is suspected of being a contributory cause of hayfever (Wodehouse 1971).

Reference

Wodehouse, R.P. (1971) Hayfever Plants. 2nd rev. edition. New York, Hafner.

Pennisetum

130 species are found in warm regions.

Pennisetum purpureum
Elephant Grass

The plant possesses sharp edged leaves capable of causing mechanical injury (Williamson 1956).

Reference

Williamson, J. (1956) Useful Plants of Malawi. ed. Greenway, P.J. Zomba, Malawi. The Government Printer. Previously publsihed as Useful Plants of Nyasaland.

Phleum

15 species are found in temperate Eurasia, North America to Mexico and temperate South America.

Phleum pratense
Timothy Grass

Dermatitis from Timothy Grass with a positive patch test reaction to the pollen was reported by Ramirez and Eller (1930).

Persons handling this grass can develop maculo-papular dermatitis especially in August and September (Schwartz et al 1957). Mitchell and Mitchell (1945) obtained positive patch tests with the albumen fraction and negative reactions with the lipid fraction of Timothy pollen in a patient with seasonal dermatitis.

Pollen extracts of Timothy grass and of Cocksfoot grass (Dactylis) produced immediate hypersensitivity skin reactions in patients with allergic rhinitis and also delayed reactions in 4/6 patients following intradermal injection. The pollen extracts also produced lymphocyte transformation and inhibition of leukocyte migration when incubated with white cells of some atopic patients (Brostoff and Roitt 1969). In a series of 2700 intradermal skin-tests to 12 common inhalant antigens, Green et al (1967) reported a 6 percent incidence of delayed skin reactions. No delayed reactions were observed in 20 children who had immediate reactions to pollen extracts of some grasses and Compositae plants (Go et al 1970).

References

Brostoff, J. and Roitt, I.M. (1969) Cell-mediated (delayed) hypersensitivity in patients with summer hay-fever. Lancet 2, 1269.

Go, S., Michaels, D.L. and Ellis, E.F. (1970) Delayed hypersensitivity to pollen. Lancet 1, 1115.

Green, G.R., Zewiman, B., Beerman, H. and Hildreth, E.A. (1967) Delayed skin reactions to inhalant antigens. J. Allergy Appl. Immunol. 40, 224.

Mitchell, J.H. and Mitchell, W.F. (1945) Seasonal Dermatitis due to the Albumin Fraction of Timothy Pollen. J. Allergy 16, 48.

Ramirez, M.A. and Eller, J.J. (1930) The "Patch test" in "Contact Dermatitis" (Dermatitis venenata). J. Allergy 1, 489.

Schwartz, L., Tulipan, L. and Birmingham, D.J. (1957) Occupational Diseases of the Skin. 3rd ed. Philadelphia. Lea and Febiger pp. 637-72.

Poa

300 species are cosmopolitan. Many are useful pasture grasses.

Poa spp. Bluegrass

The pollen of some species can cause hayfever (Wodehouse 1971).

Reference

Wodehouse, R.P. (1971) Hayfever Plants. 2nd rev. edition. New York. Hafner.

Phyllostachys

40 species are native from the Himalayas to Japan.

Phyllostachys pubescens

An outbreak of dermatitis was observed in the spring of 1971 in the Gifu district of Japan. The flower appeared to be the responsible agent in a farmer aged 35 years, who had contact dermatitis of the hands. A patch test was positive. Flowering of this plant is generally regarded as occurring once about every 60 or 120 years (Ito 1972).

Reference

Ito, K. (1972) Pers. Comm.

Rhynchelytrum

37 species are found in tropical Africa, Madagascar and from Arabia to Indochina.

Rhynchelytrum repens
(syn. Tricholaena rosea)
Natal grass

This species is cultivated for dry bouquets. The pollen may be a minor contributor to hayfever (Wodehouse 1971).

Reference

Wodehouse, R.P. (1971) Hayfever Plants. 2nd rev. edition. New York, Hafner.

Saccharum

Five species are native to tropical and subtropical regions.

Saccharum officinarum
Sugar Cane

The plant, perhaps a native of eastern Asia, is cultivated in most warm regions. Sugar is contained in the soft central tissues of the stem. The canes are cut before flowering and crushed to extract the juice. The saw-edge of the leaf is used to scarify an infant's face before tattooing (Burkill 1935). Labourers in sugar-cane fields can develop an urticarial eruption from Mucuna pruriens (Behl et al 1966) and pruritic pustular folliculitis which starts on the lower limbs and spreads to other hairy areas producing follicular atrophy and cicatricial alopecia (Pardo-Castello 1962). Workers who habitually carry cut canes develop hyperkeratosis and thickening of the skin of the shoulders (Pardo-Castello 1962). The stigma is unilateral depending on the handedness of the individual (Arnold 1968). According to Schwartz et al (1957) almost no sugar eczema occurs on plantations but, in sugar mills, squamous and tylotic eczema of the palms and thickening of the nails occurs in workers who clean the centrifuges with large quantities of water. A fungus of stored sugar canes can cause dermatitis of the exposed skin and genitals (Abstract

1921). Furunculosis, known as sugar-boils, can affect sugar, candy and ice-cream workers; crystals of sugar can scratch the skin and exert a hygroscopic effect (Sequeira 1911, Ferranini 1920, Queries and Minor Notes 1929, Downing and Welch 1932, Schwartz et al 1957). Respiratory symptoms (bagassosis) can affect workers exposed to crushed extracted sugar cane (bagasse).

Sugar is also derived from Beta. Some other reactions attributed to sugar are noted in the introduction to this family.

Saccharum spontaneum
Thatch Grass

This species can cause mechanical injury by the sharp edges of the leaves (Behl et al 1966).

References

Abstract (1921) Dermatitis among workersin cane. Il Lavoro 11, 274. Abstr. J. Industr. Hyg. 3, 103.

Arnold, H.L. (1968) Poisonous plants of Hawaii. Rutland, Vermont. Charles E. Tuttle.

Behl, P.N., Captain, R.M., Bedi, B.M.S. and Gupta, S. (1966) Skin-irritant and sensitizing plants found in India, New Delhi. P.N. Behl, Irwin Hospital.

Burkill, I.H. (1935) A Dictionary of the Economic Products of the Malay Peninsula. 2 Vols. London. Crown Agents for the Colonies.

Downing, J.G. and Welch, C.E. (1932) Industrial Dermatoses and Their Treatment: Review of 10 year's literature. New Engl. J. Med. 206, 666.

Ferranini, L. (1920) The professional stigmata of ice-cream makers. Il Lavoro 12, 97; Abstr. (1920) J. Ind. Hyg. 2, 199.

Pardo-Castello, V. (1962) Common dermatoses in agricultural workers in the Caribbean area. Industr. Med. Sug. 31, 305.

Queries and Minor Notes (1929) JAMA 93, 1407.

Sequeira, J.H. (1911) Diseases of the Skin. First ed. London. J. and A. Churchill. p. 78.

Schwartz, L., Tulipan, L. and Birmingham, D.J. (1957) Occupational Diseases of the Skin. 3rd ed. Philadelphia. Lea & Febiger. pp. 637-672.

Secale

Four species are native to regions from eastern Europe to central Asia; one species is native to southern Africa.

Secale cereale
Rye

This species is cultivated in northern Europe as a cereal and for fodder. Contact sensitivity to this species and to other plants of this family was observed by Marcussen (1937). The pollen is a minor cause of hayfever (Wodehouse 1971).

References

Marcussen, P.V. (1937) Combined eczematous and urticarial hypersensitivity to hay and straw. Acta. derm.-venereol. 18, 186.

Wodehouse, R.P. (1971) Hayfever Plants. 2nd rev. edition. New York, Hafner.

Setaria

140 species. Tropical and warm temperate. S. italica is named Italian Millet.

Setaria lutescens

Cattle which eat the plant can develop stomatitis (Bankowski et al 1956).

Setaria scandens

The leaf is irritant to the skin (Watt and Breyer-Brandwijk 1962).

Setaria verticillata

The seed can attach itself to clothing and to animals (Watt and Breyer-Brandwijk 1962).

References

Bankowski, R.A., Wichmann, R.W. and Stuart, E.E. (1956) Stomatitis of Cattle and Horses due to Yellow Bristle Grass (Setaria lutescens). J. Am. Vet. Med. Assoc. 129, 149.

Watt, J.M. and Breyer-Brandwijk, M.G. (1962) The Medicinal and Poisonous Plants of Southern Africa. 2nd ed. Edinburgh. E. & S. Livingstone.

Sorghum

60 species are found in tropical and subtropical regions. Some yield a red dye, especially when injured (Williamson 1956).

Sorghum halepense
(Johnson Grass)

In an investigation of 'weed dermatitis' in the Southern United States, an extract of this plant produced negative patch test reactions in all of 50 consecutive patients tested (Shelmire 1939). The pollen can cause hayfever (Wodehouse 1971).

Sorghum vulgare
(Millet, Guinea Corn, Broom Straw)

25 cases of dermatitis in Sorghum cutters were observed by Hoffer (1918). He was unable to decide whether the plant itself or a parasite upon it was responsible.

This plant forms the bristles of certain brooms. The particles of dust given off in the making of brooms contain a hard 'spike' which surrounds the seed; this material caused intense pruritus and eczema (Piccinini 1920), considered to be a mechanical rather than a chemical irritation (Carossi cited by White 1934). Occupational hazards in broom-making are described by Schwartz et al (1957).

References

Carossi, "Brooms" (Broom, Corn, Sorghum) Occupation and Health. Brochure 139. Geneva cited by White (1934).

Hoffer, G. (1918) Dermatitis in Sorghum cutters. Policlinico, Rome 25, 341; Abstr. JAMA 70, 1801, 1918.

Piccini (1920) cited by White (1934).

Schwartz, L., Tulipan, L. and Birmingham, D.J. (1957) Occupational Diseases of the Skin. 3rd ed. Philadelphia. Lea & Febiger. pp. 637-672.

Shelmire, B. (1939) Contact Dermatitis from Weeds; Patch Testing with their oleoresins. JAMA 113, 1085

Williamson, J. (1956) Useful Plants of Malawi. ed. Greenway, P.J. Zomba, Malawi. The Government Printer. Previously published as Useful Plants of Nyasaland.

Wodehouse, R.P. (1971) Hayfever Plants. 2nd rev. edition. New York, Hafner.

Sporobolus

150 species are found in tropical and warm temperate regions.

Sporobolus spp.
Bedgrass

The plants can cause mechanical injury (Oakes and Butcher 1962).

Reference

Oakes, A.J. and Butcher, J.O. (1962) Poisonous and injurious plants of the U.S. Virgin Islands. Misc. Publ. 882. U.S. Dept. of Agriculture, Washington, D.C.

Stenotaphrum

Seven species are found in tropical and subtropical regions.

Stenotaphrum dimidiatum
Buffalo grass

The plant can cause cuts and itchiness in humans (Aplin 1976).

Reference

Aplin, T.E.H. (1976) Poisonous garden plants and other plants harmful to man in Australia. Bull. 3964 Gov't Printer, Western Australia

Stipa

300 species are found in tropical and temperate regions. S. tenacissima (Esparto Grass) is used to make paper.

Stipa spp. Spear Grass

Early explorers of Australia noted mechanical injury from this grass. The awns can irritate the skin of humans and of sheep (Cleland 1914).

Stipa comata (Needle Grass) and S. spartea (Porcupine Grass) can produce mechanical injury (Muenscher 1951).

References

Cleland, J.B. (1914) Plants, including fungi, poisonous or otherwise injurious to man in Australia. Australasian Med. Gaz. 35, 569. idem. Tasmanian Ag. Gaz. 32, 361 and 401.

Muenscher, W.C. (1951) Poisonous plants of the United States, 2nd ed. New York. The Macmillan Co.

Themeda

Ten species are found in warm regions of Africa and Asia.

Themeda arguens

The sharp-pointed seed is used to pierce the earlobe (Burkill 1935).

Themedia triandra

The sharp callus of the mature fruit can become entangled in the wool of sheep (Watt and Breyer-Brandwijk 1962).

References

Burkill, I.H. (1935) A Dictionary of the Economic Products of the Malay Peninsula. 2 Vols. London. Crown Agents for the Colonies.

Watt, J.M. and Breyer-Brandwijk, M.G. (1962) The Medicinal and Poisonous Plants of Southern Africa. 2nd ed. Edinburgh. E. & S. Livingstone.

Triodia

35 species are native to Australia.

Triodia sp.
(possibly Festuca sp.)
Porcupine, Spinifex Grass.

Early explorers of Australia noted that the pointed leaf spines can break off under the skin (Cleland 1925).

Reference

Cleland, J.B. (1925) Plants, including fungi, poisonous or otherwise injurious to man in Australia. Med. J. Australia 2, 443.

Triticum

About 20 species are native to Europe, the Mediterranean region and western Asia. The cultivated species fall into three groups according to chromosome number.

Triticum spp. Wheat

Cultivars of these species are the principal Westernsource of flour which can cause dermatitis. See also flour, bakers' eczema.

Triticum Bakers' eczema

An insect, Trogoderma sp., which infests flour (Triticum), has irritant hairs (Swan and Papp 1972).

Reference

Swan, L.A. and Papp, C.S. (1972) The common insects of North America. New York. Harper & Row. p. 395.

Triticum

Inhalation of a fungus of wheat flour can produce wheat weevil disease, a form of allergic alveolitis (Morgan and Seaton 1975).

Reference

Morgan, W.K.C. and Seaton, A. (1975) Occupational Lung Diseases. Philadelphia, Saunders.

A fungicide applied to wheat and barley (Hordeum) (zinc and manganese ethylene bisdithiocarbamate) produced allergic contact dermatitis in a man who prepared the seed and in a farmer (Burry 1976).

Reference

Burry, J.N. (1976) Contact dermatitis from agricultural fungicide in South Australia. Contact

Dermatitis 2, 288.

Vetiveria

10 species are native to tropical Africa, Asia and Australia.

Vetiveria zizanoides
Khus-khus
(syn. Andropogon, Squarrosus)

The plant yields a volatile oil, the chemistry of which is given by Merck (1968).

Oil of Vetiver derived from this species and used in perfumes, cologne and toilet waters can produce dermatitis in hypersensitive individuals (Greenberg and Lester 1954).

Vetiver acetate of a certain grade has sensitizing properties (Opdyke 1974).

Reference

Opdyke, D.J. (1974) Monographs on Fragrance Raw Materials. Fd. Cosmet. Toxicol. 12, 1011.

Greenberg, L.A. and Lester, D. (1954) Handbook of Cosmetic Materials. New York. Interscience.

Merck Index (1968) An Encyclopedia of Chemicals and Drugs. ed. Stecher, P.D. 8th ed. Rahway, N.J. Merck and Co. Inc.

Zea

One species, originally from tropical South and Central America, is now cultivated in most tropical and subtropical regions.

Zea mays
Indian Corn, Maize

About a third of 50 corn-pickers developed eczema or papular urticaria (Goldshtein and Speranski 1962). Blighted corn (DiPrisco 1953) and an arsenic preparation applied for corn-blight (Lapysheff 1931) caused dermatitis. Dermatitis was observed in 3-7% (Seligman and Key 1968) and in 15% (Tudor 1941) of workers in corn-processing plants. The dermatitis was a low-grade irritant type almost confined to those handling wet corn during processing for canning. Szego (1965) observed positive patch tests to the leaf in a survery of agricultural workers. Corn flour was reported to cause dermatitis (Coca et al 1931) and cornstarch on sheets was reported to cause contact urticaria. Cornstarch, considered to be a known allergen, is removed from certain cosmetics (Schieffelin 1973). Corn or maize can be infested by a parasite (Ciarocchi).

The pollen can cause hay-fever (Wodehouse 1971). See also Cereals.

Contact sensitivity to maize is noted under Beta.

Contact dermatitis of the fingers from popcorn was reported by Waldbott and Shea (1948).

References

Coca, A.F., Walzer, M. and Thommen, A.A. (1931) Asthma and Hayfever. Springfield, Ill. Charles C. Thomas.

DiPrisco, L. (1952) Dermatitis in farmers due to blighted corn. Folia med. (Napoli) 35, 377.

Goldshtein, L.M. and Speranski, W.N. (1962) Maize contact dermatitis. Sborn. Nauch. Rab. Po Leprol. I Dermatol. 16, 160.

Lapysheff, D. (1931) Occupational dermatoses due to arsenic. Sovet Vest. Dermat. 9, 126; Abstr. Arch. Dermat. & Syph. (1931) 24, 1089.

Schieffelin & Co. (1973) Almay Hypo-allergenic cosmetics product formulary. 8th ed. Pharmaceutical Laboratories Division. 562. 5th Avenue, New York, N.Y. 10036.

Seligman, E.J. and Key, M.M. (1968) Corn Dermatitis. Archs. Derm. 97, 664.

Szego, L. (1965) Sensitisation by agricultural crops and crop-protection preparations. I. Studies of plant (leaf) extracts. Acta. Med. Acad. Sci. Hung. 21, 19. (Excerpta Medica XVII, 13, 3468.

Tudor, R.B. (1941) Corn dermatitis. Lancet 61, 450.

Ciarocchi, cited by White, R.P. (1934) The Dermatergoses of Occupational Affections of the Skin. 4th ed. London. H.K. Lewis.

Wodehouse, R.P. (1971) Hayfever Plants. 2nd rev. edition. New York, Hafner.

Waldbott, G.L. and Shea, J.J. (1948) Causative diagnosis of contact dermatitis II. A classification of patterns on the hands. Archs. Derm. Syph. 57, 975.

Goodacre, R.L., Clancy, R.L., Davidson, R.A. and Mullens, J.E. (1976) Cell mediated immunity to corn starch in starch-induced granulomatous peritonitis. Gut. 17,202.

Grant, J.B., Davies, J.D., Jones, J.V., Espiner, H.J. and Eltringham, W.K. (1976) The immunogencity of starch glove powder and talc. Br. J. Surg. 63, 864.

GROSSULARIACEAE

150 species in two genera are found in temperate Eurasia, north-west Africa, North and central America and Pacific South America to Fuegia.

Ribes

150 species are found in north temperate and Andine regions.

Ribes spp.
Gooseberry, Currant

The spines of these species can produce mechanical injury. Sensitivity to gooseberry was reported by Besche (1929).

Reference

Besche, A. de (1929) Serologische Untersuchungen uber "Allergische Krankheiten" beim Menschen. Acta. path. Scand. 6, 115.

GUTTIFERAE

(syn. CLUSIACEAE)

1000species in 40 genera are mostly tropical. Mammea americana is cultivated for its edible fruit.

Chemistry is recorded by Hegnauer (1966).

Reference

Hegnauer, R. (1966) Chemotaxonomy of Plants. Vol. 4. Basel, Birkhauser. p. 216.

Calophyllum

Eight species are found in Madagascar and Mauritius, 100 species in IndoMalaysia, IndoChina, the Pacific region and tropical Australia, four species in tropical America and the West Indies. C. tacamahaca yields a resin, tacamahac.

Calophyllum brasiliense
Jacareuba

The moist sawdust of jacareuba, especially that of older trees, caused persistent dermatitis and folliculitis in Brazilian woodworkers (Freise 1932, 1936). It contains a pyranoxanthone (King et al 1953) and other xanthones (Silva Pereira et al 1966).

Calophyllum inophyllum
Mast Wood, Alexandrian Laurel

The sap of this species irritates the skin and eyes (Morton 1971). An oil derived from the seeds, named Domba oil, has rubefacient and irritant properties (Quisumbing 1951). The wood can produce dermatitis (Lewin 1962).

References

Morton, J.F. (1971) Plants Poisonous to People in Florida and other warm areas. Miami, Florida. Hurricane House Publishers, Inc.

Quisumbing, E. (1951) Medicinal Plants of the Philippines. Tech. Bull. 16. Manila, Philippine Islands. Manila Bureau of Printing. 1234 pp.

Silva Pereira, M.O. da et al (1966) A quimica de gutiferas brasiloiras. IX: Constituentes xantonicas do Calophyllum brasiliense. A. acad. brasil. Cienc. 38(3/4), 425.

Freise, F.W. (1932) Gesundheitsschädigungen durch Arbeiten mit giftigen Hölzern. Beobachtungen aus brasilianischen

Gewerbebetrieben. Archiv. für Gewerbepathologie und Geweibehygiene 3, 1.

Freise, F.W. (1936) Vergiftungen durch Brasilianische. Werkholzer I, II. Sammlung der Vergiftungsfullen 7c, 1 and 61.

King, F.E., King, T.J. and Manning, K1C. (1953) The constitution of Jacareubin, a pyranoxanthone from Calophyllum brasiliense. J. Chem. Soc. 3922.

Lewin, L. (1962) Gifte und Vergiftungen. Lehrbuch der Toxologie. 5 Aufl. Ulm. K.F. Haug., cited by Hausen (1970).

Hausen, B.M. (1970) Untersuchungen über Gesundheitsschädigende Hölzer. Thesis Hamberg.

Caraipa

20 species are found in tropical South America. Some species of the genus yield medicinal balsam and useful hard timber (Shaw 1973).

Caraipa densiflora
and Caraipa spp.
Tamacoari, Laksiri

The sap of the bark and sapwood is said to be so caustic as to blister the skin (Record and Mell 1924, Record and Hess, 1943).

References

Record, S.J. and Mell, C.D. (1924) Timbers of Tropical America. New Haven, Yale.

Record, S.J. and Hess, R.W. (1943) Timbers of the New World. New Haven, Yale.

Clusia

145 species are mostly found in warm regions of America and in Madagascar and New Caledonia.

Clusia rosea
Pitch Apple, Copey

A resin obtained from the trunk and mature fruits is used in powdered form for counter-irritant purposes (Morton 1962).

Reference

Morton, J.F. (1962) Ornamental Plants with Poisonous Properties II. Proc. Florida Hort. Soc. 75, 484.

Garcinia

400 species are found in tropical regions, especially of Asia, and in Southern Africa.

Garcinia gibbsae

The exudate of this tree is said to cause blood poisoning (Cleland 1943).

Garcinia hanburyi
Gamboge

The gum resin derived from this species has an acrid taste and a powder of it excites sneezing (Wren 1968).

Garcinia mangostana
Mangosteen

The rind of the edible fruit is used for astringent purposes (Corner 1952).

Garcinia morella and other Garcinia spp.

The resin of several species is known as gamboge. Gamboge is irritant to the eye of rabbits (Duke-Elder and MacFaul 1972) and is used for an irritant effect in Chinese Medicine (Smith 1969).

References

Corner, E.J.H. (1952) Wayside Trees of Malaysia. Singapore, Government Printer.

Cleland, J.B. (1943) Plants, including fungi, poisonous or otherwise injurious to man in Australia. Series IV. Med. J. Australia. 2, 161.

Duke-Elder, S. and MacFaul, P.A. (1972) System of Opthalmology. Vol. XIV Injuries Part 2. Nonmechanical injuries. Irritant Vegetable Products pp. 1180-1196 and Self-inflicted injuries pp. 1916-1918. London. Henry Kimpton.

Smith, F.P. (1969) Chinese Materia Medica. Vegetable kingdom. 2nd ed. Rev. by Hei, P.D. Taipei, Taiwan. Ku T'ing Book House.

Wren, R.W. (1968) Potter's New Cyclopaedia of Botanical Drugs and Preparatios by Wren, R.C. Re-edit by Wren, R.W. Potter & Clarke Ltd. Health Science Press. Rustington, Sussex.

Hypericum

400 species are found in temperate regions and on tropical mountains.

Hypericum aethiopicum

A resin from the flowers is used as a rubefacient (Watt and Breyer-Brandwijk 1962).

Hypericum spp.
St. John's Wort

Farmer (1941) reported a case of contact dermatitis from St. John's Wort. A bullous patch test reaction was observed. Ingestion of the plants by animals can lead to primary photosensitisation from absorption of the plant pigment hypericin (Kingsbury 1964, Morton 1971). The idea, formerly held, that contact with the plant was responsible for the effect has been disproved (Watt and Breyer-Brandwijk 1962).The fresh flowers in olive oil are used in Herbal Medicine for application to the skin (Wren 1968). Photosensitivity from ingestion of the plants, known as hypericism, has not been observed in humans, but Nowak et al (1974) claimed success in treating vitiligo by oral administration and topical application of extracts of the plants.

References

Farmer, E.W. (1941) The patch test as means of diagnosis in contact dermatitis. Med. J. Australia 1, 9.

Kingsbury, J.M. (1964) Poisonous Plants of the United States and Canada. Englewood Cliffs, New Jersey. Prentice-Hall Inc.

Morton, J.F. (1971) Plants Poisonous to People in Florida and other warm areas. Miami, Florida. Hurricane House Publishers Inc.

Nowak, A., Woyton, A. and Baran, E. (1974) Fotodynamiczne dzialanie extractum hyperici w zastosowaniu do leczenia vitiligo. Przegl Dermatol. 61,77.

Watt, J.M. and Breyer-Brandwijk, M.G. (1962) Medicinal and poisonous plants of Southern Africa. 2nd ed. Edinburgh. E. & S. Livingstone.

Wren, R.W. (1968) Potter's New Cyclopaedia of Botanical Drugs and Preparations by Wren, R.C. Reedit. by Wren, R.W. Potter and Clarke Ltd. Health Science Press. Rustington, Sussex.

Mammea

One species is found in tropical America and the West Indies, one species in tropical Africa, 20 species in Madagascar and 27 species in IndoMalaysia and the Pacific region.

Mammea americana

This species is cultivated for its edible fruit, the mammea or San Domingo apricot. The flowers are used in preparing a liquer, eau de Créole. The wood is said by Nigerian wood-workers to cause 'skin itches' (Werndorff 1964). M. americana contains xanthones similar to those of Mesua (Chow and Quon 1968).

References

Chow, Y.L. and Quon, H.H. (1968) Chemical constituents of the heartwood of Mesua ferrea. Phytochem. 7(10), 1871.

Werndorf, G. von (1964) Pers. comm. to Woods and Calnan (1976).

Woods, B. and Calnan, C.D. (1976) Toxic Woods. Brit. J. Derm. 94, Suppl. 13, June.

Mesua

40 species are found in IndoMalaysia.

Mesua ferrea
Ironwood,
Indian rosechestnut, Na

The report of the International Labor office listed ironwood as a source of dermatitis (Senear 1933). He found that there were three woods named ironwoods viz. the above and Eusideroxylon zwageri (Borneo ironwood) and Hopea parviflora (Malabar ironwood) and that it was not possible to decide which, if any, of these botanical species was relevant.

This south-eastern Asian wood was suspected of being poisonous (Lewin 1928). It contains xanthones similar to those in Calophyllum and Mammea (Govindachari et al 1967, Chow and Quon 1968).

References

Govindachari, T.R., Pai, B.R., Subramaniam, P.S. et al (1967) Constituents of Mesua ferrea L.I. Mesuaxanthone A & B. Tetrahedron 23, 243.

Lewin, L. (1928) Gifte im Holzgewerbe. Berlin, Stilke.

Chow, Y.L. and Quon, H.H. (1968) Chemical constituents of the heartwood of Mesua ferrea. Phytochem. 7(10), 1871.

Senear, F.E. (1933) Dermatitis due to woods. JAMA 101, 1527.

Psorospermum

Between 40 and 45 species are found in tropical Africa and Madagascar.

Psorospermum corymbiferum var. corymbiferum
(syn. P. guineense)

The root-bark contains a fluorescent anthroquinonic pigment. Animals who ingest the plant become sensitive to the action of light. The pulped roots and bark are applied for skin diseases on the Ivory Coast (Irvine 1961).

Reference

Irvine, F.R. (1961) Woody plants of Ghana. Oxford University Press. London.

GYROSTEMONACEAE

16 species in five genera are found in Australia.

Codonocarpus

Three species are found in Australia.

Codonocarpus cotinifolius

The plant yields an irritant 'mustard' oil (Kjaer 1960, 1963). (see Cruciferae).

References

Kjaer, A. (1960) Naturally derived isoThiocyanates (Mustard Oils) and their parent glucosides in Progress in the Chemistry of Organic Natural Products. ed. Zechmeister, L. Vol. 18. Vienna. Springer-Verlag. pp. 122-176.

Kjaer, A. (1963). The distribution of sulphur compounds in Chemical Plant Taxonomy. ed. Swain, T. London. Academic Press. p. 453.

HAEMODORACEAE

75 species in 14 genera are found in southern Africa, Australia, North and tropical America.

Lacnanthes

One species is found in North America.

Lacnanthes caroliniana
(syn. L. tinctorum)
Paint-root

The roots yield a red dye. Reports of photodermatitis from ingestion of the plant are anecdoatal (Blum 1941).

Reference

Blum, H.F. (1941) Photodynamic action and Diseases caused by light. Am. Chem. Soc. Monograph Ser. New York Reinhold Publ. Corp.

HAMAMELIDACEAE

80 species in 22 genera are chiefly found in subtropical regions.

Chemistry is recorded by Hegnauer (1966).

Reference

Hegnauer, R. (1966) Chemotaxonomy of plants. Vol. 4. Basel. Birkhauser. p. 238.

Hamamelis

Six species are found in eastern Asia and eastern North America.

Hamamelis virginiana

Witch-hazel derived from the plant has been reported to cause contact dermatitis (Weber 1937, Genner and Bonnevie 1938, Duke-Elder 1965).

References

Duke-Elder, S. (1965) System of Opthalmology. Vol. VIII. Diseases of the outer eye. Part 1. Allergic kerato-conjunctivitis. pp. 451. London. Henry Kimpton.

Genner, V. and Bonnevie, P. (1938) Eczematous eruptions produced by leaves of trees and bushes. Arch. Derm. Syph. 37, 583.

Weber, L.F. (1937) External causes of Dermatitis. A list of irritants. Arch. Derm. Syph. 35, 129.

HERNANDIACEAE

54 species in three genera are found in tropical regions.

Chemistry is recorded by Hegnauer (1966).

Reference

Hegnauer, R. (1966) Chemotaxonomy of plants. Vol. 4. Basel, Birkhauser. p. 246.

Hernandia

24 species are found in central America, Guiana, the West Indies, West Africa, Zanzibar, the Mascarenes, IndoMalaysia and the Pacific region.

Hernandia ovigera

The seed is a skin irritant (Uhe 1974).

Hernandia peltata

The juice, if rubbed on the skin, removes the hair (Burkill 1935).

Hernandia sonora
Jack-in-the-Box, Topolite

The leaf juice has a depilatory effect (Souder 1963). The wood can cause dermatitis in wood-workers possibly from a content of podophyllotoxin acetate (Orsler 1973, King 1953).

References

Orsler, R.J. (1973) Personal communication from Forest Products Research Laboratory, Princess Risborough, Bucks, England.

Souder, P. (1963) Poisonous plants on Guam, In venomous and poisonous animals and noxious plants of the Pacific Region. ed. Keegan, H.L. and Macfarlane, W.V. Oxford. Pergamon Press. pp.15-29.

Uhe, G. (1974) Medicinal plants of Samoa. Econ. Bot. 28, 1.

King, F.E. (1953) The chemistry of wood extractives. Chem. Ind. 1325.

HIPPOCASTANACEAE

15 species in two genera are found in north temperate regions and in South America.

Chemistry is recorded by Hegnauer (1966).

Reference

Hegnauer, R. (1966) Chemotaxonomy of plants. Vol. 4. Basel, Birkhauser. p. 2-4.

Aesculus

One species is found in south-eastern Europe, five species in India and eastern Asia, seven species in North America.

Aesculus spp.
Buckeye

The flowers and young shoots of some species, especially A. octandra are said to be capable of causing contact dermatitis (Massey 1941).

Aesculus hippocastanum
Horse Chestnut

A particle of the shell of

the horse chestnut became embedded in the conjunctiva and caused necrosis and ulceration by a local toxic effect (Grant 1962).

The prickles of the horse-chestnut are said to be relatively or completely innocuous to the eye in contrast to the hairs of some other plants which can cause conjunctival nodules (Duke-Elder and MacFaul 1972).

References

Duke-Elder, S. and MacFaul, P.A. (1972) System of Opthalmology. Vol. XIV. Injuries Part 1. Mechanical Injuries. Extra-ocular foreign bodies. pp. 464-67 and Agricultural Injuries pp. 32-34. London. Henry Kimpton.

Grant, W.M. (1962) Toxicology of the eye. Springfield, Ill. Charles C. Thomas.

Massey, A.B. (1941) Plant Poisoning. Merck Reports. 50, 24.

HYDRANGEACEAE

115 species in ten genera are found in north temperate and subtropical regions and in the Andes from Mexico to southern Chile.

Hydrangea

80 species are found from the Himalayas to Japan, the Philippine islands and Java; in Atlantic North America and on the mountains of Central America to Chile.

Hydrangea sp.
Hydrangea

Two cases of vesicular contact dermatitis in florists were reported by Apted (1973). The leaf and petal produced positive patch test reactions but tests in controls were not recorded.

Hydrangea arborescens

The wood is reported to be injurious to wood-workers (Wagner 1938, Lewin 1962).

References

Apted, J.H. (1973) Phytodermatitis from Hydrangeas. Arch. Derm. 108, 427.

Hausen, B.M. (1970) Untersuchungen über Gesundheitsschädigende Hölzer. Thesis, Hamburg.

Lewin, L. (1962) Gifte und Vergiftungen. Lehrbuch der Toxologie Ulm. 5. Aufl. Verlag K.F. Haug., cited by Hausen (1970).

Wagner, E. (1938) Umgang mit giftigen Holzern. Holzmarkt 300, 1., cited by Hausen (1970).

HYDRASTIDACEAE

One or two species are found in Japan and North America.

Hydrastis

One species is found in Japan, one in eastern North America.

Hydrastis canadensis
Golden Seal

At one time, this plant grew wild in the woods of eastern North America but its medicinal use as a 'tonic' led almost to extermination from ruthless collection of the rhizomes. The plant is cultivated (Wren 1968) and is listed as an irritant without clinical details (Schwartz et al 1957).

References

Schwartz, L., Tulipan, L. and Birmingham, D.J. (1957) Occupational Diseases of the Skin. 3rd ed. Philadelphia. Lea & Febiger. pp. 637-672.

Wren, R.W. (1968) Potter's New Cyclopaedia of Botanical Drugs and Preparations by Wren, R.C. Re-edit. by Wren, R.W. Potter & Clarke Ltd. Health Science Press. Rustington, Sussex.

HYDROCOTYLACEAE

(syn. UMBELLIFERAE)

375 species in 30 genera are found in temperate regions, especially southern, and on tropical mountains.

Azorella

Seventy species found from the northern Andes to temperate south America, the Falkland and Antarctic islands are densely tufted xerophytes.

A. caespitosa of the Falklands is known as balsam bog.

Azorella spp.

In the Andes, the plants are alleged to produce blistering of the skin (Towers, G.H.N. Pers. Comm. 1978.).

Hydrocotyle

100 species are found in tropical and temperate regions.

Hydrocotyle asiata
Indian Pennywort

Ingestion of the plant produced great itching over the whole body, (Waring 1875 cited by Piffard 1881). The plant was introduced to Medicine by Dr. Boileau, himself a leper, who claimed to have cured not only himself, but also many others of the disease (Piffard 1881). The juice of the leaves or whole plant is said to be excellent for stopping the irritation due to prickly heat (several authors cited by Hurst 1942).

References

Hurst, E. (1942) The Poison Plants of New South Wales. N.S.W. Poison Plants Committee; Sydney.

Piffard, H.G. (1881) A Treatise on the Materia Medica and Therapeutics of the Skin. New York. Wm. Wood and Co.

Waring, E.J. (1875) Remarks on some of the Bazaar Medicines and common Medical Plants of India. London, cited by Piffard (1881).

HYDROCHARITACEAE

80 species in 16 genera are tropical and sub-tropical water plants.

Ottelia

40 species are found in tropical and sub-tropical regions.

Ottelia alismoides

The plant is said to be rubefacient (Quisumbing 1951).

Reference

Quisumbing, E. (1951) Medicinal Plants of the Philippines. Tech. Bull. 16. Manila, Philippine Islands. Manila Bureau of Printing. 1234 pp.

HYDROPHYLLACEAE

250 species in 18 genera have a cosmopolitan distribution, except in Australia. There are about 100 North American species, many of which are cultivated as annual or perennial garden plants. Some are native annuals of the deserts and semi-arid regions of the southwest United States. The plants are usually hairy and sometimes glandular.

Eriodictyon glutinosum (Yerba Santa) has an aromatic odour used to mask the taste of Cinchona (Quinine), (Wren 1968).

Phacelia
(Scorpion Weed)

200 species are native to North America and the Andes.

Chemistry is recorded by Hegnauer (1966).

Plants of this genus can produce a linear vesicular dermatitis resembling poison ivy dermatitis (Toxicodendron), (Munz 1932, Berry et al 1962). Walking amongst the plants and handling the flowers produced dermatitis on the lower limbs and on the hands. Patch test confirmed that the plants are allergenic (Berry et al 1962). The sap stains the skin brown (Munz 1932). The following species are recorded as capable of producing dermatitis:
Phacelia brachyloba (Munz 1932), Ph. campanularia (Munz 1932), Ph. crenulata (Desert or False Heliotrope), (Munz 1932, Berry et al 1962), Ph. grandiflora (Munz 1932, Berry et al 1962), Ph. infundibuliformia (Weber 1937), Ph. minor (California Bluebell) (Munz 1932), Ph. pedicellata (Munz 1932), Ph. parryi (Berry et al 1962), Ph. viscida (Berry et al 1962).

Some other Phacelia species did not produce dermatitis in sensitized individuals; the allergenic species were contained in three different sections of the genus and agreed only in being viscid glandular plants (Munz 1932).

References

Berry, C.Z., Shapiro, S.I. and Dahlen, R.F. (1962) Dermatitis venenata from Phacelia crenulata. Archs. Derm. (Chicago) 85, 737.

Hegnauer, R. (1966) Chemotaxonomy of plants. Vol. 4. Basel, Birkhauser. p. 271.

Munz, P.A. (1932) Dermatitis produced by Phacelia (Hydrophyllaceae). Science 76, 194.

Weber, L.F. (1937) External causes of dermatitis. A list of irritants. Arch. Derm. Syph. 35, 109.

Wren, R.W. (1968) Potter's new Cyclopaedia of Botanical Drugs and Preparations by Wren, R.C. Re-edit. by Wren, R.W. Potter and Clarke Ltd. Health Science Press. Rustington, Sussex.

Nama

40-50 species are found in the south-western United States to the West Indies and South America; one species is found in Hawaii.

Nama hispidum var spathulatum

A plant collector noted that the plant blistered the skin (Altsshul 1973).

Reference

Altschul, S. Von R. (1973) Drugs and foods from little-known plants. Cambridge, Mass. Harvard Univ. Press.

Wigandia

Six species are native to Mexico to Peru and to the West Indies.

Wigandia caracasana (Ortiga)

The leaves of the plant growing wild in Panama possess glistening stinging hairs (Allen 1943). The plant is also cultivated.

Wigandia caracasana var. macrophilla

Vesiculo-bullous dermatitis occurred in a woman who repeatedly contacted this cultivated variety. Patch tests to the leaf and stem gave inconclusive results probably indicating the effects of stinging hairs; dried plant material is probably less noxious (Anderson and Ayres 1931).

References

Allen, P.H. (1943) Poisonous and Injurious Plants of Panama. Am. J. Trop. Med. Suppl. 23, 1.

Anderson, N.P. and Ayres, S. (1931) Dermatitis venenata due to Wigandia caracasana, hitherto unrecognized cause. Report of a case. Calif. and West med. 34, 378.

HYMENOCARDIACEAE

Five species in one genus are found in tropical Africa and south-east Asia.

Hymenocardia

The distribution of the genus is that of the family. The genus was formerly placed in Euphorbiaceae.

Hymenocardia acida

The powdered leaves are used as snuff (Irvine 1961).

References

Irvine, F.R. (1961) Woody plants of Ghana. London. Oxford University Press.

ICACINACEAE

400 species in 58 genera are found in tropical regions.

Chemistry is recorded by Hegnauer (1966).

Reference

Hegnauer, R. (1966) Chemotaxonomy of plants. Vol. 4. Basel Birkhauser. p. 275.

Citronella

In a broad sense of the genus, 30 species are found in Malaysia, tropical Australia, the Pacific region and tropical America. C. gongonha provides a tea.

Citronella
(syn. Villaresia)

The wood of Villaresia moorei causes sneezing (Cleland 1943).

Reference

Cleland, J.B. (1943) Plants including fungi, poisonous or otherwise injurious to man in Australia. IV. Med. J. Australia. 11, 161.

ILLICIACEAE

42 species in one genus are found in tropical south-eastern Asia, North America and the West Indies.

Illicium

42 species are found in India, eastern Asia, western Malaysia, Atlantic North America, Mexico and the West Indies.

Illicium verum
Star-Anise

Oil of Anise derived from the fruits of this species and from Pimpinella anisum has been reported to cause dermatitis (Greenberg and Lester 1954). Anethol is said to be the responsible agent.

Illicium religiosum

Dermatitis from this species was reported by Timoshin (1958).

References

Greenberg, L.A. and Lester, D. (1954) Handbook of Cosmetic Materials. New York. Interscience.

Timoshin, A.G. (1958) Dermatitis due to Illicum religiosum. Vestn. Derm. Vener. 32, 77.

Illicium

Star anise oil produced allergic and irritant reactions. (Rudzki and Grzywa 1976).

Reference

Rudzki, E. and Grzywa, Z. (1976) Sensitizing and irritating properties of star anise oil. Contact Dermatitis 2, 305.

IRIDACEAE

800 species in 60 genera are found in tropical and temperate regions. The chief centres of distribution are southern Africa and tropical America. Crocus sativus provides saffron used for dyeing and flavouring and was formerly used in exanthematous diseases to promote the eruption.

Chemistry is recorded by Hegnauer (1963).

Reference

Hegnauer, R. (1963) Chemotaxonomy of Plants. Vol. 2. Basel, Birkhauser. p. 236.

Gladiolus

300 species are found in the Canary islands, Madeira, western and central Europe, from the Mediterranean region to south-western and central Asia and in tropical and southern Africa.

Gladiolus communis
Gladiolus

Gladiolus segetum

These species have irritant properties (Pammel 1911).

Reference

Pammel, L.H. (1911) A manual of poisonous plants. Torch Press. Cedar Rapids, Iowa. Reprinted Univ. Microfilms Inc. Ann Arbor, Mich. 1965. pp. 476-7.

Iris

300 species are found in north temperate regions.

Iris sp. Iris

Dioscorides (First Century A.D.) noted that beating the plants provoked sneezing.

Contact dermatitis from species of this genus was reported by Shelmire (1940). Application of the plant to the healthy skin produced redness, slight burning, eczematoid and urticarial eruptions (Piffard 1881).

Hjorth (1961) observed a

patient contact sensitive to a blue iris. A patch test to the petal of the blue iris was positive but to the green leaf negative; patch tests to petal and green leaf of a yellow iris were negative. The patient was also contact sensitive to Rosa.

References

Dioscorides, The Greek Herbal of: Englished by John Goodyer: A.D. 1655. Edited and first printed A.D. 1933 by R.T. Gunther 1959. New York, Hafner Publishing Co.

Hjorth, N. (1961) Eczematous allergy to Balsams, allied perfumes and flavouring agents. Copenhagen, Munksgaard.

Piffard, H.G. (1881) A treatise on the Materia Medica and Therapeutics of the skin. New York. Wm. Wood and Co.

Shelmire, B. (1940) Contact dermatitis from vegetation. South Med. J. 33, 338.

Iris florentina

Florentine, Veronese and Moroccan roots are sold; the Verona root is sold trimmed for infants' use when teething (Wren 1968).

The dried rhizome of this and other Iris spp. provides orris root which smells like violets (Viola) and yields 'essence of violets' of perfumery. The root formerly inserted into wounds as 'issue peas' produced eczematoid and urticarial eruptions (White 1887). 'Violet water' produced dermatitis on the chest of a girl; the solution has a strong odour of orris root which was the usual substitute for the genuine perfume of violets in such preparations (White 1887). Ramirez and Eller (1930) reported three cases of dermatitis from orris root. Glossitis and gingivitis resulted from a dentifrice which contained orris root (Winter 1948). Preparations containing orris root can cause pustular conjunctivitis and recurrent corneal ulceration (Duke-Elder 1965). Orris root caused dermatitis in users, salesgirls in stores and a barber; its use in adhesive plasters caused dermatitis (White 1934). Orris root can cause dermatitis in pharmaceutical chemists (Schwartz et al 1957).

Orris root was said to be allergenic for atopic dermatitis (Coca et al 1931) and to produce coryza, asthma and skin eruptions (Greenberg and Lester 1954, Klarmann 1958).

Oil of Orris root is derived from orris root. Concrete of Orris root was said to be a common allergen (Greenberg and Lester 1954). Orris root in raw form, which formerly accounted for many allergic reactions has been replaced by a refined orris root oil which is considered to be non-reactive (Burks 1962).

References

Burks, J.W. Jr. (1962) South. med. J. 55, 1006.

Coca, A.F. et al (1931) Asthma and Hayfever. Springfield, Ill. Charles C. Thomas.

Duke-Elder, S. (1965) System of Opthalmology. Vol. VIII. Diseases of the outer eye. Part 1. Allergic kerato-conjunctivitis. pp. 451, London. Henry Kimpton.

Greenberg, L.A. and Lester, D. (1954) Handbook of Cosmetic Materials. New York. Interscience.

Klarmann, E.G. (1958) Perfume dermatitis. Ann. Allergy. 16, 425.

Ramirez, M.A. and Eller, J.J. (1930) The "Patch test" in "Contact Dermatitis" (Dermatitis venenata). J. Allergy 1, 489.

Schwartz, L., Tulipan, L. and Birmingham, D.J. (1957) Occupational Diseases of the Skin. 3rd ed. Philadelphia. Lea & Febiger. pp. 637-672.

White, J.C. (1887) Dermatitis venenata: An account of the Action of External irritants upon the Skin. Boston. Cupples & Hurd.

White, R.P. (1934) The Dermatergoses or Occupational Affections of the Skin. 4th ed. London. H.K. Lewis.

Winter, G.R. (1948) Allergic manifestations caused by the use of a dentifrice containing orris root powder. J. Periodont. 19, 108.

Wren, R.W. (1968) Potter's New

Cyclopaedia of Botanical Drugs and Preparations by Wren, R.C. Re-edit by Wren, R.W. Potter and Clarke Ltd. Health Science Press. Rustington, Sussex.

Iris pseudacorus
Yellow Flag

The seeds of the plant named tiger lily seeds used as a bracelet caused dermatitis of the wrist, later of the arms and face. Patch tests to the seed and leaf produced positive reactions (Calnan 1970).

References

Calnan, C.D. (1970) Iris pseudacorus L. Contact Dermatitis Newsletter, London 8, 171.

Iris germanica

The plant is acrid and irritant (Aplin 1976).

Reference

Aplin, T.E.H. (1976) Poisonous garden plants and other plants harmful to man in Australia. Western Australian Dept. of Agriculture Bull. 3964.

Iris susiana
(or I. chalcedonica)
Turkey Floure de louce

The crushed root is irritant to the skin (Gerard 1636).

Reference

Gerard, J. (1636) The Herball or Generall Historie of Plantes. The essence thereof distilled by M. Woodward (1927) from the edition of Th. Johnson 1630. London. Gerald Howe.

Iris versicolor
Blue Flag

A sensitizing agent is present in the root and stocks and other parts of the plant (Muenscher 1951, McCord 1962).

References

McCord, C.P. (1962) The Occupational Toxicity of Cultivated Flowers. Ind. Med. Surg. 31, 365.

Muenscher, W.C. (1951) Poisonous plants of the United States, 2nd ed. New York. The MacMillan Co.

JUBULACEAE

About 815 species in four genera are world-wide in distribution, especially found in tropical and subtropical regions and rare in frigid climates. Most are epiphytes, growing on trunks and branches of trees and shrubs.

Within this family there are four genera: Frullania with nearly 800 species, Jubula with 15 and Steerea and Neohattoria, both of which are monotypic.

The family is world-wide in distribution, but rare in frigid climates; it is most richly repessented in the tropics and subtropics. A high proportion of the species are epiphytes, growing on trunks and branches of trees and shrubs. Most species are tolerant of desiccation and high illumination. Jubula is confined largely to damp shaded rock surfaces.

Frullania

Nearly 800 species have been described, mostly from tropical and subtropical regions. Frullania, like most leafy liverworts, thrives in areas where the humidity is high, but withstands desiccation. The species occur as epiphytes on trunks and branches of trees and shrubs and also on cliffs and rocks. Most are of a deep madder-red colour. They persist on the bark of fallen trees.

Chemistry

Frullania tamarisci was found to yield an allergenic sesquiterpene lactone by Knoche et al (1969), Perold et al (1972). This species was also studied by Connolly and Thornton (1973).

The principal immunochemical requisite of the lactones is a methylene group attached to the lactone ring (Mitchell et al 1970). Only one of 12 Frullania species, which were tested, was devoid of allergenic activity, suggesting that allergenicity is a common feature of species of this genus (Mitchell et al 1970). The methylene group is also responsible for some cytotoxic effects of lactones (Kupchan 1970).

Essential oil containing terpenoids is known from a liverwort (Matsuo et al 1971).

Epiphytic plants on trees were suspected as agents of contact dermatitis by Spillman (1921). The early literature was reviewed by Schulmann and Detouillon (1932). LeCoulant and Lopes (1956, 1960) incriminated Frullania and lichens in wood-cutter's eczema in France and Bancons (1966) detailed the findings in 75 cases, extended by LeCoulant et al (1966), Bancons and Maleville (1967). Mitchell et al (1969) described seven cases of Frullania dermatitis from western Canada and 70 additional cases have subsequently been observed in that area (Mitchell 1975a). Other cases have been observed in France (Graciansky and Taieb 1966, Foussereau et al 1971) and Oregon (Storrs and Mitchell 1975).

Contact dermatitis from Frullania spp. affects the exposed skin surfaces of forest-workers. We have not commonly seen the involvement of the genital region which was emphasized by LeCoulant et al (1966). Differences in climate and thus in habit of dress may explain the varied distribution patterns. Canadian workers wear rainwear suitable for a cold wet climate. Workers can become sensitized after a few weeks or only after many years in forest-work. The dermatitis appears within a day or two of contacting vegetation and clears within a few weeks after leaving such work. Attacks are more severe in wet weather and widespread dermatitis can occur if the clothing is wetted by rain. Contact sensitivity to the fungi of lichens has been observed in 25 of 75 patients (Mitchell 1969). Weakly sensitized workers can usually continue in forest-work but recurrent dermatitis occurs. Strongly sensitized workers are obliged to leave forest-work. Cross-sensitivity is observed with other plants which yield allergenic sesquiterpene lactones notably in the vascular plant families Compositae and Magnoliaceae (Mitchell et al 1970, Mitchell and Dupuis 1971, Mitchell 1975b).

Hardening has not been observed in Canadian cases but LeCoulant et al (1966) produced hyposensitisation in 70 percent of their cases by repeated application of the plant to the skin. The Canadian cases included a geologist and gardener but the great majority have been workers employed in the forest-industry, notably fallers (those who fell trees). LeCoulant et al (1966) observed dermatitis most commonly in cultivators; and in lumber jacks, pruners, forest rangers, wood merchants, truck drivers (who transport wood with the bark on it), saw-mill workers, carpenters, coopers, resin harvesters, cabinet makers and persons making wooden matches. They found that the allergen of Frullania penetrates into the bark and outer wood of trees thus contaminating lumber. The Canadian cases have not included any sawmill workers and are almost confined to those who handle the bark of trees. In the Bordeaux area of France, oak (Quercus), Chestnut (Castanea), Acacia, poplar (Populus) and beeches (Fagus) often support Frullania: in Canada, cedar (Thuja), hemlock (Tsuga), fir (Picea) and spruce (Picea) are some of the trees which support Frullania. Frullania is often abundant on shrubs in the understorey of forest areas of coastal British Columbia. The genera Vaccinium and Menziesia often have large populations of Frullania that readily break loose from the shrub and attach to the clothing. Regional botanical differences account for names such as Oak-dermatitis (France) and Cedar-poisoning (Canada), Spruce-dermatitis (Oregon) which have been misapplied to Frullania dermatitis. Contact dermatitis from Thuja (Cedar) results from contact with the heart-wood of the tree and seems to be uncommon. In view of the relatively common occurrence of Frullania dermatitis in France and Canada, it seems likely that the disorder goes unrecognized in some other forest areas.

References

Bancons, F. (1966) L'allergie au Frullania. Son role dans la "Dermite due Bois de Chene". Thesis. Bordeaux, Drouillard.

Bancons, F. and Maleville, J. (1967) Logger's dermatitis: role of Frullania. Arch. Mal. Prof. 28, 407.

Connolly, J.D. and Thornton, I.M.S. (1973) Sesquiterpenoid lactones from the liverwort Frullania tamarisci. Phytochemistry 12, 631.

Foussereau, J., Maleville, J., Heid, E. et al (1971) Allergic eczema due to Frullania. Bull Soc. franc. Derm. Syph. 78, 168.

Graciansky, P. de and Taieb, M. (1966) Sensitisation and desensitisation to Frullania. Bull. Soc. franc. Derm. Syph. 73, 55.

Knoche, H., Ourisson, G., Perold, G.W. et al (1969) Allergenic component of a liverwort: a sesquiterpene lactone. Science 166, 239.

Kupchan, S.M., Fessler, D.C., Eakin, M.A. and Giacobbe, T.J. (1970) Reactions of alpha methylene lactone tumour inhibitors with model biological necleophiles. Sciene 168, 376.

Kupchan, S.M. (1970) Recent advances in the chemistry of tumor inhibitors of plant origin. Trans. N.Y. Acid. Sci. 32, 85.

LeCoulant, P. and Lopes, G. (1956) A propos des dermites des bois. J. Med. Bordeaux 3, 245.

LeCoulant, P. and Lopes, G. (1956) A propos des dermites des bois: recherches experimentalis sur l'allergie aux muscinées. J. Med. Bordeaus 133, 245.

LeCoulant, P. and Lopes, G. (1960) Rôle pathogene des muscinées-hepatiques dans les industries du bois. Arch.Mal.Prof. 21, 370.

LeCoulant, P., Texier, L., Maleville, J. et al (1966) L'allergie au Frullania: Son role dans la "Dermite due Bois de Chene". Bull. Soc. franc. Derm. Syph. 73, 440.

Matsuo, A., Nakayama, M. and Hayashi, S. (1971) Aromatic esters from the liverwort, Isotachis japonica. Z. Naturforsch 266, 1023.

Mitchell, J.C., Schofield, W.B., Singh, B. and Towers, G.H.N. (1969) Allergy to Frullania. Allergic contact dermatitis occurring in forest workers, caused by exposure to Frullania nisquallensis. Archs. Derm. 100, 46.

Mitchell, J.C., Fritig, B., Singh, B. and Towers, G.H.N. (1970) Allergic contact dermatitis from Frullania and Compositae. The role of sesquiterpene lactones. J. Invest. Derm. 54, 233.

Mitchell, J.C., Dupuis, G. and Geissman, T.A. (1972) Allergic contact dermatitis from sesquiterpenoids of plants. Additional allergenic sesquiterpene lactones. Brit. J. Derm. 87, 235.

Mitchell, J.C. (1975a) Unpublished observations.

Mitchell, J.C. (1975b) Biochemical basis of geographic ecology. Derm. Int. 14, 239 and 301.

Perold, G.W., Muller, J.C. and Ourisson, G. (1972) Structure d'une lactone allergisante: le frullanolide - I. Tetrahedron 28, 5797.

Schulmann, E. and Detouillon, P. (1932) L'ecema du bois et la sensibilisation sylvestre. Paris Med. 83, 55.

Spillman, L. (1921) Dermite artificielle due a l'ecorce de chene. Bull. Soc. franc. Derm. Syph. 28, RS 33.

Storrs, F. and Mitchell, J.C. (1975) Contact dermatitis from a liverwort Frullania. Cutis 18,681.

JUGLANDACEAE

Fifty species in seven genera are native to north temperate and subtropical regions, south to India, IndoChina and the Andes.

Chemistry is recorded by Hegnauer (1966).

Carya

25 species are native to eastern North America. The trees (Hickory) are cultivated for their wood and for the edible fruit e.g. (Pecans, like walnuts). Some species yield juglone (Thomson 1971).

Carya pecan
(syn. C. illinoensis)
(Pecan)

Contact dermatitis occurring in a nut merchant from oil of pecan was briefly noted by Swinny (1951).

The pollen of pecan (C. pecan) and other Carya spp. can cause hayfever (Wodehouse 1971).

References

Hegnauer, R. (1966) hemotaxonomy of plants. Vol. 4. Basel, Birkhauser pg. 279.

Swinny, G. (1951) Periorbital dermatitis. Ann. Alldergy. 9,774.

Thomson, R.H. (1971) Naturally occurring quinones. 2nd ed. London. Academic Press.

Wodehouse, R.P. (1971) Hayfever Plants 2nd rev. edition. New York, Hafner.

Juglans

Fifteen species are native to the Mediterranean regions, eastern Asia, IndoChina and the Andes. Many species are cultivated for their fruit. The wood is valuable. The seeds yield oil.

A naphthaquinone, juglone, derived from J. regia, J. nigra, J. cinerea (Butternut) and from some other plants of this family is present in the green parts as a glycoside or in reduced form and has been identified in water run-off from the trees (Thomson 1971).

Reference

Thomson, R.H. (1971) Naturally occurring quinones. 2nd ed. London. Academic Press.

Juglans spp. Walnut

The pollen of some species is suspected of causing hayfever (Wodehouse 1971).

Reference

Wodehouse, R.P. (1971) Hayfever Plants. 2nd rev. edition. New York, Hafner.

Juglans nigra
Black Walnut, American walnut

The juice of the nut shells stains the skin dark brown. Schwartz (1931) stated that occupational dermatitis from this source was not known to occur. A single case of dermatitis of the finger-webs from occupational exposure was of irritant nature (Siegel 1954).

Juglans regia
European walnut

The west Asian tree is widely cultivated and naturalized. The black colour of Walnut juice has been used for centuries to stain white skin, to darken the hair and for an astringent effect (Smith 1969) Oil of Walnut is used for varnish, paint and perfumery (Greenberg and Lester 1954).

Contact-sensitivity to the wood was observed in five cases (Schürkämper 1972) and a case of contact dermatitis was reported by Schleicher (1974).

Contact sensitivity to the wood was observed in a cabinet-maker who was also contact sensitive to Turreanthus and Tectona (Calnan 1970). Cross-sensitivity to quinones was reviewed by Mitchell (1975) Juglone has irritant properties (Auyone et al 1968).

Contact senstiivity to juglone was reported by Barniske (1957). Attempts to use juglone as a topical sunscreen were abandoned because commerically available juglone was found to yield a chromatographic fraction capable of causing allergic contact dermatitis; this fraction was unstable under ordinary conditions of storage (Runge 1972). Juglone was found to be a strong sensitizer for guinea pigs (Hausen 1974).

Juglone (5-oxy-1:4-napthoquinone) is not irritant or sensitizing (Telegina 1965).

Ingestion of English walnuts has been correlated with recurrent oral ulceration (Editorial 1974).

A cabinet-maker who had extensive dermatitis showed a positive patch test reaction to walnut. He also showed positive patch test reactions to other woods, viz. Tectona and Turreanthus and other plants and allergens so that the significance of the positive reaction to walnut was considered doubtful. This patient has been receiving treatment for three years by systemic steroid administration for his illness, which was considered to be polyarteritis with pulmonary involvement. He changed his occupation and made a complete recovery from the dermatitis (Woods and Calnan 1976). It seems possible that this case was an instance of occupational skin and lung wood toxicity or allergy.

References

Woods, B. and Calnan, C.D. (1976) Toxic Woods. Brit. J. Derm. 94, Suppl. 13, June.

Auyong, T.K., Deboer, B. and Oberpriller, J.O. (1968). Effects of intradermal injection of juglone in the guinea pig. Arch. int. Pharmacodyn. 176, 298.

Barniske, R. (1957) Dermatitis bullosa, ausgelöst durch den Saft grüner Walnutschalen (*Juglans regia* L.). Derm. Wochenschr. 135, 189.

Calnan, C.D. (1970) Avodiré wood sensitivity. Contact Dermatitis Newsletter (London) 8, 190.

Hausen, B.M. (1974) Pers. comm.

Runge, W. (1972) Pers. comm.

Schleicher, H. (1974) Uber phytogene allergische Kontaktekzeme. Derm. Monatsschrift. 160, 433.

Schürkämper, H. (1972) Allergie durch tropische Hölzer. Thesis, Munich cited by Hausen, B.M. (1974) pers. comm.

Schwartz, L. (1931) Dermatitis venenata due to contact with Brazilian walnut. Publ. Health. Rep. 46, 1938.

Siegel, J.M. (1954) Dermatitis due to black walnut juice. Arch. Derm. Syph. (Chic.) 70, 511.

Mitchell, J.C. (1975) Biochemical basis of geographic ecology. International Journal of Dermatology Part 1, 14, 239; Part 2, 14, 301.

Editorial (1974) Recurrent oral ulceration. Brit. Med. J. 2, 757.

Telegina, K.A. (1965) The use of Yuglon in treatment of neurodermatitis. Sov. Med. 28, 110.

KRAMERIACEAE

25 species in one genus are found in warm regions of America. The fruits are covered with bristles or spines, often barbed.

Krameria (syn. *Ratanhia*)

25 species are found from the Southern United States to Chile.

Krameria argentea
Rhatany

Krameria triandra

Preparations of the plant were formerly officinal (Wren 1968) and produced dermatitis (Mibelli 1929, Lewith and Langecker 1930). Tincture of Krameria produced cheilitis and stomatitis (Zakon et al 1947). A preparation containing *Krameria* caused dermatitis of the anogenital skin. Positive patch test reactions to the preparation were observed. Sensitisation to *Krameria* was produced experimentally in 86% of 37 individuals (Grolnick 1938 a, b,).

One of 12 patients contact sensitive to Balsam of Peru (*Myroxylon*) showed a positive patch test reaction to the tincture (Hjorth 1961).

References

Grolnick, M. (1938a) Studies in contact dermatitis. III. Active sensitization with *Krameria* in man. J. Invest. Dermat. 1, 179.

Grolnick, M. (1938b) Dermatitis due to haemorrhoidal ointment containing *Krameria* and oil of cade. JAMA 110, 951.

Hjorth, N. (1961) Eczematous Allergy to Balsams. Munksgaard, International Booksellers and Publishers Ltd., Copenhagen.

Lewith, R. and Langecker, H. (1930) Uber einen Fall von Ratanhiadermatitis (Idiosynkrasie gegen Ratanhiagerbsaure). Derm. Wschr. 90, 477, cited by Touton(1932).

Mibelli, A. (1929) Sull' impiego dell'estratto di ratania in dermatol. Arch. ital. Dermat. 4, 281, cited by Touton (1932).

Touton, K. (1932) Hauterkrankungen durch phanerogamische Pflanzen und ihre Produkte (Toxicodermia et Allergodermia phytogenes), in Barnewitz, J. et al Angeborene Anomalien, Lichtdermatosen, Pflanzengifte, Thermische Schadigungen, Einfluss Innerer Storungen auf die Haut. Berlin, Verlag von Julius Springer.

Wren, R.W. (1968) Potter's New Cyclopaedia of Botanical Drugs and Preparation by Wren, R.C. Re-edit. by Wren, R.W. Potter and Clarke Ltd. Health Science Press. Rustington, Sussex.

LABIATAE

3500 species in 180 genera are cosmopolitan. The leaves are often hairy and possess epidermal glands which secrete volatile oils giving characteristic scents to many species. Many species are used in Herbal Medicine (Wren 1968). Some are bitter e.g. Hyssopus (Hyssop) of the Crucifixion (John XIX. 29). Many species yield essential oils.

Chemistry is recorded by Hegnauer (1966).

References

Hegnauer, R. (1966) Chemotaxonomy of plants. Vol. 4. Basel, Birkhauser. p. 289.

Wren, R.W. (1968) Potter's New Cyclopaedia of Botanical Drugs and Preparations by Wren, R.C. Re-edit. by Wren, R.W. Potter & Clarke Ltd. Health Science Press. Rustington, Sussex.

Coleus

150 species are palaeotropical. Many hybrids and forms are popular as house, greenhouse and garden plants.

Coleus sp.

A species of this genus was noted to cause dermatitis of the exposed parts (Weber 1937). Four positive patch test reactions obtained by Hjorth (1968) possibly indicate irritancy.

References

Hjorth, N. (1968) at Finsen Institute. Pers. Comm.

Weber, L.F. (1937) External causes of dermatitis. A list of irritants. Arch. Derm. Syph. 35, 129

Lavandula

28 species are native to Atlantic Islands and the Mediterranean region west to India. L. vera (Lavender) yields Oil of Lavender from the flowers; L. spica and L. stoechas are also used.

Lavandula spp.

L. officinalis yields Oil of Lavender; a hybrid of this plant and of L. latifolia yields Lavendin Oil (Arctander 1960). The oils from the various commercial plants vary considerably in chemical content.

The flower has been used as a skin irritant (Watt and Breyer-Brandwijk 1962). English Lavender powder produced a strong positive patch test reaction in a patient who had atopic eczema (Michelson 1936). Oil of Lavender is irritant to guinea pig skin (Greenberg and Lester 1954). Bath preparations containing the oil produced erythematous eruptions (Finkenrath 1941). The oil can produce dermatitis in hypersensitive individuals (Tulipan 1938, Tzanck et al 1939, Zündel 1936, Klarmann 1958, LeCoulant et al 1964, Foussereau and Benezra 1970). Lavender oil in perfumes can cause dermatitis (Schwartz and Peck 1948). Hyperpigmentation of the skin has been observed from contact with preparations containing the oil (Szántó 1929, Sandler 1939, Weber 1937). Psoralens which occur in Citrus are not known from Lavandula but the oils may be intermixed. Oil of Lavender produced nil positive patch test reactions in 312 persons tested (Fregert and Hjorth 1968) but six positive reactions in 1,147 patients tested in European Eczema Clinics (Calnan 1970).

References

Arctander, S. (1960) Perfume and Flavor materials of Natural Origin. Elizabeth, J.N. Published by the author.

Calnan, C.D. (1970) Oil of cloves, laurel, lavender, peppermint. Contact Dermatitis Newsletter 7, 148.

Finkenrath, K. (1941) Arzneischäden in der Dermatologie. Med. Klin. 37, 897.

Finkenrath, K. (1941) Arzneischäden in de Dermatologie. Schädigung durch Kosmetika. Med. Klin. 37, 1050.

Foussereau, J. and Benezra, C. (1970) Les Eczemas Allergiques Professionnels. Paris. Masson.

Fregert, S. and Hjorth, N. (1968) Results of standard patch tests with substances abandoned. Contact Dermatitis Newsletter 5, 85.

Greenwood, L.A. and Lester, D. (1954) Handbook of Cosmetic Materials. New York. Interscience.

Klarmann, E.G. (1958) Perfume dermatitis. Ann. Allergy 16, 425.

LeCoulant, P., Texier, L., Maleville, J. et Doussy, N.N. (1964) Sensibilisation a une creme antihistaminique. Bull. Soc. franc. Derm. Syph. 71, 234.

Michelson, H.E. (1936) Dermatitis due to inhalant dust. Archs. Derm. Syph. 33, 397.

Sandler, I.L. (1939) Photosensitizing agents: a brief review of the literature. JAMA 112, 2411.

Schwartz, L. and Peck, S.M. (1946) Cosmetics and Dermatitis. New York. Hoeber.

Schwartz, L., Tulipan, L. and Peck, S.M. (1947) Occupational Diseases of the Skin. Philadelphia. Lea & Febiger.

Szanto, J. (1929) Über Pigmentierungen nach Sensibilisierung der Haut mit ätherischen Ölen. Zbl. Haut.-u. GeschlKr. 28, 451.

Tulipan, L. (1938) Cosmetic irritants. Archs. Derm. Syph. 38, 906.

Tzanck, A., Sidi, E. and Dobkevitch (1939) Histamine et tests. Bull Soc. franc. Derm. Syph. 49, 879.

Watt, J.M. and Breyer-Brandwijk, M.G. (1962) The Medicinal and poisonous plants of Southern Africa. 2nd ed. Edinburgh. E. & S. Livingstone.

Zündel, W. (1936) Erfahrungen mit Hautfunktion sprüfungen an 2000 Patienten. Arch. Derm. Syph. Wien. 173, 435.

Leonotis

40 species are native to tropical and South Africa, one species is pantropical.

Leonotis nepetaefolia
Hollowstalk

The hairs of the plant are irritant and contact with the leaves can cause dermatitis in susceptible individuals (Gowanloch and Brown 1943).

References

Gowanloch, J.N. and Brown, C.A. (1943) Poisonous snakes, plants and Black Widow Spider of Louisiana. Louisiana Dept. Conserv. New Orleans, La. cited by Oakes and Butcher (1962).

Oakes, A.J. and Butcher, J. (1962) Poisonous and injurious plants of the U.S. Virgin Islands. Misc. Publ. 882. U.S. Dept. of Agriculture. Washington, D.C.

Leonurus

14 species are native to temperate Eurasia.

Leonurus cardiaca
Motherwort

Contact with the leaves can produce dermatitis (Massey 1941, Behl et al 1966) and a fragrant lemon-scented oil from the plant can cause photosensitisation (Behl et al 1966).

References

Behl, P.N., Captain, R.M., Bedi, B.M.S. and Gupta, S. (1966). Skin-irritant and sensitizing plants found in India, New Delhi. P.N. Behl, Irwin Hospital.

Massey, A.B. (1941) Plant Poisoning. Merck Reports. 50, 24.

Marrubium

40 species are native to temperate Eurasia and the Mediterranean region.

Marrubium vulgare
White Horehound

An irritant is present in the juice of the plant which can cause contact dermatitis (McCord 1962). An extract of the plant produced negative patch test reactions in 50 patients who had 'weed dermatitis' (Shelmire 1939). The plant yields a volatile oil and a bitter principle, marubiin (Merck 1968). The plant has been used to flavour beer.

References

McCord, C.P. (1962) The Occupational Toxicity of Cultivated Flowers. Ind. Med. Surg. 31, 365.

Merck Index (1968) An encyclopedia of chemicals and drugs. ed. Stecher, P.G. Rahway, New Jersey. Merck Index.

Shelmire, B. (1939) Contact Dermatitis from Weeds; Patch testing with their oleoresins. JAMA 113, 1085.

Melissa

Three species are native to regions from Europe to central Asia and Persia.

Melissa officinalis
Balm

A tea made from the plant is said to induce sweating (Grieve 1970).

Reference

Grieve, M. (1970) A Modern Herbal. Darien, Conn. Hafner Publ. Co.

Mentha

25 species are native to north temperate regions, South Africa and Australia.

Mentha citrata
Bergamont Mint

Dermatitis in two bar-tenders was attributed to contact with this species. Positive patch test reactions were obtained with *M. citrata*, negative with *M. vera*. Seven of 18 controls showed irritant reactions to an almond oil extract of *M. citrata* (Sams 1940).

Mentha piperita

Menthol, the chief constituent of Oil of Peppermint derived from this species, is irritant in high concentration especially if evaporation from the skin is prevented (Harry 1948). Perfumes and colognes containing menthol and/or Oil of Peppermint can produce dermatitis in some individuals; workers in candy factories can also be affected (Greenberg and Lester 1954). Oil of Peppermint produced positive patch test reactions in 4 of 1,147 patients tested in European Eczema Clinics (Calnan 1970).

Mentha spicata
(syn. *M. viridis*)

Oil of Spearmint is derived from this species. A finisher of chewing gum who had contact dermatitis showed positive patch test reactions to diluted spearment flavouring and to cassia (*Cinnamomum cassia*) (Morris 1954).

Mentha longifolia

The leaf is said to be irritant to the skin (Watt and Breyer-Brandwijk 1962).

Mentha pulegium
Penny Royal

The plant is used as a rubefacient (Watt and Breyer-Brandwijk 1962).

Mentha satureioides
Penny Royal

Ingestion of the plant was suspected as a cause of hepatic photosensitisation in sheep (Hurst 1942, Watt and Breyer-Brandwijk 1962).

Essential oils from these plants are noted in many reviews of cosmetic dermatitis as allergenic but the evidence is meagre.

References

Calnan, C.D. (1970) Oils of cloves, laurel, lavender, pappermint. Contact Dermatitis Newsletter 7, 148.

Greenberg, L.A. and Lester, D. (1954) Handbook of Cosmetic Materials. New York. Interscience Publishers Inc.

Harry, R.G. (1948) Cosmetic Materials. Vol. 2. London. Leonard Hill.

Hurst, E. (1942) The Poison Plants of New South Wales. N.S.W. Poison Plants Committee; Sydney.

Morris, G.E. (1954) Dermatoses among Food Handlers. Industr. Med. Surg. 23, 343.

Sams, W.M. (1940) Occupational dermatitis due to mint. Arch. Derm. and Syph. 41, 503.

Watt, J.M. and Breyer-Brandwijk, M.G. (1962) The Medicinal and poisonous plants of Southern Africa. 2nd ed. Edinburgh. E. & S. Livingstone.

Monarda

12 species are native to North America and Mexico. The leaves of some make Oswego tea.

Monarda punctata
Horsemint

This species is an infrequent skin sensitizer (Shelmire 1940).

Reference

Shelmire, B. (1940) Contact dermatitis from vegetation. South Med. J. 33, 337.

Moschosma

Seven species are found from tropical Africa to Queensland.

Moschosma polystachum

The crushed leaves can cause sores in the mouth (Burkill 1935).

Reference

Burkill, I.H. (1935) A Dictionary of the Economic Products of the Malay Peninsula. 2 Vols. London. Crown Agents for the Colonies.

Ocimum

150 species are found in tropical and warm temperate regions especially Africa.

Ocimum basilicum
Basil

The juice of the plant is sternutatory (Quisumbing 1951).

Reference

Quisumbing, E. (1951) Medicinal Plants of the Philippines. Philipp. Dep. Agr. and Nat. Resources Tech. Bull. No. 16. Manila. Bureau of Printing 1234 pp.

Ocimum gratissimum

This species yields Brazilian oil from which eugenol is derived (Bedoukian 1967). Sensitivity to eugenol is noted under Oil of Clove (Syzygium).

Reference

Bedoukian, P.Z. (1967) Perfumery and Flavoring Synthetics. 2nd ed. New York. Elsevier.

Ocimum sanctum

Systemic symptoms can occur from proximity to the plant (Morton 1969).

Reference

Morton, J.F. (1969) Some ornamental plants excreting respiratory irritants. Proc. Florida State Hort. Soc. 82, 415.

Perilla

Four or six species are found from India to Japan.

Perilla frutescens var. acuta

In one of two housewives who pickled this plant and radish (Raphanus) a patch test to 'Hi-z' emulsion used for sterilizing the vegetables produced a positive reaction (Takahashi 1967).

Perilla frutescens var. discolor

Beefsteak Plant

Dermatitis of the fingers was observed in workers who picked the leaves of this plant for food processing. The leaves have been used as a fragrant vegetable in Japan from ancient times (Nakayama 1975, pers. comm.). Women and old persons were particularly affected. Patch tests with the leaf produced irritant reactions but allergic reactions probably also occurred (Uchida 1970). Perilla oil, derived from the seeds of Perilla ocymoides (syn. P. frutescens) and P. nankinensis cultivated in China, Japan and India, is used as a drying oil similar to linseed oil (Linum) for waterproofing paper, umbrellas and for lacquerware (Howes 1974).

Perilla oil is used to make varnishes, printing ink and paints. In the United States, the oil is mixed with soy-bean oil (Glycine) to make protective paints (Usher 1974).

References

Howes, F.N. (1974) A Dictionary of Useful and Everyday Plants and their Common Names. Cambridge University Press. pp. 290.

Uchida, A. (1970) Cultivation of leaves of Perilla frutescens Britton and dermatitis. Jap. J. Hyg. 25, 164.

Takahashi, N. (1967) Dermatitis due to the handling of vegetables. Jap. J. Derm. 77, 358.

Usher, G. (1974) A dictionary of plants used by man. London. Constable.

Plectranthus

250 species are found from tropical Africa to Japan, Malaysia, Australia and the Pacific region.

Plectranthus sp.

Hjorth (1968) observed two positive patch test reactions to a species of this genus.

Reference

Hjorth, N. (1968) at Finsen Institute. Pers. Comm.

Pogostemon

40 species are native to China and IndoMalaysia.

Pogostemon heyneahus

The powdered leaves are used as a snuff to produce sneezing (Burkill 1935).

Pogostemon patchouly var. suavis

The leaves of this plant yield Oil of Patchouly (Patchouli) (Fenaroli 1971). Three of 893 patients who had eczema showed positive patch test reactions to a sample of this oil. Positive reactions were also observed to turpentine, colophony, Juniperus, Cinnamomum, wood and coal tar (Calnan 1970).

Some patients who were contact sensitive to the oil also reacted to Oil of Cinnamon (Cinnamomum), (Calnan 1970).

References

Burkill, I.H. (1935) A Dictionary of the Economic Products of the Malay Peninsula. 2 Vols. London. Crown Agents for the Colonies.

Calnan, C.D. (1970) Oil of cloves, laurel, lavender, peppermint. Contact Dermatitis Newsletter 7, 148.

Fenaroli, G. (1971) Fenaroli's Handbook of Flavor Ingredients. ed. Furia, T.E. and Bellanca, N. Cleveland, Ohio. The Chemical Rubber Co.

Patchouli oil Indonesian produced positive patch test reactions in 2/10 patients who had perfume dermatitis (Norak 1974).

Reference

Norak, M. (1974) Contact sensitization to constituents of perfume composition in antiphlogistic ointment. Cs. Derm. 49, 375.

Prostanthera

50 species are native to Australia.

Prostanthera sp.

A species of this genus was suspected to cause dermatitis (Hurst 1942).

Reference

Hurst, E. (1942) The Poison Plants of New South Wales. N.S.W. Poison Plants Committee: Sydney.

Rosmarinus

Three species are native to the Mediterranean region.

Rosmarinus officinalis
Rosemary

The plant has been used to scent soap (Collins 1964). Oil of Rosemary (Merck 1968) was a suspected agent of contact dermatitis (Klarmann 1958). The oil can irritate the skin and eyes. Bath preparations containing the oil can cause erythema; perfumes, colognes and toilet waters containing the oil can cause dermatitis in hypersensitive persons. The oil is also said to produce photosensitivity (Greenberg and Lester 1954).

References

Collins, M. (1964) Spices of the World Cookbook. Baltimore, McCormick.

Klarmann, E.G. (1958) Perfume dermatitis. Ann. Allergy 16, 425.

Merck Index (1968) An Encyclopedia of Chemicals and Drugs. ed. Stecher, P.G. Rahway, New Jersey. Merck Co.

Greenberg, L.A. and Lester, D. (1954). Handbook of Cosmetic Materials. New York. Interscience.

Salvia

70 species are found in tropical and temperate regions.

Salvia officinalis
Sage

Cheilitis and stomatitis from sage tea were reported by Zakon et al (1947). The plant has been used to treat hyperhidrosis (Merck 1968).

References

Merck Index (1968) An Encyclopedia of Chemicals and Drugs. ed. Stecher, P.G. Rahway, New Jersey, Merck Co.

Zakon, S.J., Goldberg, A.L. and Kahn, J.B. (1947) Lipstick cheilitis: Common Dermatosis. Report of 32 cases. Arch. Derm. Syph. 56,499.

Salvia sclarea

Clary sage oil from this species was irritant to abraded rabbit skin when applied under occlusion. No irritation or sensitisation was observed for humans (Opdyke 1974). In several cases of dermatitis attributed to sage, positive patch test reactions were obtained from the mucous membranes but not from the skin (Urbach and Wiethe 1931).

Clary sage oil produced positive reactions in 2/60 perfumery workers who had dermatitis (Gutman and Somov 1968).

References

Opdyke, D. (1974) Monographs on fragrance raw material. Fd. Cosmet. Toxicol. 12, 807.

Urbach, E. and Wiethe, C. (1931) Atherische Ole als Ursache von allergischen Haut-und Schleimhauterkrankungen. Munch. med. Wschr. 78, 2030.

Gutman, S.G. and Somov, B.A. (1968). Allergic reactions caused by components of perfumery preparations. Vestn. Derm. Verner. 42, 62.

Thymus

300 tp 400 species are native to temperate Eurasia. Several species provide oils.

Thymus vulgaris
Thyme

Oil of Thyme is a rubefacient (Wren 1968). This species, and other plants, yield thymol which can produce irritation of the skin (Greenberg and Lester 1954). Thymol has caused dermatitis in dentists (Schwartz et al 1957), and, when used in toothpaste, cheilitis and glossitis (Beinhauer 1940).

Oil of thyme, in bath preparations, has been reported to cause hyperemia and severe inflammation (Greenberg and Lester 1954).

References

Beinhauer, L.G. (1940) Cheilitis and glossitis from tooth-paste. Arch. Derm. & Syph. 41, 892.

Greenberg, L.A. and Lester, D. (1954) Handbook of Cosmetic Materials. New York, Interscience. Publishers Inc.

Schwartz, L., Tulipan, L. and Birmingham, D.J. (1957) Occupational Diseases of the Skin. 3rd ed. Philadelphia. Lea & Febiger pp. 637-672.

Wren, R.W. (1968) Potter's New Cyclopaedia fo Botanical Drugs and Preparations by Wren, R.C. Reedit. by Wren, R.W. Potter and Clarke, Ltd. Health Science Press. Rustington, Sussex.

LAURACEAE

2000 to 2500 species in 32 genera are found in tropical and subtropical regions.

Chemistry is recorded by Hegnauer (1966).

References

Hegnauer, R. (1966) Chemotaxonomy of plants. Vol. 4. Basel, Birkhauser. pp. 350.

Alseodaphne

25 species are native to China, south-eastern Asia and Indo-Malaysia.

Alseodaphne insignis
(syn. Persea) Medang

The bark contains fine needle like pruritogenic particles (Altschul 1973) and the inner bark, or possibly the sawdust, irritates the skin of sawyers (Burgess 1966).

References

Altschul, S. von R. (1973) Drugs and foods from little-known plants. Cambridge, Mass. Harvard Univ. Press.

Burgess, P.F. (1966) Timbers of Sabah, (Sabah Forest Records. No. 6). Sabah, Malaysia. The Forest Dept.

Aniba

40 species are native to central and tropical South America.

Aniba coto
Cotc

Cotoin derived from the bark is irritant to the mucous membrances (Merck 1968).

Aniba rosaeodora
Bois de rose femelle

Aniba duckei
Pau rosa

The wood of these species replaced Convolvulus as the main source of oil of rosewood in the 19th century. According to Woods and Calnan (1976) the rosewood which Grossmann (1910, 1920) reported as causing dermatitis and constitutional symptoms in wood workers was from this genus. Rosewood oil produced at least one irritant reaction in patch tests on healthy subjects (Katz 1946). The chemistry of rosewood oil was investigated by Mors et al (1957) and Gottlieb and Mors (1959).

References

Gottlieb, O.R. and Mors, W.B. (1959) The chemistry of Rosewood II. Isolation and identification of cotoin and pinocembrin. J. Am. Chem. Soc. 80, ii, 2263.

Grossmann, J. (1910) Gesundheitsschadliche Holzer Bayrische. Industrielle Gewerbeblott 96, (6), 51.

Grossmann, J. (1920) Gesundheitsschadliche Holzarten. Der Holzkaufer (Leipzig) 17, 529, 535, 540, 545.

Katz, A.E. (1946) Spice Mill 69, 46, 50 quoted in Chem. Abstr. 40, 7525.

Mors, W.B., Gottlieb, O.R. and Djerassi, C. (1957) The chemistry of Rosewood. Isolation and structure of anibine and 4-methoxyparacotoin. J. Am. Chem. Soc. 79, 4507.

Woods, B. and Calnan, C.D. (1976) Toxic Woods. Brit. J. Derm. 94, Suppl. 13, June.

Merck Index (1968) An Encyclopedia of Chemicals and Drugs. ed. Stecher, P.G. 8th ed. Rahway, N.J. Merck and Co. Ltd.

Beilschmiedia

Over 200 species are native to tropical regions, Australia and New Zealand.

Beilschmiedia mannii
Spicy Cedar

The fruit juice is used as a counter-irritant (Irvine 1961).

Reference

Irvine, F.R. (1961) Woody Plants of Ghana. Oxford University Press. London.

Cinnamomum

250 species are native to eastern Asia and IndoMalaysia.

Cinnamomum spp.
Cinnamon

Some 15 species yield essential oils (Gildemeister and Hoffman 1956).

Cinnamomum camphora

Camphor is distilled from the wood or young shoots. When camphor is rubbed into the skin or kept in contact with the skin and evaporation prevented, it is an irritant. When applied in alcoholic solution and allowed to evaporate, it is a refrigerant and blanches the skin. Application of Oil of Camphor to the skin produces a sensation of warmth followed by a slight degree of local anaesthesia (Greenberg and Lester 1954). The vapour is irritant to the eye (Finkenrath 1941). Oil of Camphor is said to be a contact sensitizer (Flandin et al 1937, Urbach 1942) as well as an irritant (Schwartz et al 1957). Camphor is produced from pinene; isomers are known (Merck 1968). In camphor factories, fumes of acetic acid can cause keratitis (Duke-Elder and McFaul 1972).

Cinnamomum camphora
(syn. Laurus camphora)
Camphorwood

Grossmann (1920) experienced severe headache and giddiness after working with camphorwood. The wood contains camphor and borneol. It is sometimes used for chests and cabinets.

References

Duke-Elder, S. and MacFaul (1972) System of Opthalmology. Vol.XIV. London. Henry Kimpton. P. 1180.

Finkenrath, K. (1941) Arzneischaden in der Dermatologie. Med. Klinik 37, 897; cited by Greenberg and Lester (1954).

Flandin, C., Rabeau, H. and Ukrainczyk (1937) L'intolerance a la terebenthine et aux substances du groupe des terpenes. Bull. Soc. franc. Derm. Syph. 44, 315.

Gildemeister, E. and Hoffmann, F. (1956) Vol. 4; (1959) Vol. 5; (1961) Vol. 4; (1961) Vol. 7; Die Atherischen Ole. Berlin: Akademie-Verlag. (10 volumes).

Greenberg, L.A. and Lester, D. (1954) Handbook of Cosmetic Materials. New York. Interscience Publishers Inc.

Grossmann, J. (1920) Gesundheitsschädliche Holzarten. Der Holzkäufer (Leipzig). 17, 529, 535, 540 and 545.

Merck Index (1968) An Encyclopedia of Chemicals and Drugs. ed. Stecher, P.G. 8th ed. Rahway, N.J. Merck and Co. Ltd.

Schwartz, L., Tulipan, L. and Birmingham, D.J. (1957) Occupational Diseases of the Skin. 3rd ed. Philadelphia. Lea and Febiger. pp. 637-672.

Urbach, E. (1942) Odors (osymls) as allergenic agents. J. Allergy 13, 387.

Cinnamomum spp.

Sources of Cinnamon and Cassia.

Cinnamomum cassia provides Cassia bark and Oil of Cassia (also known as Oil of Cinnamon).

Cinnamomum mercadoi is sometimes substituted for C. zeylanicum

Cinnamomum loureirii provides Saigon cinnamon bark.

Cinnamomum oliveri provides Australian cinnamon bark (Black Sassafras).

Cinnamomum tamala

(Indian Cassia) is often substituted for C.zeylanicum

Cinnamomum zeylanicum

(True Cinnamon) provides Cinnamon bark and Oil of Cinnamon.

Distilled Cinnamon leaf oil contains less cinnamic aldehyde than oil from the bark.

The botanical origin of oils of cinnamon and cassia is lacking from some published reports. The name Oil of Cinnamon used by American authors usually refers to C. cassia. A patient who was contact sensitive to C. cassia was stated to be able to handle C. zeylanicum without ill-effect (Laubach et al 1953).

Reference

Laubach, J.L., Malkinson, F.D. and Ringrose, E.J. (1953) Cheilitis caused by cinnamon (cassia) oil in tooth paste. JAMA 152, 404.

Cinnamomum

Allergic contact dermatitis from cinnamon may flare up, taking the form of pompholyx, following ingestion of cinnamon (Pirilä 1970).

Reference

Pirilä, V. (1970) Endogenic contact eczema. Allergie und Asthma 16, 15 (German).

Cinnamic aldehyde in toothpaste caused contact sensitivity (Magnusson and Wilkinson, Kirton and Wilkinson 1975).

Opportunities for contact with cinnamic aldehyde were reviewed by Collins and Mitchell (1975). Cinnamic aldehyde in perfumes can cause dermatitis (Schorr 1975).

References

Collins, F.W. and Mitchell, J.C. (1975) Aroma chemicals. Contact Dermatitis 1, 43.

Kirton, V. and Wilkinson, D.S. (1975) Sensitivity to cinnamic aldehyde in a toothpaste. 2. Further studies. Contact Dermatitis 1,77.

Magnusson, B. and Wilkinson, D.S. (1975) Cinnamic aldehyde in toothpaste I. Clinical aspects and patch tests. Contact Dermatitis 1, 70.

Schorr, W.F. (1975) Cinnamic aldehyde allergy. Contact Dermatitis 1, 108.

Cinnamomum cassia
Chinese Cinnamon, Cassia

Oil of Cinnamon (Oil of Cassia) derived from this plant is irritant and can blister the tongue; allergic contact dermatitis from the oil or from the bark and flower buds used as a spice can occur in cooks, bakers, grocers and confectioners (Tulipan 1932, Silvers 1939, Zundel and Jentsch 1939, Howell 1946, Epstein 1950, Wutrich 1970).

A girl who dipped toothpicks in Oil of Cassia to flavour them developed dermatitis of the hands and forearms. The face and lower abdomen were affected by contact with the hands (White 1887). A woman developed contact dermatitis of the lips, right cheek and right hand from a toothpaste containing cinnamon oil. Patch tests to 'synthetic' cinnamon oil 1% in alcohol and to a natural cinnamon oil 5% in olive oil produced positive reactions (Laubach et al 1953). Oil of cinnamon in toothpaste caused dermatitis of the left hand to which the toothpaste was applied; the face and lips were not affected (Cummer 1940). A candy-maker who handled cinnamon (cassia) flavouring developed dermatitis of the hands, abdomen and thighs; patch tests to the crushed candy which contained 1% cassia flavouring, to oil of cinnamon leaves 5% in olive oil and to cinnamic aldehyde 5% in petrolatum produced positive reactions; negative to Oil of Mace (Myristica), Oil of Capsicum and vanillin (Kern 1960). In a case of dermatitis of the face and hands from a toothpaste containing cinnamon oil, the buccal mucous membrane was unaffected but ingestion of the oil resulted in recurrence of dermatitis of the hands; a patch test to cinnamon oil 1% in alcohol produced a positive reaction; negative to oil of Peppermint (Mentha), Oil of Anise (Pimpinella) and methyl salicylate (Leifer 1951).

In a finisher of chewing gum who had dermatitis, patch tests to diluted cassia flavouring and to spearmint (Mentha) produced positive reactions (Morris 1954).

A candy maker who had dermatitis of the hands developed generalized dermatitis after a positive patch test reaction to cinnamon oil (Downing 1947).

A woman exposed to the vapour of cinnamon oil, used for making bubble gum, developed cheilitis; a patch test to cinnamon (cassia) oil 2% in alcohol produced a positive reaction, negative in 8 controls (Miller 1941).

The oil of Cinnamon of the United States Pharmacopoeia is the volatile oil distilled from the leaves and twigs of this plant. This oil is known as Oil of Cassia in the British Pharmaceutical Codex. Immature fruits are used for the same purposes as the bark in flavouring (Wren 1968). Oil of Cassia in perfumes can cause dermatitis (Greenberg and Lester 1954, Schwartz et al 1957) and is removed from certain cosmetics (Schieffelin 1973).

Cinnamon can cause dermatitis in pharmaceutical chemists (Schwartz et al 1957).

References

Cummer, C.L. (1940) Dermatitis due to oil of cinnamon. Arch. Derm. Syph. 42, 674.

Downing, J.G. (1947) Occupational Dermatoses (Ergodermatoses): Diagnosis, Disability and Treatment. New England J. Med. 237, 755.

Epstein, F.W. (1950) Contact dermatitis due to cinnamon. Ohio Med. J. 46, 659.

Greenberg, L.A. and Lester, D. (1954) Handbook of Cosmetic Materials. New York. Interscience Publishers, Inc.

Howell, J.B. (1946) Contact dermatitis: An analysis or tabulation of all cases proved in a single year. Arch. Derm. and Syph. 53, 265.

Kern, A.B. (1960) Contact dermatitis from cinnamon. Arch. Derm. 81, 599.

Laubach, J.L., Malkinson, F.D. and Ringrose, E.J. (1953) Cheilitis caused by cinnamon (cassia) oil in toothpaste. JAMA 152, 404.

Leifer, W. (1951) Contact dermatitis due to cinnamon. Arch. Derm. Syph. 64, 52.

Miller, J.A. (1941) Cheilitis from sensitivity to oil of cinnamon present in bubble-gum. JAMA 116, 131.

Morris, G.E. (1954) Dermatoses among Food Handlers. Industr. Med. Surg. 23, 343.

Schieffelin and Co. (1973) Almay Hypo-allergenic cosmetics product formulary. 8th ed. Pharmaceutical Laboratories Division. 562-5th. Avenue, New York, N.Y. 10036.

Schwartz, L., Tulipan, L. and Birmingham, D.J. (1957) Occupational Diseases of the Skin. 3rd ed. Philadelphia. Lea and Febiger, pp. 637-672.

Silvers, S.H. (1939) Stomatitis and dermatitis venenata with purpura, resulting from Oil of Cloves and Oil of Cassia. Dental Items Interest 61, 649.

Tulipan, L. (1932) Dermatitis from cinnamon. Arch. Derm. Syph. 25, 921.

White, J.C. (1887) Dermatitis venenata: An account of the Action of External irritants upon the Skin. Boston. Cupples and Hurd.

Wren, R.W. (1968) Potter's New Cyclopaedia of Botanical Drugs and Preparations by Wren, R.C. Re-edit. by Wren, R.W. Potter and Clarke Ltd. Health Science Press. Rustington, Sussex.

Wütrich, B. (1970) Zur Genese des Backerekzems. Hautarzt 21, 214.

Zundel, W. and Jentsch, M. (1939) Die allergischen Vorgange beim Backerekzem und ihre Deutung. Arch. Derm. Syph. (Berlin) 178, 469.

Cinnamic aldehyde is a constituent of cinnamon oils and the synthetic chemical is used for flavouring (Collins and Mitchell 1975). Cinnamic aldehyde is allergenic and cross-sensitizes with cinnamic alcohol, cinnamic acid and Balsam of Peru (*Myroxylon*) (Hjorth 1961). Cinnamic aldehyde was found to be a sensitizer in toothpaste (Magnusson and Wilkinson 1975) The chemical has been observed to cause contact urticaria (Malten 1973).

Schorr (1975) observed five patients who were contact sensitive to cinnamic aldehyde. Additional sensitivity to Jasmin Absolute (*Jasminum*) was observed. This material may contain alpha-amyl cinnamic aldehyde.

References

Collins, F.W. and Mitchell, J.C. (1975) Aroma chemicals. Contact Dermatitis 1, 43.

Malten, K. (1973) Pers. Comm.

Hjorth, N. (1961) Eczematous allergy to Balsams, Allied Perfumes and Flavouring Agents. Copenhagen: Munksgaard.

Magnusson, B. and Wilkinson, D.S. (1975) Cinnamic aldehyde in toothpaste 1. Clinical aspects and patch tests. Contact Dermatitis 1, 70.

Magnusson, B. and Wilkinson, D.S. (1975) Sensitivity to cinnamic aldehyde in a toothpaste. 2. Further studies. Contact Dermatitis 1, 77.

Schorr, W.F. (1975) Cinnamic aldehyde allergy. Contact Dermatitis 1, 108.

Cinnamomum loureirii
Saigon Cinnamon

A female employed in making fruit juices developed vesicular dermatitis to the dorsum of the right hand and forearm flexure. A patch test to an aqueous extract of the bark produced a positive reaction negative in controls (Ito 1972).

Cinnamomum mercadoi

The bark is rubefacient (Quisumbing 1951).

References

Ito, K. (1972) Director, Dept. of Dermatology, Gifu University, Japan. Personal communication.

Quisumbing, E. (1951) Medicinal Plants of the Phillipinnes. Tech. Bull. 16. Manila, Phillipinne Islands. Manila Bureau of Printing. 1234 pp.

Cinnamomum zeylanicum

15 of 1382 patients who had eczema showed positive patch test reactions to a sample of Oil of Cinnamon. Some of the patients were also contact-sensitive to Balsams of Peru and Tolu (Myroxylon), benzoin (Styrax), styrax (Liquidambar), colophony and turpentine (Pinus), patchouli (Pogostemon) and ginger (Zinziber), (Calnan 1970).

An oil from C. zeylanicum and C. cassia produced positive patch test reactions in 6 males and 15 females who had hand eczema; in 16 of the 21 persons, contact sensitivity to cinnamon appeared to be the main cause or a contributory cause of the eczema (Agrup 1969).

References

Argup, G. (1969) Hand eczema and other hand dermatoses in South Sweden. Acta. derm.-venereol 49 Suppl 61. pp. 1-91.

Calnan, C.D. (1970) Oil of Cinnamon. Contact Dermatitis Newsletter 8, 181.

Cryptocarya

200 to 250 species are found in tropical regions, except in Cental Africa, and in the subtropics. The fruits of C. moschata (Brazilian Nutmeg) are used as a spice.

Cryptocarya pleurosperma
Poison Walnut

Webb (1948) described dermatitis which started on the hands two or three days after handling the cut bark or wood, and later spreading to the face and scrotum. He did not report patch tests with the sawdust but he found that the alkaloid cryptopleurine, derived from the wood, had a blistering effect.

Cryptopleurine, isolated from the sap and bark, an alkaloid with irritant and possibly allergenic properties, has also produced dermatitis in laboratory workers (de la Lande 1948, Gellert and Riggs 1954, Cleland and Lee 1963).

According to Woods and Calnan (1976) poison walnut is used a good deal in Australia despite its known toxicity.

References

Cleland, J.B. and Lee, D.J. (1963) The poisonous and urticating plants of Australia in Venomous and Poisonous Animals and Noxious Plants of the Pacific Region. ed. Keegan, H.L. and Macfarlane, W.V. Oxford. Pergamon Press. pp.3-13.

Gellert, E. and Riggs, N.V. (1954) Cryptopleurine: An alkaloid of Cryptocarpa pleurosperma. Aust. J. Chem. 7, 113.

de la Lande, I.S. (1948) The alkaloids of Cryptocarpa pleurosperma. Austr. J. Exp. Biol. med. Sci. 26, 181.

Webb, L.J. (1948) Alkaloids in Queensland Cryptocarpa spp. Austral. J. Science 11, 26.

Woods, B. and Calnan, C.D. (1976) Toxic Woods. Brit. J. Derm. 94, Suppl. 13, June.

Dicypellium

One species is found in Brazil.

Dicypellium caryophyllatum
Fap cravo, red wood, canella, Cayenne rosewood

The bark of this tree (known as Cassia caryophyllata) is used as a substitute for cloves and cinnamon. The wood is valuable but is little exported from Brazil. Freise (1932) classed it with the toxic Nectandra and Ocotea spp.

Reference

Freise, F.W. (1932) Gesundheitsschädigungen durch Arbeiten mit giften Hölzern. Beobachtungen aux brasilianischen Gewerbebetrieben. Archiv für Gewerbepathologie und Gewerbehygiene 3,1.

Laurus

One species is native to Madeira and the Canary Islands. The other species of the genus, L. nobilis (Laurel, Sweet Bay), is native to the Mediterranean region. The common Laurel (Cherry Laurel) of English gardens is Prunus laurocerasus (Rosaceae family).

Laurus spp.

Some Laurel trees, known in Malaysia as Medang Miang, have irritant bark; the species names are not known with certainty (Corner 1952).

Laurus nobilis
Laurel, Sweet Bay

The leaved branches were used as wreaths and garlands in Ancient Rome thus providing other colloquial names, Roman or Noble Laurel. Bay leaf used as a culinary herb caused stomatitis and cheilitis (Jirasek and Skach 1962, Skach 1964). Oil of Bay (Laurel Oil) is derived from the leaves. Laurel oil in toothpastes and proprietary ointments (Spier and Sixt 1953) and in hat-bands (Gronemeyer 1953) caused dermatitis. The oil produced positive patch test reactions in 3.9% (Paschoud 1962) and in 5 of 1147 patients (Calnan 1970) in European eczema clinics. Wagner (1959) and Bandmann and Dohn (1960) referred to contact sensitivity to laurel oil.

Foussereau et al (1967 a, b) made a detailed study of contact sensitivity to laurel oil. A sensitizer present in the leaves of some races of L. nobilis is probably a sesquiterpene lactone (Asakawa et al 1974). Cross-sensitivity can occur with some other plants notably Compositae and Magnoliaceae species which yield sesquiterpene lactones (Mitchell 1975). Laurel oil 2% in petrolatum is suitable for patch testing.

References

Asakawa, Y., Benezra, C., Ducombs, G. et al (1974) Cross-sensitization between Frullania and Laurus nobilis: Archs. Derm. 110, 957.

Bandmann, J.H. and Dohn, W. (1960) Das Lorbeerol als nicht seltene Ursache allergischer Kontaktenzeme. Munch. med. Wschr. 102,680.

Calnan, C.D. (1970) Oil of cloves, laurel, lavender, peppermint. Contact Dermatitis Newsletter 7, 148.

Corner, E.J.H. (1952) Wayside trees of Malaysia. Singapore, Government Printer.

Foussereau, J., Benezra, C. and Ourisson, G. (1967a) Contact dermatitis from Laurel. I Clinical Aspects. Trans. St. John's Hosp. Derm. Soc. (Lond.) 53, 141.

Foussereau, J., Benezra, C. and Ourisson, G. (1967b) Contact dermatitis from Laurel. II Chemical Aspects. Trans. St. John's Hosp. Derm. Soc. (Lond.) 53, 147.

Gronemeyer, W. (1953) Hatband dermatitis (also a contribution on epicutaneous passive transmission Dtsch. Med. Wschr. 78, 232.

Jirasek, L. and Skach, M. (1962) Perioral contact eczema with eczematous stomatitis after the use of bay leaves (Laurus nobilis L.) in food Cs. Derm. 37, 18.

Mitchell, J.C. (1975) Contact sensitivity to sesquiterpene lactones. Derm. Int. 14, 239 and 301.

Paschoud, J.M. (1962) Critical observations on the composition of the so-called standard series for epicutaneous tests. Dermatologic (Basel) 124, 196.

Skatch, M. (1964) Eczematous type of stomatitis. Oral Medicine 18, 455.

Spier, H.W. and Sixt, I. (1953) Laurel as a hitherto little recognized allergen in contact eczema. Derm. Wschr. 128, 805.

Wagner, G. (1959) Eine Analyse von 500 allergischen Kontaktekzemen. Berufsdermatosen 7, 307.

Litsea

400 species are native to warm regions of Asia, Australia and America.

Litsea sp. Medang

The sticky sap is said to be

very irritant to the skin (Altschul 1973). The flowers are said to be irritant because of their fine hairs and the pulp of the ripe fruit is also irritant (Corner 1952).

Litsea cubeba

A balsam or oil from the plant was implicated in contact sensitivity (Rudzki and Grzywa 1976).

Reference

Rudzki, E. and Grzywa, Z. (1976) Sensitizing and irritating properties of star anise oil. Contact Dermatitis 2, 305.

Litsea polyantha

The bark is said to be very irritant (Burkill 1935).

References

Altschul, S. von R. (1973) Drugs and foods from little-known plants. Cambridge, Mass. Harvard Univ. Press.

Burkill, I.H. (1935) A dictionary of the economic products of the Malay Peninsula. 2 Vols. London. Crown Agents for the Colonies.

Corner, E.J.H. (1952) Wayside trees of Malaysia. Singapore, Government Printer.

Mezilaurus

Nine species are found in tropical South America.

Mezilaurus Itauba

This species colloquially named Itauba has not been implicated in adverse effects (see Ocotea).

Botany of Nectandra, Ocotea and Phoebe.

According to Shaw (1973):

Nectandra Roland. ex Rottb. (~ Ocotea Aubl.) 100 species are found from central to sub-tropical America. N. rodiaei Hook (greenheart) and others yield good timber.

Ocotoea Aubl. Three to four hundred species are found in tropical and subtropical America, a few in tropical and southern Africa and the Mascarenes. O. bullata E. Mey of southern Africa, yields a useful timber, stinkwood.

Phoebe Ness. 70 species are found in Indomalaysia, tropical America and the West Indies. The American species hitherto referred to Phoebe should be removed to Persea and Cinnamomum.

Reference

Shaw, H.K.A. (1973) A Dictionary of the Flowering Plants and Ferns. The late J.C. Willis. 8th ed. Cambridge University Press.

Kukachka (1970) refers to:

Ocotea rodiaei	Greenheart
Ocotea rubra	Determa
Phoebe porosa	Imbuia

Reference

Kukachka, B.F. (1970) Properties of imported tropical woods. USDA Forest Service Research Paper. FPL125 Forest Products Laboratory, Madison, Wis.

Woods and Calnan (1976) refer to:

Phoebe porosa Mez. (Ocotea porosa L. Barr.) Imbuya

Ocotea rodiaei Mez. (Nectandra rodiaei (Hook.) Schomb.) Greenheart

Ocotea barcellensis Mez. Louro inamui

Ocotea rubra Mez. Red Louro

Ocotea puberula Nees. Laurel amarillo

Ocotea usambarensis Engl. East African Camphorwood

Ocotea bullata E. Mey Stinkwood

Reference

Woods, B. and Calnan, C.D. (1976) Toxic Woods. Brit. J. Derm. 94, Suppl. 13, June.

Nectandra spp. (many are called Ocotea spp. by other botanists).

Friese (1932) divided the toxic Lauraceae woods of Brazil into three groups:

(a) Canella: Nectandra spp.

(b) Itauba: probably Ocotoea spp. but not Mezilarus which is another itauba (Record and Mell 1924).

(c) Pao cravo: Dicypellium

According to Freise (1932) all these contain apiol and at least two alkaloids which produced vomiting, diarrhoea, cramps, cardiac stimulation, headaches and dizziness. Some Nectandra spp. from northern Brazil had a strongly irritant oil in their bark, which caused persistent pyoderma in the fingerwebs and at the angles of the mouth.

References

Freise, F.W. (1932) Gesundheitsschädigungen durch Arbeiten mit giftigen Hölzern. Beobachtungen aus brasilianischen Gwerbebetrieben. Archiv für Gewerbepathologie und Gewerbehygiene 3, 1.

Record, S.J. and Mell, C.D. (1924) Timbers of Tropical America. New Haven, Yale.

Nectandra
(syn. Ocotea)

100 species are native to Central to sub-tropical South American.

Nectandra spp.
(Paracoto, Embuia, Imbuya, Brazilian Walnut)

Paracoto bark, which is used for astringent effects, contains crystalline material (Wren 1968). Schwartz 1931) observed dermatitis in cabinet makers from Brazilian Walnut wood which he thought was either Nectandra sp. or Cordia goeldiana but according to Record and Hess (1943) the wood was actually from Phoebe porosa. Patch tests to the sawdust produced positive reactions.

Nectandra rodiaei (syn. Ocotea rodiaei) Green heart

The saw-dust of this Antilles (West Indies) tree can produce respiratory symptoms in wood-workers (Handbook of Hardwoods 1956, Hanslian and Kadlec 1966, VII, Sandermann and Barghoorn 1956). The alkaloid, berberine, may be responsible (Hausen 1970).

Nectandra splendens

The hollow branches of the tree house stinging ants (Altschul 1973).

References

Altschul, S. von R. (1973) Drugs and foods from little-known plants. Cambridge, Mass. Harvard Univ. Press.

Handbook of Hardwoods (1966) Forest Products Research. Ministry of Technology. London. HMSO.

Hanslian, L. and Kadlec, K. (1966) Drevo z hlediska hygieniskeho (VII). Biologicky Silne agresivni dreviny. Drevo 21, 157.

Hausen, B.M. (1970) Untersuchungen über Gesundheitsschädigende Hölzer. Thesis, Hamburg.

Sandermann, W. and Barghoorn, A.W. (1956) Gesundheitsschadigende Holzer. HolzRoh-Werkst 14, 87.

Wren, R.W. (1968) Potter's New Cyclopaedia of Botanical Drugs and Preparations by Wren, R.C. Re-edit. by Wren, R.W. Potter and Clarke Ltd. Health Science Press. Rustington, Sussex.

Schwartz, L. (1931) Dermatitis venenata due to contact with Brazilian walnut wood. Publ. Health Rep. 46, 1938.

Record, S.J. and Hess, R.W. (1943) Timbers of the New World. New Haven, Yale.

Nothaphoebe

30 species are native to south-eastern Asia.

Nothaphoebe panduriformis

The sap is said to be vesicant (Burkill 1935).

Reference

Burkill, I.H. (1935) A dictionary of the economic products of the Malay Peninsula. 2 Vols.London. Crown Agents for the Colonies.

Ocotea (syn. Nectandra)

Most of 300-400 species are native to tropical and sub-tropical America, a few to Africa.

Ocotea spp.
Louro, Jiqua, Pisie

The South American species of this genus can cause dermatitis (Woods 1968). O. bullata is known as stink-wood.

Ocotea cyrubarum
Brazilian Sassafras

A safrole of perfumery is derived from this species (Fenaroli 1971). A derivative, heliotropin, is said to cause dermatitis (Klarmann 1958).

Ocotea porosa
(syn. Phoebe)

This species was observed to cause mucocutaneous effects in woodworkers (de Carvalho 1956). The noxious effects of this species may be from alkaloids (Hausen 1970).

Cordia goeldiana was a name given by Schwartz (1931) to Brazilian walnut but this was in fact Phoebe porosa, (Record and Hess 1943).

Ocotea rodiaei
(syn. Nectandra rodiaei)

The noxious effects of this species may be from the alkaloid berberine (Hausen 1970).

References

Record, S.J. and Hess, R.W. (1943) Timbers of the New World. New Haven, Yale.

Schwartz, L. (1931) Dermatitis venenata due to contact with Brazilian walnut wood. Publ. Hlth. Rep. (Washington) 46,1938.

de Carvalho, L.P. (1956) Occupational contact allergens. Brasilmed. 70, 77.

Fenaroli, G. (1971) Fenaroli's Handbook of Flavor Ingredients. ed. Furia, T.E. and Bellanca, N. Cleveland, Ohio. The Chemical Rubber, Co.

Hausen, B.M. (1970) Untersuchungen über Gesundheitsschädigende Hölzer.Thesis, Hamburg.

Klarmann, E.G. (1958) Perfume dermatitis. Ann. Allergy. 16, 425.

Woods, B. (1968) Principal timbers causing dermatitis in Textbook of Dermatology. ed. Rook,., Wilkinson, D.S. and Ebling, F.J.G. Oxford. Blackwell Scientific Publ. pp. 1891.

Ocotea bullata

This species was listed as a cause of dermatitis by Schwartz et al (1957) without clinical details.

Reference

Schwartz, L., Tulipan, L. and Birmingham, D.J. (1957) Occupational Diseases of the Skin. 3rd ed. Philadelphia. Lea and Febiger. pp. 637-672.

Ocotea usambarensis
East African Camphorwood

Orsler (1973) received two trade reports of skin and mucous membrane irritation from the wood.

Reference

Orsler, R.J. (1973) Personal communication from Forest Products Research Laboratory, Princess Risborough, Bucks, England.

Ocotea barcellensis
Louro inamui

Ocotea rubra
Red louro

Ocotea puberula
Laurel amarillo

Many South American species of Ocotea or Nectandra are called louro or laurel. Record and Mell (1924) describe the wood of O. puberula as peppery. Woods and Calnan (1976) described five cases of dermatitis from louro used as a veneer in a furniture factory.

Two of five patients showed positive patch test reactions to the wood, three doubtful reactions. Seventeen other men with dermatitis (query in the factory or other eczema subjects) showed negative reactions to the wood. Two of the patients were also contact sensitive to Distemonanthus but three showed negative reactions.

References

Record, S.J. and Mell, C.D. (1924) Timbers of Tropical America. New Haven, Yale.

Woods, B. and Calnan, C.D. (1976) Toxic Woods. Brit. J. Derm. 94, Suppl. 13, June.

Ocotea rodiaei
(syn. Nectandra rodiaei)
Greenheart

According to Woods and Calnan (1976) the wood of this species has sometimes been confused with the more irritating Surinam greenheart (Tabebuia). Splinters of O. rodiaei cause troublesome wounds and the dust irritates workers' throats (Grossmann 1920, Woods 1951). It contains several alkaloids (McKennis et al 1956, Hearst et al 1968).

References

Grossmann, J. (1920) Gesundheitsschädliche Holzarten Der Holzkäufer (Leipzig) 17, 529, 535, 540 and 545.

Hearst, P.J., Shamma, M., Dudock, B.S. et al (1968) Greenheart alkaloids III Sepeerine (ocoteamine) and Demararine. J. Org. Chem. 33, 1229.

McKennis, H., Jr., Hearst, P.J., Drisko, R.W. et al (1956) Isolation of a tetramethoxylated alkaloid from Demerara greenheart. J. Amer. Chem. Soc. 78, 245.

Woods, R.P. (1951) Timbers of South America. 2nd ed. Timber Development Association Ltd. London.

Woods, B. and Calnan, C.D. (1976) Toxic Woods. Brit. J. Derm. 94, Suppl, 13, June.

Phoebe porosa
(syn. Ocotea porosa)
Imbuya, imbuia

Imbuya sawdust was irritating to some workmen (Schmieg 1926). Brazilian walnut wood produced vesicular dermatitis in eleven workers. The incidence varied from 10 to 20% in different factories. Many men without dermatitis had coryzal symptoms (Schwartz 1931). He thought that the wood was Nectandra or Cordia goeldiana as had earlier writers, but Record (1929) showed that it was in fact Phoebe porosa.

References

Record, S.J. (1929) Walnut woods - true and false. Tropical woods 18, 4.

Schmieg, K. (1926) Notes on new cabinet woods from Brazil. Tropical Woods 5, 1.

Schwartz, L. (1931) Dermatitis venenata due to contact with Brazilian walnut wood. Publ. Hlth. Rep. (Washington) 46, 1938.

The fine sawdust is reported to be very irritating to certain individuals (Kukachka 1970).

Reference

Kukachka, B.F. (1970) Properties of imported tropical woods. USDA Forest Service Research Paper. FPL125 March. U.S. Dept. Agric. Forest Service. Forest Products Laboratory. Madison, Wis. U.S.A.

Persea

150 species are found in tropical regions. P. gratissima (Avocado) provides edible fruit.

Persea americana
Avocado

The seed yields a milky juice the colour of which turns from red to black and marks cloth. Powdered seed is used as a rubefacient and the seed oil is irritant when used as an injection vehicle (Watt and Breyer-Brandwijk 1962).

Reference

Watt, J.M. and Breyer-Brandwijk, M.G.

(1962) The Medicinal and Poisonous Plants of Southern and Eastern Africa. 2nd ed. Edinburgh. E. & S. Livingstone Ltd.

Phoebe

70 species are native to IndoMalaysia and the West Indies. The American species hitherto referred to *Phoebe* should be removed to *Persea* and *Cinnamomum*, (Willis 1966). Noxious effects of *Phoebe porosa* (Brazilian Walnut) are considered under *Ocotea porosa*.

Reference

Willis, J.C. (1966) A Dictionary of the Flowering Plants and Ferns. 7th Ed. Revised by Shaw, H.K.A. Cambridge, University Press.

Sassafras

Two species are native to China, one species to eastern North America.

Sassafras albidum
(syn. *S. officinale*)

Oil of Sassafras derived from this plant and from *S. variifolium* is said to produce dermatitis in hypersensitive individuals (Tulipan 1938). Heliotropin, a derivative of saffrole, used in cosmetics, has been reported to cause dermatitis (Greenberg and Lester 1954).

References

Greenberg, L.A. and Lester, D. (1954) Handbook of Cosmetic Materials. New York. Interscience.

Tulipan, L. (1938) Dosmetic irritants. Archs. Derm. Syph. 38, 906.

Umbellularia

One species is native to California.

Umbellularia californica
Oregon myrtle, bay,
Californian olive

This species produces irritation of the mucous membrane of some persons who handle it (Chittenden 1974).

The bark and leaves contain a pungent volatile oil (Record and Hess 1943).

References

Record, S.J. and Hess, R.W. (1943) Timbers of the New World. New Haven, Yale.

Chittenden, F.J. (1974) (The late) The Royal Horticultural Society Dictionary of Gardening. 2nd ed. Reprinted (with corrections) Vol. IV. Oxford. Clarendon Press.

LECYTHIDACEAE

325 species in 15 genera are native to tropical America.

Chemistry is recorded by Hegnauer (1966).

Bertholletia

Two species are native to tropical South America and the West Indies.

Bertholletia excelsa
Brazil nut tree

Workers in a candy factory developed dermatitis of the hands and upper limbs from Brazil nuts. Patch tests to the nut and its oil produced positive patch test reactions in 7 of 8 cases (Markson 1942). In a patient who had urticaria of the lips from chewing Brazil nuts, a patch test to a piece of the nut produced a local urticarial reaction (Maddin 1974).

A positive scratch test to brazil nut was observed in a foodhandler who had dermatitis (Hjorth and Roed-Petersen 1976).

References

Hjorth, N. and Roed-Petersen, J. (1976) Occupational protein contact dermatitis in food handlers. Contact Dermatitis 2, 28.

Hegnauer, R. (1966) Chemotaxonomy of plants. Vol. 4. Basel, Birkhauser. p. 381.

Maddin, W.S. (1974) Pers. Comm.

Markson, L.S. (1942) Dermatitis from seed and oil of Bertholletia excelsa (Brazil Nut). Archs. Derm. Syph. 46, 831.

Couroupita

20 species are native to tropical America and the West Indies.

Couroupita guianensis
Cannonball Tree

The large fruits are a hazard to persons who walk under the tree (Corner 1952, Menninger 1967).

Couroupita nicaraguensis

The wood has been known as grendilla and used for musical instruments (Hausen 1970).

References

Corner, E.J.H. (1952) Wayside trees of Malaysia. Singapore, Government Printer.

Hausen, B.M. (1970) Untersuchungen über Gesundheitsschädigende Hölzer. Thesis, Hamburg.

Menninger, E.A. (1967) Fantastic Trees. New York. The Viking Press.

Lecythis

50 species are native to tropical America.

Lecythis spp.
Monkey-pot

The oily seeds of some species are edible (sapucaia nuts).

The seeds are used to catch monkeys.

Ingestion of the seeds can cause alopecia from a content of mimosine (Gooderatne 1966).

Lecythis ollaria
Coco de Mono

Universal alopecia and nail changes were observed to follow ingestion of the nuts (Aronow and Kerdel-Vegas 1965).

An amino acid derivative of selenium, produced by some of the trees from pockets of selenium in the soil, has toxic properties (Kerdel-Vegas 1964, 1973, Kerdel-Vegas et al 1965).

According to Woods and Calnan (1976) the botanical name of this species is as follows: -Lecythis grandiflora Aubl. (L. ollaria L.)

Lecythis pisonis
Sapucaia

Sapucaia wood had to be soaked in a mixture of urine and soda for several days before being worked because a saponin present in the fresh wood could produce severe mucosal irritation, headache and vomiting (Freise 1932).

References

Aronow, L., and Kerdel-Vegas, F. (1965) Seleno-cystathionine, a pharmacologically active factor in the seeds of Lecythis ollaria. Nature, Lond. 205, 1185.

Gooderatne, B.W.M. (1966) Massive generalized alopecia after poisoning by Gloriosa superba. Brit. Med. J. 1, 1023.

Kerdel-Vegas, F. (1964) Generalized hair loss due to the ingestion of "Coco de Mono" (Lecythis ollaria). J. Invest. Derm. 42,91

Kerdel-Vegas, F., Wagner, T., Russell P.G. et al (1965) Structure of the pharmacologically active factor in the seeds of Lecythis ollaria. Nature, Lond. 205, 1186.

Kerdel-Vegas, F. (1973) The challenge of tropical dermatology. Trans. St. John's Hosp. Derm. Soc. 59, 1

Freise, F.W. (1932) Gesundheitsschädigungen durch Arbeiten mit giftigen Hölzern. Beobachtungen aus brasilianischen Gewerbebetrieben. Archiv. für Gewerbepathologie und Gewerbehygiene 3, 1.

Woods, B. and Calnan, C.D. (1976) Toxic Woods. Brit. J. Derm. 94, Suppl. 13, June.

Kerdel-Vegas, F. (1966) The depilatory and cytotoxic action of "Coco de Mono" (Lecthyis ollaria) and its relationship to chronic seleniosis. Econ. Bot. 20, 187.

LEGUMINOSAE (FABACEAE)

12,000 species in 60 genera are cosmopolitan, living in every soil and climate. Trees, shrubs, water plants, xerophytes and climbers are represented. The roots of most species exhibit tubercles containing bacteria of the genus Rhizobium and plants provided with these tubercles are able to take up more atmospheric nitrogen. The plants appear to consume the nitrogen-rich bacteria which live in their cells.

The family is divided into Mimosoideae and Caesalpinioideae which are mostly tropical and Lotoideae (Papilinioideae) which are both tropical and temperate (Harborne et al 1971).

Chemistry is recorded by Harborne et al (1971).

References

Harborne, J.B., Boulter, D. and Turner, B.L. (1971) Chemotaxonomy of the Leguminosae. London. Academic Press.

Sub-family Lotoideae (Papilionoideae)

Tribe Abreae

Abrus

12 species are found in tropical regions.

Chemistry

Abrin, a toxic principle of the seeds, is irritant to the mucous membranes. Ricin from Ricinus has similar but milder actions.

Abrus precatorius
Jequirity

The juice of the plant is irritant to the mucous membranes (Watt and Breyer-Brandwijk 1962).

The hard red seeds with black tips known as Crab's Eyes are strung into necklaces and rosaries and are used as weights and tourist souvenirs and in 'pea-shooters'. Dermatitis can occur on the neck of persons who wear necklaces made by piercing the seeds and threading them on a string (Behl et al 1966).

The seed material is irritant to the eye and has been used for the purpose of malingering (Burkill 1935, Somerset 1945, Somerville-Large 1947, Morton 1971). The seeds may be coated with lacquer (Rhus vernicifera).

References

Behl, P.N., Captain, R.M., Bedi, B.M.S. and Gupta, S. (1966) Skin-irritant and sensitizing plants found in India, New Delhi. P.N. Behl, Irwin Hospital.

Burkill, I.H. (1935) A Dictionary of the Economic Products of the Malay Peninsula. 2 Vols. London. Crown Agents for the Colonies.

Morton, J.F. (1971) Plants Poisonous to People in Florida and other warm areas. Miami, Florida. Hurricane House Publishers Inc.

Somerset, E.J. (1945) Self-inflicted conjunctivitis. Brit. J. Ophth. 29, 196.

Somerville-Large, L.B. (1947) Self-inflicted eye injuries. Tr. Ophth. Soc. U. Kingdom 67, 185.

Watt, J.M. and Breyer-Brandwijk, M.G. (1962) The Medicinal and poisonous plants of Southern Africa. 2nd ed. Edinburgh. E. & S. Livingstone.

Sub-family Mimosoideae

Tribe Acacieae

Acacia

Perhaps 800 species are found in tropical and sub-tropical regions. Many are armed with thorns capable of causing mechanical injury and the thorns of some house stinging ants. The common name, acacia, is applied to Robinia.

Acacia spp.

The tip of the thorn of 'acacia', possibly of this genus, retained in the ciliary body produced severe recurrent iriodocylitis (Paufique and Hugonnier 1966). The pollen is suspected of causing hayfever (Wodehouse 1971). Contact with the pollen can cause dermatitis (Rowe 1931).

Reference

Paufique, L. and Hugonnier, R. (1966) Iriodocyclite recidivante par epine d'acacia dans le corps ciliaire. Bull. Sco. Ophtal. Franc. 66, 547.

Rowe, A.H. (1931) Botanical survey of San Joaquin County in central California. J. Allergy 3, 98.

Wodehouse, R.P. (1971) Hayfever Plants. 2nd rev. edition. New York, Hafner.

Acacia aneura
Mulga

Slivers of the wood are said to have a poisonous effect and can produce cutaneous granulomas (Cleland 1943).

Reference

Cleland, J.B. (1943) Plants including fungi, poisonous or otherwise injurious to man in Australia. IV. Med. J. Australia. 11, 161.

Acacia catechu
Black Catechu

The wood yields a brown dye which is used for dyeing cloth. Catechu, also derived from Uncaria, is often adulterated. Dermatitis from dyed uniforms known as Khaki probably resulted from fabric finishes or chromate rather than from the dye itself (Peterkin 1948, Hellier 1960) although effects of the dye could not be excluded (Davies and Barker 1944).

References

Davies, J.H.T. and Barker, A.N. (1944) Textile dermatitis. Brit. J. Derm. Syph. 56, 33.

Hellier, F.F. (1960) Dermatitis purpurica after contact with textiles. Hautarzt 11, 173.

Peterkin, G.Z.G. (1948) Textile dermatitis in men. Arch. Derm. Syph. 58, 249.

Acacia cunninghamii

This species is said to cause skin irritation (Gardner and Bennets 1956).

Acacia cyperophylla
Red Mulga

Scratches from the wood are notable for festering (Cleland 1931).

Acacia dealbata

The familiar 'mimosa' of florists is usually this species. Oil of Mimosa of perfumery is said to cause contact dermatitis (Greenberg and Lester 1954).

Acacia delibrata

The pods contain a saponin which is irritant to the mucous emmbranes (Hurst 1942).

Acacia farnesiana

Cassie of perfumery is derived from this species.

Acacia greggii
Desert Catclaw

Mechanical injury can occur from the spines.

References

Cleland, J.B. (1931) Plants including fungi, poisonous or otherwise injurious to man in Australia III. Med. J. Australia 2, 775.

Gardner, C.A. and Bennets, H.W. (1956) The toxic plants of Western Australia. Perth West. Australian Newspapers Ltd.

Greenberg, L.A. and Lester, D. (1954) Handbook of Cosmetic Materials. New York. Interscience.

Hurst, E. (1942) The Poisonous Plants of New South Wales. N.S.W. Poison Plants Committee; Sydney.

Acacia harpophylla
Brigalow

The wood can cause eczema in wood-workers and the bark or possibly caterpillars on the bark have irritant effects (Cleland 1943).

Acacia implexa
Hickory

Cattle who eat the plant are said to develop dermatitis (Hurst 1942).

Acacia karroo
Kangaroo Thorn

This thorny species which is used as a barrier or hedge is capable of causing mechanical injury.

Acacia melanoxylon
Australian Blackwood

The wood can produce dermatitis and rhinorrhoea in woodworkers (Cleland 1925, Burry 1969). Patch tests produced negative results (Robertson 1926).

Acacia senegal
Acacia

This and other species furnish Gum Arabic which has been reported to cause respiratory allergy particularly in the printing trade, (Sprague 1942, Maytum and Magath 1932, Bohner et al 1941). Dermatitis from Gum Arabic (Acacia) has also been reported (Greenberg and Lester 1954, Turiaf et al 1959). A gum from cashew (*Anacardium*) may be used to adulterate Gum Arabic.

References

Bohner, C.B., Sheldon, J.M. and Trenis, J.W. (1941) Sensitivity to gum acacia, with report of 10 cases of asthma in printers. J. Allergy 12, 290.

Burry, J.N. (1969) The value of patch testing: A review of 363 cases of allergic contact dermatitis. Med. J. Australia 1, 1226.

Cleland, J.B. (1943) Plants including fungi, poisonous or otherwise injurious to man in Australia. (Series II). Med. J. Australia 2, 443.

Cleland, J.B. (1943) Plants including fungi, poisonous or otherwise injurious to man in Australia. IV. Med. J. Australia. 11, 161.

Greenberg, L.A. and Lester, D. (1954) Handbook of Cosmetic Materials. New York. Interscience.

Hurst, E. (1942) The Poisonous Plants of New South Wales. N.S.W. Poison Plants Committee; Sydney.

Maytum, C.K. and Magath, T.B. (1932) Sensitivity to acacia. JAMA 99, 2251.

Robertson, D.G. (1926) An investigation of certain health aspects in persons engaged in the wood working industries. Commonwealth Dept. of Health. (Division of Industrial Hygiene). Pub. No. 4. Melbourne. Government Printer.

Sprague, P.H. (1942) Bronchial asthma due to sensitivity to gum acacia. Canad. Med. Ass. J. 47, 253.

Turiaf, J., Tabart, J., Seneze, M., and Vernier, D. (1959) Allergy to gum arabic in printing workers. J. Franc. Med. Chir. Thor. 13, 617.

Acacia seyal

This species furnished the coffins of Ancient Egypt and the Ark of the Old Testament.

Acacia shirleyi
Lancewood

The bark or possibly caterpillars on the bark can produce irritation (Cleland 1931). Flavonols may be responsible (Hausen 1970).

Slivers of the wood, Australian lancewood, were said to cause painful wounds "like snake-bite" (Maiden 1919).

References

Cleland, J.B. (1931) Plants including fungi, poisonous or otherwise injurious to man in Australia. III. Med. J. Austr. 2, 775.

Hausen, B.M. (1970) Untersuchungen über Gesundheitsschädigende Hölzer. Thesis. Hamburg.

Maiden, J.H. (1919) Notes on Acacia. No. IV. J. Proc. Roy. Soc. New South Wales 53, 219.

Sub-family Mimosoideae

Tribe Adenanthereae

Adenanthera

8 species are found in tropical Asia, Australia and the

Pacific region.

Chemistry

Some species of this genus yield lapachol (Gibbs 1963) a sensitizer of *Tectona*.

Adenanthera pavonina
Red Sandalwood

The seeds known as Circassian beans are used in necklaces (Morton 1962).

References

Gibbs, R.C. (1963) History of Chemical Taxonomy in Chemical Plant Taxonomy. ed. Swain, T. London. Academic Press.

Morton, J.F. (1962) Ornamental Plants with Poisonous Properties. II. Proc. Florida Hort. Soc. 75, 484.

Sub-family Caesalpiniodeae

Tribe Detarieae

Afzelia

14 species are native to tropical Africa and Asia.

Afzelia africana
Doussie

This and possibly other species of this genus, notably *A. bipindensis* can produce dermatitis and respiratory symptoms in wood-workers (Raymond 1959, Irvine 1961, Zafiropoulo et al 1968, Hublet et al 1972, Hausen 1970).

References

Hausen, B.N. (1970) Untersuchungen über Gesundheitsschädigende Hölzer. Thesis, Hamburg.

Hublet, P., Sporcq, J., Oleffe, J. et al (1972) Etude sur les accidents cutanes et muqueux provoques par les bois tropicaux dans l'industrie due bois en Belgique Arch. Belges. Med. Social. 30, 314.

Irvine, F.R. (1961) Woody Plants of Ghana. Oxford. University Press. London.

Zafiropoulo, A., Audibert, A. and Charpin, J. (1968) A propos des accidents dus a la manipulation des bois exotiques. Rev. Franc. Allerg. 8, 155.

Raymond, V. (1959) Dermatoses professionnelles dan la bâtiment. Revue du Praticien 9, 2683.

Sub-family Mimosoideae

Tribe Ingeae

Albizia

100 or possibly 150 species are found in warm regions of the Old World. The fragrant wood of *A. odoratissima* is known as Ceylon Rosewood. The leaves of *A. coriaria* form a lather known as Poor Man's Soap. The bark of *A. lebbeck* contains saponins and is also used as a soap. The West African timbers are known in industry.

Albizia antihelmintica

The pollen is irritant to the eye (Watt and Breyer-Brandwijk 1962).

Albizia falcata, *A. ferruginea* *A. belleck* and *A. tanganyicensis* known as Batai, Kokko and Siris and other species of this genus have been reported to cause upper respiratory symptoms in wood-workers (Lewin 1928, Griffioen 1949, Vorreiter 1949, Farmer 1972, Sandermann and Barghoorn 1956, Hausen 1970). Some species were formerly placed in the genera *Acacia* and *Calliandra*.

References

Hausen, B.M. (1970) Untersuchungen über Gesundheitsschädigende Hölzer. Thesis, Hamburg.

Sandermann, W. and Barghoorn, A.W. (1956) Gesundheitsschädigende Nutzholzer. Holz. Roh-Werkst. 14, 37.

Watt, J.M. and Breyer-Brandwijk, M.G. (1962) The Medicinal and Poisonous Plants of Southern Africa. 2nd ed. Edinburgh. E. & S. Livingstone.

Farmer, R.H. (1972) A Handbook of Hardwoods. 2nd ed. London. H.M.S.O.

Griffioen, K. (1949) Bevat Djeungdjinghout een giftige en

irriterende Stof? Tectona 39, 175.

Lewin, L. (1928) Gifte im Holzgewerbe. Berlin, Stilke.

Vorreiter, L. (1949) Holztechnologisches Handbuck. Wien, Fromme (later edition 1958).

Albizia falcataria
(syn. A. moluccana, A. falcata)

The fine sawdust produced by machining the dry wood is said to produce sneezing and tearing in some individuals, (Kukachka 1970).

Reference

Kukachka, B.F. (1970) Properties of imported tropical woods. U.S.D.A. Forest Service Research Paper. FPL125 March. U.S. Dept. Agric. Forest Service. Forest Products Laboratory. Madison, Wis. U.S.A.

Albizzia julibrissin
Mimosa

The pollen is suspected of causing hayfever (Wodehouse 1971).

Reference

Wodehouse, R.P. (1971) Hayfever Plants. 2nd rev. edition. New York, Hafner.

Sub-family Lotoideae (Papilionoideae)

Tribe Geoffroeae

Andira

35 species are native to tropical American and Africa. Some yield lapachol (Krogh 1964) which is a sensitizer of Tectona.

Andira americana
(syn. Vouacapoua)
Acapú, wacapou

The wood of acapú causes persistent itching papules (Freise 1932).

Reference

Freise, F.W. (1932) Gesundheitsschädigungen durch Arbeiten mit giftigen Hölzern. Beobachtungen aus brasilianischen Gewerbebetrieben. Archiv für Gewerbepathologie und Gewerbehygiene 3, 1.

Andira araroba

Goa powder derived from the timber of this tree is irritant to the respiratory tract of wood-workers (White 1887). Goa powder extract was introduced for the topical therapy of psoriasis by an English dermatologist, Balmanno Squire, in 1878. Chrysarobin is a naturally occurring mixture derived from the wood. The name chrysarobin is also applied to the pure substance 1, 8-dihydroxy-3-methyl-q-anthrone which makes up about 30% of the naturally occurring mixture (Strakosch 1944, Brown 1970).

In industrial accidents, chrysophanic acid has produced conjunctivitis and keratitis (Duke-Elder and MacFaul 1972).

References

Brown, T.H. (1970) Part III Drug Index in Current Dermatologic Management. ed. Maddin, S. St. Louis. C.V. Mosby.

Duke-Elder, S. and MacFaul, P.A. (1972) System of Opthalmology. Vol. XIV Injuries Part 2. Non-mechanical injuries. Irritant Vegetable Products pp. 1180-1196. and Self-inflicted injuries pp. 1016-1018. London. Henry Kimpton.

Krogh, H.K. (1964) Contact eczema caused by true teak (Tectona grandis). A follow-up study of a previous epidemiological investigation, and a study into the sensitizing effect of various teak extracts. Brit. J. Indust. Med. 21, 65.

Strakosch, E.A. (1944) Studies on ointments. VI. Ointments containing chrysarobin. Archs. Derm. Syph. 49, 1.

White, J.C. (1887) Dermatitis venenata: An account of the Action of External irritants upon the Skin. Boston. Cupples & Hurd.

Andira inermis
Partridge-wood

The tree can cause dermatitis in wood-workers. This common name is also applied to Piratinera guianensis and Livistona inermis of the Palm family (Lewin 1928).

The wood contains an isoflavonoid which is related to dalbergiones (see Dalbergia) and biochanin A which is related to ayanin (see Distemonanthus) (Cocker et al 1962).

A report of cough and urticaria from partridge-wood by Friese in 1932 seems to refer to this species not to Pithecolobium (Woods and Calnan 1976).

References

Hausen, B.M. (1970) Untersuchungen über Gesundheitsschädigende Hölzer. Thesis, Hamburg.

Lewin, L. (1928) Gifte in Holzgewerbe. Beitrage zur Giflkunde Heft 1. Berlin. Georg Stilke Verlag. cited by Hausen (1970).

Cocker, W., Dahl, T., Dempsey, C. et al (1962) Extractives from Andira inermis. J. Chem. Soc. 4906.

Woods, B. and Calnan, C.D. (1976) Toxic Woods. Brit. J. Derm. 94, Suppl. 13, June.

Sub-family Lotoideae (Papilionoideae)

Tribe Loteae

Anthyllis

50 species are found in Europe, North Africa and Western Asia.

Anthyllis cretica
(syn. Ebenus cretica)

The wood has been known as Grenadilla and used for musical instruments (Hausen 1970).

Dermatitis from musical instruments (Stern 1891) seems to have been from Dalbergia.

References

Hausen, B.M. (1970) Untersuchungen über Gesundheitsschädigende Hölzer. Thesis, Hamburg.

Stern, E. (1891) Uber einige Hautkrankungen der Musiker. Munch. med. Wschr. 42, 739, cited by Hausen (1970).

Hausen, B.M. (1970) Untersuchungen über Gesundheitsschädigende Hölzer. Thesis, Hamburg.

Sub-family Caesalpiniodeae

Tribe Cassieae

Apuleia

Two species are native to Brazil.

Apuleia molaris
(syn. A. leiocarpa, A. ferrea) Ferro

The wood caused dermatitis in wood-workers, and one carpenter developed constitutional symptoms after contact with fresh sawdust especially on hot days. The wood, when dried, remains capable of causing dermatitis (Friese 1932, 1936). Confusion over the nomenclature of the genus was discussed by Woods and Calnan (1976). Oxyayanin A, an allergen of Distemonanthus has been isolated from the wood (Filho and Gottlieb 1968).

References

Filho, R.B. and Gottlieb, O.R. (1968) Oxianinas A: Flavonas hexaoxigenades de apuleia leiocarpa. Anais da Academia Brasileira de Ciencias 40, 151.

Freise, F.W. (1932) Gesundheitsschädigungen durch Arbeiten mit giftigen Hölzern. Beobachtungen aus brasilianischen Gewerbebetrieben. Archiv für Gewerbepathologies und Gewerbehygiene 3, 1.

Friese, F.W. (1936) Vergiftungen durch Brasilianische Werkhölzer I. II. Sammlung der Vergiftungsfallen 7C 1 & 61.

Woods, B. and Calnan, C.D. (1976) Toxic Woods. Brit. J. Derm. 94, Suppl. 13, June.

Sub-family Lotoideae (Papilionoideae)

Tribe Stylosantheae

Arachis

15 species are native to Brazil and Paraguay.

Contact dermatitis of the fingers from peanuts was reported by Waldbott and Shea (1948). Octyl gallate in peanut butter can cause dermatitis (Van Ketel 1978).

Reference

Waldbott, G.L. and Shea, J.J. (1948) Causative diagnosis of contact dermatitis II. A classification of patterns on the hands. Archs. Derm. Syph. 57, 975.

Van Ketel, W.G. (1978) Dermatitis from octyl gallate in peanut butter. Contact Dermatitis 4, 60.

Arachis hypogaea
Ground or Pea Nut

Pea Nut oil was reported to cause a local reaction and generalized urticaria when used as an injection vehicle (Chafee 1941).

Reference

Chafee, F.H. (1941) Sensitivity to peanut oil with report of a case. Ann. Int. Med. 15, 1116.

Sub-family Lotoideae (Papilionoideae)

Tribe Astragaleae

Astragalus

2,000 species are cosmopolitan except absent from Australia.

Astragalus gummifer

This and other species yield Tragacanth gum which has been reported to cause respiratory allergy (Greenberg and Lester 1954). Cross-sensitivity was observed to Gum Arabic (Acacia senegal) and to Karaya Gum (Sterculia urens).

Astragalus pectinatus
Loco Weed

Ingestion of this species, containing selenocystathionine, can cause hair-loss (Schoental 1965).

References

Greenberg, L.A. and Lester, D. (1954) Handbook of Cosmetic Materials. New York. Interscience.

Schoental, R. (1965) Toxicology of natural products. Food Cosmetic. Toxicol. 3, 609.

Sub-family Caesalpiniodeae

Genus Detarieae

Baikiaea

10 species are native to tropical Africa.

Baikiaea plurijuga
(syn. Baikea)
Rhodesian Teak

This species can cause respiratory symptoms in wood-workers (Ordman 1949).

Reference

Ordman, D. (1949) Wood dust as an inhalant allergen. South Afr. med. J. 23, 973.

Sub-family Lotoideae (Papilionoideae)

Tribe Sophoreae

Baphia

65 species are found in warm parts of Africa and Madagascar, one species in Borneo.

Baphia nitida
Camwood

A red dye derived from the wood is used as a cosmetic in Africa (Irvine 1961).

The sawdust is very pungent, like snuff (Holtzapffel and Royle 1843).

References

Irvine, F.R. (1961) Woody Plants of Ghana. Oxford. University Press. London.

Holtzapffel, C. and Royle (1843) Descriptive catalogue of the woods commonly employed in this country for the mechanical and ornamental arts. An extract from: Turning and mechanical manipulation. London, Holtzapffel quoted by Woods, B. and Calnan, C.D. (1976).

Woods, B., and Calnan, C.D. (1976) Toxic Woods. Brit. J. Derm. 94, Suppl. 13, June.

Sub-family Caesalpinioideae

Tribe Sclerolobieae

Batesia

One species is found in northern Brazil.

Batesia floribunda
Acapu rana

The woods of this species and of Campsiandra laurifolia are both colloquially named acapú rana (false acapu) or manaiara. Men sawing the wood of acapú rana suffer headaches and sometimes vomiting (Freese 1932).

Reference

Freise, F.W. (1932) Gesundheitsschädigungen durch Arbeiten mit giftigen Hölzern. Beobachtungen aus brasilianischen Gewerbebetrieben. Archiv für Gewerbepathologie und Gewerbehygiene 3, 1.

Sub-family Lotoideae (Papilionoideae)

Tribe Sophoreae

Bowdichia

Three species are native to tropical South America.

Bowdichia nitida
Sucupira

Allergic contact dermatitis was observed in a cabinet-maker from exposure to the saw-dust of this species (Heyl 1966). Positive patch test reactions were observed to 2,6-dimethoxy-para-benzoquinone and to two other quinones derived from the wood. The patient was also contact sensitive to Dalbergia and dalbergiones (Hausen et al 1972).

References

Hausen, B.M., Simatupang, M.H., and Kingreen, J.C. (1972) Untersuchungen zur Uberempfindlichkeit gegen Sucupira - und Palisanderholz. Berufsdermatosen 20, 1.

Heyl, U. (1966) Kontaktekzem bei Uberempfindlichkeit gengen Sucupira - und Palisanderholz. Berufsdermatosen 14, 239.

Sub-family Lotoideae (Papilionoideae)

Tribe Aeschynomeneae

Brya

Seven species are native to central America and the West Indies.

Brya ebenus
(syn. Amerimnum ebenus, Inga vera)
Cocus wood

During the nineteenth century cocus wood replaced boxwood as the favorite wood for flutes, though it was known to cause irritation of the lips in some players (Rockstro 1890). According to Woods and Calnan (1976) the wood of a flute made of grendadilla or red ebony which caused dermatitis of the lip and chin (Stern 1891) was almost certainly Cuban cocuswood. Flute makers who sawed cocus wood were said to develop dermatitis (Crocker 1903). Dermatitis of the face from cokus (Thompson 1914) may refer to this species. An instrument maker who had dermatitis showed a positive patch test reaction to cocus wood but evidence for contact with the wood was circumstantial (Schröpl 1935).

References

Crocker, H.R. (1903) Diseases of the skin. 3rd ed. p. 418. London, Lewis.

Rockstro, R.S. (1890) The Flute. 2nd ed. pp. 141-142. London, Rudall Carte (1928) cited by Woods and Calnan (1976).

Schröpl, E. (1934) Eczema from Grenadilla wood. Derm. Wschr. 16, 498-500. Abstr. Urol. Cutan. Rev. 39, 571 (1935).

Stern, E. (1891) Ueber einige Hautkrankheiten der Musiker. Munch.

med. Wochen. 38, 739.

Thompson, W.G. (1914) The occupational diseases. New York., Appleton.

Woods, B. and Calnan, C.D. (1976) Toxic Woods. Brit. J. Derm. 94, Suppl. 13, June.

Sub-family Caesalpiniodeae

Tribe Caesalpinieae

Bussea

Four species are native to tropical Africa and Madagascar.

Bussea occidentalis

The bark, if chewed, produces salivation, tingling of the tongue, thirst, cracked and swollen lips, itching of the scalp and a hot feeling to the face. These symptoms disappear after half to one hour (Irvine 1961).

Reference

Irvine, F.R. (1961) Woody Plants of Ghana. Oxford University Press. London.

Tribe Erythrineae

Butea

30 species are found in Indo-Malaysia and China.

Butea monosperma
(syn. *B. frondosa*)
Bastard Teak, Dhak Tree

The seeds of this tree, when pounded with lemon juice and applied locally, act as a powerful rubefacient (Unesco 1960). The red juice when dried is known as Benzal kino.

Reference

Unesco (1960) Medicinal Plants of the Arid Zones. Arid Zone Research XIII. Paris. Place de Fontenoy.

Sub-family Caesalpinioideae

Tribe Caesalpinieae

Caesalpinia

100 species are found in tropical and sub-tropical regions. Several species yield a red dye named brazilin or sappan. Several can cause mechanical injury by their thorns and are used as barrier hedges.

Caesalpinia apuleia

This tree can cause dermatitis in wood-workers (Sandermann and Barghoorn 1956).

Caesalpinia bonduc
(syn. *C. crista*)
Molucca Bean

The bark is used as a rubefacient and the pounded seeds have vesicant properties (Dalziel 1937, Quisumbing 1951).

Caesalpinia echinata
Brazilwood

Caesalpinia paraensis
Muirapixuna

Freise (1932) included these among leguminous woods which caused skin irritation. *Swartzia tomentosa* is known as muirapixuna (Record and Hess 1943).

References

Freise, F.W. (1932) Gesundheitsschädigungen durch Arbeiten mit giftigen Hölzern. Beobachtungen aus brasilianischen Gewerbebetrieben. Archiv für Gewerbepathologie und Gewerbehygiene 3, 1.

Record, S.J. and Hess, R.W. (1943) Timbers of the New World. New Haven, Yale.

Dalziel, J.M. (1937) The Useful Plants of West Tropical Africa. London. Crown Agents.

Quisumbing, E. (1951) Medicinal Plants of the Philippines. Philipp. Dep. Agr. and Nat. Resources Tech. Bull. No. 16. Manila. Bureau of Printing. 1234 pp.

Sandermann, W. and Barghoorn, A.W. (1956) Gesundheitsschädigende Nutzholzer. Holz. Roh-Werkst. 14, 37.

Sub-family Mimosoideae

Tribe Ingeae

Calliandra

100 species are found in Madagascar, and warm regions of Asia and America.

Calliandra portoricensis
Corpse-awakener

The sap is irritant to the eye and the powdered seeds are used to produce sneezing (Dalziel 1937).

Calliandra tetragona

This Mexican species is listed as a cause of dermatitis by Sandermann and Barghoorn (1956).

References

Dalziel, J.M. (1937) The Useful Plants of West Tropical Africa. London. Crown Agents.

Sandermann, W. and Barghoorn, A.W. (1956) Gesundheitsschädigende Nutzholzer. Holz. Roh-Werkst. 14, 37.

Sub-family Caesalpinioideae

Tribe Sclerolobieae

Campsiandra

Three species are found in tropical America.

Campsiandra laurifolia
Acapú rana

The woods of this species and of Batesia floribunda are both colloquially named acapú rana (false acapú) or maniara. Men sawing the wood of acapu rana suffer headaches and sometimes vomiting (Freise 1932).

Reference

Freise, F.W. (1932) Gesundheitsschädigungen durch Arbeiten mit giftigen Hölzern. Beobachtungen aus brasilianischen Gewerbebetrieben. Archiv für Gewerbepathologie und Gewerbehygiene 3, 1.

Sub-family Caesalpiniodeae

Tribe Cassieae

Cassia

500 or perhaps 600 species are found in tropical and warm temperate regions excluding Europe. Many species are cultivated for the purgative drug, senna which is said to be capable of causing dermatitis in pharmaceutical chemists (Schwartz et al 1957).

Chemistry is recorded by Thomson (1971).

Reference

Thomson, R.H. (1971) Naturally Occurring Quinones. 2nd ed. London. Academic Press.

Schwartz, L., Tulipan, L. and Birmingham, D.J. (1957) Occupational Diseases of the Skin. 3rd. ed. Philadelphia. Lea and Febiger, pp. 637-672.

Cassia acutifolia
Alexandrian Senna

This species has been reported to cause dermatitis of the face, hands and genitals (Schwartz et al 1957).

Cassia augustifolia
This species is said to be irritant (Perrot and Paris 1971).

Cassia chaemaecrista
Partridge Pea

In an investigation of 'weed dermatitis', an extract of this plant produced negative patch test reactions (Shelmire 1939).

Cassia siamea
Tagayasan

The wood of this Japanese tree contains a powder which stains the skin and can cause conjunctivitis, dermatitis, respiratory and systemic symptoms (Iwukuwa 1911, White 1934).

Cassia sophora

Contact with the bark can produce dermatitis (Uhe 1974).

References

Iwukuwa, K. (1911) Uber des entzundungserregende Pulver des japanischen Nutzholzes "Tagayasan". Arch. exp. Path. Pharm. 65, 315.

Perrot, E. and Patis, R. (1971) Les plantes medicinales. 2 vols. Paris. Presses Universitaires de France. 245 (+XXVI (index))

Schwartz, L., Tulipan, L. and Birmingham, D.J. (1957) Occupational Diseases of the Skin. 3rd. ed. Philadelphia. Lea and Febiger, pp. 637-672.

Shelmire, B. (1939) Contact dermatitis from weeds: Patch testing with their oleoresins. JAMA 113, 1085.

Uhe, G. (1974) Medicinal plants of Samoa. Econ. Bot. 28, 1.

White, R.P. (1934) The Dermatergoses or Occupational Affections of the Skin. 4th ed. London. H.K. Lewis.

Sub-family Lotoideae (Papilionoideae)

Tribe Sophoreae

Castanospermum

One species is native to sub-tropical regions of Australia.

Castanospermum australe
Moreton Bay Chestnut, Black Bean
Australian Chestnut, Queensland Red Bean

This species can produce irritation of the nasal cavity and dermatitis in wood-workers (Maiden 1909, Boas 1947). Eight men working the timber developed nasal irritation and nosebleeds (Aldersley 1925). The sawdust was reputed to cause eczema in certain sensitive persons (Cleland, J.B. in discussion of Aldersley 1925).

The wood contains an isoflavone, a phenol and saponins (Eade et al 1963).

References

Boas, I.H. (1947) The Commercial Timbers of Australia. Their Properties and Uses. Melbourne. Government Printer. Commonwealth of Australia. Council for Scientific and Industrial Research.

Maiden, J.H. (1909) On some plants which cause inflammation or irritation of the skin. Ag. Gaz. New South Wales. 20, 111 and 1073.

Eade, R.A., Hinterberger, H. and Simes, J.J.H. (1963) Afrormosin from Castanospermum australe. Cunn. et Fras. Australian J. Chem. 16, 188.

Aldersley, R.B. (1925) Sensitiveness to proteins of wood. Med. J. Australia 2, 25.

Sub-family Lotoideae (Papilionoideae)

Tribe Pterocarpeae

Centrolobium

Seven species are native to tropical America.

Centrolobium robustum
Zebra Wood

According to Hausen (1970) ill-effects from Zebra wood may refer to this species or to Astronium.

Reference

Hausen, B.M. (1970) Untersuchungen über Gesundheitsschädigende Hölzer. Thesis, Hamburg.

Sub-family Caesalpiniodeae

Tribe Cassieae

Ceratonia

One species is native to the Mediterranean region.

Ceratonia siliqua
Carob tree

The pods (algaroba, St. John's bread) are full of juicy pulp containing sugar and gum, and are used for fodder. The seeds are said to have been the original of the carats of jewellers. The pollen is suspected of causing hayfever (Wodehouse 1971).

Reference

Wodehouse, R.P. (1971) Hayfever Plants. 2nd rev. edition.

New York, Hafner.

Sub-family Lotoideae (Papilinoideae)

Tribe Vicieae

Cicer

20 species are native to North Africa, Abyssinia and the eastern Mediterranean regions to central Asia.

Cicer arietinum
Chick Pea

In France, cultivators of this food plant have been observed to develop dermatitis (Gougerot 1952). A chick-pea was used to produce a factitial eruption (Downing 1950).

References

Downing, J.G. (1950) Simulation and self infliction as encountered in industrial Dermatology. Arch. Industr. Hyg. Occup. Med. 1, 271.

Gougerot, (1952) cites a paper by Jeaume and Naroc.

Sub-family Lotoideae (Papilionoideae)

Tribe Sophoreae

Cladrastis

Four species are native to eastern Asia, one species to eastern North America. C. tinctoria, known as Yellow Wood, yields a dye.

Cladrastis lutea

Florida Box-wood

This species is listed as capable of producing dermatitis (Schwartz et al 1957).

Reference

Schwartz, L., Tulipan, L. and Birmingham, D.J. (1957) Occupational Diseases of the Skin. 3rd ed. Philadelphia. Lea & Febiger. pp. 637-672.

Sub-family Caesalpiniodeae

Tribe Detarieae

Copaifera

Twenty-five species are native to tropical America, five to tropical Africa.

Copaifera spp.
(syn. Copaiba)
Purple Heart

Several species, notably C. balsun yield resins (copals), Balsam of Copaiba and Oil of Copaiba. Balsam of Copaiba was said to produce contact urticaria (Rost 1924). Seven of 13 patients contact sensitive to Balsam of Peru (Myroxylon) showed positive patch test reactions to Balsam of Copaiba.

Copaifera bracteata

This species is listed as injurious by Hanslian and Kadlec (1966) but the wood named purpleheart which was described as toxic by Grossmann (1920) is now known to be derived from Peltogyne spp. not from Copaifera bracteata (Record and Hess 1943, Nomenclature générale 1965).

References

Hanslian, L. and Kadlec, K. (1966) Drevo z hlediska hygienickeho (Vii). Biologicky silne agresivni dreviny. Drevo 21, 157.

Rost, G.A. (1924) Dermatitis herpetiformis and the thyroid. Klin. Wschr. 3, 14. Abstr. JAMA 82, 588, 1924.

Grossmann, J. (1920) Gesundheitsschädliche Holzarten Der Holzkäufer (Leipzig) 17, 529, 535, 540 and 545.

Nomenclature générale (1965) Nomenclature générale des bois tropicaux. Association technique internationale des bois tropicaux. Nogent-sur-Marne.

Record, S.J. and Hess, R.W. (1943) Timbers of the New World. New Haven, Yale.

Sub-family Lotoideae (Papilionoideae)

Tibe Coronilleae

Coronilla

20 species are native to Europe and to the Mediterranean region.

Coronilla glanca

This horticultural shrub which is naturalized in Devon is potentially phototoxic from a content of psoralen (Pathak et al 1962).

Coronilla scorpioides

The seeds contain psoralen.

Reference

Pathak, M.A., Daniels, F. Jr., and Fitzpatrick, T.B. (1962) Presently known distribution of furocoumarins (psoralens) in plants. J. Invest. Derm. 39, 225.

Sub-family Lotoideae (Papilionoideae)

Tribe Crotolarieae

Crotalaria

Over 500 species are found in tropical and sub-tropical regions. Some yield hemp fibres.

Crotalaria spp.

Ingestion of C. aridicola and C. trifoliastrum can cause ulceration of the oesophagus of horses (Everist 1972).

Ingestion of some species, notably C. burkeana, can cause laminitic crotalism in some animals. Some species of animals appear to be unaffected. The disease is characterized by inflammation of the horn-forming membrane and thickening of the hoof to form a type of onychogryphosis (Watt and Breyer-Brandwijk 1962, Verdcourt and Trump 1969).

References

Everist, S.L. (1972) Queensland Herbarium, Brisbane, Australia. Personal communication concerning plants recorded in Australia as having caused dermatitis or other contact injury to man or livestock.

Verdcourt, B. and Trump, E.C. (1969) Common Poisonous Plants of East Africa. London. Collins.

Watt, J.M. and Breyer-Brandwijk, M.G. (1962) The Medicinal and poisonous plants of Southern Africa. 2nd ed. Edinburgh. E. & S. Livingstone.

Sub-family Lotoideae (Papilionoideae)

Tribe Galegeae

Cyamopsis

Three or four species are found in tropical and sub-tropical regions of Africa, Arabia and India.

Cyamopsis tetragonoloba
(syn. C. psoraliodes)
Cluster Bean

Dermatitis of the hands, face and exposed skin surfaces has been observed in farmers who cultivate this plant (Behl et al 1966).

References

Behl, P.N., Captain, R.M., Bedi, B.M.S. and Gupta, S. (1966). Skin-irritant and sensitizing plants found in India. New Delhi. P.N. Behl. Irwin Hospital.

Sub-family Lotoideae (Papilionoideae)

Tribe Cytiseae

Cytisus

25 or perhaps 30 species are found on Atlantic islands and in Europe and the Mediterranean region.

Cytisus laburnum
(syn. Laburnum vulgare)
Laburnum

This species is listed as injurious to the skin in several reviews. Systemic toxicity from the alkaloid, cytisin, is documented. Orsler (1973) lists the wood as producing dermatitis and respiratory symptoms.

Cytisus scoparius

The plant yields a medicinal material, scoparius (Merck 1968).

References

Merck Index (1968) An Encyclopedia of Chemicals and Drugs. ed. Stecher, P.G. 8th ed. Rahway, N.J. Merck and Co. Inc.

Orsler, R.J. (1973) Personal communication from Forest Products Research Laboratory, Princess Risborough. Bucks. England.

Sub-family Lotoideae (Papilionoideae)

Tribe Dalbergieae

Dalbergia

300 species are found in tropical and sub-tropical regions and in South Africa. Many species yield valuable timber e.g.

D. grenadillo — Mexico
Cocobolo, Grenadilla

D. hypoleuca — Costa Rica, Nicaragua
Cocobolo

C. latifolia — India
East Indian Rosewood, Blackwood

D. melanoxylon — Africa
Blackwood

D. nigra — Brazil
(syn., Amerimnon)
Rosewood, Caviuna

D. retusa — Panama
Cocobolo

D. sissoo — India
Sissoo, Shisham

D. stevensonii — Honduras
Rosewood

The colloquial and trade names of the woods from these species are confusing. Pallisander and Jacaranda are other common names for Dalbergia; Jacaranda is also a botanical genus name. The species used in industry and the trade names are listed by Beekman (1964). Caviuna as a cause of dermatitis (Rotberg 1938) may refer to Amerimnon (syn. Dalbergia). Barroso (1947) refers to this common name for D. nigra.

Like many other woods of this family, cocobolo possesses to a very high degree, the valuable characteristics of density, colour and durability. Strong, hard, compact and fairly heavy, easily worked, of extreme durability, it is naturally in high favour with the cutlery and turnery trade. In colour the wood varies from a light reddish-orange to a deep rich red or rose, beautifully marked with numerous, irregular, concentric markings of deep or black purple. An oily substance present in the wood not only makes it susceptible of a high degree of finish, but also tends to waterproof it and make it resistant to the influence of moisture, even when left in contact with water indefinitely. It is this latter characteristic which is mainly responsible for the supreme position that cocobolo holds in the cutlery trade. It is used for knife handles, brush backs and small tool handles, chessmen, musical and scientific instruments, butts of billiard cues, etc. (Garrett 1922).

The saw-dust can cause contact dermatitis in wood-workers (Garratt 1922, Rothberg 1938) and is among the six common causes of such dermatitis in France (Zafiropoulo et al 1968). An instrument-maker developed dermatitis of the exposed skin surfaces from wood-dust derived from a room adjoining that in which he worked (Schröpl 1934). In another instance, the wood-dust responsible for the dermatitis was derived from an adjacent factory (Findley 1972).

Cross-sensitivity to Machaerium scleroxylon was observed (Heyl 1966, Hausen et al 1972). The allergenic chemicals are dalbergiones (Schulz and Dietrichs 1962). The chemistry of these compounds is recorded by Ollis (1968), Harborne et al (1971), Seshadri (1972). The finished wood can also produce dermatitis at sites of contact. Flute-players developed dermatitis of the lips from wooden mouthpieces (Stern 1891, Meister 1934, Griebel 1935). Wooden knife-handles caused dermatitis of the hands (Levin 1939, Howell and Blair 1950). Hair-brushes caused dermatitis of the hands (Mackee 1913). Carving a knitting bag handle produced dermatitis (Abramowitz and Swarts 1938). Bracelets and necklaces produced dermatitis at the contact sites (Blaisdell

1924 , Levin and Behrman 1939, Howell and Blair 1950, Leider and Schwartzfeld 1950). Botanical identification of finished wood is a difficult task. Reports of dermatitis from Cocobolo, Pallisander and Jacaranda may refer to Dalbergia (Tottie 1939, Escartefigue 1935, Modlmayr 1931, Touraine et al 1934). Some other reports of dermatitis from bracelet, brooch and knife (Hollander 1941) may refer to these woods.

Patch testing with wood-shavings and with an ether extract of the wood diluted with corn oil was recommended (Howell and Blair 1950). Several authors report flares of dermatitis following patch-testing.

Cross-sensitivity between Primula and Dalbergia results from a chemical relationship between primin and dalbergiones (Hjorth et al 1969).

Hausen (1970) cites references for the individual species:

Dalbergia latifolia (Stern 1891, Sternberg 1908, Garratt 1922) Chemistry (Eyton et al 1962, 1965).

Dalbergia melanoxylon (Grobmann 1910, Nestler 1924, Meister 1934).

Dalbergia nigra (Escartefigue 1935, Touraine et al 1934, Schulz 1962). Chemistry (Eyton et al 1965).

Dalbergia retusa (Abramowitz and Swarts 1938, Blaisdel 1924, Grobmann 1910, Lewin 1928, Moll 1950, Nordin 1947, Record and Garratt 1923, Howell 1950, Leider and Schwartzfeld 1950, Levin 1941, Levin and Behrman 1939, Moldmayer 1931, Meister 1934, Schulz and Dietrichs 1962).

Dalbergia variabilis, D. lanceolaria, D. toxicaria are also noted.

References

Abramowitz, E.W. and Swarts, W.B. (1938) Dermatitis due to cocobolo wood. Archs. Derm. Syph. 37, 441.

Barroso, C. (1947) Dermatite eczematosa de tipo dermocontacto provocaca pela serragem de caviuna (Dalbergia nigra). Hospital, Rio de Janeiro 31, 291.

Beekman, W.B. (1964) Elsevier's Wood Dictionary in Seven Languages. 2 Vols. Amsterdam. Elsevier.

Blaisdell, J. H. (1924) Case histories in Dermatology. Urol. Cut. Rev. 28, 665.

Escartefigue, M.M. (1935) Eczematoid dermatitis of neck and forearms from wearing necklace and bracelet of palisandre wood. Bull. Soc. franc. Derm. Syph. 42, 670. (French).

Eyton, W.B., Ollis, W.D., Sutherland, I.O. et al (1962) Dalbergiones: a new group of natural products. Proc. chem. Soc. 301 (no vol. no.)

Eyton, W.B., Ollis, W.D., Sutherland, I.O. et al (1965) The neoflavonoid group of natural products. I. Dalbergiones, a new class of quinones. Tetrahedron 21, 2683.

Findley, L.J. (1972) An unusual case of Rosewood dermatitis of the genus Dalbergia (East Indian Roeswood). Brit. J. Industr. Med. 29, 343.

Garratt, G.A. (1922) Poisonous Woods. J. Forestry, 20, 479.

Griebel, C.R. (1935) Concerning a rare form of allergy. Ztschr. f. Laryng. Rhin. Otol. 26, 99 (German).

Grobmann, J. (1910) Gesundheitsschadliche Holzer. Bayr. Indust. Gewerbebelt 96, 51.

Harborne, J.B., Boulter, D.and Turner, B.L. (1971) Chemotaxonomy of the Leguminosae. London. Academic Press.

Hausen,B.M. (1970) Untersuchungen über Gesundheitsschädigende Hölzer. Thesis, Hamburge.

Hausen, B.M. Simatupange, M.Y. and Kingreen, J.C. (1972) Untersuchungen zur Überempfindlichkeit gegen Sucupira - und Palisanderholz. Berufsdermatosen 20, 1.

Heyl, V. (1966) Kontaktekzem bei Überemfindlichkeit gegen sucupira und Palisander-Holz. Berufsdermatosen 14, 239.

Hjorth, N., Fregert, S. and Schildknecht, H. (1969) Cross-sensitisation between synthetic primin and related quinones. Acta derm.-venereol. 49, 552.

Hollander, L. (1941) Dermatitis due to stain on the wooden handle of a kitchen knife. Archs. Derm. Syph. 43, 381.

Howell, J.B. and Blair, D.S. (1950) Eczema of the hands from wooden-handled objects. Archs. Derm. Syph. 62, 400.

Leider, M. and Schwartzfeld, H.K. (1950) Allergic eczematous contact type dermatitis caused by Cocobolo wood, (Dalbergia). Archs. Derm. 62, 125.

Levin, S.J. (1941) Cocobolo wood dermatitis. J. Allergy 12, 489.

Levin, O.L. and Behrman, H.T. (1939) Bracelet dermatitis. New York State J. Med. 39, 1877.

Lewin, L. (1928) Gifte in Holzgewerbe. Beitrage zur Giftkunde. Heft 1. Berlin. Georg Stilke.

McKee, G.M. (1913) Dermatitis venenata from cocobolo wood. J. Cutan. Dis. 31, 582.

Meister, H. (1934) Über eine neue Atiologie für Gesichtsekzeme. Schweiz. med. Wschr. II, 993.

Meister, H. (1934) New etiology of facial eczema. JAMA 103, 2058.

Modlmayer (1931) Palisander. bzw. Cocoboloholz-dermatitis. Zbl. Haut.-Geschlkrkh. 36, 728.

Moll, F. (1950) Giftiges Holz und Gewerbekrankheiten. "Holz" 4, 77.

Nestler, A. (1924) Hautreizende Hölzer. Die Umschau 17, 860.

Nordin, J. (1947) Yrkessjukdomar (Gewerbekrankheiten). Uppsala. Ed. 2. p. 605-11.

Ollis, W.D. (1968) New structural variants among the isoflavonoid and neo-flavanoid classes, in Recent Advances in Phytochemistry. Vol. 1. ed. Mabry, T. New York. Appleton-Century-Crofts.

Record, S.J. and Garrat, G.A. (1923) Cocobolo-wood. Yale Univ. School For. Bull. 8, 35.

Rotberg, A. (1938) Dermatitis due to hypersensitivity to caviuna. Arch. Dermat. Sao Paulo 2, 141.

Schröpl, E. (1934) Eczema from Grenadilla wood. Derm. Wschr. 16, 498 (German) Abstr. Urol. Cutan. Rev. 39, 571, 1935.

Schulz, K.-H. (1962) Chemische Struktur und allergene Wirkung. Editio Cantor KG. Aulendorf/Württ.

Schulz, K. -H and Dietrichs, H.H. (1962) Quinone as sensitizing component of Rio-Pallisander (Dalbergia nigra) and Cocobolo (Dalbergia retusa) woods. Allergie u. Asthma 8, 125 (German)

Stern, E. (1891) Über einige Hautkrankheiten der Musicker: ein Beitrag zu den professionellen Dermatosen. Munch. med. Wchnschr. 42, 739.

Sternberg, M. (1908) Aus dem Gebiete der Berufskrankheiten. Med. Klin. 14, 479.

Tottie, M. (1939) Jacaranda als Ursache von Dermatitiden. Acta derm.-venereol 19, 235.

Touraine, A., Ménétrel, B. and Jouenne, M. (1934) Eczematous dermatitis from pallisander. Bull. Soc. franc. Derm. Syph. 41, 1969 (French)

Zafiropoulo, A., Audibert, A. and Charpin, J. (1968) A propos des accidents dus a la manipulation des bois exotiques. Rev. franc. Allerg. 8, 155.

Seshadri, T.R. (1972) Polyphenols of Pterocarpus and Dalbergia woods. Phytochemistry 11, 881.

Dalbergia

Woods and Calnan (1976) give the following botanical species and skin-reactive articles and notes as represented in the papers of various authors. The wood was previously confused with Coccoloba, cocus (Brya) and other woods.

They reported eight patients contact sensitive to rosewood (*Dalbergia* spp.), seven men and one woman, aged from 46-60 years. Their occupations were musical instrument maker, wood machinist (2), cabinet-maker (2), timber yard foreman, veneer preparer and housewife. Some of them reacted to other woods, probably by multiple specific sensitivity. All eight patients showed positive patch test reactions to rosewood dust; two who were tested to dalbergione, 0.1% in petrolatum, showed positive reactions. Three who were tested to *Primula* showed negative reactions. *Primula* and *Dalbergia* can cross-react.

Dalbergia retusa

Cocobolo, granadillo, nambar, palo negro, foseholz, red fox-wood, rosewood

Dalbergia granadillo
(syn. *Amerimnon granadillo*)
same common names as *D. retusa*
Dalbergia hypoleuca and
Dalbergia spp.

Nestler (1912) - moist sawdust; alcohol and benzol extracts of sawdust.

Mackee (1913) - sandpapering of cocobolo hairbrushes.

Pittier (1918) - botanical source of cocobolo

Record and Hess (1943) - botanical source of cocobolo

Record and Garratt (1923) - botany. American trade reports of dermatitis gave an incidence of 10-30 percent in wood-workers exposed to the fine dust. The eruption began on the face and hands and in severe cases, became generalized with conjunctivitis. The fine dust was responsible, mainly in hot weather.

Levin (1941), Leider and Schwartzfeld (1950), Howell and Blair (1950) - localized dermatitis from contact with knife-handles, bracelets, recorders and other finished articles made of cocobolo wood.

Anon (1933), Steinbrinck (1950), Hausen (1970), Meister (1934) - wood of the musical instrument, the recorder, causing dermatitis of the face.

Eaton (1973) - nasal irritation in workers finishing and sanding cocobolo wood.

D. retusa contains S-4'-hydroxy-4-methoxy dalbergione, R-4-methoxy dalbergione and other quinones and phenols (Schulz and Dietrichs, 1962; Hausen 1970).

References

Anon (1933) Erkrankungen bei Benutzung von Cocobolo - Blöckfloten. Collegium musicum (Bärenreiter) 1, 13.

Eaton, K.K. (1973) Respiratory allergy due to exotic wood dust. Clinical Allergy 3, 307.

Hausen, B.M. (1970) Untersuchungen über Gesundheitsschädigende Hölzer. Thesis, Hamburg.

Meister, H. (1934) Ueber eine neue Aetiologie für Gesichtsekzeme Schweiz. med. Wochen. ii, 993.

Nestler, A. (1912) Die hautreizende Wirkung des Cocoboloholzes. Berichte der deutschen botanischen Gesellschaft 30, 120.

Pittier (1918) cited by Record and Hess (1943), cited by Woods and Calnan (1976).

Record, S.J. and Hess, R.W. (1943) Timbers of the New World. Yale, New Haven.

Record, S.J. and Garratt, G.A. (1923) Cocobolo. Yale University School of Forestry Bulletin. No. 8. New Haven.

Steinbrinck, W. (1950) Besondere Beobachtungen an allergischen Krankheiten. Zeitschrift für die gesamte innere Medizin. 5, 311.

Schulz, K.H. and Dietrichs, H.H. (1962) Chinone als sensibilisierende Bestandteile von Rio-Palisander (*Dalbergia nigra*) und Cocobolo (*D. retusa*) Holz. Allergie u. Asthma. 8, 125.

Woods, B. and Calnan, C.D. (1976) Toxic Woods. Brit. J. Derm. 94, Suppl. 13, June.

Dalbergia nigra
Brazilian rosewood, jacaranda, pallisandre Brésil, Rio or Bahia rosewood, caviuna, palisander, jacaranda pardo

same common names: Dalbergia cubilquitzensis; Dalbergia spruceana

Gougerot and Blamoutier (1922) - Cabinet maker working with pallisandre developed dermatitis of the face and hands.

Gougerot and Delay (1932) - Pallisandre dermatitis associated with lacrimation, sneezing and coughing. The botanical source of the wood was not stated.

Touraine et al (1934) - identified the 'palissandre des Indies' in their case as D. nigra but according to Woods and Calnan (1976) their botanical remarks are not impressive and its origin suggests D. latifolia.

Tottie (1938) - dermatitis in three carpenters using Jacaranca envaco which is a Brazilian name for D. nigra not to be confused with Jacaranda.

Freise (1932) - dermatitis in forestry workers handling various kinds of jacaranda.

Barroso (1947) - dermatitis from caviuna (D. nigra).

Gronomeyer and Fuchs (1957) Asthma from D. nigra.

D. nigra contains R-4-methoxydalbergione and other quinones (Schulz and Dietrichs 1962).

D. nigra is now in short supply, and the more irritant Machaerium scleroxylon is sometimes substituted for it (Eyton et al 1965).

References

Barrosso, C. (1947) Dermatite eczematoso de tipo dermocontacto provocada pela serragem de caviuna (Dalbergia nigra). O Hospital (Rio) 31, 291.

Eyton, W.B., Ollis, W.D., Sutherland, I.O. et al (1965) The Neoflavanoid group of natural products I-III Tetrahedron 31, 2683.

Freise, F.W. (1932) Gesundheitsschädigungen durch Arbeiten mit giftigen Hölzern. Beobachtungen aus brasilianischen Gewerbebetrieben. Archiv für Gewerbepathologie und Gewerbehygiene 3, 1.

Gougerot and Blamoutier (1922) Dermite eczémateuse professionnelle du à la poudre de pallisandre. Bull. Soc. méd. Hôp. Paris 46, 739.

Gougerot and Delay (1932) Eczéma par sensibilisation au bois de palissandre. Bull. Soc. franc. Derm. 39, 1339.

Gronemeyer, W. and Fuchs, E. (1967) Krankteiten durch inhalative Allergen-invasion. In: Lehrbuch der klinischen Allergie. ed. Hansen, K. and Werner, M. Stuttgart. Thieme.

Schulz, K.H. and Dietrichs, H.H. (1962) Chinone als sensibilisierende Bestandteile von Rio-Palisander (Dalbergia nigra) und Cocobolo (D. retusa) Holz. Allergie u. Asthma. 8, 125.

Tottie, M. (1938) Jacaranda als Ursache von Dermatitiden. Acta. derm.-venereol 19, 235.

Touraine, Hesse, J. and Golé (1932) Vingt cas de dermatite par bois satine ('Peroba grande amarella'). Bull. Soc. franc. Derm. Syph. 39, 1392.

Woods, B. and Calnan, C.D. (1976) Toxic Woods. Brit. J. Derm. 94, Suppl. 13, June.

Dalbergia latifolia

Palissandre Asie, Indian rosewood, East Indian rosewood, Bombay blackwood.

Dalbergia sissoo

Sissoo, shisham

Dalbergia oliveri
Burma tulipwood, pinkwood, bois de rose

Dalbergia greveana
Madagascar rosewood, French rosewood

Dalbergia cochinchinensis

Madagascar rosewood, French rosewood, Thailand rosewood, chin chan

The above species are trade named Palissandre Asie.

Sternberg (1908) - urticarial rashes and swellings in carpenters working with Indian rosewood.

Escartefigue (1935) - Dermatitis from necklace and bracelet of Madagascar palissandre.

Findley (1972) - Dermatitis in a man who had only indirect contact with D. latifolia sawdust.

D. latifolia and D. cochinchinensis contain R-4-methoxy dalbergione and other quinones (Dempsey and Donnelly 1963; Donnelly et al 1968, Donnelly et al 1969).

References

Dempsey, C.B. and Donnelly, D.M.X. (1963) Extractives of Dalbergia latifolia. Chem. Ind. 23.3.63. p. 491.

Donnelly, D.M.X., Nangle, B.J., Prendergast, J.P. et al (1968) Isolation of R-5-o-methyllatifolin from Dalbergia cochinchinensis Pierre. Phytochemistry 7, 647.

Donnelly, B.J., Donnelly, D.M.X., O'Sullivan, A.M. et al (1969) The isolation and structure of melanoxin, a new dihydrobenzfuran from Dalbergia melanoxylon. Tetrahedron 25, 4409.

Escartefique, M. (1935) Dermo-épidermite eczématiforme ... de palissandre. Bull. Soc. franc. Derm. Syph. 42, 670.

Findley, L.J. (1972) An unusual case of rosewood dermatitis of the genus Dalbergia (East Indian rosewood). Brit. J. Industr. Med. 29, 343.

Sternberg, M. (1908) Aus dem Gebiete der Berufskrankheiten. Med. Klin. 14, 479.

Dalbergia retusa
Cocabolla

Respiratory allergy occurred from the wood (Eaton 1973).

Reference

Eaton, K.K. (1973) Respiratory allergy to exotic wood dust. Clinical Allergy 3, 307.

Dalbergia stevensonii

Honduras rosewood, Nagaed wood, palssandre Honduras

Orsler (1973) received trade reports of dermatitis from this wood. It is used to make the musical instrument, xylophone. It contains a dalbergione (Hausen 1970).

References

Hausen, B.M. (1970) Untersuchungen über Gesundheitsschädigende Hölzer. Thesis, Hamburg.

Orsler, R.J. (1973) Personal communication from Forest Products Research Laboratory, Princess Risborough, Bucks, England.

Dalbergia melanoxylon

African blackwood, mpingo, Mozambique or Senegal ebony, ébène, African grenadilla.

According to Woods and Calnan (1976), in England, clarinets are usually made of African blackwood. This wood is often used for flutes and other instruments, especially in Germany. Moll (1950) noted that the wood was known, in the trade, to be irritant. Woods and Calnan (1976) reported two cases of contact dermatitis from D. melanoxylon (African blackwood). Both of them were employed in making the musical instrument, clarinet. Patch tests to the wood-dust produced positive reactions. One of the patients was also patch test positive to the wood-dust of Tectona. Control tests were not recorded.

D. melanoxylon contains several quinones including S-4'-hydroxy-4-methoxy dalbergione (Donnelly et al 1969) and S-4-methoxy dalbergione (Hausen 1970) which is also found in D. violacea (Eyton et al 1965).

References

Eyton, W.B., Ollis, W.D., Sutherland, I.O. et al (1965) The Neoflavanoid group of natural products I-III. Tetrahedron 31, 2683.

Donnelly, B.J., Donnelly, D.M.X. O'Sullivan, A.M. et al (1969) The isolation and structure of melanoxin, a new dihydrobenzfuran from Dalbergia melanoxylon. Tetrahedron 25, 4409.

Moll, F. (1950) Giftiges Holz und Gewbekrankheiten. Holz (Munchen) 4, 76.

Woods, B. and Calnan, C.D. (1976) Toxic Woods. Brit. J. Derm. 94, Suppl. 13, June.

Dalbergia variabilis

Brazilian tulipwood, bois de rose

Dalbergia oliveri

Dalbergia cearensis

Kingwood, bois de violette, violet wood, violetta.

According to Woods and Calnan (1976) citing Record and Hess (1943) D. caerensis is probably the 'kingswood' which Freise (1932) called Machaerium violaceum Ducke. He described it as a very severe skin-irritant, often leading to persistent ulceration.

References

Freise, F.W. (1932) Gesundheitsschädigungen durch Arbeiten mit giftigen Hölzern. Beobachtungen aus brasilianischen Gewerbebetrieben. Archiv für Gewerbepathologie und Gewerbehygiene 3, 1.

Record, S.J. and Hess, R.W. (1943) Timbers of th New World. New Haven, Yale.

Woods, B. and Calnan, C.D. (1976) Toxic Woods. Brit. J. Derm. 96, Suppl. 13, June.

Chemistry of Dalbergia spp.

Earlier workers, summarized by Sandermann and Barghoorn (1936) blamed flavones, saponins and glycosides for the irritant effects of rosewood, but the discovery of sensitizing quinones in other woods such as teak and mansonia led Schulz and Dietrichs (1962) to look for similar substances in D. nigra and D. retusa. They found three quinones which they called Dalbergia-quinones A, B and C, and demonstrated by patch tests on patients that these were the sensitizers, the strongest being R-3,4-dimethoxydalbergione. Eyton et al (1956) have studied the chemistry of this 'neoflavanoid' group of quinones in detail. They have now been found in other Dalbergia spp., Machaerium, Peltogyne and Goniorrhachis (Hausen 1970).

References

Eyton, W.B., Ollis, W.D., Sutherland, I.O. et al (1965) The Neoflavanoid group of natural products I-III. Tetrahedron 31, 2683.

Hausen, B.M. (1970) Untersuchungen über Gesundheitsschädigende Hölzer. Thesis, Hamburg.

Sandermann, W. and Barghoorn, A.W. (1956) Gesundheitsschadigende Nutzhölzer. Holz. Roh-Werkst. 14, 37 and 87.

Schulz, K.H. and Dietrichs, H.H. (1962) Chinone als sensibilisierende Bestandteile von Rio-Palisander (Dalbergia nigra) und Cocobolo (D. retusa) Holz. Allergie u. Asthma. 8, 125.

Natural dalbergenones (dalbergiquinones) of these species were reviewed by Seshadri (1972).

Reference

Seshadri, T.R. (1972) Polyphenols of Pterocarpus and Dalbergia woods. Phytochemistyr 11, 881.

Sub-family Caesalpiniodeae

Tribe Detarieae

Daniellia

Eleven species are native to tropical West Africa.

Daniellia spp.

Balsam Tree

African Copaiba derived from

species of this genus has been used to adulterate Copaiba derived from Copaifera.

Sub-family Lotoideae (Papilionoideae)

Tribe Lonchocarpeae

Derris

80 species are found in tropical regions.

Derris spp.
Tuba, Cubé

Workers who prepare an insecticide from the roots and florists who use the insecticide can develope dermatitis. The clinical features suggest an irritant effect from the powder for the skin and eye rather than allergic contact dermatitis (Racouchot 1939, Dorne and Friedman 1940, Simons 1948, Schwartz et al 1957, Thienes and Haley 1972).

References

Dorne, M. and Friedman, T.B. (1940) Derris root dermatitis. JAMA 115, 1268.

Racouchot, J. (1939) Dermatose professionelle. Plantes a Rotenone. Arch. mal. prof. 2, 149.

Schwartz, L., Tulipan, L., and Birmingham, D.J. (1957) Occupational Diseases of the Skin. 3rd. ed. Philadelphia. Lea and Febiger pp. 637-672.

Simons, C.P. (1948) A tropical occupational disease due to derris. Acta derm.-venereol. 28, 601 (Abstr. Brit. J. Indust. Med. 6, 265, 1949).

Thienes, C.H. and Haley, T.J. (1972) Clinical Toxicology. 5th ed. Philadelphia. Lea & Febiger.

Sub-family Mimosoideae

Tribe Mimoseae

Desmanthus (syn. Acuan)

40 species are native to America and Madagascar. A. illinoensis was investigated for a role in weed dermatitis' with negative results (Shelmire 1939).

Reference

Shelmire, B. (1939) Contact dermatitis from Weeds; Patch testing with their oleoresins. JAMA 113, 1085.

Sub-family Mimosoideae

Tribe Adenanthereae

Dichrostachys

20 species are found in southern tropical regions.

Dichrostachys spp.
Marabou Thorn

The spines of some African species are said to produce irritant or poisonous effects if they penetrate the skin (Irvine 1961, Watt and Breyer-Brandwijk 1962).

References

Irvine, F.R. (1961) Woody Plants of Ghana. Oxford. University Press. London.

Watt, J.M. and Breyer-Brandwijk, M.G. (1962) The Medicinal and poisonous plants of Southern Africa. 2nd ed. Edinburgh. E. & S. Livingstone.

Sub-family Caesalpinioideae

Tribe Cassieae

Dicorynia

Two species are native to Guiana and the Amazon basin.

Dicorynia guianensis
Angélique

This species is said to have injurious effects from the tryptamin which it contains (Hausen 1970).

The wood is reported to be toxic (Baumer 1955). Alkaloids are present in the wood (Sandermann and Lange 1967).

Reference

Hausen, B.M. (1970) Untersuchungen über Gesundheitsschädigende Hölzer. Thesis, Hamburg.

Baumer, M. (1955) Que fait-il croire de la toxicité de certains bois tropicaux? Bois et Forêts des Tropiques 43, 27.

Sandermann, W. and Lange, W. (1967) Chemische Untersuchung des Holzes von Angélique (Basralocus - Dicorynia guianensis Amsh.) Holzforschung 21, 154.

Sub-family Lotoideae (Papilionoideae)

Tribe Sophoreae

Diplotropis

Twelve species are native to tropical America.

Diplotropis purpurea

This wood is named sucupira as is Bowdichia nitida. The sucupira wood reported by Heyl (1966) to cause dermatitis was identified by Hausen et al (1972) as Bowdichia nitida. Ferreirea spectabilis is named yellow sucupira.

References

Hausen, B.M., Simatupang, M.H. and Kingreen, J.C. (1972) Untersuchungen zur Überempfindlichkeit gegen Sucupira - und Palisanderholz. Berufsdermatosen 20, 1.

Heyl, U. (1966) Kontaktekzem bei Überempfindlichkeit gengen Sucupira - und Palisanderholz. Berufsdermatosen 14, 239.

Sub-family Lotoideae (Papilionoideae)

Tribe Geoffroeae

Dipteryx

Some species of the genus Coumarouna and of the genus Taralea are included in this tropical American genus.

Dipteryx odorata
Tonquin

The red coloured sawdust of this tree caused a workman's hair, when wetted, to turn to a bright grass-green colour (Thompson 1914 cited by Garratt 1922, Bernhard-Smith 1923). Tonquin beans are a commercial source of coumarin (Thompson 1914).

Woods and Calnan (1976) refer to a trade report of 'poisoning' in a furniture factory from handling tonquin wood from the Phillipines.

References

Bernhard-Smith, A. (1923) Poisonous Plants of All Countries. 2nd ed. London. Bailliere, Tindall and Cox.

Thompson cited by Garratt, G.A. (1922) Poisonous Woods. J. Forestry 20, 479.

Thompson, W.G. (1914) The occupational diseases. New York. Appleton.

Woods, B. and Calnan, C.D. (1976) Toxic Woods. Brit. J. Derm. 94, Suppl. 13, June.

Sub-family Caesalpiniodeae

Tribe Cassieae

Distemonanthus

One species is native to tropical West Africa.

Distemonanthus benthamianus
Ayan, Nigerian Satinwood

This tree is sometimes named African or Yellow Satinwood and thus confused with Afrormosia laxiflora which it resembles and which bears the same vernacular name. The yellow pigment from the wood stains clothes (Irvine 1961).

A male coffin manufacturer, aged 56 years, developed contact dermatitis from sawdust and shavings, affecting the upper limbs, chest, legs, groins and dorsa of the feet. Patch test reactions were strongly positive to the flavonoid compounds, oxyayanin A and oxyayanin B, weakly positive to ayanin and distemonanthin, negative in one control. Two varieties of ayan wood are known, one rich in oxyayanin B, the other rich in distemonanthin; the former seems more likely to cause sensitisation. A variation in extractive content such as this may account for the sporadic occurrence of ayan dermatitis (Morgan and Thomson 1967).

Ayanin is the orange 3,7,4'-trimethyl ether of quercetin (Dean 1963), and thus related to rutin, one of the best studied glycoside-flavonoids. The above report is the first implicating members of this group of compounds in plant dermatitis. Flavonoid compounds are widely distributed in plants (Geissman and Crout 1969, Harborne 1966).

Eight of 22 furniture makers who had dermatitis showed positive patch test reactions to ayan. The wooddust may be irritant in factory conditions of heat and sweating (Woods and Calnan 1976).

References

Dean, F.M. (1963) Naturally occurring oxygen ring compounds. London. Butterworths.

Geissman, T.A. and Crout, D.H.G. (1969) Organic Chemistry of Secondary Plant Metabolism. San Francisco. Freeman, Cooper Co.

Harborne, J.B. (1966) The evolution of flavonoid pigments in plants in Comparative Phytochemistry. ed. Swain, T. London. Academic Press.

Irvine, F.R. (1961) Woody Plants of Ghana. Oxford University Press. London.

Morgan, J.W.W. and Thomson, J. (1947) Ayan dermatitis. Brit. J. Industr. Med. 24, 156.

Woods, B. and Calnan, C.D. (1976) Toxic Woods. Brit. J. Derm. 94, Suppl. 13, June.

Echirospermum

This generic name refers to a mixture of Cassia, Caesalpinia, etc.

Echirospermum balthazarii
Vinhatico

Several woods are known as vinhatico, e.g. Plathymenia sp., Chloroleucon vinhatico and E. balthazarii. The wood which was reported by Freise (1932) to irritate the nose, eyes and other mucous membranes and identified by him as E. balthazarii was more likely the Brazilian species Plathymenia reticulata (Woods and Calnan 1976).

References

Freise, F.W. (1932) Gesundheitsschädigungen durch Arbeiten mit giftigen Hölzern. Beobachtungen aus brasilianischen Gewerbebetrieben. Archiv für Gewerbepathologie und Gewerbehygiene 3, 1.

Woods, B. and Calnan, C.D. (1976) Toxic Woods. Brit. J. Derm. 94, Suppl 13, June.

Sub-family Mimosoideae

Tribe Adenanthereae

Entada

30 species are found in warm regions.

Entada phaseoloides

The juice of the bark causes conjunctivitis and irritation of the eye (Burkill 1935, Watt and Breyer-Brandwijk 1962).

References

Burkill, I.H. (1935) A Dictionary of the Economic Products of the Malay Peninsula. 2 Vols. London. Crown Agents for the Colonies.

Watt, J.M. and Breyer-Brandwijk, M.G. (1962) The Medicinal and poisonous plants of Southern Africa. 2nd ed. Edinburgh. E. & S. Livingstone.

Sub-family Mimosoideae

Tribe Ingeae

Enterolobium

Ten species are native to tropical America and the West Indies.

Enterolobium cyclocarpum
Guanacasta

The sawdust is 'irritant' (Thiébault 1965) for the respiratory tract (Orsler 1973).

The fine dust arising from machining the dry wood causes irritation of the mucous membranes of most individuals (Kukachka 1970).

References

Kukachka, B.F. (1970) Properties of

imported tropical woods. USDA Forest Service Research Paper. FPL125 March. U.S. Dept. Agric. Forest Service. Forest Products Laboratory. Madison, Wis. U.S.A.

Orsler, R.J. (1973) Personal communication from Forest Products Research Laboratory. Princess Risborough, Bucks, England.

Thiébault, A. (1965) Nomenclature Generale des Bois Tropicaus. L'Association Technique Internationale des Bois Tropicaux. 45, bis Avenue de la Belle-Gabrielle, Nogent-sur Marne, France.

Sub-family Lotoideae (Papilionoideae)

Tribe Erythrineae

Erythrina

100 species are found in tropical and subtropical regions.

Erythrina spp.

Some are thorny and used as barrier hedges (Corner 1952, Williamson 1956).

Erythrina crista-galli
Cry-Baby

The copious nectar which drips from the flower of this small tree accounts for the colloquial name. Other 'Rain-trees' are noted under Acer. The plant yields cystisin and related alkaloids (Pichard and Luco 1944).

Erythrina corallodendron

The wood of this tropical American tree is noted as injurious from a content of alkaloid (Hausen 1970).

Erythrina fusca

The alkaloids of Erythrina are described by Folkers and Koninsky, (1940).

References

Corner, E.J.H. (1952) Wayside Trees of Malaysia. Singapore, Government Printer.

Folkers, K. and Koninsky, F. (1940) Erythrina alkaloids X. J. Am. Chem. Soc. 62, 1677.

Hausen, B.M. (1970) Untersuchungen über Gesundheitsschädigende Hölzer. Thesis, Hamburg.

Pichard, R. and Luco, J.V. (1944) A pharmacological study of an extract of Erythrina crista galli. J. Pharmacol. 80, 62.

Williamson, J. (1956) Useful Plants of Malawi. ed. Greenway, P.J. Zomba, Malawi. The Government Printer. Previously published as Useful Plants of Nyasaland.

Sub-family Caesalpinioideae

Tribe Dimorphandreae

Erythrophleum

17 species are found in Africa, the Seychelle Islands, tropical and eastern Asia and Australia.

Erythrophleum guineense
Ordeal Tree, Doom Bark
(West Africa)

The bark is irritant to the eye and nasal cavity and has a local anaesthetic action in the mouth (Irvine 1961, Watt and Breyer-Brandwijk 1962).

The saw-dust can produce dermatitis and sneezing in woodworkers (Watt and Breyer-Brandwijk 1962).

An extract of the wood produced vomiting, respiratory symptoms, headache, dizziness and bradycardia (Lewin 1928). Hausen (1970) found alkaloids in the bark (but not in the wood). E. laboucheri in Australia and E. coumiga in Madagascar are probably also toxic (Golse 1937, Hausen 1970).

References

Irvine, F.R. (1961) Woody Plants of Ghana. Oxford University Press. London.

Watt, J.M. and Breyer-Brandwijk, M.G. (1962) The Medicinal and poisonous plants of Southern Africa. 2nd ed. Edinburgh. E. & S. Livingstone.

Golse, M.J. (1937) Les plates toxiques des Colonies. Bull. Trav. Soc. Pharm. Bordeaux. 75, 102.

Hausen, B.M. (1970) Untersuchungen über Gesundheitsschädigende Hölzer. Thesis, Hamburg.

Lewin, L. (1928) Gifte im Holzgewerbe. Berlin, Stilke.

Sub-family Lotoideae (Papilionoideae)

Tribe Psoralieae

Eysenhardtia

14 species are native to the south-eastern United States south to Guatemala.

Eysenhardtia amorphoides

The source of Lignum Nephriticicum was uncertain for a long time. The history is recorded by Stapf (1909).

The wood, which was used medicinally as Lignum nephriticum (Howes 1974), may be that described as irritant by Senear (1933) and Weber (1937).

References

Howes, F.N. (1974) A Dictionary of Useful Everyday Plants and their Common Names. Cambridge University Press. pp. 290.

Senear, F.E. (1933) Dermatitis due to Woods. JAMA 101, 1527.

Weber, L.F. (1937) External causes of Dermatitis. A list of irritants. Arch. Derm. Syph. 35, 129.

Stapf, O. (1909) XXXIX - Lignum Nephriticum. Kew Bull. (No. 7) pg. 293.

Sub-family Lotoideae (Papilionoideae)

Tribe Sophoreae

Ferreirea

Two species are native to Brazil and Paraguay.

Ferreira spectabilis

The wood is said to cause dermatitis (Orsler 1973, Hausen 1970), possibly from anthraquinones.

King et al (1952) found chrysophanic anthranol in the wood but Simatupang et al (1967) could not confirm this finding and suggested that King's material came from Vatairea lundelli which is similar microscopically.

References

Hausen, B.M. (1970) Untersuchungen über Gesundheitsschädigende Hölzer. Thesis, Hamburg.

Orsler, R.J. (1973) Personal communication from Forest Products Research Laboratory, Princess Risborough, Bucks, England.

King, F.E., Grundon, M.F. and Neill, N.G. (1952) Constituents of the heartwood of Ferreira spectabilis. J. Chem. Soc. 4580.

Simatupang, M.H., Dietrichs, H.H. and Gottwald, H. (1967) Über die hautreizenden Stoffe in Vatairea guianensis Aubl. Holzforschung 21, 89.

Sub-family Caesalpinioideae

Tribe Caesalpinieae

Gleditsia

Eleven species are found in tropical and sub-tropical regions.

Gladitsia chinensis and G. japonica are irritant. The thorny plant may be confused with Prosopis (Smith 1969).

Reference

Smith, F.P. (1969) Chinese Materia Medica. Vegetable kingdom. 2nd ed. Rev. by Hei, P.D. Taipei, Taiwan. Ku T'ing Book House.

Sub-family Lotoideae (Papilionoideae)

Tribe Glycineae

Glycine

Ten species have been recognized from tropical and warm temperate regions of Africa and Asia.

Glycine max (syn. G. hispida)
Soy Bean

The hairs on the pods are irritant to the mouth and gut and have been used for criminal poisoning (Burkill 1935).

The plant is used for green fodder and yields soya beans. An oil is obtained from the seeds. A 'milk' made from the ground beans (Soya) can have goitrogenic effects (Kingsbury 1964).

Soybean meal was reported to cause respiratory allergy (Virchow 1965). Oil of Soya Bean has caused an acneiform folliculitis in industrial workers (Greenberg and Lester 1954). The beans when deliberately infected with Aspergillus are used to make Soy-Sauce. Ketchup (Catsup) is derived from a Malaysian word, kechap: various flavours are added to ketchups and the fungus which is added may be derived from Hibiscus (Burkill 1935). Some yield aflatoxin.

References

Burkill, I.H. (1935) A Dictionary of the Economic Products of the Malay Peninsula. 2 Vols. London. Crown Agents for the Colonies.

Greenberg, L.A. and Lester, D. (1954) Handbook of Cosmetic Materials. New York. Interscience.

Kingsbury, J.M. (1964) Poisonous Plants of the United States and Canada. Englewood Cliffs, New Jersey. Prentice-Hall Inc.

Virchow, C. (1965) Allergy to soybean. Allergie u Asthma 11, 57.

Sub-family Lotoideae (Papilionoideae)

Tribe Astragaleae

Glycyrrhiza

18 species are found in temperate and sub-tropical America, temperate Eurasia, North Africa and south-east Australia.

Glycyrrhiza glabra
Liquorice

This and other species furnish liquorice. Excessive consumption of liquorice can produce symptoms similar to those of aldosteronism (Conn et al 1968).

Reference

Conn, J.W., Rovner, D.R. and Cohen, E.L. (1968) Licorice-induced pseudo aldosteronism. JAMA 205, 492.

Sub-family Caesalpiniodeae

Tribe Detarieae

Goniorrhachis

One species is found in south-eastern Brazil.

Goniorrhachis marginata
Guarabu, Itapicuru

The heartwood contains the known allergen 4-methoxydalbergione (of Dalbergia spp.). (Sousa et al 1967).

Reference

Sousa, J.R. de, Gottlieb, O.R. and Magalhaes, M.T. (1967) Neo-flavanoides mos gêneros Goniorrhachis e Peltogyne Anais da Academia brasileira de Ciencias 39, 227.

Sub-family Lotoideae (Papilionoideae)

Tribe Milletieae

Goodia

Two species are native to South Australia.

Goodia latifolia
Golden Tip, Clover Tree

Cattle are said to eat the plant greedily and as a result to develop 'black scours'. The tongues become black and the hides acquire a bluish tint and become rough and bound (Maiden 1895).

Reference

Maiden, J.H. (1895) Botanical notes. Is Goodia poisonous to stock? Agr. Gaz. New South Wales 6, 306.

Sub-family Caesalpiniodeae

Tribe Detarieae

Gossweilerodendron

One species is native to tropical Africa.

Gossweilerodendron balsamiferum
Agba, Tola Branca, Pink Mahogany

The tree is reported to cause

dermatitis in woodworkers (Zafiropoulo et al 1968, Hausen 1970, Hublet et al 1972). Splinters (slivers) are known in the industry to be particularly prone to cause "festering" sores in the skin (Wilkinson 1971). The pink resin of the tree is burnt as an illuminant in Africa (Dalziel 1937). Respiratory irritation from the wood has not been noted (Orsler 1969).

According to Woods and Calnan (1976) the wood 'tola' which was reported by Symanski (1957) to produce asthma was probably this species rather than Oxystigma oxyphyllum.

They reported two cases of dermatitis in machinists from agba with positive patch test reactions to the wood; one of the machinists also showed a positive patch test reaction to Distemonanthus.

References

Dalziel, J.M. (1937) The Useful Plants of West Tropical Africa. London. Crown Agents.

Hausen, B.M. (1970) Untersuchungen über Gesundheitsschädigende Hölzer. Thesis, Hamburg.

Hublet, P., Sporcq, J., Oleffe, J. et al (1972) Etude sur les accidents cutanes et muqueux provoques par les bois tropicaux dans l'industrie due bois en Belgique. Arch. Belges. Med. Social. 30, 314.

Orsler, R.J. (1969) The effects of irritant timbers. Woodworking Industry 26, 28.

Wilkinson, D.S. (1971) Dermatitis from Khaya mahoganies in the furniture industry. 'Atti' del symposium sulla preventione delle dermatose professionali. Monte Porzio Cantone, 1960 and personal communication (1971).

Zafiropoulo, A., Audibert, A. and Charpin, J. (1968) A propos des accidents dus a la manipulation des bois exotiques. Rev. Franc. Allerg. 8, 155.

Symanski, H.J. (1957) Opticuatrophic nach Verarbeitung von exotischen Hölzern. Medizinische Klinik 52, 198.

Woods, B. and Calnan, C.D. (1976) Toxic Woods. Brit. J. Derm. 94, Suppl. 13, June.

Sub-family Caesalpinioideae

Tribe Detarieae

Guibourtia

Four species are native to tropical America, eleven to tropical Africa.

Guibourtia copallifera (syn. Copaifera)

A gum copal, derived from the tree, is used in pharmacy, for varnishes, lacquers and sealing wax and in the preparation of patent leather (Dalziel 1937, Oliver 1959).

References

Dalziel, J.M. (1937) The Useful Plants of West Tropical Africa. London. Crown Agents.

Oliver, B. (1959) Nigeria's Useful Plants. Nigerian Field 24, 70.

Sub-family Caesalpinioideae

Tribe Caesalpineae

Haematoxylum

Three species are native to Mexico, Central America, the West Indies and South-West Africa.

Haematoxylum campechianum
Logwood

The heart-wood contains haematoxylin, used for dyeing and for making ink and microscopical stains. Dermatitis of the hands was said to be caused by haematoxylin in gloves. Patch tests to the glove gave positive reactions. The dye itself was not used for patch testing (Sezary and Deval 1932). Hypersensitivity to natural dyes can occur but dermatitis is rare among dyers or weavers of dyed furs (Schwartz et al 1957). These authors also discussed skin hazards in the manufacture of ink, tannin, sumac (Rhus), Cutch (Acacia catechu), Fustic (Chlorophora tinctoria), cashew nut oil (Anacardium) and turpentine (Pinus).

Reference

Schwartz, L., Tulipan, L. and Birmingham, D.J. (1957) Occupational Diseases of the Skin. 3rd ed. Philadelphia. Lea & Febiger. pp. 637-672.

Sézary, A. and Deval, L. (1932) Dermite artificielle causée par des gants noirs. Bull. Soc. franc. Derm. Syph. 39, 1370.

Sub-family Caesalpinioideae

Tribe Detarieae

Hymenaea

25 species are native to Mexico, Cuba and tropical South America.

Hymenaea sp.

The wood is valuable. The wood causes skin irritation (Freise 1932).

Hymenaea courbaril

A resin (copal or anime) exudes from the stem and is often found in lumps underground near the trees, as in *Agathis* and *Trachylobium*. Dermatitis from copal resin is noted under *Agathis*. Copal resins are used in varnishes.

Reference

Freise, F.W. (1932) Gesundheitsschädigungen durch Arbeiten mit giftigen Hölzern. Beobachtungen aus brasilianischen Gewerbebetrieben. Archiv für Gewerbepathologie und Gewerbehygiene 3, 1.

Sub-family Lotoideae (Papilionoideae)

Tribe Indigoferaeae

Indigofera

700 species are found in warm regions.

Chemistry is recorded by Thomson (1971).

Reference

Thomson, R.H. (1971) Naturally Occurring Quinones. 2nd ed. London. Academic Press.

Indigofera spp.
Indigo

Several species provide the dye, indigo. Dermatitis is common in the indigo dyeing process of textiles but there is no evidence that indigo or its derivatives are responsible (White 1934). Women employed in shelling indigo develop an exceptionally long right thumb nail (Schwartz et al 1957). Indigo appears to be, at the most, only mildly irritant to the eye (Grant 1962).

References

Grant, W.M. (1962) Toxicology of the eye. Springfield, Ill. Charles C. Thomas.

Schwartz, L., Tulipan, L., and Birmingham, D.J. (1957) Occupational Diseases of the Skin. 3rd ed. Philadelphia. Lea and Febiger. pp. 637-672.

White, R.P. (1934) The Dermatoses or Occupational Affections of the Skin. 4th ed. London. H.K. Lewis.

Sub-family Mimosoideae

Tribe Ingeae

Inga

200 species are native to tropical and sub-tropical America and the West Indies.

Inga vera
Grenadilla

The authenticity of a report of dermatitis from this wood (Schwartz et al 1957) is doubtful since the colloquial name Grenadilla is also applied to *Brya* and *Dalbergia*.

Reference

Schwartz, L., Tulipan, L. and Birmingham, D.J. (1957) Occupational Diseases of the Skin. 3rd ed. Philadelphia. Lea and Febiger. pp. 637-672.

Sub-family Caesalpinioideae

Tribe Detarieae

Instia

Nine species are native to Madagascar and islands off tropical East Africa and to tropical Asia and Malaysia.

Instia palembanica
Merbau

The hands of wood-workers become stained black from handling the wood (Burgess 1966). Lapachol, a sensitizer of Tectona is reported from some species (Thomson 1971, Krogh 1964). Orsler (1973) received unconfirmed reports of irritation from this species and from I. bijuga.

References

Burgess, P.F. (1966) Timbers of Sabah (Sabah Forest Records No. 6). Sabah, Malaysia. The Forest Department.

Krogh, H.K. (1964) Contact eczema caused by true teak (Tectona grandis). A follow-up study of a previous epidemiological investigation and a study into the sensitizing effect of various teak extracts. Brit. J. Industr. Med. 21, 65.

Orsler, R.J. (1973) Personal communication from Forest Products Research Laboratory. Princess Risborough, Bucks, England.

Thomson, R.H. (1971) Naturally Occurring Quinones. 2nd ed. London. Academic Press.

Sub-family Caesalpinioideae

Tribe Cassieae

Koompassia

Four species are native to Malaysia, Borneo and New Guinea.

Koompassia excelsa
Tualang, Sialang

The sap is irritant to the skin and produces an inflammation like erysipelas (Burkill 1935). The hard timber of the felled tree is highly inflammable, more so when fresh than dead (Corner 1952).

References

Burkill, I.H. (1935) A Dictionary of the Economic Products of the Malay Peninsula. 2 Vols. London. Crown Agents for the Colonies.

Corner, E.J.H. (1952) Wayside Trees of Malaysia. Singapore, Government Printer.

Sub-family Lotoideae (Papilionoideae)

Tribe Aeschynomeneae

Kotschya

Thirty species are native to tropical Africa.

Kotschya ochreata
(syn. Smithia)

The plant has haemostatic properties (Irvine 1961).

Reference

Irvine, F.R. (1961) Woody plants of Ghana. Oxford University Press. London.

Sub-family Lotoideae (Papilionoideae)

Tribe Laburneae

Laburnum

In a strict sense of the genus, two species are found in central Europe; in a broad sense, four species are found in Europe, northern Africa and western Asia.

Laburnum anagyroides
Common Laburnum
(syn. L. vulgare, Cystisus laburnum)

Exposure to the sawdust was said to cause constitutional symptoms (Lewin 1928). The wood and the seeds contain the poisonous alkaloid, cytisine.

Reference

Lewin, L. (1928) Gifte im Holzgewerbe. Berlin, Stilke.

Sub-family Lotoideae (Papilionoideae)

Tribe Vicieae

Lathyrus

130 species are found in north temperate regions and on mountains of tropical America and South America. Lathyrus odoratus is the Sweet Pea of horticulture.

Lathyrus hookeri

Photosensitivity is reported from ingestion of the plant (North 1967).

Lathyrus sativus

Guinea pigs which are fed the seeds develop alopecia, slight dermatitis and ulcers on the hind legs (North 1967). The human disease, lathyrism, was reviewed by Watt and Breyer-Brandwijk (1962) and Kingsbury (1964).

References

Kingsbury, J.M. (1964) Poisonous Plants of the United States and Canada. Englewood Cliffs, New Jersey. Prentice-Hall Inc.

North, P.M. (1967) Poisonous Plants and Fungi in Colour. London. Blandford Press Ltd.

Watt, J.M. and Breyer-Brandwijk, M.G. (1962) The Medicinal and poisonous plants of Southern Africa. 2nd ed. Edinburgh. E. & S. Livingstone.

Sub-family Mimosoideae

Tribe Mimoseae

Leucaena

50 species are native to tropical America, one to Polynesia and one is pantropical.

Leucaena glauca

West Indian Lead Tree, Horse Tamarind.

The young pods are eaten as a vegetable by Malays and the mature dried seeds are eaten raw (Burkill 1935, Corner 1952). Ingestion of the plant can cause alopecia in some animals, particularly in horses and pigs; some other animals appear to be unaffected (Morris 1896, Hurst 1942, Irvine 1961, Watt and Breyer-Brandwijk 1962). The toxic principle is mimosine (Kingsbury 1964). McKee (1958) and Owen (1958) refer to loss of hair in humans. Young rats fed the leaves and seeds can develop cataracts (Grant 1962). The biological action of mimosine was investigated by Crounse et al (1962).

References

Burkill, I.H. (1935) A Dictionary of the Economic Products of the Malay Peninsula. 2 Vols. London. Crown Agents for the Colonies.

Corner, E.J.H. (1952) Wayside Trees of Malaysia. Singapore. Government Printer.

Crounse, R.G., Maxwell, J.D. and Blank, H. (1962) Inhibition of growth of hair by mimosine. Nature 194, 694.

Grant, W.M. (1962) Toxicology of the eye. Springfield, Ill. Charles C. Thomas.

Hurst, E. (1942) The Poisonous Plants of New South Wales. N.S.W. Poison Plants Committee; Sydney.

Irvine, F.R. (1961) Woody Plants of Ghana. Oxford University Press. London.

Kingsbury, J.M. (1964) Poisonous Plants of the United States and Canada. Englewood Cliffs, New Jersey. Prentice-Hall Inc.

McKee, H.S. (1958) South Pacific Comm. Quart. Bull. 8, 62 cited by Biology Data Book (1964) ed. Altman, P.L. and Dittmer, D.S. Washington, D.C. Fed. Amer. Soc. Exp. Biol.

Morris, D. (1896) On the singular effect produced on certain animals in the West Indies feeding on the young shoots, leaves and seeds of the wild Tamarind or Junibai plant (Leucaena glauca Benth.). Brit. Ass. Adv. Sci. Rep. 1017.

Owen, L.N. (1958) Hair loss and other toxic effects of Leucaenia glauca ("Jumbey"). Veterinary Record 70, 454.

Watt, J.M. and Breyer-Brandwijk, M.G. (1962) The Medicinal and poisonous plants of Southern Africa. 2nd ed. Edinburgh. E. & S. Livingstone.

Sub-family Lotoideae (Papilionoideae)

Tribe Lespedezeae

Lespedeza

100 species are found in regions from the Himalayas to China and Japan and in Australia and temperate North America.

Lespedeza frutescens
Bush Clover

Animals fed mouldy hay of this plant can develop a bleeding syndrome (Kingsbury 1964). The plant was observed to have no allergenic effect in an investigation of 'weed dermatitis' (Shelmire 1939).

References

Kingsbury, J.M. (1964) Poisonous Plants of the United States and Canada. Englewood Cliffs, New Jersey. Prentice-Hall Inc.

Shelmire, B. (1939) Contact Dermatitis from Weeds; Patch Testing with Their Oleoresins. JAMA 113, 1085.

Sub-family Lotoideae (Papilionoideae)

Tribe Dalbergieae (ambiguous)

Lonchocarpus

150 species are found in tropical America, the West Indies, Africa and Australia.

Lonchocarpus costillai

The wood is said to be irritant (Orsler 1973).

Lonchocarpus cyanescens
Yoruba Indigo

The ground roots are applied to the skin to produce irritation (Irvine 1961).

Lonchocarpus nicou
Stinkwood

The crude plant preparation and rotenone derived from the plant can cause dermatitis, conjunctivitis and rhinitis (Thienes and Haley 1972).

References

Irvine, F.R. (1961) Woody Plants of Ghana. Oxford University Press. London.

Orsler, R.J. (1973) Personal communication from Forest Products Research Laboratory. Princess Risborough, Bucks, England.

Thienes, C.H. and Haley, T.J. (1972) Clinical Toxicology. 5th ed. Philadelphia. Lea & Febiger.

Sub-family Lotoideae (Papilionoideae)

Tribe Lupineae

Lupinus

200 species are native to America and the Mediterranean region.

Lupinus spp. Lupin

Hepatic photosensitisation can occur in animals from ingestion of some species (Kingsbury 1964). Hjorth (1968) obtained negative patch test reactions to lupin.

Lupinus termis

Thrombocytopenic purpura was observed in a male child who ate the beans (Lavy 1964).

References

Hjorth, N. (1968) at Finsen Institute. Pers. Comm.

Kingsbury, J.M. (1964) Poisonous Plants of the United States and Canada. Englewood Cliffs, New Jersey, Prentice-Hall Inc.

Lavy, R. (1964) Thrombocytopenic purpura due to Lupinus termis bean. J. Allergy 35, 386.

Sub-family Mimosoideae

Tribe Ingeae

Lysiloma

35 species are native to regions from the south-western United States to tropical America and to the West Indies.

Lysiloma sabicu

Sabicu, Horse-flesh Mahogany

The wood was said to cause coryza-like symptoms (Legge 1907). Cuban sabicu is Peltophorum adnatum. The wood of L. bahamensis contains an alkaloid (Virtanen and Gmelin 1959).

References

Legge, T.M. (1907) Report of the Chief Inspector of Factories and Workshops. 1907, 248, London.

Virtanen and Gmelin (1959) Unreferenced by Woods and Calnan (1976).

Woods, B. and Calnan, C.D. (1976) Toxic Woods. Brit. J. Derm. 94, Suppl. 13. June.

Sub-family Lotoideae (Papilionoideae)

Tribe Pterocarpeae

Machaerium

150 species are native to regions from Mexico to tropical South America and to the West Indies. Some of the jacaranda or rosewood timbers are provided by species of this genus and by Dalbergia.

Machaerium pedicellatum

Dalbergiones derived from the wood were found to be responsible for allergic contact dermatitis in machinists (Ogiyama and Yasue 1973).

Machaerium schomburgkii

This species is now known as Paramacherium schomburgki (Woods and Calnan 1976).

The wood is listed as capable of producing dermatitis (Hanslian and Kadlec 1966) probably from Grossmann (1910).

According to Woods and Calnan (1976) the wood implicated may actually have been one of the woods named snakewood, possibly Piratinera guianensis.

References

Hanslian, L. and Kadlec, K. (1966) Drevo z hlediska hygienickeho (Vii). Biologicky silne agresivni dreviny. Drevo 21, 157.

Ogiyama, K. and Yasue, M. (1973) Constituents of Machaerium pedicellatum heartwood. Phytochemistry 12, 2544.

Grossmann, J. (1910) Gesundheitsschädliche Hölzer Bayrische Industrielle Gewerbeblatt 96 (6), 51.

Woods, B. and Calnan, C.D. (1976) Toxic Woods. Brit. J. Derm. 94, Suppl. 13 June.

Machaerium scleroxylon

Jacaranda, Pao Ferro, Caviuna vermelha

The literature concerning contact dermatitis from the wood of this species was reviewed by Morgan et al (1968). They observed an outbreak of dermatitis in a furniture factory. The hands, cheeks, lips, forehead, neck and the exposed skin surfaces were affected in seven of 24 workers at risk. Dalbergiones were found to be the allergenic components of the wood. Cross-sensitivity to Dalbergia was observed but D. nigra was a weaker sensitizer.

Patch-testing with petroleum extracts of the wood and with 3,4-dimethoxydalbergione can produce active sensitisation. This chemical may be used in a concentration 0.1% in petrolatum unless further observations in a larger number of individuals indicate that the concentration should be further reduced (Maibach 1970).

Dermatitis from the wood has been reported from Brazil (Miranda Bastos and Matos Filho 1962) and Germany (Hausen 1970). The species is sometimes mixed with shipments of Dalbergia nigra which is becoming commercially scarce (Phillips 1966, Farmer 1972).

References

Farmer, R.H. (1972) A Handbook of Hardwoods. 2nd ed. London. H.M.S.O.

Hausen, B.M. (1970) Untersuchungen über Gesundheitsschädigende Hölzer. Thesis, Hamburg.

Miranda Bastos, A.D. and Matos

Filhos, A. de (1962) A 'Jacaranda' timber causing dermatitis. Proc. 5th Forest. Congr. 3, 1414.

Phillips, E.W.J. (1966) Dermatitis caused by a rosewood substitute. Wood 31, 44.

Maibach, H.I. (1970) Active sensitisation to wood extracts. Contact Dermatitis Newsletter, London. 7, 149.

Morgan, J.W.W., Orsler, R.J. and Wilkinson, D.S. (1968) Dermatitis due to the wood dusts of Khaya anthotheca and Macherium scleroxylon. Brit. J. Ind. Med. 25, 119.

Machaerium violaceum

Orelha d'Onca

This species is listed as a cause of dermatitis by Sandermann and Barghoorn (1956) probably from Freise (1932) who listed the species with the common name orelha d'onca. According to Woods and Calnan (1976) the species may actually have been Dalbergia cearensis.

References

Sandermann, W. and Barghoorn, A.W. (1956) Gesundheitsschädigende Nutzhölzer Holz Roh-Werkst 14, 37.

Freise, F.W. (1932) Gesundheitsschädigungen durch Arbeiten mit giftigen Hölzern. Beobachtungen aus brasilianischen Gewerbebetrieben. Archiv für Gewerbepathologie und Gewerbehygiene 3, 1.

Woods, B. and Calnan, C.D. (1976) Toxic Woods. Brit. J. Derm. 94, Suppl 13, June.

Sub-family Lotoideae (Papilionoideae)

Tribe Trifoleae

Medicago

100 species are native to temperate Eurasia, the Mediterranean region and South Africa.

Medicago spp.

Species of this genus have hooked fruits which attach themselves to animals (Howes 1974).

Medicago denticulata
(syn. M. hispida)
Bur Clover, Medick, Trefoil

The spiny pods are capable of producing mechanical injury.

Photosensitisation from ingestion of the plant by animals is documented (Hurst 1942, Watt and Breyer-Brandwijk 1962) but a record of a similar effect in man from contact with the plant is not substantiated (Mathews 1937).

Medicago sativa

Alfalfa, Lucerne

This fodder plant has been suspected of causing photosensitivity in animals who ingest it (Mathews 1937, Watt and Breyer-Brandwijk 1962) and its use for guinea pig feed may interfere with experiments concerning photosensitivity (Urbach 1972). Contact dermatitis (Anderson 1944) and eczema from ingestion of a tea (Kaufman 1954) have been reported.

Lucerne caused rhinitis, asthma and urticaria especially when it was handled in the dry state, during baling the hay or milling it into powder. The pollen is suspected of causing hayfever (Wodehouse 1971). Injection of an infusion of alfalfa seed as a nostrum for arthritis produced oedematous eruptions in two cases (Kaufman 1954).

References

Anderson, C.R. (1944) Contact dermatitis from alfalfa and bur clover. Arch. Derm. Syph. 5, 201.

Hurst, E. (1952) The Poisonous Plants of New South Wales. N.S.W. Poison Plants Committee; Sydney.

Kaufman, W.H. (1954) Alfalfa Seed Dermatitis. JAMA 155, 1058.

Mathews, F.P. (1937) Photosensitisation and the photodynamic diseases of man and the lower animals. Arch. Path. 23, 399.

Urbach, F. (1972) Temple University, School of Medicine. In discussion American Academy of Dermatology, December 1972.

Watt, J.M. and Breyer-Brandwijk, M.G. (1962) The Medicinal and poisonous plants of Southern Africa. 2nd ed. Edinburgh. E. & S. Livingstone.

Howes, F.N. (1974) A Dictionary of Useful and Everyday Plants and their Common Names. Cambridge University Press. pp. 290.

Wodehouse, R.P. (1971) Hayfever Plants. 2nd rev. edition. New York, Hafner.

Sub-family Caesalpinioideae

Tribe Sclerolobieae

Melanoxylon

Three species, native to tropical South America, provide useful timber.

Melanoxylon brauna

This wood is said to cause dermatitis (Hanslian and Kadlec 1966). Hausen (1970) cites Friese (1932) for an injurious effect of the wood. He described pustules and necrotizing inflammation from the sawdust especially when it contacted minor wounds on the legs.

References

Freise, F.W. (1932) Gesundheitsschädigungen durch Arbeiten mit giftigen Hölzern. Beobachtungen aus brasilianischen Gewerbebetrieben. Arch. Gewerbepath.-hyg 3, 1.

Hanslian, L. and Kadlec, K. (1966) Drevo z hlediska hygienickeho (VIII). Biologicky ucinne a malo ucinne dreviny. Drevo 21, 229.

Hausen, B.M. (1970) Untersuchungen über Gesundheitsschädigende Hölzer. Thesis, Hamburg.

Sub-family Lotoideae (Papilionoideae)

Tribe Trifolieae

Melilotus

25 species are native to temperate and subtropical Eurasia and the Mediterranean region.

Melilotus alba

White Sweet Clover

Ingestion of the plant in the form of hay can cause a bleeding tendency and haemorrhages into the skin from a content of dicoumarol. In an investigation of 'weed dermatitis', the plant produced negative patch test reactions (Shelmire 1939).

Melilotus arvensis

The plant is ingested by Chinese people to impart a fragrance to the body (Smith 1969).

Melilotus officinalis

Yellow Sweet Clover

Haemorrhagic skin necroses in animals can occur from ingestion of the mouldy plant; dicoumarol is responsible (Kingsbury 1964). Dicoumarol has been implicated in alopecia (Cornbleet and Hoit 1957).

References

Cornbleet, T. and Hoit, L. (1957) Alopecia from coumarin. Arch. Derm. 75, 440.

Kingsbury, J.M. (1964) Poisonous Plants of the United States and Canada. Englewood Cliffs, New Jersey. Prentice-Hall Inc.

Shelmire, B. (1939) Contact Dermatitis from Weeds; Patch Testing with their oleoresins. JAMA 113, 1085.

Smith, F.P. (1969) Chinese Materia Medica. Vegetable kingdom. 2nd ed. Rev. by Hei, P.D. Taipei, Taiwan. Ku T'ing Book House.

Sub-family Caesalpinioideae

Tribe Amherstieae

Microberlinia

Two species are found in west equatorial Africa.

Microberlinia spp.

Zebrawood

The wood is said to be irritant (Zafiropoulo et al 1968) but the name zebrawood is also applied to Astronium.

References

Zafiropoulo, A., Audibert, A. and Charpin, J. (1968) A propos des accidents dus a la manipulation des bois exotiques. Rev. Franc. Allerg. 8, 155.

Sub-family Lotoideae (Papilionoideae)

Tribe Millettieae

Millettia

180 species are found in tropical and subtropical regions.

Millettia spp.

Several species notably M. ferruginea yield rotenone, the cutaneous effects of which are noted under Derris.

Millettia laurentii

Wenge

Splinters of wenge cause persistent inflammation and exposure to the sawdust can cause abdominal cramps.

This species can cause mucocutaneous reactions in wood-workers (Hublet et al 1972). Hausen (1974) was able to sensitize guinea pigs to ethanol/chloroform extracts of the wood.

Millettia megasperma

Native Wisteria

The exudation of the cut vine of this Australian species is very astringent from a high content of tannin and yields a kino (Maiden 1891).

Millettia stuhlmannii

Panga-Panga

This species has been implicated in asthma of wood-workers (Ordman 1949).

References

Hausen, B.M. (1974) Pers. Comm.

Hublet, P., Sprocq, J., Oleffe, J. et al (1972) Etude sur les accidents cutanes et muqueux provoques par les bois tropicaux dans l'industrie due bois en Belgique. Arch. Belges. Med. Social 30,314.

Maiden, J.H. (1891) On two undescribed exudations from the Leguminosae. Proc. Linn. Soc. New South Wales. 6, 679.

Ordman, A. (1949) Bronchial asthma caused by the inhalation of wood dust. Ann. Allergy. 7, 492.

Sub-family Mimosoideae

Tribe Mimoseae

Mimosa

Perhaps 500 species are found in tropical and sub-tropical America, a few in Africa and Asia. They are frequently thorny.

Mimosa pigra

(syn. M. asperata)

Thorn of Blood

The roots are irritant (Irvine 1961).

Mimosa pudica

Sensitive plant

This thorny plant is injurious to the gut of animals which eat it (Burkill 1935). Mimosine is derived from the plant; the effects of this chemical are noted under Leucaena.

References

Burkill, I.H. (1935) A Dictionary of the Economic Products of the Malay Peninsula. 2 Vols. London. Crown Agents for the Colonies.

Irvine, F.R. (1961) Woody Plants of Ghana. Oxford University Press. London.

Mimosa

The caterpillar of the flannel moth which haunts mimosa trees in the southern United States can cause contact dermatitis (Grater 1975). The common name mimosa can refer to Mimosa and to some species of Acacia (Howes 1974).

References

Grater, W.C. (1975) Report on weed dermatitis in Dermatology in Practice 8, 2 (Lederle Labs.)

Howes, F.N. (1974) A Dictionary of Useful and Everyday Plants and their Common Names. Cambridge University Press. pp. 290.

Sub-family Caesalpinioideae

Tribe Dimorphandreae

Mora

Ten species are native to tropical South America and the West Indies.

Mora excelsa

The wood-dust is acrid and irritant to the respiratory tract (Handbook of Hardwoods 1956, Orsler 1973). M. gonggrijpii appears to have a similar effect.

Mora spp.

Mora, Morabukea, Nato

The fine sawdust produces a bitter taste on the lips (Kukachka 1970).

References

Handbook of Hardwoods (1956) Forest Products Research. Ministry of Technology. London. HMSO.

Orsler, R.J. (1973) Personal communication from Forest Products Research Laboratory, Princess Risborough, Bucks, England.

Kukachka, B.F. (1970) Properties of imported tropical woods. USDA Forest Service Research Paper. FPL125 March. U.S. Dept. Agric. Forest Service. Forest Products Laboratory. Madison, Wis. U.S.A.

Sub-family Lotoideae (Papilionoideae)

Tribe Erythrineae

Mucuna

120 species are found in tropical and sub-tropical regions. Some have stinging hairs on the pods.

Mucuna spp. Cowitch

The English name 'cowitch' came into being by attempts to force a meaning (i.e. itching) into a distorted form, first 'ke-whage' and then 'kowhage' of the Hindu name 'Kewach' (Burkill 1935). Labourers in sugar-cane fields developed urticarial reactions from the plants (Behl et al 1966). The hairs of the wild species of Mucuna sting when the plants themselves are long dead (Burkill 1935). Various authors report the following species as having irritant hairs: M atropurpurea, M. coriacea, M. flagellipes, M. gigantea, M. hirsuta, M. melanocarpa, M. monosperma, M. nigricans, M. poggei, M. pruriens, M. quadrilata, M. sloanei, M. stans, M. urens. The hairs of M. urens were noted to be air-borne and capable of producing irritation at a distance (Allen 1943).

References

Allen, P.H. (1943) Poisonous and injurious plants of Panama. Am. J. Trop. Med. Suppl. 23, 1.

Behl, P.N., Captain, R.M., Bedi, B.M.S. and Gupta, S. (1966) Skin-irritant and sensitizing plants found in India, New Delhi. P.N. Behl, Irwin Hospital.

Burkill, I.H. (1935) A Dictionary of the Economic Products of the Malay Peninsula. 2 Vols. London. Crown Agents for the Colonies.

Mucuna pruriens

Buffalo Bena, Pica-Pica, Cowhage

The velvety surface of the crooked pods is made up of thousands of rigid, brittle barbed hairs which are easily detached on contact with the skin. Penetration of the skin by the hairs produces itching (Allen 1943).

Cowhage hairs were formerly used in an ointment, Ung. urticans (White 1887). The stinging hairs have been used in Africa to simulate leprosy, being first applied to the skin which is then rubbed with the latex of a Euphorbia. This causes swelling and numbness, persistent for several weeks (Dalziel 1937).

Labourers were observed to develop urticaria; some developed conjunctivitis and keratitis. Dried hairs mixed in the soil can irritate the feet (Dao 1967).

The active pruritogenic principle is a proteolytic enzyme,

mucunain (Shelly and Arthur 1955, Arthur and Shelley 1955).

References

Allen, P.H. (1943) Poisonous and Injurious Plants of Panama. Am. J. Trop. Med. Suppl. 23, 1.

Arthur, R.P. and Shelley, W.B. (1955) The role of proteolytic enzymes in the production of pruritus in man. J. Invest. Derm. 25, 341.

Dalziel, J.M. (1937) The Useful Plants of West Tropical Africa. London. Crown Agents.

Dao, L. (1967) Dermatitis por plantas en los llanos de Venezuela. Derm. Int. (Philadelphia) 6, 77.

Shelly, W.B. and Arthur, R.P. (1955) Studies on Cowhage (Mucuna pruriens) and it's pruritogenic proteinase, mucunain. Archs. Derm. 72, 399.

White, J.C. (1887) Dermatitis venenata: An account of the action of External irritants upon the skin. Boston. Cupples and Hurd.

Sub-family Lotoideae (Papilionoideae)

Tribe Tephrosieae

Mundulea

30 species are native to Madagascar, one to tropical Africa, southern India and Ceylon.

Mundulea sericea

This species yields rotenone (Irvine 1961), the cutaneous effects of which are noted under Derris.

Reference

Irvine, F.R. (1961) Woody Plants of Ghana. Oxford University Press. London.

Tribe not listed

Myrocarpus

Four species of southern Brazil and Paraguay yield a balsam like balsam of Peru (Myroxylon).

Myrocarpus frondosus

The wood of this Brazilian species yields Cabreuva oil from which is derived nerolidol and hence, the sesquiterpene alcohol, farnesol. Man himself uses farnesol, which occurs in his own surface lipid, as a perfume (Nicolaides 1965).

Reference

Nicolaides, N. (1965) Skin Lipids IV Biochemistry and Function. American Oil Chemists Society Journal 42, 708.

Sub-family Lotoideae (Papilionoideae)

Tribe Sophoreae

Myroxylon

Two species are native to tropical South America.

Myroxylon balsamum var. pereirae yields Balsam of Peru.

M. balsamum var. balsamum yields Balsam of Tolu. The tree is beaten, then scorched with a torch to cause part of the bark to separate from the trunk. Within a few days, the bark drops and the balsam exudes from the exposed wood. This is soaked off with rags and boiled in water. Contact sensitivity to wood of the tree was observed by de Carvalho (1956).

Contact dermatitis from Balsam of Peru was recognized in Germany in 1880 and France in 1889 (Cummer 1927, Touton 1932). Early authors described systemic toxicity from absorption of the balsam which had been applied for treatment of scabies and to the nipples of a nursing mother (Cummer 1927). Albuminuria was noted by Hazen (1914) after treatment of scabies.

Balsam of Peru is a mixture of many different substances and as a rule sensitisation leads to a complicated pattern of multiple allergies which vary from one patient to another (Hjorth 1959). Balsam of Peru contains a number of simple chemicals (cinnamic acid, benzyl cinnamate, vanillin, benzylbenzoate and benzoic acid) which constitute 60 percent of the total while the remaining 40 percent consists of resins. Patch tests with the low molecular weight ingredients yield inconstant positive reactions and half of the patients studied by Hjorth (1959) showed negative reactions to all:

Results of patch tests with low molecular weight ingredients of Balsam of Peru (103 cases) (from Hjorth 1959).

Ingredient	Positive reaction
Cinnamic acid	27 cases
Benzyl cinnamate	19 cases
Vanillin	15 cases
Benzyl benzoate	12 cases
Benzoic acid	10 cases
One or more positive	54 cases
All negative	49 cases

He therefore concluded that the important allergens must be found in the resinous fractions. The exact composition of these resins is unknown but they are thought to be polymers of esters of coniferyl alcohol with benzoic acid and cinnamic acid. In his series 70 patients (85 percent) showed positive patch tests to coniferyl benzoate and sometimes the patch test was followed by a clinical aggravation (a focal flare) and sensitisation induced by patch testing was observed in nine of 27 patients. These observations supported the assumption that this substance is one of the most important allergens in Balsam of Peru. By dry heat, coniferyl benzoate is decomposed, among other compounds to isoeugenol and eugenol. Hjorth (1959) found that isoeugenol gave positive reactions in 83 of 132 patients examined (63 percent). Vanillin, Vanilla, is also related to coniferyl benzoate, and although reactions to pure vanillin are uncommon 34 of 63 patients showed positive patch tests to natural Vanilla (Bourbon). Cross-sensitisation is also seen between Balsam of Peru and cinnamon, Cinnamomum, benzoin-storax, Styrax and orange peel Citrus; in the last named instance, the resinous fraction of orange peel is possibly responsible, since limonene, linalool and the coloring matter do not appear to be causative.

Hjorth (1961) provided a comprehensive monograph on eczematous allergy to Balsam of Peru. The presently known cross-reactions are tabulated (Table). The constituents of Balsam of Tolu were investigated by Wahlberg et al (1971).

24% of 101 children who had dermatitis and 6% of 284 adults who had dermatitis showed positive patch test reactions to Balsam of Peru (Fregert and Moller 1963).

14/64 patients with leg ulcers showed positive patch test reactions to Balsam of Peru (Van Dijk et al 1973). 64 (18 males and 46 females) of 712 individuals showed positive patch test reactions to Balsam of Peru. In 18 of 64, contact sensitivity to the balsam was considered to be the main cause or a contributory cause of hand eczema (Agrup 1969).

References

Agrup, G. (1969) Hand Eczema and other hand dermatoses in South Sweden. Acta. Derm.-venereol 49 Suppl. 61. pp. 1-91.

Cummer, C.L. (1927) Dermatitis produced by Balsam of Peru. Arch. Derm. Syph. 16, 44.

de Carvalho, L.P. (1956) Occupational contact allergens. Brasil-med. 70, 77.

Fregert, S. and Moller, H. (1963) Contact allergy to Balsam of Peru in children. Brit. J. Derm. 75, 218.

Hazen, H.H. (1914) Industrial skin diseases. J. Cutan. Dis. 32, 487.

Hjorth, N. (1959) Eczematous allergy to Balsam of Peru and allied natural resins. Presentation to the European Congress of Allergy. London. Sept. 3.

Hjorth, N. (1961) Eczematous allergy to Balsams, Allied Perfumes and Flavouring Agents. Copenhagen. Munksgaard.

Touton, K. (1932) Hauterkrankungen durch phanerogamische Pflanzen und ihre Produkte (Toxicodermia et Allergodermia phytogenes), in Barnewitz, ᵀ. et al. Angeborene Anomalien, Lichtdermatosen, Pflanzengifte, Thermische Schadigungen, Einfluss Innerer Störungen auf die Haut. Berlin, Verlag von Julius Springer.

Van Dijk, E., Neering, H. and Vitanyi, B.E.J. (1973) Contact hypersensitivity to sesame oil in patients with leg ulcers and eczema. Acta derm.- venereol 53, 133.

Wahlberg, I. et al (1971) Constituents of commercial Tolu Balsam. Acta. chem. Scand. 25, 3285.

Cross-reactions and sources of allergic contact dermatitis from Balsam of Peru and cross-reacting materials (Collins and Mitchell 1975).

Cross-reactions

Plant Materials

Cinnamon	*Cinnamomum*
Clove	*Eugenia*
Orange peel	*Citrus*
Storax	*Liquidambar*
Benzoin	*Styrax*
Rosin	*Pinus*
Vanilla	*Vanilla*
Balsam of Tolu	*Myroxylon*

Chemicals

Cinnamic aldehyde

Cinnamic acid

Cinnamic alcohol

Cinnamates

Benzoic acid

Benzyl benzoate

Benzyl alcohol

Eugenol

Balsam of Peru

Sources of Exposure:

Therapeutic and over-the-counter applications, suppositories, liquids in dentistry, essential oils, cosmetics, hair tonics and lotions, perfumes, flavours, cough mixtures, throat lozenges, balsams of pine and spruce (*Pinaceae*), pastries and cakes with essences, Danish pastries, caramels, cola-type drinks (*Cola*), toothpaste, some wines and liquers (Vermouth, Curacao), poplar buds (*Populus*) for bee-keepers.

References

Collins, F.W. and Mitchell, J.C. (1975) Aroma Chemicals. Reference sources for perfume and flavour ingredients with special reference to cinnamic aldehyde. Contact Dermatitis 1, 43.

Fisher (1974) discussed the clinical significance of positive patch test reactions to Balsam of Peru, referring to perfume dermatitis, occupational dermatitis in dentists, bakers, bee-keepers, painters, violinists and laboratory technicians, to dermatitis from topical medications and sunscreens, flavoring agents, orange and vanilla and cross-sensitivity with resorcinol monobenzoate used in certain cellulose ester plastics (steering wheel, sunglasses, hearing aids and ball-point pens).

Reference

Fisher, A.A. (1974) The clinical significance of positive patch test reactions to Balsam of Peru. Cutis. 13, 909.

Although Balsam of Peru has been less used in medications in recent years in Europe, contact sensitivity to the balsam and to wood tars (*Pinaceae*) has increased suggesting that other sources of sensitisation (perfumes in toilet soaps and cosmetics) are relevant (Olholm-Larsen and Heydenreich 1976).

Reference

Olholm-Larsen, O. and Heydenreich, G. (1976) Allergy to balsam of Peru and wood tars: an increasing problem? Contact Dermatitis 2, 293.

Cinnamic alcohol produced positive patch test reactions in 13/60 perfumery workers who had dermatitis (Gutman and Somov 1968). The other positive reactions were to Kumarin (4/60), citronellol (2/60), orange oil (3/60), hydroxycitronellal (2/60), clary sage oil (2/60), vanillin (2/60), acetylanizol (2/60), lemon oil (1/60), phenylethylalcohol (1/60).

Reference

Gutman, S.G. and Somov, B.A. (1968) Allergic reactions caused by components of perfumery preparations. Vestn. Derm. Vener. 42, 62.

Of 36 patients contact sensitive to Balsam of Peru 22 (61%) showed positive reactions to wood tars (Ebner 1974).

Reference

Ebner, H. (1974) Perubalsam and Parfüms. Hautarzt 25, 123.

Individuals contact sensitive to Balsam of Peru can also be contact sensitive to resorcinol monobenzoate (Calnan 1975).

Reference

Calnan, C.D. (1975) Resorcinol monobenzoate. Contact Dermatitis 1, 59.

Active sensitisation by patch testing with Balsam of Peru was recorded by Calnan (1975).

Reference

Calnan, C.D. (1975) Active sensitixation to para and Balsam of Peru. Contact Dermatitis 1, 126.

In some balsams and essential oils are found benzyl alcohol, benzyl benzoate, benzyl cinnamate and benzyl salicylate. The adverse skin effects of these compounds were reviewed by Opdyke (1973).

Reference

Opdyke, D.L.J. (1973) Monographs on fragrance raw materials. Fd. Cosmet. Toxicol. 11, 1011-1030.

Immediate reactions to Balsam of Peru were cited by Rudzki and Grzywa (1976) and Friis and Hjorth (1973).

References

Friis, B. and Hjorth, N. (1973) Immediate reactions to patch tests with balsam of Peru. Contact Dermatitis Newsletter 13, 389.

Rudzki, E. and Grzywa, Z. (1976) Immediate reactions to balsam of Peru, cassia oil and ethyl vanillin. Contact Dermatitis 2, 360.

4.8% of patients with leg ulcers were contact sensitive to Balsam of Peru (Angelini et al 1975).

Reference

Angelini, G., Tantuccio, F. and Meneghini, C.L. (1975) Contact dermatitis in patients with leg ulcers. Contact Dermatitis 1,81.

Sub-family Lotoideae (Papilionoideae)

Tribe Phaseoleae

Neorautanenia

10 species are native to southern tropical Africa.

Neorautanenia pseudopachyrrhiza

The tuber of a plant, which is probably this species, produces an eczematous eruption if rubbed over the body (Watt and Breyer-Brandwijk 1962).

Reference

Watt, J.M. and Breyer-Brandwijk, M.G. (1962) The Medicinal and poisonous plants of Southern Africa. 2nd ed. Edinburgh. E. & S. Livingstone.

Sub-family Lotoideae (Papilionoideae)

Tribe Hedysareae

Onobrychis

120 species are found in regions from Europe and the Mediterranean to central Asia. *O. viciaefolia* (syn. *O. sativa*) known as Holy Clover is grown for forage.

Onobrychis sativa

Esparsetteklee

Dermatitis from this species was reported by Matras (1931).

Reference

Matras (1931) Phytogene Dermatitis durch Esparsetteklee (Onobrychis). Zbl. Hautkrkh 36, 163, cited by Touton (1932).

Touton, K. (1932) Hauterkrankungen durch phanerogamische Pflanzen und ihre Produkte (Toxicodermia et Allergodermia phytogenes), in Barnewitz, J. et al. Angeborene Anomalien, Lichtdermatosen, Pflanzengifte, Thermische Schädigungen, Einfluss Innerer Störungen auf die Haut. Berlin, Verlag von Julius Springer.

Sub-family Caesapliniodieae

Tribe Caesalpinieae

Oxystigma

Eight species are native to tropical Africa.

Oxystigma oxyphyllum

The wood is said to produce asthma (Hausen 1970).

The wood implicated may have been Gossweilerodendron.

Reference

Hausen, B.M. (1970) Untersuchungne über Gesundheitsschädigende Hölzer. Thesis, Hamburg.

Paramacherium

Three species are found in Panama and tropical South America.

Paramacherium schomburgkii

(syn. Macherium schomburgkii)

The wood is noted under Macherium.

Sub-family Mimosoideae

Tribe Adenanthereae

Parapiptadenia

(syn. Piptadenia)

Two species are native to tropical America. P. rigida yields a gum.

Piptadenia africana

Dahoma

Naso-pharyngeal irritation from the wood-dust is noted under Piptadeniastrum.

Piptadenia peregrina

Cojoba

Injection of an extract of the seeds into humans produced a syndrome resembling carcinoid (Turner and Merlis 1959).

Reference

Turner, W.J. and Merlis, S. (1959) Effect of some indolealkylamines on man.Arch. Neur. Psych. 81, 121.

Sub-family Miminsoideae

Tribe Parkieae

Parkia

40 species are found in tropical regions. The seeds of P. africana are eaten. P. bicolor provides a useful wood. The fruit pods of P. speciosa, when eaten, cause the body to smell of garlic (Allium) (Corner 1952, Irvine 1961).

References

Corner, E.J.H. (1952) Wayside Trees of Malaysia. Singapore, Government Printer.

Irvine, F.R. (1961) Woody Plants of Ghana. Oxford University Press. London.

Sub-family Caesalpiniodeae

Tribe Caesalpinieae

Parkinsonia

Two species are native to tropical America and South Africa.

Parkinsonia aculeata

Jerusalem Thorn

This spiny plant, which is used for hedging, is capable of producing mechanical injury (Oakes and

Butcher 1962, Irvine 1961).

References

Irvine, F.R. (1961) Woody Plants of Ghana. Oxford University Press. London.

Oakes, A.J. and Butcher, J.O. (1962) Poisonous and injurious plants of the U.S. Virgin Islands. Misc. Publ. 882. U.S. Department of Agriculture, Washington, D.C.

Sub-family Caesalpinioideae

Tribe Detarieae

Peltogyne

25 species are native to tropical South America. Some yield dyes.

Peltogyne sp. Roxingho

The wood can cause dermatitis (Hanslian and Kadlec 1966). Hausen (1974) was able to sensitize guinea pigs to an ethanol/chloroform extract of the wood.

Peltogyne densiflora

Pao Roxo, Bois de Violette, Purpleheart

Dalbergiones have been isolated from the wood (De Sousa et al 1967). Such chemicals from Dalbergia are allergenic.

The smell of the wood when worked is unpleasant and causes nausea and anorexia (Grossman 1920). Cough and urticaria can occur in workers who polish the wood (Freise 1932).

References

Hanslian, L. and Kadlec, K. (1966) Wood from the standpoint of hygiene (VIII). Species with some or little biological effect. Drevo 21, 229.

Hausen, B.M. (1974) Pers. Comm.

DeSousa, J.R., Gottlieb, O.R. and Magalhaes, M.T. (1967) Neoflavanoides mos generos Goniorrhachis e Peltogyne. Anais da Academia brasileira de Ciencias. 39, 227.

Freise, F.W. (1932) Gesundheitschädigungen durch Arbeiten mit giftigen Hölzern. Beobachtungen aus brasilianischen Gewerbebetrieben. Archiv für Gewerbepathologie und Gewerbehygiene 3, 1.

Grossman, J. (1920) Gesundheitsschädliche Holzarten. Der Holzkäufer (Leipzig) 17, 529, 535, 540 and 545.

Sub-family Caesalpinioideae

Tribe Caesalpineae

Peltophorum

Twelve species are native to tropical Africa.

Peltophorum adnatum

Untoward effects are attributed to this wood (Hausen 1970).

Peltophorum pterocarpum

Yellow Flame

A dye from the wood is used for batik (Corner 1952).

Peltophorum violacea

(syn. Brasilettia)

A report of dermatitis from the wood was received by Orsler (1973).

References

Corner, E.J.H. (1952) Wayside Trees of Malaysia. Singapore, Government Printer.

Hausen, B.M. (1970) Untersuchungen über Gesundheitsschädigende Hölzer. Thesis, Hamburg.

Orsler, R.J. (1973) Personal communication from Forest Products Research Laboratory, Princess Risborough, Bucks, England.

Sub-family Lotoideae (Papilionoideae)

Tribe Sophoreae

Pericopsis

(syn. Afrormosia)

Five species native to tropical Africa yield afrormosia wood. One species native to Ceylon yields a cabinet wood known as nedun. One species is found on the Palau and Carolina islands.

Pericopsis elata

(syn. Afrormosia elata)

Afrormosia

The wood can produce dermatitis and respiratory symptoms (Hausen 1970, Hublet et al 1972, Orsler 1969).

Gronemeyer and Fuchs (1967) mention asthma from the wood.

Splinters of afrormosia are said to be troublesome and often become septic. In a furniture factory where afrormosia was being used an outbreak of dermatitis occurred. Twenty men were tested to the wood with only one doubtful positive reaction (Woods and Calnan 1976). In one case Tectona seemed to be the main sensitizer although a patch test to afrormosia produced a possibly false positive reaction.

References

Hausen, B.M. (1970) Untersuchungen über Gesundheitsschädigende Hölzer. Thesis, Hamburg.

Hublet, P., Sporcq, J., Oleffe, J. et al (1972) Etude sur les accidents cutanes et muqueux provoques par les bois tropicaux dans l'industrie due bois en Belgique. Arch. Belges. Med. Social. 30, 314.

Orsler, R.J. (1969) The effects of irritant timbers. Woodworking Industry 26, 28.

Gronemeyer, W. and Fuchs, E. (1967) Krankheiten durch inhalative Allergen-Invasion. In Lehrbuch der klinischen Allergie ed. Hansen, K. and Werner, M. Stuttgart, Thieme.

Woods, B. and Calnan, C.D. (1976) Toxic Woods. Brit. J. Derm. 94, Suppl. 13, June.

Sub-family Lotoideae (Papilionoideae)

Tribe Phaseoleae

Phaseolus

200 or more species are found in tropical and sub-tropical regions chiefly in America. Some cultivated species are P. coccineus, Scarlet Runner, P. lunatus, Lima bean and P. vulgaris, Kidney Bean.

Dermatitis in bean-pickers (Sneid 1955, Schwartz et al 1957) and in housewives is of rare occurrence (Behl et al 1966). Parasitic bites can occur in persons who harvest beans (White 1934). Shellers of beans and of peas (Pisum) can develop paronychia and atrophy of the nails (White 1934).

References

Behl, P.N., Captain, R.M., Bedi, B.M.S. and Gupta, S. (1966) Skin-irritant and sensitizing Plants found in India, New Delhi. P.N. Behl, Irwin Hospital.

Schwartz, L., Tulipan, L. and Birmingham, D.J. (1957) Occupational Diseases of the Skin. 3rd ed. Philadelphia. Lea and Febiger. pp. 637-672.

Sneid, P. (1955) Occupation health on the farm. Indust. Med. 24, 117.

White, R.P. (1934) The Dermatergoses or Occupational Affections of the Skin. 4th ed. London. H.K. Lewis.

Ingestion of beans and of 'ersatz' flour (Triticum) in war-time conditions of poor nutrition was said to be the cause of Riehl's melanosis (Arzt 1948, Kerl 1921, Riehl 1917, Reiches 1953). The food was thought to form a skin photosensitiser. A preponderance in women is difficult to explain on the basis of endogenous causes. The effects of sunlight were generally agreed.

References

Arzt, L. (1948) Weiterer Beitrag zur "Melanosis Riehl". Wien. klin. Wchnschr. 60, 594.

Kerl, W. (1921) Über die "Melanose (Riehl)". Arch. Dermat. u. Syph. 130, 436.

Reiches, A.J. (1953) Occupational melanosis. Arch. Derm. Syph. 67, 616.

Riehl, G. (1917) Über eigenartige Malanose. Wien. Klin. Wchnschr. 30, 780.

In the Balkan countries, it was the practice to catch bed-bugs on Phaseolus leaves, the insect's legs being impaled on the hooked epidermal hairs (Richardson 1943).

Reference

Richardson, H.H. (1943) The action of bean leaves against the bed-bug. J. Econ. Entomol. 36, 543.

Sub-family Lotoideae (Papilionoideae)

Tribe Phaseoleae

Physostigma

Five species are native to tropical Africa.

Physostigma venenosum

Ordeal Bean

Physostigmine (eserine), derived from the seeds and used medicinally can produce allergic contact dermatitis, keratitis (Duke-Elder 1965) and depigmentation of the eyelids (Jacklin 1965).

References

Duke-Elder, S. (1965) System of Ophthalmology. Vol. VIII. Diseases of the Outer eye. Part I. Allergic kerato-conjunctivitis. pp. 451. London. Henry Kimpton.

Jacklin, H.N. (1965) Depigmentation of the eyelids in eserine allergy. Amer. J. Ophthal. 59, 89.

Sub-family Mimosoideae

Tribe Adenanthereae

Piptadeniastrum

One species is native to tropical Africa.

Piptadeniastrum africanum

(syn. Piptadenia africana)

Dabema, Dahoma, Agboin

The wood dust is irritant to the eyes, nose and throad (MacKenna and Horner 1954, Irvine 1961, Thiebault 1965, Hausen 1970).

The freshly sawn wood has an ammoniacal smell which disappears when the wood is seasoned.

References

Hausen, B.M. (1970) Untersuchungen über Gesundheitsschädigende Hölzer. Thesis, Hamburg.

Irvine, F.R. (1961) Woody Plants of Ghana. Oxford University Press. London.

Thiebault, A. (1965) Nomenclature Generale des Bois Tropicaux. L' Association Technique Internationale des Bois Tropicaux. 45 bis Avenue de la Belle-Gabrielle, Nogent-sur Marne, France.

MacKenna, R.M.B. and Horner, S. (1954) Occupational skin diseases in Industrial Medicine and Hygiene. ed. Merewether, E.R.A. London. Butterworth.

Sub-family Lotoideae (Papilionoideae)

Tribe: Lonchocarpeae

Piscidia

Ten species are native to Florida, Mexico and the West Indies.

Piscidia erythrina

West Indian Dogwood

The wood is said to be irritant (Schwartz et al 1957) and to be toxic to humans (Lewin 1962).

The wood is used as a fish poison.

Reference

Schwartz, L., Tulipan, L. and Birmingham, D.J. (1957) Occupational Diseases of the Skin. 3rd. ed. Philadelphia. Lea and Febiger. pp. 637-672.

Lewin, L. (1962) Gifte und Vergiftungen. Ulm, Haug.

Sub-family Lotoideae (Papilinoideae)

Tribe Vicieae

Pisum

Six species are native to the Mediterranean region and western Asia.

Pisum sativum

Garden Pea

Men employed in unloading sacks of peas suffered parasitic bites (Hudelo and Dumet 1924). Absorption of water by ingested dried peas can lead to intestinal obstruction (Cleland 1931).

References

Cleland, J.B. (1931) Plants including fungi, poisonous and otherwise injurious to man in Australia III. Med.J.Australia 2, 775.

Hudelo and Dumet (1924) Dermatosis from the bites of pediculoides ventricosus in grain loaders. Bull. Soc. franc. Derm. Syph. 31, 405.

Asthma from green peas is noted under Spinacia.

Sub-family Mimosoideae

Tribe Ingeae

Pithecellobium

(syn. Pithecolobium)

200 species are found in tropical regions. Several species have been reported to cause mechanical injury by their thorns.

Pithecellobium arboreum

Bahama sabicu,
Black Tamarind

According to Woods and Calnan (1976) the identification of the angelim (partridge wood), which produced irritation, as Pithecolobium (Freise 1932) is improbable. Lysiloma is also known as sabicu.

The wood dust can cause dermatitis (Garratt 1922).

Pithecellobium dulce

Madras Thorn,
Manila Tamarind

The bark is irritant to the eye and the sap can irritate the skin (Morton 1962). The pulp around the seeds is said to be edible (Corner 1952); the root-shoots and seedlings are as thorny as barbed wire (Morton 1962).

Pithecellobium ellipticum

The tree, in Malaysia, usually harbours the nests of red ants (Corner 1952).

Pithecellobium filicifolium

The wood is said to produce dermatitis (Schwartz et al 1957).

Pithecellobium saman

This species is a 'rain-tree' of South America (Meninger 1967). 'Rain trees' are discussed under Acer.

References

Corner, E.J.H. (1952) Wayside Trees of Malaysia. Singapore, Government Printer.

Garratt, G.A. (1922) Poisonous woods. J. Forestry 20, 479.

Menninger, E.A. (1967) Fantastic Trees. New York. The Viking Press.

Morton, J.F. (1962) Ornamental Plants with Poisonous Properties II. Proc. Florida Hort. Soc. 75, 484.

Schwartz, L., Tulipan, L. and Birmingham, D.J. (1957) Occupational Diseases of the Skin. 3rd ed. Philadelphia. Lea and Febiger. pp. 637-672.

Freise, F.W. (1932) Gesundheitsschädigungen durch Arbeiten mit giftigen Hölzern. Beobachtungen aus brasilianischen Gewerbebetrieben. Archiv für Gewerbepathologie und Gewerbehygiene 3, 1.

Woods, B. and Calnan, C.D. (1976) Toxic Woods. Brit. J. Derm. 94, Suppl. 13, June.

Sub-family Mimosoideae

Tribe Adenanthereae

Plathymenia

Three species native to Brazil and Argentina provide good timber.

Plathymenia reticulata

Vinhatico

Vinhatico was reported to cause dermatitis in woodworkers (De Carvalho 1956).

Respiratory irritation from this wood may have been incorrectly attributed to Echirospermum.

Reference

DeCarvalho, L.P. (1956) Dos alergenos de contato nas profissoes. Brasil-med 70, 77.

Sub-family Mimosoideae

Tribe Adenanthereae

Prosopis

40 species are found in warm America, one in tropical Africa and two from the Caucasus to India. Some are xerophytic, without leaves; many are thorny.

The pollen can cause hayfever (Wodehouse 1971).

Reference

Wodehouse, R.P. (1971) Hayfever Plants. 2nd rev. edition. New York, Hafner.

Prosopis africana

An irritant alkaloid is present in the leaves (Hausen 1970).

Reference

Hausen, B.M. (1970) Untersuchungen über Gesundheitsschädigende Hölzer. Thesis, Hamburg.

Prosopis juliflora

var. glandulosa Mesquite

The wood used in the fire-place produced dermatitis in a farmer (Fox 1941) and a man who worked with the seasoned wood developed dermatitis (Stewart 1940). Patch tests produced positive reactions but controls were not recorded. Shelmire (1940) observed dermatitis from the wood.

Mesquite gum (Sonora gum) has irritant properties (Behl et al 1966). The wax on the thorn, if it penetrates the eye, is responsible for severe damage (Brunner and Bieberdorf 1950).

Prosopis spicigera

A kino gum from the tree is irritant (Behl et al 1966).

References

Behl, P.N., Captain, R.M., Bedi, B.M.S. and Gupta, S. (1966) Skin-irritant and sensitizing plants found in India, New Delhi. P.N. Behl, Irwin Hospital.

Brunner, H. and Bieberdorf, F.W. (1950) The effects of the mesquite thorn on the human eye. Trans. Am. Acad. Opthal. 54, 595.

Fox, E.C. (1941) Mesquite wood dermatitis. Arch. Derm. Syph. 44, 1098.

Shelmire, B. (1940) Contact dermatitis from vegetation. South Med. J. 33, 338.

Stewart, C.D. (1940) Mesquite wood dermatitis. Arch. Derm. Syph. 42, 937.

Sub-family Lotoideae (Papilionoideae)

Tribe Psoralieae

Psoralea

130 species are found in tropical and sub-tropical regions. P. esculenta of North America (Prairie turnip) has an edible tuberous root. P. decumbens is used in Africa for a tea.

Chemistry is recorded by Dean (1963) and Harborne et al (1971). The plant yields psoralen (Pathak et al 1962).

References

Dean, F.M. (1963) Naturally occurring oxygen ring compounds. London. Butterworth.

Harborne, J.B., Boulter, D. and Turner, B.L. (1971) Chemotaxonomy of the Leguminosae. London. Academic Press.

Pathak, M.A., Daniels, F., Jr. and Fitzpatrick, T.B. (1962) Presently known distribution of furocoumarins (Psoralens) in plants. J. Invest. Derm. 39, 225.

Psoralea corylifolia

Bavachee

The plant has been used for a phototoxic effect in the treatment of vitiligo since about 1400 B.C. (Pathak et al 1971, Behl et al 1966, Singh et al 1974). The seeds are currently so used but can cause severe reactions (Behl et al 1966).

References

Behl, P.N., Captain, R.M., Bedi, B.M.S. and Gupta, S. (1966) Skin-irritant and sensitizing plants found in India, New Delhi. P.N. Behl, Irwin Hospital.

Pathak, M.Z., Toda, K. and Fitzpatrick, T.B. (1971) Psoralens and cutaneous photosensitisation. Scientific Exhibit. American Academy of Dermatology. Chicago. December.

Singh, G., Ansari, Z. and Dvivedi, R.N. (1974) Vitiligo in Ancient Indian Medicine. Arch. Derm. 109, 913.

Psoralea

Addition of water to a vehicle containing methoxsalen enhanced the phototoxic activity of the compound (Suhonen 1976).

Reference

Suhonen, R. (1976) Phototoxicity of methoxsalen in various vehicles. Contact Dermatitis 2, 264.

Sub-family Lotoideae (Papilionoideae)

Tribe Pterocarpeae

Pterocarpus

100 species are found in tropical regions. Several provide kino, astringent resins (Dalziel 1937, Irvine 1961). Some provide red dyes. One such, Saunders Red (Merck 1968) is used to colour Tincture of Lavender (Lavandula) (Wren 1968). Tincture Kino was formerly officinal.

Pterocarpus sp. Padouk

Nestler (1924, 1926) found that an ether extract of padouk, possibly P. indicus, caused irritation of his skin in less than 2 hours. The wood dust can produce dermatitis (Zafiropoulo et al 1968). The chemistry was studied by Bevan (1958).

The flavanoid and neoflavanoid constituents of Pterocarpus spp. and Dalbergia spp. were reviewed by Seshadri (1972).

Pterocarpus angolensis

Muninga, Keejat, African Teak, Sealing Wax Tree

The wood dust can cause dermatitis and respiratory symptoms, (Schweisheimer 1952, Timber Technology 1957, Ordman 1949). One of Ordman's two patients was also affected by Thuja plicata and by a Congo hardwood identified by Schweisheimer (1951) as Lovoa klaineana. A young woman packed the sawdust into her vagina to make her husband 'hot' (Watt and Breyer-Brandwijk 1962).

Pterocarpus indicus

Angsana

Lignum nephriticum, a remedy of earlier times, was derived from this species (Burgess 1966). The wood dust is listed as a cause of dermatitis (Hanslian and Kadlec 1966).

Pterocarpus santalinus

Ceylon mahogany, possibly this species, caused conjunctival irritation and vomiting (Hausen 1970).

Artocarpus intergrifolia had also been called Ceylon Mahogany.

Refernces

Bevan, C.W.L. (1958) Wood extractives. West Afr.J.Biol. Chem. 2, 36.

Hausen, B.M. (1970) Untersuchungen über Gesundheitsschädigende Hölzer. Thesis, Hamburg.

Nestler, A. (1924) Hautreizende Hölzer. Umschau 28, 1007.

Nestler, A. (1926) Die hautreizende Wirkung des sogenannten 'Padouk-Holzes'. Planta (Archiv für wissenschaftliche Botanica) 2, 537, cited by Woods and Calnan (1976).

Schweisheimer, W. (1952) Wood dust and respiratory diseases. Wood 17, 181.

Woods, B. and Calnan, C.D. (1976) Toxic Woods. Brit. J. Derm. 94, Suppl. 13, June.

Burgess, P.F. (1966) Timbers of Sabah. (Sabah Forest Records, No. 6). Sabah, Malaysia. The Forest Dept.

Dalziel, J.M. (1937) The Useful Plants of West Tropical Africa. London. Crown Agents.

Hanslian, L. and Kadlec, K. (1966) Wood from the standpoint of hygiene VII. Species with a highly aggressive biological effect. Drevo. 21, 157.

Irvine, F.R. (1961) Woody plants of Ghana. Oxford University Press. London.

Merck Index (1968) An Encyclopedia of Chemicals and Drugs. ed. Stecher, P.G. 8th ed. Rahway, N.J. Merck and Co. Inc.

Ordman, D. (1949) Bronchial asthma caused by inhalation of wood dust. Ann. Allergy. 7, 492.

Ordman, D. (1949) Wood dust as an inhalant allergen. South Afric. med. J. 23, 972.

Schweisheimer, W. (1952) Wood dust and respiratory diseases. Wood 17, 181.

Timber Technology (1957) Wood dust and the wood worker. (Editorial) 65, 205.

Watt, J.M. and Breyer-Brandwijk, M.G. (1962) The Medicinal and poisonous plants of Southern Africa. 2nd ed. Edinburgh. E. & S. Livingstone.

Wren, R.W. (1968) Potter's New Cyclopaedia of Botanical Drugs and Preparations by Wren, R.C. Re-edit by Wren, R.W. Potter and Clarke, Ltd. Health Science Press. Rustington, Sussex.

Zafiropoulo, A., Audibert, A. and Charpin, J. (1968) A propos des accidents dus a la manipulation des bois exotiques. Rev. Franc. Allerg. 8, 155.

Seshadri, T.R. (1972) Polyphenols of Pterocarpus and Dalbergia woods. Phytochemistry. 11, 881.

Sub-family Lotoideae (Papilionoideae)

Tribe Robineae

Robinia

20 species are native to eastern North America and Mexico.

Robinia pseudacacia

False Acacia, Locust

The blossom, which yields a volatile oil, has been used as a condiment (Watt and Breyer-Brandwijk 1962). The bark is poisonous and the plant, when used for fodder, is said to produce stomatitis in animals. The honey is said to be toxic. Chinese people who drank a concoction of the plant were said to develop rigors and swelling of the subcutaneous tissues especially of the extremities. The plant yields an allergenic toxalbumin, robin. Some discrepancies in the literature are discussed by Watt and Breyer-Brandwijk (1962) and Kingsbury (1964). The plant emits biologically active volatile emanations (Morton 1971). Dubreuilh (1931) and Schulmann and Detouillon (1932) refer to dermatitis from the wood as a cause of woodcutter's eczema (now recognized as caused by lichens and Frullania). Woods and Calnan (1976) refer to fearsome thorns of the plant disliked by the woodman. Hausen (1970) notes reports by Wagenfuhr (1961, 1967). Heliotropin derived from the plant has been reported to cause contact dermatitis (Greenberg and Lester 1954).

Robinia zambesica

The plant is reported to cause 'schleimhaut-reizung' (Codd cited by Hausen 1970).

References

Codd, L.E.W. (1951) Trees and shrubs of the Kruger National Park. Bot.

Surv. Mem. 26, 1. Pretoria.

Dubreuilh, W. (1931) L'eczéma des boucherons. Ann. Derm. 2, 199.

Greenberg, L.A. and Lester, D. (1954) Handbook of Cosmetic Materials. New York. Interscience.

Hausen, B.M. (1970) Untersuchungen über Gesundheitsschädigende Hölzer. Thesis, Hamburg.

Kingsbury, J.M. (1964) Poisonous Plants of the United States and Canada. Englewood Cliffs, New Jersey. Prentice-Hall Inc.

Morton, J.F. (1971) Plants Poisonous to People in Florida and other warm areas. Miami. Florida. Hurricane House Publishers Inc.

Schulmann, E. and Detouillon, P. (1932) L'eczéma du bois et la sensibilisation sylvestre. Paris med. 83, 55.

Wagenfuhr, R. (1961) Gift es giftige Holzer? Mobel u. Wohnr. 4, 120.

Wagenfuhr, R. (1967) Kann Holz giftig sein? Wiss. Fortschr. 6, 279.

Watt, J.M. and Breyer-Brandwijk, M.G. (1962) The Medicinal and poisonous plants of Southern Africa. 2nd ed. Edinburgh. E. & S. Livingstone.

Woods, B. and Calnan, C.D. (1976) Toxic Woods. Brit. J. Derm. 94, Suppl. 13, June.

Pseudacacia zambesica

A report concerning this wood is noted under Robinia (p. 426).

Sub-family Mimosoideae

Tribe Ingeae

Samanea

20 species are native to regions from Mecixo to tropical South America and to tropical Africa.

Samanea dinklagei

(syn. Cathormion)

The dry sawdust is irritant to the respiratory tract (Dalziel 1937).

The bark is pounded and used as soap suggesting the presence of saponins.

Reference

Dalziel, J.M. (1937) The Useful Plants of West Tropical Africa. London. Crown Agents.

Sub-family Caesalpiniodeae

Tribe Casealpinieae

Schotia

18 species are native to tropical and southern Africa.

Schotia brachypetala

The wood-dust is said to irritate the eyes (Watt and Breyer-Brandwijk 1962).

Reference

Watt, J.M. and Breyer-Brandwijk, M.G. (1962) The Medicinal and poisonous plants of Southern Africa. 2nd ed. Edinburgh. E. & S. Livingstone.

Sub-family Lotoideae (Papilionoideae)

Tribe Sophoreae

Sophora

50 species are found in tropical and warm temperate regions.

Sophora spp.

The seeds contain cytisins (see Cytisus and Laburnum) and related alkaloids (Briggs 1946).

Sophora japonica

Pagoda tree

The bark has a strong smell which affects those who prune it. Four turners had colic and diarrhoea after working with freshly cut wood but the dry wood is said to be harmless (Hamel 1811, Loudon 1844).

Sophora tetraptera

Kowhai

The wood is listed as

injurious from a content of alkaloid (Hausen 1970). Two persons who ate from spoons made of kowhai wood became seriously ill (Aston 1923). The bark is intensely bitter.

Sophora tomentosa
Silver Bush

The plant which has been used in Chinese Medicine as a haemostatic since ancient times yields rutin (Vitamin P), (Kariyone 1971).

References

Hausen, B.M. (1970) Unterschungen über Gesundheitsschädigende Hölzer. Thesis, Hamburg.

Kariyone, T. (1971) Atlas of Medicinal Plants. Osaka, Japan. Takeda Chemical Industries.

Aston, B.C. (1923) The poisonous, suspected and medicinal plants of New Zealand. New Zealand J. Agric. 26,78 and 149.

Briggs, L.H. (1946) Plant products of New Zealand. J. Proc. Roy. Soc. New South Wales 80, 151.

Du Hamel, H. L. (1811-1816) Traité des Arbres et Arbustes qui se cultivent en France et pleine Terre. Paris, Michel. New edition cited by Woods and Calnan (1976).

Loudon, J.C. (1844) Arboretum et Fructicetum Britannicum. 2nd ed. London, Longman cited by Woods and Calnan (1976).

Woods, B. and Calnan, C.D. (1976) Toxic Woods. Brit. J. Derm. 94, Suppl. 13, June.

Sub-family Caesalpiniodeae

Tribe Swartzieae

Swartzia

100 species are found in tropical America and Africa.

Swartzia sp.

The colloquial name muirapixuna is also used for Caesalpinia paraensis.

Swartzia madagascariensis

Dermatitis from the wood was reported to Orsler (1973).

Swartzia tomentosa

The wood dust is said to produce dermatitis (Lewin 1928).

References

Hausen, B.M. (1970) Untersuchungen über Gesundheitsschädigende Hölzer. Thesis, Hamburg.

Lewin, L. (1928) Gifte in Holzgewerbe. Beiträge zur Giftkunde. Heft. 1 Berlin. Stilke cited by Hausen (1970)

Orsler, R.J. (1973) Personal communication from Forest Products Research Laboratory, Princess Risborough, Bucks, England.

Sub-family Caesalpiniodeae

Tribe Amherstieae

Tamarindus

One species is native to tropical Africa.

Tamarindus indica
Tamarind

The tree was cultivated in Ancient Egypt for its fruits and is widely distributed in the tropics.

The pulp around the seeds is eaten. The powdered dry leaf has a caustic effect. The bark is astringent. Ground tamarind seed, used as a sizing for cloth can cause asthma (Murray et al 1957). A textile worker developed dermatitis from the flour (Cirla et al 1970).

References

Cirla, A.M., Nava, C. and Limonta, A. (1970) A case of occupational allergy to tamarind flour. Med. Lav. 61, 447.

Murray, R., Dingwall-Fordyce, I. and Lane, R.E. (1957) An outbreak of Weaver's cough associated with tamarind seed powder. Brit. J. Industr. Med. 14, 105.

Sub-family Lotoideae (Papilionoideae)

Tribe Galegeae

Tephrosia

300 species are found in tropical and subtropical regions.

Tephrosia virginiana

The crude plant preparation or rotenone derived from it may cause dermatitis, conjunctivitis and rhinitis (Thienes and Haley 1972).

Tephrosia vogelii

Fish Poison Plant

The people wading in the poisoned water to drive or catch the fish, generally complain of deadness in the legs or roughness of the skin (Dalziel 1937).

The leaves of this plant and the roots of T. toxicaria yield deguelin which can cause skin irritation; the chemistry is given by Merck (1968). Deguelin is also derived from Derris, Leguminosae.

References

Dalziel, J.M. (1937) The Useful Plants of West Tropical Africa. London. Crown Agents.

Merck, Index (1968) An Encyclopedia of Chemicals and Drugs. ed. Stecher, P.G. 8th ed. Rahway, N.J. Merck and Co. Inc.

Thienes, C.H. and Haley, T.J. (1972) Clinical Toxicology. 5th ed. Philadelphia. Lea and Febiger.

Sub-family Caesalpinioideae

Tribe Amherstieae

Trachylobium

One species, found in tropical east Africa, Madagascar and Mauritius, yields copal resin, which is dug up from the soil near the roots or in a half-fossilised condition from places where trees once existed.

Copal is derived from this tree and from Hymenaea courbaril, Leguminosae. Copal is known as resin copal, gum copal, animé (soft copal), kaurie or cowrie and occurs as hard or soft copal (Merck 1968).

The chemistry is given by Merck (1968). Hypersensitivity has been reported and dermatitis occurs in its use in manufacture (Greenberg and Lester 1954, Ferrand et al 1937, Schwartz et al 1957).

References

Ferrand, M., Rabeau, H. and Ukrainczyk (1937) Intolérance aux résines chez un artiste peintre. Tests cutanés. Bull. Soc. Franc. Derm. Syph. 44, 77.

Greenberg, L.A. and Lester, D. (1954) Handbook of Cosmetic Materials. New York. Interscience.

Merck Index (1968) An Encyclopedia of Chemicals and Drugs. ed. Stecher, P.G. 8th ed. Rahway, N.J. Merck and Co. Inc.

Schwartz, L., Tulipan, L. and Birmingham, D.J. (1957) Occupational Diseases of the Skin. 3rd ed. Philadelphia. Lea & Febiger.pp. 637-672.

Trachylopium hornemannianum

This species furnishes a copal resin which is dug from the remains of trees long dead. A variety of plants yield copals e.g. Agathis, Bursera, Canarium, Copaifera, and Hymenaea, (Usher 1954).

Contact sensitivity to copal has been reported (Ferrand et al 1937) and dermatitis can occur in workers in its manufacture (Schwartz et al 1947).

References

Ferrand, M., Rabeau, H. and Ukrainczyk (1937) Intolérance aux résines chez un artiste peintre. Tests cutanés. Bull. Soc. franc. Derm. Syph. 44, 77.

Schwartz, L., Tulipan, L. and Peck, S.M. (1947) Occupational Diseases of the Skin. Philadelphia. Lea & Febiger.

Usher, G. (1974) A Dictionary of Plants used by Man. London. Constable.

Sub-family Lotoideae (Papilionoideae)

Tribe Trifolieae

Trifolium

300 species are found in temperate land subtropical areas (not South East Asia or Australia).

Trifolium spp.

Clover, Trefoil, Shamrock

Trifoliosis or Bighead, a photosensitivity syndrome in animals which occurs from eating Trifolium spp. is reviewed by Kingsbury (1964), Watt and Breyer-Brandwijk (1962). Whether photosensitization by alsike, Trifolium hybridum, is primary or hepatogenous is not clear. The skin surfaces most likely to show the effects of photosensitivity are those which contact moisture when the animals are at pasture, namely the muzzle and the feet; for this reason, the disorder has been known as 'dew poisoning'. Stomatitis and ulceration of the tongue, i.e. sites not exposed to light, can also occur. In Australia the condition has been known as Aphis poisoning but it is not due to ingestion of this parasite but results from photosensitization due to the ingestion of compounds present in Trifolium. For photosensitivity see also Tribulus. Clover is also a common name for Melilotus.

Trifolium arvense

Rabbit-Foot Clover

Mechanical injury can occur from the hairy calyx on ingestion by animals, forming together with other objects, 'hair balls' (phytobezoars) (Muenscher 1951).

Trifolium hybridum

Alsike Clover

This species grows naturalized by roadsides throughout the British Isles; contains photosensitising agents. See also Trifolium spp. Ingestion of the plant causes photodermatitis in animals (Mathews 1937, Watt and Breyer-Brandwijk 1962), see also Medicago. According to Mathews (1937), Edwards (1941) and Muenscher (1951) contact with this plant can cause photodermatitis in man; according to Hardin and Arena (1969) contact with the leaves can cause dermatitis. The listing of this plant as a cause of dermatitis by Gardner and Bennetts (1956) in Australia gives no details.

Trifolium incarnatum

Crimson Clover

The hairy inflorescences form phytobezoars (Hurst 1942). Mechanical injury by hairy calyx can occur (Muenscher 1951).

Trifolium pratense

Red Clover

This species is reported to cause 'urticaria or skin irritation' without clinical details (Gardner and Bennetts 1956). The flowers are used in a plaster in Herbal Medicine (Wren 1968).

Trifolium repens

White Clover

Hjorth (1968) recorded 0 positive patch tests from this plant. The plant is thought to favour the formation of phytobezoars. Some strains of the plant contain a cyanogenetic glucoside which has goitrogenic effects for animals on ingestion; the presence of this compound and its relevant enzyme is genetically determined and a non-cyanogenetic strain has been evolved (Watt and Breyer-Brandwijk 1962).

References

Edwards, J.K. (1941) Proc. S. Dakota Acad. Sci. 21, 22, quoted by Watt and Breyer-Brandwijk (1962).

Gardner, C.A. and Bennetts, H.W. (1956) The Toxic Plants of Western Australia. Perth West. Australian Newspapers Ltd.

Hardin, J.W. and Arena, J.M. (1969) Human Poisoning from native and cultivated plants. Durham, North Carolina. Duke University Press.

Hjorth, N. (1968) at Finsen Institute. Pers. Comm.

Hurst, E. (1942) The Poison Plants of New South Wales. N.S.W. Poison Plants Committee; Sydney.

Kingsbury, J.M. (1964) Poisonous Plants of the United States and Canada. Englewood Cliffs, New Jersey. Prentice-Hall Inc.

Mathews, F.P. (1937) Photosensitisation and the photodynamic diseases of man and the lower animals. Arch. Path. 23, 399.

Muenscher, W.C. (1951) Poisonous plants of the United States. 2nd ed. New York. The MacMillan Co.

North, P.M. (1967) Poisonous Plants and Fungi in Colour. London. Blandford Press. Ltd.

Watt, J.M. and Breyer-Brandwijk, M.G. (1962) The Medicinal and poisonous plants of Southern Africa. 2nd ed. Edinburgh. E. & S. Livingstone.

Wren, R.W. (1968) Potter's New Cyclopaedia of Botanical Drugs and Preparations by Wren, R.C. Re-edit by Wren, R.W. Potter and Clarke Ltd. Health Science Press. Rustington, Sussex.

Sub-family Lotoideae (Papilionoideae)

Tribe Trifolieae

Trigonella

135 species are found in the Mediterranean region, Europe, Asia, South Africa and Australia.

Trigonella foenum-graecum

Fenugreek

The plant is used as an ingredient in curry-powders and to perfume butter (Watt and Breyer-Brandwijk 1962). A principal constituent is anethole (Fenaroli 1971). Anethole is the chief constituent of Oil of Anise (Pimpinella or Illicium) and Oil of Fennel (Foeniculum). A case of sensitivity (stomatitis) due to a denture cream containing Oil of Anise which was 90% anethole has been reported (Loveman 1938).

References

Fenaroli, G. (1971) Fenaroli's Handbook of Flavor Ingredients ed. Furia, T.E. and Bellanca, N. Cleveland, Ohio. The Chemical Rubber Co.

Loveman, A.B. (1938) Stomatitis venenata. Report of a case of sensitivity of the mucous membranes and the skin to oil of anise. Arch. Derm. Syph. 37, 70.

Watt, J.M. and Breyer-Brandwijk, M.G. (1962) The Medicinal and poisonous plants of Southern Africa. 2nd ed. Edinburgh. E. & S. Livingstone.

Sub-family Lotoideae (Papilionoideae)

Tribe Pterocarpeae

Vatairea

Seven species are found in tropical South America.

Vatairea araroba

(syn. Andira)

Yields the compounds noted under V. guianensis (Simatupang et al 1967).

Vatairea guianensis

Quassia, partridge wood

The wood caused dermatitis and conjunctivitis when imported into Germany among some other South American timbers (Simatupang et al 1967). The wood contains chrysophanic acid and physcion and their anthranols which are irritant, see Andira.

Vatairea lundelli

Yields chrysophanic acid (Simatupang et al 1967).

Reference

Simatupang, M.H., Dietrichs, H.H. and Gottwald, H. (1967) Uber die hautreizenden Stoffe in Vatairea guinanensis Aubl. Holzforschung 21, 89.

Sub-family Lotoideae (Papilionoideae)

Tribe Dalbergieae

Vataireopsis

Three species are found in Brazil.

<u>Vataireopsis araroba</u>

Angelim amarello

(syn. <u>Andira araroba</u>)

The sawdust irritates the eyes of workmen (Record and Hess 1943). The bark and the wood are the source of goa powder from which chrysarobin is derived (see <u>Andira</u>).

<u>Reference</u>

Record, S.J. and Hess, R.W. (1943) Timbers of the New World. New Haven, Yale.

Sub-family Lotoideae (Papilionoideae)

Tribe Vicieae

<u>Vicia</u>

150 species are found in North temperate and South America.

<u>Vicia faba</u>

Broad-Bean (has many cultivated variants)

Favism is an acute disorder resulting either from the ingesting of the broad bean or the inhalation of its pollen, resulting in an acute haemolytic anaemia and acute hepatitis (Watt and Breyer-Brandwijk 1962). The disorder is genetically determined as a glucose-6-phosphate dehydrogenase deficiency (Kingsbury 1964). Symptoms may appear within minutes after inhalation of the pollen or after 5 - 24 hours after eating the bean.

<u>Vicia sativa</u>

Common Vetch, Tare

This species contains a photosensitising principle (North 1967).

<u>References</u>

Kingsbury, J.M. (1964) Poisonous Plants of the United States and Canada. Englewood Cliffs, New Jersey. Prentice-Hall Inc.

North, P.M. (1967) Poisonous Plants and Fungi in Colour. London. Blandford Press Ltd.

Watt, J.M. and Breyer-Brandwijk, M.G. (1962) The Medicinal and poisonous plants of Southern Africa. 2nd ed. Edinburgh. E. & S. Livingstone.

Sub-family Lotoideae (Papilionoideae)

Tribe Phaseoleae

<u>Vigna</u>

80 - 100 species are found especially in Africa and Asia.

<u>Vigna ungiculata</u>

(<u>V. sinensis</u>)

Horse Gram, Cherry-Bean. Cow-Pea, Garter Plant

This plant of tropical Asia forms pods which are eaten like French beans or used as horse or cattle-fodder. Dermatitis reported from this plant is probably due to the batata louse (<u>Trombiculum</u> species), (Simons 1952).

<u>Reference</u>

Simons, R.D.G. (1952) Handbook of Tropical Dermatology. New York. Elsevier.

Sub-family Caesalpinioideae

Tribe Sclerolobieae

<u>Vouacapoua americana</u>

(<u>Andira</u>)

This species is listed as an irritant wood (causing dermatitis), (Orsler 1973).

A report of dermatitis from <u>V. americana</u> is listed under <u>Andira</u>.

<u>Reference</u>

Orsler, R.J. (1973) Personal communication from Forest Products Research Laboratory, Princess Risborough, Bucks, England.

Sub-family Papilionoideae

Tribe Galegeae

<u>Whitfordiodendron</u>

Nine species are found in Formosa, China and West Malaysia.

Whitfordiodendron sp.

This genus is very intimately related to Millettia. Some, like species of the latter genus, have irritant properties possibly for the skin (Burkill 1935).

Whitfordiodendron erianthum

The fruits are very acid (Burkill 1935).

Reference

Burkill, I.H. (1935) A Dictionary of the Economic Products of the Malay Peninsula. 2 Vols. London. Crown Agents for the Colonies.

Sub-family Lotoideae (Papilionoideae)

Tribe: Millettieae

Wisteria

Ten species are found in East Asia and East North America.

Wisteria sp.

McCord (1962) noted that an extract of this plant was available commercially for patch testing. Dermatitis from the plant has apparently not been reported.

Reference

McCord, C.P. (1962) The Occupational Toxicity of Cultivated Flowers. Ind. Med. Surg. 31, 365.

Sub-family Papilionoideae

Tribe Sophoreae

Xanthocercis

(syn. Pseudo-Acacia)

Two species are found in tropical east Africa and Madagascar.

Pseudo-Acacia zambesiaca

Nyala

Wood-workers may develop severe irritation of the nose and throat (Watt and Breyer-Brandwijk 1962).

The wood is a strong mucosal irritant (Codd 1951).

References

Codd, L.E.W. (1951) Trees and shrubs of the Kruger National Park. Pretoria, Department of Agriculture.

Watt, J.M. and Breyer-Brandwijk, M.G. (1962) The Medicinal and poisonous plants of Southern Africa. 2nd ed. Edinburgh. E. & S. Livingstone.

Sub-family Mimosoideae

Tribe Adenanthereae

Xylia (syn. Esclerona)

15 species are native to tropical Africa, Madagascar and tropical Asia. Some yield good timber.

Xylia dolabriformis

Pyinkado

This Phillipine wood is reported to be injurious (Heilig 1957).

Xylia xylocarpa

(syn. X. dolabriformis)

Pyinkado

The sawdust causes sneezing (Laslett 1894, Boulger 1908).

References

Hausen, B.M. (1970) Untersuchungen über Gesundheitsschädigende Hölzer. Thesis, Hamburg.

Heilig, P.M. (1957) Ziekten veroorzaakt door bewerking van. zekere houtscorten. Vakbl. moubelind 38, 1440, cited by Hausen (1970).

Boulger, G.S. (1908) Wood. 2nd ed. London, Arnold cited by Woods and Calnan (1976).

Laslett, T. (1894) Timber and timber trees. 2nd ed. p. 226. London, MacMillan, cited by Woods and Calnan (1976).

Woods, B. and Calnan, C.D. (1970) Toxic Woods. Brit. J. Derm. 94, Suppl. 13, June.

Sub-family Caesalpinioideae

Tribe Swartzieae

Zollernia

Ten species are found in central and tropical South America.

Zollernia paraensis

This Brazilian species is listed as a wood that can produce dermatitis by Hanslian and Kadlec (1966). Hausen (1970) cited Friese (1932) for a report of dermatitis from the wood.

References

Friese, F.W. (1932) Gesundheitsschädigungen durch Arbeiten mit giftigen Hölzern. Arch. Gewerbepath-hyg. 3, 1.

Hanslian, L. and Kadlec, K. (1966) Wood from the standpoint of hygiene (VIII). Species with some or little biological effect. Drevo. 21, 229.

Hausen, B.M. (1970) Untersuchungen über Gesundheitsschädigende Hölzer. Thesis, Hamburg.

LEMNACEAE

40 species in four genera are cosmopolitan water-plants. The family is related to Araceae.

Lemna minor

Ill-defined possibly irritant properties are ascribed to this species (Smith 1969).

References

Smith, F.P. (1969) Chinese Materia Medica. Vegetable kingdom. 2nd ed. Rev. by Hei, P.D. Taipei, Taiwan. Ku T'ing Book House.

Wolffia

10 species are found in tropical and temperate regions. W. arrhiza is the smallest known flowering plant.

Wolffia arrhiza

Water infested with this plant has been strongly suspected of tainting coffee (Coffea) (Wild 1961).

Reference

Wild, H. (1961) Harmful aquatic plants in Africa and Madagascar. Kirkia 2, 1.

LEONTICACEAE

15 species in three genera are found in north temperate regions.

Caulophyllum

Two species are native to north-eastern Asia and North America.

Caulophyllum thalictroides
Blue Cohosh

The dust of the root is irritant to the mucous membranes (Lloyd). Reports of dermatitis from handling the root stock (Muenscher 1951, Weber 1937, etc.) apparently refer to this note.

References

Lloyd, cited by White (1887) Dermatitis venenata: An account of the Action of External irritants upon the Skin. Boston. Cupples & Hurd. Lloyd was a wholesale dealer in medicinal plants.

Muenscher, W.C. (1951) Poisonous plants of the United States. 2nd ed. New York. The Macmillan Co.

Weber, L.F. (1937) External causes of Dermatitis. A list of irritants. Arch. Derm. Syph. 35, 129.

LICHENS

Some 17,000 lichen species are distributed from the equator to the Arctic and Antarctic and from sea level to mountains. A lichen plant body is composed of an alga and a fungus, usually an Ascomycete. A classification of the fungi is provided by Ainsworth (1971) and of the algae by Ahmadjian (1967).

Chemistry is recorded by Asahina and Shibata (1954) and Culberson (1969). The unique chemicals generally known as 'lichen substances' e.g. usnic acid are derived from the fungi of lichens. Fungal isolates retain a capacity to produce them in culture (Ahmadjian and Reynolds 1961).

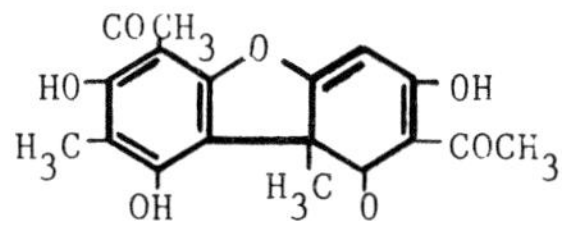

Usnic Acid

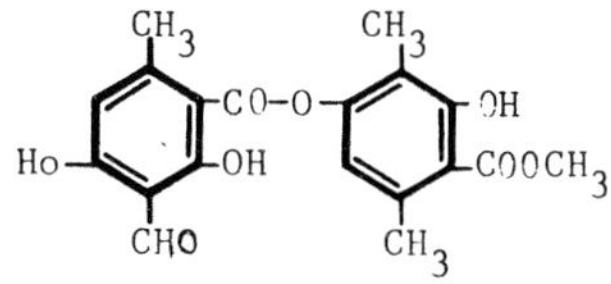

Atranorine

Woodcutter's eczema

Spillmann (1921) described dermatitis on the ear and side of the neck in a man who had carried freshly-cut oak logs on his shoulder. He suggested that fungi on the bark might be responsible. Tommasi (1929) reported similar cases from Italy and suspected an 'idiosyncrasy' because attacks often followed returning to work with wood. Dubreuilh (1931) described six cases of 'woodcutter's eczema' and emphasized the role of the bark. Schulmann and Détouillon (1932) distinguished between chronic lichenified eczema of the hands, perhaps due to resin, and acute 'sylvestro-sensibilization' of face, hands and genitals. Conjunctivitis was often associated with the dermatitis (Lagrange 1923).

Exposures to Oak (Quercus), beech (Fagus), chestnut (Castanea), poplar (Populus), acacia (Robinia), plane (Platanus), elm (Ulmus) and conifers could all produce dermatitis (Senear 1933). Tenchio (1948) then obtained positive patch tests with Parmelia caperata, found growing on the bark of firs (Abies), larches (Larix) and chestnuts (Castanea).

Ghillini (1954) reported dermatitis from the same lichen growing on oak (Quercus) and Ilex. LeCoulant and Lopès (1956) found that other lichens and mosses also contained the allergen, but much the strongest reactions were obtained with Frullania and other liverworts of the Jungermannales. These liverworts were found on the bark of most deciduous trees in South-western France, and on undergrowth and rocks even among conifers, on the bark of which lichens prevail. In their review LeCoulant et al (1966) concluded that liverworts were the main cause of woodcutter's eczema, and were in fact responsible for 2-4% of all contact dermatitis in that part of France. According to Philippe et al (1965) they also cause rhinitis, asthma and urticaria, with positive intradermal tests. Knoche et al (1969) showed that sesquiterpene lactones similar to those widespread in the Compositae were the sensitizers in Frullania tamarisci.

Mitchell (1965) investigated 'cedar-poisoning' in British Columbia lumbermen, obtaining positive patch tests with bark lichens and the usnic acid they contain, but negative results with the wood itself (Mitchell and Armitage 1965). Champion (1965) found similar usnic acid sensitivity in an English woodcutter's wife who had only indirect contact with ash bark through her husband's working clothes. Since then he has seen patients with contact sensitivity to lichens who did not react to usnic acid. Several atopic patients had exacerbations of eczema as well as rhinitis and asthma after contact with lichens and algae, especially on apple (Malus) trees. Three of them had positive patch tests with lichens (mainly Lecanora spp.), but algae gave only positive prick tests (Champion, 1971). Mitchell et al (1969) now consider that in America as in Europe Frullania is a more frequent cause of dermatitis than lichens, and have studied cross-sensitivity between liverworts and Compositae (Mitchell et al 1970, 1972).

References

Champion, R.H. (1965) Wood-cutter's Disease: Contact Sensitivity to Lichen. Brit. J. Dermat. 77, 285.

Champion, R.H. (1971) Atopic sensitivity to Algae and Lichens. Brit. J. Derm. 85, 551.

Dubreuilh, W. (1931) L'eczéma des bûcherons. Ann. Derm. Syph. 7, S.2, 199.

Ghillini, C.A. (1954) Un lichene causa di Allergosi cutanea. Rivista de Anatomia e Patologica. Oncologia 8, 755.

Knoche, H., Ourisson, G., Perold, G.W., Foussereau, J. and Maleville, J. (1969) Allergenic component of a liverwort: a sesquiterpene lactone. Science 166, 239.

Lagrange, H. (1923) Conjonctivite d'origine anaphylactique. Presse médicale 31, 112.

LeCoulant, P. and Lopes, G. (1956) Allergie aux lichens: recherches experimentales preliminaries, extraction d'un allergene a pouvoir antibiotic probable. J. Med. Bordeaux. 133, 869.

LeCoulant, M.P. et al (1966) L'allergie au *Frullania*: Son role dans la "Dermite du Bois de Chene". Bull. Soc. franc. Derm. Syph. 73, 440.

Mitchell, J.C. (1965) Allergy to Lichens. Archs. Derm. 92, 142.

Mitchell, J.C. and Armitage, J.S. (1965) Dermatitis Venenata from Lichens. Archs. Environ. Health 11, 701.

Mitchell, J.C., Scholfield, W.B., Singh, B. and Towers, G.H.N. (1969) Allergy to *Frullania*. Allergic contact dermatitis occurring in forest workers caused by exposure to *Frullania nisqualensis*. Archs. Derm. 100, 46.

Mitchell, J.C., Fritig, B., Singh, B. Towers, G.H.N. (1970) Allergic contact dermatitis from *Frullania* and Compositae. The role of sesquiterpene lactones. J. Invest. Derm. 54, 233.

Mitchell, J.C., Dupuis, G., Geissman, T.A. (1972) Allergic contact dermatitis from sesquiterpenoids of plants. Additional Allergic Sesquiterpene Lactones and Immunological specificity of Compositae, liverworts and lichens. Brit. J. Derm. 87, 235.

Philippe, J., Guibert, L. and Combes, R. (1965) Considérations sur les allergies sylvaines. Revue francaise d'Allergie 5, 95.

Schulmann, E. and Detouillon, P. (1932) L'eczema du bois et la sensibilisation sylvestre. Paris Med. 83, 55.

Senear, F.E. (1933) Dermatitis due to woods. JAMA 101, 1527.

Spillman, L. (1921) Artificial dermatitis due to the action with oak. Bull. Soc. franc. Derm. Syph. 6, 33.

Tenchio, F. (1948) Etiologie de l'eczema des bucherons, Dermatologica 97, 72.

Tommasi, L. (1929) Dermite dei boscaiuoli de ipersensibilita. Giornale italiano di Dermatologie. 70, 1223.

Alectoria, *Cetraria*, *Cladonia*, *Lecanora*, *Parmelia*, *Physica*, *Usnea* and *Xanthoria* species have been reported allergenic.

So-called 'cedar-poisoning' in Canada and 'pine-poisoning' in the north-west U.S.A. are principally due to occupational contact with epiphytes, lichens and *Frullania*. The dermatitis affects principally the exposed skin surfaces. Lichen substances, which were tested, were found to have no phototoxic activity (Mitchell 1966). Less obvious distribution patterns are found when lichens fall inside an open shirt and lodge at the waist-line or when the clothes are wetted by rain. Usnic acid is insoluble in water but is carried down from trees by rainwater and is present in soil, until degradation occurs.

Dermatitis occurring in woodworkers in Canada was found to be due to usnic acid present in *Usnea* spp. and other lichens present on trees (Mitchell 1965). d-Usnic acid was allergenic but l-usnic acid was inactive (Mitchell 1966). Some depsides of lichens viz. atranorine, evernic and perlatolic acids were also allergenic (Mitchell and Shibata 1969). Some individuals who are contact sensitive to lichens show negative patch test reactions to usnic acid (Champion 1971).

Contact dermatitis from lichens occurring in forest-workers is often accompanied by multiple specific sensitivity to *Frullania*

(Liverwort). The algae of lichens can produce Type I hypersensitivity reactions (Champion 1965), Algae. Opportunity for contact with lichens was discussed by Mitchell and Armitage (1965). Lichens are susceptible to air-pollution and tend to disappear from urban areas (LeBlanc 1961, Gilbert 1965) probably because they can accumulate extraneous chemicals (Smith 1962, Oddoze and Puissant 1963). Lichenized fungal spores and portions of the lichen body (thallus) can be air-borne (Petterrson 1940, Garrett 1971). Evernia prunastri (Oak Moss) is used in perfumery (Arctander 1960) and various lichens have been used for dyeing cloth (Bulletin 1935). Usnic acid is marketed as an antibiotic ointment (Mitchell 1966).

References

Ahmadjian, V. and Reynolds, J.T. (1961) Production of biologically active compounds by isolated lichenized fungi. Science 133, 700.

Ahmadjian, V. (1967) A guide to the algae occurring as lichen symbionts: isolation, culture, cultural physiology and identification. Phycologia 6, 127.

Ainsworth, G.C. (1971) Ainsworth and Bisby's Dictionary of the Fungi. 6th ed. Kew. Commonwealth Mycological Institute.

Arctander, S. (1960) Perfume and Flavor Materials of Natural Origin. Elizabeth, N.J. Publ. by author.

Asahina, Y. and Shibata, S. (1954) Chemistry of Lichen Substances. Tokyo. Japanese Society Promotion of Science.

Bulletin (1935) Home dyeing with natural dyes. Bull. 230. U.S. Dept. Agriculture.

Champion, R.H. (1971) Atopic sensitivity to algae and lichens. Brit. J. Derm. 85, 551.

Culbertson, C.F. (1969) Chemical and Botanical Guide to Lichen Products. Chapel Hill. Univ. Carolina Press.

Garrett, R.M. (1971) Studies on some aspects of ascospore liberation and dispersal in lichens. Lichenologist 5, 33.

Gilbert, O.L. (1965) Lichens as indicators of air pollution in the Tyne Valley in Ecology and the Industrial Society ed. Goodman G.T. et al. Oxford, Blackwell. p. 35.

LeBlanc, F. (1961) Influence de l'atmosphérè polluée des grandes agglomérations urbaines sur les épiphytes corticoles. Rev. Canada Biol. 20, 823.

Mitchell, J.C. (1965) Allergy to lichens. Archs. Derm. 92, 142.

Mitchell, J.C. and Armitage, S. (1965) Dermatitis venenata from lichens. Arch. Environ. Hlth. 11, 701.

Mitchell, J.C. (1966) Absence of psoralen-type phototoxicity from usnic acid, some lichens, and lichen substances. J. Invest. Derm. 47, 61.

Mitchell, J.C. (1966) Stereoisomeric specificity of usnic acid in delayed hypersensitivity. J. Invest. Derm. 47, 167.

Mitchell, J.C. and Shibáta, S. (1969) Immunological activity of some substances derived from lichenized fungi. J. Invest. Derm. 52, 517.

Oddoze, L. and Puissant, A. (1963) Of lichens, caribou, and tuna. Canad. Med. Ass. J. 88, 1038.

Petterrson, B. (1940) Experimentelle Untersuchungen über die evenemochore Verbreitung der Sporenflanzen. Acta. Bot. Fenn. 25, 1.

Usnea barbata

Resinoid Mousse de Chene produced positive patch test reactions in 2/10 patients who had perfume dermatitis (Novak 1974).

Evernia furfuracea

is known as Oak Moss.

Reference

Novak, M. (1974) Contact sensitisation to constituents of perfume composition in antiphlogistic ointment. Cs. Derm. 49, 375.

Two dealers in firewood developed contact dermatitis from the spores of Parmelia caperata on firewood logs (Leonardi 1954). Laria rufimana was implicated by Ciambellotti (1927, 1928).

References

Ciambellotti, E. (1927) Atti. R. Accad. Fisiocritici in Siena Series X, 2, 109 and Arch. Ital. di. Dermatol 3, 41 (1928) cited by Leonardi (1954).

Leonardi, G. (1954) Spore di lichens boschivo (Palmeria caperata) causa di allergosi cutanea. Folia Allerg 1, 219.

A patient who was contact sensitive to Evernia could not tolerate perfumes. Evernia enters into the composition of various perfumes (oak moss, cuir de Russie, Chypre type perfumes) (Favennec M.-J and Favennec, F. 1976).

Reference

Favennec, M.-J. and Favennec, F. (1976) Les maladies cutanes en agriculture. L'Ouest Médical 29(5), 395-402.

Favennec, F. (1974) Sensibilisation su Lichen, à la Candidine et a Frullania. L'Ouest Médical 27 (18) 1647.

Krauskopf, J. (1974) Phytodermatoses caused by lichens. Cesk Dermatol 49, 383.

Immediate hypersensitivity to lichens was reported by (Philippe et al 1965).

Reference

Philippe, J., Guibert, L. and Combes, R. (1965) Considérations sur les allergies sylvaines. Rev. Franc. Allerg. 5, 95.

LILIACEAE

This very large family containing about 3,700 species in 250 genera, is as a whole cosmopolitan, but certain groups are of limited distribution.

Very few of the Liliaceae are of economic importance, except for their ornamental qualities, but plants with outstanding horticultural merit such as autumn crocus, tulips and hyacinths belong to this family. Urginea, Colchicum, Aloe and Veratum are sources of drugs.

Because of the size of the family and the wide differences between different genera in their botanical properties and their influence on the skin, the genera are here considered separately and are arranged in alphabetical order rather than in accordance with their botanical affinities.

Chemistry

Slob, A. et al (1975) On the occurrence of tuliposides in the Liliiflorae. Phytochemistry 14, 1997. (Tuliposide, A. was detected in Erythronium, Tulipa, Gagea, Bomarea and Alstroemeria. alpha-methylene-gamma-butyrolactone is derived from tuliposide A.).

Agapanthus

Five species are native to southern Africa.

Agapanthus orientalis

African blue lily

The sticky acrid sap in the leaves can cause severe ulceration of the mouth (Aplin 1976).

Reference

Aplin, T.E.H. (1976) Poisonous garden plants and other plants harmful to man in Australia. Western Australian Dept. of Agriculture Bull. 3964.

Aloe

About 275 species are found in tropical and southern Africa, 42 in Madagascar, and 12-15 in Arabia, the Cape Verde Islands and India.

Aloes were long cultivated for their bitter sap, which was used medicinally (Flückiger and Hanbury 1874) and various species were introduced commercially to the Mediterranean region and the East and West Indies. Aloes are still used in medicine as a purgative. Powdered aloe leaf or its ash is a frequent ingredient of snuff in South Africa, but is suspected of carcinogenic effects on the paranasal sinuses

(Watt and Breyer-Brandwijk 1962).

Some species are decorative and are cultivated particularly for the beauty of their foliage, in the open where the climate is favourable, and under glass elsewhere.

The gelatinous material inside the leaf of *Aloë* sp. was recommended in ancient Herbals for the alleviation of inflammatory changes in the skin. More recently it has been advocated in the treatment of radiodermatitis (Wright 1936, Harry 1948, Gjerstad and Riner 1968) and of leg ulcers (El Zawahry et al 1973). However beneficial effects coult not be confirmed experimentally in rats (Rowe 1940).

Those most exposed to a dermatitis risk are those handling the drug in the pharmaceutical industry.

Chemistry

To obtain the drug aloe, the leaves are sliced and the sap is evaporated. Aloes consist of a variable mixture of aloin, aloe-emodin and other substances (Merck Index 1968). Aloin, an anthraquinone which was found in about half of one hundred species examined (McCarthy 1969) must be regarded as a potential sensitizer (Cronin 1968).

Dermatitis

In a case of allergic dermatitis caused by Aloes, the sensitizer was found to be emodin (Jadassohn 1926).

Two patients with contact dermatitis from Compound Tincture of Benzoin showed a positive patch test reaction to Tincture of Aloes and Tincture of Storax (Steiner and Leifer 1949). One of 18 patients sensitive to Balsam of Peru showed a positive patch test reaction to Aloes (Hjorth 1961).

The sharp tenticles on the leaf margin of species such as *Aloë ferox* are a source of mechanical injury.

References

Cronin, E. (1968) Studies in Contact Dermatitis. XVIII. Dyes in Clothing. Trans. a. Rep. St John's Hosp. derm. Soc. Lond. 54, 156.

El Zawahry, M., Hegazy, M.R. and Helal, M. (1973) Use of Aloe in Treating Leg Ulcers and Dermatoses. Derm. Internat. 12, 68.

Flückiger, F.A. and Hanbury, D. (1874) Pharmacographin. London, Macmillan pp. 616-627.

Gjerstad, G. and Riner, T.D. (1968) Current Status of Aloe as a Cure-all. Am. J. Pharm. 140, 58.

Harry, R.G. (1948) Cosmetic Materials, Vol. 2. London, Leonard Hill.

Hjorth, N. (1961) Eczematous Allergy to Balsams, Allied Perfumes and Flavouring Agents. Copenhagen, Munksgaard.

Jadassohn, W. (1926) Quoted by Touton, K., *in* Handbuch der Haut und Geschlechtskrankheiten, Vol. 4, Pt. 1. Berlin, Springer.

McCarthy, T.J. (1969) Distribution of Glycosyl Compounds in South African *Aloë* Species. Planta Medica, 17, 1.

Merck Index (1968)

Rowe, T.D. (1940) Effect of Fresh *Aloe vera* Jell in the Treatment of Third-degree Roentgen Reactions on White Rats. J.Am. Pharm. Ass. 29, 348.

Steiner, K. and Leifer, W. (1949) Investigation of Contact-type Dermatitis due to Compound Tincture of Benzoin. J. invest. Derm. 13, 351.

Watt, J.M. and Breyer-Brandwijk, M.G. (1962) The Medicinal and Poisonous Plants of Southern and Eastern Africa. 2nd Edit. Edinburgh, E. and S. Livingstone Ltd.

Wright, C.S. (1936) *Aloe vera* in treatment of roentgen ulcers and telangiectasis. JAMA 106, 1363.

Asparagus

The 300 or so species of this genus are widely distributed over the Old World. Several species are of horticultural value, particularly as foliage for bouquets, e.g. *Asparagus sprengeri*, *A. plumosus* and

A. medeoloides. Other species are cultivated for the beauty of their flowers.

The young shoots of A. officinalis are highly esteemed as a vegetable and cultivators, canners and cooks handling them are exposed to the risk of dermatitis. A decoction of the fruit is used in African folk medicine, particularly as a diuretic.

Chemistry is recorded by Hegnauer (1963).

Asparagus officinalis contains asparagin, coniferin and the glucoside vanillin, according to Hurst (1942); other workers have not confirmed the presence of coniferin but have isolated a second glucoside (Merck 1968). The allergic sensitizer has not been identified. It is apparently not asparagin or vanillin (see below).

Reference

Hegnauer, R. (1963) Chemotaxonomy of Plants. Vol. 2. Basel. Birkhauser pp. 336-338.

Dermatitis

Prolonged and repeated exposure is usually necessary to induce dermatitis. Possibly the first recorded cases (Güntz 1880) were two patients, who prepared asparagus in a restaurant, who developed vesicular dermatitis of hands, arms, neck and face, and also conjunctivitis. Brenning's (1920) patient had handled asparagus for 8 years before she developed dermatitis, and Schoenhof's 1924) for 18 years.

The tendency for all exposed skin to be affected to some degree and to be papular or vesicular was again demonstrated by Sternthal's (1925) patient. A vegetable cook in a large hotel (Urbach 1929) had an extensive dermatitis of hands, forearms and face, and gave bullous patch test reactions on the skin and on the gums. She developed itching and blisters after eating asparagus. However another woman with asparagus dermatitis could eat asparagus without discomfort (Courmont 1930). Dermatitis of the hands and arms developed in a worker on an asparagus farm (Hajos and Mohrmann 1929). Progressive desensitization appeared to follow repeated application of the plant to the skin.

In Brunswick, Germany, where much asparagus was grown and canned, dermatitis was well known to those engaged in the industry (Sternthal 1925). Halberg (1932) also reported cases in a canning factory; he obtained positive patch-test reactions with the juice, i.e. the fluid in which the asparagus had been cooked, but not with asparagin.

It is only the young shoots which are tender and gastronomically desirable, and it is normally only these that are gathered and prepared. There is some evidence that only the young shoots cause dermatitis (Hardin and Arena 1969). A patient reported by Stewart (1972) reacted to young shoots but could handle the mature plants with impunity. Patch tests confirmed the clinical observations. Since asparagus is known to contain vanillin, the patient was also patch-tested with Balsam of Peru; there was no reaction. The same author usefully confirmed that in normal subjects a patch test with young asparagus shoots provokes at the most a transitory irritant reaction.

References

Brenning, C. (1920) A case of dermatitis due to Asparagus. Derm. Wschr. 71, 851.

Courmont, P. (1930) Anaphylaxie cutanee au suc d'asperges. Lyon Med. 145, 184.

Güntz, J.-E. (1880) Miliaria - Ausschlag in Folge var Berührung mit roham Spargel (Asparagus officinalis). Vierteljahrresschrift Derm. Syph. 7, 65.

Hajos, B. and Mohrmann, B.H.U. (1929) Spargelidiosyncrasie. Klin. Wschr. 8, 1024.

Halberg, V. (1932) Five cases of asparagus dermatitis. Hospitalstidende, 75, 1235.

Hardin, J.W, and Arena, J.M. (1969) Human Poisoning from Native and Cultivated Plants. Durham, North Carolina, Duke University Press.

Hurst, E. (1942) The Poison Plants of New South Wales. N.S.W. Poison Plants Committee, Sydney.

Merck Index (1968)

Schoenhof, S. (1924) Asparagus dermatitis. Derm. Wschr. 79, 1221.

Sternthal, A. (1925) Asparagus dermatitis. Derm. Wschr. 80, 254.

Stewart, W.D. (1972) Personal Communication.

Urbach, E. (1929) Epidermale und epimucöse Spargeldermatitis. Zentralblatt für U.u.G., 32, 35.

Chemistry

Yanagawa, H., Kato, T. and Kitahara, Y. (1972) Asparagusic acid, dihydroasparagusic acid and S-acetyldihydroasparagusic acid. A new plant growth inhibitor in etiolated young *Asparagus officinalis*. Tetrahedron Letters 25, 2549.

Asphodelus

About 12 species of this plant are distributed over a large area extending from the Mediterranean region to India. Some species are extremely abundant.

Dermatitis

Reports of dermatitis in man (Gardner and Bennetts 1956) and in cattle (Hurst 1942) lack detail. *A. fistulosus* is suspected.

References

Gardner, C.A. and Bennetts, H.W. (1956) The Toxic Plants of Western Australia. Perth. West. Australian Newspapers Ltd.

Hurst, E. (1942) The Poison Plants of New South Wales. N.S.W. Poison Plants Committee, Sydney.

Bowiea

The two species placed in this genus are natives of south and East Africa. *B. volubilis* is sometimes cultivated. The bulb is said to irritate the damp skin (Watt and Breyer-Brandwijk 1962).

Reference

Watt, J.M. and Breyer-Brandwijk, M.G. (1962) The Medicinal and Poisonous Plants of Southern and Eastern Africa. 2nd Edit. Edinburgh, E. and S. Livingstone.

Colchicum

The 60 or more species of *Colchicum* are found in Europe, Central Africa and Northern India. Many species are cultivated for the beauty of their crocus-like flowers (autumn crocus). The poisonous properties of the corm of *Colchicum autumnale* (Autumn Crocus or Meadow Saffron) impressed early physicians more than its therapeutic virtues; it appeared in the London Pharmacopoeia from 1618 to 1639 and then was omitted until the 1788 edition (Flückiger and Hanbury 1874). Other species, notably *C. luteum*, are also used medically.

Chemistry

Colchicum is employed in the treatment of gout and as a topical antimitotic agent. Demecolcine is used in leukaemia.

Dermatitis

The cutaneous manifestation induced by colchicum derivatives administered medicinally are beyond the scope of this book and are well covered in texts on drug reactions. Demecolcine is irritant to the intact skin (Randazzo 1957).

The fresh corms of *C. autumnale*, *C. luteum*, and probably other species are irritant to the skin and mucous membranes. (Dispensatory 1884, Behl et al 1966, North 1967). The leaves are said to cause dermatitis (Muenscher 1951, McCord 1962).

Ingestion of *C. autumnale* has been followed by alopecia (Gooneratne 1966).

References

Behl, P.N., Captain, R.M., Bedi, B.M.S. and Gupta, S. (1966) Skin-irritant and Sensitizing Plants Found in India. New Delhi, P.N. Behl, Irwin Hospital.

Dispensatory, The National (1884) Philadelphia, Stille and Maisch. Cited by White, J.C. (1887)

Flückiger, F.A. and Hanbury, D. (1874) Pharmacographia. London, Macmillan.

Gooneratne, B.W.M. (1966) Massive Generalized Alopecia after Poisoning by Gloriosa superba. Br. med. J. i, 1023.

McCord, C.P. (1962) The Occupational Toxicity of Cultivated Flowers. Ind. Med. Surg. 31, 365.

Muenscher, W.C. (1951) Poisonous Plants of the United States. 2nd. Edit. New York, The Macmillan Co.

North, P.M. (1967) Poisonous Plants and Fungi in Colour. London, Blandford Press Ltd.

Convallaria

C. majalis (Lily of the Valley), the only species in this genus, occurs throughout temperate Europe, Asia and North America. It is a popular cultivated flower. Although it is so frequently handled by florists and gardeners, fully authenticated cases of dermatitis are rare. The leaves appear to be mildly irritant (Muenscher 1951, McCord 1962).

References

McCord, C.P. (1962) The Occupational Toxicity of Cultivated Flowers. Ind. Med. Surg. 31, 365.

Muenscher, W.C. (1951) Poisonous Plants of the United States. 2nd Edit. New York, The Macmillan Co.

Drimia

About 45 species of Drimia are known in tropical and South Africa. The generic name, which is derived from a Greek word meaning acrid, appropriately labels plants the bulbs of which are intensely irritant. This property is attributed to raphides of calcium oxalate.

As none of the species so far described is of much horticultural merit, human contact with these bulbs is limited.

Eremurus

Some fifty species of Eremurus are distributed over Western and Central Asia, and are particularly numerous in Iran. The stately beauty of many species and hybrids ensures theit cultivation wherever ornamental horticulture flourishes. Personal experience has given no indication that these so-called Foxtail Lilies are irritant, and the report of two cases of contact dermatitis of the face and arms attributed to Eremurus awaits confirmation (Sidi 1962).

Reference

Sidi, E. (1962) Personal communication to Epstein, S. Newer Contact Sensitizers in the Home. In Dermatoses due to Environmental and Physical Factors, edit. Rees, R.B. Springfield, Ill., Charles C. Thomas, p. 227.

Erythronium

Of some 25 species in this genus, one, E. dens-canis (Dog tooth violet) is distributed through Europe, temperate Asia and Japan; the remaining species occur in North America. Many species are cultivated E. dens-canis is frequent in gardens in Western Europe.

Chemistry

Some species have been shown to contain α-methylene-γ-butyrolactone, which is an allergen in Tulipa, a related genus. This allergen may also be present in species not yet investigated.

Dermatitis

Only a few workers in specialist nurseries are likely to come sufficiently frequently into contact with Erythronium for this plant to be a primary sensitizer. However it may well induce reactions in those already sensitized to the ubiquitous tulip.

Fritillaria

This north temperate genus contains over 80 species, many of which are cultivated. Two of the most popular, F. meleagris (Snake's head) and F. imperialis (Crown imperial), are said to be irritant (Pammel 1911).

Reference

Pammel, L.H. (1911) A Manual of Poisonous Plants. Cedar Rapids

Iowa, Torch Press. Reprinted Univ. Microfilms Inc., Ann Arbor, Mich., 1965, pp. 476-7.

Gloriosa

The five species are natives of Africa and tropical Asia, but are grown in glass houses elsewhere as they are highly decorative.

Chemistry

The tubers yield colchicine, gloriosine and related alkaloids (Hegnauer 1963).

The tubers have been used for criminal poisoning, but have also been ingested accidentally on account of their resemblance to those of the sweet potato (Ipomoea batatas).

Dermatitis

The tubers are irritant. If they are eaten they cause numbness of the lips and tongue (Hardin and Arena 1969) which has been followed in one reported case by generalized alopecia (Gooneratne 1966).

References

Gooneratne, B.W.M. (1966) Massive Generalized Alopecia after Poisoning by Gloriosa superba. Br. med. J., i, 1023.

Hardin, J.W. and Arena, J.M. (1969) Human Poisoning from Native and Cultivated Plants. Durham, North Carolina, Duke University Press.

Hegnauer, R. (1963) Chemotaxonomy of Plants. Vol. 2. Basel. Birkhauser pp. 295-297.

Hyacinthus

The 30 or so species in this horticulturally important genus are mainly natives of the Eastern Mediterranean region, but a few occur in tropical and South Africa. Several species are cultivated, but by far the most popular is H. orientalis, which was first developed by artificial selection in Turkey and subsequently in Holland (Gorer 1970). H. orientalis, the so-called common hyacinth, is now one of the most commonly cultivated bulbs for indoor and outdoor decoration, and workers in the bulb industry, gardenders, florists and housewives may all be exposed in some degree to a dermatitis hazard. H. romanus (Roman hyacinth) is also quite frequently cultivated.

Chemistry

Needle shaped crystals of calcium oxalate, 2.5-5 mm in length, are abundant in the bulb scales and have long been recognised as a cause of skin irritation (Morris 1896). About 6% of calcium oxalate is present in bulb scales and a similar concentration has been found in the dust on tables used for sorting and packing (Hjorth and Wilkinson 1968).

Hyacinths also probably contain allergenic substances, which have not been identified (Van der Werff 1959). Fungi, parasites, fungicides and pesticides must also be considered (Van der Werff 1959).

Oil of Hyacinth, which is used in perfumes, has caused allergic dermatitis (Varga 1936). Hyacinthin is phenylacetaldehyde (Fenaroli 1971). The chemistry of Hyacinthus is recorded by Hegnauer (1963) and Oil of Hyacinth contains some known sensitisers.

Dermatitis

(Harrison 1906, Schwartz et al 1957, McCord 1962).

Hyacinth bulb dermatitis is predominantly of irritant type, and is very familiar to nurserymen. However the irritant properties of the bulbs are such that it is often difficult to confirm the suspected coexistence of allergic dermaitis, sometimes suggested by the clinical features.

The commonest clinical picture is dry fissured scaling and erythema of the finger tips, often with hyperkeratosis beneath the nails (Kranenburg 1930, Johnson 1935). Sometimes a more extensive eczematous dermatitis involves hands, arms and face (Freeman 1897).

Dust contaminated with oxalate crystals can pass beneath clothing and cause irritable patchy erythema and oedema, often most marked around the waist and in the anogenital region (Van der Werff 1969).

Bulb growers are often aware that some cultivars of H. orientalis are more likely to cause trouble than others: L'Innocence, Marconi, Carnegie and City of Harlem were considered particularly liable to cause dermatitis (Van der Werff 1969). The variety albulus of H. romanus has been regarded as exceptionally irritant (Maiden 1909).

Patch tests with bulb scales should be interpreted with caution. A positive patch test to a fragment of leaf is probably evidence of sensitization.

References

Fenaroli, G. (1971) Fenaroli's Handbook of Flavor Ingredients. Ed. Furia, T.E. and Pellanea, M. Cleveland, Ohio, The Chemical Rubber Co.

Freeman, W.T. (1897) A Note on the Skin Irritation Caused by Handling Hyacinth Bulbs. Br. J. Derm. 9, 66.

Gorer, R. (1970) The Development of Garden Flowers. London, Eyre and Spottiswode, p. 79.

Harrison, A.J. (1906) Dermatitis from without and Dermatitis from within. Bristol med. clin. J. 24, 325.

Hjorth, N. and Wilkinson, D.S. (1968) Contact Dermatitis IV. Tulip Fingers, Hyacinth Itch and Lily Rash. Br. J. Derm. 80, 696.

Johnson, D.W. (1935) Dermatitis Due to Hyacinth Bulbs. Archs. Derm. 32, 289.

Kranenburg, W.R.H. (1930) Juckreiz und Dermatitis nach Verarbeitig von Hyacinthen und Tulpen. Z. Gewerbehyg. 17, 73.

McCord, C.P. (1962) The Occupational Toxicity of Cultivated Flowers. Ind. Med. Surg. 31, 365.

Maiden, J.H. (1909) On Some Plants Which Cause Inflammation or Irritation of the Skin. Ag. Gaz. New South Wales, 20, 1073.

Morris, D. (1896) Proc. Linn. Soc. 5 Nov. (Cited by Maiden, 1909)

Schwartz, L., Tulipan, L. and Birmingham, D.J. (1957) Occupational Diseases of the Skin. 3rd Ed. Philadelphia, Lea & Febiger, pp. 637-672.

Van der Werff, P.J. (1969)

Varga, A.V. (1936) Acute Generalized Eczema Caused by Hyacinth Oil. Derm. Wschr. 1, 104.

Lilium

Very many of the 80 species of this north temperate genus are stately and beautiful plants and are widely cultivated, yet fully authenticated accounts of undesirable effects on the skin are rare. L. longiflorum and L. superbum (Turk's cap Lily) have been listed as irritant (Weber 1937).

Reference

Weber, L.F. (1937) External Causes of Dermatitis. A List of Irritants. Archs. Derm. 35, 129.

Muscari

There are about 60 species, all natives of the Mediterranean region. Many species are popular garden plants, known collectively as Grape Hyacinths.

M. racemosum is reported to be irritant (Pammel, 1911).

Reference

Pammel, L.H. (1911) A Manual of Poisonous Plants. Cedar Rapids, Iowa, Torch Press. Reprinted Univ. Microfilms Inc., Ann Arbor, Mich., 1965, pp. 476-7.

Narthecium

Five of six species are natives of the temperate regions of the Northern Hemisphere: one occurs in Japan.

N. ossifragum, the bog asphodel, is said to have caused photosensitization in sheep (North 1967).

Reference

North, P.M. (1967) Poisonous Plants and Fungi in Colour. London, Blandford Press Ltd.

Ornithogalum

About 150 species are distributed over Europe, Asia and Africa. Many are decorative and are frequently cultivated.

Chemistry

Some species contain an alkaloid, probably related to colchicine (Kingsbury 1964). Hegnauer (1963) reviewed the chemistry.

Many species contain raphides of calcium oxalate, which may cause intense irritation when the bulbs or leaves are handled, e.g. *O. caudatum* (Pohl 1965). Raphides are present but less abundant in *O. thyrsoides* and *O. saundersiae*, which are not reported to be irritant.

References

Kingsbury, J.M. (1964) Poisonous Plants of the United States and Canada. Englewood Cliffs, New Jersey, Prentice-Hall Inc.

Pohl, R.W. (1965) Contact Dermatits from the Juice of *Ornithogalum caudatum*. Toxicon. 3, 167.

Hegnauer, R. (1963) Chemotaxonomy of Plants. Vol. 2. Basel. Birkhauser. pp. 333 - 334.

Scilla

There are 80 - 100 species, natives of Europe, Asia and Africa. Many are beautiful and are widely cultivated.

Several species are irritant (Hoffman 1904 a,b., Chevalier 1933). *S. indica* (Behl et al 1966), *S. maritima* and *S. rubra* (Schwartz et al 1957), *S. bifolia* (the common Scilla of horticulture) (Pammel 1911), *S. festalis*, *S. nonscripta* (Common Bluebell) have been specifically recorded as such.

Chemistry is recorded by Hegnauer (1963).

References

Behl, P.N., Captain, R.M., Bedi, B.M.S. and Gupta, S. (1966) Skin-irritant and Sensitizing Plants Found in India. New Delhi, P.N. Behl, Irwin Hospital.

Chevalier, A. (1933) Scilles à Bulbes Comestibles ou Vénéneux. Rev. Bot. appl. 13, 469.

Hoffman, E. (1904 a) Ueber die Primelkrankheit und andere durch Pflanzen venursachte Hautentzündungen Münch. med. Wschr. 51, 1966.

Pammel, L.H. (1911) A Manual of Poisonous Plants. Cedar Rapids Iowa, Torch Press. Reprinted Univ. Microfilms Inc., Ann Arbor, Mich., 1965, pp. 476-7.

Schwartz, L., Tulipan, L. and Birmingham, D.J. (1957) Occupational Diseases of the Skin. 3rd Ed. Philadelphia, Lea and Febiger, pp. 637-672.

Hegnauer, R. (1963) Chemotaxonomy of Plants. Vol. 2. Basel. Birkhauser. pp. 329-336.

Hoffman, E. (1904b) Ueber durch Pflanzen bedingte arteficielle Dermatitiden (mit Demonstration mikroskopischer Präparate der Scilla-dermatitis.) Berlin. Klin. Wochen. 41, 960.

Tulipa

There are about 100 species, widely distributed through Europe, West and Central Asia and North Africa. However tulips are cultivated in most countries in which the climate is suitable. The original development of garden tulips took place in Turkey, whence they were introduced to Western Europe in the 16th century. Their subsequent development has been largely the work of Dutch horticulturalists, who by selection and hybridisation have produced an immense range of types and cultivars. The natural species from which modern garden tulips were derived are still a matter for speculation. Although the hybrid garden tulips account for the great bulk of the tulip bulb trade, many of the species have a more refined beauty and are often cultivated.

Those most exposed to the risk of dermatitis from tulip bulbs are the collectors, sorters and packers in the large bulb nurseries of Holland and Cambridgeshire and Lincolnshire in England. The incidence of dermatitis is high, although few of those affected may seek medical advice, for what is regarded as a known hazard of the occupation. In one nursery 8 of 12 employees were affected (Klaschka et al 1964). Florists and flower arrangers as well as nurseries may have frequent contact with the cut flowers.

Chemistry

By using paper chromatography to isolate ethanol-soluble fractions and then patch-testing with the chromatograms, Verspyck Mijnssen (1967) was able to detect an allergenic principle, but it could not be obtained in crystalline form. Brongersma-Oosterhoff (1967) isolated the compound and identified it as α-methylene-γ-butyrolactone. In the plant this is bound as a glycoside. It is probable that in this glycoside-enzymes-glucose + lactone system, only the lactone is allergenic. The same substance was independently isolated by Bergman et al (1967) in a study of a fungicidal substance formed during the early stages of bulb development. Other antibiotic lactones have been isolated (Tschesche et al 1968), but there is evidence of only one allergen in tulips (Verspyck Mijnssen 1969).

The concentration of allergen is highest in the bulb, less in stem and leaves, and least in the petals. The main site of the allergen in the bulb is the epidermis of the scales. The content of the allergen diminishes rapidly in the outermost scales during the last weeks of growth, immediately before harvest. During this period the outermost scale forms the leathery brown skin, which is not allergenic. In the second and deeper layer of scale, which remains white and fleshy, the allergen persists during storage (Bergman 1968).

Experienced florists have often found that some cultivars cause dermatitis more frequently than others, e.g. "Preludium" and "Rose Copeland" (Van Der Werff 1959). Bertwistle (1937) also found the latter cultivar to be more irritant than others. Some florists who have become sensitized to tulips find that they can handle some cultivars but not others (Rook 1961). Bulb patch tests with nine cultivars (Klaschka et al 1964) showed no differences between the reactions. Patch-testing supplemented by gas chromatography (Verspyck Mijnssen 1969) showed that only one cultivar ("Red Emperor" = "Madame Lefeber") contained less bulb allergen than the other eleven studied. However not only quantitative factors are involved in the causation of plant dermatitis; structural variations may well influence the release of the allergen from damaged plant tissues; it would be premature to dismiss practical observations which may solve employment problems.

Dermatitis

Three main clinical syndromes are recorded. The first is an irritant reaction affecting bulb handlers. Investigations in Britain (Bertwistle 1937) indicated that up to 85% of workers were affected by tingling and tenderness of the finger-tips, about 12 hours after slicing the bulbs. Granulation tissue formed beneath the nail, followed by onycholysis, transverse splitting of the nail plate, and in severe cases by subungual abscesses (see also Overton 1926). This irritant effect is a component of the classical syndrome known as "tulip fingers". Patch tests with pure tulip allergen 1:600 gave positive reactions in all control subjects. However all patients with tulip fingers gave positive reactions also to a test with a one in 20,000 dilution of the allergen, to which controls did not react, (Hjorth and Wilkinson 1968). In tulip fingers the changes described above are combined with those attributable to the allergic reaction: erythema and scaling, later complicated by hyperkeratosis and fissuring, develop in a pattern determined by the precise manner in which the individuals occupation requires him to handle the bulb.

Other patients develop a more extensive eczematous dermatitis on the hands, with some dissemination to arms, face and genitalia. These more extensive patterns occur in some bulb handlers (Verspyck Mijnssen 1968, Rappaport and Walker 1936, Caulfield 1936) but are seen particularly in those who handle the cut flowers. Further reports on the observed manifestations are provided by Baefverstidt 1936, Touraine and Neret 1938, Flandin and Ukrainczyk 1938, Osborne and Putnam 1932 and Gore 1962.

The dust in tulip sheds may precipate conjunctivitis, rhinitis and asthma and reaginic responses to tulip antigens can occur (Van der Werff 1959).

Patch Testing

As the pure tulip allergen is not readily available, patch tests may be performed with outermost bulb scales, after removal of the brown skin. To obviate dependence on seasonal supplies extracts may be prepared from bulbs which have been tested for allergenicity. The cultivar "Apeldoorn" is recommended (Hjorth and Wilkinson 1968). The following extracts are suitable:

1. 96% ethanol extract of tulip bulbs, which is stable for some months in a refrigerator; or preferably
2. an extract prepared by shaking fresh bulbs for 90 minutes in 80% acetone in water. 1% of this extract in 70% ethanol is used for patch testing.

Management

Severely affected workers may have to change their occupation as piece workers seldom find it satisfactory to work in gloves. It should be remembered that the tulip allergen is present also in Alstromeria, and Erythronium.

References

Beafverstidt, B. (1936) Occupational Dermatosis in a Gardener. Dermatologische Gesellshaft (Stockh.), Oct. 14.

Bergman, B.H.H., et al (1967) Isolation and Identification of α-methylene-γ-butyrolactone, a Fungitoxic Substance from Tulips. Recl. Trav. chim. Pays-Bays, 86, 709.

Bergman, B.H.H., et al (1968) A Fungitoxic Substance Extracted from Tulips and its Possible Role as a Protectant against Disease. In Proceedings of an International Symposium on Physiological and Biochemical Aspects of Host-pathogen Interactions. Neth. J. Plant Path. 74, 157.

Bertwistle, A.P. (1937) "Tulip fingers". Brit. med. J. 2, 255.

Brongersmo-Oosterhoff, U.W. (1967) Structure Determination of the Allergenic Agent, Isolated from Tulip Bulbs. Recl. Trav. chim. Pays.-Bas, 86, 705.

Caulfield, A.H.W. (1936) Report of the Investigation and Successful Treatment (Prevention) of Dermatitis Resulting from the Handling of Tulip Bulbs. J. Allergy, 8, 181.

Gore, H.C., Jr. (1962) "Tulip Fingers" (Dermatitis Venenata due to Constituent in Tulip Bulb). Archs. Derm. 85, 798.

Hjorth, N. and Wilkinson, D.S. (1968) Contact Dermatitis IV. Tulip Fingers, Hyacinth Itch and Lily Rash. Br. J. Derm. 80, 696.

Klaschka, F., Grimm, W. and Beiersdorff, H.U. (1964) Tulip Contact Eczema as Occupational Dermatosis. Hautarzt, 15, 317.

Osborne, E.D. and Putnam, E.D. (1932) Industrial Dermatoses. J. Am. med. Ass. 99, 972.

Overton, S.G. (1926) Dermatitis from Handling Flower Bulbs. Lancet, 2, 1003.

Rabeau, H. and Ukrainczyk, F. (1938) Two Cases of Occupational Dermatitis in Flower Handlers. Bull. Soc. franc. Derm. Syph. 45, 595.

Rappaport, B.Z. and Walker, W.H. (1937) Tulip Bulb Dermatitis. J. Allergy, 8, 379.

Rook, A.J. (1961) Plant Dermatitis. The Significance of Variety-specific Sensitisation. Br. J. Derm. 73, 283.

Touraine, A. and Neret (1938) Occupational Dermatitis from Tulips. Bull. Soc. franc. Derm. Syph. 45, 1017.

Tschesche, R., Kammerer, J.J., Wulff, G. and Schonbeck, F. (1968) Über die Antibiotisch Wirksame Substanzen der Tulpe (Tulipa Gesneriana). Tetrahedron Letters, (6), 701.

Van der Werff, P.J. (1959) Occupational Diseases Among Workers in the Bulb Industries. Acta. allerg. 14, 338.

Verspyck Mijnssen, G.A.W. (1967) Patch Testing with Paper Chromatograms. A Method for Isolating Allergenic Agents Applied to the Investigation of Tulip Eczema. (173rd Meeting Netherl. Soc. Derm. Leiden 1966). Dermatologica, 134, 379.

Verspyck Mijnssen, G.A.W. (1968) De pathogenese en aetiologie van de "tulpenvingers". Groningen, Wolters-Noordhoff. n.v.

Verspyck Mijnssen, G.A.W. (1969) Pathogenesis and Causative Agent of "Tulip Finger". Br. J. Derm. 81, 737.

Additional Reference

Bleumink, E. and Nater, J.P. (1973) Contact dermatitis to garlic: cross reactivity between garlic, onion and tulip. Arch. Dermatol. Forsch. 247, 117.

Urginea

There are about 100 species of *Urginea*, natives of the Mediterranean region, Africa and India. Some species are cultivated in gardens, but are not of great horticultural merit. *U. maritima* formerly known as *U. Scilla* and *Scilla maritima*) is the source of squill which was used medicinally from a very early period and remained in use until recently (Stannard 1974). Other species are used as substitutes for *U. maritima* and have similar properties (Flückiger and Hanbury 1874).

Chemistry

Squill contains glycosides scillarin A and B, with properties somewhat similar to digitalis (Gemmill 1974). The chemistry is recorded by Hegnauer (1963).

Dermatitis

Many species are irritant. Powdered squill caused severe keratoconjunctivitis and iritis (Achermann 1928).

References

Achermann, E. (1928) Kerato-iritis durch Scilla-staub (Scilla-Reintaisnoid). Klin. Mbl. Augenheilk. 81, 196.

Flückiger, F.A. and Hanbury, D. (1874) Pharmacographia. London, Macmillan, p. 627.

Gemmill, C.C. (1974) The Pharmacology of Squill. Bull. N.Y. Acad. Med. 50, 747.

Stannard, J. (1974) Squill in Ancient and Medieval Materia Medica. Bull. N.Y. Acad. Med. 50, 684.

Hegnauer, R. (1963) Chemotaxonomy of Plants. Vol. 2. Basel, Birkhauser pp. 329-336.

Veratrum

The 25 species of *Veratrum* are natives of the North temperate region. They are rarely cultivated. Few genera illustrate more impressively the futility of employing popular plant names in scientific writing. The popular name Hellebore is applied to two species and is also applied to the botanically unrelated *Helleborus* species (Ranunculaceae). In the American West the name Skunk Cabbage is appled to species of *Veratrum*; in the American East Skunk cabbage is applied to an arum.

The rhizomes of some *Veratrum* species are powdered and sold as a Hellebore Powder for the destruction of lice and caterpillars. The powder is intensely irritating (Wren 1968).

Chemistry

Veratrin is present throughout the plant, but is most abundant in the rhizomes. The chemistry is recorded by Hegnauer (1963).

Dermatitis

All species are irritant (Pammel 1911, Weber 1937, Schwartz et al. 1957, Muenscher 1951).

References

Muenscher, W.C. (1951) Poisonous Plants of the United States. 2nd Ed. New York, The Macmillan Co.

Hegnauer, R. (1963) Chemotaxonomy of Plants. Vol. 2. Basel. Birkhauser pp. 291-293.

Pammel, L.H. (1911) A Manual of Poisonous Plants. Cedar Rapids, Iowa, Torch Press. Reprinted Univ. Microfilms Inc., Ann Arbor, Mich., 1965, pp. 476-7.

Schwartz, L., Tulipan, L. and Birmingham, D.J. (1957) Occupational Diseases of the Skin. 3rd Ed. Philadelphia, Lea and Febiger, pp. 637-672.

Weber, L.F. (1937) External Causes of Dermatitis. A List of Irritants. Archs. Derm. 35, 129.

Wren, R.W. (1968) Potter's New Cyclopaedia of Botanical Drugs and Preparations by Wren, R.C. Re-edit. by Wren, R.W. Rustington, Sussex, Potter and Clarke ltd., Health Science Press.

LIMNANTHACEAE

Eleven species in two genera are native to North America.

Limnanthes

Ten species are native to Pacific North America.

Limnanthes douglasii

The seeds contain a 'mustard oil' thioglucoside (Kjaer 1960) such as produce irritant effects from Cruciferae species.

References

Kjaer, A. (1960) Naturally derived isoThiocyanates (Mustard oils) and their parent glucosides in Progress in the Chemistry of Organic Natural Products. ed. Zechmeister, L. Vol. 18. Vienna. Springer-Verlag. pp. 122-176.

LINACEAE

290 species in 12 genera are cosmopolitan.

Chemistry is recorded by Hegnauer (1966).

Linum

230 species are found in temperate and subtropical regions especially in the Mediterranean region.

Linum usitatissimum

The fibre of this species furnishes flax from which linen is made.

The seeds (linseed) yield an oil by pressure and the remaining 'cake' is used for cattle-feed. Dermatitis and ulceration on the dorsa of the feet in gatherers of flax was attributed to contact with chamomile (Anthemis or Matricaria, Compositae) growing in the fields (D'Agostino 1927). Positive patch tests to the leaf of Linum were observed by Szego (1965). The sharp points of the seeds can cause mechanical injury. Insect parasites can cause pseudophytodermatitis in flax gatherers. Irritant oils of mustard and rape (Cruciferae) can contaminate the flax (Barnes 1931). Flax seed hair tonic caused contact dermatitis (Ramirez and Eller 1930). Burlap sugar bags (of jute, Tiliaceae) in which the linseed is shipped irritated longshoremen (Schwartz et al 1957). Linseed oil produced a positive patch test in one of 45 painters investigated for contact dermatitis; three-quarters of them were contact sensitive to turpentine (Pirila 1947). Acne-form folliculitis in linen mills can result from linseed oil or oils used on the machinery (Purdon 1885, Leloir 1885 cited by White 1934). Workers with flax in the moist state can develop allergic contact dermatitis of the exposed parts (White 1934). Flax-spinners can develop exfoliation of the skin of the hands and finally ulceration (Downing et al 1932). Flax-soakers can develop vesicular dermatitis of the hands probably from the hot chemical solutions employed (Downing et al 1932). An intradermal test with linseed 'cake' produced urticaria (Rajka 1948). Linseed cake can produce dermatitis in extractors of linseed oil; the dermatitis occurs on the extensor surfaces of the hands and forearms, occasionally on the upper arms and face and on the legs (Vokoun 1927). Seeds, used for pressing, from South America and India, were found to be more liable to cause dermatitis than seeds from Canada and the United States. Ingestion of Linseed 'cake' (flax meal) induced Type I hypersensitivity and the meal also irritated the skin (Black 1930 cited by White 1934). The incidence of linseed dermatitis varies with the source of the seed and the season of the year; the oil may produce a follicular eruption (Barnes 1931). Linen spinners can develop traumatic lesions of the hands and hyperkeratosis of the palms, paronychia and vasomotor disturbances of the hands together with irritation from the chemicals used in hot solutions for washing the fibres (Meneghini and Gianotti 1953). Flax in cigarette paper produced dermatitis; the flax fibre, cooked and bleached, prior to the paper-making process, also produced positive patch test reactions (Tye 1950). Linseed oil may be irritant and occasionally sensitizing (Schwartz et al 1957). Pure linseed oil was found to be non-irritant by patch test (Greenberg and Lester 1954). Linseed oil can be contaminated with rape seed oil (Brassica napus). Flax-workers are subject to irritant dermatitis from paraffin and coarse raw hemp can irritate the skin (Kinnear et al 1955). Subcutaneous nodules followed a sixth injection of mercury salicylate in linseed oil (Sutton 1923). Flaxseed applied as a poultice caused urticaria (Derbes and Coleman 1972). Linseed can be infested with a mite which can produce pseudophytodermatitis (Thomas 1944). Type I hypersensitivity to flax was demonstrated by Nicholson (1927).

Occupational contact sensitivity to flax seed and to linseed oil was reported in a seaman exposed to flax products; he was also contact sensitive to Ambrosia (ragweed) and other Compositae species (Jordan et al 1942).

Oil of Linseed, considered to be a known allergen, is removed from certain brand-name cosmetics (Schieffelin 1973).

Flax-seeds can cause conjunctival reactions (Duke-Elder and MacFaul 1972, Humphrey 1970).

References

Barnes, M.H. (1931) Linseed dermatitis. J. Industr. Hyg. 13, 49.

Black, W.C. (1930) Flax hypersensitiveness. JAMA 94, 1064.

D'Agostino, M. (1927) Flax dermatitis. Semana Med. 34, 643. Abstr. JAMA 89, 2148. 1927.

Derbes, V.J. and Coleman, W.P. (1972) Urticaria due to inhalants. Cutis 9, 847.

Downing, J.G. and Welch, C.E. (1932) Industrial Dermatoses and their Treatment: Review of 10 year's literature. New Eng. J. Med. 206, 666.

Duke-Elder, S. and MacFaul (1972) System of Opthalmology. Vol. XIV. Injuries Part I. Mechanical Injuries. Extra-ocular foreign bodies. pp. 464-67 and Agricultural Injuries pp. 32-34. London. Henry Kimpton.

Greenberg, L.A. and Lester, D. (1954) Handbook of Cosmetic Materials. New York. Interscience.

Hegnauer, R. (1966) Chemotaxonomy of Plants. Vol. 4. Basel, Birkhauser pp. 393.

Humphrey, W.T. (1970) Flax seeds in opthalmic folk medicine. Amer. J. Ophthal. 70, 287.

Jordon, J.W., Campbell, P.C. and Osborne, E.D. (1942) Ragweed dermatitis among workers in the flour and grain industries. Arch. Derm. Syph. 46, 721.

Kinnear, J., Rogers, J., Finn, O.A. and Mair, A. (1955) Dermatoses in jute workers. Brit. J. Industr. Med. 12, 36.

Leloir (1885) cited by White (1934).

Meneghini, C.L. and Gianotti, F. (1953) Contribution to the knowledge of cutaneous pathology in the working of linen and hemp. Med. D. Lavoro. 44, 538.

Nicholson, D. (1927) Cutaneous reactions to flax and linen in five cases of bronchial asthma and two of hayfever with poor results from specific treatment. Canad. Med. Ass. J. 17, 552.

Nixon, J.A. (1944) Cheese itch and "Itchy Cargoes" in reference to Workmen's Compensation Proc. Roy. Soc. Med. 37, 405.

Pirila, V. (1947) On occupational diseases of the skin among paint factory workers, painters, polishers and varnishers in

Finland. Acta. derm.-venereol. 17, Suppl. 16.

Purdon (1885) cited by White (1934).

Rajka, O. (1948) Occupational dermatitis from Sunflower seed and linseed. Orvosok Lapja (Budapest) 4, 158.

Ramirez, M.A. and Eller, J.J. (1930) The "Patch test" in "Contact Dermatitis", (Dermatitis venenata). J. Allergy 1, 489.

Schieffelin & Co. (1973) Almay Hypo-allergenic cosmetics product formulary. 8th ed. Pharmaceutical Laboratories Division 562 Fifth Avenue, New York, N.Y. 10036.

Schwartz, L., Tulipan, L. and Birmingham, D.J. (1957) Occupational Diseases of the Skin. 3rd ed. Philadelphia, Lea & Febiger.

Sutton, I.C. (1923) Tumor formation after injection of mercuric salicylate in vegetable oil. Archs. Derm. 7, 223.

Szego, L. (1965) Sensitization by agricultural crops and crop-protection preparations I. Studies of plant (leaf) extracts. Acta Med. Acad. Sci. Hung. 21, 19 (Excerpta Medica XVII, 13, 3468).

Thomas, P. (1944) in discussion of Nixon (1944).

Tye, M.J. (1950) Cigarette paper dermatitis. J. Invest. Derm. 14, 77.

Vokoun, F.J. (1927) Linseed oil dermatitis. JAMA 89, 20.

White, R.P. (1934) The Dermatergoses or Occupational Affections of the Skin. 4th ed. London, H.K. Lewis.

LOASACEAE

250 species in 15 genera are mostly found in tropical and subtropical regions of America. Some are cultivated. Many species possess grapnel or stinging hairs.

Chemistry is recorded by Hegnauer (1966).

Blumenbachia

Sting Lily

Three species are native to temperate South America. Some cultivated forms, some previously known as *Caiophora* or *Loasa*, have irritant properties.

Caiophora

65 species are native to South America. Some species possess stinging hairs (Uphof and Hummeh 1962).

Gronovia

Two species, native to Mexico, Venezuela and Ecuador possess grapnel or stinging hairs.

Gronovia scandens

The plant is covered with barbed stinging hairs (Allen 1943).

Loasa

100 species, native to Mexico and temperate South America, possess stinging hairs. Allen (1943) lists three species with stinging properties for man. A patch test to *L. tricolor* produced a negative result (Leipold 1936).

References

Allen, P.H. (1943) Poisonous and injurious plants of Panama. Am. J. Trop. Med. Suppl. 23, 1.

Hegnauer, R. (1966) Chemotaxonomy of plants. Vol. 4. Basel, Birkhauser. pp. 402.

Leipold (1936) Dermatitis of the hands and face due to hypersensitivity to chrysanthemum and camonile. Report: 62. Tagund d. Vereinig. Suedwest deutsch Dermat. Heidelberg, Nov. 14.

Uphof, J.C.T. and Hummeh, K. (1962) Plant hairs. In Encyclopedia of Plant Anatomy. Vol. 4., Part V., Berlin-Nikolassen: Gebruden Borntraegen.

Cevallia

One species is found in the south-western United States and Mexico.

Cevallia spp.

Stinging hairs are known in species of this genus (Thurston and Lersten 1969).

Reference

Thurston, E.L. and Lersten, R.N. (1969) The morphology and toxicology of plant stinging hairs. Botan. Rev. 35, 393.

Eucnide

Ten species are found in the south-western United States and Mexico.

Eucnide spp.

Stinging hairs are known in species of this genus (Thurston and Lersten 1969).

Reference

Thurston, E.L. and Lersten, N.R. (1969) The morphology and toxicology of plant stinging hairs. Botan. Rev. 35, 393.

Fuertesia

One species is found in the West Indies (southern Domingo).

Fuertesia spp.

This species possesses stinging hairs (Thurston and Lersten 1969).

Reference

Thurston, K.L. and Lersten, N.R. (1969).

Reference

Thurston, E.L. and Lersten, N.R. (1969) The morphology and toxicology of plant stinging hairs. Botan. Rev. 35, 393.

Mentzelia

70 species are native to tropical and subtropical America and the West Indies. Stinging hairs appear to be absent from this genus.

Mentzelia oligosperma

The rough barbed hairs of the plant can irritate the skin (White 1887).

Mentzelia ornata

The hooked hairs of this and other species of the genus are irritant (Pammel 1911).

References

Pammel, L.H. (1911) A Manual of Poisonous plants. Torch Press. Cedar Rapids, Iowa. Reprinted Univ. Microfilms Inc. Ann Aror, Mich. 1965.

White, J.C. (1887) Dermatitis venenata: An account of the Action of External irritants upon the Skin. Boston. Cupples & Hurd.

LOGANIACEAE

130 species in seven genera are mostly found in the tropics, a few in warm temperate regions.

Chemistry is recorded by Hegnauer (1966).

Gelsemium

One species is native to eastern Asia, two species to the southeastern United States and northern Mexico.

Gelsemium sempervirens

Yellow Jessamine

Many collectors of the root complain of its poisonous effects upon the skin (Cheney 1887). Subsequent reports of dermatitis from the plant probably refer to this note. The plant yields poisonous honey (Morton 1964).

References

Cheney cited White, J.C. (1887) Dermatitis venenata: An account of the Action of External irritants upon the Skin. Boston. Cupples and Hurd.

Cheney was a dealer in vegetable drugs.

Hegnauer, R. (1966) Chemotaxonomy of plants. Vol. 4. Basel, Birkhauser pp. 414.

Morton, J.F. (1964) Honeybee plants of South Florida. Proc. Florida

State Horticult. Soc. 77, 415.

LORANTHACEAE (VISCACEAE)

1300 species, in 36 or more genera, found in tropical and temperate regions, are parasitic or semi-parasitic plants which have green leaves. The parasitic root of *Viscum* branches within the tissues of the host.

Chemistry is recorded by Hegnauer (1966).

Phoradendron

About 190 species are native to America and the West Indies.

Phoradendron flavescens

American Mistletoe

A case of vesicular striate dermatitis from gathering the plant was reported by O'Farrel (1943). A patch test to the leaf produced a positive reaction; control tests were not recorded.

Viscum

60 or 70 species are native to warm regions of the Old World.

Viscum album

European Mistletoe

This species of folk-lore appeared in the British Pharmaceutical Codex of 1934. A sticky substance from the plant, known as Bird-Lime, was used on fly-papers. Astringent and irritant properties are ascribed to *Viscum* spp. (Pammel 1911, Watt and Breyer-Brandwijk 1962).

References

Hegnauer, R. Chemotaxonomy of Plants. Vol. 4. Basel, Birkhauser. pp. 429.

O'Farrell, N.M. (1943) Dermatitis Venenata due to Mistletoe. Arch. Derm. Syph. 43, 416.

Pammell, L.H. (1911) A Manual of Poisonous plants. Torch Press. Cedar Rapids, Iowa. Reprinted Univ. Microfilms Inc. Ann Arbor. Mich. 1965. pp. 476-7.

Watt, J.M. and Breyer-Brandwijk, M.G. (1962) The Medicinal and poisonous plants of Southern Africa. 2nd ed. Edinburgh. E. & S. Livingstone.

LYCOPODIACEAE

The species of this family are mostly saprophytic.

Lycopodium

Club-Moss

450 species are found in tropical and temperate regions.

The spores form a fine yellowish powder used for dusting pills, suppositories and rubber gloves. Granulomatous reactions in wounds can occur from its use for surgical gloves (Antopol 1933, Erb 1935). The inflammable powder can cause burns (Whitebread 1941). The powder used in powders, soaps and shampoos has been reported to cause dermatitis (Greenberg and Lester 1954).

References

Antopol, W. (1933) Arch. Path. 16, 326, cited by Boyd (1956).

Boyd, W. (1956) Pathology for the Surgeon. Philadelphia pp. 36.

Erb, I.H. (1935) Surg. Gynec. Obst. 60, 40 cited by Boyd (1956).

Greenberg, L.A. and Lester, D. (1954) Handbook of Cosmetic Materials. New York. Interscience.

Whitebread, C. (1941) Beware of *Lycopodium*. Am. Fern. J. 31, 100.

Lycopodium clavatum and

L. complanatum

Theatrical persons and pharmacists had hayfever from the powder (Salén 1951).

Reference

Salén, E.B. (1951) *Lycopodium* allergy. Acta. Allergol. 4, 308.

LYTHRACEAE

500 species in 25 genera are found in all except frigid zones.

Chemistry is recorded by Hegnauer (1966).

Reference

Hegnauer, R. (1966) Chemotaxonomy of Plants. Vol. 4. Basel, Birkhauser. pp. 438.

Ammania

30 species are cosmopolitan.

Ammania spp.

The leaves of some species are used for blistering the skin. A. multiflora is apparently innocuous after drying since the plant is eaten (Bailey 1906-7).

Ammania baccifera

The plant is acrid and vesicant (Burkill 1935). Application of the leaf to the skin for half an hour will produce a blister (Quisumbing 1951). The plant is common in rice-fields and has irritant properties (Behl et al 1966).

Ammania senegalensis

(syn. A. auriculata).

The plant is used as a blistering agent (Uphof 1959, Behl et al 1966).

References

Bailey, F.M. (1906-7) Weeds and suspected poisonous plants of Queensland, Brisbane quoted by Hurst (1942).

Behl, P.N., Captain, R.M., Bedi, B.M.S. and Gupta, S. (1966) Skin-irritant and sensitizing plants found in India, New Delhi. P.N. Behl. Irwin Hospital.

Burkill, I.H. (1935) A Dictionary of the Economic Products of the Malay Peninsula. 2 Vols. London. Crown Agents for the Colonies.

Hurst, E. (1942) The Poison Plants of New South Wales. N. S. W. Poison Plants Committee; Sydney.

Quisumbing E. (1951) Medicinal Plants of the Phillipines. Tech. Bull. 16. Manila, Phillipine Islands. Manila Bureau of Printing 1234 pp.

Uphof, J.C. Th. (1959) Dictionary of the Economic Plants. New York. Hafner Publ. Co.

Cuphea

250 species are native to America. Many are covered with sticky glandular hairs.

Cuphea urens

This species has irritant properties (Pardo-Castello 1923).

Reference

Pardo-Castello, V. (1923) Dermatitis venenata. Arch. Derm. Syph. 7, 80.

Lawsonia

One species is found in palaeotropical distribution. Botanical varieties are recognized.

Lawsonia inermis

(syn. L. alba)

The powdered leaves form henna, used in the East to stain the finger nails to a red colour. For relatively permanent dyeing with henna, the pH must be about 5.5; this may be achieved by the addition of citric, boric and adipic acid (Merck 1968). When used as a dye for the eyebrows and eyelashes there is a risk of injury to the eyes, possibly from an astringent effect of tannin present in the leaves (Irvine 1961). The leaves are applied, topically, to control perspiration (Oliver 1959). Extraction of the leaves with weak alkali yields 2-hydroxynaphthaquinone (lawsone) (Merck 1968). Imported powdered leaves are often contamined. For dyeing, henna is often combined with indigo (Indigofera). Contact reactions attributed to henna dye (Abramowicz 1930, Bab 1933, Touton 1932) were possibly due to paraphenylenediamine also present in the dye solution (Greenberg and Lester 1954, Grant 1962). Lawsone has been used as a topical sunscreen (Johnson et al 1973). Behl et al (1966) observed contact dermatitis of the palms and soles from henna applied for cosmetic purposes and henna dust can irritate the face and exposed skin surfaces. Henna may be adulterated with other acrid and vesicant plants.

References

Abramowicz, I. (1930) Klinische und experimentelle Untersuchungen über Augenschädigungen durch das Haarfarbmittel Henna. Klin. oczna 8, 153 (Abstr. Zbl. f. g. Ophth. 25, 674. 1931).

Bab, W. L. (1933) Schädigung des Auges durch Wimpernfärbung. Deutsche. med. Wchnschr. 59, 1041.

Irvine, F. R. (1961) Woody Plants of Ghana. Oxford University Press.London.

Behl, P.N., Captain, R.M., Bedi, B.M.S. and Gupta, S. (1966) Skin-irritant and sensitizing plants found in India, New Delhi. P.N. Behl, Irwin Hospital.

Johnson, J.A., Czaplewski, R. R. and Fusaro, M.M. (1973) Protection against long ultraviolet light with dihydroxyacetone-naphthoquinone. Dermatologica 147, 104.

Merck Index (1968) An Encyclopedia of Chemicals and Drugs. ed. Stecher, P.G. 8th ed. Rahway, N.J. Merck and Co. Inc.

Oliver, B. (1959) Nigeria's Useful Plants. Nigerian Field 24, 70.

Touton, K. (1932) Hauterkrankungen durch phanerogamische Pflanzen und ihre Produkte (Toxicodermia et Allergodermia phytogenes), in Barnewitz, J. et al Angeborene Anomalien, Lichtdermatosen, Pflanzengifte, Thermische Schädigungen, Einfluss innerer Störungen auf die Haut. Berlin, Verlag von Julius Springer.

Nesaea

50 species are found in tropical and South Africa, Madagascar, Ceylon, Australia and South America.

Nesaea salicifolia

Ingestion of the plant is said to cause violent perspiration (Bailey 1906-7).

References

Bailey, F.M. (1906-7) Weeds and suspected poisonous plants of Queensland. Brisbane, quoted by Hurst 1942.

Hurst, E. (1942) The Poison Plants of New South Wales, N. S. W. Poison Plants Committee; Sydney.

MAGNOLIACEAE

This family consists of 230 species in 12 genera found in temperate and tropical eastern Asia and America. Oil passages are present in the tissues of the plants.

Liriodendron

One species, native to eastern North America, is planted as an ornamental, reaching 60m in height. The timber is known in commerce as Canary Whitewood. The tree is grown as a shade tree in Vancouver and is sometimes named Magnolia when offered for sale in Europe.

Liriodendron tulipifera
Tulip Tree, Yellow Poplar

Dermatitis from the wood, which was used for making pianos, was reported by Brezina in 1912 (Hausen 1973). Two patients had dermatitis of the hands and face from whitewood sawdust; in one of them, a patch test to the sawdust produced a positive reaction, negative in ten controls (Hausen 1970). Four of five individuals who were contact-sensitive to sesquiterpene lactones of Compositae species and of Frullania showed positive patch test reactions to the leaf (Mitchell 1975). The sesquiterpene lactones, liperolide and gamma-liriodenolide from the leaf (Doskotch et al 1972) and tulipinolide and costunolide from the bark (Doskotch and El-Feraly 1969) are potentially allergenic (Mitchell and Dupuis 1971). Costunolide is probably an allergen of Saussurea (Mitchell and Epstein 1974). These findings suggest that the allergens of Liriodendron may be sesquiterpene lactones. In two cases, quinones seemed to be the allergens of the wood (Hausen, B.M. Pers. Comm. 1974).

References

Doskotch, R.W. and El-Feraly, F.S. (1969) Antitumor agents II: Tulipinolide, a new germacranolide sesquiterpene, and costunolide. Two cytotoxic substances from Liriodendron tulipifera L. J. Pharm. Sci. 58, 877.

Doskotch, R.W., Keely, S.L. Jr. and Hufford, C.D. (1972) Lipiferolide, a cytotoxic germacranolide and gamma-liriodenolide, two new sesquiterpene lactones from Liriodendron tulipifera. Chem. Comm. (Chem. Soc. J. Lond.) 20, 1137.

Hausen, B.M. (1973) Holzarten mit gesundheitsschadigenden Inhaltsstoffen Stuttgart. DRW-Verlags-GmbH.

Mitchell, J.C. and Dupuis, G. (1971) Allergic contact dermatitis from sesquiterpenoids of the Compositae family of plants. Brit. J. Derm. 8, 139.

Mitchell, J.C. and Epstein, W.L. (1974) Contact hypersensitivity to a perfume material, Costus Absolute. Arch. Derm. 110, 871.

Mitchell, J.C. (1975) Contact sensitivity to sesquiterpene lactones and some perfume materials. (in) Derm. Int. 14, 301 (see p. 312).

Hausen, B.M. (1970) Untersuchungen uber Gesundheitsschadigende Holzer. Thesis, Hamburg.

Magnolia

80 species are found from the Himalayan mountains east to Japan, Borneo and Java and in eastern North America and the West Indies south to Venezuela. Magnolia kobus provides an essential oil, the principal constituents of which are citral, eugenol and cineol (Kariyone 1971). A phenolic compound, magnolol, is sometimes found as fine crystals in the bark of some Magnolia species (Kariyone 1972). Illicium verum provides Star Anise oil used in flavouring and perfumery (Arctander 1960). The bark of Magnolia species is used to adulterate cinnamon (Smith 1969).

Magnolia grandiflora

An essential oil of perfumery has been derived from the plant (Arctander 1960). The leaves were boiled to make a dye. A dyer developed contact dermatitis of the hands from this work, subsequently of the face, possibly from exposure to the vapour. A patch test produced a positive reaction, negative in controls. Patch test dermatitis appeared at the sites of contact with the cut edge and pin prick holes in the leaf indicating that damage to the leaf was necessary to release the allergenic principle (Genner and Bonnevie 1938). Five individuals who were contact sensitive to sesquiterpene lactones of Compositae species and of *Frullania* showed positive patch test reactions to cut pieces of the leaf of *Magnolia grandiflora* (Mitchell 1975). The finding that damage to the plant tissues was necessary to release the allergen was confirmed. A sesquiterpene lactone, parthenolide, has been isolated from this species (Wiedhopf et al 1973). Parthenolide was found to produce positive patch test reactions in individuals who were contact-sensitive to various Compositae species and sesquiterpene lactones (Mitchell and Dupuis 1971). These findings suggest that such lactones may be the allergens of *Magnolia*. Parthenolide is also derived from *Michelia champaca* of this family.

Magnolia hypoleuca

In the case of contact dermatitis described by Genner and Bonnevie (1938), a dry leaf of this plant produced a positive patch test reaction, weaker in degree than that produced by *Magnolia grandiflora*.

Magnolia virginiana

This species is used in Herbal Medicine. The bark is irritating to the tongue (Wren 1968).

References

Arctander, S. (1960) Perfume and Flavor Materials of Natural Origin. Elizabeth, N.J. Published by the author.

Genner, V. and Bonnevie, P. (1938) Eczematous eruptions produced by leaves of trees and bushes. Arch. Derm. Syph. 37, 583.

Kariyone, T. (1971) Atlas of Medicinal Plants. Osaka, Japan. Takeda Chemical Industries.

Mitchell, J.C. and Dupuis, G. (1971) Allergic contact dermatitis from sesquiterpenoids of the Compositae family of plants. Brit. J. Derm. 84, 139.

Mitchell, J.C. (1975) Contact sensitivity to sesquiterpene lactones and some perfume materials. (in) Derm. Int. 14, 301 (see p. 312).

Smith, F.P. (1969) Chinese Materia Medica. Vegetable kingdom. 2nd ed. Rev. by Hei, P.D. Taipei, Taiwan. Ku T'ing Book House.

Wiedhopf, R.M., Young, M., Bianchi, E. and Cole, J.R. (1973) Tumor inhibitory agent from *Magnolia grandiflora* (Magnoliaceae). J. Pharm. Sci. 62, 345.

Wren, R.W. (1968) Potter's New Cyclopaedia of Botanical Drugs and Preparations by Wren, R.C. Re-edit. by Wren, R.W. Potter and Clarke Ltd. Health Science Press, Rustington, Sussex.

Michelia

Fifty species are found in tropical Asia and China. Several species provide useful timber. In Malaysia, the fragrant flowers are used for adorning the hair and neck (Corner 1952).

Michelia champaca

The flowers yield oil of champaca of perfumery (Arctander 1960) which contains esters of benzoic acid, benzaldehyde, benzyl alcohol and isoeugenol (Merck Index 1968). Biochemical information is given by Hegnauer (1964). The bark is used to adulterate cinnamon (Smith 1969). Four of five individuals who were contact sensitive to sesquiterpene lactones of Compositae species and of *Frullania* showed positive patch test reactions to oil of champaca (Mitchell 1975). In one of five cases the leaf produced a positive patch test reaction. The root of the plant yields parthenolide (Govindachari et al 1964).

Michelia lanuginosa

The bark of the tree yields parthenolide and some other

sesquiterpene lactones (Talapatra et al 1973). Parthenolide has been found to produce positive patch test reactions in individuals who were contact sensitive to various Compositae species and sesquiterpene lactones (Mitchell and Dupuis 1971).

These findings suggest that such lactones may be the allergens of Michelia (Mitchell 1975).

References

Corner, E.J.H. (1952) Wayside trees of Malaysia. Singapore, Government Printer.

Govindachari, T.R., Joshi, B.S. and Kamat, V.N. (1964) Revised structure of parthenolide. Tetrahedron Letters 52, 3927.

Hegnauer, R. (1969) Chemotaxonomie der Pflanzen. Vol. 5. Basel. Birkhauser Verlag. pp. 11-21.

Merck Index (1968) An Encyclopedia of Chemicals and Drugs. ed. Stecher, P.G. 8th ed. Rahway, N.J. Merck & Co. Ltd.

Mitchell, J.C. and Dupuis, G. (1971) Allergic contact dermatitis from sesquiterpenoids of the Compositae family of plants. Brit. J. Derm. 84, 139.

Mitchell, J.C. (1975) Contact sensitivity to sesquiterpene lactones and some perfume materials. (in) Derm. Int. 14, 301 (see p. 312).

Smith, F.P. (1969) Chinese Materia Medica. Vegetable kingdom. 2nd ed. Rev. by Hei, P.D. Taipei, Taiwan. Ku T'ing Book House.

Talapatra, S.K., Patra, A. and Talapatra, B. (1973) Parthenolide and a new germacranolide. 11,13-dehydrolanuginolide from Michelia lanuginosa. Phytochemistry 12, 1827.

MALPIGHIACEAE

800 species in 60 genera are found in tropical regions especially in South America. The plants are usually covered with branched unicellular hairs. Heteropterys leona is used as a pediculicide (Irvine 1961). Chemistry is recorded by Hegnauer (1969).

Gaudichaudia

Fifteen species are native to Mexico and Central America.

Gaudichaudia schiedeana

The hairs on the plant are very irritating (Altschul 1973).

Malpighia

35 species are found in tropical America and the West Indies. Some have stinging, some spine-toothed hairs (Chittenden 1974).

Malpighia linearis

The lower surface of the leaf bears fine irritant hairs (Altschul 1973).

Malpighia polytricha

Pain is produced when the hairs on the lower sides of the leaves enter the skin (Altschul 1973).

Malpighia suberosa

The prickles on the leaves are a possible source of injury (Altschul 1973).

Malpighia urens
Touch-me-not

This plant was listed as a cause of mechanical injury by Oakes and Butcher (1962).

Malpighia urens
Cowitch Cherry

This species possesses stinging hairs (Chittenden 1974) and was noted to produce skin reactions (Pardo-Castello 1923).

Sphedamnocarpus

Twenty species are found in tropical and southern Africa and Madagascar.

Sphedamnocarpus pruriens

The fruit of this plant possesses intensely irritating,

bifurcated hairs (Watt and Breyer-Brandwijk 1962).

References

Altschul, S. von R. (1973) Drugs and foods from little-known plants. Cambridge, Mass. Harvard Univ. Press.

Chittenden, F.J. (1974) The Royal Horticultural Society Dictionary of Gardening. 2nd ed. Vol. 3. Oxford. Clarendon Press.

Hegnauer, R. (1969) Chemotaxonomy of plants. Vol. 5. Basel. Birkhauser. pp. 23-29.

Irvine, F.R. (1961) Woody plants of Ghana. London. Oxford University Press.

Oakes, A.J. and Butcher, J.O. (1962) Poisonous and injurious plants of the U.S. Virgin Islands. Misc. Publ. 882. U.S. Department of Agriculture. Washington, D.C.

Pardo-Castello, V. (1923) Dermatitis venenata. A study of the tropical plants producing dermatitis. Arch. Derm. 7, 81.

Watt, J.M. and Breyer-Brandwijk, M.G. (1962) The Medicinal and Poisonous Plants of Southern and Eastern Africa. 2nd ed. Edinburgh. Livingstone.

MALVACEAE

1000 species in 75 genera are found in tropical and temperate regions.

Abutilon

Over 100 species are found in tropical and subtropical regions. Abutilon avicennae provides a useful fibre named Chinese jute.

Abutilon species

The leaves of some species can produce irritant patch test reactions. Reactions registered as allergic should be accepted with caution (Hjorth 1968, Agrup 1969).

Abutilon indicum
Indian Mallow

In two cases of contact dermatitis attributed to Indian Mallow, strong positive patch test reactions were observed (Underwood and Gaul 1948).

References

Agrup, G. (1969) Hand eczema and other hand dermatoses in South Sweden. Acta derm.-venereol. 49, Suppl. 61.

Hjorth, N. (1968) at the Finsen Institute. Personal communication.

Underwood, G.B. and Gaul, L.E. (1948) Overtreatment dermatitis in dermatitis venenata due to plants. JAMA 138, 570.

Althaea

Twelve species are distributed from western Europe to northeastern Siberia. Althaea officinalis (Marshmallow) has been used for treating skin diseases (Huriez and Fagez 1968, Wren 1968).

Althaea rosea
Hollyhock

The hairy leaves, stems and pollen are irritant (McCord 1962). Hjorth (1968) observed irritant patch test reactions from the plant, and noted that reactions registered as allergic should be accepted with caution. In two cases of contact dermatitis attributed to Hollyhock, strong positive patch test reactions were observed.

References

Hjorth, N. (1968) at the Finsen Institute. Personal Communication.

Huriez, C. and Fagez, C. (1968) On the association of Althea and dexamethasone - Dexalta ointment. Lille Med. 13, 121 (Suppl.).

McCord, C.P. (1962) The Occupational Toxicity of Cultivated Flowers. Ind. Med. Surg. 31, 365.

Underwood, G.B. and Gaul, L.E. (1948) Overtreatment dermatitis in dermatitis venenata due to plants. JAMA 138, 570.

Wren, R.C. (1956) Potter's new cyclopaedia of botanical drugs and preparations. 7th ed. New York. Pitman.

Gossypium

Some 20 species are found in tropical and subtropical regions. Cultivated forms are grown in Old and New Worlds to provide cotton which consists of long hairs covering the seeds. Cotton-seed oil is obtained by crushing the seeds and the oil-cake, following expression, is used for cattle feed.

Gossypium species
Cotton

Commercial cotton may be derived from four main species (Howes 1974). The hairs of cotton plants are irritant (Behl et al 1966). Pseudophytodermatitis can result from contact with cotton and its derivatives.

Cotton, like cereals and straw (Gramineae), can be infested with a mite, *Pyemotes* (*Pediculoides*)(Van Thiel 1953). This mite was found to be an agent of 'cotton-seed dermatitis' in dock-labourers (Nixon 1915, O'Donovan 1921). Agricultural chemicals (Karimov 1970), a varnish used in cotton mills (Schwartz and Pool 1933), and chromates present in cotton used in upholstery (Nixon 1915) have been implicated.

Type I hypersensitivity reactions to cotton seed oil (Brown 1929, Spies et al 1942, Bernton et al 1949, Figley 1949, Harris and Shure 1950, Plymyer 1959) are probably attributable to a water soluble proteinaceous fraction of the oil. Cotton seed was implicated in a death from allergy testing by intradermal injection of 0.02ml of an extract (Harris and Shure 1959). Atopic patients scratch-test sensitive to cotton seed protein were found to be unaffected by ingestion of cottonseed oil (Bernton et al 1949). In discussion of this paper, reference was made to mouth ulceration and oedema of the lips from ingestion of the oil in a sensitive individual. However, patch tests with the oil in sensitive atopic patients were negative. Taub (1945) listed sources of contact with cotton seed oil which was formerly much used in topical therapy and in cosmetics.

Cross-sensitivity was observed to Kapok (*Ceiba*, Bombacaceae) (Brown 1929). Respiratory diseases (byssinosis) can occur in cotton textile workers (Merchant et al 1972).

Cancer of the scrotum in cotton spinners was reviewed by Brockbrank (1941).

References

Behl, P.N., Captain, R.M., Bedi, B.M.S. and Gupta, S. (1966) Skin-irritant and sensitizing plants found in India, New Delhi. P.N. Behl.

Bernton, H.S., Coulson, E.J. and Stevens, H. (1949) On allergy to Cotton seed oil. JAMA 140, 869.

Brockbrank, E.M. (1941) Mule Spinner's Cancer. Epithelioma of the Skin in Cotton Spinners. London. H.K. Lewis.

Brown, G.T. (1929) Cotton seed and kapok sensitisation. JAMA 93, 370.

Figley, K.D. (1949) Sensitivity to edible vegetable oils. J. Allergy 20, 198.

Harris, C. and Shure, N. (1950) Sudden death due to allergy tests. J. Allergy 21, 208.

Howes, F.N. (1974) A Dictionary of Useful and Everyday Plants and their common names. Cambridge University Press.

Karimov, A.M. (1970) Occupational skin diseases in cotton growers caused by chemical poisons, and measures for their prevention. Gig. Tr. Prof. Zabol. 14, 35.

Merchant, J.A. et al (1972) Byssinosis and chronic bronchitis among cotton textile workers. Ann. Int. Med. 76, 423.

Nixon, J.A. (1915) Cotton-seed dermatitis. Brit. J. Derm. 27, 122.

Nixon, J.A. (1915) Cotton seed dermatitis. Proc. Roy. Soc. Med. 8, 112.

O'Donovan, W.J. (1921) Dermatitis due to Carpoglyphus passularum. Brit. J. Derm. 32, 297.

Plymyer, R.E. (1959) Cottonseed allergy. Univ. Mich. Med. Bull. 25, 220.

Schwartz, L. and Pool, C.L. (1933) An outbreak of dermatitis in cotton mills due to varnish. J. Indust. Hyg. 15, 214.

Spies, J.R., Chambers, D.C., Bernton, H.S. and Stevens, H. (1942) The chemistry of allergens VII. The nature of the unidentified allergens of cotton seed. J. Allergy 14, 7.

Taub, S.J. (1945) Cotton seed allergy. JAMA 183, 334.

Van Thiel, P.H. (1953) Arthropods and other animals in relation to Dermatology, in Handbook of Tropical Dermatology and Medical Mycology. ed. Simons, R.D.G. Amsterdam Elsevier Publ. Co. Vol. II. p, 908.

Hibiscus

300 species are found in tropical and subtropical regions. Hibiscus abelmoschus (Musk-mallow) is used as an insecticide and in herbal medicine as a topical remedy for itching (Wren 1968). This species provides Ambrette seed of perfumery (Arctander 1960). Hibiscus rosa-sinensis is used to blacken the eyebrows and shoes and the young leaves are eaten as spinach (Irvine 1961). Hibiscus sabdariffa is used for making jelly (Behl et al 1966).

Hibiscus species

Hjorth (1965) observed allergic contact dermatitis from species of the genus with significant positive patch test reactions. A case of periocular eczema was traced to Hibiscus (Kaalund-Jorgenson 1951).

Hibiscus elatus
Blue mahoe, majagua

The wood smells peppery when worked and causes sneezing (Stone 1924, Record and Mell 1924).

Hibiscus esculentus
(syn. Abelmoschus esculentus)
Ochra, Ladies' fingers, Gumbo

The plant provides a common vegetable in warm climates, much used in soups and stews (Howes 1974). The hairs on the plant are a common source of inflammation and itching (Morton, J.F. 1975, pers. comm.).

The immature mucilaginous fruit is the vegetable named okra. Weber (1937) included this species among plants known to cause dermatitis. Behl et al (1966) observed allergic contact dermatitis in gardeners and housewives from this species. In a housewife working in a kitchen garden, dermatitis affected the left index finger and thumb. A positive patch test reaction was obtained.

Hibiscus irritans

Practically all parts of the plant are covered with sharp stellate hairs which can penetrate and become embedded in the skin (Watt and Breyer-Brandwijk 1962).

Hibiscus panduriformis

The stem is thickly covered with short white hairs amongst which are irritating bristles (Watt and Breyer-Brandwijk 1962).

References

Arctander, S. (1960) Perfume and Flavor Materials of Natural Origin. Elizabeth, N.J. Published by the author.

Behl, P.N., Captain, R.M., Bedi, B.M.S. and Gupta, S. (1966) Skin-irritant and sensitizing plants found in India, New Delhi. P.N. Behl.

Hjorth, N. (1965) Contact sensitivity to plants and balsams.

Europ. Congr. Allergy. Acta. Derm.-venereol. 65.

Irvine, F.R. (1961) Woody Plants of Ghana. London. Oxford University Press.

Kaalund-Jorgensen, O. (1951) Eczema perioculare (Dermatitis of the eyelids). Acta derm.-venereol. 31, 83.

Watt, J.M. and Breyer-Brandwijk, M.G. (1962) The Medicinal and Poisonous Plants of Southern and Eastern Africa. 2nd ed. Edinburgh. Livingstone.

Weber, L.F. (1937) External causes of Dermatitis. A list of irritants. Archs. Derm. Syph. 35, 129.

Wren, R.W. (1968) Potter's New Cyclopaedia of Botanical Drugs and Preparations by Wren, R.C. Re-edit. by Wren, R.W. Potter and Clarke Ltd. Health Science Press. Rustington, Sussex.

Record, S.J. and Mell, C.D. (1924) Timbers of Tropical America. New Haven, Yale.

Stone, H. (1924) The timbers of commerce. London. Rider.

Howes, F.N. (1974) A dictionary of useful and everyday plants and their common names. Cambridge. University Press.

Malachra

Six species are found in warm regions of America and in the West Indies. The plants have rough hairs.

Malachra alceifolia
Wild Okra

This species was listed as a cause of mechanical injury (Oakes and Butcher 1962).

Malachra urens

This species was reported to produce dermatitis (Pardo-Castello 1923).

References

Oakes, A.J. and Butcher, J.O. (1962) Poisonous and injurious plants of the U.S. Virgin Islands. Misc. Publ. 882. U.S. Department of Agriculture. Washington, D.C.

Pardo-Castello, V. (1923) Dermatitis venenata. A study of the tropical plants producing dermatitis. Archs. Derm. 7, 81.

Sida

200 species are found in warm regions, especially in America. Some have spines. Sida rhombifolia provides a fibre.

Sida urens

This species was listed as an irritant by Pammel (1911).

Reference

Pammel, L.H. (1911) A Manual of Poisonous plants. Torch Press. Cedar Rapids, Iowa. Reprinted Univ. Microfilms Inc. Ann Arbor, Mich., 1965.

Thespesia

15 tropical species are known as trees or tall herbaceous plants.

Thespesia populnea
Polynesian Rosewood

This plant was listed as vesicant for the skin by Quisumbing (1951). The leaves are used for counter-irritant purposes.

Reference

Quisumbing, E. (1951) Medicinal Plants of the Philippines. Philipp. Dept. Agr. and Nat. Resources. Tech. Bull. No. 16. Manila. Bureau of Printing. 1234 pp.

MARANTACEAE

400 species in 30 genera are found in tropical regions chiefly in America.

Chemistry is recorded by Hegnauer (1963).

Reference

Hegnauer, R. (1963) Chemotaxonomy of Plants. Vol. 2. Basel.

Birkhauser. P. 359.

Maranta

23 species are native to tropical America.

Maranta arundinacea

This species furnishes West Indian Arrowroot. The starch of the root is said to produce respiratory allergy (Greenberg and Lester 1954).

Thaumatococcus

One species is native to West Africa.

Thaumatococcus danielli

The pulp around the seed has a sweetening effect on the taste similar to that produced by Synsepalum, Sapotaceae (Dalziel 1937).

References

Dalziel, J.M. (1937) The Useful Plants of West Tropical Africa. London. Crown Agents.

Greenberg, L.A. and Lester, D. (1954) Handbook of Cosmetic Materials. New York. Interscience.

MARTYNIACEAE

13 species in 3 genera are native to tropical and subtropical America.

Chemistry is recorded by Hegnauer (1969)

Reference

Hegnauer, R. (1969) Chemotaxonomy of Plants. Vol. 5. Basel, Birkhauser. P. 48.

Martynia

One species is native to Mexico.

Species of this genus have hooked fruits which attach themselves to animals (Howes 1974).

Martynia lutea
Devil's Claws, Ram's Horn

The fruit has two long curved thorns suitable for animal distribution. Those who cut the plants are subject to extreme dizziness (Froggatt cited by Cleland 1925).

References

Howes, F.N. (1974) A Dictionary of Useful and Everyday Plants and their Common Names. Cambridge University Press. pp. 290.

Froggatt cited by Cleland, J.B. (1925) Plants including fungi, poisonous or otherwise injurious to man in Australia. (Series II) Med. J. Australia 2, 443.

MELASTOMATACEAE

3000 species in 240 genera are found in tropical and subtropical regions. Thr fruit of Melastoma blackens the mouth.

Miconia

700 species are found in tropical America and the West Indies, one species in West Africa.

Miconia sp.

The wood yields primin, an allergen of Primula obconica (Marini-Bettolo et al 1971).

Reference

Marini-Bettolo et al (1971) Gez. chim. Ital. 101, 41, cited by Hausen (1975), unpublished observations.

MELIACEAE

1400 species in 50 genera are found in warm regions. The seeds of several species provide oils. Aglaia odorata (Mock lime) is used to provide a scent for clothing and tea (Corner 1952, Arctander 1960).

Chemistry is recorded by Hegnauer (1969).

References

Arctander, S. (1960) Perfume and Flavor Materials of Natural Origin. Published by the author. Elizabeth, N.J.

Corner, E.J.H. (1952) Wayside Trees of Malaysia. Singapore, Government Printer.

Hegnauer, R. (1969) Chemotaxonomy of Plants. Vol. 5. Basel, Birkhauser. p. 54.

Amoora

Amoora polystachya
Tasua

Amoora cucullata

25 species are native to Indo Malaysia. The wood of some species can produce respiratory symptoms (Orsler 1973) and skin irritation (Altschul 1973).

Carapa

Seven species are found in tropical regions.

Carapa guianensis
Brazilian mahogany

This species was listed as a source of dermatitis by Senear (1933).

Carapa procera
Monkey Cola

The sawdust was used as a rubefacient and can produce dermatitis (Irvine 1961).

References

Altschul, S. von R. (1973) Drugs and foods from little-known plants. Cambridge, Mass. Harvard Univ. Press.

Irvine, F.R. (1961) Woody plants of Ghana. Oxford University Press. London.

Orsler, R.J. (1973) Personal communication from Forest Products Research Laboratory, Princess Risborough, Bucks, England.

Senear, F.E. (1933) Dermatitis due to woods. JAMA 101, 1527.

Cedrela

Six or seven species are found from Mexico to South America. Some yield valuable timber known as Stinking Mahogany or Citron. Cedrela odorata, used for cigar boxes is known as West Indian Cedar. The wood dust of some species can produce dermatitis (Hanslian and Kadlec 1966) especially C. tooni (Orsler 1973).

References

Hanslian, L. and Kadlec, K. (1966) Drevo z heediska hygienickeho (VIII). Biologicky ucinne a malo ucinne dreviny. Drevo 21, 229.

Orsler, R.J. (1973) Personal communication from Forest Products Research Laboratory, Princess Risborough, Bucks, England.

Dysoxylum
(Dysoxylon)

200 species are native to Indo Malaysia. Some are known as Australian Mahogany and Indian Cedar.

Dysoxylum muelleri
Red bean, stavewood, miva mahogany, Australian blackwood

Furniture workers who worked with the wood of red bean for 4 or 5 days developed influenza-like symptoms, vomiting and nose bleeds. The more seasoned the wood, the worse it became (Maiden 1909). After sawing the wood Bisset (1949) developed similar symptoms with painful breathing, headache and loss of appetite. The wood can cause eczema (Maiden 1909). A man developed rhinorrhoea, and asthma after working with any wood (query including this species) (Pulleine 1925).

Dysoxylum richii
Maotamea

This species was said to cause eczema and irritation of the eye and throat (Maiden 1909). Stavewood is a common name for a tree of this genus which is said to irritate the skin (Thiebault 1965).

References

Pulleine, R.H. (1925) in discussion of Aldersley, R.B. (1925).

Aldersley, R.B. (1925) Sensitiveness to proteins of wood. Med. J. Australia 2, 25.

Bisset, I.J.W. (1949) Irritant properties of Miva mahogany. Forest Products Newsletter no. 178, p. 3.

Maiden, J.H. (1909) On some plants which cause inflammation or irritation of the skin. Agric. Gaz. New South Wales 20, 1073.

Thiebault, A. (1965) Nomenclature Generale des Bois Tropicaux. L'Association Technique Internationale des Bois Tropicaux. 45, bis Avenue de la Belle-Gabrielle, Nogent-sur Marne, France.

Ekebergia

15 species are found in tropical and South Africa and in Madagascar.

Ekebergia senegalensis

The charred powdered roots cause violent sneezing (Irvine 1961).

Reference

Irvine, F.R. (1961) Woody plants of Ghana. Oxford University Press. London.

Entandrophragma

35 species found in tropical and South Africa. Some are known in the lumber trade as Cedar or Mahogany.

Entandrophragma angolense
Tiama

A few cases of dermatitis from the wood of this species have been observed in the furniture industry (Wilkinson 1972).

Entandrophragma candolei
Sipo

The wood irritates the skin and mucous membranes (Hublet et al 1972).

Entandrophragma cylindricum
Sapele

Brezina (1921) described a scarlatina-like eruption on the arms which followed polishing 'sapeli-mahogany'. No patch tests were recorded and the botanical identity of the wood was not certain.

Entandrophragma utile
Utile

Woods and Calnan (1976) reported two cases of dermatitis from the wood dust. A machinist had dermatitis and swelling of the eyelids. The dermatitis spread to face, neck, scalp, elbow flexures, groins, popliteal skin and feet. Another patient was also contact sensitive to Dalbergia. They comment that the wood is extensively used and the incidence of 'toxic' effects probably low.

References

Woods, B. and Calnan, C.D. (1976) Toxic Woods. Brit. J. Derm. 94, suppl. 13, June.

Brezina, E. (1921) Internationale Ubersicht uber Gewerbekrankheiten uber des Jahr 1913. ed. by Teleky, L. and Brezina, E. Berlin, Springer.

Hublet, P., Sporcq, J., Oleffe, J. et al (1972) Etude sur les accidents cutanes et muqueux provoques par les bois tropicaux dan l'industrie du bois en Belgique. Arch. Belges, Med. Social. 30, 314.

Wilkinson, D.S. (1973) Personal communication.

Guarea

150 species are found in tropical America and 20 species in Africa.

Guarea cedrata
Bossé

All the men in contact with this West African wood in a factory complained of severe irritation of the nose and throat (MacKenna and Horner 1954). Orsler (1973) received trade reports of skin and nasal irritation from the wood.

Other species known as Obobo and Nigerian Pear Wood, notably Guarea thompsonii have been implicated (Hausen 1970) but the chemicals responsible are unknown.

Guarea thompsonii

The wood is said to be more irritating than that of G. cedrata (Farmer 1972).

Guarea trichilioides and other Guarea spp.

The bark of this American tree smells of musk and, when powdered, has emetic and haemostatic properties (Record and Hess 1943).

References

Hausen, B.M. (1970) Undersuchungen uber Gesundheitsschadigende Holzer. Thesis, Hamburg.

Orsler, R.J. (1973) Personal communication from Forest Products Research Laboratory, Princess Risborough, Bucks, England.

Record, S.J. and Hess, R.W. (1943) Timbers of the New World. New Haven, Yale.

Farmer, R.H. (1972) A Handbook of Hardwoods. 2nd ed. HMSO London.

MacKenna, R.M.B. and Horner, S. (1954) Occupational skin diseases in Industrial Medicine and Hygiene. ed. Merewether, E.R.A. London, Butterworth.

Khaya

Eight species are native to tropical Africa and Madagascar.

Khaya anthotheca
African mahogany, acajou

Khaya euryphylla

Khaya ivorensis
(syn. K. kalainei)
African mahogany, acajou

Khaya nyasica
East African mahogany

Khaya senegalensis
Bissilom

The species are difficult to distinguish, especially after felling. They are often imported mixed though K. ivorensis provided the bulk of the timber (Rendle 1956).

Reference

Rendle, B.J. (1956) Variation in the quality of African mahogany. Wood 21, 349.

Khaya spp.
African Mahogany

The wood can produce dermatitis in wood-workers (Morgan and Wilkinson 1965, Morgan and Orsler 1967, Wilkinson 1968, 1970, Morgan et al 1968). Contact dermatitis from the wood-dust can ressemble seborrhoeic dermatitis or neurodermatitis. The dermatitis affected the face, neck and ears but the postauricular skin was spared and the bald rather than the hairy area of the scalp was affected in workmen who did not wear caps. The hands usually escaped (Wilkinson 1973). The outer heart-wood freshly prepared as wood dust in a concentration 10% in petrolatum was satisfactory for patch-testing. Khaya wood dust was not irritant by patch test in contrast to Tectona. Khaya is not a strong sensitiser; 10% of exposed workers were affected and the dermatitis was not severe. A sensitizing component of the wood is anthothecol which can be tested at a concentration 0.5% or 0.1% in petrolatum. Higher concentrations produce a risk of active sensitisation. The wood dust does not appear to affect the respiratory tract.

Other woods, introduced into shipments of K. anthotheca, can be distinguished by chemical tests. Several may also produce sensitisation but some are inactive. West African Mahogany is a name given to a variety of hardwoods and patch tests should be carried out with botanically identified woods in addition to samples supplied from the work area.

In respiratory disease from Khaya, fungus growth in the wood was suspected (Dantin-Gallego et al 1952).

Zafiropoulo et al (1968)

and Hausen (1970) describe dermatitis from the species. Bevan et al (1963) discuss the chemistry.

K. anthotheca cross-reacts with K. euryphylla but not with K. ivorensis.

An American report of asthma from mahogany (Sosman et al 1969) may refer to Khaya spp. or to Swietenia sp. 'Mahogany from Congo and Ghana' which caused dermatitis in 15 of 68 furniture makers (Shevlyakov 1969) seems to have been Khaya spp. rather than Swietenia sp.

Khaya senegalensis

This species was included in a list of toxic timbers by Czimatis and Hagemann (1910).

References

Bevan, C.W.L., Rees, A.H. and Taylor, D.A.H. (1963) West African timbers Part VII. Anthothecol - an extractive from Khaya anthotheca. J. Chem. Soc. 938.

Dantin-Gallego, J., Armayor, A.F. and Fiesco, J. (1952) Some new toxic woods: some new manifestations of toxicity. Industr. Med. Surg. 21, 42.

Hausen, B.M. (1970) Undersuchungen uber Gesundheitsschadigende Holzer. Thesis, Hamburg.

Morgan, J.W.W. and Wilkinson, D.S. (1965) Sensitization to Khaya anthotheca. Nature, Lond. 207, 1101.

Morgan, J.W.W. and Orsler, R.J. (1967) Simple test to distinguish Khaya anthotheca from K. ivorensis and K. grandifolia. J. Invest. Med. Sci. 18, 61.

Morgan, J.W.W., Orsler, R.J. and Wilkinson, D.S. (1968) Dermatitis due to the wood dusts of Khaya anthotheca and Macherium scleroxylon. Brit. J. Ind. Med. 25, 119.

Wilkinson, D.S. (1968) Wood Dermatitis. Sensitization to Khaya anthotheca (African Mahogany). Brit. J. Derm. 80, 195.

Wilkinson, D.S. (1970) Dermatitis from Khaya mahoganies in the furniture industry. Symposium sulla prevenzione delli dermatosi professionali tenutose. Monte Porzio Cantone.

Wilkinson, D.S. (1973) Personal communication.

Zafiropoulo, A., Audibert, A. and Charpin, J. (1968) A propos des accidents dus a la manipulation des bois exotiques. Rev. Franc. Allerg. 8, 155.

Czimatis and Hagemann (1910) Ueber Erkrankungen durch Holzstaub. Hygienische Rundschau 20, 761.

Shevlyakov, L.V. (1969) On dermatitis caused by tropic species of wood. Vestn. Derm. Vener. 43, 73.

Sosman, A.J., Schlueter, D.P., Fink, J.N. et al (1969) Hypersensitivity to wood dust. New Eng. J. Med. 281, 977.

Lovoa

Eleven species are native to tropical africal

Lovoa
Dibetou, African Walnut

Some species notably L. klaineana (African Walnut) and L. trichiliodes can cause dermatitis, respiratory symptoms and possibly systemic effects in woodworkers (Zafiropoulo et al 1968, Schweisheimer 1952, Ordman 1949, Allemany-Vall 1958, Symanski 1957).

One man who had dermatitis showed positive patch test reactions to L. klaineana and to Mansonia sp. (Woods and Calnan 1976).

References

Allemany-Vall, R. (1958) Rhinitis and dermatitis caused by exotic woods. Occupational Allergy, Leiden p. 273-277.

Ordman, D. (1949a) Bronchial asthma caused by the inhalation of wood dust. Ann. Allergy 7, 492.

Ordman, D. (1949b) Wood dust as an inhalant allergen. South Africa Med. J. 23, 973.

Schweisheimer, W. (1952) Wood dust and respiratory diseases. Wood 17, 181.

Symanski, H.F. (1957) Opticusatrophie nach Verarbeitung tropischer Holzer? Med. Klin. 52, 198.

Zafiropoulo, A., Audibert, A. and Charpin, J. (1968) A propos des accidents dus a la manipulation des bois exotiques. Rev. Franc. Allerg. 8, 155.

Woods, B. and Calnan, C.D. (1976) Toxic Woods. Brit. J. Derm. 94, Suppl. 13, June.

Melia

Possibly two or as many as 15 species are known from tropical and subtropical regions. Some yield useful timber.

Melia azedarach
Chinaberry

Eating the fruits causes stomatitis (Verdcourt and Trump 1969, Morton 1971) and the oil from the fruits is irritant (Simpson and Lim 1935).

Melia excelsa

The fruit smells like garlic (*Allium*) and the leaves are intensely bitter.

Melia indica
Nim or Margosa Tree

The plant, which smells like garlic, is used medicinally, as an insecticide and is incorporated into soap, lotions and toothpaste (Corner 1952).

References

Corner, E.J.H. (1952) Wayside Trees of Malaysia. Singapore, Government Printer.

Morton, J.F. (1971) Plants Poisonous to People in Florida and other warm areas. Miami, Florida. Hurricane House Publishers, Inc.

Simpson, I.A. and Lim, E.C. (1935) Margosa fruit suspected to be cause of a case of fatal poisoning. Malayan Med. J. 10, 138.

Verdcourt, B. and Trump, E.C. (1969) Common Poisonous Plants of East Africa. London. Collins.

Sandoricum

Ten species are native to Mauritius and Indo Malaysia. Some have edible fruit.

Sandoricum indicum
(syn. *S. nervosum*)

MacKenna and Horner (1954) described sneezing, epistaxis, tightness of the chest, body-aches, 'marked mental dimness' and bradycardia which affected four men sawing the wood and to a lesser degree other men nearby and the investigating physician. There was no dermatitis. The heart-wood contains a triterpene, katonic acid (King and Morgan 1960).

References

King, F.E. and Morgan, J.W.W. (1960) The constitution of Katonic acid, a triterpene from *Sandoricum indicum*. J. Chem. Soc. 4738.

MacKenna, R.M.B. and Horner, S. (1954) Occupational skin diseases in Industrial Medicine and Hygiene. ed. Merewether, E.R.A. London, Butterworth.

Swietenia
American Mahogany, Acajou

Seven or eight species are native to tropical America and to the West Indies where the timber was used by Raleigh to repair his ships in Elizabethan times. The wood was used for cabinet work in England in 1680 and the seeds reached India in 1795.

Sweitenia macrophylla
American mahogany
Honduras mahogany
Tabasco mahogany
Baywood, Acajou amérique

Swietenia mahogani
American, Cuban, West Indian or Spanish Mahogany, Acajou amérique

American mahogany used for cabinet work has become scarcer and largely replaced by Khaya. Some authors have not distinguished between these sources of mahogany (Hausen 1970).

Dermatitis from the wood was reported by Herxheimer (1912). Schwartz and Russell (1941) and Steiner and Schwartz (1944) reported dermatitis from use of the woods in boat and airplane manufacture. The botanical species are not clearly defined and over 60 species of varied botanical origin have been offered as Mahogany (Burkill 1935). The chemicals responsible are unknown (Hausen 1970).

'Mahogany from Congo and Ghana' which caused dermatitis in 15 of 68 furniture makers (Shevlyakov 1969) seems to have been Khaya sp. rather than Swietenia sp.

References

Burkill, I.H. (1935) A Dictionary of the Economic Products of the Malay Peninsula. 2 Vols. London Crown Agents for the Colonies.

Hausen, B.M. (1970) Untersuchungen uber Gesundheitsschadigende Holzer. Thesis, Hamburg.

Herxheimer, H. (1912) On industrial diseases of the skin. Deutsch. med. Wochenschr. 38, 18.

Schwartz, L. and Russell, J.P. (1941) Skin hazards in airplane manufacture. Publ. Health Rep. 56, 1581.

Steiner, S.D. and Schwartz, L. (1944) Dermatitis from Mahogany wood (Swietenia macrophylla). Industr. Med. 13, 234.

Shevlyakov, L.V. (1969) On dermatitis caused by tropic species of wood. Vestn. Derm. Vener. 43, 73.

Toona
(syn. Cedrela)

Fifteen species are found in tropical Asia and Australia.

Toona sureni

Toona spp.

Orsler (1973) received trade reports of skin irritation from this wood.

Reference

Orsler, R.J. (1973) Personal communication from Forest Products Research Laboratory, Princess Risborough, Bucks, England.

Turraeanthus

Six species are native to tropical Africa.

Turraeanthus africanus
Avodiré

The wood has produced dermatitis and asthma in wood-workers (Hausen 1970, Calnan 1970, Zafiropoulo et al 1968, Kerharo and Bouquet cited by Irvine 1961, Hublet et al 1972).

The sawdust is said to make wood-cutters spit blood (Irvine 1961).

References

Calnan, C.D. (1970) Avodiré wood sensitivity. Contact Dermatitis Newsletter (London) 8, 190.

Hausen, B.M. (1970) Untersuchungen uber Gesundheitsschadigende Holzer. Thesis, Hamburg.

Hublet, P., Sporcq, J., Oleffe, J. et al (1972) Etude sur les accidents cutanes et muqueux provoques par les bois tropicaux dan l'industrie due bois en Belgique. Arch. Belges. Med. Social. 30, 314.

Kerharo, J. and Bouquet, A., cited by Irvine, F.R. (1961) Woody Plants of Ghana. Oxford University Press. London.

Zafiropoulo, A., Audibert, A. and Charpin, J. (1968) A propos des accidents dus a la manipulation des bois exotiques. Rev. Franc. Allerg. 8, 155.

MENISPERMACEAE

350 species in 65 genera are found in warm regions.

A few species are medicinal on account of a bitter principle in the root.

Chemistry is recorded by Hegnauer (1969).

Reference

Hegnauer, R. (1969) Chemotaxonomy of Plants. Vol. 5. Basel, Birkhauser, p. 73.

Anamirta

One species is found in Indo Malaysia.

Anamirta cocculus

The fruits are used as a fish-poison. Cavities in the plants are inhabited by mites (acarodomatia). Application of the plant to the scalp was said to produce a scarlet eruption on the body and arms (Allen 1874-1879 cited by Piffard 1881).

Reference

Piffard, H.G. (1881) A treatise on the Materia Medica and Therapeutics of the Skin. New York. Wm. Wood and Co.

Burasaia

Four species are found in Madagascar.

Burasaia madagascariensis

The alkaloids of the wood may be injurious to wood-workers (Pernet 1957, Hausen 1970).

References

Hausen, B.M. (1970) Undersuchungen uber Gesundheitsschadigende Holzer. Thesis, Hamburg.

Pernet, R. (1957) Les plantes medicinales malgaches. Catalogue de nos connaissances chimiques et pharmacologiques. Mem. Inst. Sci. Madagascar B8, 1.

Coscinium

Eight species are found in Indo Malaysia and Indo China.

Coscinium fenestratum (syn. Menispermum fenestratum) Columbo-wood

The wood of this Ceylonese tree may be injurious to wood-workers from a content of berberine (Hausen 1973). Reactions to berberine are noted under Berberis.

In Ceylon a dye and a bitter tonic are extracted from the wood. Vorreiter (1958) lists it as a toxic wood causing vomiting, diarrhoea and cramps. The plant is only a climber and produces no timber (Gamble 1902).

References

Hausen, B.M. (1973) Holzarten mit Gesundheits-schadigenden inhaltsstoffen DRW Verlags GmbH Stuttgart.

Gamble, J.S. (1902) A Manual of Indian Timbers. 2nd ed. Reprinted by Bishen Singh Mahendra Pal Singh, Dehra Dun, 1972.

Vorreiter, L. (1949) Holztechnologisches Handbuch. Wien, Fromme (later edition 1958).

Menispermum Moonseed

Three species are found in temperate eastern Asia, Atlantic North America and Mexico.

Menispermum canadense Yellow Pirila

The root of this plant like that of sarsaparilla (Smilax) has been used in Herbal Medicine for skin diseases (Wren 1968).

The rough sharp ridges of the fruit pips can cause mechanical injury (Der Marderosian 1966).

Reference

Wren, R.W. (1968) Potter's New Cyclopaedia of Botanical Drugs and Preparations by Wren, R.C. Re-edit. by Wren, R.W. Potter and Clarke Ltd. Health Science Press. Rustington, Sussex.

Der Marderosian, A. (1966) Poisonous plants in and around the home. American Journal of Pharmaceutical Education 30, 115.

Penianthus

Six species are found in tropical West Africa.

Penianthus zenkeri

The root shavings, when put on wounds, produce a burning sensation (Irvine 1961).

Reference

Irvine, F.R. (1961) Woody plants of Ghana. Oxford University Press. London.

Sphenocentrum

One species is found in tropical West Africa.

Sphenocentrum jollyanum

The roots are acid in the mouth but cause things eaten thereafter to taste sweet (Dalziel 1937). This property is also noted with Synsepalum and Maranta.

Reference

Dalziel, J.M. (1937) The Useful Plants of West Tropical Africa. London. Crown Agents.

MONTINIACEAE

Four species in two genera are found in south-western and tropical East Africa and in Madagascar.

Montinia

One species is found in southern Africa. The leaf contains an acrid, pungent principle (Watt and Breyer-Brandwijk 1962).

Reference

Watt, J.M. and Breyer-Brandwijk, M.G. (1962) The Medicinal and poisonous plants of Southern Africa. 2nd ed. Edinburgh. E.& S. Livingstone.

MORACEAE

This family includes about 1400 species in 53 genera. Most are trees or shrubs of the tropics or subtropics, but a few species are indigenous to temperate regions.

Lac (shellac) is produced on several species by the punctures of an insect.

Antiaria

There are four species in tropical Africa and Indo Malaysia.

Antiaria africana
Timber: Antiaria

This tree yields a useful timber for general constructional purposes, and is exported to Europe in small quantities (Hausen 1973). Whilst it shares to some extent the toxic properties of A. toxicaria, it is by no means so aggressively irritant.

Antiaria toxicaria
Upas tree

This tree of legendary ill repute was believed to kill all who came near it (White 1887, Menninger 1967). It contains cardioactive glucosides (Hausen 1973, Hegnauer 1969, Wehrli et al 1962) which have been used as arrow-poisons. The use of the timber is limited by its toxicity. The bark is made into a fabric which may irritate the skin, unless the bark-fibre is thoroughly cleaned of all traces of latex (Burkill 1935, Osol and Farrer 1955).

A severe dermatitis has been reported in those felling or handling the tree (Van Hasselt 1862, Grossman 1920, Bernhard-Smith 1923). The sap is said to be harmless on unbroken skin (Gimlette 1929) but may irritate scratches (Irvine 1961).

References

Bernhard-Smith, A. (1923) The Poisonous Plants of All Countries. 2nd ed. London, Bailliere, Tindall & Cox.

Burkill, I.H. (1935) A Dictionary of the Economic Products of the Malay Peninsula. 2 Vols. London, Crown Agents for the Colonies.

Grossman, J. (1920) Gesundheits-schadliche Holzarten Der Holzkaufer (100-103) 17, 519-30; 540-51; 545-46.

Hegnauer, R. (1969) Chemotaxonomy of Plants. Vol. 5. Basel, Birkhauser. pp. 107-128.

Menninger, E.A. (1967) Fantastic Trees. New York, The Viking Press.

Osol, A. and Farrer, G.E. (Ed.) (1955) Dispensatory of the .S.A. Philadelphia, J.B. Lippincott.

Van Hasselt (1862) Handbuch der Figtlehre Braunschweig. Cited by White (1887).

White, J.C. (1887) Dermatitis venenata: an Account of the Action of External Irritants Upon the Skin. Boston, Cupples and Hurd.

Hausen, B. (1973) Holzarten mit gesundheits-schadigenden Inhaltsstoffen. Stuttgart. DRW-Verlags-GmbH.

Gimlette, J.D. (1929) Malay Poisons and Charm Cures. 3rd ed. London, Churchill.

Irvine, F.R. (1961) Woody plants of Ghana. London, Oxford University Press.

Wehrli, W., Schindler, O. and Reichstein, T. (1962) Die Glykoside des Milchsaftes von *Antiaris toxicaria* Lesch. aus Malaya sowie von *A. africana*. Engl. aus Kenya. Helv. Chim. Acta 45, 1183.

Shellac

Shellac is lac melted and run into thin plates (Oxford English Dictionary). Shellac is a resinous excretion of the insect *Laccifer* (*Tachardia*) *lacca* produced on certain trees (Estrin 1973). Shellac can produce allergic contact dermatitis (Fisher 1973).

References

Estrin, N.F. (1973) Cosmetic Ingredient Dictionary. 1st ed. Washington, D.C. Cosmetic, Toiletry and Fragrance Ass. Inc.

Fisher, A. (1973) Contact Dermatitis. 2nd ed. Lea and Febiger.

Artocarpus

Forty-seven species are found in south-eastern Asia and Indo Malaysia. Several species are cultivated all over the tropics e.g. *A. altilis* (bread-fruit) and *A. heterophyllus* (jak). The timber is useful and that of *A. integrifolia* has been called Ceylon Mahogany (see *Pterocarpus santalinus*). The fruits of some species weigh as much as 10 kg. Such species are not recommended for planting at roadsides or in gardens.

Brosimum

Some 50 species are natives of temperate and tropical South America. Some yield a drinkable latex, others edible achenes.

Brosimum gaudichaudii
Mamica de cadela

The root yields bergapten, psoralen and other coumarins, the photosensitizing capacity of which has been investigated (Martins et al 1974).

Brosimum guianense
(syn. *Piratinera guianensis*)

Brosimum paraense
(syn. *Piratinera paraensis*)

The wood contains quinones chemically related to those found in *Piratinera guianensis* (Hausen 1970)

Guinea pigs could be sensitised to an ethanol/chloroform extract of the wood (Hausen 1974).

A report of toxicity from

the wood of bois de Feroles (Czimatis and Hagemann 1910) seems to refer to B. paraense and not to Ferolia spp. (Woods and Calnan 1976 citing Record and Hess 1943).

References

Hausen, B.M. (1974) Personal communication.

Czimatis and Hagemann (1910) Ueber Erkrankungen durch Holzstaub. Hygienische Rundschau 20, 761.

Record, S.J. and Hess, R.W. (1943) Timbers of the New World. New Haven, Yale.

Woods, B. and Calnan, C.D. (1976) Toxic Woods. Brit. J. Derm. 94, Suppl. 13, June.

Hausen, B.M. (1970) Untersuchungen uber Gesundheitsschadigende Holzer. Thesis, Hamburg.

Martins, J.E.C., Puzetti, G.L. and Sodre, M. (1974) Effects of Psoralen and Bergapten on irradiated Skin. Derm. Int. 13, 124.

Brounsettia

Seven or eight species are native to eastern Asia. The bark of B. papyrifera (paper mulberry) provides a fibre used for paper and cloth.

Brounsettia spp.

The pollen of some species can cause hayfever (Wodehouse 1971).

Reference

Wodehouse, R.P. (1971) Hayfever Plants. 2nd rev. edition. New York, Hafner.

Chlorophora

There are twelve species in the tropics of America, Africa and Madagascar. Several of the species yield a valuable timber, which, on account of its superficial resemblance to oak or to teak, has been sold under a confusing multiplicity of names. The most important species is Chlorophora excelsa, and "Chlorophora" without specific identification usually refers to this tree.

Chlorophora excelsa
Iroko, Kambala,
African Teak, Moreira,
Moule

The timber is strong, durable and weather resistant and is much used for outdoor and indoor constructional work, including boat building.

Chemistry

The alkaloid chlorophorin is an allergic sensitizer (Schulz 1957, 1960, 1962, 1967). The molecule is composed of a four-fold oxidized stilbene nucleus and an aliphatic side chain, and is chemically related to the allergenic compounds of Toxicodendron (King and Grundon 1950).

Dermatitis

Dermatitis affects carpenters, joiners and other wood workers, rather than those felling the trees. The sawdust was recognized as causing dermatitis of eyelids and genitalia, in Breslau over 60 years ago (Czimatis and Hagemann 1910). Iroko is amongst the six commonest causes of dermatitis from woods in France (Zafiropoulo et al 1968). However the latex oozing from the freshly felled timber appears to be irritant and has caused acute, followed by chronic, dermatitis in East African workers (Piorkowski 1944).

There are numerous reports of dermatitis in wood workers; taken together the reports provide a graphic picture of a severe dermatitis, sometimes associated with ocular and respiratory symptoms, and assuming almost epidemic proportions particularly where high temperature and humidity favour eccrine sweating.

The earliest clinical and chemical studies were made in Germany and France (Hubinot 1928, Frei 1931, 1932, Loro 1923). In an outbreak of dermatitis in a joiners' workshop Jung (1967) noted positive patch test reactions to the sawdust. Goessens (1936) reported a case of generalized dermatitis caused by the sawdust. Frei (1932) obtained positive patch test reactions with sawdust and Ragot and Brun (1948) with an aqueous extract.

Thienemann (1941) noted the development of dermatitis in a proportion of workers approximately ten weeks after this wood was first introduced. He gave a good description of the distribution of the dermatitis, which involved the arms, the face and chest and the scrotom. The incidence of dermatitis in some workshops has been very high: in one machine shop all of the more than 50 workers were affected in some degree, though only 9 had severe dermatitis, sometimes accompanied by upper and lower respiratory tract symptoms (Davidson 1941). This variation in the clinical picture was noted also by Langelez (1950); some workers developed only a mild papular prurigo of exposed or covered skin, a few developed dermatitis particularly of the neck and ears, and some in each group had conjunctivitis and asthma.

This variation suggests that the sawdust both irritates and sensitizes, and the investigation of a case of dermatitis in a machinist supported this assumption. Patch tests with the dry dust were positive in the patient and in 4 of 5 control subjects, but tests with 0.1% chlorophorine in soft paraffin were positive only in this patient (Beer 1970).

Respiratory symptoms may be severe. Obstructive rhinitis without asthma occurred in men handling Iroko and Bété and both rhinitis and asthma in another who worked with Iroko, Obèche, *Triplochiton* and Framiré (Zafiropoulo et al 1968). In reporting 11 cases of asthma in men exposed to the dust of Iroko and Teak (*Tectona*), Ganse (1968) noted that only a proportion of these patients gave positive scratch test reactions and that inhalation tests were sometimes positive when these were negative. It is not established whether the respiratory symptoms are purely irritant in origin or whether a reaginic antibody is implicated.

For patch testing, 1% chlorophorin in soft paraffin is probably suitable, unless this concentration is proved to sensitize some subjects (Maibach 1970). In one patient patch tests with 0.1% chlorophorin were negative, whilst tests to 0.5% and 1.0% were positive (Wilkinson 1969).

Thiel (1960) reported contact sensitivity to the wood.

Mucocutaneous reactions from this species in the wood working industry was reported by Hublet et al (1972).

Chlorophora tinctoria
Old Fustic, Mora

This wood was formerly used almost exclusively as the source of the yellow dye, morin. Now that morin has been largely replaced by synthetic dyes, the timber is being used for the manufacture of furniture and musical instruments (Hausen 1970).

It is said to have irritant and sensitizing properties (Peche 1947) similar to those of *C. excelsa*, but as it has been relatively little used as timber, no reliable assessment of its hazards is yet possible.

References

Beer, W.E. (1970) Sensitivity to Iroko wood in a wood machinist. Personal communication. Contact Dermatitis Newsletter 7, 159 (January).

Czimatis and Hagemann (1910) Uber Erkrankungen durch Holzstaub. Hyg. Rundsch. 20, 761.

Davidson, J.M. (1941) Toxic Effects of Iroko. An African Wood. Lancet 1, 38.

Frei, (1931) Dermatitiden durch sogenanntes afrikanisches Teakholz ("Kambala-Teak"). Derm. Ztschr. 62, 187.

Frei, (1932) Dermatitis durch afrikanisches Teakholz (Kambala-Teak). Derm. Wschr. 94, 27.

Ganse, W. van (1968) Respiratory Allergies of Occupational Origin Provoked by Exotic Woods. (French) Arch. Mal. prof. 29, 205.

Goessens, (1936) Concerning Intoxications Due to Exotic Wood. Rev. Path. Phys. Trav. 12, 314.

Hausen, B.M. (1970) Undersuchungen uber Gesundheitsschadigende Holzer. Thesis, Hamburg.

Hubinot, G. (1928) Titel u. Zschr. wie Goessens (1936) 12, 318.

Jung, H.-D. (1967) Berufliche Kontaktekzeme durch Kambala-Teak-Holz. Dtsch. Gesundheitsw. 22, 2141.

King, F.E. and Grundon, F.M. (1949) The Constitution of Chlorophorin, a Constituent of Iroko, the Timber of Chlorophora excelsa. J. Chem. Soc. Lond. 3348 and (1950) 3547.

Langelez, A. (1950) Dermatitis due to Kambala Wood. (French) Rev. Bois, 4, 26.

Maibach, H.I. (1970) Active sensitization to Wood Extracts. Personal communication. Contact Dermatitis Newsletter 7 (Jan.), p. 149.

Peche, F. (1947) Bois congolais et dermatoses. Bull. Compt. Ven. Bois Cong. 8, 2.

Loro, H.-A.-M. (1923) L'urticaire de l'Iroko. Arch. Med. Pharm. Nav. 114, 136.

Piorkowski, F.O. (1944) Woodworker's Dermatitis in East Africa. East Afr. med. J. 21, 60.

Schulz, K.H. (1957) Allergische Kontaktdermatitis durch exotische Holzer, insbesonders durch Kambala-Teakholz. Berufsdermatosen 5, 238.

Schulz, K.H. (1960) Uber die sensibilisierende Wirkung von Inhaltsstoffen tropischer Holzer, 1 Symposium Dermatologorum Pragae. Prague, Vytvarny atelie Novinarskych savodu Mir, 2, 318.

Schulz, K.H. (1937) Berufsdermatosen - ausgewahlte Kapital. Z. haut-u. GeschlKr., 42, 499.

Thienemann, K. (1941) Kambala Teakwood Dermatoses. (German) Arch. f-Derm. Syph. 182, 551.

Wilkinson, D.S. (1969) Sensitivity to Iroko Wood in a Boat Builder. Personal Communication. Contact Dermatitis Newsletter 6, 142 (July).

Zafiropoulo, A., Audibert, A. and Charpin, J. (1968) A propos des accidents dus a la manipulation des bois exotiques. Rev. Franc. Allerg. 8, 155.

Ragot, A. and Brun, J.R. (1948) Les dermatoses professionelles du bois d'Iroko. 9th Internat. Congr. Industr. Med. pp. 354-8. Bristol, Wright.

Thiel, A. (1960) A propos de 7 cas de sensibilisation au bois de Kambala, 1 Symposium Dermatologorum Pragae, 1960, Vytvarny atelier Novinarskych zavodu Mir, 1962, 2, 315.

Hublet, P., Sprocq, J., Oleffe, J. et al (1972) Etude sur les accidents cutanes et muqueux provoques par les bois tropicaux dan l'industrie du bois en Belgique. Arch. Belges. Med. Social. 30, 314.

Fatoua

One species is found in Madagascar: one species in the eastern Pacific region.

Fatoua pilosa

The plant causes itching of mild degree (Altschul 1973).

Reference

Altschul, S. von R. (1973) Drugs and foods from little-known plants. Cambridge, Mass. Harvard Univ. Press.

Ficus

Some 800 species are widely distributed throughout the warmer regions of the world. When the word fig is used without qualification it refers to Ficus carica, which has been cultivated for millenia and has been very widely dispersed from its point of origin which was probably in the area of which Syria is the centre (Candolle 1886), in which the fig grows wild. The fig is cultivated wherever the climate is suitable, and survives, although it does not prosper, even in Northern Europe.

Some other species of Ficus yield edible figs. Others are cultivated as ornamental plants.

Ficus asperifolia
Sandpaper Tree

The rough leaves are used as an abrasive by carpenters in Africa, and the sap is used as a gloss for blackening boots and shoes (Irvine 1961). It is not reported whether it shows the irritant or photosensitizing properties of some other species.

Ficus atrox

This plant is reported as irritant (Burkill 1935).

Ficus carpraefolia

The rough leaves are used as an abrasive (Williamson 1956).

Ficus carica

The fig and the tree which bears it have for so long formed such an important component of man's environment in the Mediterranean region, the Near and Middle East and parts of India, that its products have come to occupy a place in ancient and in modern indigenous medicine. Man comes into intimate contact with the fruit as cultivator, gatherer, packer or consumer, or even as a carpenter, although the timber is of limited value and is mainly used locally for boxes and other small articles (Hausen 1970).

The fig itself may be regarded as a head of flowers turned outside in, and highly specialized pollination mechanisms have been evolved (Corner 1952).

The pollens of native species of North America are suspected of causing hayfever (Wodehouse 1971).

Chemistry

The latex contains a proteolytic enzyme, ficin (Merck 1968) which is irritant to inflamed skin and to the conjunctiva (Watt and Breyer-Brandwijk 1962). It has pruritogenic properties similar to those of mucunain (Arthur and Shelley 1955) and is irritating to skin and eye (Grant 1962).

The latex yields also ficusin, a psoralen, and 8-methoxypsoralen (Pathak et al 1962). The sap of peel, fruit and leaves was a photosensitizer in all test subjects (Kitchevatz 1934, Kitchevatz 1936).

Medicinal Applications

"But ye vitiligines albae are cataplasmed with ye leaues or ye boughes of ye Black Figge" (Dioscorides c. 50 A.D.). It appears therefore that the capacity of the sap of the fig to induce pigmentation was known almost 2000 years ago. The sap was used as a counterirritant in Southern Europe by the 13th century (Straton 1912) and probably earlier. It is used in India in the treatment of eczema and psoriasis (Behl et al 1966).

Dermatitis

The precise causes of the various clinical syndromes are debatable. Conflicting statements concern in particular the direct irritancy of the sap. In such a widely established species with numerous named cultivars and spontaneously developed varieties, it could be predicted that such properties as the irritancy of the sap would be very variable. In many reports of patch tests the possibility that an irritant reaction might occur has been ignored. On the present evidence it is fair to say that figs cause irritant dermatitis, but vary in their capacity to do so. Whether figs can also cause an allergic contact dermatitis is uncertain. Figs can also cause a photodermatitis, but by what mechanism is not known - a possible role of psoralens is not clearly defined; there is no convincing evidence that an immunological process is concerned.

Dermatitis occurring in young children picking figs is believed to be due to small hairs on the leaves (Davidson 1899); as this author points out the fig-leaf seems to be a most unsuitable choice for an article of clothing. Whilst some authors find the fig itself non-irritant (Davidson 1899) others, e.g. Maiden (1909) say that the peel irritates the mouth and that some individuals develop dermatitis from gathering green figs. However contact with the latex could presumably not be completely excluded in this case, and this is certainly the principal cause of dermatitis in fig-gatherers. It has been reported from Turkey (Behcet et al 1938) and from California (Legge 1921): some immediate discomfort is experienced and vesicles develop after 3 or 4 hours.

The therapeutic applications of the sap may be followed by ulceration (Straton 1912) and, in India, by bullous dermatitis, ulceration, hyperpigmentation, depigmentation and even keloidal scars (Behl et al 1966).

Straton (1912) noted that contact with fig sap could result in pigmentation lasting as long as 30 years; the pigmentation could be prevented by washing the hands soon after contact. The role of sunlight in provoking the reactions to fig sap was noted by Vigne and Ponthieu (1936) and was investigated by Behcet et al (1938, 1939) in Turkey. Behcet had earlier (1933) reported that dermatitis could be induced with either the sap or a decoction of the leaves. The methods of investigators then available were limited, but it could be shown that whilst some patients had a true photodermatitis, provoked by sunlight, others developed a bullous reaction to an alcoholic extract of fig even if protected from light.

Berlin (1930) reported that fig dermatitis was common in Palestine during the summer months, and affected mainly boys aged 6 to 12. A bullous eruption developed on exposed skin, mainly on the limbs and around the mouth, and was followed by pigmentation. Fig sap produced a bullous reaction on the author's arm after 48 hours.

Photodermatitis from contact with the fresh figs or foliage was reported by Kuske (1938, 1940) and Rossetti (1947). The cases of bullous dermatitis reported by Paionne (1938) were probably light-induced. On the other hand Furtado (1951) observed photodermatitis of the hands and arms, followed by streaky hyperpigmentation, after the use of an extract of fig leaves as a shampoo; a patch test was negative. Five other patients with a similar reaction had earlier been reported (Aleixo 1935) but were not patch tested. An infusion of fig leaves reputed to remove stains caused dermatitis in two patients who used it to wash clothes (Pershangov 1965).

Those engaged in drying, packing or cooking figs sometimes develop a chronic eczema of the fingers and hands, which may be associated with paronychia (Behl et al 1966), but even in these occupations the clinical picture is variable. Six candy-makers, and a housewife who cooked figs, all developed a bullous photodermatitis with pigmentation (Popoff and Zaharieff 1935). An elderly labourer who was employed in drying figs developed after 24 hours an irritable eruption of face and neck and axillae, of uncertain causation (Emido 1940).

The diagnosis of fig dermatitis is further complicated by the fact that dried figs, like other stored foods, may harbour a mite, Carpoglyphus, which may give rise to an extensive papular eruption (O'Donovan 1920, Belisario 1948, Pirila 1951, Rokstad 1943).

References

Aleixo, A. (1935) Dermatitis due to Extract of Fig Leaves. Brasil-med. 49, 553.

Arthur, R.P. and Shelley, W.B. (1955) The Role of Proteolytic Enzymes in the Production of Pruritus in Man. J. Invest. Derm. 25, 341.

Behcet, H.D., Ottenstein, K., Lion, K. and Dessauer, F. (1938) On the Question of Fig Dermatitis. Deri Hast. ve Frengi Klinigi Ars. 5, No. 23-26.

Behcet, H.D., Ottenstein, B., Lion, K. and Dessauer, F. (1939) Fig Dermatitis. Experiments on the Chemical, Physical, and Allergic Factors which may Provoke Fig Dermatitis (French) Ann. Derm. Syph. 10, 32 and 125.

Behl, P.N., Captain, R.M., Bedi, B.M.S. and Gupta, S. (1966) Skin-irritant and Sensitizing Plants Found in India, New Delhi. P.N. Behl, Irwin Hospital.

Belisario, J.C. (1948) Some Aspects of Occupational Dermatitis in Australia. Proc. Br. Med. Ass. Excerpta Medica Sect. 13 (1948) 3, Abstr. 2808, p. 590.

Berlin, C. (1930) Figtree Dermatitis (German) Derm. Wschr. 90, 733.

Burkill, I.H. (1935) A Dictionary of the Economic Products of the Malay Peninsula. 2 Vols. London, Crown Agents for the Colonies.

Candolle, A. de (1886) Origin of Cultivated Plants. 2nd ed. (Reprint 1959), p. 295. Hafner, New York.

Corner, E.J.H. (1952) Wayside Trees of Malaysia. Singapore, Government Printer.

Davidson, A. (date uncertain, quoted 1899) Therap. Gaz. 22, 86 quoted in Pharm. J. 4th Series, 8, 335. Apr. 15, 1899, quoted by Maiden (1909).

Dioscorides (c. 50 A.D.) The Greek Herbal of. Englished by John Goodyer: A.D. 1855. Edited and first printed A.D. 1933 by R.T. Gunther 1959. New York, Hafner Publishing Co.

Emodi, G. (1940) Dermatitis due to Dry Figs. Ungarische Dermatologische Gasellschaft, Budapest. Offizieller Bericht 9, XI.

Furtado, T.A. (1951) Dermatitis Caused by an Extract of Fig Leaves (Portuguese) Ann. Brasil Derm. Sif. 26, 121.

Grant, W.M. (1962) Toxicology of the Eye. Springfield, Ill., Charles C. Thomas.

Hausen, B.M. (1970) Untersuchungen uber Gesundheitsschadigende Holzer. Thesis, Hamburg.

Irvine, F.R. (1961) Woody Plants of Ghana. London. Oxford University Press.

Kitchevatz, M. (1934) Etiology and Pathogenesis of Dermatitis due to Contact with Figs: Role of Light. Bull. Soc. Franc. Dermat. et Syph. 41, 1751.

Kitchevatz, M. (1936) Nouvelles recherches sur la photosensibilisation de la peau. Bull. Soc. Franc. Derm. Syph. 43, 581.

Kuske, H. (1938) Experimentelle Untersuchungen zur Photosensibilisierung der Haut durch pflanzliche Wirkstoffe; lichtsensibilisierung durch Furocumarine als Ursache verschiedener phytogener Dermatosen. Arch. Derm. Syph. 178, 112.

Kuske, H. (1940) Perkutane Photosensibilisierung durch pflanzliche Wirkstoffe. Dermatologica 82, 273.

Legge, R.T. (1921) Occupational diseases of the skin and hands in California industry. Calif. State J. Med. 19, 461.

Maiden, J.H. (1909) On Some Plants Which Cause Inflammation or Irritation of the Skin. Agr. Gaz. New South Wales 20, 111, 1073.

Merck Index (1968) ed. Stecher, P.G. 8th ed. Rahway, N.J. Merck and Co.

O'Donovan, W.J. (1920) Dermatitis due to Carpoglyphus passularum. Br. J. Derm. 32, 297.

Paionne, J. (1938) Papulobullous Dermatosis due to Fig Juice. Brasil-med. 52, 347.

Pathak, M.A., Daniels, F. Jr. and Fitzpatrick, T.B. (1962) Presently Known Distribution of Furocoumarins (Psoralens) in Plants. J. Invest. Derm. 39, 225.

Pershangov, A.B. (1965) Dermatitis Caused by Fig. Vestn. Derm. Vener. 39, 73.

Pirila, V. (1951) On Cheese and Fig Mite Dermatitis. Act. derm.-vener. (Stockh.) 31, 630.

Popoff, L. and Zaharieff, B. (1935) Uber die Dermatitis bullosa, striata and pigmentose (Feigenbaumdermatitis). Jb. Univ. Sofia Med. Fak. 14, 153 (abstr. Zentralb. f. Haut.-u. Geschlectskr. 54, 21, 1937).

Rokstad, I. (1943) Endemic outbreaks of skin eruption caused by mites from food stuff (figs) and tobacco. Acta derm.-venereol. 24, 113.

Rossetti, N. (1947) Vegetable sensitizers; hyperchromic photodermatitis caused by fig tree. An brasil de dermat. e sif 22, 177 abstr. Year Book of Dermatology and Syphilology (1948) p. 163.

Straton, C.R. (1912) Dermatitis venenata. Br. med. J., ii, 1139.

Vigne, P. and Ponthieu (1936) Dermite du figuier. Bull. Soc. franc. Derm. Syph. 43, 710.

Watt. J.M. and Breyer-Brandwijk, M.G. (1962) The Medicinal and Poisonous Plants of Southern and Eastern Africa. 2nd ed. Edinburgh. E.& S. Livingstone, Ltd.

Williamson, J. (1956) Useful Plants of Malawi. ed. Greenway, P.J. Zomba, Malawi, The Government Printer. Previously published as Useful Plants of Nyasaland.

Wodehouse, R.P. (1971) Hayfever Plants. 2nd rev. edition. New York, Hafner.

Ficus edelfeltii

This plant is reported as irritant (Burkill 1935).

Reference

Burkill, I.H. (1935) A Dictionary of the Economic Products of the Malay Peninsula. 2 Vols. London, Crown Agents for the Colonies.

Ficus elastica
India rubber plant

This species is popular as a house-plant and is much favoured for the decoration of waiting-rooms and offices: it is a possible cause of allergic dermatitis; a patch test to a leaf was positive in one patient (Agrup 1969).

Reference

Agrup, G. (1969) Hand eczema and Other Hand Dermatoses in South Sweden. Acta derm.-vener. (Stockh.) 49, Suppl. 61, pp. 1-91.

Ficus exasperata

The leaves are used as an abrasive (Irvine 1961).

Reference

Irvine, F.R. (1961) Woody Plants of Ghana. London. Oxford University Press.

Ficus fulva
Stinging fig

The twigs, leaves and figs are set with short stinging bristles (Corner 1951). It is not clear whether the 'sting' is mechanical or chemical.

Reference

Corner, E.J.H. (1952) Wayside Trees of Malaysia. Singapore. Government Printer.

Ficus hispida

Ingestion of the dried unripe fruit and application of

powder to the skin produced a lowered minimal erythema dose by irradiation with an ultraviolet lamp (Ansari et al 1975).

Reference

Ansari, Z., Dioivedi, R.M. and Singh, G. (1975) Phototoxic properties of Ficus hispida (Kath Cular). Ind. J. Derm. Venereol. 41, XVII.

Ficus macrophylla
Australian banyan,
Moreton Bay Fig

This plant is irritant; a patch test was positive in 8 of 38 persons (Fregert and Hjorth 1969).

Reference

Fregert, S. and Hjorth, N. (1969) Results of Standard Patch Tests with Substances Abandoned. Personal Communication. Contact Dermatitis Newsletter 5, 85. (February)

Ficus mallotocarps

The leaves are abrasive (Williamson 1956).

Reference .

Williamson, J. (1956) Useful Plants of Malawi. ed. Greenway, P.J. Zomba, Malawi, The Government Printer. Previously published as Useful Plants of Nyasaland.

Ficus pumila
(syn. Ficus scandens,
Ficus repens,
Ficus stipulata)
Climbing Fig

According to Maiden (1920) the sap of this plant can cause intense irritation of the eye.

Reference

Maiden, J.H. (1920) Plants which Produce Inflammation or Irritation of the Skin. Ag. Gaz. New Wouth Wales, 3i, 386.

Ficus septica

The leaves are irritant to workers who chop them up and mix them with opium (Burkill 1935).

Reference

Burkill, I.H. (1935) A Dictionary of the Economic Products of the Malay Peninsula. 2 Vols. London, Crown Agents for the Colonies.

Ficus tumila
Wild Fig of Australia

The sap can cause bullous dermatitis and severe eye complications, which may lead to permanent impairment of vision. Patch tests were positive, but tests in control subjects were not mentioned (English and Grey 1943).

Reference

English, P.B. and Grey, L.P. (1943) Sap Dermatitis and Conjunctivitis Caused by the Wild Fig (Ficus tumila). Medical Journal of Australia, 1, 578.

Ficus venenata

The sap is strongly irritant (Burkill 1935).

Reference

Burkill, I.H. (1935) A Dictionary of the Economic Products of the Malay Peninsula. 2 Vols. London, Crown Agents for the Colonies.

Maclura

There are about 12 species in the warmer parts of America, Africa and Asia.

Maclura pomifera
(syn. M. aurantiaca,
Toxylon pomiferum)
Osage Orange, Bow wood

This plant is used as an ornamental hedge in America, Australia and India. The wood is used for bows and carriage poles and by turners and cabinet makers (Hausen 1970). The bark yields tannic acid and a yellow dye which has been used as a substitute for fustic from Chlorophora. The inedible fruit, known as the horse apple, is irritant (Schur 1932).

An antifungal chemical constituent is maclurin, an alkaloid (Barnes and Gerber 1965).

The tree can cause mechanical injury by its spines, and dermatitis by contact with its latex. Reports are brief (Schwartz et al 1957, Hurst 1942, Muenscher 1951, Gardner and Bennetts 1956) and it is by no means clear whether the latex is irritant or sensitizing, or both. The pollen can cause hayfever (Wodehouse 1971).

Maclura tinctoria
(syn. Chlorophora tinctoria)

The sap contains tetrahydroxystilbene which is chemically related to chlorophorin of Chlorophora (Laidlaw and Smith 1959).

References

Barnes, R.A. and Gerber, N.N. (1965) The antifungal agent from Osage orange wood. J. Amer. Chem. Soc. 77, 3259.

Gardner, C.A. and Bennetts, H.W. (1956) The Toxic Plants of Western Australia. Perth, West. Australian Newspapers Ltd.

Hausen, B.M. (1970) Untersuchungen uber Gesundheitsschadiegende Holzer. Thesis, Hamburg.

Schur, A. (1932) Dermatitis venenata. Report of a case due to Osage orange (Maclura pomifera). Archs. Derm. 26, 312.

Laidlaw, R.A. and Smith, G.A. (1959) Heartwood extractives of some timbers of the family Moraceae. Chemistry and Industry, 1604.

Hurst, E. (1942) The Poison Plants of New South Wales. N.S.W. Poison Plants Committee, Sydney.

Muenscher, W.C. (1951) Poisonous Plants of the United States. 2nd ed. New York, Macmillan.

Schwartz, L., Tulipan, L. and Birmingham, D.J. (1957) Occupational Diseases of the Skin. 3rd ed. Philadelphia, Lea and Febiger, pp. 637-672.

Wodehouse, R.P. (1972) Hayfever Plants. 2nd rev. edition. New York, Hafner.

Morus

There are about 10 species widely distributed in North and South America, tropical Africa and southwest Asia. Several species are cultivated for their edible fruit, the mulberry, or for their leaves, which are fed to silkworms.

Morus alba
White Mulberry

Morus nigra
Common Mulberry

Morus rubra
Red Mulberry

These three species are used to feed silkworms (as are various other trees). The leaves of M. rubra are said to cause dermatitis (Hardin and Arena 1969), but no documented reports of dermatitis from any part of the tree have been discovered. Disorders of eyes, skin or respiratory tract, which affected one half of the workers on a silkworm farm, were attributable to the hairs and scales of the moths, Bombyx mori (Marconi et al 1951, Paun et al 1964) and to a toxic substance from the cocoons (Kochergin 1957). Cresol was incriminated by Goodman in 1933.

Potton (Bull. de l'Acad de Med. 17, 803 cited by White 1887) under the title Mal de vers, described an inflammatory affection of the hands among silk weavers who unwind the silk from the cocoons. He attributed the disease to the presence of the worm in its cocoon, to its decomposition and to changes which gradually take place in its interior.

The pollen of some species can cause hayfever (Wodehouse 1971).

References

Hardin, J.W. and Arena, J.M. (1969) Human Poisoning from Native and Cultivated Plants. Durham, N. Carolina, Duke University Press.

Kochergin, V.N. (1957) Protective Paste for Prophylaxis of Dermatitides and Burns of Workers in Silk Winding Mills. From the Symposium. Vopr. Derm. I. Vener. (Tashkent), 161-164.

Marconi, F., Sansoni, I. and Coli, S. (1951) Allergy to the Moths of the Silkworm. Accad. Med. Genova 66, 158.

Paun, R., Popescu, I.G., Gheorghiu, T., Zamfirescu-Gheorghiu, M., Claru, C., Iota, C.G. and Molner, C. (1964) Studies on Occupational Allergy in a Silkworm Cultivation Station. Rev. Roum. Med. Interne 1, 413.

Potton. Bull. de l'Acad de Med. 17, 803 cited by White, J.C. (1887) Dermatitis venenata: An account of the Action of External irritants upon the Skin. Boston. Cupples and Hurd.

Wodehouse, R.P. (1971) Hayfever Plants. 2nd rev. edition. New York, Hafner.

Piratinera

The twelve species are natives of tropical America.

Piratinera guianensis (syn. Brosimum guainense) Snakewood, Amourette

The wood is so extremely hard that it will not accept nails, but it has some uses and is imported to Europe in limited quantities (Hausen 1970).

Workers with the wood of this species developed headache, irritation of the nose and throat, nausea and skin inflammation (Grossmann 1920). The sawdust produced salivation and severe thirst and all parts of the tree were very irritating to the skin where it was thin (Freise 1932). This author rubbed a powder of the bark into his own forearm; a burning inflammation developed and left a stain which persisted for some weeks. Hausen (1970) found evidence of quinones in the wood, chemically related to those of *Brosimum paraense*.

Two coumarins have been isolated from the wood, but phototoxic effects have not been reported as such (Hausen 1970). Alcohol/chloroform extracts of the wood produced sensitization in guinea pigs (Hausen 1974).

References

Freise, F.W. (1932) Gesundheitsschadigungen durch Arbeiten mit giftigen Holzern. Beobachtungen aus brasilianischen Gewerbebetrieben. Archiv fur Gewerbepathologie und Gewerbehygiene 3, 1.

Grossmann, J. (1920) Gesundheitsschadliche Holzarten Der Holzkaufer (Leipzig). 17, 529, 535, 540 and 545.

Hausen, B.M. (1970) Untersuchungen uber Gesundheitsschadigende Holzer. Thesis, Hamburg.

Hausen, B.M. (1974) Personal Communication.

Streblus

There are 22 species in Madagascar, South-east Asia and Indo Malaysia. The taxonomy of this and related genera is confusing.

Streblus, *Phyllochlamys*, *Pseudomorus* and *Taxotrophis* are accepted as synonyms.

Streblus brunoniana Whalebone tree

Maiden (1920) reported the statement of a correspondent that the sap was severly irritant to the eyes. Subsequent authors have cited this apparently isolated report (e.g. Hurst 1942).

References

Hurst, E. (1942) The Poison Plants of New South Wales. N.S.W. Poison Plants Committee, Sydney.

Maiden, J.H. (1920) Plants which produce Inflammation or Irritation of the Skin. Ag. Gaz. New South Wales 31, 386.

MYRICACEAE

40 species in four genera are of cosmopolitan distribution.

Chemistry is recorded by Hegnauer (1969).

Reference

Hegnauer, R. (1969) Chemotaxonomy of Plants. Vol. 5. Basel, Birkhauser. p. 138.

Myrica

35 species are almost cosmopolitan.

Myrica cerifera

This species yields bay berry wax which has been reported to be irritant and sensitizing (Greenberg and Lester 1954).

Reference

Greenberg, L.A. and Lester, D. (1954) Handbook of Cosmetic Materials. New York. Interscience.

MYRISTICACEAE

300 species in 18 genera are found in tropical regions especially in Asia.

Cephalosphaera

One species is found in tropical Africa.

Cephalosphaera usambarensis

The tree provides a hardwood timber. A fat obtained from the dried fruit causes dermatitis in 'susceptible' persons (Watt and Breyer-Brandwijk 1962).

Reference

Watt, J.M. and Breyer-Brandwijk, M.G. (1962) The Medicinal and Poisonous Plants of Southern Africa. 2nd ed. Edinburgh. E.& S. Livingstone.

Myristica

120 species are found in tropical regions. Myristica argentea provides a form of Mace.

Myristica fragrans

The seed provides the spice named Nutmeg, and the aril which is around the seed provides the spice named Mace. Oils of Nutmeg and of Mace do not appear to have been used for patch testing; they contain some sensitizers (Stecher 1968). Myristic acid is present in nutmeg butter and in palm seed fats (Palmae). Isopropyl myristate is used in cosmetics and topical preparations (Stecher 1968), and has been reported to cause allergic contact dermatitis (Calnan 1968). Sensitization appears to be rare since none of 100 and of 230 consecutive eczematous patients patch tested to isopropyl myristate, 5 per cent in petrolatum, showed positive patch test reactions (Rantuccio and Meneghini 1970, Meneghini 1970). Possible cross-sensitivity between isopropyl myristate, turpentine and tars reported in a preliminary note by Wilkinson (1969) requires confirmation. Ingestion of nutmegs can cause poisoning. The syndrome includes redness of the skin, dryness of the mouth and hallucinations (Hardin and Arena 1969). The narcotic properties of nutmegs may result from the transformation of myristicin into an amphetamine derivative (Schlemmer et al 1973).

References

Calnan, C.D. (1968) Isopropyl myristate sensitivity. Contact Dermatitis Newsletter, London 3, 41.

Hardin, J.W. and Arena, J.M. (1969) Human Poisoning from Native and cultivated plants. Durham, North Carolina. Duke University Press.

Meneghini, C.L. (1970) Cosmetic constituents. Contact Dermatitis Newsletter, London 8, 182.

Rantuccio, F. and Menghini, C.L. (1970) Results of patch testing with cosmetic components in consecutive eczematous patients. Contact Dermatitis Newsletter, London. 7, 156.

Schlemmer, R.F., Farnsworth, N.R., Cordell, G.A. et al (1973) Nutmeg Pharmacognosy. New Eng. J. Med. 289, 922.

Stecher, R.H. (1968) Merck Index. 8th ed. Rahway, N.J. Merck and Co. Inc.

Wilkinson, D.S. (1969) Isopropyl myristate. Contact Dermatitis Newsletter, London. 6, 144.

Pycnanthus

Eight species are found in tropical Africa.

Pycnanthus angolensis
Ilomba

The wood of this West African tree has been reported injurious in the trade, said to produce nausea and vomiting (Hausen 1970).

Reference

Hausen, B.M. (1970) Untersuchungen uber Gesundheitsschadigende Holzer. Thesis, Hamburg.

Staudtia

Two or three species are found in West Africa.

Staudtia stipitata
Niove

Niove is listed as a skin irritant (Alemany-Vall 1958).

Reference

Alemany-Vall, R. (1958) Rhinitis and dermatitis caused by exotic woods. in Occupational Allergy. p. 273. Leiden, Stenfert-Kroese.

MYRTACEAE

3000 species in 100 genera are found in warm regions, chiefly in Australia and tropical America. Many have edible fruits.

Chemistry is recorded by Hegnauer (1969).

Reference

Hegnauer, R. (1969) Chemotaxonomy of Plants. Vol. 5. Basel, Birkhauser. p. 171.

Backhousia

Seven species are found in eastern Australia. Backhousia citriodora yields an essential oil.

Backhousia myrtifolia
(syn. B. australis)
Australian lancewood, grey myrtle

Since splinters of Australian lancewood, Acacia shirleyi, were said to cause painful wounds (Maiden 1919) other lancewoods viz. B. myrtifolia, Curtisia dentata, and Oxandra lanceolata have been included in lists of toxic woods without any published evidence (Woods and Calnan 1976).

References

Maiden, J.H. (1919) Notes on Acacia, no. IV. J. Proc. Roy. Soc. New South Wales 53, 219-200 (whole paper 171-238 + plates).

Woods, B. and Calnan, C.D. (1976) Toxic Woods. Brit. J. Derm. 94, Suppl. 13, June.

Eucalyptus

500 species are found in Australia and two or three species in Indo Malaysia. The barks of the trees of this family vary considerably but, being easily recognized, are an aid in classification and account for some of the common names. The most common kind is smooth bark (Gum trees) which exfoliates in patches. Other kinds have scaly bark (Blood-woods, etc.), thick and fibrous bark (Stringy-barks), hard furrowed bark, often black with age (Iron barks). Eucalyptus oils vary in chemical composition.

Eucalyptus camaldulensis

The decaying cocoon of a moth found under the loose bark produces intense itching when it comes into contact with sweating skin (Watt and Breyer-Brandwijk 1962).

Reference

Watt, J.M. and Breyer-Brandwijk, M.G. (1962) The Medicinal and poisonous plants of Southern Africa. 2nd ed. Edinburgh. E.& S. Livingstone.

Eucalyptus divaricata

Eucalyptus globulus
Blue Gum

Eucalyptus hemiphloia
White Gum

Eucalyptus leucoxylon
Blue Gum

Eucalyptus macrorrhyncha
Red Stringy Bark

Eucalyptus maculata
Spotted Gum

Eucalyptus marginata
Jarrah

Eucalyptus microcorys

Eucalyptus pilularis

The bark or wood of these species have been reported to produce dermatitis (Maiden 1909, Cleland 1925, Hanslian and Kadlec 1966). Sensitive persons are said to develop urticaria from handling the foliage (Watt and Breyer-Brandwijk 1962). Behl et al (1966) observed that the irritant and sensitizing properties are slight but that eucalyptus oil is rubefacient and that ingestion of the oil can produce skin eruptions in some individuals. Irritant effects of the oils have been reported (Galewsky 1904, 1905, Macpherson 1923). The composition of the oils (Watt and Breyer-Brandwijk 1962) suggests possible allergenecity but evidence for such an effect is scanty (Lowenfeld 1932, Greenberg and Lester 1954).

The oil is poisonous when ingested (MacPherson 1925, Cleland 1925).

Eucalyptus diversicolor
Karri

The wood or possibly arsenic used to treat the wood caused skin irritation (Cleland 1925).

Eucalyptus hemiphloia

The bark irritates the skin (Cleland 1925).

Eucalyptus leucoxylon

The sawdust causes spasmodic rhinorrhea (Cleland 1925).

Eucalyptus macrorrhyncha

The bark irritates the skin (Cleland 1925).

Eucalyptus maculata
Spotted gum

In some parts of Queensland timber-getters and sawyers had 'spotted-gum rash' but in other areas of the country the disorder did not seem to occur (Maiden 1909).

Eucalyptus saligna
'Rio Rosewood', 'Pao Ferro'

Three carpenters developed erythema multiforme after working with the wood stated to be of this genus probably of this species, with Dalbergia nigra, and with Macherium scleroxylon respectively (Holst et al 1976).

Behl, P.N., Captain, R.M., Bedi, B.M.S. and Gupta, S. (1966) Skin-irritant and sensitizing plants found in India, New Delhi. P.N. Behl, Irwin Hospital.

Cleland, J.B. (1925) Plants including fungi, poisonous or otherwise injurious to man in Australia. (Series II) Med. J. Australia 2, 443.

Galewsky (1904) Uber Eukalyptus-Dermatitis. Derm. Ztschr. 11, 752.

Galewsky (1905) Uber Eukalyplus-dermatitiden. Derm. Ztschr. 12, 36.

Greenberg, L.A. and Lester, D. (1954) Handbook of Cosmetic Materials. New York. Interscience.

Hanslian, L. and Kadlec, K. (1966) Drevo z hlediska hygienickeho (VIII). Biologicky ucinne a malo ucinne dreviny. Drevo. 21, 229.

Holst, R., Kirby, J. and Magnusson, B. (1976) Sensitisation to tropical woods giving erythema multiforme-like eruptions. Contact Dermatitis 2, 295.

Loewenfeld, W. (1932) Ekzematose Uberempfindlichkeit gegen Eukalyptusol. Derm. Wschr. 95, 1281.

MacPherson, J. (1923) Dermatitis from Eucalyptus trees. Med. J. Austr. 2, 265.

MacPherson, J. (1925) The toxicology of Eucalyptus oil. Med. J. Australia 2, 108.

Maiden, J.H. (1909) On some plants which cause inflammation or irritation of the skin. Agric. Gaz. New South Wales 20, 1073.

Watt, J.M. and Breyer-Brandwijk, M.G. (1962) The Medicinal and poisonous plants of Southern Africa. 2nd ed. Edinburgh. E.& S. Livingstone.

Eugenia

1000 species are found in tropical and subtropical regions. Many have edible fruit. The flower buds of some species are used as cloves (Syzygium).

Reported allergenicity of eugenol was reviewed by Opdyke (1975).

Eugenia caryophyllata

Oleum Caryophylli refers to Oil of Cloves (Syzygium).

Eugenia jambolana
Jambul

The seeds are used for astringent purposes (Wren 1968).

Eugenia myritifolia

Contact sensitivity to this plant and to Medicago was reported by Anderson (1944).

References

Anderson, C.R. (1944) Contact dermatitis from alfalfa and bur clover. Arch. Derm. Syph. 5, 201.

Wren, R.W. (1968) Potter's New Cyclopaedia of Botanical Drugs and Preparations by Wren, R.C. Re-edit. by Wren, R.W. Potter and Clarke, Ltd. Health Science Press. Rustington, Sussex.

Opdyke, D.L.J. (1975) Monographs on Fragrance raw materials. Rd. Cosmet. Toxicol. 13, 545.

Eugenia uniflora

Respiratory symptoms can result from trimming the plant (Morton 1969).

Reference

Morton, J.F. (1969) Some ornamental plants excreting respiratory irritants. Proc. Florida State Hort. Soc. 82, 415.

Melaleuca

One species is native to Indo Malaysia, 100 species to Australia and the Pacific region.

Melaleuca leucadendron
Paperbark, Cajeput

Paperbark refers to the shedding of the bark which remains partially attached to the tree.

Contact with the roots, branches and seedpods can cause dermatitis; volatile emanations from the tree, when in bloom, can also produce dermatitis without direct contact (Morton 1971).

Oil of Cajeput contains a phenolic compound which chelates copper from the distillation vessels and changes from a yellow to a green colour (Lowry 1973). Artificial colouring may be added to produce a desired green colour (Nasution et al 1973).

The chemistry of the oil is given by Merck (1968); eucalyptol (cineol) is a major constituent. The oil has irritant properties and can produce dermatitis and folliculitis when used for massage (Greenberg and Lester 1954).

A patient who had contact dermatitis from application of the oil was sensitive to eucalyptol (Sezary and Horowitz 1935).

Tiger Balsam, a commonly used balm in the Orient, probably contains this oil and Oil of Wintergreen (Betula) and turpentine (Nasution et al 1973).

The bark is used as a rubefacient in India (Behl et al 1966). Cajeput oil can cause dermatitis and folliculitis (Simons 1953).

References

Greenberg, L.A. and Lester, D. (1954) Handbook of Cosmetic Materials. New York. Interscience.

Lowry, J.B. (1973) A new constituent of biogenetic, pharmacological and historical interest from Melaleuca cajeputi oil. Nature 241, 61.

Merck Index (1968) An Encyclopedia of Chemicals and Drugs. ed. Stecher, P.G. 8th ed. Rahway, N.J. Merck and Co. Inc.

Morton, J.F. (1971) Plants Poisonous to People in Florida and other warm areas. Miami, Florida. Hurricane House Publishers, Inc.

Nasution, D., Klokke, A.H. and Nater, J.P. (1973) A survey of occupational dermatoses in Indonesia. Berufsdermatosen 21, 215.

Sezary, A. and Horowitz, A. (1935) Intolerance cutanee (eczema artificial) au gomenol. Bull. Soc. franc. Derm. Syph. 42, 425.

Behl, P.N., Captain, R.M., Bedi, B.M.S. and Gupta, S. (1966) Skin-irritant and sensitizing plants found in India, New Delhi. P.N. Behl, Irwin Hospital.

Simons, R.D.G. (1953) Handbook of Tropical Dermatology and Medical Mycology. Vol. 2. pp. 1444-1452. Amsterdam, Elsevier.

Melaleuca linariifolia
Tea Tree

The bark or a caterpillar under the bark caused irritation in persons who climbed the tree (Maiden 1916).

Melaleuca nodosa

Handling the leaves, twigs and bark was said to produce irritation (Cleland 1925).

Melaleuca styphelioides

Maiden (1916) refers to a report of irritation by this species.

Melaleuca viridiflora

Oil of Niaouli is derived from this species (Merck 1968); a major constituent is eucalyptol (cineol).

References

Cleland, J.B. (1925) Plants including fungi, poisonous or otherwise injurious to man in Australia (Series II) Med. J. Australia 2, 443.

Maiden, J.H. (1916) On some plants which cause irritation of the skin. Ag. Gaz. New South Wales 27, 39.

Merck Index (1968) An Encyclopedia of Chemicals and Drugs. ed. Stecher, P.G. 8th ed. Rahway, N.J. Merck and Co. Inc.

Melaleuca quinquenervia (syn. M. leucadendron)

Respiratory symptoms can occur from proximity to the plant (Morton 1969).

Reference

Morton, J.F. (1969) Some ornamental plants excreting respiratory irritants. Proc. Florida State Hort. Soc. 82, 415.

Myrtus

100 species are native to tropical and subtropical regions expecially of America.

Myrtus communis
Myrtle

This West Asian tree which figures in the Old Testament has long been naturalized in Europe. The leaves are used to make a tea

(Wren 1968).

Reports of dermatitis from myrtle lack detail (Genner and Bonnevie 1938), and may refer to other plants with this common name viz. Backhousia myrtifolia and Nothofagus cunninghamii. The chemistry of Oil of Myrtle is given by Merck (1968).

References

Genner, V. and Bonnevie, P. (1938) Eczematous eruptions produced by leaves of trees and bushes. Arch. Derm. Syph. 37, 583.

Merck Index (1968) An Encyclopedia of Chemicals and Drugs. ed. Stecher, P.G. 8th ed. Rahway, N.J. Merck and Co. Inc.

Wren, R.W. (1968) Potter's New Cyclopedia of Botanical Drugs and Preparations by Wren, R.C. Re-edit. by Wren, R.W. Potter and Clarke, Ltd. Health Science Press. Rustington, Sussex.

Pimenta

18 species are native to tropical America and the West Indies. The West Indian genus Amomis is within this genus.

Pimenta acris
Bayberry Wild Clove, Wild Cinnamon

Bay rum derived from the leaves and fruits of this species and from other ingredients used in hairdressing caused dermatitis of the face and scalp (White 1887).

Oil of Bay, derived from this species and from Myrcia acris, has been reported to cause dermatitis in hypersensitive individuals (Greenberg and Lester 1954). The chemistry of the oil is given by Merck (1968); among the constituents are eugenol and phellandrene. Contact sensitivity to these chemicals was reported by Woeber and Krombach (1969). Photodermatitis from Bay rum is not substantiated.

References

Greenberg, L.A. and Lester, D. (1954) Handbook of Cosmetic Materials. New York. Interscience.

Merck Index (1968) An Encyclopedia of Chemicals and Drugs. ed. Stecher, P.G. 8th ed. Rahway, N.J. Merck and Co. Inc.

White, J.C. (1887) Dermatitis venenata: An account of the Action of External irritants upon the Skin. Boston. Cupples and Hurd.

Woeber, K. and Krombach, M. (1969) Zur Frage der Sensibilisierung durch atherische Ole (Vorlaufige Mitteilung). Berufsdermatosen. 17, 320.

Pimenta officinalis
Jamaica Pepper

The unripe fruits of this species form allspice. Allspice is irritant to the skin (White 1887); it was used like Capsicum in rubefacient plasters. Oil of Pimenta has irritant properties. The chemistry is given by Merck (1968). 19 of 408 patients who had hand eczema (Agrup 1969) and a salad maker (Hjorth and Weisman 1972) showed positive patch test reactions to allspice.

References

Agrup, G. (1969) Hand Eczema and other hand dermatoses in South Sweden. Acta derm.-venereol. 49 Suppl. 61. pp. 1-91.

Hjorth, N. and Weisman, K. (1972) Occupational dermatitis in Chefs and Sandwich Makers. Contact Dermatitis Newsletter, London 11, 301.

Merck Index (1968) An Encyclopedia of Chemicals and Drugs. ed. Stecher, P.G. 8th ed. Rahway, N.J. Merck and Co. Inc.

White, J.C. (1887) Dermatitis venenata: An account of the Action of External irritants upon the Skin. Boston. Cupples and Hurd.

Psidium

140 species are native to America and the West Indies.

Psidium guajava
Guava

The fruits are used to make Guava jelly, a type of jam. The bark and roots are astringent from the tannin which they contain (Irvine 1961).

Reference

Irvine, F.R. (1961) Woody Plants of Ghana. Oxford University Press. London.

Rhodomyrtus

20 species are found from India to Australia.

Rhodomyrtus macrocarpa
Finger Cherry, Loquat

Ingestion of the fruits can cause blindness (Flecker 1944, Walsh 1957).

References

Flecker, H. (1944) Sudden blindness after eating "finger cherries"; (Rhodomyrtus macrocarpa). Med. J. Australia 2, 183.

Walsh, F.B. (1957) Clinical Neuro-Ophthalmology. Baltimore. Williams and Wilkins.

Syncarpia

Five species are native to Queensland.

Syncarpia glomulifera

The wood can cause dermatitis (Mair 1968).

Reference

Mair, K. (1968) Director, Royal Botanic Gardens, Sydney, Australia, personal communication from records of the Herbarium.

Syzygium

500 species are found in palaeotropical regions. The genus has distinctions from Eugenia. The dried flower buds of S. aromaticum form the spice, cloves (Schmid 1972). Oil of Cloves, used in perfumery, can produce irritation (Greenberg and Lester 1954). Contact dermatitis, cheilitis and stomatitis have been reported from the oil (Sternberg 1937, Zakon et al 1947, Silvers 1939, Gaul 1963).

The oil produced a positive patch test reaction at concentration 1% in petrolatum, negative in 8 controls (Gaul 1963). 14 of 1147 eczema patients showed positive patch test reactions to the oil 1% in petrolatum; some were sensitive to other essential oils (Agrup 1969). One of 380 eczema patients showed a positive patch test reaction to the oil (Meneghini et al 1971).

The chemistry of Oil of Cloves is given by Merck (1968); the constituents include eugenol, caryophyllene and vanillin.

Oil of Cloves and eugenol can produce dermatitis in dentists (Schwartz et al 1957). Eugenol has sensitizing properties (Greenberg and Lester 1954, Hjorth 1961).

References

Agrup, G. (1969) Hand Eczema and other hand dermatoses in South Sweden. Acta derm.-venereol. 49 Suppl. 61. pp. 1-91.

Gaul, L.E. (1963) Dermatitis of the hands from oil of cloves. Skin. 2, 314.

Greenberg, L.A. and Lester, D. (1954) Handbook of Cosmetic Materials. New York. Interscience.

Hjorth, N. (1961) Eczematous allergy to Balsams, Allied Perfumes and Flavouring Agents. Copenhagen. Munksgaard.

Meneghini, C.L., Rantuccio, F. and Lomuto, M. (1971) Additives, vehicles and active drugs of topical medicaments as causes of delayed-type allergic dermatitis. Dermatologica 143, 137.

Merck Index (1968) An Encyclopedia of Chemicals and Drugs. ed. Stecher, P.G. 8th ed. Rahway, N.J. Merck and Co. Inc.

Silvers, S.H. (1939) Stomatitis and dermatitis venenata with purpura resulting from Oil of Cloves and Oil of Cassia. Dental Items Interest 61, 649.

Sternberg, L. (1937) Contact dermatitis. J. Allergy 8, 185.

Zakon, S.J., Goldberg, A.L. and Kahn, J.B. (1947) Lipstick cheilitis: Common dermatosis: Report of 32 cases. Arch. Derm. Syph. 56, 499.

Schmid, R. (1972) A resolution of the Eugenia - Syzygium controversy. Amer. J. Bot. 59, 423.

Syzygium aromaticum

Clove oil contains eugenol which has sensitizing properties (Koch et al 1971, Woeber and Krombach 1969).

References

Koch, G., Magnusson, B. and Nyguist, G. (1971) Contact allergy to medicaments and materials used in dentistry. II. Sensitivity to eugenol and colophony. Odontol. Rev. 22, 275.

Woeber, K. and Krombach, M. (1969) Zur Frage der Sensibilisierung durch atherische Ole. Berufsdermatosen 17, 320.

NAJADACEAE

50 species in one genus are cosmopolitan submerged fresh water plants.

Najas

The distribution and habit of the genus is that of the family.

Najas spp
(syn. Naias spp.)
Pondweed, Stonewort

The prickly siliceous needles of these weeds can produce irritation followed by secondary infection of the hands and feet of rice-field workers (Behl et al 1966).

Reference

Behl, P.N., Captain, R.M., Bedi, B.M.S. and Gupta, S. (1966) Skin-irritant and sensitizing plants found in India, New Delhi. P.N. Behl, Irwin Hospital.

NAUCLEACEAE
(~ RUBIACEAE)

200 species in 10 genera occur in tropical regions as trees or shrubs.

Mitragyna

Twelve species are found in tropical Africa and Asia.

Mitrgyna ciliata
Abura

Mitragyna stipulosa

The partially seasoned wood has a pungent smell and some workers find the sawdust to be irritating (Titmuss 1965). A silia content of up to 0.24 per cent has been reported for M. ciliata (Kukachka 1970). There are occasional trade complaints of dermatitis and nasal irritation in England (Orsler 1973) and in Nigeria (Woods and Calnan 1976). Wilkinson (1973) observed a case of dermatitis from the wood; a patch test produced a positive reaction. Nagenfuhr (1961) noted that the sawdust was said to cause mucosal irritation and vomiting in Germany. Alkaloids are found in the wood of some species (Hausen 1970).

References

Kakachka, B.F. (1970) Properties of imported tropical woods. USDA Forest Service Research Paper. FPL125 March. U.S. Dept. Agric. forest Service. Forest Produces Laboratory. Madison, Wis. U.S.A.

Orsler, R.J. (1973) Personal communication from Forest Products Research Laboratory, Princess Risborough, Bucks, England.

Wagenfuhr, R. (1961) Gift es giftige Holzer. Mobel and Wohnraum 4, 120.

Wilkinson, D.S. (1973) Personal Communication.

Woods, B. and Calnan, C.D. (1976) Toxic Woods. Brit. J. Derm. 94, Suppl. 13, June.

Nauclea
(syn. Sarcocephalus, in a strict sense)

35 species are found in tropical Africa, Asia and Polynesia. This genus has been placed in a family, Naucleaceae.

Nauclea diderrichii
(syn. Nauclea trillesii)
(syn. Sarcocophalus diderrichii)
Bilinga, Opepe

Workers with this wood developed a yellow colour of the skin, a camphor odour of the breath and alkaloidal poisoning (Dispensatory 1926, White 1934, Henry 1949, Hausen 1970). The timber has been known as West African Boxwood and confused with Gonioma (Hausen 1970).

According to Woods and Calnan (1976) it is impossible now to tell how far this wood was responsible for the outbreaks of toxic effects in shuttle-makers described under Gonioma. They noted dermatitis and nasal irritation sometimes with fever and headaches from Nauclea trillesii (Sarcocephalus diderrichii) in Nigeria. The bark contains alkaloids (McLean and Murray 1970).

Nauclea subdita
Bur-Flower Bush

The root-bark yields an intensely yellow dye (Corner 1952).

References

Corner, E.J.H. (1952) Wayside Trees of Malaysia. Singapore. Government Printer.

Dispensatory of the U.S.A. (1926) 21st ed. Philadelphia. J.B. Lippincott Co. pp. 600-601, cited by Siegel (1954)

Hausen, B.M. (1970) Untersuchungen uber Gesundheitsschadigende Holzer. Thesis, Hamburg.

Henry, T.A. (1949) The Plant Alkaloids. London, p. 447, cited by Irvine (1961).

Irvine, F.R. (1961) Woody Plants of Ghana. London. Oxford University Press.

Siegel, J.M. (1954) Dermatitis due to black walnut juice. Archs. Derm. Syph. 70, 511.

White, R.P. (1934) The dermatergoses or occupational affections of the skin. 4th ed. London. H.K. Lewis.

McLean, S. and Murray, D.G. (1970) Isolation of indole (beta-carboline), pyridine and indole-pyridine alkaloids from Nauclea diderrichi. Canad. J. Chem. 48, 867.

Woods, B. and Calnan, C.D. (1976) Toxic Woods. Brit. J. Derm. 94, Suppl. 13, June.

NYCTAGINACEAE

Mirabilis

290 species in 30 genera are mostly tropical. Sixty species are found in America.

Mirabilis jalapa
Four o'clock, False Jalap, Marvel of Peru

The root and seed (containing the alkaloid trigonelline) are irritant to the skin and mucosa (Der Marderosian 1966). The tuberous roots were formerly used as jalap (Ipomoea, Convolvulaceae).

Reference

Der Marderosian, A. (1966) Poisonous plants in and around the home. American Journal of Pharmaceutical Education 30, 115.

OCHNACEAE

600 species in 40 genera are found in tropical regions.

Chemistry is recorded by Hegnauer (1969).

Reference

Hegnauer, R. (1969) Chemotaxonomy of plants. Vol. 5. Basel, Birkhauser. p. 219.

Lophira

Two species are found in tropical western Africa.

Lophira lanceolata
(syn. L. alata)
African Oak, Azobé

The wood is reported to produce itching (Briefwechsel 1966).

References

Briefwechsel (1966) Brief der Norddeutschen Holzberufs-genossenschoft an die BFA in Reinbek vom. 6.10.1966, cited by Hausen (1970).

Briefwechsel (1966) Brief des Centre Technique Forestier Tropical. Nogent-sur-Marne an die BFA in Reinbek vom. 21.11.1966, cited by Hausen (1970).

Hausen, B.M. (1970) Untersuchungen uber Gesundheitsschadigende Holzer. Thesis, Hamburg.

OLACACEAE

250 species in 25 genera are found in tropical regions. Ochanostachys (Corner 1952), Olax (Irvine 1961) and Scorodocarpus sp. (Burkill 1935, Corner 1952) have an odour of garlic (Allium).

Chemistry is recorded by Hegnauer (1969).

Reference

Hegnauer, R. (1969) Chemotaxonomy of plants. Vol. 5. Basel, Birkhauser. p. 277.

Coula

Three species are found in tropical western Africa.

Coula edulis

The wood can produce dermatitis and asthma in wood-workers (Dantin-Gallego et al 1952).

References

Burkill, I.H. (1935) A Dictionary of the Economic Products of the Malay Peninsula. 2 Vols. London. Crown Agents for the Colonies.

Corner, E.J.H. (1952) Wayside Trees of Malaysia. Singapore, Government Printer.

Dantin-Gallego, J., Armyor, A.F. and Riesco, J. (1952) Some new toxic woods. Some new manifestations of toxicity. Ind. Med. Surg. 21, 41.

Irvine, F.R. (1961) Woody plants of Ghana. Oxford University Press. London.

Ongokea

Two species are found in western equatorial Africa.

Ongokea gore
(syn. O. klaineana)

The sap is used as a styptic and the oil of the kernels is used to anoint the body (Irvine 1961).

Reference

Irvine, F.R. (1961) Woody plants of Ghana. Oxford University Press. London.

Ximenia

Between ten and fifteen species are found in tropical America, tropical and southern Africa and tropical Asia and Australia. Ximenia spp. are thorny shrubs or small trees more or less parasitic on other plants (Corner 1952).

Ximenia americana
Wild olive, Wild Lime,
Citron de Mer

The oil of the kernels of this valuable timber tree smells of garlic (Allium) and is used to anoint the body and hair in Africa (Irvine 1961).

Ximenia caffra

The wood dust is irritating to the nose and throat and may produce violent sneezing (Watt and Breyer-Brandwijk 1962).

References

Corner, E.J.H. (1952) Wayside Trees of Malaysia. Singapore, Government Printer.

Irvine, F.R. (1961) Woody plants of Ghana. Oxford University Press. London.

Watt, J.M. and Breyer-Brandwijk, M.G. (1962) The Medicinal and poisonous plants of Southern Africa. 2nd ed. Edinburgh. E.& S. Livingstone.

OLEACEAE

600 species in 29 genera are of cosmopolitan distribution, especially found in temperate and tropical Asia.

Chemistry is recorded by Hegnauer (1969).

Reference

Hegnauer, R. (1969) Chemotaxonomy of plants. Vol. 5. Basel, Birkhauser. p. 231.

Forsythia

One species is found in south-eastern Europe, six species in eastern Asia.

McCord (1962) noted the availability of a commercial extract of the plant for patch-testing. Hjorth (1968) observed two positive patch test reactions to the plant.

References

Hjorth, N. (1968) At Finsen Institute. Personal Communication.

McCord, C.P. (1962) The Occupational Toxicity of Cultivated Flowers. Ind. Med. Surg. 31, 365.

Fraxinus

70 species are found in the northern hemisphere especially in eastern Asia, North America and the Mediterranean region.

Fraxinus spp.
Ash

Dermatitis from ash was observed by Weber (1953) and Shalupenko (1962). Champion (1965) reported dermatitis in a wood-cutter's wife, due to contact with her husband's working clothes. She was sensitive to the lichen Lecanora conizaeoides growing on ash bark, but not to the wood itself.

The pollen of some species can cause hayfever (Wodehouse 1971).

Fraxinus excelsior
European Ash

The wood was listed as capable of causing dermatitis (Hanslian and Kadlec 1966).

References

Hanslian, L. and Kadlec, K. (1966) Wood from the standpoint of hygiene VIII. Species with some or little biological effect. Drevo. 21, 229.

Shalupenko, V.N. (1962) Dermatitis arising from contact with Fraxinus. Vestn. Derm. Vener. 36, 82.

Weber, L.F. (1953) Dermatitis venenata from native woods. Arch. Derm. Syph. 67, 388.

Champion, R.H. (1965) Wood-cutter's disease: contact sensitivity to lichens. Brit. J. Derm. 77, 285.

Wodehouse, R.P. (1971) Hayfever Plants. 2nd rev. edition. New York, Hafner.

Jasminum

300 species are found in tropical and subtropical regions of the Old World.

Jasminum officinale
var. grandiflorum
(syn. J. grandiflorum)

Schwartz et al (1957) referred to dermatitis from the plant.

Handling or wearing the flowers can cause contact dermatitis (Behl et al 1966). Occupational dermatitis was observed in a flower seller; the eruption affected the fingers of a man who picked and sold the flowers during the flowering season which in India is March to August. A patch test to a portion of the flower produced a positive reaction (Bedi 1971).

Jasmine used as bracelet around the wrist and garland around the neck produced dermatitis in a woman (Behl et al 1966).

Jasmine may have both irritant and sensitizing properties; the fresh juice applied to corns is supposed to soften them; the leaves contain salicylic acid (Quisumbing 1951, Behl et al 1966).

Oil of Jasmine may cause dermatitis in hypersensitive individuals (Greenberg and Lester 1954).

Jasmin oil (20 percent in petrolatum) was found to produce positive patch test reactions in 19/103 Japanese persons who had dermatitis from cosmetics; such positive reaction was found in 1/49 controls who had other dermatitis and in 0/42 healthy controls (Nakayama 1973 Pers. Comm. and Nakayama et al 1974).

In a case of dermatitis attributed to a jasmine bouquet type of perfume the offending agent was found to be benzylidene acetone (Bloom 1944).

Jasminum Absolute produced positive patch test reactions in some patients who were contact sensitive to cinnamic aldehyde. Jasmine Absolute may contain alpha-amyl cinnamic aldehyde (Schorr 1975).

Methylheptine carbonate used for the production of artificial jasmine odours is a sensitizer (Tulipan 1938, Whitacre and Parsil 1950). An allergen of synthetic Jasmine used in perfumes is alpha-amyl cinnamic aldehyde (Schorr 1975).

References

Bedi, B.M.S. (1971) Jasmine flower-contact dermatitis (report of a case). Ind. J. Derm. 16, 61.

Behl, P.N., Captain, R.M., Bedi, B.M.S. and Gupta, S. (1966) Skin irritant and sensitizing plants found in India, New Delhi. P.N. Behl.

Bloom, D. (1940) Eczema venenatum. Archs. Derm. Syph. 42, 968.

Greenberg, L.A. and Lester, D. (1954) Handbook of Cosmetic Materials. New York. Interscience.

Nakayama, H., Hanaoka, H. and Ohshiro, A. (1974) Allergen controlled system (ACS). p. 42. Tokyo, Kanehara Shuppan.

Quisumbing, E. (1951) Medicinal Plants of the Philippines. Tech. Bull. 16. Manila, Philippine Islands. Manila Bureau of Printing. 1234 pp.

Schorr, W.F. (1975) Cinnamic aldehyde allergy. Contact Dermatitis 1, 108.

Schwartz, L., Tulipan, L. and Birmingham, D.J. (1957) Occupational Diseases of the Skin. 3rd ed. Philadelphia. Lea and Febiger. pp. 637-672.

Tulipan, L. (1938) Cosmetic irritants. Archs. Derm. Syph. 38, 906.

Whitacre, F.M. and Parsil, R.C. (1950) Cosmetic sensitizers. Ann. Allergy. 8, 670.

Ligustrum

Between 40 and 50 species are found from Europe to northern Persia, in eastern Asia and from Indo Malaysia to New Guinea and Queensland.

Ligustrum
Privet

Dermatitis occurred in a person who trimmed a privet hedge (Davies 1939).

Ligustrum amurense
Amoor Privet

This species was said to cause dermatitis (Shelmire 1940, McCord 1962).

Ligustrum lucidum
Privet

A wax produced by an insect from the plant is used as beeswax (see Populus)(Smith 1969).

The pollen can cause hay-fever (Wodehouse 1971).

Ligustrum vulgare

This species has irritant properties (Pammel 1911). Respiratory symptoms can occur from proximity to the plant (Morton 1969).

References

Davies, J.H.T. (1939) Contact dermatitis. Practitioner 142, 636.

McCord, C.P. (1962) The Occupational Toxicity of Cultivated Flowers. Ind. Med. Surg. 31, 365.

Morton, J.F. (1969) Some ornamental plants excreting respiratory irritants. Proc. Florida State Hort. Soc. 82, 415.

Pammel, L.H. (1911) A Manual of Poisonous plants. Torch Press. Cedar Rapids, Iowa. Reprinted Univ. Microfilms Inc. Ann Arbor, Mich. 1965. pp. 476.

Shelmire, B. (1940) Contact dermatitis from vegetation. South Med. J. 33, 338.

Smith, F.P. (1969) Chinese Materia Medica. Vegetable kingdom. 2nd ed. Rev. by Hei, P.D. Taipei, Taiwan. Ku T'ing Book House.

Wodehouse, R.P. (1971) Hayfever Plants. 2nd rev. edition. New York, Hafner.

Olea

Twenty species are widely distributed. Olea europaea is cultivated. Several species yield good timber.

Olea eurbpaea
Olive

The wood has been reported to cause dermatitis (Koelsch 1910, McCord 1958, Senear 1933). Irritation by 'olivewood' is mentioned by Legge (1907). Smith (1920) identifies this as Elaeodendron sp. (olive plum) but according to Woods and Calnan (1976) who cite Boulger (1908), Olea sp. seems more likely. Contact dermatitis from olive oil, which is often adulterated, was noted by White (1934), Greenberg and Lester (1954). Injection of olive oil into the eye of animals produces an inflammatory reaction (Grant 1972). Oleic acid was reported to cause dermatitis among stenographers handling stencil sheets (Hailey 1923). Oleic acid has irritant properties and has been suspected as a sensitizer (Greenberg and Lester 1954).

Contact dermatitis of the fingers from olives was reported by Waldbott and Shea (1948).

References

Grant, W.M. (1962) Toxicology of the eye. Springfield, Ill. Charles C. Thomas.

Greenberg, L.A. and Lester, D. (1954) Handbook of Cosmetic Materials. New York. Interscience.

Hailey, W.H. (1923) Dermatitis from oleic acid. Arch. Derm. Syph. 8, 530.

Hausen, B.M. (1970) Untersuchungen uber Gesundheitsschadigende Holzer. Thesis, Hamburg.

Koelsch, F. (1910) "Tagesgeschicitliche Notizen" in Munch. med. Wschr. 5, 179, cited by Hausen (1970).

McCord, C.P. (1958) The toxic properties of some timber woods. Ind. Med. Surg. 27, 202.

Senear, F.E. (1933) Dermatitis due to woods. JAMA 101, 1527.

Waldbott, G.L. and Shea, J.J. (1948) Causative diagnosis of contact dermatitis II A classification of patterns on the hands. Archs. Derm. Syph. 57, 975.

White, R.P. (1934) The Dermatergoses or Occupational Affections of the Skin. 4th ed. London. H.K. Lewis.

Boulger, G.S. (1908) Wood. 2nd ed. London, Arnold.

Legge, T.M. (1907) Report of the Chief Inspector of Factories and Workshops. p. 248, London.

Smith, E.P. (1920) Plant dermatitis. J. Bot. 58, 130.

Woods, B. and Calnan, C.D. (1976) Toxic Woods. Brit. J. Derm. 94, Suppl. 13, June.

Syringa

30 species are found from south-eastern Europe to eastern Asia.

Syringa vulgaris
Lilac

The plant is said to cause dermatitis (Schwartz et al 1957, McCord 1962).

The odour of lilac can cause hayfever (Biederman 1937).

References

McCord, C.P. (1962) The Occupational Toxicity of Cultivated Flowers. Ind. Med. Surg. 31, 365.

Schwartz, L., Tulipan, L. and Birmingham, D.J. (1957) Occupational Diseases of the Skin. 3rd ed. Philadelphia. Lea and Febiger.

Biederman, J.B. (1937) Sensitivity to flowers. Laryngoscope 47, 825.

ONAGRACEAE

640 species in 21 genera are found in temperate and tropical regions.

Circaea

Twelve species found in northern temperate and arctic regions have fruits covered with hooked bristles. Species of this genus have hooked fruits which attach themselves to animals (Howes 1974).

Reference

Howes, F.N. (1974) A Dictionary of Useful and Everyday Plants and their Common Names. Cambridge University Press.

Fuchsia

100 species are found in New Zealand, Tahiti and central and South America.

Fuchsia

Positive patch test reactions to a hybrid of this genus and also to *Streptocarpus* were reported by Agrup and Fregert (1968), Agrup (1969).

References

Agrup, G. and Fregert, S. (1968) Patch test reactions to *Streptocarpus*. Contact Dermatitis Newsletter 4, 72.

Agrup, G. (1969) Hand Eczema and other hand dermatoses in South Sweden. Acta Derm.-venereol. 49 Suppl. 61. pp. 1-91.

Gaura

18 species are found in North America, Mexico and Argentina.

Guara parviflora
Lizard's Tail

In an investigation of 'weed dermatitis' this species produced a positive patch test reaction in one of 50 patients tested (Shelmire 1939).

Reference

Shelmire, B. (1939) Contact Dermatitis from Weeds; Patch Testing with Their Oleoresins. JAMA 113, 1085.

Hartmannia
(syn. *Oenothera*)

15 species are found from North America to Bolivia and in the West Indies.

Hartmannia speciosa
Showy Evening Primrose

In an investigation of 'weed dermatitis' this species produced a positive patch test reaction in one of 50 patients tested (Shelmire 1939).

Reference

Shelmire, B. (1939) Contact Dermatitis from Weeds; Patch testing with Their Oleoresins. JAMA 133, 1085.

Oenothera

80 species are found in America (especially in temperate regions) and in the West Indies.

Oenothera biennis
Evening Primrose

Maiden (1909) received a report that this species produces eczema in humans. It is possible that his correspondent was referring to Primula.

Reference

Maiden, J.H. (1909) On some plants which cause inflammation or irritation of the skin. Ag. Gaz. New South Wales. 20, 111 and 1073.

OPILIACEAE

60 species in eight genera are found in tropical regions, especially in Asia.

Chemistry is recorded by Hegnauer (1969)

Reference

Hegnauer, R. (1969) Chemotaxonomy of plants. Vol. 5. Basel, Birkhauser. p. 248.

Agonandra

Ten species are found from Mexico to tropical South America.

Agonandra brasiliensis
(brasileira)
Pao marfim

This satinwood substitute contains a saponin which irritates mucous membranes (Freise 1932). According to Woods and Calnan (1976) the common name pao marfim more often refers to Aspidosperma vargasii.

References

Freise, F.W. (1932) Gesundheiteschadigungen durch Arbeiten mit giftingen Holzern. Beobachtungen aus brasilianischen Gewerbebetrieben Arch. Gewerbepath.-hyg. 3, 1 (1970).

Woods, B. and Calnan, C.D. (1976) Toxic Woods. Brit. J. Derm. 94, Suppl. 13, June.

Opilia

22 species are found in palaeotropical regions.

Opilia celtidifolia

Chewing the leaves causes the saliva to turn red and produces a special sensation in the throat (Irvine 1961).

Reference

Irvine, F.R. (1961) Woody plants of Ghana. Oxford University Press. London.

ORCHIDACEAE

17,000 species in 735 genera are of cosmopolitan distribution, abundant in the tropics but rare in arctic regions.

Cypripedium

50 species are found in north temperate regions.

Cypripedium reginae
(C. spectabile)

Cypripedium calceolus
var. pubescens
Lady's Slipper Orchid

Dermatitis of the hands and face occurred in a botanist who collected the plants. He observed that his hands were stained with the purplish secretion of the glandular hairs which densely clothed the stems and leaves (McNair 1923, Pammel 1911). The dermatitis resembled Toxicodendron dermatitis. Other species of this genus have been incriminated (Mackoff and Dahl 1951). The plants are most liable to cause dermatitis when fruiting. Tests with the leaf hairs suggest an allergenic effect (Nestler 1907, 1908).

References

McNair, J.B. (1923) Rhus Dermatitis. Chicago, Ill. University of Chicago Press.

Mackoff, S. and Dahl, A.O. (1951) A botanical consideration of the weed oleoresin problem. Minn. Med. 34, 1169.

Nestler, A. (1907) Das Sekret der Drusenhaare der Gattung Cypripedium mit besonderer Berucksichtigung seiner hautreizenden Wirkung. Ber. dtsch. bot. Ges cited by Touton (1932).

Nestler, A. (1908) Das Hautgift der Cypripedien. Wiesner-Feskschrift. p. 200, cited by Touton (1932).

Pammel, L.H. (1911) A Manual of Poisonous plants. Torch Press. Cedar Rapids, Iowa. Reprinted Univ. Microfilms Inc. Ann Arbor, Mich. 1965. pp. 476-7.

Touton, K. (1932) Hauterkrankungen durch phanerogamische Pflanzen und ihre Produkte (Toxicodermia et Allergodermia phytogenes), in Barnewitz, J. et al Angeborene Anomalien, Lichtdermatosen, Pflanzengifte, Thermische Schadigungen, Einfluss Innerer Storungen auf die Haut. Berlin, Verlag von Julius Springer.

Vanilla

90 species are found in tropical and subtropical regions. The spice, vanilla, is obtained from the pods of species of this genus.

Vanilla griffithi

This wild plant, common in the Malay Peninsula contains a slightly milky latex, which when dropped on the hand or arm produces a very unpleasant irritation of the skin, as I know by experience (Ridley 1921). The latex is used by native girls, mixed with oil to strengthen and thicken the hair, much as cantharides (sic) is used in Europe.

Vanilla planifolia

Workers who handled the pods developed dermatitis of the hands and face. The action of a mite or of cardol was suspected. Cardol derived from Anacardium was said to be applied to the pods to darken them (White 1887). Workers who clean, pack and sort the pods can develop dermatitis (White 1934, Downing 1939). Dermatitis from vanilla is known in the perfume and confectionery industries (Greenberg and Lester 1954, Schwartz et al 1957). Hutchinson (1892) termed the dermatitis 'vanillaism'. Conjunctivitis and a partially generalized pustular eruption followed handling vanilla pods (Hiley 1909). A mold which covers the pods and chemicals applied to the pods have been suspected. Vanilla in a hair lotion produced dermatitis; the patient carried out a patch test to vanilla with a positive result (Leggett 1914).

In an outbreak of contact dermatitis in workers with vanilla, 20% of those exposed were affected but they recovered in three weeks and were never troubled again; probably some transient contaminant was responsible (Gougerot and Basset 1939). Irritation occurring in persons who cut the vines was attributed to calcium oxalate crystals in the juice. The juice also irritates the mouth (Morton 1962). A positive patch test to vanilla was observed in a sandwich maker who had contact-dermatitis (Hjorth and Weisman 1972). Contact dermatitis from vanilla may present as erythema only, without eczematous changes (Sidi and Hincky 1964). Vanillin has sensitizing properties and cross-sensitivity is observed with some constituents of Balsam of Peru (Myroxylon) (Hjorth 1961). Eating vanilla caused a flare of eczema in a patient who was contact sensitive to the balsam (Pirila 1970). Vanilla and vanillin used in perfumery have caused dermatitis (Greenberg and Lester 1954).

References

Downing, J.G. (1939) Cutaneous eruptions among industrial workers. Archs. Derm. Syph. 39, 12.

Gougerot, H. and Basset, A. (1939) Occupational eczema due to vanilla. Bull. Soc. franc. derm. 46, 1329.

Greenberg, L.A. and Lester, D. (1954) Handbook of Cosmetic Materials. New York. Interscience.

Hiley, R.F. (1909) Dermatitis due to Vanilla. Lancet 1, 1433 and 1907, Feb 16 and 1906, Nov. 24.

Hjorth, N. (1961) Eczematous Allergy to Balsams. Munksgaard, International Booksellers and Publishers Ltd., Copenhagen.

Hjorth, N. and Weismann, K. (1972) Occupational dermatitis in Chefs and Sandwich Makers. Contact Dermatitis Newsletter, London 11, 301.

Hutchinson, J. (1892) Arch. Surgery 4, 49 cited by White (1934).

Leggett, W. (1914) Vanilla as a skin irritant. Brit. Med. J. 1, 1351.

Morton, J.F. (1962) Ornamental Plants with Poisonous Properties II. Proc. Florida Hort. Soc. 75, 484.

Pirila, V. (1970) Endogenic Contact Eczema. Allergie Asthma 16, 15.

Ridley, H.N. (1921) Addendum to Sprague, T.A. (1921) Plant dermatitis. Journal of Botany 59, 309-310.

Schwartz, L., Tulipan, L. and Birmingham, D.J. (1957) Occupational Diseases of the Skin. 3rd ed. Philadelphia. Lea and Febiger. pp. 637-672.

Sidi, E. and Hincky, M. (1964) Unusual clinical appearances of allergic contact dermatitis. Rev. Clin. Esp. 1, 209.

White, J.C. (1887) Dermatitis venenata; An account of the Action of External irritants upon the skin. Boston. Cupples and Hurd.

White, R.P. (1934) The Dermatergoses or Occupational Affections of the Skin. 4th ed. London. H.K. Lewis.

OXALIDACEAE

875 species in three genera are mostly found in tropical and subtropical regions.

Chemistry is recorded by Hegnauer (1969).

Reference

Hegnauer, R. (1969) Chemotaxonomy of Plants. Vol. 5. Basel, Birkhauser. p. 255.

Oxalis

800 species are of cosmopolitan distribution. Several species have become troublesome weeds. The tubers of *O. deppei* and other species are used as food.

Oxalis spp.
Wood Sorrel

The sap of most members of the family is sour from the presence of oxalic acid or its potassium salt (Corner 1952). Oxalic acid is a strong irritant (Greenberg and Lester 1954).

Oxalis repens

The sap has escharotic properties and is used to remove corns (Quisumbing 1951).

References

Corner, E.J.H. (1952) Wayside Trees of Malaysia. Singapore, Government Printer.

Greenberg, L.A. and Lester, D. (1954) Handbook of Cosmetic Materials. New York. Interscience.

Quisumbing, E. (1951) Medicinal Plants of the Philippines. Tech. Bull. 16. Manila, Philippine Islands. Manila Bureau of Printing. 1234 pp.

PAEONIACEAE

33 species in one genus are found in north temperate regions. The family is related to Ranunculaceae.

Chemistry is recorded by Hegnauer (1969).

Reference

Hegnauer, R. (1969) Chemotaxonomy of plants. Vol. 5. Basel, Birkhauser, p. 258.

Paeonia
Peony

Several species including *P. officinalis* are used in Herbal

Medicine (Grieve 1970, Wenzel and Haskell 1952). Schwartz et al (1957) list the genus as capable of causing dermatitis without clinical details.

References

Grieve, M. (1970) A Modern Herbal. Darien, Conn. Hafner Publ. Co.

Schwartz, L., Tulipan, L. and Birmingham, D.J. (1957) Occupational Diseases of the Skin. 3rd ed. Philadelphia. Lea and Febiger. pp. 637-672.

Wenzel, D.G. and Haskell, A.R. (1952) Pharmacological action of Paeonia officinalis (var. number 4 pink). J. Amer. Pharm. Ass. 42, 162.

PALMAE
(syn. ARECACEAE)

2500 species in 217 genera are found in tropical and sub-tropical regions. The family furnishes many of the necessaries of life in the tropics.

Sharp-tipped palm fronds lying beneath trees in places that children use for play can cause injuries which usually occur at the knee. When no puncture wound is discernible, the foreign body reaction which ensues can mimic various bone, joint and soft tissue disorders. In one case one thorn was removed but persistent swelling resulted from other thorns which were not at first suspected to be present (Cozen and Fonda 1953).

Inhalation of moldy thatch dust can produce Papua or New Guinea lung, a form of allergic alveolitis (Morgan and Seaton 1975).

References

Cozen, L. and Fonda, M. (1953) Palm Thorn Injuries. Difficulty in diagnosis of late sequelae. Calif. Med. 79, 40.

Morgan, W.K.C. and Seaton, A. (1975) Occupational Lung Diseases. Philadelphia, Saunders.

Acrocomia

30 species are found in tropical America and the West Indies.

Acrocomia aculeata

The leaves and the spathes which enclose the flowers possess long needle-like black spines which can penetrate the skin (Allen 1943). He listed 14 other species of the genus which have this property.

Reference

Allen, P.H. (1943) Poisonous and injurious plants of Panama. Am. J. Trop. Med. Suppl. 23, 1.

Areca

54 species are found in Indo Malaysia, the Solomon and Bismarck Islands and Northern Australia.

Areca catechu

This species is cultivated in tropical Asia for its seeds, areca or betel nuts. The seed is cut into slices and rolled up in a leaf of betel pepper (Piper betle) with a little lime; when chewed it turns the saliva bright red. The habit is an ancient one and the variations complex (Burkill 1935, Muir and Kirk 1960). Acacia catechu may be added to the quid as well as various spices.

Betel-chewers maintain that the chewing keeps the gums healthy but continual betel-chewing ultimately destroys the teeth (Burkill 1935). Muir and Kirk (1960) concluded from their observations that cancer of the mouth occurring in habitual chewers is due to tobacco (Nicotiana) added to the chew. Cheilitis can occur in chewers (Mendelson 1924). There are many ill-defined races of the palm which are cross-pollinated by insects. Some of the races of palm are unsuitable for the betel nut chewer producing an unpleasant sensation of tightness in the throat with profuse secretion of mucus. The nuts of such races are called by the Malays 'pinang mengkelan' (the pinang which chokes). Therefore when a good tree is recognized it is well cared for (Burkill 1935).

References

Burkill, I.H. (1935) A dictionary of the Economic Products of the

Malay Peninsula. 2 Vols. London. Crown Agents for the Colonies.

Mendelson, R.W. (1924) Tinea labialis (Betel-nut dermatitis of the lips). J. Trop. Med. 27, 284.

Muir, C.S. and Kirk, R. (1960) Betel, Tobacco and Cancer of the Mouth. Brit. J. Cancer 14, 597.

Arenga

Eleven species are found in Indo Malaysia, except in Guinea, and in the Caroline and Christmas islands. The plants yield sugar, sago and fibre.

Arenga obtusifolia

This species which has been said to be irritating is inconstantly so in Hawaii (Arnold 1968).

Arenga pinnata

The fruit-wall is full of needle-crystals and is exceedingly irritant to the mouth. There is a story of the capture of the town of Surabaya in 1545 A.D. by means of the artifice of throwing the pulped fruits of this palm with carcasses into the river which supplied drinking water to the inhabitants. The pulped fruit brings fish to the surface of a pond; crushed fruit is placed along the margins of fish-ponds both to discourage poachers whose bare feet are irritated by the fruit-walls and to discourage the fish from approaching the edge of the pond (Burkill 1935). The fruit (nut) contains microscopic stinging crystals (Souder 1963).

Arenga westerhoutii

The fruit is poisonous from the irritant needle-crystals in its tissues. The Malays may give the juice in coffee for criminal purposes and irritation and swelling of the mouth and throat results (Burkill 1935).

References

Arnold, H.L. (1968) Poisonous plants of Hawaii. Rutland, Vermont. Charles E. Tuttle.

Burkill, I.H. (1935) A dictionary of the economic products of the Malay Peninsula. 2 Vols. London. Crown Agents for the Colonies.

Souder, P. (1963) Poisonous plants on Guam. In venomous and poisonous animals and noxious plants of the Pacific Region. ed. Keegan, H.L. and Macfarlane, W.V. Oxford. Pergamon Press. pp. 15-29.

Astrocaryum

50 species are found in tropical America. Several species yield fibre and oil.

Astrocaryum alatum

The mid-ribs of the leaves, particularly towards their base, are covered with flattened brown or black needle-like spines which can penetrate the skin (Allen 1943). He listed eight other species of the genus which have this property.

Astrocaryum standleyanum

The trunks possess long, flat, black, needle-like spines. The leaves are also armed with spines which can penetrate the skin of the feet through light walking shoes (Allen 1943).

Reference

Allen, P.H. (1943) Poisonous and injurious plants of Panama. Am. J. Trop. Med. Suppl. 23, 1.

Bactris

Between 180 and 250 species have been described from America and the West Indies. B. minor (peach palm) provides edible fruit.

Bactris augustinea

A heavy armature of spines on the canes and leaf petioles often inflict painful wounds on the forest traveller (Allen 1943). He lists 35 other species of the genus having this property.

Reference

Allen, P.H. (1943) Poisonous and injurious plants of Panama.

Am. J. Trop. Med. Suppl. 23, 1.

Astrocaryum spp.,
Bactris spp., etc.
Palms

Dermatitis of the arms and general constitutional symptoms occurred in men working with palm wood in Brazil. Patch tests with a wax extracted from the wood produced positive reactions (Freise 1937).

Reference

Freise, F.W. (1937) Vergiftungen durch Brasilianische Werkholzer III Sammlung ver Vergiftungsfallen 8c, 13.

Calamus

375 species are found in palaeotropical regions.

Calamus spp.

The plants are troublesome in tropical forests because the hooks of the plant catch on clothing. The stripped stems (rattan canes) are used for making chair bottoms, baskets, cables, etc.

Rotan (Rattan) dermatitis was described by Simons (1952) who contracted it in a Japanese prisoner of war camp. The disease most frequently occurs on the lower arms and backs of the thighs. It is characterized by urticaria, papules and sometimes also by prurigo. It is caused by the varnish or by the bites of insects, usually the common bed bugs living in the twisted curls of used cane chairs.

Calamus caesius

Scrapings from the canes, which have glossy coats from the presence of silica, are irritant to the mucous membranes and have been used for criminal poisoning together with powdered glass (Burkill 1935).

Calamus rotang
Elanewel, Pontyanac

The hands of basket-makers are sometimes covered by a white mold which is shaken out by splitting, hammering and cutting the canes. The palms of the hands develop painful longitudinal fissures which curiously tend to spare the palmar and digital flexural areas. The fungus present on the canes is thought to be the cause of these changes (White 1934).

References

Burkill, I.H. (1935) A dictionary of the economic products of the Malay Peninsula. 2 Vols. London. Crown Agents for the Colonies.

Simons, R.D.G. (1952) Handbook of Tropical Dermatology. New York. Elsevier.

White, R.P. (1934) The Dermatergoses or Occupational affections of the skin. 4th ed. London. H.K. Lewis.

Caryota

12 species are found in Ceylon, Indo Malaysia, the Solomon islands and north-eastern Australia.

Caryota aequatorialis

Irritant crystals are present in the plant tissues (Burkill 1935).

Caryota mitis
Tufted Fishtail Palm

The fruit pulp and juice of the plant are irritant to the skin from the presence of stinging crystals. Persons in Florida who cleaned the seeds for propagation have found that such skin inflammation lasts for some hours (Morton 1962).

Caryota urens
Toddy Fishtail Palm

This species yields palm sugar, sago, fibre and wood.

The fruits contain irritant needle-like crystals (Burkill 1935). Eating the crushed berries can produce stomatitis. The fruit pulp and juice have (Allen 1943) an effect on the skin similar to that of C. mitis (Morton 1962). The fibres at the bases of the leaf-stalks are a source of dermatitis (Arnold 1968). Flecker (1945) refers to an injurious effect of the plant.

A gardener, when carrying the ripe fruit on both forearms, immediately felt an acute stinging pain which lasted five hours at the sites of contact (Flecker 1945).

References

Allen, P.H. (1943) Poisonous and injurious plants of Panama. Am. J. Trop, Med. Suppl. 23, 1.

Arnold, H.L. (1968) Poisonous plants of Hawaii. Rutland, Vermont. Charles E. Tuttle.

Burkill, I.H. (1935) A dictionary of the economic products of the Malay Peninsula. 2 Vols. London. Crown Agents for the Colonies.

Flecker, H. (1945) Injuries produced by plants in tropical Queensland. Med. J. Australia 1, 636.

Morton, J.F. (1962) Ornamental Plants with poisonous properties. II. Proc. Florida Hort. Soc. 75, 484.

Cocos

The single species in this genus probably originated in tropical Asia or Polynesia and is now cultivated throughout the tropics.

Cocos nucifera
Coconut

This species is the world's chief producer of vegetable fat at the present time.

The fruits falling from the trees can inflict blunt injury. In Florida, they are left on the trees as a tourist attraction but removed at the time of a hurricane warning.

The tar obtained by burning the shell is used as a rubefacient (Quisumbing 1951).

Copra itch is not an allergy to copra (dried coconut flesh) but an infestation (Simons 1952, Laarman 1952, Nasution et al 1973). Copra mite dermatitis, seen in workers in copra mills and dock-workers, presents an eruption resembling scabies but without burrows (Schwartz et al 1957). It is localized on the hands, arms and legs. Sometimes the whole body, except the face, is affected. The lesions are fairly numerous, itch extremely and consist of papules, papulo-pustules, pustules, crusts and excoriations. The eruption begins on the hands and spreads to the arms, legs and trunk. There is no tendency to heal spontaneously as long as the patient continues at work (Whitfield 1915, Cleveland 1940, Nixon 1944).

Saturated acids of lower molecular weight (caproic, caprylic and capric acids) in coconut oil used in soap are skin irritants. As the molecular weight rises above that of capric acid, the irritant action becomes less (Blank 1939). Coconut oil and soaps made from it produce dermatitis in some persons (Greenberg and Lester 1954). Lauric acid is derived from coconut oil; lauryl gallate, used in fats, can cause dermatitis (Brun 1964).

Application of Coconut oil, probably impure and possibly perfumed, can cause hyperpigmentation of the face in Indians (Khare and Naik 1973).

References

Blank, I.H. (1939) Action of soap on skin. I. Patch test with fatty acids. Archs. Derm. Syph. 39, 811.

Brun, R. (1964) Kontaktekzem auf Laurylgallat und p-Hydroxybenzoesaureester. Berufsdermatosen 12, 281.

Cleveland, D.E.H. (1940) Mite dermatitis (copra itch; cheese mite itch). Archs. Derm. Syph. 41, 831.

Greenberg, L.A. and Lester, D. (1954) Handbook of Cosmetic Materials. New York. Interscience.

Khare, K.C. and Naik, G.D. (1973) Oil dermatitis. Ind. J. Derm. Vener. 39, 203.

Laarman, J.J. (1952) Copra itch in the Netherlands. Documenta de morbis tropicis. No. 4.

Nasution, D., Klokke, A.H. and Nater, J.P. (1973) A survey of occupational dermatoses in Indonesia. Bemfsdermatosen 21, 215.

Nixon, J.A. (1944) Cheese itch and "Itchy Cargoes" in reference to Workmen's Compensation. Proc. Roy. Soc. Med. 37, 235.

Quisumbing, E. (1951) Medicinal plants of the Philippines. Tech. Bull. 16. Manila, Philippine Islands. Manila Bureau of Printing. 1234 pp.

Schwartz, L., Tulipan, L. and Birmingham, D.J. (1957) Occupational Diseases of the Skin. 3rd ed. Philadelphia. Lea and Febiger. pp. 637-672.

Simons, R.D.G. (1952) Handbook of Tropical Dermatology. New York. Elsevier.

Whitfield, A. (1915) Copra itch. Brit. J. Derm. 27, 122.

Copernicia

30 species are found in tropical America and the West Indies.

Copernicia cerifera
Wax or Carna-Uba palm

Carnuba wax, derived from the leaves of this species, has been reported to produce dermatitis (Kohn 1913, Greenberg and Lester 1954). Carnauba wax is often used together with candellila wax derived from Euphorbia and Pedilanthus (Merck Index 1968). Candellila wax has not been reported to cause dermatitis (Greenberg and Lester 1954). Esparto wax derived from Stipa, etc. may be used as a substitute or extender for carnauba wax (Greenberg and Lester 1954). Negative reactions were obtained in all of 968 persons patch tested to Carnauba wax, 10% in vaseline (Fregert and Hjorth 1968).

References

Fregert, S. and Hjorth, N. (1968) Results of Standard Patch tests with substances abandoned. Contact Dermatitis Newsletter, London 5, 85.

Greenberg, L.A. and Lester, D. (1954) Handbook of Cosmetic Materials. New York. Interscience.

Kohn, D. (1913) Glattolin als Ursache einer hartnackigen Dermatitis colli. Munch. med. Wschr. No. 22 cited by Touton (1932).

Merck Index (1968) An Encyclopedia of Chemicals and Drugs. ed. Stecher, P.G. 8th ed. Rahway, N.J. Merck and Co. Inc.

Touton, K. (1932) Hauterkrankungen durch phanerogamische Pflanzen und ihre Produkte (Toxicodermia et Allergodermia phytogenes), in Barnewitz, J. et al Angeborene Anomalien, Lichtdermatosen, Pflanzengifte, Thermische Schadigungen Einfluss Innerer Storungen auf die Haut. Berlin, Verlag von Julius Springer.

Daemonorops

100 species are found in Indo Malaysia.

Daemonorops

A kino derived from the fruit and used for colouring varnishes, etc. is known as Dragon's Blood. This name is also used for a product of Dracaena (Howes 1950). A Dragon's Blood produced negative patch test reactions in 13 individuals who were contact sensitive to Balsam of Peru (Myroxylon) (Hjorth 1961).

References

Hjorth, N. (1961) Eczematous allergy to Balsams, Allied Perfumes and Flavouring Agents. Copenhagen: Munksgaard.

Howes, F.N. (1950) Age-old resins of the Mediterranean region and their uses. Economic Botany 4, 307.

Desmoncus

65 species found in tropical America are climbing palms with hooks like Calamus.

Desmoncus horridus

The canes are heavily armed with black needle-like spines. The terminal pairs of leaflets have been transformed into recurved barbs, fashioned as the barbs of an arrow, which may tear the clothing and inflict dangerous wounds (Allen 1943). He listed six other species of this genus with these characteristics.

Reference

Allen, P.H. (1943) Poisonous and Injurious Plants of Panama. Am. J. Trop. Med. Suppl. 23, 1.

Guilielma
(syn. Bactris)

Seven species are found in tropical South America.

Guiliema utilis

The entire plant, particularly the trunks and leaf bases are covered with spines which are a ready source of skin injury and infection (Allen 1943).

Reference

Allen, P.H. (1943) Poisonous and Injurious Plants of Panama. Am. J. Trop. Med. Suppl. 23, 1.

Hexopetion
(syn. Astrocaryum)

One species is found in Mexico.

Hexopetion americanum

This species is armed with spines which can penetrate the skin (Allen 1943).

Reference

Allen, P.H. (1943) Poisonous and Injurious Plants of Panama. Am. J. Trop. Med. Suppl. 23, 1.

Jessenia

Six species are found in Trinidad and tropical South America.

Jessenia batana

The long spines of this palm are used for darts in blow pipes (Howes 1974).

Reference

Howes, F.N. (1974) A Dictionary of useful and everyday plants and their common names. Cambridge. University Press.

Phoenix

17 species are found in warm regions of Africa and Asia. P. dactylifera is the date palm.

Phoenix canariensis
Canary Date Palm

Phoenix loureiri
Pigmy Date Palm

Punctures by sharp thorns on the petioles of these palms are commonly experienced by nursery and landscape gardeners in Florida. The spine-tip may be broken off and serve as a foreign body but a chemical irritant may also be present in the thorns (Morton 1962). A date-palm thorn produced a bony reaction simulating Ewing's sarcoma of bone; no puncture wound could be found (Maylahn 1952). Women handling damaged dates have been infested with a mite (Oppenheim and Taglicht 1925, cited by White 1934, Schwartz et al 1957).

References

Maylahn, D.J. (1952) Thorn induced "Tumors" of bone. J. Bone Joint Surg. 34A, 386.

Morton, J.F. (1962) Ornamental Plants with Poisonous Properties II. Proc. Florida Hort. Soc. 75, 484.

White, R.P. (1934) The Dermatergoses or Occupational Affections of the Skin. 4th ed. London. H.K. Lewis.

Schwartz, L., Tulipan, L. and Birmingham, D.J. (1957) Occupational Diseases of the Skin. 3rd ed. Philadelphia. Lea and Febiger, pp. 637-672.

Sabal

25 species are found in warmer regions of America and the West Indies. The leaves of Sabal palmetto, thatch or palmetto palm

are used for thatching.

Sabal palmetto
Cabbage palmetto

This species was listed as an irritant plant without clinical details (Schwartz et al 1957).

Reference

Schwartz, L., Tulipan, L. and Birmingham, D.J. (1957) Occupational Diseases of the Skin. 3rd ed. Philadelphia. Lea and Febiger. pp. 637-672.

Wallichia

Six species are found from the eastern Himalayas to southern China.

Wallichia disticha

The berries and perhaps the leaves of this species have irritant properties (Burkill 1935, Behl et al 1966).

References

Behl, P.N., Captain, R.M., Bedi, B.M.S. and Gupta, S. (1966) Skin-irritant and sensitizing plants found in India, New Delhi. P.N. Behl, Irwin Hospital.

Burkill, I.H. (1935) A dictionary of the economic products of the Malay Peninsula. 2 Vols. London. Crown Agents for the Colonies.

PANDANACEAE

700 species in three genera are characteristic plants of the Old World tropics but a few are found in warm temperate regions.

Pandanus
Screw-Pine

600 species are found in palaeotropical regions. Several species have sweetly scented flowers or leaves which are used for ornament in the East.

Pandanus sp.

Eating the fruits caused sore lips and blistered tongue; boiled fruits were innocuous (Cleland 1925).

Pandanus tectorius
(syn. P. odoratissimus)

The sharp serrated leaves of the plant can cause mechanical injury. Indian women habitually use the male inflorescence, which is a long spike of strongly scented flowers without petals or sepals, to adorn the hair. The outer part of the flower and the blossoms yield an essential oil. The flowers and leaves can cause dermatitis in housewives and florists (Behl et al 1966).

References

Behl, P.N., Captain, R.M., Bedi, B.M.S. and Cupta, S. (1966) Skin-irritant and sensitizing plants found in India, New Delhi. P.N. Behl, Irwin Hospital.

Cleland, J.B. (1925) Plants including fungi, poisonous or otherwise injurious to man in Australia. (Series II) Med. J. Australia 2, 443.

PAPAVERACEAE

200 species in 26 genera are chiefly found in north temperate regions.

Chemistry is recorded by Hegnauer (1969).

Reference

Hegnauer, R. (1969) Chemotaxonomy of Plants. Vol. 5. Basel, Birkhauser. p. 264.

Argemone

Ten species are found in the western and eastern United States, Mexico and the West Indies.

Argemone mexicana
Thistleroot, Mexican Poppy

The prickles on the leaves and fruiting capsules can cause mechanical injury to humans and grazing animals (Oakes and Butcher 1962). The acrid yellow sap has slightly corrosive properties (Dalziel 1937, Quisumbing 1951) and the plant can cause dermatitis in some individuals (Behl et al 1966).

The seed is a common adulterant of mustard seed (Brassica) either by chance or for profit. Ingestion of Argemone seed oil has caused epidemic dropsy in humans in Africa and India with hyperpigmentation of the skin and 'sarcoidal' angiomatous swellings and glaucoma (Watt and Breyer-Brandwijk 1962).

Berberine, one of the alkaloids derived from the plant, produces intense pain when infiltrated into the conjunctiva for the treatment of trachoma or into the skin for the treatment of Leishmaniasis (Watt and Breyer-Brandwijk 1962). Berberine, when injected as a local anaesthetic, occasionally produces hyperpigmentation at the site of injection (Seery and Bieter 1940). Reactions to berberine are also noted under Berberis.

Argemone platyceras
Prickly Poppy

This species can produce mechanical injury (Meunscher 1951).

References

Behl, P.N., Captain, R.M., Bedi, B.M.S. and Gupta, S. (1966) Skin-irritant and sensitizing plants found in India, New Delhi. P.N. Behl, Irwin Hospital.

Dalziel, J.M. (1937) The useful plants of west tropical Africa. London. Crown Agents.

Meunscher, W.C. (1951) Poisonous plants of the United States. 2nd ed. New York. The Macmillan Co.

Oakes, A.J. and Butcher, J.O. (1962) Poisonous and injurious plants of the U.S. Virgin Islands. Misc. Publ. 882. U.S. Department of Agriculture, Washington, D.C.

Quisumbing, E. (1951) Medicinal Plants of the Philippines. Tech. Bull. 16. Manila, Philippine Islands. Manila Bureau of Printing. 1234 pp.

Seery, T.M. and Bieter, R.N. (1940) A contribution to the pharmacology of Berberine. J. Pharmacol. 69, 64.

Watt, J.M. and Breyer-Brandwijk, M.G. (1962) The medicinal and poisonous plants of Southern Africa. 2nd ed. Edinburgh. E.& S. Livingstone.

Bocconia

Ten species are found in warm regions of Asia and the West Indies.

Bocconia sp.

Injection of an extract of the plant produces local anaesthesia but there is also an irritant effect (Martinez 1969).

Reference

Martinez, M. (1969) The Medicinal Plants of Mexico. 5th ed. Mexico City. Andres Botas.

Chelidonium

One species is found in temperate and sub-arctic Eurasia.

Chelidonium majus
Tetterwort, Greater Celandine, Rock Poppy

Dioscorides (First Century A.D.) referred to a bitter and biting nature of the plant. The fresh juice, when applied to the skin, is acrid, irritant and vesicant and even escharotic (Loudon 1855, Van Hasselt 1862, Oesterlen 1856, U.S. Dispensatory 1884, Cheney 1887, cited by White 1887, Piffard 1881). The juice was used for treating warts and the plant was familiar as a medicinal in the Middle Ages. The plant, commonly found near old walls and ruins in most parts of England and Wales, can produce dermatitis (North 1967). Hardin and Arena (1969) refer to dermatitis from the plant which is established in moist soil from Canada to North Carolina and Missouri.

The yellow-red sap of the plant is irritating to the eye (Hilbert 1916).

Chelidonic acid derived from this plant is an acrid irritant which has been used to treat warts. Repeated subcutaneous injections for the treatment of an epithelioma of the eyelid produced much reaction and pain after each injection and the lids sloughed and scarred up to the orbital margin (Duke-Elder and MacFaul 1972).

Sanguinarine has been identified as one of the alkaloids of this plant and of Sanguinaria.

The Lesser Celandine is a common name for Ranunculus.

References

Cheney (1887) Personal communications to White (1887). Mr. Cheney was a wholesale dealer in medicinal vegetable drugs.

Dioscorides, The Greek Herbal of: Engliahse by John Goodyer: A.D. 1655. Edited and first printed A.D. 1933 by R.T. Gunther 1959. New York. Hafner Publishing Co. 2, 206.

Duke-Elder, S. and MacFaul, P.A. (1972) System of Opthalmology. Vol. XIV. Injuries Part 1. Mechanical Injuries. Extraocular foreign bodies pp. 464-67 and Agricultural Injuries pp. 32-34. London. Henry Kimpton.

Hardin, J.W. and Arena, J.M. (1969) Human Poisoning from native and cultivated plants. Durham, North Carolina. Duke University Press.

Loudon (1855) Encyclopedia of Plants. London. Cited by White (1887).

Hilbert, R. (1916) Iritis durch Einwirkung des Milchsaftes von Chelidonium majus L. Zbl Brakt Augenh 40, 142.

North, P.M. (1967) Poisonous plants and fungi in colour. London. Blandford Press. Ltd.

Oesterlen (1956) Handbuch der Heilmittellehre. Tubingen cited by White (1887).

Piffard, H.G. (1881) A treatise on the Materia Medica and Therapeutics of the skin. New York. Wm. Wood and Co.

U.S. Dispensatory, The National (1884) Philadelphia. Stille and Maisch. cited by White (1887).

Van Hasselt (1862) Handbuch der Giftlehre Braunschweig cited by White (1887).

White, J.C. (1887) Dermatitis venenata: an account of the Action of External irritants upon the skin. Boston. Cupples and Hurd.

Glaucium

25 species are found in Europe, southwestern and central Asia.

Glaucium flavum

This species has irritant properties (Pammel 1911).

Reference

Pammel, L.H. (1911) A Manual of Poisonous Plants. Torch Press. Cedar Rapids, Iowa. Reprinted Univ. Microfilms Inc. Ann Arbor, Mich. 1965. pp. 476-7.

Papaver

100 species are found in Europe, Asia, southern Africa, Australia and America.

Papaver dubuim

This species can cause contact dermatitis (Gardner and Bennetts 1956).

Papaver somniferum
Opium Poppy

Opium, the dried latex of the unripe capsule, yields about 20 alkaloids including morphine. Contact dermatitis occurred in workers in a morphine factory (Levin 1908), and in nurses who made morphine tablets (Dore and Thomas 1944, Jordon and Osborne 1939). Crude morphine produced dermatitis in factory-workers and patch tests with morphine hydrochloride produced negative results (Dore and Thomas 1944, Green 1944). Morphine itself has produced strong sensitivity; a nurse showed a positive patch test reaction to morphine solutions diluted to 1 in 1,000,000 and exposure to the air in a ward produced clinical symptoms (Jordon and Osborne 1939). Ethylmorphine can cause dermatitis of the eyelids (Duke-Elder 1965, Cummer 1931). Opium applied to the skin caused dermatitis of the genitals (Heller 1931). Contact dermatitis from morphine or its unidentified impurities is most likely to occur at the factory level where mechanical handling is avoided and the compounds are worked largely by hand. Panniculitis can occur in morphine addicts (Lopez et al 1961).

The plant was cultivated as a source of cooking oil by Egyptians as early as 1500 B.C. The seed which is free of narcotic properties provides oil and the treated seed is used as a condiment for poppy-seed cake and bread.

Papaver rhoeas

The plant has irritant properties (Pammel 1911).

References

Cummer, C.L. (1931) Dermatitis of the eyelids caused by Dionin. Arch. Derm. Syph. 23, 68.

Dore, S.E. and Thomas, E.W.P. (1944) Contact dermatitis in a morphine factory. Brit. J. Derm. Syph. 56, 177.

Duke-Elder, S. (1965) System of Opthalmology. Vol. VIII. Diseases of the outer eye. Part 1. Allergic kerato-conjunctivitis. pp. 451. London. Henry Kimpton.

Gardner, C.A. and Bennetts, H.W. (1956) The Toxic Plants of Western Australia. Perth West. Australian Newspapers Ltd.

Green, G.C. (1944) The occurrence of "Morphia Rash" in the manufacture of morphine salts from opium. Brit. J. Derm. Syph. 56, 182.

Heller, N.B. (1931) Acute dermatitis due to opium preparations. Archs. Derm. Syph. 24, 417.

Jordon, J.W. and Osborne, E.D. (1939) Contact dermatitis from opium derivatives. JAMA 113, 1955.

Levin (1908) Med. Klin. 4, 1633, cited by White (1934).

Lopez, P.B., Baquero, G.F. and De la Solana, J.G. (1961) Subcutaneous fatty necrosis (Panniculitis in a morphine addict). Bol. Soc. Cuba, Derm. Sif. 18, 35.

Pammel, L.H. (1911) A Manual of Poisonous plants. Torch Press. Cedar Rapids, Iowa. Reprinted Univ. Microfilms Inc. Ann Arbor, Mich. 1965. pp. 476-7.

White, R.P. (1934) The Dermatergoses or Occupational Affections of the skin. 4th ed. London. H.K. Lewis.

Roemeria

Seven species are found from the Mediterranean region to central Asia and Afghanistan.

Roemeria violacea

This species has irritant properties (Pammel 1911).

Reference

Pammel, L.H. (1911) A Manual of Poisonous plants. Torch Press. Cedar Rapids, Iowa. Reprinted Univ. Microfilms Inc. Ann Arbor, Mich. 1965. pp. 476-7.

Sanguinaria

One species is found in Atlantic North America.

Sanguinaria canadensis
Blood Root

The plant contains blood-red juice which the North American Indians used to stain the skin of their bodies. The taste of the root is bitter and acrid and, if chewed, burning occurs in the mouth and throat (Schermeister et al 1967). The root 'poisons' those who handle it (Cheney 1887, cited by White 1887) and the dust of the root is irritant to the mucous membranes (Lloyd 1887 cited by White 1887).

A female laboratory worker developed a vesicular eruption on the fingers, face, neck and chest one day after handling Sanguinaris powder. It is possible that she had been exposed to poison ivy (Toxicodendron) three days previously (Fox 1921).

References

Cheney (1887) Pers. Comm. to White (1887). Mr. Cheney was a wholesale dealer in medicinal vegetable drugs.

Fox, H. (1921) Dermatitis venenata from Oriental cashew nut. Arch. Derm. Syph. 3, 202.

Schermeister, L.J. et al (1967) Common Poisonous Plants of the Northern Plains Dangerous to Man. Fargo, North Dakota. North Dakota Institute for Regional Studies.

White, J.C. (1887) Dermatitis venenata: An account of the Action of External irritants upon the Skin. Boston. Cupples and Hurd.

PEDALIACEAE

50 species in 12 genera are found in tropical and southern Africa, Madagascar and Indo Malaysia.

Chemistry is recorded by Hegnauer (1969).

Reference

Hegnauer, R. (1969) Chemotaxonomy of plants. Vol. 5. Basel, Birkhauser. p. 299.

Harpagophytum

Eight species are found in southern Africa and Madagascar.

Harpagophytum grandidiere
Grapple Tree

The seed pod is a shell-like capsule constructed like so many interlaced fish-hooks which fastens itself to animals and to clothing (Menninger 1967).

Harpagophytum procumbens
Grapple Plant

The fruit, which is beset with large woody grapples about 2.5cm long pointed and barbed, is troublesome to wool-growers. It can cripple and, on gaining access to the mouth, it can firmly hook itself to the two jaws leading to death by starvation (Watt and Breyer-Brandwijk 1962).

References

Menninger, E.A. (1967) Fantastic Trees. New York. The Viking Press.

Watt. J.M. and Vreyer-Brandwijk, M.G. (1962) The Medicinal and poisonous plants of Southern Africa. 2nd ed. Edinburgh. E.& S. Livingstone.

Sesamum

30 species are found in tropical and southern Africa and ir Asia.

Sesamum elatum

The seed of this species used as a food is sometimes adulterated with that of Ceratotheca sesamoides.

Sesamum indicum
Sesame, Gingili

The plant is cultivated, especially in India, for the oil (Sesame, Ben or Teel oil) from its seeds.

Cattle fed excessively on sesame meal develop eczema associated with loss of hair and itching (Watt and Breyer-Brandwijk 1962). Immediate (Type I) hypersensitivity reactions to sesame oil can occur (Batterman et al 1958, Tornsey 1964). Sesame oil is used as a substitute for olive oil and other oils in cosmetic creams (Greenberg and Lester 1954) and in oleomargarine, iodized oil and cosmetics (Merck Index 1968). Foods containing the oil were listed by Tornsey (1964).

Sesame oil, a constituent of an officinial zinc oxide liniment, was found to be the cause of contact dermatitis in 15/98 patients with leg ulcers for which the liniment was used. In one patient a positive patch test to crude oleic acid was observed as well as a positive patch test to sesame oil. As the patients did not react to peanut oil (Arachis) nor to olive oil (Olea) it was considered that triglycerides were not responsible for the dermatitis but rather the unsaponifiable fraction of the oil (which constitutes about 2% of the oil). This fraction contains sesamol, sesamolin and sesamin (Van Dijk et al 1972, 1973).

In 100 cases of leg ulcers, 11 of 100 patients showed positive patch test reactions to a paste containing 40% sesame oil and a higher proportion showed positive reactions to 100% sesame oil (Malten 1972).

The principal allergens of sesame oil are sesamin and sesamolin (Neering et al 1975).

Sesamum schenckii

Contact with the leaves can produce vesication (Watt and Breyer-Brandwijk 1962).

References

Batterman, R.C., Grossman, A.J., Leifer, P. (1958) Skin eruption with gold therapy: influence of sesame oil. Arthr. Rheum. 1, 167.

Greenberg, L.A. and Lester, D. (1954) Handbook of Cosmetic Materials. New York. Interscience.

Malten, K.E. (1972) Sesamoil contact hypersensitivity in leg-ulcer-patients. Contact Dermatitis Newsletter, London. 11, 251.

Merck Index (1968) An Encyclopedia of Chemicals and Drugs. ed. Stecher, P.G. 8th ed. Rahway, N.J. Merck and Co. Inc.

Neering, H., Vitányi, B.E.J., Malten, K.E. et al (1975) Allergens in sesame oil contact dermatitis. Acta Dermatovener 55, 31.

Torsney, P.J. (1964) Hypersensitivity to sesame seed. J. Allergy 35, 514.

Van Dijk, E., Neering, H., and Vitányi, B.E. (1972) Contact hypersensitivity to sesame oil in zinc oxide ointment. Ned. Tijdschr. Geneeskd. 116, 2255.

Van Dijk, E., Neering, H. and Vitányi, B.E.J. (1973) Contact hypersensitivity to sesame oil in patients with leg ulcers and eczema. Acta derm.-venereol. 53, 133.

Watt, J.M. and Breyer-Brandwijk, M.G. (1962) The Medicinal and poisonous plants of Southern Africa. 2nd ed. Edinburgh. E.& S. Livingstone.

PEPEROMIACEAE

1000 species in four genera are found in tropical regions.

Peperomia

Over 1000 species have been described from tropical and subtropical regions especially from America.

Peperomia sp.

Hjorth (1968) recorded two positive patch test reactions to species of this genus. In 21 consecutive cases, negative reactions were recorded. Strong irritancy therefore appears to be unlikely.

Peperomia pellucida

The plant has a strong mustard-like ocour. Pulling the weed can cause asthma-like symptoms (Morton 1969).

References

Hjorth, N. (1968) at Finsen Institute. Pers. comm.

Morton, J.F. (1969) Some ornamental plants excreting respiratory irritants. Proc. Florida State Hort. Soc. 82, 415.

PERIPLOCACEAE

200 species in between 45 and 50 genera are found in tropical and warm temperate regions of the Old World especially in tropical Africa. This family was formerly included in the family Asclepiadaceae.

Cryptostegia

Two species are found in Madagascar.

Cryptostegia grandiflora
Rubber Vine,
Purple Allamande

When the vine is dry, a fine powdery dust which emerges

causes violent coughing, swelling of the nose and blistering of the eyelids. Not all individuals are affected (White 1923). Dried trimmings of the plant give off a dust that is exceedingly irritating to the eyes, nose and throat (Morton 1958). The acrid, sticky milky sap is a drastic irritant to the skin. Gloves should be worn when pruning or working with the plants (Oakes and Butcher 1962).

Cryptostegia madagascarensis
Rubber Vine

Contact with all parts of the plant can cause dermatitis (Hardin and Arena 1969).

References

Hardin, J.W. and Arena, J.M. (1969) Human Poisoning from native and cultivated plants. Durham, North Carolina. Duke University Press.

Oakes, A.J. and Butcher, J.O. (1962) Poisonous and injurious plants of the U.S. Virgin Islands. Misc. Publ. 882. U.S. Department of Agriculture, Washington, D.C.

White, C.T. (1923) Weeds of Queensland, the rubber vine (Cryptostegia grandiflora) Queensland Agric. J. 19, 286.

Parquetina

One species is found in West Equatorial Africa.

Parquetina nigrescens
(syn. Periploca nigrescens)

The latex turns black when dry (Irvine 1961). The leaves when applied to the skin produce a burning sensation (Walker 1953).

References

Irvine, F.R. (1961) Woody plants of Ghana. Oxford University Press. London.

Walker, A. (1953) Usages pharmaceutiques des plates spontanees de Gabon. Bull. de l'Institut d'Etudes Centrafricaines Nos. 4, 5, 6, cited by Irvine (1961).

Periploca

Ten species are found in northern and tropical Africa and the Orient notably eastern Asia.

Periploca graeca
Windenholz

This small tree has long been considered poisonous (Loudon 1844) and this may include the little used wood (Lewin 1928). It contains the cardiac glycoside, periplocin (Hausen 1970). Woods and Calnan (1976) refer to the related plant Sarcostemma australe of the Asdepiadaceae family as having irritant sap.

References

Hausen, B.M. (1970) Untersuchungen uber Gesundheitsschadigende Holzer. Thesis, Hamburg.

Lewin, L. (1928) Gifte im Holzgewerbe. Berlin, Stilke.

Loudon, J.C. (1844) Aboretum et Fruticetum Britannicum. 2nd ed. London, Longman, cited by Woods and Calnan (1976).

Woods, B. and Calnan, C.D. (1976) Toxic Woods. Brit. J. Derm. 94, Suppl. 13, June.

PHYTOLACCACEAE

100 species in 12 genera are chiefly found in tropical America and southern Africa.

Chemistry is recorded by Hegnauer (1969).

Reference

Hegnauer, R. (1969) Chemotaxonomy of plants. Vol. 5. Basel, Birkhauser p. 305.

Gallesia

Two species are found in Peru and Brazil.

Gallesia gorazema

Gallesia integrifolia

The plants smell like onions (Allium)(Thiébault 1965).

Reference

Thiébault, A. (1965) Nomenclature Générale des Bois Tropicaux. L'Association Technique Internationale des Bois Tropicaux. 45 bis Avenue de la Belle-Gabrielle, Nogent-sur Marne, France.

Phytolacca

35 species are found in tropical and subtropical regions.

Phytolacca spp.

In general, the leaf of species of this genus has an acrid taste and 'burns' the tongue (Watt and Breyer-Brandwijk 1962).

Phytolacca acinosa

The oil of the plant is used externally as a rubefacient and can cause irritant dermatitis (Chopra et al 1958).

Phytolacca decandra
(syn. P. americana)
Pokeberry, Pokeweed, Garget

The plant was formerly officinal. An ointment made from it was applied for haemorrhoids. The dust of the dried root is irritant to the eye and produces sneezing. The symptoms of poisoning from ingesting of the plant include burning in the mouth.

The green plant and root often produce inflammation of the skin (communication to White 1887, Lloyd 1887 cited by White 1887). An ointment made from the plant excites a sense of heat and smarting; it is stimulating when applied to the skin, frequently producing an eschar (Bigelow 1917, cited by White 1887). The juice or a strong decoction of the root applied to the skin when tender or abraded, causes smarting or a burning pain (Dispensatory 1884). The action of the fresh plant on workmen in a laboratory was similar to that of Podophyllum causing serious inflammation of the eyelids (Lloyd 1887 cited by White 1887).

Phytolacca dioica
Ombu, Umbu

The tree at night gives off a vile odour (Menninger 1967). Accidental application of the juice of the root to the eyeball produced blindness lasting as long as 48 hours (Watt and Breyer-Brandwijk 1962).

Phytolacca dodecandra

The juice is used as a styptic but produces a marked burning sensation in wounds (Watt and Breyer-Brandwijk 1962).

Phytolacca octandra
Inkweed, Pokeweed

"I took hold of it with my bare hand to break it off, as it is very brittle, with the result that my arms became saturated with the juice which looked like blood. It commenced to burn, and small pimples appeared on the skin and I found relief by bathing it in water" (Hansen in Anon 1913). "All parts of the plant possess acrid properties" The juice of the fresh plant, or strong decoction of the root, applied locally may strongly irritate the skin, especially if tender or abraded" (Dr. Johnson in Anon 1913).

The plant is referred to (Anon 1913) as P. octandra but the references quoted it in concerning the poisonous nature of the plant, refer to P. decandra.

The Maoris used P. octandra as ink and the plant provides a useful wood-stain (Anon 1913). The plant is used as a soap substitute in Mexico (Watt and Breyer-Brandwijk 1962).

References

Anon (1913) Inkweed: its value as a poison. New Zealand J. Agricult. 7, 369.

Bigelow (1917) American Medical Botany. Boston: (1824) Florula Bostoniensis. Boston, cited by White (1887).

Chopra, R.N., Cyopra, I.C., Handa, K.L. and Kapur, L.D. (1958). Chopra's Indigenous Drugs of India. Ed. 2. U.N. Dhur & Sons Ltd., Calcutta.

Dispensatory, The National (1884) Philadelphia. Stille and Maisch., cited by White (1887).

Menninger, E.A. (1967) Fantastic Trees. New York. The Viking Press.

Watt, J.M. and Breyer-Brandwijk, M.G. (1962) The Medicinal and poisonous plants of Southern Africa. 2nd ed. Edinburgh. E.& S. Livingstone.

White, J.C. (1887) Dermatitis venenata: An accound of the Action of External irritants upon the Skin. Boston. Cupples and Hurd.

PINACEAE

250 species in 10 genera are found in the northern hemisphere, south to Sumatra, Java, central America and the West Indies.

Numerous common names are used for species of this family (Handbook of Softwoods 1957, Sargent 1965, Elsevier 1964).

References

Elsevier's Wood Dictionary (1964) by Beekman, W.B. 2 vols. Elsevier Publ. Co. Amsterdam.

Handbook of Softwoods (1957) Forest Products Research. Ministry of Technology. London. HMSO.

Sargent, C.S. (1965) Manual of the trees of North America (excluding Mexico). 2 vols. New York, Dover Publications Inc.

Abies
Fir

50 species are found in north temperate regions and central America.

Abies spp.
Fir

Species of this genus are commonly named Fir or Whitewood and, in Great Britain, European silver pine, etc. (Handbook of Softwoods 1957).

An extract of Fir made by the method of Fregert and Rorsman (1963) was used to investigate 125 patients for dermatitis suspected to be caused by woods. Positive patch test reactions were observed in six males and two females. In these eight patients, a commercial extract of Fir obtained from Hollister-Stier Laboratories, Spokane, Washington produced positive patch test reactions in two cases. Contact sensitivity to fir was considered significant in four of the males, three forest-workers and a farmer. The farmer bedded his cattle on fir shavings; when he changed his bedding to straw, his hand dermatitis cleared (Mitchell 1970).

At the Finsen Institute from 1935 to 1963, 12 cases of contact dermatitis from 'fir' wood were observed (Hjorth 1965).

Some firs cause woodcutters' eczema from lichens or *Frullania* growing on the bark (Tenchio 1948).

Abies alba
(syn. *A. pectinata*)
Silver fir

This species yields Alsatian turpentine.

Farmers who felled the sawed silver fir during the winter developed recurrent dermatitis of the hands and arms spreading to the face and neck at that season only. Patch tests to fir resin gave strong positive reactions (Ganzoni 1929). Siemens (1929) reported dermatitis from the foliage of silver fir; patch tests were not recorded.

Abies balsamea
Balsam Fir

This species yields Canada Balsam which has been reported to produce dermatitis when used in perfumery (Greenberg and Lester 1954). A laboratory worker who was sensitized in her work to Canada Balsam showed positive patch test reactions to Canada Balsam and to lavender oil (*Lavandula*), eucalyptus oil (*Eucalyptus*), clove oil (*Eugenia*), Balsam of Peru (*Myroxylon*), styrax (*Liquidambar*) and to eugenol, isoeugenol, nerolidol and farnesol (Rudzki and

Kielak 1972).

A florist developed contact dermatitis from the foliage of balsam fir; a patch test produced a positive reaction (Kappes 1948).

Abies canadensis
Hemlock Spruce

The resin named Canada Pitch derived from this species is irritant (White 1887).

Abies grandis

The foliage and bark of the tree produced positive patch test reactions in one case; patch tests to the wood produced negative reactions (Suskind 1967).

Abies pectinata

This species is listed as injurious (Hanslian and Kadlec 1966).

Abies sibirica

This species yields Siberian Pine Oil which is used as a rubefacient (Wren 1968).

References

Fregert, S. and Rorsman, H. (1963) Simultaneous Hypersensitivity to Balsam of Pine and to Balsam of Peru. Acta derm.-venereol. 42, 21.

Greenberg, L.A. and Lester, D. (1954) Handbook of Cosmetic Materials. New York. Interscience.

Handbook of Softwoods (1957) Forest Products Research. Ministry of Technology. London. HMSO.

Hanslian, L. and Kadlec, K. (1966) Wood from the standpoint of hygiene VIII. Species with some or little biological effect. Drevo 21, 229.

Hjorth, N. (1965) Contact sensitivity to plants and balsams in Symposium on Allergic Contact czema in Theory and Practice. ed. Skog, E. (Europ. Congr. Allergy) Acta derm-venereol. and Contact Dermatitis Newsletter 6, 131, 1969.

Rudzki, E. and Kielak, D. (1972) Sensitivity to some compounds related to balsam of Peru. Contact Dermatitis Newsletter 12, 335.

Mitchell, J.C. (1970) Patch test results - screening set and plants. Contact Dermatitis Newsletter, London 8, 177.

Suskind, R.R. (1967) Dermatitis in the Forest Product Industries. Arch. Environ. Health 15, 322.

Wren, R.W. (1968) Potter's New Cyclopaedia of Botanical Drugs and Preparations by Wren, R.C. Re-edit. by Wren, R.W. Potter and Clarke Ltd. Health Science Press. Rustington, Sussex.

Kappes, L.O. (1948) Balsam as a cause of contact dermatitis in a florist. Ann. Allergy 6, 21.

Ganzoni, M. (1929) Das Ekzem als Arbeitsschadigung und seine rechtliche Stellung in der Versicherung. Schweizer medizinische Wochenschrift 59, 1169.

Siemens, H.W. (1929) Strichformige akute Dermatitis. Dermatologische Zeitschrift 55, 257.

Tenchio, F. (1948) Etiologie de l'eczema des bucherons. Dermatologica 97, 72.

Cedrus
True Cedar

Four species are recognized.

Cedrus libani
Cedar of Lebanon

Cedrus atlantica
Atlantic Cedar (Algeria)

Cedrus brevifolia
from Cyrpus

Cedrus deodara
Deodar (Himalayas)

Other botanical species which are commonly named Cedar are Libocedrus and Thuja.

Handling the wood or cones and contact with the odorous gummy sap of these trees is likely to cause irritation of the skin of wood-cutters, foresters and carpenters (Chopra et al 1958). Woodcutters who saw timber from these trees are liable to dermatitis (Behl et al 1966).

C. deodara, in India, provides a turpentine which can cause dermatitis (Behl et al 1966).

The native cedar of the United States named as a source of dermatitis (Weber 1953) probably refers to Thuja.

The wood dust of cedar of Lebanon can produce asthma (Greenberg 1972).

References

Behl, P.N., Captain, R.M., Bedi, B.M.S. and Gupta, S. (1966) Skin-irritant and sensitizing plants found in India, New Delhi. P.N. Behl, Irwin Hospital.

Chopra, R.N., Chopra, I.C., Handa, K.L. and Kapur, L.D. (1958) Chopra's Indigenous Drugs of India. 2nd ed. Calcutta. U.S. Dhur and Sons Ltd.

Greenberg, M. (1972) Respiratory symptoms following brief exposure to cedar of Lebanon dust. Clin. Allergy 2, 219.

Weber, L.F. (1953) Dermatitis venenata from native woods. Arch. Derm. Syph. 67, 388.

Larix

Ten or twelve species are found in Europe, northern Asia and North America.

Larix spp.

The wood can cause woodcutters' eczema (Schulmann and Detouillon 1932). Tenchio (1948) noted the presence of lichens and liverworts (Frullania) on larch trees. These are responsible for woodcutters' eczema.

References

Schulmann, E. and Detouillon, P. (1932) L'eczéma du bois et al sensivilisation sylvestre. Pris. Med. 1, 55.

Tenchio, F. (1948) Etiologie de l'eczema des Bucherons. Dermatologica 97, 72.

Larix americana
Tamarack

The bark is used for an astringent effect in Herbal Medicine (Wren 1968).

Larix decidua
(syn. L. europaea)
Larch

A furniture-maker developed occupational urticaria from wood-dust of this tree. The dust concentration during the grinding of the wood in the mill exceeded 10 mg/m^3. Epicutaneous tests to larch veneer and to a petroleum ether extract of untreated larch wood produced positive results. α-Pinene, β-pinene and delta-3 carene were demonstrated in the extract (Hanslian and Kadlec 1964). A scarlatiniform eruption was attributed to ingestion of Venice turpentine which is derived from this species (Angus 1913).

Larix leptolepis

This species was listed as an irritant wood capable of producing dermatitis (Orsler 1973).

References

Angus, W. (1913) Scarlatiniform rash due to Venice turpentine. Brit. Med. J. 1, 712.

Hanslian, L. and Kadlec, K. (1964) Allergy caused by Larch wood. Pracov. Lek. 16, 362.

Orsler, R.J. (1973) Personal communication from Forest Products Research Laboratory, Princess Risborough, Bucks, England.

Wren, R.W. (1968) Potter's New Cyclopaedia of Botanical Drugs and Preparations by Wren, R.C. Re-edit. by Wren, R.W. Potter and Clarke Ltd. Health Science Press. Rustington, Sussex.

Picea

50 species are found in north temperate regions especially in eastern Asia.

Picea spp.
Spruce

Dermatitis from spruce was mentioned by White (1917) Workers who cut up the wood and women who sanded it developed vesicular and bullous dermatitis (Hebblewaite cited by White 1934). In a sawmill worker who had asthma, intradermal tests to spruce and pine (*Pinus*) produced positive reactions, negative in controls (Bahn 1928). An instrument maker who had dermatitis of the hand showed positive patch test reactions to spruce and casein glue (Woods and Calnan 1976).

Contact sensitivity to Balsam of Pine (*Pinus*) or spruce was found in 5.5% of 1247 patients; the majority reacted to both balsams. Many of the patients were also contact sensitive to Balsams of Tolu and Peru (*Myroxylon*), Storax (*Liquidambar*) or benzoin (*Styrax*). Only in a minor number of cases could exposure to oil of turpentine and rosin (colophony)(*Pinus*) be held responsible. Hydroxystilbenes which have been isolated from balsam of pine were postulated as the sensitizing agents (Fregert and Rorsman 1963). Persons contact sensitive to Balsam of Peru (*Myroxylon*), balsam of pine (*Pinus*) and balsam of spruce are often contact sensitive to diethylstilboestrol and nearly all persons sensitive to the latter are sensitive to the balsams (Fregert and Rorsman 1960). Some coumarins are related to oestrogenic substances (Soine 1964).

35 of 712 patients showed positive patch test reactions to a mixture of balsams of spruce and pine, 15% of each. In 12 of the 35 patients, contact sensitivity to the balsams were considered to be the main or a contributory cause of hand eczema. The sources of exposure were considered to be handling spruce and pine twigs and freshly cut pine trees, wood-working, florists' work, handicrafts and dressing Christmas Trees (Agrup 1969). Dermatitis from a balsam (query *Abies balsamea*) occurred in a florist (Kappes 1948). Dermatitis from balsams usually arises from therapeutic use of popular medicaments; cross-sensitivity with Balsam of Peru (*Myroxylon*) is frequently observed (Hjorth 1961).

Picea abies
(syn. *Picea excelsa* and *Abies excelsa*)
Norway spruce
Spruce-fir

The resin which exudes from this tree is named Burgundy pitch. When applied to the skin in the form of a plaster and worn for varying periods, the plaster causes redness, itching papules and on delicate skins, even pustules and ulcers (White 1887).

Picea mariana

Two asthmatic patients became sensitive to the needles; intradermal tests produced positive reactions (Cobe 1930).

References

Cobe, H.M. (1930) Sensitivity due to Christmas trees. Journal of Allergy 1, 442.

White, J.C. (1887) Dermatitis venenata: An account of the action of external irritants upon the skin. Boston. Cupples and Hurd.

White, R.P. (1934) The Dermatergoses or Occupational Affections of the Skin. 4th ed. London. H.K. Lewis.

White, C.J. (1917) Two modern methods to be employed in the treatment of chronic eczema. JAMA 68, 81.

Bahn, K. (1928) Beitrag zur Frage der Allergie bei Holzsagereiarbeitern. Klinische Wochenschrift 7, 1963.

Agrup, G. (1969) Hand Eczema and other hand dermatoses in South Sweden. Acta derm.-venereol. 49 Suppl. 61. pp. 1-91.

Fregert, S. and Rorsman, H. (1960) Hypersensitivity to Diethylstilbestrol: Cross-sensitization to Dienestrol, Hexestrol, Bisphenol A., p-Benzyl-Phenol, Hydroquinone-monobenzylether and p-Hydroxybenzoic-Benzylester, Acta Dermatovener (Stockholm) 40, 206.

Fregert, S. and Rorsman, H. (1963) Hypersensitivity to Balsam of Pine and Spruce. Archs. Derm. 87, 693.

Hjorth, N. (1961) Eczematous Allergy to Balsams. Munksgaard, International Booksellers and Publishers Ltd., Copenhagen.

Kappes, L.O. (1948) Balsam as a cause of contact dermatitis in a florist. Ann. Allergy 6, 21.

Soine, T.O. (1964) Naturally occurring coumarins and related physiological activities. J. Pharm. Sci. 53, 231.

Woods, B. and Calnan, C.D. (1976) Toxic Woods. Brit. J. Derm. 94, Suppl. 13, June.

Pinites

Pinites succinifera

This extinct species furnishes a fossil resin, Amber. Oil of Amber has been used as a rubefacient (Greenberg and Lester 1954).

Reference

Greenberg, L.A. and Lester, D. (1954) Handbook of Cosmetic Materials. New York. Interscience.

Pinus

Between 70 and 100 species are found in north temperate regions and on mountains in the northern tropics.

Pinus spp.
Pine

Although species of this genus are extensively cut for wood and resins, dermatitis in forest-workers appears to be uncommon. Two of 125 forest-workers who had dermatitis showed positive patch test reactions to an acetone extract of pine wood (Mitchell 1970). Shavings of the wood produced dermatitis in wood-workers (Peri 1910). Workers can develop dermatitis from the oil of pine chips used for making rope (Schwartz et al 1957).

Five carpenters who had contact dermatitis showed positive patch test reactions to pine wood sawdust and extracts (Wilkinson, D.S. 1973, Pers. Comm). It is not known whether the sensitizer is a stilbene such as pinosylvine (King 1953), delta-3-carene as in turpentine or some other compound. Woodcutter's eczema from pine trees is caused by lichens or liverworts (Frullania) on the bark.

Dermatitis occurred in foresters working on pines infested with a caterpillar, Thaumatopoea pinivora. Patch tests to the caterpillar hairs produced positive reactions, negative to the pulped cocoon (Katzenellenbogen 1955). Some caterpillar hairs are irritant.

References

Katzenellenbogen, I. (1955) Caterpillar dermatitis as an occupational disease. Dermatologica 111, 99.

King, F.E. (1953) The chemistry of wood extractives. Chem. Ind. 1325.

Woods and Calnan (1976) reported six wood-workers who had dermatitis and positive patch test reactions to deal or pine.

Pinus sylvestris is known as red deal. In one of them, positive patch test reactions were observed to pinosylvin, anthothecol, colophony, formalin and turpentine. Two also reacted to Tectona, one of these to lapachol and anthothecol.

Reference

Woods, B. and Calnan, C.D. (1976) Toxic Woods. Brit. J. Derm. 94, Suppl. 13, June.

Pinus radiata

Three cases of contact dermatitis from this wood were reported by Burry (1969).

The wood is used in Australia in the building industry, for box making, as fencing posts and in furniture manufacture. Nine male patients developed dermatitis from exposure to the sawdust, the wood or the tree. Four were reactive to adhesive plaster, three to wood turpentine and one to colophony (Burry 1976).

Pinus sylvestris

Three cases of contact dermatitis from this wood - in two workers in wood-yards and in a messenger in a wood research establishment - were observed by Wilkinson (1973, pers. comm.).

Derivatives of Pinus can produce dermatitis. Contact sensitivity to Balsam of Pine is noted under Picea.

Exacerbation of turpentine dermatitis occurred in a painter after he ate sweets made from pine buds (Jadassohn 1960).

A joiner's mate who had eczema of the hands was found to show positive patch test reactions to dry and moist pine dust and to colophony resin (Beer 1970).

Pine wood extract, applied as a topical remedy for ringworm of the toes, produced dermatitis (Goodman 1933).

References

Beer, W.E. (1970) Sensitivity to Iroko wood in a wood machinist. Internat. Contact Newsletter 7, 159.

Goodman, H. (1933) Silk Handlers' Disease of the Skin. New York. Medical Lay Press.

Jadassohn, W. (1960) Eczema due to known chemical substances. Acta Allerg. (Kbh.) 15 (Suppl. 7), 185.

Mitchell, J.C. (1970) Patch test results - screening set and plants. Contact Dermatitis Newsletter, London 8, 177.

Schwartz, L., Tulipan, L. and Birmingham, D.J. (1957) Occupational Diseases of the Skin. 3rd ed. Philadelphia. Lea and Febiger.

White, R.P. (1934) The Dermatergoses or Occupational Affections of the Skin. 4th ed. London. H.K. Lewis.

Peri, A. (1910) La lavorazione della corda di truciolo di pino nelle fonderie di tuba di ghisa. Le lesioni cutanee delle mani delle cordaie. Il Ramazzini (Firenze) 4, 383.

Burry, J.N. (1976) Contact dermatitis from radiata pine. Contact Dermatitis 2, 262.

Turpentine and Colophony (Rosin)

Sources of turpentine are recorded by Usher (1974).

Turpentine gum, oil, spirit	Pinus palustris
Turpentine, Austrian	Pinus nigra
Turpentine, Bordeaux	Pinus pinaster
Turpentine, Canada	Abies balsamea
Turpentine, China	Pistacia terebinthis
Turpentine, French Oil	Pinus pinaster
Turpentine, Greek	Pinus halepensis
Turpentine, Hungarian	Pinus cembra
Turpentine, Indian	Pinus longifolia
Turpentine, Japanese	Larix dahurica
Turpentine, Jura	Picea excelsa
Turpentine, Strassburg	Abies pectinata
Turpentine, Venice	Larix decidua

Botanical sources of turpentine are listed for South Africa by Watt and Breyer-Brandwijk (1962) and for New Zealand by Williams and Bannister (1962).

Turpentines derived from different geographical locations can vary in their chemical composition. Fresh turpentine can vary in chemical composition from aged turpentine (Anon 1971).

Colophony (Rosin) is derived

principally from Pinus palustris.

Garland (1886) reported a case of contact dermatitis from turpentine applied for a sprained wrist followed by recurrence at the contact site (focal flare) and partially generalized dermatitis after ingesting turpentine for treatment of bronchitis. Dermatitis of the face from turpentine used by painters to clean pallets and brushes was reported by White (1887). Oil of turpentine has long been used as a rubefacient.

Early reports of dermatitis from turpentine were reviewed by White (1934).

References

Anon (1971) Turps and Turps. Trans. St. John's Hosp. Dermatol. Soc. 57, 223.

Garland, O.H. (1886) Terebene rash. Lancet 1, 1005.

Usher, G. (1974) A dictionary of plants used by man. London. Constable.

Watt, J.M. and Breyer-Brandwijk, M.G. (1962) The Medicinal and poisonous plants of Southern Africa. 2nd ed. Edinburgh. E.& S. Livingstone.

White, J.C. (1887) Dermatitis venenata: An account of the Action of External irritants upon the Skin. Boston. Cupples and Hurd.

White, R.P. (1934) The Dermatergoses or Occupational Affections of the Skin. 4th ed. London. H.K. Lewis.

Williams, A.L. and Bannister, M.H. (1962) Composition of gum turpentines from twenty-two species of pines grown in New Zealand. J. Pharm. Sci. 51, 970.

Pirila (1968) provided the following information: -

Oil of turpentine is a variable mixture of numerous terpenoid compounds and is derived from various sources; for instance, from the balsam of pine trees and as a by-product in the manufacture of sulphate cellulose. The main components, 2 pinene (=α-pinene), 2(10)-pinene (=β-pinene), 3-carene (δ3-carene), and dipentene (d- and l-limonene) are monoterpenes, which have a common chemical formula $C_{10}H_{16}$, but different structures.

Practically all oils of turpentine contain large amounts of l-pinene. On the other hand, the 3-carene content varies in the different types, being high (30-40 percent) in most sulphate oils and low or negligible in many balsam oils, e.g. French oil of turpentine.

The Finnish oils of turpentine, mostly sulphate oils, contain large amounts of both 3-carene and 2-pinene. 3-carene has been shown and convincingly confirmed by us to have a stronger eczematogenic effect than the other terpenes. Moreover, 3-carene is much more rapidly oxidized than the other terpenes. The easier oxidizability of 3-carene is in good conformity with our observation that the addition of small amounts of this terpene markedly increases the eczematogenic effect of the others. This phenomenon explains also most of the positive reactions we obtained with different commercial brands of 2-pinene containing minute amounts of carene only.

However, not all the positive reactions to other terpenes appeared to be due to carene impurities. Therefore, with the earlier observation that the eczematogenic effect of 3-carene depends on its hydroperoxide content as a basis, we compared the degree of sensitivity to different terpenes in a total of 106 patients sensitized to oil of turpentine. The more the other terpenes were purified of 3-carene, the lower, as a rule, were the eczematogenic effects of their oxidation products. The sole obvious exception was 2-carene, which was included in the study since it presumably has hydroperoxides in common with 3-carene. On the other hand, positive eczematous reactions to the other terpenes were obtained in a few cases only. Thus, four of forty-five patients tested with sufficiently purified samples of 2-pinene and one of sixteen patients tested with limonene reacted only at test concentrations 20 times higher than the threshold for 3-carene. In these cases the reactions to 2-pinene and limonene have to be considered specific. Moreover, some of the other reactions may be due to weak but specific sensitivity to 2-pinene, 2(10)-pinene or limonene. However, in the majority of our cases the hypersensitivity was obviously directed towards 3- and 2-carenes alone, or more accurately, in our opinion, towards one or more carene hydroperoxides.

Since several hydroperoxides of 3- and 2-carene are, at least theoretically, common to both and since the Finnish oils of turpentine do not contain significant amounts of 2-carene, it is reasonable to conclude that the reactions to the latter are due to some of their common hydroperoxides. On the other hand, the chemical structures of the other terpenes differ so much from that of 3-carene that they cannot be expected to have any hydroperoxides in common. Moreover, since sensitivity to other terpenes than carene was the exception rather than the rule and always weaker than to 3-carene, true cross-sensitivity does not appear probable; but simultaneous, independent sensitization to different terpenes may preferably be considered. The almost negligible role played by terpenes other than 3-carene in Finland can be attributed both to the markedly stronger eczematogenic effect of 3-carene and to the predominant exposure to its hydroperoxides as a result of the considerable carene content of the Finnish oils of turpentine and of the rapid oxidation of 3-carene.

The patterns of sensitivity to different terpenes can be expected to vary according to the exposure. In fact, in a subject experimentally sensitised to French balsam oil of turpentine containing small amounts of 3-carene only, the sensitivities to 2-pinene and 3-carene were of approximately equal degree. Furthermore, the pattern appears to be different elsewhere; for instance, in Germany (Grimm and Gries 1967). Therefore, a comparative study, with the same test substances, would be advisable among patients from areas where different types of oil of turpentine are used. However, even as such, our results allow conclusions on the specificity and patterns of hypersensitivity to different terpenes.

This subject was reviewed by Pirila et al (1969). The incidence of turpentine contact dermatitis has declined in countries where legislation has resulted in the substitution of other solvents.

References

Grimm, W. and Gries, H. (1967) Studies on turpentine oil allergy. I. Berufsdermatosen 15, 253.

Pirila, V. (1968) Pattern of sensitivity to different terpenes. Contact Dermatitis Newsletter, London 3, 48.

Pirila, V., Kilpio, O., Olkkonen, A. et al (1969) On the chemical nature of the eczematogens in Oil of Turpentine. V. Pattern of sensitivity to different terpenes. Dermatologica 139, 183.

Colophony (Rosin)

Rosin (Colophony, abietic anhydride) is the residue left after distilling off the volatile oil from the oleoresin obtained from *Pinus sylvestris* and other species. Rosin occurs as wood rosin obtained from pine stumps: gum rosin is the exudate from incisions in the living trees, *Pinus palustris* and *P. caribaea*: Tall Oil (Liquid rosin) is a by-product of the wood pulp industry. (Tall is a Swedish name for pine). Rosin is chiefly produced in the United States. Its constituents are about 90% resin acids and 10% neutral matter. Of the resin acids about 90% are isomeric with abietic acid; the other 10% is a mixture of dihydroabietic acid and dehydroabietic acid. Rosin oil is obtained by dry distillation of rosin.

Ester gums are combinations of natural resins (such as rosin) with glycerine. Emulsions of acid ester gums may be used as fabric finishers and produce allergic contact dermatitis from clothing. The probable main sensitizing agent in such a finish was abietic acid or one of its derivatives (Schwartz et al 1940). Although this paper has been frequently cited, abietic acid was not actually proven allergenic.

Rosin produced contact dermatitis in a violinist (Ramirez and Eller 1930). Rosin in hair lacquer and adhesive plaster caused dermatitis (Greenberg and Lester 1954). Colophony gave positive patch test reactions in 6/16 persons contact sensitive to adhesive plaster (Jirasek and Kvicalova 1965). 19 of 712 persons (250 males and 462 females) tested showed positive patch tests to colophony. In 13 of the 19 cases, allergy to this material was considered to be the main cause or a contributory cause of hand eczema. Products most often suspected as causative were adhesive tape, furniture polish and saw-dust (Agrup 1969).

Fregert et al (1969) gave the incidence of sensitivity to colophony in various European Eczema Clinics.

Six patients in a spinal injuries centre showed positive patch test reactions to colophony (Walshe 1975); she discussed the sources of exposure. Physiotherapy wax contaminated with colophony produced dermatitis (Hambly and Wilkinson 1975). 5 of 306 patients with leg ulcers were contact sensitive to colophony (Angelini et al 1975). Colophony rosin applied to a belt to increase friction produced dermatitis in an engineer (Wilkinson and Calnan 1975). Colophony in soap may have caused dermatitis (Cooke and Kurwa 1975). A pre-wash dirt remover used on a collar produced dermatitis of the neck. The remover contained colophony. The patient was patch test positive to colophony and rosin powder (Kirk 1976).

References

Agrup, G. (1969) Hand Eczema and other hand dermatoses in South Sweden. Acta derm.-venereol. 49 Suppl. 61 p. 1-91.

Angelini, G., Rantuccio, F. and Meneghini, C.L. (1975) Contact dermatitis in patients with leg ulcers. Contact Dermatitis 1, 81.

Cooke, M.A. and Kurwa, A.R. (1975) Colophony sensitivity. Contact Dermatitis 1, 192.

Fregert, S., Groth, O., Hjorth, N. et al (1969) Alcohol dermatitis. Acta derm.-venereol. 49, 493.

Greenberg, L.A. and Lester, D. (1954) Handbook of Cosmetic Materials. New York. Interscience.

Hambly, E.M. and Wilkinson, D.S. (1975) Dermatitis from contaminated physiotherapy wax. Contact Dermatitis 1, 53.

Jirasek, L., and Kvicalova, E. (1965) The irritating effect of adhesive plaster. Derm. Wschr. 151, 384.

Kirk, J. (1976) Colophony collar dermatitis. Contact Dermatitis 2, 294.

Ramirez, M.A. and Eller, J.J. (1930) The "Patch test" in "Contact Dermatitis" (Dermatitis venenata). J. Allergy 1, 489.

Schwartz, L., (1940) An outbreak of dermatitis from new resin fabric finishes. JAMA 115, 906.

Walshe, M.M. (1975) Contact dermatitis in a spinal injuries centre. Contact Dermatitis 1, 3.

Wilkinson, D.S. and Calnan, C.D. (1975) Rosin used for belt-drive machine. Contact Dermatitis 1, 64.

Wood tars

Wood tars are obtained by the destructive distillation of the woods of various botanical species (e.g. pine (*Pinus*), beech (*Fagus*), birch (*Betula*) and juniper *Juniperus*)). Such therapeutic tars are refined to a lesser or greater degree. Pine tar contains many substances present in colophony (rosin) so that these products can give concomitant reactions.

Positive patch test reactions to wood tars are of importance in directing attention to many other substances encountered in daily life. In 1831 consecutive patients with dermatitis, 88 (4.8%) showed positive patch tests to wood tars. 35 per cent of patients sensitive to wood tars were also sensitive to perfumes of popular toilet soaps and detergents (Hjorth 1965).

Wood creosote derived from wood tar differs in composition from Coal tar. Application of Burgundy pitch derived from *Pinus abies* can produce an eczematous eruption (Piffard 1881).

alpha-pinene in Boot Polish

Boot polish may consist of a mixture of paraffin wax, carnauba wax (*Copernicia*), modified Montan wax (obtained from lignite), a microcrystalline wax, a dye (Nigrosine in the case of black polish) and two solvents white spirit and alpha-pinene. The last named produced a positive patch test in a patient who was contact sensitive to boot polish (Hindson 1972). A perfume compound (Violet 3567) caused allergic contact dermatitis from shoe polish (Broughton 1969). Ekblad (1956) placed shoe polish at the head of his list of eczematous sensitizers and stated that one particular brand was usually the offender; it seems likely that he was patch testing at an irritant concentration.

References

Broughton, R.H. (1969) An unusual case of shoe polish contact dermatitis. J. Roy. Nav. Med. Serv. 55, 54 and personal communication 1972 (Contact Dermatitis Newsletter, London 6, 115.

Ekblad, G. (1956) Contact sensitivities. Bull. Ass. Mil. Dermat. 5, 2.

Hindson, T.C. (1972) Personal Communication. (Contact Dermatitis Newsletter, London 6, 116.)

Hjorth, N. (1965) Contact sensitivity to plants and balsams in Symposium on Allergic Contact Eczema in Theory and Practice. ed. Skog, E. (Europ. Congr. Allergy) Acta derm.-venereol. and Contact Dermatitis Newsletter 6, 131.

Piffard, H.G. (1881) A treatise on the Materia Medica and Therapeutics of the skin. New York. Wm. Wood and Co.

Pine pollen

Pine pollen, which has acid-fast staining characteristics similar to those of the tubercle bacillus, has been suggested for a role in the aetiology of sarcoidosis (Cummings and Hudgins 1958). They investigated several species identified only by common name. The hypothesis seems dubious (Scadding 1967).

Pine pollen has been suspected of causing hayfever (Wodehouse 1971).

References

Cummings, M.M. and Hudgins, P.C. (1958) Chemical constituents of pine pollen and their possible relationship to sarcoidosis. Am. J. Med. Sci. 236, 311.

Scadding, J.G. (1967) Sarcoidosis. London. Eyre and Spottiswode. p. 483.

Wodehouse, R.P. (1971) Hayfever Plants. 2nd rev. edition. New York, Hafner.

Paper

Paper is obtained from pine trees and from other species. The pulp undergoes many processes of purification during which tars, oils and resins are separated. Allergic contact dermatitis can occur from exposure to pine tar, colophony and essential oils (Schwartz et al 1957). Various chemicals are added to the refined product according to the requirements of the finished paper. Irritation from alkalis, calcium bisulphite, sodium hydroxide and other chemicals can occur. Paper which has been sized by resin caused contact dermatitis of the hands; abietic acid and resins containing colophony were implicated by patch testing (Wikstrom 1969). Cigarette paper caused dermatitis (Tye 1950). Paper containing formalin did not produce positive patch test reactions in persons contact sensitive to formaldehyde (Fisher et al 1962).

References

Fisher, A.A., Kanof, N.B. and Biondi, E.M. (1962) Free formaldehyde in textiles and paper. Archs. Derm. 86, 753.

Schwartz, L., Tulipan, L. and Birmingham, D.J. (1957) Occupational Diseases of the Skin. 3rd ed. Philadelphia. Lea & Febiger. pp. 637-672.

Tye, M.J. (1950) Cigarette paper dermatitis. J. Invest. Derm. 14, 77.

Wikstrom, K. (1969) Allergic contact dermatitis caused by paper. Acta derm.-venereol. 40, 547.

Pseudotsuga

Seven species are found in eastern Asia and western North America.

Pseudotsuga menziesii (syn. P. taxifolis) Douglas Fir

This species is variously known as Oregon Pine, Columbian Pine and Douglas spruce or Red Fir (Sargent 1965). Two patients were reported to be contact sensitive to Douglas fir; only in one of them was the sensitivity considered relevant to the clinical dermatitis (Suskind 1967). Wilkinson (pers. comm. 1973) observed a wood-worker who was contact sensitive to the wood of this species.

A messenger at the Forest Products Research Laboratory with slight exposure to many woods developed severe dermatitis of the exposed skin. Patch test to Douglas fir produced strong positive reactions, negative to several other woods (Wilkinson, D.S. Pers. comm. 1973).

Trade complaints are received of septic splinter wounds (Orsler 1973, Nordin 1947). Neudorffer (1902) reported a case of general symptoms after wreath-making with Douglas fir. The wood yields alpha-pinene and the resin delta-3-carene (Hancock and Swan 1965).

References

Hancock, M.V. and Swan, E.P. (1965) The petroleum ether soluble extractives ... of Douglas fir. Phytochemistry 4, 791.

Neudorffer, R. (1902) Ein Fall von Vergiftung durch die Douglasfichte (Tsuga douglasii) Centralblatt fur innere Medizin 23, 993.

Nordin, J. (1947) Yrkessjunkdomar (Industrial diseases) 2, 605 Uppsala.

Orsler, R.J. (1973) Personal communication from Forest Products Research Laboratory, Princess Risborough, Bucks, England.

Sargent, C.S. (1965) Manual of the trees of North America (excluding Mexico). 2 vols. New York, Dover Publications Inc.

Suskind, R.R. (1967) Dermatitis in the Forest Product Industries. Arch. Environ, Health 15, 322.

Tsuga

15 species are found in the Himalayas, eastern Asia and North America.

Tsuga canadensis Hemlock spruce

This wood is valued for its wood, bark (used in tanning) and pitch (Canada pitch). The wood is often shipped from British Columbia under the name Alaska Pine. One of 125 forest-workers who had dermatitis showed a positive patch test reaction to a commercial acetone extract of this wood (Mitchell 1970).

Tsuga heterophylla

This tree is said to cause dermatitis (Orsler 1973).

References

Mitchell, J.C. (1970) Patch test results - screening set and plants. Contact Dermatitis Newsletter, London 8, 177.

Orsler, R.J. (1973) Personal communication from Forest Products Research Laboratory, Princess Risborough, Bucks, England.

PIPERACEAE

Over 2000 species in four genera are found in tropical regions.

Chemistry is recorded by Hegnauer (1969).

Reference

Hegnauer, R. (1969) Chemotaxonomy of plants. Vol. 5. Basel, Birkhauser p. 311.

Piper

2000 species are found in tropical regions.

Piper angustifolium
Matico

The leaves of this species and varieties are used for their astringent and styptic properties in Herbal Medicine. Oil of Matico is derived from the plant (Wren 1968).

Piper bantamense

This and some other Piper spp. are rubefacient and are used as counter-irritants (Burkill 1935).

Piper cubeba
Java Pepper, Cubebs

The dried unripe fruit forms the condiment, cubebs. Oil of Cubeb, derived from the plant is used in cosmetics (Greenberg and Lester 1954).

Piper betle
Betel Pepper

The leaf is chewed with the betel nut, Areca.

Piper guineense
Black Pepper, West African

The berries were brought from Liberia to Europe in the 14th and 15th centuries but they do not appear to have been accepted as a substitute for P. nigrum, a pepper which is more aromatic (Dalziel 1937). The dried black berries (Dalziel 1937) and the seeds (Irvine 1961) are used for counter-irritant purposes.

Piper methysticum
Kawa, yangona

The powdered root of this plant, prepared so as to form a beverage, is drunk on festive occasions among the Polynesians and Fijians. Over-indulgence induces a state of exhilaration with loss of power in the legs. Chronic addiction induces a marked coarsening and roughening of the skin, with wasting and debility (Cilento 1944).

Piper nigrum
Pepper

To obtain black pepper, the berries are picked before they are fully ripe; they turn black and shrivel when dried. To obtain white pepper, the berries are allowed to ripen before harvesting and the outer shell is removed leaving a greyish-white kernel (Collins 1969). The fruit has a rubefacient effect (Watt and Breyer-Brandwijk 1962) and is irritant to the nose and eyes (Burkill 1935). Ground pepper applied to the skin causes severe pain and redness and sometimes vesication (White 1887). Dilute 'white pepper oil' was observed to produce three positive patch test reactions in 406 persons investigated for hand eczema (Agrup 1969).

References

Agrup, G. (1969) Hand Eczema and other hand dermatoses in South Sweden. Acta derm.-venereol. 49 Suppl. 61. pp. 1-91.

Burkill, I.H. (1935) A Dictionary of the Economic Products of the Malay Peninsula. 2 vols. London. Crown Agents for the Colonies.

Cilento, R. (1944) Some poisonous plants, sea and land animals of Australia and New Guinea. Brisbane. W.R. Smith and Patterson Pty. Ltd. (University of Queensland Library Q.L. 100 C5. 1944. 3. Biol.)

Collins, M. (1969) Spices of the World Cook Book. Baltimore, Maryland. McCormick.

Dalziel, J.M. (1937) The useful plants of west tropical Africa. London. Crown Agents.

Greenberg, L.A. and Lester, D. (1954) Handbook of Cosmetic Materials. New York. Interscience.

Irvine, F.R. (1961) Woody plants of Ghana. Oxford University Press. London.

Watt, J.M. and Breyer-Brandwijk, M.G. (1962) The medicinal and poisonous plants of Southern Africa. 2nd ed. Edinburgh. E.& S. Livingstone.

White, J.C. (1887) Dermatitis venenata: An account of the action of external irritants upon the skin. Boston. Cupples and Hurd.

Wren, R.W. (1968) Potter's new cyclopaedia of botanical drugs and preparations by Wren, R.C. Re-edit. by Wren, R.W. Potter and Clarke Ltd. Health Science Press. Rustington, Sussex.

PISTACIACEAE

10 species in one genus are found from the Mediterranean region to Afghanistan, from eastern Asia to Malaysia and in warm regions of North America. The family differs from Anacardiaceae with which it is usually associated.

Pistachia

Ten species are found from the Mediterranean region to Afghanistan, from south-eastern and eastern Asia to Malaysia and in the southern United States, Mexico and Guatemala.

Pistachia sp.

The genus was included in a list of anacardiaceous plants which can cause dermatitis (Blank 1957) but there is no evidence of cross-sensitivity with Toxicodendron.

Pistachia khinjuk

This species is irritant (Pammel 1911).

Pistachia lentiscus
Mastic

According to Schwartz et al (1957) mastic and other natural resins can cause dermatitis. Oil of Mastic is used in cosmetics (Greenberg and Lester 1954).

Pistachia terebinthus

Chian turpentine derived from this plant has rubefacient properties. The plant is said to be irritant (Schwartz et al 1957).

Pistachia vera

The edible pistachio nut stains the lips, tongue and skin to a red colour.

References

Blank, H. (1957) Dermatitis from Anacardiaceae. Proc. Florida Mango Forum. 17th Annual Meeting Miami, Oct. 16th.

Greenberg, L.A. and Lester, D. (1954) Handbook of Cosmetic Materials. New York. Interscience.

Pammel, L.H. (1911) A Manual of Poisonous plants. Torch Press. Cedar Rapids, Iowa. Reprinted Univ. Microfilms Inc. Ann Arbor, Mich. 1965. p. 476-7.

Schwartz, L., Tulipan, L. and Birmingham, D.J. (1957) Occupational Diseases of the Skin. 3rd ed. Philadelphia. Lea and Febiger.

PITTOSPORACEAE

200 species in nine genera are found from tropical Africa to the Pacific region. Eight genera are found in Australia.

Chemistry is recorded by Hegnauer (1969). Furanocoumarins

have been isolated from this family (Hegnauer 1971)

References

Hegnauer, R. (1969) Chemotaxonomy of plants. Vol. 5. Basel Birkhauser p. 325.

Hegnauer, R. (1971) Chemical patterns and relationships of Umbelliferae in The Biology and Chemistry of the Umbelliferae ed. Heywood, V.H. Suppl. 1. to Bot. J. Linnaean Soc. Vol. 64. London. Academic Press. pp. 267-277.

Bursaria

Three species are found in Australia.

Bursaria spinosa
Australian boxthorn

A man developed squamous carcinoma of the skin of the forehead at the site of a boxthorn prickle puncture injury. Tetanus followed a penetrating wound by a boxthorn prickle (Cleland 1925). Boxthorn is also a common name for *Buxus*.

The Australian boxthorn mentioned by Cleland (1925) is probably *Bursaria spinosa* (Woods and Calnan 1976).

References

Cleland, J.B. (1925) Plants including fungi, poisonous or otherwise injurious to man in Australia. (Series II) Med. J. Australia 2, 443.

Woods, B. and Calnan, C.D. (1976) Toxic Woods. Brit. J. Derm. 94, Suppl. 13, June. They cite Cleland (1914) but probably refer to Cleland (1925).

Pittosporum

150 species are found in tropical and subtropical Africa, Asia, Australia, New Zealand and the Pacific region.

Pittosporum eugenoides
Hedge Laurel, Lemon Wood

The wood is said to have produced dermatitis (Schwartz et al 1957).

Reference

Schwartz, L., Tulipan, L. and Birmingham, D.J. (1957) Occupational Diseases of the Skin. 3rd ed. Philadelphia. Lea and Febiger. pp. 637-672.

PLANTAGINACEAE

270 species in three genera are found in cosmopolitan distribution.

Chemistry is recorded by Hegnauer (1969).

Reference

Hegnauer, R. (1969) Chemotaxonomy of plants. Vol. 5. Basel, Birkhauser. p. 330.

Plantago

265 species are found in cosmopolitan distribution.

Plantago sp.

Plantago seed may cause sensitisation and dermatitis (Greenberg and Lester 1954). The material is known as Flea seed (Merck Index 1968).

Plantago major
Greater Plantain

The green parts of a plant, possibly this species, yield a mustard oil type of thioglucoside related to those of Cruciferae (Kjaer 1960, 1963).

Plantago ovata

This plant yields medicinal psyllium which can cause sensitization and dermatitis when used in permanent wave solutions (Greenberg and Lester 1954).

Plantago psyllium

The mucilage of the seeds is used in paper, cotton and silk sizing.

References

Greenberg, L.A. and Lester, D. (1954) Handbook of Cosmetic Materials. New York. Inter-Science.

Kjaer, A. (1960) Naturally derived isoThiocyanates (Mustard Oils) and their parent glucosides in Progress in the Chemistry of Organic Natural Products. ed. Zechmeister, L. Vol. 18. Vienna. Springer-Verlag pp. 122-176.

Kjaer, A. (1963) The distribution of sulphur compounds in Chemical Plant Taxonomy. ed. Swain, T. London. Academic Press. p. 453.

Merck Index (1968) An Encyclopedia of Chemicals and Drugs. ed. Stecher, P.G. 8th ed. Rahway, N.J. Merck and Co. Inc.

PLATANACEAE

Ten species in one genus are found in northern temperate regions. The under-surfaces of the leaves and the young parts of the plant are often clothed with an evanescent or more or less persistent felt of stellate of simple hairs. The fruit is a globose head surrounded by a tuft of long bristly pappose hairs.

Chemistry is recorded by Hegnauer (1969)

Reference

Hegnauer, R. (1969) Chemotaxonomy of plants. Vol. 5. Basel, Birkhauser. p. 338.

Platanus
Plane, Sycamore, Cottonwood

Ten species are recognized.

Platanus orientalis is found from south-eastern Europe to northern Persia. P. kerrii is found in Indo-China. P. occidentalis is found in eastern North America. Seven species are found in the southwestern United States and Mexico. The hybrid x P. hispanica (P. orientalis x P. occidentalis) is widely planted.

Platanus sp.
'Platanos'

'The Lanugo of the leaves and ye Pilulae (falling into the ears and eyes) doth hurt the hearing and the sight' (Dioscorides, First Century A.D.). Hayfever and asthma occurring in a male individual, who pruned the tree, was attributed to downy material which was found on the leaves and 'seed balls' during the summer. Other trees did not affect him nor did plane trees at other times of the year. Scratch tests with a watery suspension of the downy material from the leaves produced positive reactions (Zacharin 1933).

Platanus acerifolia

The tree is a cause of woodcutter's eczema (Schulman and Detouillon 1932) now recognized as caused by lichens and Frullania.

Platanus occidentalis

The bristly fruits can produce mechanical injury in animals (Meunscher 1951).

Platanus orientalis

A specimen of this tree on the island of Kos, Greece, is reputed to be the Tree of Hippocrates, the Father of Medicine. A seedling of this tree grown in Canada produced conjunctival and naso-pharyngeal irritation in four workers from its leaf hairs. Type I hypersensitivity could not be demonstrated by scratch tests (Ross and Mitchell 1974).

References

Dioscorides, The Greek Herbal of: Englished by John Goodyer: A.D. 1655. Edited and first printed A.D. 1933 by R.T. Gunther 1959. New York. Hafner Publishing Co. 2, 206.

Muenscher, W.C. (1951) Poisonous plants of the United States. 2nd ed. New York. The Macmillan Co.

Ross, A.F. and Mitchell, J.C. (1974) Respiratory irritation by leaf hair of the tree Platanus. Ann. Allerg. 32, 94.

Schulmann, E. and Detouilloun, P. (1932) L'eczema du bois et al sensibilisation sylvestre. Paris med. 83, 55.

Zacharin, D. (1933) Plane tree leaves a cause of seasonal asthma and hay fever. Med. J.

Australia 1, 467.

PLUMBAGINACEAE

775 cosmopolitan species in 19 genera are especially found on salt steppes and sea coasts.

Chemistry is recorded by Hegnauer (1969).

Reference

Hegnauer, R. (1969) Chemotaxonomy of plants. Vol. 5. Basel, Birkhauser. p. 341.

The yellow naphthoquinone pigment, plumbagin (methyl juglone) occurs in a colourless combined form and is liberated from root tissue by acid treatment. Plumbagin appears to be characteristic of plants of the tribe Plumbagineae (Harborne 1966).

Tribe: Plumbagineae

(20-30 species)

Root. Plumbagin present in 8/8 species examined.

Tribe: Staticeae

(150-300 species)

Root. Plumbagin absent in all of 28 species examined.

Organ	*P. capensis*	*P. europea*
Petal	-	+
Leaf	-	+
Root	+	+

Organ	*P. pulchella*	*P. rosea*
Petal	-	-
Leaf	+	-
Root	+	+

Organ	*P. zeylanica*
Petal	-
Leaf	-
Root	+

Plumbagin is also found in some species of the families Droseraceae, Ebenaceae, and Euphorbiaceae (Thomson 1971).

Plumbagin has an irritating odour and causes sneezing; it stains the skin to a purple colour and has a vesicant action. The compound was found to be present in a paste of Babink or Babini root (botanically unidentified) used in Turkey to produce false evidence of violence by way of purplish discoloration of the skin indistinguishable from bruising. Following cases of alleged assault, the Turkish police instigated an investigation of the composition of the root and plumbagin was isolated and identified. The same purple stain was produced by application of the crystalline material to the skin accompanied by pain and later by vesication (Hisar and Wolff 1954, 1955).

References

Harborne, J.B. (1966) The evolution of flavonoid pigments in plants in Comparative Phytochemistry. Ed. Swain, T. London. Academic Press.

Hisar, R.S. and Wolff, R.E. (1954, 1955) Sur l'identification de cristaux vesicants extraits des racines de Babink. Bull. Soc. Chim. France 33, ibid 507.

Thomson, R.H. (1971) Naturally Occurring Quinones. 2nd ed. London. Academic Press.

Ceratostigma
(syn. *Plumbago*)

Eight species are found in eastern tropical Africa, Tibet, the Himalayas, China, Burma and Siam.

Ceratostigma spp.

Some species yield plumbagin (Thomson 1971).

Limonium

300 cosmopolitan species are especially found from the Mediterranean region to central Asia in steppes and salt marshes.

Limonium carolinianum
Sea Lavender,
Marsh Rosemary

The taste of the root is bitter and astringent. The plant is used in Herbal Medicine for its astringent properties (Wren 1968).

Plumbagella
(syn. Plumbago)

One species is found in Central Asia.

Plumbagella sp.

This species yields plumbagin (Morton 1971).

References

Morton, J.F. (1971) Plants Poisonous to People in Florida and other warm areas. Miami, Florida. Hurricane House Publishers Inc.

Thomson, R.H. (1971) Naturally Occurring Quinones. 2nd ed. London. Academic Press.

Wren, R.W. (1968) Potter's New Cyclopaedia of Botanidal Drugs and Preparations by Wren, R.C. Re-edit. by Wren, R.W. Potter and Clarke Ltd. Health Science Press. Rustington, Sussex.

Plumbago

Twelve species are found in warm regions.

Plumbago spp.

Plants of this genus have vesicant properties (Burkill 1935).

Plumbago capensis
Cape Plumbago, Leadwort

Contact with the roots, leaves and stems of the plant (especially the roots) can blister the skin of 'sensitive' individuals (Morton 1962). The roots yield plumbagin (Thomson 1971).

Plumbago coerulea

This species yields plumbagin (Thomson 1971).

Plumbago europaea

The plant reddens and vesicates healthy skin (Piffard 1881) and is used as a counter-irritant (Burkill 1935). The plant was formerly used by beggars in southern Europe to produce sores on the skin with the intention of inciting pity. The roots, leaves and flowers yield plumbagin (Thomson 1971).

Plumbago indica
(syn. P. rosea)

The plant is mentioned by Sanskrit writers as a vesicant. The dried roots are less active than the fresh root (Burkill 1935). The root is used in several caustic preparations, particularly by malingerers (Behl et al 1966, Quisumbing 1951).

Plumbago pulchella
Yerba del Diablo

The plant has a vesicant and caustic effect (Martinez 1969). This species yields plumbagin (Thomson 1971).

Plumbago rosea

The fresh bark of the root rubbed into a paste and applied to the skin causes pain and ultimately blisters (Waring 1875).

Plumbago scandens

The root has a vesicant action on healthy skin (Wibmer 1841-42). The plant yields plumbagin (Thomson 1971).

Plumbago zeylanica
Ceylon Leadwort

In ancient Sanscrit and Mohammedan literature this plant is described as vesicant for the skin.

The leaves and roots have a vesicant and caustic effect on the skin (Watt and Breyer-Brandwijk 1962, Irvine 1961, Chopra 1933, Quisumbing 1951). The plant is employed in the same manner as cantharides. The root is ground with a little flour and water and applied to the skin. In five minutes there is a pricking sensation; in 15 minutes pain and after 12 to 15 hours a bulla forms. The pain associated with the blistering is greater than that from application of cantharides (Burkill 1935). The plant is used as an abortefacient by introducing it into the vagina to produce an irritant action (Burkill 1935) and in India by malingerers (Chopra 1933). Lewis (1922) reported the death of an African woman who was rubbed all over the body with the bark of this species. Masai girls of southern Africa use the irritant effect of the plant to produce post-inflammatory hyperpigmentation for cosmetic purposes as did the natives of Hawaii (Watt and Breyer-Brandwijk 1962).

References

Behl, P.N., Captain, R.M., Bedi, B.M.S. and Gupta, S. (1966) Skin-irritant and sensitizing plants found in India, New Delhi. P.N. Behl, Irwin Hospital.

Burkill, I.H. (1935) A dictionary of the economic products of the Malay Peninsula. 2 vols. London. Crown Agents for the Colonies.

Chopra, R.N. (1933) Indigenous Plants of India: Their medical and economic aspects. Calcutta. The Art Press.

Irvine, F.R. (1961) Woody plants of Ghana. Oxford University Press. London.

Lewis, J. (1922) Some observations on South African toxicology. South Afr. Med. Rec. 20, 350.

Martinez, M. (1969) The Medicinal Plants of Mexico. 5th ed. Mexico City. Andres Botas.

Morton, F.J. (1962) Ornamental Plants with Poisonous Properties II. Proc. Florida Hort. Soc. 75, 484.

Quisumbing, E. (1951) Medicinal plants of the Philippines. Tech. Bull. 16. Manila, Philippine Islands. Manila Bureau of Printing. 1234 pp.

Thomson, R.H. (1971) Naturally Occurring Quinones. 2nd ed. London. Academic Press.

Piffard, H.G. (1881) A treatise on the Materia Medica and Therapeutics of the Skin. New York. Wm. Wood and Co.

Waring, E.J. (1875) Remarks on some of the Bazaar Medicines and Common Medical Plants of India. London. cited by Piffard (1881).

Watt, J.M. and Breyer-Brandwijk, M.G. (1962) The Medicinal and poisonous plants of Southern Africa. 2nd ed. Edinburgh. E.& S. Livingstone.

Wibmer, K. (1841-42) Die Wirkung der Arzneimittel und Gifte in gesunden Thierischen Korper. 5 volumes. Munchen. cited by Piffard (1881).

Statice

This genus comprizes *Armeria* and *Limonium*.

Statice limonium
English Sea Lavender

The plant has properties similar to those of *Limonium* and is used in the same fashion (Wren 1968).

Reference

Wren, R.W. (1968) Potter's New Cyclopaedia of Botanical Drugs and Preparations by Wren, R.C. Re-edit. by Wren, R.W. Potter and Clarke Ltd. Health Science Press. Rustington, Sussex.

PODOCARPACEAE

125 species in six genera are found mostly in the southern hemisphere extending north to Japan, central America and the West Indies.

Dacrydium

Between 20 and 25 species are found in Indo Malaysia, Tasmania, New Zealand, New Caledonia, Fiji and Chile.

Dacrydium cupressinum
Red Pine, Rimu

The wood of this useful New Zealand timber tree is irritating to the nose (Cleland 1925).

Podocarpus

100 species are found from tropical to temperate regions of the soughern hemisphere north to the Himalayas and Japan.

Podocarpus milanjianus var. gracilior
Yellow wood

The wood of this species produced allergic contact dermatitis in wood-workers and also conjunctivitis and rhinitis (Piorkowski 1944). Positive patch test reactions were observed to an ether-alcohol extract of the wood.

References

Cleland, J.B. (1925) Plants including fungi, poisonous or otherwise injurious to man in Australia. (Series II) Med. J. Australia 2, 443.

Piorkowski, F.O. (1944) Woodworkers' dermatitis in East Africa. East Afric. Med. J. 21, 60.

PODOPHYLLACEAE

20 species in six genera are found in north temperate regions especially in eastern Asia and eastern North America.

Podophyllum

Ten species are found in the Himalayas and eastern Asia, one species in eastern North America.

Podophyllum emodi

This species has counter-irritant effects and is used in Herbal Medicine (Wren 1968).

Podophyllum peltatum
May Apple, American Mandrake

The pulp of the ripe fruit is edible, being used in preserves and beverages (Grey's Manual 1970). Persons handling the powdered root in commercial operations can develop ulcerative skin lesions, conjunctivitis and keratitis (Dispensatory 1884, White 1887, O'Donovan 1935, Kingsbury 1964, Schwartz et al 1957, Nelson 1953). The root yields podophyllin resin which is a varying mixture of 16 or more physiologically active compounds (Hartwell and Schrecker 1958). Podophyllin (Kaplan 1942) and crystalline derivatives named peltatins (Sullivan and Hearin 1952) have a destructive effect on condylomata (soft warts).

References

Dispensatory, The National (1884) Philadelphia. Stille and Maisch. cited by White (1887).

Gray's Manual of Botany (1970) 8th ed. by Fernald, M.L. New York. Van Nostrand Reinhold.

Hartwell, J.L. and Schrecker, A.W. (1958) The Chemistry of Podophyllum. Fortschritte der Chemie Organischer Naturstoffe. 15, 83.

Kaplan, I.W. (1942) Condylomata acuminata. New Orleans Med. Surg. J. 94, 388.

Kingsbury, J.M. (1964) Poisonous plants of the United States and Canada. Englewood Cliffs, New Jersey. Prentice-Hall Inc.

Nelson, L.M. (1953) Use of podophyllin (Podophyllum resin) in Dermatology. Archs. Derm. Syph. 67, 488.

O'Donovan, W.J. (1935) Dermatitis due to podophyllum resin. Brit. J. Dermat. 47, 13.

Schwartz, L., Tulipan, L. and Birmingham, D.J. (1957) Occupational Diseases of the Skin. 3rd ed. Philadelphia. Lea and Febiger. pp. 637-672.

Sullivan, M. and Hearin J.T. (1952) Treatment of condyloma acuminatum with peltatins. Archs. Derm. Syph. 66, 706.

White, J.C. (1887) Dermatitis venenata: An account of the Action of External irritants upon the Skin. Boston. Cupples and Hurd.

Wren, R.C. (1968) Potter's New Cyclopaedia of Botanical Drugs and Preparations by Wren, R.C. Re-edit. by Wren, R.W. Potter and Clarke Ltd. Health Science Press. Rustington, Sussex.

POLEMONIACEAE

300 species in 15 genera are found chiefly in North America, a few in Chile, Peru, Europe and northern Asia. Phlox is cultivated.

Chemistry is recorded by Hegnauer (1969).

Reference

Hegnauer, R. (1969) Chemotaxonomy of plants. Vol. 5. Basel, Birkhauser. p. 349.

Polemonium

50 species are found in temperate Eurasia, North America and Mexico; two species in Chile.

Polemonium coeruleum
Jacob's Ladder,
Greek Valerian

The plant is used in Herbal Medicine for its astringency (Wren 1968).

Reference

Wren, R.W. (1968) Potter's New Cyclopaedia of Botanical Drugs and Preparations by Wren, R.C. Re-edit. by Wren, R.W. Potter and Clarke Ltd. Health Science Press. Rustington, Sussex.

POLYGALACEAE

800 species in 12 genera are of cosmopolitan distribution excepting New Zealand, Polynesia and the arctic zone.

Chemistry is recorded by Hegnauer (1969).

Reference

Hegnauer, R. (1969) Chemotaxonomy of plants. Vol. 5. Basel, Birkhauser. p. 352.

Carpolobia

Ten species are found in tropical West Africa.

Carpolobia lutea

The powdered bark, which is used as snuff, produces tearing and sneezing (Irvine 1961).

Reference

Irvine, F.R. (1961) Woody plants of Ghana. Oxford University Press. London.

Polygala

The distribution of the genus is that of the family.

Polygala alba

Polygala boykini

These species have irritant effects (Pammel 1911).

Polygala senega
Senega Snake-root

The root which is used in Herbal Medicine is acrid and acid with a rancid odour (Wren 1968). The plant is irritant (Pammel 1911).

Polygala senega
var. latifolia

The root which is used as an expectorant contains methyl salicylate (Kariyone 1971).

References

Kariyone, T. (1971) Atlas of Medicinal Plants. Osaka, Japan. Takeda Chemical Industries.

Pammel, L.H. (1911) A Manual of Poisonous plants. Torch Press. Cedar Rapids, Iowa. Reprinted Univ. Microfilms Inc. Ann Arbor, Mich. 1965.

Wren, R.W. (1968) Potter's New Cyclopaedia of Botanical Drugs and Preparations by Wren, R.C. Re-edit. by Wren, R.W. Potter and Clarke Ltd. Health Science Press. Rustington, Sussex.

Securidaca

80 species are found in tropical regions except in Australia.

Securidaca longipedunculata

The powdered root is numbing to the tongue, produces cheilitis, and, when inhaled produces sneezing. The flower has the gragrance of the violet (Viola). Insertion of the root into the vagina is the accepted means of suicide for the Luvale women of southern Africa; in addition to local caustic effects, necrosis of the liver occurs. Methyl salicylate is present in the root (Watt and Breyer-Brandwijk 1962). The powdered root causes violent sneezing. The sap is irritating and the powdered bark can blind the eyes (Irvine 1961).

References

Irvine, F.R. (1961) Woody plants of Ghana. Oxford University Press. London.

Watt, J.M. and Breyer-Brandwijk, M.G. (1962) The Medicinal and poisonous plants of Southern Africa. 2nd ed. Edinburgh. E.& S. Livingstone.

POLYGONACEAE

800 species in 40 genera are chiefly found in north temperate regions, a few in tropical, arctic and southern regions. The fruits of some species possess hooks.

Chemistry is recorded by Hegnauer (1969).

Reference

Hegnauer, R. (1969) Chemotaxonomy of plants. Vol. 5. Basel, Birkhauser. p. 361.

Coccoloba

150 species are found in tropical and subtropical America.

Coccoloba rheifolia

The wood is said to be capable of producing dermatitis (Orsler 1973).

Coccoloba laurifolia

Coccoloba utifera
Sea Grape

Twenty workmen in Strasbourg were said to have irritation of the eyes and nose after working with coccoloba in 1904. As investigations into the cause were unsuccessful, nothing was published at the time but Czimatis and Hagemann (1910) refer to the incident. Hausen (1970) who elucidated this, noted that he had heard of irritation by the wood in Guadeloupe but found no case-reports. He found several alkaloids in the wood. According to Woods and Calnan (1976) the strong sensitizer cocobolo was not finally identified as Dalbergia spp. till 1918, and was long confused with similarly named woods such as Coccoloba, Cocos and cocus (Wiesner 1903). Cocobolo seems the likeliest cause of the Strasbourg outbreak, as Coccoloba has never been much exported (Boulger 1908, Record and Hess 1943).

References

Hausen, B.M. (1970) Untersuchungen uber Gesundheitsschadigende Holzer. Thesis, Hamburg.

Orsler, R.J. (1972) Personal communication from Forest Products Research Laboratory, Princess Risborough, Bucks, England.

Boulger, G.S. (1906/7) Familiar Trees. London. Cassele.

Czimatis and Hagemann (1910) Ueber Erkrankungen durch Holzstaub. Hygienische Rundschau 20, 761.

Record, S.J. and Hess, R.W. (1943) Timbers of the New World. New Haven, Yale.

Wiesner, J. (1903) Die Rohstoffe des Pflanzenreiches. 2nd ed. Leipzig, Engelmann.

Woods, B. and Calnan, C.D. (1976) Toxic Woods. Brit. J. Derm. 94, Suppl. 13, June.

Emex

Two species are found in the Mediterranean region, southern Africa and Australia.

Emex australis
Double gee

The spiny fruits can cause injuries to humans and livestock (Aplin 1976).

Reference

Aplin, T.E.H. (1976) Poisonous garden plants and other plants harmful to man in Australia. Bull. 3964. Western Australian Department of Agriculture. W.C. Brown. Govt. Printer, Western Australia.

Fagopyrum

Fifteen species are found in temperate Eurasia.

Fagopyrum esculentum
Buck-wheat

This species is widely cultivated especially in North America. The plant is used for green fodder and provides good honey. The seeds are used to make flour.

Fagopyrism is a form of primary photosensitivity which occurs in animals which ingest the young flowers and the seeds. Pigments with an absorption band about 590 nm are responsible for photosensitisation (Watt and Breyer-Brandwijk 1962, Kingsbury 1964). Fagopyrin and related fluorescent chemicals are related to those of Hypericum (Bigger 1959). Buck-wheat has been reported to cause contact irritation of the skin (Watt and Breyer-Brandwijk 1962, Meunscher 1951). Photosensitivity has been reported to occur in humans who ingest buck-wheat (Pammel 1911, Bruce 1927, Sheard et al 1928, Mathews 1937, Meunscher 1951, Behl et al 1966). Buck-wheat can produce Type I hypersensitivity reactions (Blumstein 1935). According to Blumstein (1935) and Blum (1941) most, if not all, cases of buck-wheat poisoning in man are not examples of photosensitisation but are allergic reactions. Hjorth (1968) recorded one positive patch test reaction to the plant and negative reactions in five cases.

Using the method of Daniels (1965), the seeds of F. esculentum, both with the husk on and dehusked, did not produce psoralen-type phototoxicity for Candida albicans (Mitchell 1972, unpublished observation). Fagopyrism has also been attributed to ingestion of Polygonum (Mathews 1937).

Use of the straw as a head rest caused asthma and rhinitis (Matsumura et al 1964). Injection of the allergen caused sudden death (Lamson 1924).

Fagopyrum tartaricum

This species has been implicated in photosensitization of animals.

References

Behl, P.N., Captain, R.M., Bedi, B.M.S. and Gupta, S. (1966) Skin-irritant and sensitizing plants found in India, New Delhi. P.N. Behl, Irwin Hospital.

Biggers, J.D. (1959) Photodynamic compounds in plants in The Pharmacology of Plant Phenolics. ed. Fairbairn, J.W. London. Academic Press. p. 71-79.

Blum, H.F. (1941) Photodynamic action of diseases caused by light. Am. Chem. Soc. Monograph Ser. New York Reinhold Publ. Corp.

Blumstein, G.L. (1935) Buckwheat sensitivity. J. Allergy 7, 74.

Bruce, E.A. (1927) Astrogalus campestris and other stock-poisoning plants of British Solumbia. Dominion of Canada Dept. Agr. Bull. 88.

Daniels, F. Jr. (1965) A simple microbiological method for demonstrating phototoxic compounds. J. Invest. Derm. 44, 259.

Hjorth, N. (1968) at Finsen Institute. Pers. Comm.

Meunscher, W.C. (1951) Poisonous plants of the United States. 2nd ed. New York. The Macmillan Co.

Kingsbury, J.M. (1964) Poisonous plants of the United States and Canada. Englewood Cliffs, New Jersey. Prentice-Hall Inc.

Mathews, F.P. (1937) Photosensitization and the photodynamic diseases of man and the lower animals. Arch. Path. 23, 399.

Pammel, L.H. (1911) A Manual of Poisonous plants. Torch Press. Cedar Rapids, Iowa. Reprinted Univ. Microfilms Inc. Ann Arbor, Mich. 1965. p. 476-7.

Sheard, C., Caylor, H. and Schlotthauer, C. (1928) Photosensitization of animals after injestion of buckwheat. J. Exp. Med. 47, 1013.

Watt, J.M. and Breyer-Brandwijk, M.G. (1962) The Medicinal and poisonous plants of Southern Africa. 2nd ed. Edinburgh. E.& S. Livingstone.

Lamson, R.W. (1924) Sudden death associated with the injection of foreign substance. J. Am. Med. Ass. 82, 1091.

Matsumura, T., Tateno, K., Yugami, S. et al (1964) Six cases of buckwheat asthma induced by buckwheat flour attached to buckwheat chaff in pillows. J. Asthma res. 1, 219.

Oxygonum

30 species are found in tropical and southern Africa.

Oxygonum atriplicifolium

The three spined fruits stick to the feet when walking (Williamson 1956).

Reference

Williamson, J. (1956) Useful Plants of Malawi. ed. Greenway, P.J., Zomba, Malawi. The Government Printer. Previously published as Useful Plants of Nyasaland.

Polygonum

In a broad sense, 300 species are recognized, of cosmopolitan distribution but especially found in temperate regions. In a strict sense, 50 cosmopolitan species are recognized. Some are xerophytic.

Polygonum acre

The juice of the plant is acrid (White 1887) and irritant (Pammel 1911).

References

Pammel, L.H. (1911) A Manual of Poisonous plants. Torch Press. Cedar Rapids, Iowa. Reprinted Univ. Microfilms Inc. Ann Arbor, Mich. 1965. pp. 476-7.

White, J.C. (1887) Dermatitis venenata: An account of the Action of External irritants upon the Skin. Boston. Cupples and Hurd.

Polygonum aviculare
Wire Weed, Knot Grass

The plant is used to make a tea (Weidermannscher or Homeriana tea) and contains tannic acid and a trace of volatile oil. The plant is used for topical application as an astringent and styptic and has been reported to cause contact dermatitis in horses and sheep due to the presence of an acid or 'smarting' substance which may be salicic acid (Watt and Breyer-Brandwijk 1962). Contact with the plant has caused contact dermatitis in 'susceptible' individuals (Muenscher 1951).

Ingestion of the plant was said to produce dermatitis in animals (Gates 1930, Sampson and Malmsten 1935). The plant was listed as a source of contact dermatitis without clinical details (Gardner and Bennetts 1956). The plant was not irritant by patch test in one patient (Moslein 1963). A gardener developed dermatitis of the opposing surfaces of the right forefinger and thumb and of the intervening finger web. Two days previously he had pulled P. aviculare which was a prevalent weed. He applied an ointment to his finger and thumb. Five months later, he developed dermatitis of the forearm and trunk. This dermatitis was attributed to a re-use of the ointment at these sites. The juice of the plant was considered to have contaminated the ointment. Patch tests were not recorded (Lloyd 1914).

References

Gardner, C.A. and Bennetts, H.W. (1956) The Toxic Plants of Western Australia. Perth West. Australian Newspapers Ltd.

Gates, F.C. (1930) Principal poisonous plants in Kansas. Kansas Agr. Exp. Stat. Tech. Bull. 25.

Lloyd, G.W. (1914) Dermatitis venenata. Brit. Med. J. 2, 837.

Moslein, P. (1963) Pflanzen als Kontakt-Allergene. Berufsdermatosen 11, 24.

Meunscher, W.C. (1951) Poisonous plants of the United States. 2nd ed. New York. The Macmillan Co.

Sampson, A.W. and Malmsten, H.E. (1935) Stock poisoning plants of California. Univ. California, Coll. Agr. Expt. Stat. Bull. 593.

Watt, J.M. and Breyer-Brandwijk, M.G. (1962) The Medicinal and poisonous plants of Southern Africa. 2nd ed. Edinburgh. E.& S. Livingstone.

Polygonum barbatum

The juice of the plant is acrid. The root is astringent and the sap is applied to wounds as an 'antiseptic' (Watt and Breyer-Brandwijk 1962).

Reference

Watt, J.M. and Breyer-Brandwijk, M.G. (1962) The Medicinal and poisonous plants of Southern Africa. 2nd ed. Edinburgh. E.& S. Livingstone.

Polygonum convolvulus
Black Bindweed

Mechanical injury can occur from ingestion of the hard, trigonous, pointed fruits (Long 1924). The plant was not irritant by patch test in one patient (Moslein 1963).

References

Long, H.C. (1924) Plants Poisonous to Livestock. 2nd ed. Cambridge University Press.

Moslein, P. (1963) Pflanzen als Kontakt-Allergene. Berufsdermatosen 11, 24.

Polygonum cuspibatum

This perennial species which has become popular in Danish gardens caused a typical streaky plant dermatitis of the arms in a gardener. Patch test to the plant produced a strong vesicular reaction; one of ten controls also had a positive reaction (Hjorth and Mitchell 1973). Although patch tests to the leaves could produce an irritant reaction, the history and clinical findings left no doubt of an allergic contact dermatitis.

Reference

Hjorth, N. and Mitchell, J.C. (1973) Polygonum dermatitis. Contact Dermatitis Newsletter, London 15, 426.

Polygonum erectum
Russian Knotgrass

The plant is used in Herbal Medicine for an astringent effect (Wren 1968).

Reference

Wren, R.W. (1968) Potter's New Cyclopaedia of Botanical Drugs and Preparations by Wren, R.C. Re-edit. by Wren, R.W. Potter and Clarke Ltd. Health Science Press. Rustington, Sussex.

Polygonum fagopyrum

This botanical name was previously applied to Fagopyrum esculentum (syn. F. sagittatum). Fagopyrism has been attributed to ingestion of Polygonum sp. (Mathews 1937).

Reference

Mathews, F.P. (1937) Photosensitisation and the photodynamic diseases of man and the lower animals. Arch. Path. 23, 399.

Polygonum flaccidum

This species has irritant properties (Pammel 1911).

Reference

Pammel, L.H. (1911) A Manual of Poisonous plants. Torch Press. Cedar Rapids, Iowa. Reprinted Univ. Microfilms Inc. Ann Arbor, Mich. 1965. p. 476-7.

Polygonum histerta

The plant was not irritant by patch test in one patient (Moslein 1963).

Reference

Moslein, P. (1963) Pflanzen als Kontakt-Allergene. Berufs-dermatosen 11, 24.

Polygonum hydropiper
Smartweed, Water Pepper

The plant irritates the hands and face of persons who collect it, producing burning and itching (White 1887). The plant has irritant properties (Pammel 1911). The leaves have a biting pungent taste (Wren 1968). The acrid juice is irritant and the bruised leaves and the seeds, when employed as a poultice, blister the skin (Behl et al 1966). Other authors (Mac-Dougal 1894, Coulter 1904, Weber 1937, Muenscher 1951, Schwartz et al 1957) who refer to the irritant properties of the plant for humans do not add any clinical details other than a note of irritation of the eyes and nostrils by the juice of the plant. Some colloquial names for this plant indicate older knowledge of its properties viz. Biting Persicaria, Bity Tongue, Pepper Plant, Red Knees (Grieve 1970). The plant is used for application to haemorrhoids in Herbal Medicine probably accounting for the names Smartass and Arse-smart; another name is Culrage possibly indicating an unfavorable response in an afflicted patient.

Unfavourable effects from the plant have also been observed in animals. It is difficult to define whether contact dermatitis, dermatitis from ingestion or photo-sensitivity from ingestion actually occurred.

In 1931, this species was present in pastures in New South Wales in which a number of cows developed dermatitis (Hurst 1942).

This plant and other species of Polygonum contain acrid smarting substances which may cause dermatitis in stock if ingested (Gates 1930). The juice is acrid, causing irritation and smarting, especially when in contact with the eyes and nostrils of animals and is possibly a cause of dermatitis (Long 1924).

References

Behl, P.N., Captain, R.M., Bedi, B.M.S. and Gupta, S. (1966) Skin-irritant and sensitizing plants found in India, New Delhi. P.N. Behl, Irwin Hospital.

Coulter, S. (1904) The poisonous plants of Indiana. Proc. Indiana. Acad. Sci. 51-63.

Gates, F.C. (1930) Principal poisonous plants in Kansas. Kansas Agr. Expt. Stat. Tech. Bull. 25.

Grieve, M. (1970) A Modern Herbal. Darien, Conn. Hafner Publ. Co.

Hurst, E. (1942) The Poison Plants of New South Wales. N.S.W. Poison Plants Committee; Sydney.

Long, H.C. (1924) Plants Poisonous to Livestock. 2nd ed. Cambridge University Press.

MacDougal, D.T. (1894) Poisonous influences of various species of cyptipedium. Minesota Botan. Studies pp. 32 and 450.

Muenscher, W.C. (1951) Poisonous plants of the United States. 2nd ed. New York. The Mac-millan Co.

Pammel, L.H. (1911) A Manual of poisonous plants. Torch Press. Cedar Rapids, Iowa. Reprinted Univ. Microfilms Inc. Ann Arbor, Mich. 1965. pp. 476-7.

Schwartz, L., Tulipan, L. and Birmingham, D.J. (1957) Occupational Diseases of the Skin. 3rd ed. Philadelphia. Lea and Febiger.

Weber, L.F. (1937) External causes of dermatitis. A list of irritants. Arch. Derm. Syph. 35, 129.

White, J.C. (1887) Dermatitis venenata: An account of the Action of external irritants upon the skin. Boston. Cupples and Hurd.

Wren, R.W. (1968) Potter's New Cyclopaedia of Botanical Drugs and Preparations by Wren, R.C. Re-edit. by Wren, R.W. Potter and Clarke Ltd. Health Science Press. Rustington, Sussex.

Polygonum lapathifolium
Pale Knotweed

Ingestion of the plant is considered to cause dermatitis in cattle at some times (Hurst 1942).

Reference

Hurst, E. (1942) The Poison Plants of New South Wales. N.S.W. Poison Plants Committee; Sydney.

Polygonum minus
Slender Knotweed

This species is stated to be free from the 'biting taste' characteristic of many species of Polygonum; it was suspected of causing dermatitis in a cow in New South Wales (Hurst 1942).

Reference

Hurst, E. (1942) The Poison Plants of New South Wales. N.S.W. Poison Plants Committee; Sydney.

Polygonum nodosum
Knotgrass

Positive patch tests were observed to the whole plant, to the blossom and less strongly to the leaf and stem in one patient who had contact dermatitis. Negative patch tests to the blossom were observed in four controls. Negative patch tests were observed to P. histerta, P. persicaria, P. aviculare, P. convolvulus and P. viviparum (Moslein 1963).

Reference

Moslein, P. (1963) Pflanzen als Kontakt-Allergene. Berufsdermatosen 11, 24.

Polygonum hydropiperoides

This species is irritant (Pammel 1911).

Reference

Pammel, L.H. (1911) A Manual of poisonous plants. Torch Press. Cedar Rapids, Iowa. Reprinted Univ. Microfilms Inc. Ann Arbor, Mich. 1965. pp. 476-7.

Polygonum orientale

The plant has irritant properties (Pammel 1911). This species was considered on field evidence to have caused dermatitis of the udder and perineum of dairy cattle but on testing by external application to the skin of a steer and a calf, no observable ill-effect was produced (Hurst 1942). White (1937) states that in Queensland, the loss of five young pigs was attributed to this plant and that the symptoms of poisoning were swelling of the ears, face and eyelids with considerable irritation of the affected parts. However, feeding experiments produced negative results (Hurst 1942).

References

Hurst, E. (1942) The Poison plants of New South Wales. N.S.W. Poison Plants Committee; Sydney.

Pammel. L.H. (1911) A Manual of Poisonous Plants. Torch Press. Cedar Rapids, Iowa. Reprinted Univ. Microfilms Inc. Ann Arbor, Mich. 1965. pp. 476-7.

White, C.T. (1937) Ann. Report Govt. Botanist, Queensland.

Polygonum persicaria

The plant has a very acrid juice which can cause smarting and irritation especially when in contact with the eyes and nostrils of animals (Pammel 1911, Gates 1930). The plant was not irritant by patch test in one patient (Moslein 1963). The plant can produce dermatitis in 'susceptible' individuals (Muenscher 1951, Schwartz et al 1957). Ingestion of the plant was said to produce photosensitivity in animals (Mathews 1937).

References

Gates, F.C. (1930) Principal poisonous plants in Kansas. Kansas Agr. Expt. Stat. Tech. Bull. 25.

Mathews, F.P. (1937) Photosensitisation and the photodynamic diseases of man and the lower animals. Arch. Path. 23, 399.

Moslein, P. (1963) Pflanzen als Kontakt-Allergene. Berufsdermatosen 11, 24.

Muenscher, W.C. (1951) Poisonous plants of the United States. 2nd ed. New York. The Macmillan Co.

Pammel, L.H. (1911) A manual of poisonous plants. Torch Press. Cedar Rapids, Iowa. Reprinted Univ. Microfilms Inc. Ann Arbor, Mich. 1965. pp. 476-7.

Schwartz, L., Tulipan, L. and Birmingham, D.J. (1957) Occupational Diseases of the Skin. 3rd ed. Philadelphia. Lea and Febiger. pp. 637-672.

Polygonum prostratum
Trailing Knotweed

The plant was suspected of causing necrotic dermatitis in animals in New South Wales (Hurst 1942) and is listed as a cause of dermatitis in Australia without clinical details (Gardner and Bennetts 1957).

References

Gardner, C.A. and Bennetts, H.W. (1956) The Toxic Plants of Western Australia. Perth West. Australian Newspapers Ltd.

Hurst, E. (1942) The Poison Plants of New South Wales. N.S.W. Poison Plants Committee; Sydney.

Polygonum punctatum
Smartweed, Poor Man's Pepper, Water Pepper

The colloquial names of this species suggest an irritant effect. The leaves of the plant which is common in damp places in Britain have rubefacient properties (White 1934). The plant is listed as irritant (Weber 1937). The juice of the plant has irritant properties (Coulter 1904, Maiden 1909). The crushed leaves and stems are irritant (Allen 1943).

References

Allen, P.H. (1943) Poisonous and injurious plants of Panama. Am. J. Trop. Med. Suppl. 23, 1.

Coulter, S. (1904) The poisonous plants of Indiana. Proc. Indiana Acad. Sci. 51-63.

Maiden, J.H. (1909) On some plants which cause inflammation or irritation of the skin. Ag. Gaz. New South Wales 20, 111 and 1073.

Weber, L.F. (1937) External causes of dermatitis. A list of irritants. Arch. Derm. Syph. 35, 129.

White, R.P. (1934) The Dermatergoses or Occupational Affections of the Skin. 4th ed. London. H.K. Lewis.

Polygonum pulchrum

The rhizome of this species contains an acrid resin (Watt and Breyer-Brandwijk 1962).

Reference

Watt, J.M. and Breyer-Brandwijk, M.G. (1962) The Medicinal and poisonous plants of Southern Africa. 2nd ed. Edinburgh. E.& S. Livingstone.

Polygonum salicifolium

A paste made of the leaves is applied to sores by the Zulus (Watt and Breyer-Brandwijk 1962).

Reference

Watt, J.M. and Breyer-Brandwijk, M.G. (1962) The Medicinal and poisonous plants of Southern Africa. 2nd ed. Edinburgh. E.& S. Livingstone.

Polygonum viviparum

The plant was not irritant by patch test in one patient (Moslein 1963). The fleshy root stock can be cooked and eaten as a substitute for nuts and raisins because of its almond flavour (Szczawinski and Hardy 1972).

References

Moslein, P. (1963) Pflanzen als Kontakt-Allergene. Berufs-dermatosen 11, 24.

Szczawinski, A.F. and Hardy, G.A. (1972) Guide to Common Edible Plants of British Columbia. Handbook No. 20. Dept. of Recreations and Conservation. Government of British Columbia, Victoria, B.C.

Rheum

50 species are found in temperate and subtropical Asia.

Rheum officinale

This plant which furnishes medicinal rhubarb is listed as irritant (Schwartz et al 1957). Chrysophanic acid an irritant of Andira is derived from the plant.

Rheum palmatum

This species furnishes medicinal rhubarb. Chrysophanic acid is derived from this plant and from Rumex, senna (Cassia), cascara sagrada (Rhamnus). Related com-poinds are derived from Andira.

Rheum rhaponticum

The leaf stalk furnishes the vegetable, rhubarb. The leaf blade can cause dermatitis possibly from a content of oxalic acid and oxalates (Meunscher 1951, McCord 1962). Anapylaxis from ingestion of rhubarb was reported by Delcourt (1924).

Idiosyncrasy was suspected in the case of a clergyman who died of oxalic acid poisoning from ingesting rhubarb leaves as a substitute for spinach (Spinacia) or cabbage (Brassica) (Gardner 1917).

References

Delcourt (1924) Un cas d'anaphylaxie pour la rhubarb. Le Scalpel 77, 594.

Gardner (1917) Medical News. Brit. Med. J. 1, 635 (668 and 752).

McCord, C.P. (1962) The Occupational Toxicity of Cultivated Flowers. Ind. Med. Surg. 31, 365.

Muenscher, W.C. (1951) Poisonous plants of the United States. 2nd ed. New York. The Mac-millan Co.

Schwartz, L., Tulipan, L. and Birmingham, D.J. (1957) Occupational Diseases of the Skin. 3rd ed. Philadelphia. Lea and Febiger. pp. 637-672.

Rumex

In a broad sense 200 species are recognized, of cosmo-politan distribution especially in north temperate regions. Some species yield chrysophanic and oxalic acids.

Oxalic acid is a strong local irritant and caustic. The chemical causes gangrenous ulcera-tions. The nails turn blue, become brittle and may fall off leaving an ulcerated nail bed (Greenberg and Lester 1954).

Oxalic acid is considered to be a known allergen and is therefore removed from certain brand name cosmetics (Schieffelin 1973).

Rumex acetosa
Sour Dock, Sorrel

The taste of the plant is acrid and astringent (Wren 1968). Ingestion of the plant produces burning in the mouth and poisoning (Watt and Breyer-Brandwijk 1962). When eaten as pot-herbs or greens, the plant can produce dermatitis in 'susceptible' individuals (Allen 1943, Muenscher 1951, Behl et al 1966).

Rumex acetosella
Sheep Sorrel, Field Sorrel

The taste of the plant is acrid and astringent (Wren 1968). Ingestion of the plant produces burning in the mouth and poisoning (Watt and Breyer-Brandwijk 1962). When eaten ad pot-herbs or greens, the plant can produce dermatitis in 'susceptible' individuals (Allen 1943, Muenscher 1951, Behl et al 1966).

The acrid smarting juice is thought to be a cause of dermatitis in horses and sheep (Gates 1930). Reports of contact dermatitis in humans from the plant lack clinical details (Allen 1943, Schwartz et al 1957, Gardner and Bennetts 1956, Behl et al 1966).

Rumex aquaticus
Water Dock, Bloodwort

The root is used in Herbal Medicine for an astringent effect (Wren 1968).

Rumex crispus
Yellow Dock, Curled Dock

The plant contains oxalic acid, oxalates, chrysophanic acid, emodin, tannin and other chemicals (Watt and Breyer-Brandwijk 1962). Horses and sheep which ingest the plant in large quantities can develop dermatitis (Hurst 1942, Gates 1930, Watt and Breyer-Brandwijk 1962). Dermatitis attributed to the plant is said to be from a content of rumicin which can have rubefacient properties (Watt and Breyer-Brandwijk 1962). Rumicin is a name for chrysophanic acid. The effects of chrysophanic acid and its derivatives are noted under Andira.

In an investigation of 'weed dermatitis' an extract of the plant produced negative patch test reactions in all of 50 patients tested (Shelmire 1939). The plant is said to produce dermatitis in 'susceptible' individuals (Meunscher 1951).

Rumex hymenosepalus
Caraigre

The roots are used for tanning.

Rumex nepalensis

The root is used as an astringent and for dyeing from its content of tannin (Watt and Breyer-Brandwijk 1962).

Rumex obtusifolius

This species which yields chrysophanic acid has been used in Herbal Medicine for skin diseases (Watt and Breyer-Brandwijk 1962).

References

Allen, P.H. (1943) Poisonous and Injurious Plants of Panama. Am. J. Trop. Med. Suppl. 23, 1.

Behl, P.N., Captain, R.M., Bedi, B.M.S. and Gupta, S. (1966) Skin-irritant and sensitizing plants found in India, New Delhi. P.N. Behl, Irwin Hospital.

Gardner, C.A. and Bennetts, H.W. (1956) The Toxic Plants of Western Australia. Perth West. Australian Newspapers Ltd.

Gates, F.C. (1930) Principal poisonous plants in Kansas. Kansas Agr. Expt. Stat. Tech. Bull. 25.

Greenberg, L.A. and Lester, D. (1954) Handbook of Cosmetic Materials. New York. Interscience.

Hurst, E. (1942) The Poisonous Plants of New South Wales. N.S.W. Poison Plant Committee; Sydney.

Muenscher, W.C. (1951) Poisonous plants of the United States. 2nd ed. New York. The Macmillan Co.

Schieffelin and Co. (1973) Almay Hypo-allergenic cosmetics product formulary. 8th ed. Pharmaceutical Laboratories Division, 562 Fifth Avenue, New York, N.Y. 10036.

Schwartz, L., Tulipan, L. and Birmingham, D.J. (1957) Occupational Diseases of the Skin. 3rd ed. Philadelphia. Lea and Febiger. pp. 637-672.

Shelmire, B. (1939) Contact Dermatitis from Weeds; Patch Testing with Their Oleoresins. JAMA 113, 1085.

Watt, J.M. and Breyer-Brandwijk, M.G. (1962) The Medicinal and Poisonous plants of Southern Africa. 2nd ed. Edinburgh. E.& S. Livingstone.

Wren, R.W. (1968) Potter's New Cyclopaedia of Botanical Drugs and Preparations by Wren, R.C.

Re-edit, by Wren, R.W. Potter and Clarke Ltd. Health Science Press. Rustington, Sussex.

POLYPODIACEAE

The species in about 50 genera are of cosmopolitan distribution and especially found in wet tropical regions.

Polypodium

Abouy 75 species are of cosmopolitan distribution.

Polypodium leucotomos
Calaguala

The rhizomes contain a saponin with anti-tumour effects (Horvath 1967) and have been used topically for psoriasis (Padilla et al 1974).

References

Horvath, A., Alvarado, F. et al (1967) Metabolic effects of Calagualine and antitumoral saponine from Polypodium leucotomos. Nature 214, 5094.

Padilla, H.C., Lainez, H. and Pacheco, J.A. (1974) A new agent (Hydrophilic fraction of Polypodium leucotomos) for management of psoriasis. Derm. Int. 13, 276.

PORTULACACEAE

580 species in 19 genera are of cosmopolitan distribution and especially found in America.

Chemistry is recorded by Hegnauer (1969).

Reference

Hegnauer, R. (1969) Chemotaxonomy of plants. Vol. 5. Basel, Birkhauser. p. 383.

Lewisia

20 species are found in western North America.

Lewisia rediviva
Bitter-root

The root of this xerophytic plant is intensely bitted when raw. The root when cooked was an important food of western North American Indians (Medsger 1939).

Reference

Medsger, O.P. (1939) Edible Wild Plants. New York. The Macmillan Co.

Portulaca

200 species are found in tropical and subtropical regions.

Portulaca oleracea
Purslain

Purslain is said to allay the cutaneous effects of the mature pine processionary caterpillar (Thaumatopoeida)(Rostenburg and Solomon 1968).

Reference

Rostenberg, A. Jr. and Solomon, L.M. (1968) Jean Henri Fabre and the patch test. Archs. Derm. 98, 188.

Talinum

50 species are found in warm regions of America, especially in Mexico and in Africa and Asia.

Talinum polyandrum

The sap is acrid (Pammel 1911).

Reference

Pammel, L.H. (1911) A Manual of Poisonous plants. Torch Press. Cedar Rapids, Iowa. Reprinted Univ. Microfilms Inc. Ann Arbor, Mich. 1965. pp. 476-7.

POTALIACEAE

70 species in four genera are found in tropical regions. The family is related to Strychnaceae.

Anthocleista

Eleven species are found in tropical Africa, three species in Madagascar.

Anthocleista spp.

Nearly all these trees have vicious thorns. At a certain stage in their development, they lose their bark and leaves but retain their thorns on the trunk and come to resemble a thorny naked pole (Menninger 1967).

Reference

Menninger, E.A. (1967) Fantastic Trees. New York. The Viking Press.

Fagraea

35 species are found in Indo Malaysia, south-eastern Asia, northern Australia and the Pacific region.

Fagraea fragrans
Tembusu, Kingwood

The flowers open about susset and scent the city of Singapore. Flying-foxes gorge upon the fruits by night. The fallen flowers have a sour rotting smell (Corner 1952). The plant is known to produce dermatitis in Malaya (Kochumman 1972). Hausen (1970) refers to dermatitis from the wood.

Several men had recurrent irritation of exposed skin when sawing a fresh log with its bark on; the heartwood caused no irritation (Hon 1967). An alkaloid derived from the wood is irritant (Grossmann 1920).

References

Hon, L.Y. (1967) Skin irritation caused by Tembusu (Fagraea fragrans). Malayan Forester 30, 234.

Grossmann, J. (1920) Gesundheitsschadliche Holzarten. Der Holzkaufer (Leipzig) 17, 529, 535, 540 and 545.

Corner, E.J.H. (1952) Wayside Trees of Malaysia. Singapore, Government Printer.

Hausen, B.M. (1970) Untersuchungen uber Gesundheitsschadigende Holzer. Thesis, Hamburg.

Kochummen, K.M. (1972) Forest Botanist. Forest Research Institute. Kepong, Selangor, Malaya. Personal communication.

POTAMOGETONACEAE

About 100 cosmopolitan species in two genera are submerged or floating fresh water plants.

Potamogeton

About 100 species are cosmopolitan.

Potamogeton densus
Water Caltrops

Potamogeton crispus

The common name of these plants refers to their capacity to entangle swimmers. The name, caltrop, is noted under Tribulus.

Potamogeton illinoiensis

Skin irritation by this plant while fishing is known to Fish and Wildlife authorities (Morton, J.F. Pers. Comm 1976).

A man and wife who fished from a boat in a freshwater lake in Florida noted irritation after removing weeds from their fishing tackle. This species was identified as the cause of the reaction.

PRIMULACEAE

1000 species in 20 genera are of cosmopolitan distribution especially found in north temperate regions.

Chemistry is recorded by Hegnauer (1969).

Reference

Hegnauer, R. (1969) Chemotaxonomy of plants. Vol 5. Basel, Birkhauser. p. 387.

Anagallis

28 species are found in western Europe, Africa and Madagascar. One species is pantropical and two species are found in South America.

Anagallis arvensis
Scarlet Pimpernel

The plant which has a bitter acrid taste and yields a pungent acrid volatile oil, has long been used in Herbal Medicine

(Wren 1968). The plant yields saponins and a proteolytic enzyme (Watt and Breyer-Brandwijk 1962). The plant has irritant properties (Pammel 1911, Meunscher 1951). The leaves can cause dermatitis in persons working in fields and forests (Behl et al 1966). About 6% of individuals are sensitive and develop dermatitis when handling the flowers or leaves (Arnold 1968); he noted its relationship to Primula.

References

Arnold, H.L. (1968) Poisonous Plants of Hawaii. Rutland, Vermont. Charles E. Tuttle.

Behl, P.N., Captain, R.M., Bedi, B.M.S. and Gupta, S. (1966) Skin-irritant and sensitizing plants found in India, New Delhi. P.N. Behl, Irwin Hospital.

Muenscher, W.C. (1951) Poisonous plants of the United States. 2nd ed. New York. The Macmillan Co.

Pammel, L.H. (1911) A Manual of Poisonous plants. Torch Press. Cedar Rapids, Iowa. Reprinted Univ. Microfilms Inc. Ann Arbor, Mich. 1965.

Watt, J.M. and Breyer-Brandwijk, M.G. (1962) The Medicinal and poisonous plants of Southern Africa. 2nd ed. Edinburgh. E.& S. Livingstone.

Wren, R.W. (1968) Potter's New Cyclopaedia of Botanical Drugs and Preparations by Wren, R.C. Re-edit. by Wren, R.W. Potter and Clarke Ltd. Health Science Press. Rustington, Sussex.

Cortusa
(syn. Corthusa)

Ten species are found on mountains from central Europe to Japan and Sakhalin.

Cortusa matthioli

The plant frequently produces irritant patch test reactions which probably result from a combination of mechanical injury and chemical irritation (Nestler 1912, Woods 1962).

References

Nestler, A. (1912) Cortusa Matthioli L. eine stark. hautreizende Pflanze. Ber. dtsch. bot. Ges. 30, 330.

Woods, B. (1962) Irritant plants. Trans. St. John's Hosp. derm. Soc. 48, 75.

Bomarea

Gagea

Some species of these genera yield tuliposide-A from which alpha-methylenegammabutyrolactone, the allergen of Tulipa, is derived. Tuliposide-B is inactive in this respect (Slob et al 1975).

Reference

Slob, A., Jekel, B., de Jong, B. et al (1975) On the occurrence of tuliposides in the Liliiflorae. Phytochemistry 14, 1997.

Cyclamen

15 species are found in Europe and from the Mediterranean region to Persia.

Cyclamen sp.

A species of this geuns produced a positive patch test reaction in one patient, negative in nine patients (Hjorth 1968).

Cyclamen persicum

A positive patch test reaction to the leaf was observed in one patient (Agrup 1969).

Cyclamen persicum hybridum

A woman showed a positive patch test reaction to this hybrid and to Streptocarpus (Agrup and Fregert 1968).

References

Agrup, G. (1969) Hand Eczema and other hand dermatoses in South Sweden. Acta derm.-venereol. 49 Suppl. 61. pp. 1-91.

Agrup, G. and Fregert, S. (1968) Patch test reactions to Streptocarpus. Contact

Dermatitis Newsletter 4, 72.

Hjorth, N. (1968) at Finsen Institute. Pers. Comm.

Lysimachia

200 species are cosmopolitan, especially found in eastern Asia and North America.

Lysimachia vulgaris

Yellow Loosestripe

This plant dyes the hair yellow and kills flies and knats in the house (Dioscorides, 1st Century, A.D.). The plant is used in Herbal Medicine as an astringent and styptic (Wren 1968).

References

Dioscorides, the Greek Herbal of: Englished by John Goodyer: A.D. 1655. Edited and first printed A.D. 1933 by R. T. Gunther 1959. New York, Hafner Publishing Co.

Wren, R. W. (1968) Potter's New Cyclopaedia of Botanical Drugs and Preparations by Wren, R.C. Re-edit. by Wren, R.W. Potter and Clarke Ltd. Health Science Press. Rustington, Sussex.

Primula

500 species are found in the northern hemisphere especially in hilly districts. A few species are found elsewhere e.g. at the Strait of Magellan.

A few of the better known species are:

Primula sinensis - Chinese Primrose

Primula japonica

Primula eliator - Oxlip

Primula vulgaris (syn. P. acaulis) Primrose

Primula veris (syn. P. officinalis) Cowslip

Primula farinosa

Primula auricula - Auricula

A great many hybrids occur.

The following species were found to have no irritating action:

P. auriculata, P. capitata,

P. clusiana, P. farinosa,

P. floribunda, P. hirsuta,

P. japonica, P. megaraefolia,

P. minima, P. officinalis, and

P. rosea (Nestler 1904).

Reference

Nestler, A. (1904) Hautreizende Primeln. Untersuchungen uber Entstehung, Eigenschaften und Wirkungen des Primelhautgiftes. Berlin. Gebruder Borntrager p.6-7

Origin of Primula obconica

In 1880 Hance described Primula obconica as a new species collected around Ichang, province of Hupeh, China by T. Watters in 1879.

Reference

Hance, H.F. (1880) Stirpium duranum novarum e Primulacearum familia characteres. Journ. Bot. 18, 234.

Primin in Primula species

Sixteen of 82 species of the Primulaceae family which were investigated by the Craven screening test were found to contain primin, including P. alpicola var. alba, P. apennina, P. denticulata, P. eliator ssp. elatior, P. hirsuta, P. malacoides, P. minima, P. muscarioides, P. rosea, P. praenitens (syn. P. sinensis), P. veris ssp. veris and P. vulgaris spp. vulgaris. In all the remaining species, other quinoid compounds were detectable.

The occurrence of primin is determined by origin, temperature, light, moisture, manuring, soil pH (content of lime), habitat and season, etc. The finding of primin in P. praenitens (syn. P. sinensis), P. eliator ssp. eliator and P. veris (syn. P. officinalis) appears to explain occasional reports of dermatitis, from these species e.g. cowslip (P. veris). The 'Primula farinosa' reported by Sharpe (1912) to cause dermatitis appears to have been, in fact, P. mistassinica. This plant contains a yellow quinone.

The petals (corollas) of P. obconica, contain primin. The 'secon allergen' of Cairns (1964) is a quinhydrone (Hausen 1978). For precise botany the original paper of Hausen (1978) should be consulted.

Anagallis hirta, Dionysia aretiodes and Glaux maritima were found to contain primin (Hausen 1978).

These findings from a sensitive screening test were not in keeping with a supposition that primin was restricted to P. obconica but further extraction studies were in progress.

References

Cairns, R. (1964) Plant dermatoses: some chemical aspects and results of patch testing with extracts of Primula obconica. Trans. St. John's Hosp. Derm. Soc. 50, 137.

Hausen, B.M. (1978) On the occurrence of the contact allergen primin and other quinoid compounds in species of the family of Primulaceae. Arch. Derm. Res. 261, 311.

Sharpe, H.A. (1912) Primula dermatitis - its occurrence in rural districts. JAMA 59, 2148.

Primula cortusoides

This species has a mild skin-irritant effect (Nestler 1904). The plant can produce irritant patch test reactions (Rook and Wilson 1965).

References

Nestler, A. (1904) Hautreizende Primeln. Untersuchungen uber Entstehung, Eigenschaften und Wirkungen des Primelhautgiftes. Berlin. Gebruder Borntrager. P. 6-7.

Rook, A.J. and Wilson, H.T.H. (1965) Primula dermatitis. Brit. Med. J. 1, 220.

Primula farinosa

Cases of milkers' eczema were attributed to handling the udders of cows that had walked among the dew-laded flowers of this plant (Sharpe 1912). Since patch tests were not recorded, the association is suspect.

See Primin P. 546.

Reference

Sharpe, H.A. (1912) Primula dermatitis. Its occurrence in rural districts. JAMA 59, 2148 (Dec. 14).

Primula malacoides

This species can produce irritant patch test reactions (Hjorth 1968). The plant has never been proved to cause allergic contact dermatitis (Rook and Wilson 1965).

References

Hjorth, N. (1968) at Finsen Institute. Pers. Comm.

Rook, A.J. and Wilson, H.T.H. (1965) Primula dermatitis. Brit. Med. J. 1, 220.

Primula poculiformis

A woman was contact sensitive to this species and to P. obconica. Her gardener was unaffected (White 1934).

Reference

White, R.P. (1934) The Dermatergoses or Occupational Affections of the Skin. 4th ed. London. H.K. Lewis.

Primula sieboldii

This species has skin-irritant properties (Nestler 1904).

Reference

Nestler, A. (1904) Hautreizende Primeln. Untersuchungen uber Entstehung, Eigenschaften und Wirkungen des Primelhautgiftes. Berlin. Gebruder Borntrager. p. 6-7.

Primula sinensis

Dermatitis from the plant was reported by Gillett (1896). This species has skin irritant properties (Nestler 1904). The plant can produce irritant patch test reactions (Hjorth 1968). Only 1.4% of 277 persons who were patch tested to the leaf showed positive reactions (Fregert and Hjorth 1968). These authors concluded that the plant is a potential irritant by patch test. P. sinensis has been shown to cause allergic contact dermatitis at the most very rarely (Rook and Wilson 1965).

References

Fregert, S. and Hjorth, N. (1968) Results of Standard Patch tests with substances abandoned. Contact Dermatitis Newsletter, London 5, 85.

Hjorth, N. (1968) at Finsen Institute. Pers. Comm.

Gillett, J.F. (1896) The Poison of the Primula. Lancet 1, 1040.

Nestler, A. (1904) Hautreizende Primeln. Untersuchungen uber Entstehung, Eigenschaften und Wirkungen des Primelhautgiftes. Berlin. Gebruder Borntrager. p. 6-7.

Rook, A.J. and Wilson, H.T.H. (1965) Primula dermatitis. Brit. Med. J. 1, 220.

Primula suaveolens

Sensitisation to this species which is said to be indigenous to Oviedo, Spain, was reported by De Argumosa (1951).

Reference

De Argumosa, J.A. (1951) Sensitization to Primula suaveolens. Rev. Clin. esp. 41, 261.

Primula veris
Cowslip

This plant is a common wild flower in the woods of all parts of Great Britain. Hjorth (1968) recorded two positive patch test reactions to the plant. Allergenicity is not proven.

Reference

Hjorth, N. (1968) at the Finsen Institute. Pers. Comm.

Primula vulgaris
Primrose

The plant and root were used in Herbal Medicine: 'Of the leaves of Primroses is made as fine a salve to heal wounds as any that I know. Do not see your poor neighbour to go with wounded limbs when an halfpenny cost will heal them' (Culpeper 1653).

Reference

Culpeper, N. (1653) The Complete Herbal. Birmingham. Kynoch Press Imperial Chemical (Pharmaceuticals) Ltd.

Odour of Primula root

The various species of Primula can be divided into four groups according to the odour which comes from the root when injured. The odours resemble anise (Pimpinella), methyl salicylate and the disagreeable odour of bed bugs. A fourth group has no odour. Primula obconica belongs to the methyl salicylate group (Goris 1950, cited by Watt and Breyer-Brandwijk 1962).

References

Goris, A. (1950) Industr. Perfum. 5, 121, 177: 1950 Chem. Abstr. 44, 8062, cited by Watt and Breyer-Brandwijk (1962).

Watt, J.M. and Breyer-Brandwijk, M.G. (1962) The Medicinal and poisonous plants of Southern Africa. 2nd ed. Edinburgh. E.& S. Livingstone.

Sensitization by application of Primula obconica to the skin

Kirk (1899) produced sensitization by applying the plant repeatedly to irritated skin under occlusive dressings. Low (1935) sensitized himself and one of seven other subjects by rubbing the juice of the leaf into the abraded skin. Bloch and Steiner-Wourlisch (1926) rubbed a strong extract of the plant into the unbroken surface of the skin of twelve subjects and produced sensitization in all of them. In a previous study by the same workers in which a weaker perparation was rubbed into the abraded skin, only 10 of the 24 subjects (41%) were sensitized.

Three nonsensitive individuals were sensitized by the continuous application of fresh

Primula leaves to the forearm. The leaves were changed every 2 days. Sensitisation resulted in all three cases in 16, 17 and 29 days respectively. The skin of the face was found to react more strongly than the skin on other parts of the body. The author demonstrated a positive reaction of the oral mucous membrane to Primula on himself (Helmke 1937).

References

Bloch, B. and Steiner-Wourlisch, A. (1926) Production of Primula sensitivity and its importance for the problem of idiosyncracy. Archs. f. Dermat. u. Syph. 152, 283.

Helmke, R. (1937) On the production of Primula hypersensitiveness of the skin and mucous membranes. Med. Klin. 33, 1303.

Kirk, R. (1899) On the effects of Primula obconica on the skin. Lancet 1, 1630.

Low, R.C. (1935) Anaphylaxis and sensitisation. New York. Wm. Wood.

Variety and cultivar allergenic specificity

Hjorth (1966) found some differences in degree of allergenicity among eight named cultivars of this species. Pink forms of the plant give stronger patch test reactions than blue forms (Kirton, V. 1974, Pers. comm.). In a male horticulturalist, only one single variety of primula out of 17 species tested was allergenic (Davies 1939).

References

Davies, J.H.T. (1939) Contact dermatitis. Practitioner 142, 636

Hjorth, N. (1966) Primula dermatitis. Trans. St. John's Hosp. Derm. Soc. Lond. 52, 207.

Pollen of Primula obconica

The damp pollen is allergenic and can cause dermatitis not only from contact but also by being in its vicinity without any direct contact (Rook 1961).

Reference

Rook, A. (1961) Plant dermatitis. Botanical aspects. Trans. St. John's Hosp. Derm. Soc. 46, 41.

Cultivation of Primula species in Great Britain

The species of *Primula* which are most commonly grown as house-plants are *P. obconica* and *P. malacoides*. *P. sinensis* is retailed in smaller quantities while *P. kewensis*, *P. floribunda*, *P. denticulata* and *P. mollis* also appear in florists' shops from time to time. Other potentially allergenic species are unlikely to be contacted outside the larger botanical gardens (Rook and Wilson 1965).

Reference

Rook, A. and Wilson, H.T.H. (1965) Primula dermatitis. Brit. Med. J. 1, 220.

Primula spp. in Japan

In Japan, dermatitis from *Primula* is very rare except in occupational cultivators. In a greenhouse worker who developed dermatitis of the hands and face, patch tests to the leaves and flowers (including calyces), diluted ten times, produced positive reactions with *P. obconica*, *P. malacoides* and *P. sinensis* (Harada and Masuda 1972).

A woman gardener who carried out the pollination of *P. obconica* developed dermatitis of the face and back of hand. Patch tests to stamens, calyces, leaf backs and stems produced positive reactions (Endo, M. and Honda, M. 1972, in discussion of Masuda 1972).

Reference

Harada, S. and Masuda, T. (1972) Dermatitis due to primrose. Jap. J. Derm. 82, 578.

Primula spp. in Europe

Dermatitis from *Primula obconica* has become less common in Denmark and possibly in Europe generally as awareness of the allergenicity of the plant has spread and horticulture of the plant has diminished. In contrast, the plant is becoming more commonly sold in California thus reversing the historical trend of interest in this plant.

Breeding of species of Primula obconica

Because of the commercial importance of *P. obconica* a wealth of new varieties has been cultivated by selection, hybridization and some by mutation. As a result the plants at present available are entirely different from the original lilac variety imported from China (Maurer and Storck 1935).

The direct descendants of *P. obconica* are termed *grandiflora*. An attempt to obtain larger and longer lasting flowers by hybridization between *P. obconica* and *P. megaseafolia* resulted in the popular *P. obconica gigantea*. *P. megaseafolia* is non-allergenic, but it appeared that the allergenic properties were inherited as a dominant trait so, unfortunately, *P. obconica gigantea* varieties tend to be more sensitizing than the original *grandiflora* (Maurer and Storck 1935).

Arends, a German horticulturalist, was successful, by hybridising, in breeding a primin-free *Primula obconica* x but, unfortunately a reduction in primin content also involved a lessening of the beauty of the flowers.

Reference

Maurer, E. and Storck, A. (1935) Untersuchungen zur Zuchtung einer giftfreien Primel vom 'Obconica'-Typus. Gartenbauwissenschaft 10, 1.

Primula obconica - conditions of growth

External conditions are known to have a marked effect upon the development of the oil of the glandular hairs, so that a person who has hitherto been immune, may, on coming into contact with plants in another locality, be badly poisoned (Weydahl 1908).

References

Weydahl (1908) "Influence of different conditions of life on toxic formation of hairs in Primula obconica". Gartenflora 55, 449, cited by Smith (1920).

Smith, E.P. (1920) Plant Dermatitis. I. Journal of Botany 58, 130: II, 58, 173.

Primula obconica - Clinical features

Rook and Wilson (1965) made a detailed study of a series of 25 patients - 24 females and one male.

The age at which sensitivity began ranged from 15 to 79, with an average of 51.6 years. The length of history before a diagnosis was made varied from 2 weeks to 10 years, with an average of 17.27 months. The sites principally involved (Table below) were the face, particularly round the mouth and on the eyelids, which were often red and swollen, the neck, arms and hands. Rarely, patches occurred on the ears, thighs, buttocks, or ankles. The affected areas itched, burned, and appeared red, often oedematous, and frequently blistered. A distinctive pattern was often seen, particularly on the arms and forearms, consisting of blotches and linear streaks. This appearance is very characteristic of plant dermatitis, and in Britain is nearly always due to contact with a primula.

Site Affected by Primula Dermatitis

Sites Affected	Total	%
Eyelids	13	52
Cheeks and chin	16	64
Neck	14	56
Ears	1	4
Fingers	12	48
Hands	9	36
Arms	14	56
Ankles	1	4
Thighs and buttocks	2	8
Tongue	1	4

On the sides of the fingers quite large blisters sometimes formed after the patient had pulled dead leaves off the plant. Mucosal lesions were rare, but one patient complained of soreness of the lips and tongue, while another suffered not only from an extensive rash but from pyrexia, coryza, and conjunctivitis as a result of contact with a plant.

Less easy to recognize was the occasional mild case in which the only sign of primula sensitivity consisted in a single transient itching red patch, usually on the chin or the side of the neck, or recurrent irritation, redness, and swelling of the eyelids.

In severe cases, which may occur when the diagnosis is overlooked and the patient continues to handle the plants, the eruption may become very extensive and the face grossly oedematous, and fever and constitutional symptoms may develop. In one of the patients, not included in the present series, an attack of erythema multiforme complicated the already widespread dermatitis.

Hjorth (1970) reported that the degree of sensitivity and the intensity of exposure determine the pattern of dermatitis.

Removal of dead flowers by a housewife with a low degree of sensitivity may produce a vesicular eruption on the sides of the fingers, indistinguishable from a dyshidrotic eczema. The textbook picture of plant dermatitis with vesicles in linear patterns or violent erythema and oedema occurs in half of the cases only (Bonnevie 1939).

The resinous excretion adheres to the fingers and a highly sensitive patient's activity and agility determines further dissemination. If a patient dresses after nursing her flowerpots, indistinct streaking fingermarks develop on the shoulders and the thorax. Allergen sticking to the fingertips may cause eruptions mainly localized to the ano-genital region, the ears or the nostrils. (Bonnevie 1939, Hjorth 1966). Sometimes the initial diagnoses have been neurodermatitis of the neck or acute seborrheic eczema of the scalp.

Erythema multiforme and id-like papular universal eruptions mistaken for scabies are uncommon but have been observed by several authors (Bonnevie 1939, Rook and Wilson 1965, Hjorth 1966). The latter types of eruption suggest a haematogenous dissemination or possibly a reaction to allergen inhaled with the dust.

If patch tests with primula are performed only in clinically suspected cases, the patterns of dermatitis observed must of necessity comply with the textbook of descriptions of plant dermatitis. Where standard patch tests serve as a clue to diagnosis, the atypical patterns will be observed. In such cases the origin of the dermatitis is only revealed by detailed interrogations prompted by the positive patch tests (Bonnevie 1939, Hjorth 1966).

Conjunctivitis, keratitis and iritis have been reported in association with primula dermatitis (Grant 1962).

References

Bonnevie, P. (1939) Aetiologic und Pathogenese der Ekzemkrankheiten. Copenhagen. Nyt Nordisk Forlag.

Grant, W.M. (1962) Toxicology of the eye. Springfield, Ill. Charles C. Thomas.

Hjorth, N. (1966) Primula dermatitis: sources of error in patch testing. Trans. St. John's Hosp. Derm. Soc. 52, 207.

Hjorth, N. (1970) Primula dermatitis in Current Problems in Dermatology Vol. 3. Basel S. Karger p. 31-50.

Rook, A. and Wilson, H.T.H. (1965) Primula dermatitis. Brit. med. J. 1, 220.

Primula obconica - Historical Aspects

Primula obconica was introduced to Britain from China in 1880 and rapidly became established as a popular greenhouse plant throughout Europe and the United States. The first accounts incriminating this plant as a cause of dermatitis were published in horticultural journals (White 1888, Gardeners Chronicle 1889), and were received sceptically in England; one indignant gardener vigourously condemned "this vegetable viper". A year or two later reports began to appear in the medical journals first in England (Oldacres 1889) then in America (White 1890). Reports rapidly accumulated in England (Sym 1890, Clarke 1890, Lee 1890, Southern 1891, Swan 1891, Pooley 1893, Ackland 1893) and appeared in countries in Europe (Touton 1932). Ferguson (1890) suspected the hairs on the plant as the cause of the dermatitis. So numerous were the papers that it was predicted (Cooper 1899) that such a poisonous plant would be grown less and less frequently; but this prophecy has not been fulfilled. In 1906, Harrison called the plant the 'fatted calf' of Harley Street and this primula remains the commonest cause of plant dermatitis in Great Britain (Rook 1961).

In Germany anxiety about primula dermatitis was voiced in a question on the subject in the Reichstag; and in the United States cases were sufficiently numerous for a report by Foerster (1910) to be based on personal experience of 40 to 50 patients. These statistics are a measure of the plant's popularity, for most people are able to handle the leaves of the primula with impunity; and Shelmire (1939), who found an incidence of 8% among florists, was unable to discover a single case among 251 students tested against the leaves. Low (1924) was able to sensitize himself and his brother to *P. obconica* but failed to sensitize six other subjects.

References

Ackland, C.K. (1893) Poisoning by *Primula obconica*. Lancet 2, 289.

Clarke, F.H. (1890) Eczema caused by *Primula obconica*. Brit. Med. J. 2, 789.

Cooper, B. (1899) A case of poisoning by the *Primula obconica*. Brit. Med. J. 2, 1543.

Ferguson, J. (1890) The *Primula obconica*. Brit. Med. J. 2, 955.

Foerster, O.H. (1910) Primula dermatitis. JAMA 55, 642.

Gardeners Chronicle (1889) Aug. 3. cited by Oldacres (1889).

Harrison, A.J. (1906) Dermatitis from without and dermatitis from within. Bristol Med. Chir. J. 24, 325.

Lee, C.N. (1890) Eczema caused by *Primula obconica*. Brit. Med. J. 2, 790.

Low, R.C. (1924) Anaphylaxis and Sensitisation with special reference to the skin and its diseases. Edinburgh, Green p. 175.

Oldacres, C.E. (1889) Toxic symptoms produced by handling *Primula obconica*. Brit. Med. J. 2, 719 (Sept.)

Pooley, E.B. (1893) Poisoning by *Primula obconica*. Lancet 2, 195.

Rook, A. (1961) Plants dermatitis. Botanical aspects. Trans. St. John's Hosp. Derm. Soc. 46, 41.

Shelmire, B. (1939) Contact dermatitis from weeds. Patch testing with their oleoresins. JAMA 113, 1085.

Southern, G. (1891) Urticaria due to *Primula obconica*. Lancet 1, 112.

Swan, S.A.L. (1891) Poisonous properties of *Primula obconica*. Lancet 1, 960.

Sym, A.C. (1890) Eczema caused by *Primula obconica*. Brit. Med. J. 2, 686.

White, J.C. (1890) Oral communications on primrose dermatitis. Boston Med. Surg. J. 122, 425.

White, J.C. (1888) Note in Gardener and Forest 2, 94 (5 May) cited by White (1934).

White, R.P. (1934) The Dermatergoses or Occupational Affections of the Skin. 4th ed. London. H.K. Lewis.

Relevance of Primula dermatitis for hand eczema

An ether extract of *Primula obconica* leaves produced 20 positive reactions (4 male, 16 female) in 431 persons (153 males, 278 females) investigated for hand eczema (Agrup 1969). In 4 of the 20 cases, allergy to *Primula* was considered the main cause or a contributory cause of the hand eczema (Agrup 1969).

Reference

Agrup, G. (1969) Hand Eczema and other hand dermotases in South Sweden. Acta dermvenereol. 49 Suppl. 61. pp. 1-91.

Primula dermatitis in a blind person

An eruption from *Primula obconica* affected the skin of the nose and around the eyes. The patient who was blind had been smelling the plant (Carman 1912).

Reference

Carman, J.H. (1912) in discussion of Zeisler, J. (1910) Some uncommon and often unrecognized forms of Tosic dermatitis. JAMA 58, 2024.

Differential diagnosis of Primula dermatitis

Early writers noted a resemblance of *Primula* dermatitis to seborrhoeic eczema and ringworm (Jamieson 1893), erysipelas (Pooley 1893) and urticaria (Southern 1891, Freeman 1897). Hjorth (1966) observed 453 individuals sensitive to *P. obconica* during a six year period in Copenhagen. In some instances, the eruption resembled urticaria, erythema multiforma and scabies. He noted that the eruptions which are observed may not primarily or mainly affect the skin sites apparently in maximum contact with the plant. In eight cases *Primula* dermatitis affected the eyelids only (Kaalund-Jorgensen 1951).

References

Freeman, W.T. (1897) A note on the skin irritation caused by handling hyacinth bulbs. Brit. J. Derm. 9, 66.

Hjorth, N. (1966) Primula dermatitis. Trans. St. John's Hosp. Derm. Soc. Lond. 52, 207.

Jamieson (1893) Brit. J. Derm. 5, 140, cited by White (1934).

Kaalund-Jorgensen, O. (1951) Eczema perioculare (Dermatitis of the eyelids). Acta derm.-venereol. 31, 83.

Pooley, E.B. (1893) Poisoning by *Primula obconica*. Lancet 2, 195.

Southern, G. (1891) Urticarie due to *Primula obconica*. Lancet 1, 112.

White, R.P. (1934) The Dermatergoses or Occupational Affections of the Skin. 4th ed. London. H.K. Lewis.

Primula Dermatitis
in Current Problems in Dermatology.
Vol. 3. Basel. S. Karger.
pp. 31-50.

N. Hjorth
Department of Dermatology,
Amtssygehuset, Hellerup, Denmark

For sixty years, P. obconica has remained the predominant cause of plant dermatitis in Europe. The typical eruption is recognized by all dermatologists, but since primula dermatitis often presents atypical patterns, the frequency of the condition is generally underestimated.

Primula obconica

The primula family comprises 22 genera and 600 species, and the genus primula over 200 species (Rook and Wilson 1965). Those most commonly used for indoor decoration in Europe are P. obconica, P. malacoides, and the less popular P. sinensis. A number of primula species are grown in gardens.

Although single instances of dermatitis from several primula species have been reported, primula dermatitis is nearly always caused by P. obconica.

P. obconica was introduced from China into England in 1880 and brought onto the market in all European countries within the next twenty years. Very soon reports of dermatitis appeared everywhere. Because of the commercial importance of P. obconica a wealth of new varieties have been cultivated by selection, hybridization and some by mutation. As a result the plants at present available are entirely different from the original lilac variety imported from China (Maurer and Storck 1935).

The direct descendants of P. obconica are termed grandiflora. An attempt to obtain larger and longer lasting flowers by hybridization between P. obconica and P. megaseafolia resulted in the popular P. obconica gigantea. P. megaseafolia is non-allergenic, but it appeared that the allergenic properties were inherited as a dominant trait so, unfortunately, P. obconica gigantea varieties tend to be more sensitizing than the original grandiflora (Maurer and Storck 1935).

The allergen of P. obconica is formed in minute (0.05 to 0.3mm long) glandular hairs consisting of 3-5 cells, visible through a magnifying glass. The allergen accumulates between the cuticula and the cell membrane of the outmost cell. Eventually, the cuticula may burst and then the concentrated allergen accumulates as irregular resinous drops on the top and sides of the hair. P. obconica also has easily visible long hairs which measure between 1 and 3mm. These do not contain the primula allergen, and an impression of hairiness does not give any indication of the site of allergen in the various parts of the plants (Nestler 1904). The leaf stem, for example, appears hairy but contains less allergen than other organs.

The short hairs are of the same size all over the plant. Their number does not increase once a leaf has been formed so that the density is higher on small young leaves than on large ones. The density of glandular hairs is highest on the calyx and decreases in the following order: flower stalk, carpel, leaf, leaf stem and inflorescent stem. The upper surface of the petals has few scattered short hairs. On the leaves the short hairs are found with equal density on the upper and the lower surfaces. On the lower surface, which also has long hairs, the glandular hairs are situated between the ribs and especially along the margin (Henning 1935, Maurer and Storck 1935).

Different varieties of P. obconica have largely the same density of glandular hairs (Maurer and Storck 1935). In spite of this, however, some varieties form less allergen than others. This is considered to be a consistent characteristic, independent of the year of growth, and incidentally, also of the colour of the flower.

The allergen content of a particular specimen of P. obconica is subject to wide variations. It increases if the plant is growing in light and warmth (Klein and

Trothandl 1929) and rises acutely after nitrogen manuring (Henning 1935, Weydahl 1907). The sticky excretion on the surface of the hairs can be removed mechanically by touching, dusting or watering of the plant. As a result the allergen content decreases, although only temporarily.

These botanical findings have a bearing on the pattern and the incidence of primula dermatitis. Primula owes its popularity to the capacity for developing new leaves and flowers. Removal of a dead flower involves immediate contact with the most allergenic part of the plant, the calyx and the flower stalk. This is probably how most housewives, nurserymen and florists become sensitized. Careful nursing of a plant provides optimal conditions for production of the allergen, and a specimen bought in early spring gradually becomes more allergenic with increasing sun hours. Due to the low allergen production in early spring a few vesicles on the right hand fingers may be the only signs of sensitization. When the allergen content increases during the summer a widespread dermatitis may develop by a mere touch of the leaves.

Some extremely sensitive patients may develop an eruption if they stay in a room with P. obconica in spite of careful avoidance of direct contact with the plant. Although the allergen sublimes at 110°C, the vapour concentration in the air will be insufficient to provoke an eruption. Primula allergen, however, can spread by indirect contact, for example, via a doorhandle, a table top, or a handshake with a person who has touched a primula (Nestler 1904). Possibly the allergen is carried by dust particles.

Chemistry of the Allergen

Between 1900-1904 Nestler performed a systematic study of a number of primula species summarized in his monograph 'Hautreizende Primeln'. He found skin irritant substances in P. obconica, P. sinensis and two P. cortuisoides, namely P. sieboldi and P. mollis, while all other species examined were found to be innocuous. Ethyl ether poured over a P. obconica leaf would dissolve a crystalline substance, which sublimed at 110 C and was soluble in alcohol, ether, chloroform and benzene, but insoluble in water at 20 C.

Karrer (Bloch and Karrer 1927) succeeded in purifying the allergen by water vapour distillation of a crude ether extract. Although he used 2,000 specimens of P. obconica, the total yield was only 100mg. The melting point of the golden yellow crystals was 62-63°C. The approximate molecular formula was $C_{14}H_{18}O_3$ or $C_{14}H_{20}O_3$. The calculated molecular weight of the substance according to these formulae was 234.1 or 236.1, while the molecular weight found was 214. The biological activity of the substance, called primin, was confirmed by Bloch, who used it for experimental sensitization of man and guinea-pigs (Bloch and Steiner 1927, 1931). The primin was found to be a primary irritant in a concentration of 1%. Highly sensitive persons would react to 20μg. The study had to be abandoned because Bloch himself became excessively sensitive to primin, which prevented further studies in his dermatology department.

By paper chromatography Brachtendorff (1956) showed primin to have an RF-value of 0.77 on paper SS 598 G using acetone water 45-55 as a developer, and Fischer's base for visualization of the spot.

The structural formula of primin remained unknown until recent years when Schildknecht et al (1964, 1967) found it to be 2-methoxy-6-n-pentyl-p-benzoquinone. In accordance with Karrer's findings the yellow crystals first obtained had a melting point of 62.0°C. Paper chromatography, however, revealed an unknown colourless fluorescent impurity and further purification increased the melting point to 66.7-66.8°C. The molecular weight of the substance is 222 or a multiple of this. The chemical configuration suggested by a variety of investigative methods was confirmed by Schildknecht et al by a systhesis of primin. The properties of the synthetic primin were later studied by Fregert et al (1968) who showed that all patients clinically sensitive would react to 10μg on a filter under an occulsive patch test.

A solution of pure primin for patch testing can be produced by a convenient method described by Agrup et al (1968). Approximately 60 g of leaves and stems from a P. obconica harvested in spring was dipped in 100ml ethyl ether and then immediately afterwards sprayed with a further 100ml of ethyl ether. The 200ml were evaporated to 50ml at room temperature and the resulting solution used for patch testing. The purity and approximate amount of primin in the extract was determined by gas chromatography, in which the extract was compared with a solution of synthetic primin of known concentration.

Clinical Patterns of Primula Dermatitis

The degree of sensitivity and the intensity of exposure determine the pattern of dermatitis.

Removal of dead flowers by a housewife with a low degree of sensitivity may produce a vesicular eruption on the sides of the fingers, indistinguishable from a dyshidrotic eczema. The textbook picture of plant dermatitis with vesicles in linear patterns or violent erythema and oedema occurs in half of the cases only (Bonnevie 1939).

The resinous excretion adheres to the fingers and a highly sensitive patient's activity and agility determines further dissemination. If a patient dresses after nursing her flowerpots, indistinct streaky fingermarks develop on the shoulders and the thorax. Allergen sticking to the fingertips may cause eruptions mainly localized to the ano-genital region, the ears or the nostrils (Bonnevie 1939, Hjorth 1966). Sometimes the initial diagnoses have been neurodermatitis of the neck or acute seborrheic eczema of the scalp.

Erythema multiformeand id-like papular universal eruptions mistaken for scabies are uncommon but have been observed by several authors (Bonnevie 1939, Rook and Wilson 1965, Hjorth 1966). The latter types of eruption suggest a haematogenous dissemination or possibly a reaction to allergen inhaled with the dust.

If patch tests with primula are performed only in clinically suspected cases, the patterns of dermatitis observed must of necessity comply with the textbook descriptions of plant dermatitis. Where standard patch tests serve as a clue to diagnosis, the atypical patterns will be observed. In such cases the origin of the dermatitis is only revealed by detailed interrogations prompted by the positive patch tests (Bonnevie 1939, Hjorth 1966).

Incidence of Primula Sensitivity

Few dermatological departments include primula in their standard patch tests, so the incidence of positive reactions among patients outside Scandinavia is unknown. In 1934 Bonnevie (1939) found 8.8% of all patients examined sensitive to primula. Ninety per cent of the patients with positive reactions were women.

Since 1935 all patients with dermatitis referred to the Finsen Institute, Copenhagen, have been examined by a series of standard patch tests including Primula obconica. Between 1935 and 1964, an $8x8mm^2$ of a primula leaf was used for testing. Among 48,423 patients examined between 1935 and 1961, 2206 patients developed a positive reaction to primula leaf. In the analysis it appeared that 1825 patients (3.7%) had developed a positive reaction on the 1st to 7th day after application of the patch test, while 381 (0.8%) developed a reaction after a week or more (Hjorth 1966). Such late flares usually indicate active sensitization from the patch tests.

The incidence of sensitivity has varied, but, although it is declining from a peak in the post-war years primula sensitivity is still very common. The incidence of positive reactions have a distinct seasonal variation with a maximum from April to August and with the minimum in February. This has an influence on the percentage of positive reactions obtained by the total standard series. Disregarding primula, positive reactions occur rather uniformly throughout the year, Figs. 1, 2, pages 565, 566.

Bonnevie (1939) also found an accumulation of cases in the summer months and ascribed it to a high sale of primula at that season. Later studies, however, revealed that in Denmark the sale of primula of any species is high during early spring but very low during the peak of occurrence of dermatitis. The increase in the incidence of primula sensitivity during the summer months seems to parallel the number of sun hours (Hjorth 1967).

The seasonal variations established are, however, also influenced by the occurrence of false negative reactions to primula leaf in winter. In a study comprising 882 cases tested between September 1964 and April 1965 fresh leaves gave positive reactions in 2.5% of the patients, while the actual incidence of sensitivity as found by parallel patch tests with deep-frozen leaves harvested in May was 5.5%. The incidence of sensitivity recorded above must accordingly represent a minimum figure, as the possible occurrence of false negative reactions was unknown in the period of study.

By use of patch tests with a primula extract in an allergen of constant strength, Agrup et al (1968) found smaller differences in the incidence of positive reactions in winter and in summer than in the study reported above. Agrup et al's study is also of particular interest by demonstrating the high incidence of primula sensitivity among dermatological patients in Lund, Sweden; among 1308 females 117 had positive reactions, among 1149 males 23 reacted. In Lund, primula dermatitis has been considered quite rare until a primula extract was introduced in standard patch test series. However, the incidence of primula sensitivity in Scandinavia may be higher than elsewhere owing to the universal tradition of keeping flowerpots in window sills.

Primula dermatitis has been reported in the Uniter States, but most dermatologists consider it to be rare. 149 dermatological patients in California showed negative reactions throughout (Epstein 1969). Among 99 normal men in the U.S.A. one was found to have an unexplained sensitivity by patch test with primula extract 1:10,000 (Maibach 1969).

Methods of Patch Testing

Primula dermatitis with atypical patterns will be missed unless P. obconica is tested routinely. The frequency of dermatitis would seem to warrant routine patch tests in Europe on female patients seen between March and October. Patch tests with primula should otherwise be performed if primula dermatitis can be at all suspected.

Several methods of patch testing have been used:

1. Blumenthal and Jaffe (1933) and Urbach and Gottlieb (1946) recommended a 25% of sap from a primula leaf for patch testing. No systematic studies of the reliability of this extract have been published, but as a pulp of the leaves tends to give false negative reactions the sap will presumably also prove unreliable for testing.

2. A square of primula leaf will lead to a reliable result, provided a patient has brought her own specimen and the testing serves for confirmation of a clinical suspicion. However, the offending plant may have been discarded or causal contact with primula may have occurred unnoticed. In such cases a primula kept at a patch test laboratory must supply the paterial for testing. The variety used for such tests is usually selected by the florist. The consequences of his choice was illustrated by testing 85 patients with eight different varieties of P. obconica grown under identical conditions. One variety gave nine positive reactions, another only three. Any laboratory specimen will give false negative reactions in about half the sensitive patients who are tested during winter, and in summer a certain number of patch test sensitizations. False positive reactions probably also occur, but the frequency of these has not been evaluated. The strength of reaction to leaves appear from table I.

Table I. Strength of positive reactions to P. obconica developed between day 2-7 and later.

Strength of reaction	Before 7 days	Flare-up
+	117 (26.1%)	41 (26.6%)
++	155 (34.7%)	74 (48.0%)
+++	158 (35.4%)	39 (25.4%)
++++	17 (3.8%)	0
Total	447 cases	154 cases

The staff at a patch test laboratory who apply patch tests with primula leaves are exposed to sensitization if they handle the leaves with their fingers. If several different plants are tested at the same time, a primula sensitive patient may show false positive reactions to other plants since the allergen is carried by the fingers of the nurse from the primula leaf to leaves of other plants tested. Sometimes the adhesive tape may be contaminated.

In view of the many hazards mentioned the traditional test with primula leaf should be abandoned.

3. Extracts of primula prepared according to the method described by Agrup et al (1968) are useful both for routine testing and for testing of any patient with atypical plant dermatitis.

25ml of the extract should be applied to a circular disc of filter paper of 10mm diameter. After evaporation of the ether the test unit is wrapped in aluminium foil, and under these conditions the allergen is stable for at least three years if kept in a refrigerator. The allergen content of the extract obviously varies depending on the plant used. The presence of allergen can be proved by testing a few individuals known to be sensitive, but if such patients are not available during the preparation of the extract, the presence of allergen and the approximate strength can be confirmed by chemical spot tests, which also give a crude measure of the strength of the extract (Agrup et al 1968).

Brachtendorf's (1956) test:

Reagents: (a) 100ml of a 1% solution of 1,3,3-trimethyl-5-methoxy-2-methylene indoline in ethanol is freshly prepared and 1ml of saturated bromine water added. (b) Equal parts of 2N ammonium hydroxide and 2N sodium carbonate.

Test procedure: Two drops of solution (a) are applied on the prepared filter paper. Hot air is blown onto the patch for some seconds. Two drops of solution (b) are applied, and hot air is blown onto the paper again. In the presence of primin a blue colour develops within 10 sec. The intensity of the colour is roughly proportional to the amount of primin present. With a high content of primin the colour tends to develop very rapidly.

Craven's (1931) test:

Reagents: equal parts of ethanol and ammonium hydroxide (d = 0.880) to make 2ml. Three drops of ethylcyanoacetate are added to the mixture.

Test procedure: Two drops of the freshly prepared reagent are added to the prepared filter paper. In the presence of primin a blue colour develops within seconds.

4. Synthetic primin would be an ideal test material because of the known and well-defined concentration. At present it is, unfortunately, available in very limited quantities and for experimental purposes only. Fregert et al (1968) showed that all patients with a clinical sensitivity will show positive reactions to a dilution of 1:50,000 applied on Al-TEST (IMECO). A concentration of 1:100 invariably causes primary irritant reaction. Such reactions are also common with a concentration of 1:1,000. A concentration of 1:10,000 will give rise to

patch test sensitization but not to primary irritant reactions (Agrup et al 1969).

5. Open patch tests with 25µl of 0.01% primin give stronger and more extensive reactions than those obtained by close patch tests. This demonstrates that primin readily permeates through intact skin. Since the reactions to open tests were stronger than those to close tests, a considerable amount of the primin applied to the filter paper must be retained by the test unit (Fregert et al 1968).

Patch Test Sensitizations

Most substances included in standard patch tests are used in a concentration adapted to minimize the risk of active sensitization. With primula leaves the strength of the allergen varies beyond control, resulting in false negative and false positive reactions and possibly in patch test sensitization. Such active sensitization may be detectable, either by flare-up reactions developed seven days or later after the test, or by conversion from a negative to a positive reaction demonstrable at repeated testing.

A flare-up reaction is caused by allergen remaining in the skin in sufficient quantity to give positive reaction once the sensitivity has been caused by the amount absorbed. The reaction develops after a minimum of 6-7 days and often starts with follicular papules, which coalesce into a confluent, oedematous, but rarely vesicular reaction. The number of flare-up reactions recorded depends on the period of observations after the application of patch tests. At the Finsen Institute, Copenhagen, in 1950 only 25% of the patients returned for reading of the tests one week or more after the application. In 1958 half of the patients appeared for repeated readings after the seventh day. So although the development of an itching flare-up reaction may induce a patient to return to the clinic, the number of flare-up reactions must still be a minimum figure.

Among 48,423 patients tested with primula leaf of varying allergen content, flare-up reactions were noted in 381 (0.78%). These reactions accounted for 17% of all positive reactions to primula leaves (Hjorth 1966).

The allergen content of the average *Primula obconica* is highest between April and August and, as might have been expected, flare-up reactions preferentially occur during this period. In particular periods the variety or specimen of primula used for testing must have been exceptionally virulent. The patch test examination has sometimes doubled the number of persons sensitive, Figs. 3, 4, pages 566a & b.

The time of reaction was analysed in a study comprising 932 petients. Half the patients developed a reaction within 48 hours and 77 within six days. Very long periods of reaction may be due to insufficient observation, since some of the patients may have attended the patch test laboratory in connection with an appointment with the out-patients department.

Professor D. de Solla Price, Yale University, made an interpretation of a graph of the time of reaction to patch tests to *P. obconica* leaf in 932 patients, Fig.5, page 566a.

'The cumulative graph showing the time distribution of reactions falls into two distinct portions under analysis. A total of 635 cases react very rapidly; of them 50% in 1.5 days, 98% by the 4th day, all by the 5th day. A remainder of 297 cases react at a very steady rate of 12.6 cases per day, the rate beginning to slacken exponentially on the 19th day, to half the rate by the 23rd day, the totality being achieved by about the 35th day. Presumably this steady rate of 12.6 per day begins from the first day, some 63 cases of this type occurring by the time that the 635 cases of rapid reactions have occurred by the fifth day'. Some of the 63 patients may have been in the process of sensitization from contact with primula when they were examined by patch tests.

The majority of patients with pre-existing primula sensitivity, i.e. with positive reactions between the first and sixth day after application of patch tests are women. Women also predominate among those showing flare-up reactions (table II). This might suggest that the late reactions were not patch test sensitizations but rather expressions of a lost allergy boosted by the test. Lost sensitivity would preferentially be found among old persons. The average age of those with flare-up reactions, however, was lower than of those who reacted on day 2-6 after testing. If women predominate by those sensitized by the test, the explanation could be that casual contact with primula predisposed them for later sensitization.

Table II. Sex distribution of 25,576 patients with positive patch test reactions to P. obconica (adapted from Hjorth 1966)

	% Males tested	% Females tested
Positive day 1-7	1.41	5.07
Flare-up 7th day or later	0.36	1.26

This assumption was corroborated by a comparative study of patch test sensitizations conducted at the same time and with the same technique in Lund, Sweden, and in San Francisco. On re-examination of 234 persons tested with primin 1:10,000 Agrup et al (1969b) found 10% to have developed reaction at the second test.

In San Francisco Maibach (Maibach and Hjorth) performed repeated patch tests with primin 1:10,000 on 23 males who had been tested one year before. None had developed a positive reaction. In Lund primula sensitivity is common while it is non-existent or extremely rare in California (Epstein 1969, Maibach 1969). The differences in the sensitization rates can, therefore, be ascribed to the extent of previous exposure to the allergen.

In Copenhagen 3,372 patients with recurring or chronic dermatitis have been examined twice or more by standard patch tests including P. obconica. The patients who showed a positive reaction at the second test can be divided into three groups: 1. persons who suffered from primula dermatitis in the interval between the tests, 2. those sensitive at the first examination, and 3. those sensitized by the first patch test. The latter group might be expected to lead to a higher incidence of primula sensitivity at re-testing. However, the incidence of sensitivity was the same at the first and second test. If active sensitization, which must have occurred in connection with the first test, did not increase the total incidence of positive reactions, some sensitivities must have been lost. Loss of sensitivities is known to occur if an allergen is carefully avoided, and primula is an avoidable allergen. As a result actively induced sensitization from patch tests may vanish over a period of years.

In the author's experience patch test sensitization with primula very rarely causes a recurrence of dermatitis. In the event of a flare-up reaction a patient is carefully warned against any future contact with the plant, and for the person who can recognize a primula the risk of accidental exposure is negligible.

Relevance of Patch Test Reactions

Usually, a patch test is considered to be relevant only of contact with the allergen can be confirmed during the interview with the patient. The dermatologist must be able to describe the allergen in terms which can be understood by the patient. It is, therefore, necessary that the dermatologist should know the available varieties of P. obconica and be able to distinguish them from other species of primula.

The offending primula may be impossible to trace if contact happened at the place of work or in public offices. The general ignorance of the characteristics of P. obconica further tends to reduce the number of cases with proven primula dermatitis. Most patients conceive of P. obconica as a plant with a definite colour, size of flowers and shape of petals. These characteristics, however, vary. The shape of the green leaves is decisive.

A series of colour photos of at least eight common varieties of P. obconica and the various common species of primula should be available in any dermatological clinic in order to secure a reliable history.

Since few patients are able to recognize a primula, the relevance of a positive patch test must sometimes be decided on circumstantial evidence, such as a streaky vesicular eruption or an acute oedematous dermatitis.

Among 302 patients seen in 1941, 1947 and 1951 with a positive patch test to primula 100 (33%) were able to trace a primula in their surroundings.

82 patients had a primula at home, 18 traced it at the place of work or with friends. Sixty patients had a clinical plant dermatitis, but although they were unable to find the primula, the paucity of other Danish plants capable of causing such an eruption led by exclusion to a diagnosis of primula dermatitis. If these patients are included, half the patients with a positive patch test to primula had an actual primula dermatitis. Among 161 patients, who showed a positive patch test to primula in the years 1964-1967, 45 (28%) either had a primula at home or could remember contact with a primula elsewhere immediately before the eruption of dermatitis. Thus, the percentage of patients with a relevant reaction has not changed much. On the other hand, the two series are not strictly comparable as patients in the last group were all shown a series of colour photos of ten varieties of P. obconica. This useful supplement to the interview decisively increases the number of patients who admit a contact with primula. Forty-nine percent of the patients with positive reactions knew they were sensitive to primula. These included six of the 45 patients with primula dermatitis. In a recent study Agrup et al (1969) patch tested 411 patients with hand dermatitis, with ether extract of P. obconica. Twenty had positive reactions, but in only four contact with primula was considered to be the cause of the present eczema, and only two of them were not aware of the allergy. They, therefore, conclude that routine tests cannot be recommended. This is in contrast with the recent findings in Copenhagen reported above.

Specificity of Sensitivity

Among 100 patients sensitive to P. obconica 70% had no reactions to other substances in the standard series. Twenty-four per cent had positive reactions to two substances including primula and 6% reacted to three or more (Hjorth and Fregert 1968).

The sensitivity to primin usually extends to other quinones with a longer or shorter side-chain, although the degree of sensitivity decreases by changes in the molecular structure (Hjorth et al 1969). Persons strongly sensitive to primin also react to substances with a side-chain comprising five or six carbon atoms in the 5-position (fig. 1 and table III). p-Benzoquinone gives negative reactions throughout, and cross-sensitivity to other quinones such as hydroquinone monobenzyl ether cannot be demonstrated.

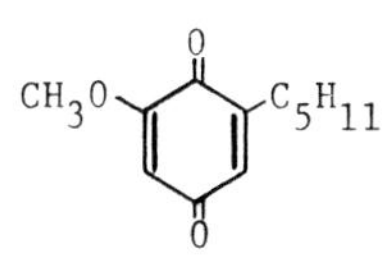

Primin

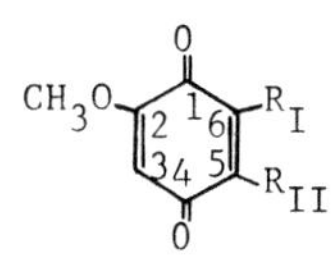

Fig. 1. Structural formula of primin and related quinones, cf. table III.

Nestler (1904) found several species of primula (P. sinensis, P. sieboldi and P. corrusoides) to contain a toxic substance assumed to be identical with the P. obconica allergen although occurring in smaller quantities. Hening also stated to have isolated primin from P. sinensis, but Klein and Trothandel could not confirm this finding. In a recent study Fregert and Hjorth (1969) have been

Table III. Reactions to primin ($R_1 = C_5H_{11}$) and related quinones (cf. fig. 1) (adapted from Hjorth, Fregert and Schildknecht, 1969)

R_1	CH_3	C_2H_5	C_3H_7	C_4H_9	C_5H_{11}	C_6H_{13}	H	H
R_{11}	H	H	H	H	H	H	C_5H_{11}	C_6H_{13}
No. tested	20	20	20	20	20	19	19	20
No. positive	1	5	9	19	20	17	6	7

unable to find primin species other than P. obconica. Standard patch tests with P. sinensis and P. obconica gave no support for an assumption of identical allergens in the two species. Eleven of consecutive patients reacted to patch tests with P. sinensis, five out of 445 to P. malachoides and five out of 196 to P. variabilis. All reactions were supposed to be of irritant nature, and only in exceptional cases coincided.

It is of great practical importance that P. malachoides may give false positive reactions but rarely sensitizes and has not been shown to cross-sensitize with P. obconica.

Many primula species are known to contain irritant substances such as saponins. Simpson (1917) found one ether soluble allergen and a water soluble irritant substance identified as a glycoside. Other authors (Klein and Trothandel 1929) suggest that the irritant substances in P. sinensis are flavones.

Dermatitis from P. malachoides, P. kewensis and several species of garden primula has been reported (Bonnevie 1939). Although these species do not contain primin, it cannot be excluded that their allergens may also occur in P. obconica, since it is unknown whether P. obconica contains any allergens other than primin. This problem deserves attention in the future.

Cross-sensitivity between plant and chemicals can occur not only between related species, but also between plants of different families. For example, balsam of Peru contains allergens which are closely related to those of benzoin and of vanilla, although these substances derive from plants belonging to different families.

P. obconica cross-sensitizes to rosewood (Hjorth and Fregert 1968), to macherium and to teak (Schulz 1969). During a short period an extract of rosewood was included in a patch test series, which also contained P. obconica (Hjorth 1965). Among 25 patients sensitive to primula nine were also sensitive to rosewood extract. At the time of study the allergen of primula was unknown, but a later investigation has confirmed the immunochemical relationship between primin and dalbergione, the allergen of rosewood. Among ten patients with a positive reaction to 0.01% of primin, five gave positive reactions to dalbergione, 1.0%. In patients with a primary sensitization from primula the degree of sensitivity to dalbergione is much lower than to primin. Persons with a primary sensitivity to rosewood gave negative reactions to primin. Aequimolar concentrations, however, cannot be used for testing since patch test with primin 0.1 or 1.0% gives irritant reactions and carries a great risk of sensitization (Hjorth, Fregert and Wilkinson in press). Another tropical wood, macherium scleroxylon, contains 2,3-dimethoxy-dalbergione and cross-sensitizes to dalbergione. Three out of the patients with a primary sensitivity to primin also reacted to dimethoxy-dalbergione, but persons with a primary sensitivity to the latter do not react to primin (Wilkinson 1969). In animal experiments, however, cross-sensitivity between primin and the dalbergiones has been found to be reciprocal (Schulz 1969).

The cross-sensitivity between primin and tropical woods rarely has any practical implication. It is fortunate indeed that occupational contact with sawdust of rosewood is rare among women and that a sensitizing exposure to P. obconica is rare in men (table III).

Prophylaxis

Education of the public has hardly brought any reduction of primula dermatitis. If the sale has declined it is due rather to the florist's reluctance to carry P. obconica in their shops although some customers would insist on buying it.

The plant is undeniably pretty, easy to grow, and bursts with new crops of flowers month after month. Housewives who know they tolerate it understandably buy new every year.

The equally pretty P. sinensis and P. malachoides have shorter flowering periods. But if it has been possible to forbid paraphenylenediamine as a hairdye, it is difficult to see why P. obconica should be allowed to cause numerous cases of dermatitis every year treated at state expense. The cost of medical fees and steroid ointments used for this preventable disease are considerable.

References

Agrup, G., Fregert, S., Hjorth, N. and Ovrum, P. Routine patch testing with ether extract of Primula obconica. Brit. J. Derm. 80, 497-502 (1968).

Agrup, G., Fregert, S. and Rorsman, H. Sensitization by routine patch testing with ether extract of Primula obconica. Brit. J Derm. 81 (1969).

Bloch, B. and Karrer, P. Chemische und biologische Untersuchungen uber die Primelidiosynkrasie. Beibl. schweiz. naturforsch. Ges., Zurich 72, 1-27 (1927).

Bloch, B. and Steiner-Wourlisch, A. Die willkurliche Erzeugung der Primeluberempfindlichkeit. beim Menschen und ihre Bedeutung fur das Idiosynkrasieproblem. Arch. Derm. Syph., Berlin. 152, 283-303 (1927a). Die Sensibilisierung des Meerschweinchens gegen Primeln. Arch. Derm., Syph., Berlin. 162, 349 (1931b).

Blumenthal, F. und Jaffe, K. Ekzem und Idiosynkrasie (Karger, Berlin 1933)

Bonnevie, P. Aetiologie und Pathogenese der Ekzemkrankheiten (Nyt Nordisk Forlag, Copenhagen 1939).

Brachtendorf, J. Untersuchungen zum Nachweis des Primins bei Primula obconica. Zuchter 26, 161-168 (1956).

Epstein, E. Personal communication (1969).

Fregert, S. and Hjorth, N. unpublished data.

Fregert, S., Hjorth, N. and Schulz, K.H. Patch testing with synthetic primin in persons sensitive to Primula obconica. Arch. Derm., Chicago 98, 144-147 (1968).

Hennig, K. Untersuchungen uber den Primingehalt verschiedener Primelarten. Gartenbauwissenschaft 9, 427-431 (1935).

Hjorth, N. and Fregert, S. Contact dermatitis; in Rook and Wilkinson: Textbook of Dermatology (Blackwell, Oxford 1968).

Hjorth, N. Contact sensitivity to plants and balsams. Proc. Europ. Congr. Allergy. Acta derm.-vener. 65, 65-79 (1965). Primula dermatitis: sources of errors in patch test sensitization. Trans. St. John's Hosp. Derm. Soc. 52, 207-219. (1966) - seasonal variations in contact dermatitis. Acta. derm.-vener. 47, 409-418 (1967).

Hjorth, N., Fregert, S. and Schildknecht, H. Cross- sensitization between synthetic primin and related quinones. Acta. derm.-vener. 49, 552-555 (1969)

Hjorth, N., Fregert, S. and Wilkinson, D.S. Cross sensitization between primin and tropical woods (To be published).

Klein, G. and Trothandl, O. Nachweis, Verteilung und Verbreitung des Primelgiftes in der Pflanze. Beitr. Biol. Pflanzen 17, 221-230 (1929).

Maibach, H. and Hjorth, N. Contact Dermatitis Newsletter, London (in print).

Maurer, E. and Storck, A. Untersuchungen zur Zuchtung einter giftfreien Primel vom 'Obconica' - Typus. Gartenbauwissenschaft 10, 1-50 (1935).

Nestler, A. Hautreizende Primeln (Borntrager, Berlin 1904).

Rook, A.J. and Wilson, H.T.H. Primula dermatitis. Brit. med. J. i, 220-222 (1965).

Schulz, K. H. Personal communication (1969).

Schildnecht, H. Struktur des Primelgijtstoffes. Z. Naturforsch 22b, 36-41 (1957). - Abwehrstoffe hoherer Pflanzen. Angew. Chem. 76, Suppl. 112, 117 (1964).

Simpson, C. A. Primrose dermatitis and its relation to anaphylaxis J. Amer. med. Ass. 69, 96-98 (1917).

Urbach, E. and Gottleib, P. M. Allergy (Grune and Stratton, New York 1946).

Weydahl, K. Uber dne Einflub der verschiedenen Lebensbedingungen auf die Gifthaarbildung bei Primula obconica Hance. Gratenflora 55, 449-445.

Wilkinson, D. S. Personal communication (1969).

Primin in Primula and other plants

Recently, Hausen has detected primin or other quinoid compounds, in species of Primula and in some other plants, Presumably the quantity present is rarely clinically significant, but further clinical investigation is required.

Reference

Hausen, B. M. (1977) Hamburg. Personal communication.

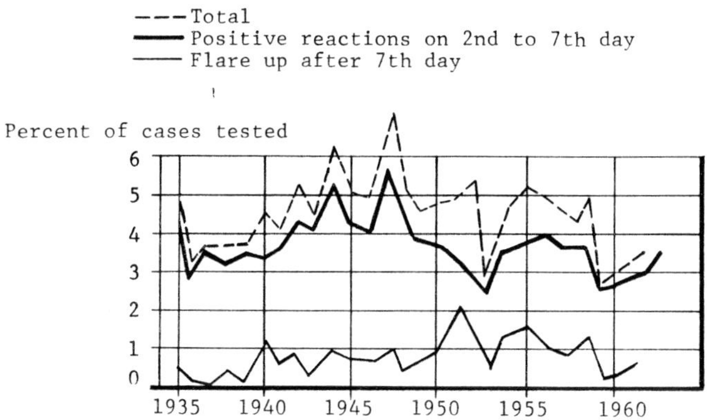

Fig. 1. Annual incidence of positive patch test reactions to P. *obconica* leaf in Copenhagen (from Hjorth, 1966).

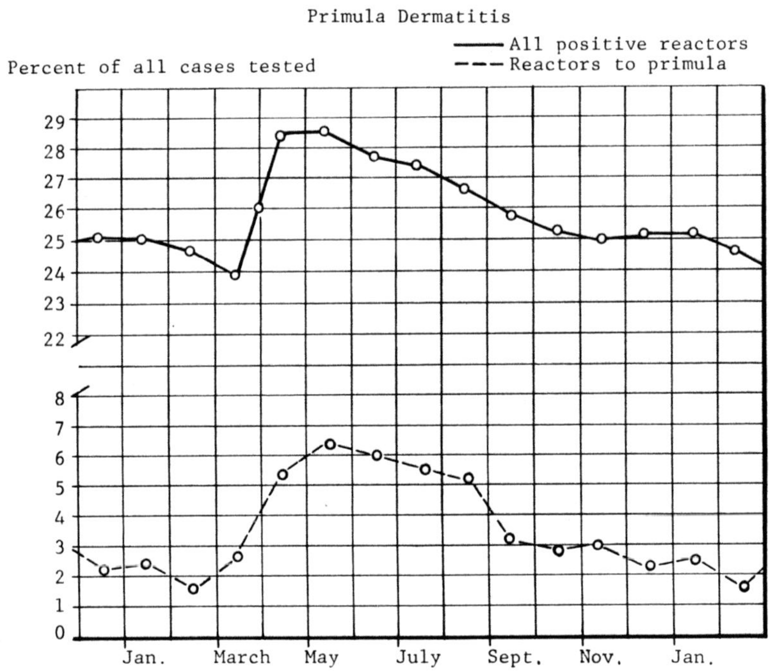

Total number examined	48,423
Total number with one or more positive reaction	12,611
Total number with positive reaction to primula	1,825

Fig. 2. Seasonal incidence of positive patch test reactions.

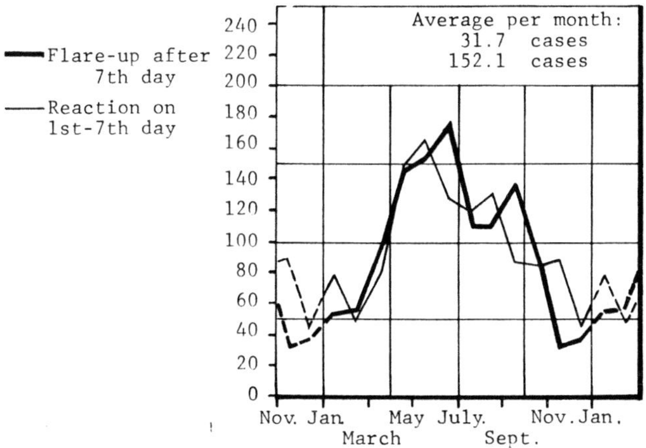

Fig. 3. Seasonal variations in flare-up reactions to *P. obconica* leaf (from Hjorth, 1966).

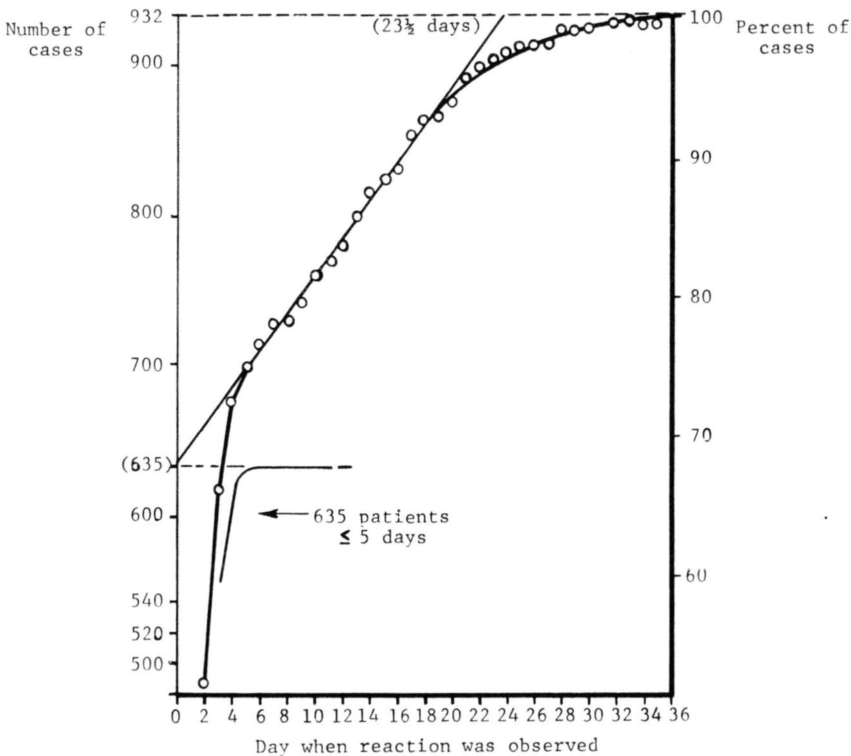

Fig. 5. Time of reaction to patch tests with *P. obconica* leaf (from Hjorth, 1966).

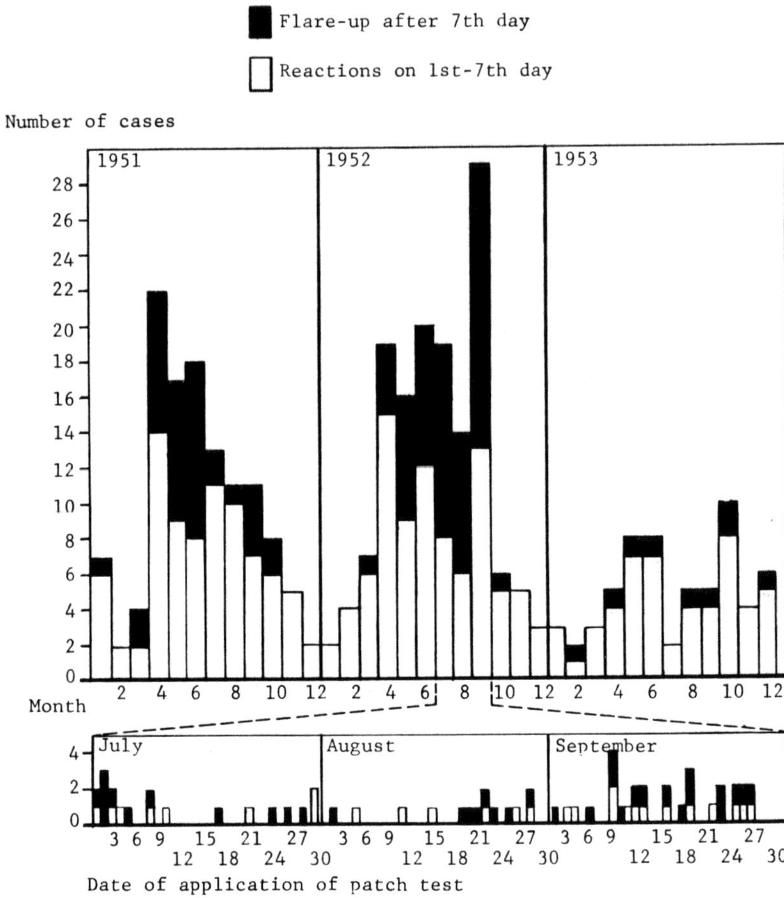

Fig. 4. Accumulation of flare-up reactions (from Hjorth, 1966).

Chemical prevention of Primula dermatitis

Helmke (1938) found that washing the area of skin exposed to a primrose leaf with a 25 per cent solution of ammonia prevented a dermatitis if it was done within 15 minutes. After longer periods or in weaker solutions the preventive property was much less marked. If a primrose leaf is soaked in a 25 percent solution of ammonia for 24 hours the dermatitis producing property is entirely lost.

Reference

Helmke, R. (1938) The prevention of primrose dermatitis by the use of ammonia. Dermat. Wchnschr. 106, 669.

PROTEACEAE

1050 species in 62 genera are found in tropical Asia, Malaysia, Australia, New Caledonia, New Zealand, tropical South America, Chile, on the mountains of tropical Africa and in southern Africa and Madagascar.

Vases containing the flowers of Lomatia silaifolia (Wild parsley) are often surrounded by dead flies (Macpherson 1932).

Chemistry is recorded by Hegnauer (1969).

References

Hegnauer, R. (1969) Chemotaxonomy of plants. Vol. 5. Basel, Birkhauser. p. 403.

Macpherson, J. (1932) Plants injurious to man in Australia. Med. J. Australia 1, 281.

Cardwellia

One species is found in Queensland.

Cardwella sublimis
Silky Oak

Cleland (1943) received several reports of dermatitis from contact with undried wood of this species. Only some of those exposed were affected. Webb (1948) refers to the properties of the wood; sawyers and others handling the fresh timber may contract dermatitis (H.C. Whibley, Cairns, personal communication to Webb 1948).

References

Cleland, J.B. (1943) Plants including fungi, poisonous or otherwise injurious to man in Australia. IV. Med. J. Australia 11, 61.

Webb. L.J. (1948) Guide to the medicinal and poisonous plants of Queensland. CSIRO Bull. 232, 1. Melbourne.

Webb, L.J. (1949b) The blistering alkaloid in "poison walnut". For. Prod. Newsletter 169, 1.

Conospermum

35 species are found in Australia.

Conospermum teretifolium

The root of the plant yields lapachol (Thomson 1971), a sensitizing agent of Tectona.

Reference

Thomson, R.H. (1971) Naturally occurring quinones. 2nd ed. London. Academic Press.

Grevillea

190 species are found in eastern Malaysia, New Hebrides, New Caledonia and Australia. Some yield useful timber.

Grevillea spp.

Leichhardt (1847) cited by Hurst (1942) referred to the vesicating property of the glutinous secretion of the seed vessels of a drooping species of Grevillea. The skin turned black in colour as from the effects of silver nitrate and was raised in painful blisters. This property was discovered accidentally and was traced to Grevillea by means of experimental application of the capsules to the skin, when the same effect was produced.

The passage, which preceded the introduction of the patch test to Dermatology by nearly half a century is as follows:

'John Murphy having no pockets in his trousers, put the seeds which he found during the stage into his bosom, close to the skin, where he had already deposited a great number of Sterculia, and was much inconvenienced by starry prickles which surround the seeds. Afterwards, finding the drooping Grevillea in fruit, he gathered some capsules and placed them as before stated. Upon arriving at the camp he felt great pain and, on examining the place, he saw, to his greatest horror, that the whole of the skin of the epigastric region was coloured black and raised into a great number of painful blisters. Upon his showing it to me, I thought that it was caused by the Sterculia prickles having irritated the skin and rendered it more sensitive to the sharp properties of the exudation of the seed vessels of Grevillea. Brown, however, merely touched the skin of his arm with the matter when blisters immediately rose, showing clearly its properties. The discoloration of the skin was like the effects of nitrate of silver.'

The natives of north-west Australia were observed to use the sap of two species of Grevillea to scarify their bodies and produce scars (Cleland 1925).

Grevillea banksii
Kahili, Rain Flower,
Silky Oak Tree

The blossoms of this tree were a common cause of contact dermatitis in the Hawaiian Islands. A study was carried out by Arnold (1942). He found that women were more frequently affected than men. Dermatitis appeared two to three days after exposure and most often affected the dorsa of the hands, wrists, face and neck. Open patch tests with various parts of the plant produced marked reactions to the fresh flower and to ether extracts of the flower. Only a few slight reactions were obtained from closed patch tests with the leaf. The lesion detail of the dermatitis was typical of plant dermatitis viz. linear erythema and/or vesicles. The blossoms are made into bouquets and leis (neck garlands) which possibly accounts for the predominance in women (6/1). The calyx, anther and style of both the red and yellow varieties of blossom contained the allergenic principle. Cross-sensitivity to the blossom of G. robusta did not appear to occur. He observed no case in which dermatitis appeared in less than 24 hours after exposure. Patch tests in control individuals were negative. Exacerbation of pre-existing dermatitis occurred in some cases following patch testing. Three of 26 patients showed some sensitivity to extracts of mango leaf (Mangifera, Anacardiaceae) probably by multiple specific sensitivity rather than by cross-sensitivity.

Kahili is also a colloquial name in Hawaii for Hedychium.

Grevillea mimosoides

The sticky secretion on the fruits of this tree in Queensland causes blistering of the skin as is well known by bushmen (Mair 1968a).

Grevillea pilulifera

Two persons who walked through the shrubs developed an intense rash (Aplin 1976).

Grevillea robusta
Australian Silky Oak

This species is now extensively employed as a shade and timber tree in Ceylon and elsewhere.

The sap irritates the eyes of men who prune the tree (Maiden 1913). The tree is used to line streets for shade purposes and in Los Angeles "Grevillea poisoning" is well known to telephone linemen and pruners (May 1960).

Some of the laboratory staff most directly involved in handling and testing of specimens of this wood were affected with skin and eye irritation. Others as directly involved in this work were not affected. The irritation developed after handling green wood or exposure to sawdust or exuded sap. It was not observed as a result of handling the dry prepared specimens (U.S. Forest Service Research Note 1964).

A male, developed vesicobullous dermatitis of the skin of the neck, arms, trunk and genital area, two days after he sawed a limb off a specimen of this tree. Sawdust fell on his face, neck and down into his clothing. A patch test to the sawdust produced a bullous response at 36 hours; tests in controls were not recorded (May 1960).

The major phenolic constituent of the wood is grevillol (5-n-tridecylresorcinol)(Cannon et al 1970).

G. robusta, *G. pyramidalis* and *Persoonia elliptica* have been found to yield 5-n-alkyl and 5-n-alkenylresorcinols. The major constituent of the vesicant exudate on the seed pods of *Grevillea pyramidalis* has been identified as 5-pentadec-10-enylresorcinol and traces of the same substance have been shown to be present in the wood of *G. robusta* (Ritchie et al 1965, Occolowitz and Wright 1962, Ridley et al 1968).

These compounds are chemically related to the sensitizing compounds of *Toxicodendron*.

References

Aplin, T.E.H. (1976) Poisonous garden plants and other plants harmful to man in Australia. Western Australian Dept. of Agriculture Bull. 3964.

Arnold, H.L. (1942) Dermatitis due to the Blossom of *Grevillea banksii*. A newly recognized and common entity in Hawaii. Arch. Derm. Syph. 45, 1037.

Cannon, J.R., Chow, P.W., Metcalf, B.W. and Power, A.J. (1970) The structure of Robustol, a novel phenol from *Grevillea robusta* A. Cunn. Tetrahedron Letters 4, 325.

Cleland, J.B. (1925) Plants including fungi, poisonous or otherwise injurious to man in Australia. (Series II) Med. J. Australia 2, 443.

Hurst, E. (1942) The Poison plants of New South Wales. N.S.W. Poison Plants Committee; Sydney.

Mair, K. (1968a) Director, Royal Botanic Gardens, Sydney Australia, personal communication from records of the Herbarium.

May, S.B. (1960) Dermatitis due to *Grevillea robusta* (Australian Silky Oak). Archs. Derm. 82, 1008.

Occolowitz, J.L. and Wright, A.S. (1962) 5-(10-pentadecnyl)-resorcinol from *Grevillea pyramidalis*. Aust. J. Chem. 15, 858.

Ridley, D.D. et al (1968) Some further constituents of *Grevillea robusta*. Aust. J. Chem. 21, 2979.

Ritchie, E. et al (1965) Chemical studies of the Proteaceae. I. *Grevillea robusta* A. Cunn. and *Orites excelsa* R. Br. Aust. J. Chem. 18, 2015.

U.S. Forest Service Research Note (1964) FPL-074 U.S. Forest Products Laboratory. U.S. Department of Agriculture, November. Hardness, density and shrinkage cnaracteristics of silk-oak from Hawaii.

Grevillea pyramidalis
(North West Australia)

Grevillea viscidula
(Northern Territory)

Both species have a sticky secretion which can cause blistering on contact with the skin. Danger also exists from drops of the secretion when sitting under the tree (Francis and Southcott 1967, Cleland and Lee 1963).

References

Cleland, J.B. and Lee, D.J. (1963) The Poisonous and Urticating Plants of Australia in Venomous and Poisonous Animals and Noxious Plants of the Pacific Region. ed. Keegan, H.L. and Macfarlane, W.V. Oxford. Pergamon Press. pp. 3-13.

Francis, D.F. and Southcott, R.V. (1967) Plants harmful to man in Australia. Misc. Bull. No. 1. Botanic Garden, Adelaide, Australia.

Persoonia

60 species are found in Australia and New Zealand.

Persoonia elliptica

An ether extract of this wood was found to be vesicant to human skin: the volatile portion of the extract was responsible and blisters appeared within 10 hours of application to the skin of the forearm. 5-n-undecylresorcinol and (Z) - 5-undec-3-enylresorcinol (persoonol) were isolated from the extract (Cannon and Metcalf 1971).

Reference

Cannon, J.R. and Metcalf, B.W. (1971) Phenolic constituents of *Persoonia elliptica* (Proteaceae). Aust. J. Chem. 24, 1925.

PSILOXYLACEAE

One species in one genus is recognized in the Mascarenes. The family is closely related to Myrtaceae.

Psiloxylon

One species is found in Mauritius and Réunion.

Psiloxylon mauritianum
Scratchwood,
bois à gratter

Dust from the crumbling bark causes itching and gives the wood its name (Stone 1921).

Reference

Stone, H. (1921) A textbook of wood. London, Rider.

PTAEROXYLACEAE

About three species in two genera are found in tropical and southern Africa and Madagascar.

Ptaeroxylon

One species is found in southern Africa.

Ptaeroxylon obliquum
(syn. *P. utile*)
Sneezewood, Cape Mahogany

The sawdust of umtati has strong peppery smell and causes violent sneezing, which restricts its commercial use (Boulder 1908, Chalk et al 1935). The substance responsible is the hydroxycoumarin nieshoutol (McCabe et al 1967, Murray and Ballantyne 1969).

References

Boulger, G.S. (1908) Wood. 2nd ed. London, Arnold.

Chalk, L., Chattaway, M.M., Burt Davy, J. et al (1935) Fifteen S. African High Forest Timber Trees. Oxford, Clarendon.

McCabe, P.H., McCrindle, R. and Murray, R.D.H. (1967) Constituents of sneezewood, *Ptaeroxylon obliquum* (Thunb.) Radlk. Part 1: chromones. J. Chem. Soc. 145.

Murray, R.D.H. and Ballantyne, M.M. (1969) Nieshoutol, a sternutatory hydroxycoumarin from sneezewood. Tetrahedron Lett. 46, 4031.

PUNICACEAE

Two species in one genus are found from south-eastern Europe to the Himalayas and on the island of Socotra.

Chemistry is recorded by Hegnauer (1969).

Reference

Hegnauer, R. (1969) Chemotaxonomy of Plants. Vol. 5. Basel, Birkhauser. p. 413.

Punica

The distribution is that of the family. The plant is cultivated.

Punica granatum
Pomegranate

The flowers are astringent and have styptic properties. If dried, pulverized, mixed with iron and taken for a year they cause the hair to turn white (Smith 1969).

Reference

Smith, F.P. (1969) Chinese Materia Medica. Vegetable kingdom. 2nd ed. Rev. by Hei, P.D. Taipei, Taiwan. Ku T'ing Book House.

PYROLACEAE

30 species in three genera found in cold north temperate and Arctic regions are evergreen perennials.

Moneses

One species is found in boreal and Arctic regions. This species is also noted under Pyrola.

Moneses uniflora
Single Delight

This plant, held on the skin with shredded undyed cedar bark as a poultice, was strong enough to cause blisters to form on the skin. The blisters were opened with broken mussel shells and smeared with catfish oil (Densmore 1939, Boas 1966, Turner and Bell 1973, Turner 1973).

References

Boas, F. (1966) Kwakiutl Ethnobotany. Ed. Codere, H. Chicago. The University of Chicago Press.

Densmore, F. (1939) Nootka and Quileute Music. Bureau of American Ethnology. Bull. 24. Smithsonian Institution, Washington, D.C.

Turner, N. and Bell, M.A.M. (1973) The ethnobotany of the southern Kwakiutl Indians of British Columbia. Econ. Bot. 27, 257.

Turner, N. (1973) The ethnobotany of the Bella Coola Indians of British Columbia. Syesis 6, 193.

Chimaphila

Eight species are found in Eurasia, north and central America and the West Indies.

Chimaphila sp.

A naphthaquinone, chimaphilin, is derived from a species of this genus (Thomson 1971).

Chimaphila maculata
Princess Blue

This species is said to be irritant (Schwartz et al 1957).

Chimaphila umbellata
Pipsissewa, Rheumatism Weed, Pine Tulip

The bruised leaves, when externally applied, sometimes induce redness, vesication and desquamation of the skin (Piffard 1881, Bigelow 1817 cited by White 1887). Piffard (1881) noted a report of successful treatment of a skin cancer by application of the plant.

References

Bigelow (1817) American Medical Botany. Boston: (1824) Florula Bostoniensis. Boston cited by White (1887).

Piffard, H.G. (1881) A treatise on the Materia Medica and Therapeutics of skin. New York. Wm. Wood and Co.

Schwartz, L., Tulipan, L. and Birmingham, D.J. (1957) Occupational Diseases of the Skin. 3rd ed. Philadelphia. Lea and Febiger. pp. 637-672.

Thomson, R.H. (1971) Naturally occurring Quinones 2nd ed. London. Academic Press.

White, J.C. (1887) Dermatitis venenata: An account of the action of external irritants upon the skin. Boston. Cupples and Hurd.

Pyrola

20 species are found in north temperate regions.

Pyrola sp.

A naphthaquinone is derived from a species of this genus (Thomson 1971).

Pyrola rotundifolia
(syn. P. media)

The plant is bruised and applied as a styptic (Smith 1969).

Pyrola uniflora
(syn. Moneses uniflora)

This species is noted under Moneses.

References

Smith, F.P. (1969) Chinese Meteria Medica. Begetable kingdom. 2nd ed. Rev. by Hei, P.D. Taipei, Taiwan. Ku T'ing Book house.

Thomson, R.H. (1971) Naturally Occurring Quinones. 2nd ed. London. Academic Press.

RANUNCULACEAE

1900 species in 50 genera, chiefly distributed in north temperate regions, are mostly herbaceous perennials with rhizomes (condensed rootstocks).

Chemistry is recorded by Hegnauer (1973). Tribes are those given by Shaw (1973). Alternative classifications are given by Ruijgrok (1966).

Many members of the family are acrid and caustic in the highest degree (Turnbull 1838). In the laboratory during the extraction of anemonin, all the plants yielding this compound were troublesome to handle (Lloyd 1887).

References

Hegnauer, R. (1973) Chemotaxonomy of plants. Vol. 6. Basel. Birkhauser. p. 10.

Lloyd (1887) cited by White (1887).

Ruijgrok, H.W.L. (1966) Distribution of ranunculin and cyanogenetic compounds in the Ranunculaceae in Comparative Phytochemistry. ed. Swain, T. London. Academic Press. p. 175.

Shaw, H.K.A. (1973) Dictionary of the flowering plants and ferns. The late J.C. Willis. 8th ed. Cambridge University Press.

Turnbull, A. (1831) The Medical Properties of the Natural Order Ranunculaceae and more particularly of the uses of Sabadilla seeds, Delphinium staphisagria and Aconitum napellus and their alcaloids. Philadelphia. Haswell, Barrington and Haswell.

White, J.C. (1887) Dermatitis venenata: An account of the action of external irritants upon the skin. Boston. Cupples and Hurd.

Phytochemical aspects

Several genera in the family Ranunculaceae possess irritant properties from the presence of an innocuous glycoside, ranunculin, which readily breaks down in bruised plant tissue by enzyme action to release protoanemonin which is a volatile, strongly irritant, unstable oil (Shearer 1938, Hill and van Heyingen 1951). Protoanemonin spontaneously undergoes polymerization yielding innocuous anemonin. Dried buttercup hay or boiled leaves are harmless on this account.

Anemonin ($C_{10}H_8O_4$) is a crystalline compound chemically related to the monoterpene cantaridin (derived from the insect Cantharis vesicatoria). Protoanemonin inhibits mitosis in plant cells (Erickson 1948). The compound produces subepidermal blistering of the skin, which agrees with its sulphydryl-binding capacity; like other subepidermal vesicants, protoanemonin is capable of inhibiting the acantholytic effect of cantharidin (Burbach 1963).

Bergman (1944) studied various species of Ranunculus for vesicant action on the skin in a search for those plants which might therefore be supposed to contain a non-irritant precursor of the irritant compound, protoanemonin.

The presence of ranunculin in a plant can be taken to indicate that such a species of Ranunculaceae may well be irritant to the skin under certain conditions e.g. adequate exposure of the skin; contact with fresh bruised plant paterial and an adequate concentration of the compound in the part of the plant to which the skin is exposed, etc.

The amount of protoanemonin in buttercups varies widely with the species of plant and its stage of growth, the highest content being at the time of flowering (Shearer 1938).

A list of species which have been found to contain ranunculin was provided by Ruijgrok (1966). Plant specimens of botanical species name may vary considerably in protoanemonin content and Ranunculus acris is very variable and has been divided into a number of subspecies or varieties (Harper 1957) in which a varied ranunculin content cannot be excluded.

Ranunculin has only been detected in the group of genera bearing the R type caryotype, that is in the two tribes Helleboreae and Anemoneae of the Ranunculaceae. Helleborus, Anemone, Clematis, Ranunculus, Ceratocephalus and Myosurus provide species which contain ranunculin (Ruijgrok 1966). Another ranunculin-like constituent is present in some species; the structure of this glycoside is not yet known (Ruijgrok 1966).

In respect to alleged photodermatitis from species of this family, (Pseudophytophotodermatitis), it is of interest that Eranthus hiemalis yields the furanochromones, visnagin and khellin, which are also present in Ammi visnaga, Umbelliferae. These furanochromones are not photoreactive but they are chemically related to psoralen.

References

Bergmann (1944) Vergleichende Untersuchungen uber die Anatomie schweizerischer Ranunculus-Arten und deren Gehalt an Anemonol und Saponin. Ber. Schweiz. Bot. Ges. 54, 399.

Burbach, J. (1963) The blistering effect of buttercups. Ned. T. Geneesk. 107, 1128.

Erickson, R.O. (1948) Protoanemonin as a mitotic inhibitor. Science 108, 533.

Harper, J.L. (1957) Biological Flora of the British Isles. Ranunculus acris L. (R. acer auct. plur.) J. Ecol. 45, 289.

Hill, R. and van Heyingen, R. (1951) Ranunculin: The precursor of the vesicant substance of the Buttercup. Biochem. J. 49, 332.

Ruijgrok, H.W.L. (1966) Distribution of ranunculin and cyanogenetic compounds in the Ranunculaceae in Comparative Phytochemistry. ed. Swain; T. London. Academic Press. p. 175.

Shearer, G.D. (1938) Some observations on the poisonous properties of buttercups. Vet. J. 94, 22.

White, J.C. (1887) Dermatitis venenata: An account of the action of external irritants upon the skin. Boston. Cupples and Hurd.

Winter, J.B. (1976) Severe urticarial reaction in a dog following ingestion of tall field buttercup. Vet. Med. Small Anim. Clin. 71(3), 307.

Tribe: Delphineae

Aconitum

300 species are found in north temperate regions.

Aconitum lycoctonum
(?Ranunculus)

Gerard (1636) stated that chewing a few of the flowers caused burning and swelling of the gums and tongue. He reported the case of a medical student who tasted a root that hogs had turned up; the student's mouth, tongue and lips swelled very extremely so that he could not speak.

Aconitum napellus
Monkshood, Wolfsbane

Application of ointment made from the plant to the intact skin produces itching and prickling without redness, (Dispensatory 1884) or redness and vesicles (Piffard 1881). The plant produced severe dermatitis in pharmaceutical workers (Lloyd 1887). When the juice is rubbed into the skin or applied to the mucous membranes, it causes a characteristic prickling and tingling sensation due to the presence of the alkaloid, aconitine (Swanson et al 1938, Behl et al 1966).

Among the symptoms of poisoning by ingestion of the plant are tingling and a burning sensation in the tongue, throat and skin (Sollman 1957). The alkaloids of the plants are described by Willaman and Schubert (1961).

References

Behl, P.N., Captain, R.M., Bedi, B.M.S. and Gupta, S. (1966) Skin-irritant and sensitizing plants found in India, New Delhi. P.N. Behl, Irwin Hospital.

Dispensatory (United States) (1884) cited by White (1887).

Gerard, J. (1636) The Herball or Generall Historie of Plantes. The essence thereof distilled by M. Woodward (1927) from the edition of Th. Johnson (1630). London. Gerald Howe.

Lloyd (1887) cited by White (1887). Lloyd was a dealer in medicinal plants.

Piffard, H.G. (1881) A treatise on the Materia Medica and Therapeutics of the Skin. New York. Wm. Wood and Co.

Sollman, T.H. (1957) A manual of pharmacology. 8th ed. Philadelphia. W.B. Saunders Co.

Swanson, E.E., Youngken, H.W., Zufall, C.V. et al (1938) Aconitum. Am. Pharmaceut. Assoc. Monogr. 1.

White, J.C. (1887) Dermatitis venenata: An account of the action of external irritants upon the skin. Boston. Cupples and Hurd.

Willaman, J.J. and Schubert, B.C. (1961) Alkaloid-bearing plants and their contained alkaloids. U.S. Department of Agr. Tech. Bull. 1234.

Aconitum neomontanum

The plant when applied to the skin has a vesicant action (Piffard 1881).

Reference

Piffard, H.G. (1881) A treatise on the Materia Medica and Therapeutics of the skin. New York. Wm. Wood and Co.

Tribe: Helleboreae

Actaea

Ten species are found in north temperate regions.

Actaea alba
White baneberry

Actaea rubra
Red baneberry

The root stock, sap and berries of the plants are markedly irritant when eaten (Youngken and Karas 1964).

Actaea spicata
Herb Christopher,
Bane berry

The rhizome was formerly officinal as Radix Christophorianae for the treatment of skin disease. The plant has a vesicant effect (Piffard 1881).

References

Piffard, H.G. (1881) A treatise on the Materia Medica and Therapeutics of the skin. New York. Wm. Wood and Co.

Youngken, H.W. Jr. and Karas, J.S. (1964) Common Poisonous Plants of New England. Publ. Health Service Publ. No. 1220. U.S. Gov't Printing Office. Washington, D.C.

Tribe: Ranunculeae

Adonis

20 species are found in northern palaeotemperate regions.

Adonis aestivalis

A. amurensis

A. vernalis

These species were noted to be irritant by Pammel (1911). *A. vernalis* was formerly used as a cardiac stimulant (Merck Index 1968).

References

Merck Index (1968) An Encyclopedia of Chemicals and Drugs. ed. Stecher, P.G. 8th ed. Rahway, N.J. Merck and Co. Inc.

Pammel, L.H. (1911) A Manual of Poisonous plants. Torch Press. Cedar Rapids, Iowa. Reprinted Univ. Microfilms Inc. Ann Arbor, Mich. 1965. pp. 476-7.

Tribe: Anemonaea

Anemone

150 species are cosmopolitan. The achenes of many species have hairs which aid wind dispersal. Gerard (1597) noted that "All the kinds of Anemones are sharp, biting the tongue..."

Anemone apennina

Anemone coronaris

These species are irritant (Pammel 1911). Anemone cernua is noted under Pulsatilla.

Anemone cylindrica (and probably also A. multifida)

A poultice made of the plant causes violent blistering when applied to the skin for 10-20 minutes (Turner and Bell 1973).

Anemone hepatica (syn. Hepatica) Liver leaf

The plant which is used in Herbal Medicine (Wren 1968) is listed as irritant (Schwartz et al 1957).

Anemone narcissiflora

The leaves are eaten as cress, soured or prepared in oil by the Eskimos of King Island, Alaska (Uphof 1959).

Anemone nemorosa
Wood anemone, Windflower

Four cases of severe vesicular dermatitis were observed following application of the leaves to the skin for rheumatism (Frenzl 1937). The plant ground and applied to the knees for rheumatism produced second degree "burns" and residual hyperpigmentation (Spengler 1946). The plant is irritant (Builliard 1780, Piffard 1881, Pammel 1911, Dufke 1930). Piffard (1881) cited authors who stated that A. nemorosa (and also A. patens) were capable of producing redness, vesicles and even ulcers when applied to the skin. White (1887) stated that he had not known this plant to cause trouble to anyone handling it although it was of wide occurrence and one of the earliest and most plucked wildflowers of spring.

Anemone obtusifolia
Wind-flower

The root of the plant, which is very acrid, is used as a blistering agent in India (Behl et al 1966).

Anemone patens

The leaves are mashed up and put on boils and bruises for an irritant (blistering) effect. The plant burns the mouth (Turner 1975).

References

Behl, P.N., Captain, R.M., Bedi, B.M.S. and Gupta, S. (1966) Skin-irritant and asnsitizing plants found in India, New Delhi. P.N. Behl, Irwin Hospital.

Builliard (1780) Histoire des Plantes Veneneuses et Suspectes de la France. Paris. cited by Woods, B. (1962).

Dufke (1930) Dermatitis externa nach Buschwindroschen. Med. Klin. 2, 1060, cited by Touton (1932).

Frenzl, F. (1937) Artificial dermatitis caused by Anemone nemorosa. Casop. lek. cesk. 76, 1831.

Gerard, J. (1597) The Historie of Plantes. London. cited by Woods, B. (1962).

Pammel, L.H. (1911) A Manual of Poisonous plants. Torch Press. Cedar Rapids, Iowa. Reprinted Univ. Microfilms Inc. Ann Arbor, Mich. 1965. pp. 476-7.

Piffard, H.G. (1881) A treatise on the Materia Medica and Therapeutics of the Skin. New York. Wm. Wood and Co.

Schwartz, L., Tulipan, L. and Birmingham, D.J. (1957) Occupational Diseases of the Skin. 3rd ed. Philadelphia. Lea and Febiger. pp. 637-672.

Spengler, F. (1946) Die therapeutische Verwend ung der _Anemone nemorosa_ des Buschwindroschers. Pharmazie _1_, 222.

Touton, K. (1932) Hauterkrankunden durch phanerogamische Pflanzen und ihre Produkte (Toxicodermia et Allergodermia phytogenes), in Barnewitz, J. et al Angeborene Anomalien, Lichtdermatosen, Pflanzengifte, Thermische Schadidgungen, Einfluss Innerer Storungen auf die Haut. Berlin, Verlag von Julius Springer.

Turner, N.C. and Bell, M.A.M. (1973) The ethnobotany of the southern Kwakiutl Indians of British Columbia. Economic Botany _27_, 257.

Turner, N. (1975) Ethnobotany of the Upper Kootenay Indians of Cranbrook and Tobacco Plains, British Columbia (by personal communication).

Uphof, J.C.Th. (1959) Dictionary of Economic Plants. New York. Hafner Publ. Co.

White, J.C. (1887) Dermatitis venenata: An account of the action of external irritants upon the skin. Boston. Cupples and Hurd.

Woods, B. (1962) Irritant plants. Trans. St. John's Hosp. Derm. Soc. _48_, 75.

Wren, R.W. (1968) Potter's New Cyclopaedia of Botanical Drugs and Preparations by Wren, R.C. Re-edit. by Wren, R.W. Potter and Clarke Ltd. Health Science Press. Rustington, Sussex.

Anemone patens
var. _wolfgangiana_
(syn. _Pulsatilla_)
Pasque flower, Wild Crocus

Aaron and Muttitt (1964) provided a detailed case-report of bullous dermatitis which resulted from compresses of the leaves. Patch tests to the plant applied for 20-60 minutes produced vesicular reactions in volunteers. Hyperpigmentation appeared at the test sites. They also noted irritation of the conjunctiva and nasal mucosa from the vapour of the crushed stems and leaves. The plant yields a vesicant substance, previously named anemone camphor, soluble in ether and chlorophorm and possessing an intensely irritant vapour (British Pharmaceutical Codex 1934). Pammel (1911) and Murphy (1959) noted irritation from the plant. Pulsatilla, a preparation of _Anemone_ spp. (Merck Index 1968) was formerly used medicinally and had irritant effects (Oesterlen 1856, Piffard 1881, Dispensatory 1884).

References

Aaron, T.H. and Muttitt, E.L.C. (1964) Vesicant dermatitis due to prairie crocus (_Anemone patens_ L.). Archs. Derm. _90_, 168.

British Pharmaceutical Codex (1934) London. Pharmaceutical Society of Great Britain.

Dispensatory (United States)(1884) cited by White (1887).

Merck Index (1968) An Encyclopedia of Chemicals and Drugs. ed. Stecher, P.G. 8th ed. Rahway, N.J. Merck and Co. Inc.

Murphy, E.V.A. (1959) Indian uses of native plants. Desert Printers Inc. Palm Desert, Calif.

Oesterlen (1856) Handbuch der Heilmittellehre. Tubigen, cited by White (1887).

Pammel, L.H. (1911) A Manual of Poisonous plants. Torch Press. Cedar Rapids, Iowa. Reprinted Univ. Microfilms Inc. Ann Arbor, Mich. 1965. pp. 476-7.

Piffard, H.G. (1881) A treatise on the Materia Medica and Therapeutics of the Skin. New York. Wm. Wood and Co.

White, J.C. (1887) Dermatitis venenata: An account of the action of external irritants upon the skin. Boston. Cupples and Hurd.

Anemone pratensis

The bruised fresh plant, when rubbed on the skin, is irritant and even vesicant (Dispensatory 1884).

Anemone pulsatilla
(syn. Pulsatilla vulgaris)

The plant is irritant (Pammel 1911, Perrot and Paris 1971).

Anemone quinquefolia

The plant is irritant (Weber 1930, 1937, Schwartz et al 1957).

Anemone ranunculoides

Anemone sylvestris

These species are listed as irritant (Pammel 1911).

References

Dispensatory (United States) (1884) cited by White (1887).

Pammel, L.H. (1911) A manual of poisonous plants. Torch Press. Cedar Rapids, Iowa. Reprinted Univ. Microfilms Inc. Ann Arbor, Mich. 1965. pp. 476-7.

Perrot, E. and Paris, R. (1971) Les plantes medicinales. 2 vols. Paris. Presses Universitaires de France. 245 (+XXVI(index)) pp.

Schwartz, L., Tulipan, L., and Birmingham, D.J. (1957) Occupational Diseases of the Skin. 3rd ed. Philadelphia. Lea and Febiger. pp. 637-672.

Weber, L.F. (1930) A list of cutaneous irritants. Archs. Derm. Syph. 21, 761.

Weber, L,F, (1937) External causes of dermatitis. A list of irritants. Archs. Derm. Syph. 35, 129.

White, J.C. (1887) Dermatitis venenata: an account of the action of external irritants upon the skin. Boston. Cupples and Hurd.

Tribe: Helleboreae

Aquilegia

100 species are found in north temperate regions.

Aquilegia vulgaris
Columbine

The plant is said to be irritant (Pammel 1911, Schwartz et al 1957).

References

Pammel, L.H. (1911) A manual of poisonous plants. Torch Press. Cedar Rapids, Iowa. Reprinted Univ. Microfilms Inc. Ann Arbor, Mich. 1965. pp. 476-7.

Schwartz, L., Tulipan, L. and Birmingham, D.J. (1957) Occupational Diseases of the Skin. 3rd ed. Philadelphia. Lea and Febiger. pp. 637-672.

Tribe: Helleboreae

Caltha

20 species are found in Arctic and north temperate regions, 12 in New Zealand and temperate South America.

Caltha palustris
Marsh Marigold, Kingcup

The juice is acrid and vesicant (Schwartz et al 1957, Behl et al 1966). Sniffing the bruised stems induces sneezing (Behl et al 1966).

Rutherfurd (undated) reported irritation in a girl who dressed her knee with a marsh-marigold instead of marsh-mallows.

References

Behl, P.N., Captain, R.M., Bedi, B.M.S. and Gupta, S. (1966) Skin-irritant and sensitizing plants found in India, New Delhi. P.N. Behl, Irwin Hospital.

Rutherfurd, N.J. (undated) An essay on the History and Pharmacology of the Ranunculaceae (unpublished) quoted by White (1934).

Schwartz, L., Tulipan, L. and Birmingham, D.J. (1957) Occupational Diseases of the Skin. 3rd ed. Philadelphia. Lea and Febiger. pp. 637-672.

White, R. (1934) The Dermatergoses or Occupational affections of the skin. 4th ed. London. H.K. Lewis.

Tribe: Clematideae

Clematis

250 species are cosmopolitan, chiefly temperate.

Clematis spp.

All the species of the genus are acrid and irritant (Dispensatory 1884, White 1887, Greshoff 1909). Lloyd (1887) stated that "in working Clematis for anemonin, our hands were blistered several times". Sniffing the powdered leaf or bruised stem induces sneezing (Watt and Breyer-Brandwijk 1962, Behl et al 1966).

References

Behl, P.N., Captain, R.M., Bedi, B.M.S. and Gupta, S. (1966) Skin-irritant and sensitizing plants found in India, New Delhi. P.N. Behl, Irwin Hospital.

Dispensatory (United States) (1884) cited by White (1887).

Greshoff, M. (1909) Phytochemical investigations at Kew. Kew Bull. 10, 397.

Lloyd (1887) cited by White (1887). Lloyd was a dealer in medicinal plants.

Watt, J.M. and Breyer-Brandwijk, M.G. (1962) The medicinal and poisonous plants of Southern Africa. 2nd ed. Edinburgh. E.& S. Livingstone.

White, J.C. (1887) Dermatitis venenata: an account of the action of external irritants upon the skin. Boston. Cupples and Hurd.

Clematis brachiata

When chewed, the leaf produces a burning sensation in the mouth (Watt and Breyer-Brandwijk 1962).

Reference

Watt. J.M. and Breyer-Brandwijk, M.G. (1962) The medicinal and poisonous plants of Southern Africa. 2nd ed. Edinburgh. E.& S. Livingstone.

Clematis caripensis

This species is irritant (Pammel 1911).

Reference

Pammel, L.H. (1911) A manual of poisonous plants. Torch Press. Cedar Rapids, Iowa. Reprinted Univ. Microfilms Inc. Ann Arbor, Mich. 1965. pp. 476-7.

Clematis dioica

The crushed leaves have vesicant properties and proximity to the plant can cause dermatitis in "susceptible" individuals (Allen 1943).

Reference

Allen, P.H. (1943) Poisonous and injurious plants of Panama. Am. J. Trop. Med. Suppl. 23, 1.

Clematis erecta

The plant is acrid and irritant (Dispensatory 1884).

Reference

Dispensatory (United States) (1884) cited by White (1887).

White, J.C. (1887) Dermatitis venenata: an account of the action of external irritants upon the skin. Boston. Cupples and Hurd.

Clematis erecta

Application of the plant to the skin caused vesicles and ulcers (Piffard 1881).

Clematis vitalba

Application of the plant to the skin produces redness, vesication and ulcers (Piffard 1881).

Reference

Piffard, H.G. (1881) A treatise on the Materia Medica and Therapeutics of the skin. New York. Wm. Wood and Co.

Clematis florida

This species is irritant (Pammel 1911).

Reference

Pammel, L.H. (1911) A manual of poisonous plants. Torch Press. Cedar Rapids, Iowa. Reprinted Univ. Microfilms Inc. Ann Arbor, Mich. 1965. pp. 476-7.

Clematis glycinoides

The plant produces vesication on prolonged contact with the skin and is irritant to the nasal passages if inhaled (Hurst 1942, Everist 1972).

References

Everist, S.L. (1972) Queensland Herbarium, Brisbane, Australia. Personal communication concerning plants recorded in Australia as having caused dermatitis or other contact injury to man or livestock.

Hurst, E. (1942) The poisonous plants of New South Wales. N.S.W. Poison Plants Committee; Sydney.

Clematis gouriana

The plant is irritant (Pammel 1911). The juice of freshly crushed leaves and stems has a vesicant action (Behl et al 1966).

References

Behl, P.N., Captain, R.M., Bedi, B.M.S. and Gupta, S. (1966) Skin-irritant and sensitizing plants found in India, New Delhi. P.N. Behl, Irwin Hospital.

Pammel, L.H. (1911) A manual of poisonous plants. Torch Press. Cedar Rapids, Iowa. Reprinted Univ. Microfilms Inc. Ann Arbor, Mich. 1965. pp. 476-7.

Clematis grandiflora (?C. grandifolia)

The juice of the plant is irritant (Dalziel 1937) and the leaves are used as a vesicant in Africa (Irvine 1961).

References

Dalziel, J.M. (1937) The useful plants of West Tropical Africa. London. Crown Agents.

Irvine, F.R. (1961) Woody plants of Ghana. Oxford University Press. London.

Clematis lanuginosa

This species is irritant (Pammel 1911).

Reference

Pammel, L.H. (1911) A manual of poisonous plants. Torch Press. Cedar Rapids, Iowa. Reprinted Univ. Microfilms Inc. Ann Arbor, Mich. 1965. pp. 476-7.

Clematis microphylla

The natives of the Encounter Bay region of Australia are said to have known of the capacity of this plant to produce irritation. Poultices of the leaves were used by European settlers as counter-irritants. If applied for too long (e.g. seven instead of three minutes) such poultices caused irritation and then blistering which appeared 12 hours after the application (Cleland 1931).

Reference

Cleland, J.B. (1931) Plants including fungi, poisonous or otherwise injurious to man in Australia III. Med. J. Australia 2, 775.

Clematis nepaulensis

Clematis orientalis

The juice of freshly crushed leaves and stems of these species has vesicant properties (Behl et al 1966).

Reference

Behl, P.N., Captain, R.M., Bedi, B.M.S. and Gupta, S. (1966) Skin-irritant and sensitizing plants found in India, New Delhi. P.N. Behl, Irwin Hospital.

Clematis paniculata

The plant was used to produce blisters for counter-irritant purposes in indigenous New Zealand Medicine (Brooker and Cooper 1961).

Reference

Brooker, S.G. and Cooper, R.C. (1921) New Zealand Medicinal Plants. Economic Botany 15, 1.

Clematis recta

The plant was used as a vesicant (Turnbull 1838).

Reference

Turnbull, A. (1838) The Medicinal Properties of the Natural Order Ranunculaceae and more particularly of the uses of sabadilla seeds, Delphinium staphisagria and Aconitum napellus and their alcaloids. Philadelphia. Haswell, Barrington and Haswell.

Clematis sinensis

In the Congo, the leaf is use as a counter irritant (Watt and Breyer-Brandwijk 1962).

Reference

Watt, J.M. and Breyer-Brandwijk, M.G. (1962) The medicinal and poisonous plants of Southern Africa. 2nd ed. Edinburgh. E.& S. Livingstone.

Clematis triloba

The juice of freshly crushed leaves and stems has vesicant properties (Behl et al 1966).

Reference

Behl, P.N., Captain, R.M., Bedi, B.M.S. and Gupta, S. (1966) Skin-irritant and sensitizing plants found in India, New Delhi. P.N. Behl, Irwin Hospital.

Clematis virginiana
Virgin's Bower

Twelve cases of recurrent eczematous dermatitis were attributed to this plant. Bullous patch test reactions were observed as early as eight hours (Lancaster 1937).

Reference

Lancaster, A.H. (1937) Clematis dermatitis. South Med. J. 30, 207.

Clematis vitalba
Traveller's Joy,
Old Man's Beard

The juice, when rubbed on the skin, will raise blisters and chewing the leaves produces ulcers in the mouth (North 1967).

This plant has increased tremendously in the United Kingdom in recent years and few chalkland hedgerows are now free of it. It seems to thrive on careless stubble burning, judging by the way it colonises scorched hedges (Seymour 1973).

References

North, P.M. (1967) Poisonous plants and fungi in colour. London. Blandofr Press Ltd.

Seymour, W. (1973) Five foes of the forester. Country Life 158, 510.

Clematis (syn. Naravelia) spp are suspected of poisonousness (Burkill 1935).

Reference

Burkill, I.H. (1935) A dictionary of the economic products of the Malay Peninsula. 2 Vols. London. Crown Agents for the Colonies.

Tribe: Delphinieae

Delphinium

250 species are found in north temperate regions.

Delphinium spp.

The seeds have long been used as an insecticide (Watt and Breyer-Brandwijk 1962). Willaman and Schubert (1961) describe the alkaloids from the plants.

References

Watt, J.M. and Breyer-Brandwijk, M.G. (1962) The Medicinal and poisonous plants of Southern Africa. 2nd ed. Edinburgh. E.& S. Livingstone.

Willaman, J.J. and Schubert, B.G. (1961) Alkaloid-bearing plants and their contained alkaloids. U.S. Dept. of Agr. Tech. Bull. 1234.

Delphinium ajacis
Larkspur

The powdered seeds are found in some commercial lice remedies (Youngken and Karas 1964). A fluid extract of the plant, which is used as a parasiticide in India, produced local irritation (Chopra et al 1958). Both seed and leaf can produce dermatitis (Watt and Breyer-Brandwijk 1962, Behl et al 1966).

References

Behl, P.N., Captain, R.M., Bedi, B.M.S. and Gupta, S. (1966) Skin-irritant and sensitizing plants found in India, New Delhi. P.N. Behl, Irwin Hospital.

Chopra, R.N., Chopra, I.C., Handa, K.L. and Kapur, L.D. (1958) Chopra's Indigenous Drugs of India. ed. 2. U.S. Dhur & Sons Ltd., Calcutta.

Watt, J.M. and Breyer-Brandwijk, M.G. (1962) The Medicinal and poisonous plants of Southern Africa. 2nd ed. Edinburgh. E.& S. Livingstone.

Youngken, H.W. Jr. and Karas, J.S. (1964) Common poisonous plants of New England. Publ. Health Service Publ. No. 1220. U.S. Gov't Printing Office, Washington, D.C.

Delphinium brunonianum

Delphinium caeruleum

The leaves and seeds of these species are irritant (Chopra et al 1958).

Reference

Chopra, R.N., Chopra, I.C., Handa, K.L. and Kapur, L.D. (1958) Chopra's Indigenous Drugs of India. Ed. 2. U.N. Dhur and Sons Ltd. Calcutta.

Delphinium consolida

A tincture of the seeds, used to destroy head lice, is bitter and acrid (Wren 1968).

An extract from the plant was vesicant (Van Hasselt 1862) and produced great burning and inflammation when applied to the skin (Oesterlen 1856). An ointment containing 'delphinin' derived from the plant, when rubbed upon the skin, caused burning, prickling and a transitory redness such as veratrin occasioned (Dispensatory 1884). (Veratrine is derived from *Schoenocaulon*.)

References

Dispensatory (United States) (1884) cited by White (1887).

Oesterlen (1856) cited by White (1887).

Van Hasselt (1862) cited by White (1887).

White, J.C. (1887) Dermatitis venenata: An account of the action of external irritants upon the skin. Boston. Cupples and Hurd.

Wren, R.W. (1968) Potter's New Cyclopaedia of Botanical Drugs and Preparations by Wren, R.C. Re-edit. by Wren, R.W. Potter and Clarke Ltd. Health Science Press. Rustington, Sussex.

Delphinium elatum

The leaves and seeds can produce dermatitis (Chopra et al 1958).

Reference

Chopra, R.N., Chopra, I.C., Handa, K.L. and Kapur, L.D. (1958) Chopra's Indigenous Drugs of India. Ed. 2. U.N. Dhur and Sons Ltd. Calcutta.

Delphinium staphisagria
Staves-acre

The juice has been used as an insecticide since Ancient times. The taste of the seeds is bitter and tingling (Wren 1968). An alcoholic solution from the seeds was applied to the heads of several children as a pediculicide. One child developed acute dermatitis of the face and hands three days after the application (Shattuck, no date).

References

Shattuck, F.C. Personal communication to White (1887).

White, J.C. (1887) Dermatitis venenata: An account of the action of external irritants upon the skin. Boston. Cupples and Hurd.

Wren, R.W. (1968) Potter's New Cyclopaedia of Botanical Drugs and Preparations by Wren, R.C. Re-edit. by Wren, R.W. Potter and Clarke Ltd. Health Science Press. Rustington, Sussex.

Delphinium vestatum

The leaves and seeds can produce dermatitis (Chopra et al 1958).

Reference

Chopra, R.N., Chopra, I.C., Handa, K.L. and Kapur, L.D. (1958) Chopra's Indigenous Drugs of India. ed. 2. U.N. Dhur and Sons Ltd. Calcutta.

Delphinium uncinatum

The plant is irritant (Pammel 1911).

Reference

Pammel, L.H. (1911) A Manual of Poisonous plants. Torch Press. Cedar Rapids, Iowa. Reprinted Univ. Microfilms Inc. Ann Arbor, Mich. 1965. pp. 476-7.

Tribe: Helleboreae

Eranthis

Seven species are found in north palaeotemperate regions.

Eranthis hyemalis
Winter Aconite

The burning taste of the plant often prevents animals from eating it (North 1967).

Reference

North, P.M. (1967) Poisonous Plants and Fungi in Colour. London. Blandford Press Ltd.

Tribe: Helleboreae

Helleborus
Hellebore

20 species are found from Europe and the Mediterranean region to the Caucasus; one species is found in western China.

The common name Hellebore has given rise to confusion since Ancient times. Theophrastus (300 B.C.) stated that "The white and black Hellebore appear to have nothing in common except the name." White or False Hellebore is Veratrum, Liliaceae. It turns out that the plants have in common a content of biologically active alkaloids (Osol and Farrar 1955).

Helleborus niger
Black Hellebore,
Christmas Rose

Dioscorides (1st Century A.D.), Cornevin (1887), Piffard (1881) and Meunscher (1951) refer to an irritant action of the bruised root-stocks and of the leaves.

Helleborus odoris

The powdered root is irritant to the eye (Duke-Elder and MacFaul 1972).

References

Cornevin, C. (1887) Des Plantes Venenueses et des Empoisonments qu'elles determinent. Paris. Firmin-Didot.

Dioscorides, The Greek Herbal Of: Englished by John Goodyer: A.D. 1655. Edited and First printed A.D. 1933 by R.T. Gunther. 1959. New York. Hafner Publishing Co.

Duke-Elder, S. and MacFaul (1972) System of Opthalmology Vol. XVI. Injuries Part 2. Non-mechanical injuries. Irritant Vegetable Products, pp. 1180-1196, and Self-inflicted injuries, pp. 1016-1018. London. Henry Kimpton.

Muenscher, W.C. (1951) Poisonous plants of the United States. 2nd ed. New York. The Macmillan Co.

Osol, A. and Farrar, G.E. (1955) The Dispensatory of the United States of America. 25th ed. Philadelphia. Lippincott.

Piffard, H.G. (1881) A treatise on the Materia Medica and Therapeutics of the Skin. New York. Wm. Wood and Co.

Tribe: Ranunculeae

Knowltonia

Ten species are found in South Africa.

Knowltonia rigida

The plant has vesicant properties (Watt and Breyer-Brandwijk 1962).

Knowltonia transvaalensis

The plant has vesicant properties but the leaf, when dried, loses its irritant property (Watt and Breyer-Brandwijk 1962).

Knowltonia vesicatoria

The plant is used as a vesicant (Turnbull 1838).

References

Thrubull, A. (1838) The Medical Properties of the Natural Order Ranunculaceae and more particularly of the uses of Sabadilla seeds, Delphinium staphisagria and Aconitum napellus and their alkaloids. Philadelphia. Haswell, Barrington and Haswell.

Watt. J.M. and Breyer-Brandwijk, M.G. (1962) The Medicinal and poisonous plants of Southern Africa. 2nd ed. Edinburgh. E.& S. Livingstone.

Tribe: Helleboreae

Nigella

20 species are found from Europe and the Mediterranean region to Central Asia.

Nigella sativa
Black Cumin

The plant when blown into the nose through a tube, induces sneezing. This species was reported to be the ultimate therapeutic agent for according to the Arabian proverb, "In the black seed is the medicine for everything except death" (Levey and Al-Khaledy 1967).

Reference

Levey, M. and Al-Khaledy, N. (1967) The Medical Formulary of Al-Samarqandi and the relation of early Arabic simples to those found in the indigenous medicine of the near East and India. Philadelphia. University of Pennsylvania Press.

Pulsatilla
(syn. Anemone)

30 species are found in temperate Eurasia.

Pulsatilla cernua
(syn. Anemone cernua)

Anemomin was first isolated and named from this plant (Kariyone 1971).

Pulsatilla is noted under Anemone patens.

Pulsatilla vulgaris is noted under Anemone pulsatilla.

Reference

Kariyone, T. (1971) Atlas of Medicinal Plants. Osaka, Japan. Takeda Chemical Industries.

Tribe: Ranunculeae

Ranunculus

400 species are found in temperate and cold regions and on tropical mountains. R. asiaticus has been developed in horticulture in many varieties which make superb cut flowers.

Ranunculus spp.
Buttercup, Crowfoot

"Ranunculus...of this there are many kinds, but ye facultie is one, sharpe and too much exulcerating" (Dioscorides, 1st Century A.D.). Culpeper (1653) noted that the Common Crowfoot was sharp and biting to the taste and blistered the tongue; an ointment of the leaves or flowers would produce a blister on the skin. He described the untoward results of application of the juice to the scalp for the treatment of alopecia. Beggars used the plants to ulcerate their feet to arouse sympathy (North 1967). Sniffing the bruised stems induces sneezing (Behl et al 1966). Buttercups and mustard plants (Cruciferae) were suggested as the agents of a case of Oppenheim's meadow dermatitis (Ullmo 1930); probably irritancy rather than photosensitivity was responsible. Kuske (1937) reported a pemphigus-like eruption from a kind of Ranunculus.

Irritation from Ranunculus spp. was reported by Lacassagne and Joly (1927), Munch (1917) and Rodziewicz and Wlodarczyk (1961).

References

Behl, P.N., Captain, R.M., Bedi, B.M.S. and Gupta, S. (1966) Skin-irritant and sensitizing plants found in India, New Delhi. P.N. Behl, Irwin Hospital.

Culpeper, N. (1653) The Complete Herbal. Birmingham. Kynoch Press. (Imperial Chemical Ltd.).

Dioscorides, The Greek Herbal of: Englished by John Goodyer: A.D. 1655. Edited and first printed A.D. 1933 by R.T. Gunther. 1959. New York. Hafner Publishing Co. 2, 206.

Kuske, H. (1937) Etiology and pathogenesis of meadow plant dermatitis. Schweiz. med. Wchnschr. 67, 117.

North, P.M. (1967) Poisonous plants and fungi in colour. London. Blandford Press Ltd.

Ullmo, A. (1932) Dermatitis bullosa striata pratensis. Ann. Derm. Syph. Paris 3, 31.

Lacassagne, J. and Joly, H. (1927) La Jambe de Dieu. - Les ulceres des queux au XVI siecle. J. Med. Lyon 8, 177, 297.

Munch, W.A. (1917) Dermatitis bullosa durch Hahnenfubgift. Schweiz. Korresp. bl. Nr. 8, cited by Touton (1932).

Touton, K. (1932) Hauterkrankungen durch phanerogamische Pflanzen und ihre Produkte (Toxicodermia et Allergodermia phytogenes), in Barnewitz, J. et al Angeborene Anomalien, Lichtdermatosen, Pflanzengifte, Thermische Schadidgungen, Einfluss Innerer Storungen auf die Haut. Berlin, Verlag von Julius Springer.

Rodziewicz, J. and Wlodarczyk, S. (1961) Cutaneous changes caused by buttercups. Przegl. Derm. 48, (Suppl.) 429.

Ranunculus acer

This species was implicated in two cases of dermatitis (Wendlberger 1935).

Reference

Wendlberger, L.J. (1935) Successful passive transmission of hypersensitivity to Ranunculus acer. Dermat. Wchnschr. 100, 141.

Ranunculus acris
Common Buttercup,
Blister Plant

The sap is vesicant (White 1887). Napoli (1917) described a factitial skin eruption simulating pemphigus seen among Italian troops. The extensor surfaces of the legs were most commonly affected, sometimes the arms or face, only once the back. Bullae were observed, varying in size from a hazel-nut to a turkey's egg, generally tense and full of lemon-yellow fluid, in some cases opalescent, never haemorrhagic, rarely purulent. Mingled with the bullae were small vesicles, in some cases confluent, in others disseminated over large patches of papular erythema resembling eczema. The affection lasted a week or longer if secondary infection occurred. The affection which appeared in epidemic form among men from the same region was found to be produced by the application of a paste made by the trituration of R. acris which was growing abundantly in the territory occupied by the regiments in which the eruption appeared. The leaves and seeds are used externally as blisters and counter-irritants in Chinese Medicine (Smith 1969). The burning sensation produced on the skin by this plant is more severe than that produced by Trautvetteria (Smith 1928).

References

Napoli, F. de (1917) Artificial pemphigus. Policlinico June 10, 1917. abstr. Brit. Med. J. 2, 14, 1917.

Smith, F.P. (1969) Chinese Materia Medical Vegetable kingdom, 2nd ed. Rev. by Hei, P.D. Taipei, Taiwan. Ku T'ing Book House.

Smith, H.I. (1928) Materia Medica of the Bella Coola and neighbouring tribes of British Columbia. Bull. No. 56 National Museum of Canada. Ottawa. King's Printer. pp. 47-68.

White, J.C. (1887) Dermatitis venenata: An account of the action of external irritants upon the skin. Boston. Cupples and Hurd.

Ranunculus arvensis
Field Crowfoot

In India, professional beggars and malingerers often use this plant to disfigure themselves with blisters (Behl et al 1966).

Reference

Behl, P.N., Captain, R.M., Bedi, B.M.S. and Gupta, S. (1966) Skin-irritant and sensitizing plants found in India, New Delhi. P.N. Behl, Irwin Hospital.

Ranunculus bulbosus

The sap (North 1967), leaves, flowers, buds and roots are irritant (White 1887). Spillman and Weiss (1931) implicated this species in Oppenheim's meadow dermatitis but probably irritancy rather than photosensitivity was responsible.

References

North, P.M. (1967) Poisonous plants and fungi in colour. London. Blandford Press Ltd.

Spillman, L. and Weiss (1931) Dermites vesicantes d'origine végétale. Bull. Soc. franc. Derm. Syph. 38, 1095.

White, J.C. (1887) Dermatitis venenata: An account of the action of external irritants upon the skin. Boston. Cupples and Hurd.

Ranunculus californicus

The plant is irritant (Weber 1937).

Reference

Weber, L.F. (1937) External causes of Dermatitis. A list of irritants. Archs Derm. Syph. 35, 129.

Ranunculus bulbosus

Vesicles and bullae occurred on the lower limbs of a girl, aged 5 years, who took a handful of buttercups to bed with her. The crushed plants were discovered between the bed-sheets (Garraway 1861).

Reference

Garraway, E. (1861) Cutaneous eruption produced by buttercups. Brit. Med. J. 1, 874.

Ranunculus cassius

Ranunculus falcatus

These species are used in the same way as R. arvensis (Behl et al 1966).

Reference

Behl, P.N., Captain, R.M., Bedi, B.M.S. and Gupta, S. (1966) Skin-irritant and sensitizing plants found in India, New Delhi. P.N. Behl, Irwin Hospital.

Ranunculus ficaria
Pilewort

The sap is irritant (North 1967). The British Pharmaceutical Codex (1934) contained a formulae for Pilewort ointment. The plant is applied to haemorrhoids for an astringent effect (Wren 1968).

References

British Pharmaceutical Codex (1934) London. Pharmaceutical Society of Great Britain.

North, P.M. (1967) Poisonous plants and fungi in colour. London. Blandford Press Ltd.

Wren, R.W. (1968) Potter's New Cyclopaedia of Botanical Drugs and Preparations by Wren, R.C. Re-edit. by Wren, R.W. Potter and Clarke Ltd. Health Science Press. Rustington, Sussex.

Ranunculus flammula
Sciatic weed

A woman developed inflammation and ulceration of the skin of the thigh after applying this plant to the part (Rutherfurd, unpublished quote by White 1928). The sap is irritant (North 1967, Hurst 1942).

References

Hurst, E. (1942) The Poison plants of New Wouth Wales. N.S.W. Poison Plants Committee; Sydney.

North, P.M. (1967) Poisonous plants and fungi in colour. London. Blandford Press.

White, R.P. (1928) The dermatergoses or occupational affections of the skin. 3rd ed. London. H.K. Lewis and Co. Ltd.

Ranunculus glaberrimus

The leaves, smashed up and dampened with water, caused blistering when applied to sore joints (Turner 1975).

Reference

Turner, N.J. (1975) Ethnobotany of the upper Kootenay Indians of Cranbrook and Tobacco Plains, British Columbia (in preparation).

Ranunculus multifidus

The plant is acrid and burning, when chewed, and irritant to the skin and eyes. It produces stomatitis in animals who eat it (Watt and Breyer-Brandwijk 1962).

Reference

Watt, J.H. and Breyer-Brandwijk, M.G. (1962) The medicinal and poisonous plants of Southern Africa. 2nd ed. Edinburgh. E.& S. Livingstone.

Ranunculus muricatus
Routh-seeded Buttercup

This species is regarded as intensely acrid (Ewart 1909).

Reference

Ewart, A.J. (1909) The weeds, poison plants and naturalized aliens of Victoria. Melbourne, quoted by Hurst (1942).

Hurst, E. (1942) The Poison plants of New South Wales. N.S.W. Poison Plants Committee; Sydney.

Ranunculus occidentalis
sp. occidentalis

The plant has vesicant properties (Turner 1970).

Reference

Turner, N. (1970) The ethnobotany of the Haida Indians of the Queen Charlotte Islands. Unpublished thesis.

Ranunculus parviflorus
Small-flowered Buttercup

The plant is irritant (Hurst 1942).

Reference

Hurst, E. (1942) The Poison plants of New South Wales. N.S.W. Poison Plants Committee; Sydney.

Ranunculus pennsylvanicus
Great Spearwort

The plant is used in the same way as *R. arvensis* (Behl et al 1966).

Reference

Behl, P.N., Captain, R.M., Bedi, B.M.S. and Gupta, S. (1966) Skin-irritant and sensitizing plants found in India, New Delhi. P.N. Behl, Irwin Hospital.

Ranunculus petiolaris

The irritant action of the plant is similar to that of cantharidin but more delayed (Martinez 1969).

Reference

Martinez, M. (1969) The medicinal plants of Mexico. 5th ed. (Quinta edicion 5th Mexican language). Mexico City. Andres Botas.

Ranunculus repens

The sap is irritant (North 1967). Inflammation of the skin of the palms can result from pulling the plant by hand (White 1887).

References

North, P.M. (1967) Poisonous plants and fungi in colour. London. Blandford Press Ltd.

White, J.C. (1887) Dermatitis venenata: An account of the action of external irritants upon the skin. Boston. Cupples and Hurd.

Ranunculus sceleratus
Cursed Crowfoot,
Celery-leaved Buttercup

The plant is vesicant and has been used as a medicinal vesicatory since Ancient times; cattle will not eat the fresh plants; when dried in hay they produce no harm (White 1887).

The plant is intensely irritant and can produce violent blistering particularly of the lips and tongue and also of the skin (Shelmire 1940, Weber 1937, Pammel, 1911, Georgia 1914, Fyles 1920, Lander 1926). The plant can be mistaken for parsley (*Petroselinum*) or celery (*Apium*) and eaten with untoward results (North 1967). The plant is used as a counter-irritant and for the treatment of vitiligo in Egypt. The leaves and stem of fresh plants yield seven tryptamine derivatives, one of which is 5-hydroxytryptamine (Bhargava et al 1965).

References

Bhargava, K.P. et al (1965) Identification of tryptamine derivatives in *Ranunculus sceleratus* L. Brit. J. Pharmacol. 25, 743.

Fyles, F. (1920) Principal poisonous plants of Canada. Dominion of Canada, Dept. Agr. Expt. Farms Bull. ser. 2, 39.

Georgia, A. (1914) Manual of Weeds. New York, cited by Hurst (1942).

Hurst, E. (1942) The poison plants of New South Wales. N.S.W. Poison Plants Committee; Sydney.

Lander, G.D. (1926) Veterinary Toxicology. 2nd ed. London, cited by Hurst (1942).

North, P.M. (1967) Poisonous plants and fungi in colour. London. Blandford Press Ltd.

Pammel, L.H. (1911) A manual of poisonous plants. Torch Press. Cedar Rapids, Iowa. Reprinted Univ. Microfilms Inc. Ann Arbor, Mich. 1965. pp. 476-7.

Saber, A.H., Mahran, G.H. and El-Alfy, T. (1968) Phytochemical investigation of Ranunculus sceleratus L. Planta Medica 16, 231.

Shelmire, B. (1940) Contact dermatitis from vegetation. South Med. J. 33, 338.

Weber, L.F. (1937) External causes of Dermatitis. A list of irritants. Archs. Derm. Syph. 35, 129.

White, J.C. (1887) Dermatitis venenata: An account of the action of external irritants upon the skin. Boston. Cupples and Hurd.

Tribe: Ranunculeae

Thalictrum

150 species are found in north temperate regions, tropical South America, tropical and southern Africa.

Thalictrum spp.

Some species of this genus are irritant (Schwartz et al 1957). Ranunculin has not been found in Thalictrum spp. (Ruijgrok 1966).

Thalictrum foliolosum
Meadow Rue

Thalictrum minus

These species are irritant (Behl et al 1966).

References

Behl, P.N., Captain, R.M., Bedi, B.M.S. and Gupta, S. (1966) Skin-irritant and sensitizing plants found in India, New Delhi. P.N. Behl. Irwin Hospital.

Schwartz, L., Tulipan, L. and Birmingham, D.J. (1957) Occupational Diseases of the Skin. 3rd ed. Philadelphia. Lea and Febiger. pp. 637-672.

Ruijgrok, H.W.L. (1966) Distribution of ranunculin and cyanogenetic compounds in the Ranunculaceae in Comparative Phytochemistry. ed. Swain, T. London. Academic Press. p. 175.

Trautvetteria

One species is found in eastern Asia, Pacific North America and Mexico.

Trautvetteria caroliniensis
(syn. T. grandis)
False Bugbane

The roots when pounded with water and applied to the skin produce an intense burning sensation (Smith 1928).

Reference

Smith, H.I. (1928) Materia Medica of the Bella Coola and neighbouring tribes of British Columbia. Bull. No. 56. Natural Museum of Canada. Orrawa. King's Printer. pp. 47-68.

RESEDACEAE

70 species in 6 genera are chiefly found in the Mediterranean region but also from Europe to central Asia and India and in southern Africa and California.

The family is botanically related to Cruciferae and Cleomaceae which yield mustard oils.

Chemistry is recorded by Hegnauer (1973).

Reference

Hegnauer, R. (1973) Chemotaxonomy of plants. Vol. 6. Basel. Birkhauser, p. 51.

Reseda

60 species are found in Europe and from the Mediterranean region to central Asia. R. lutea (Dyer's Weed) yields a yellow dye.

Reseda odorata
Mignonette

The plant has rubefacient properties (Burkill 1935). This

plant and also R. lutea, R. luteola, and R. alba contain thioglucosides from which irritant 'mustard oils' (isothiocyanates) are derived (Kjaer 1960). Allergenicity of the plants is a possibility cf. Raphanus.

References

Burkill, I.H. (1935) A Dictionary of the Economic Products of the Malay Peninsula. 2 Vols. London. Crown Agents for the Colonies.

Khaer, A. (1960) Naturally derived isoThiocyanates (Mustard Oils) and their parent glucosides in Progress in the Chemistry of Organic Natural Products. ed. Sechmeister, L. Vol. 18. Vienna. Springer-Verlag. pp. 122-176.

RHAMNACEAE

900 species in 58 genera are cosmopolitan. Many are thorny.

Chemistry is recorded by Hegnauer (1973).

Reference

Hegnauer, R. (1973) Chemotaxonomy of plants. Vol. 6. Basel, Birkhauser. p. 56.

Alphitonia

20 species are found in Malaysia, Australia and Polynesia.

Alphitonia zizyphoides

The leaves, which are used as a substitute for soap, produce anhidrosis (Uhe 1974).

Reference

Uhe, G. (1974) Medicinal Plants of Samoa. Econ. Bot. 28, 1.

Ceanothus

55 species are found in North America. The root of C. americanus is used in Herbal Medicine for astringent effects. The thorns can cause mechanical injury.

Ceanothus velutinus
Sticky Laurel, Tea Bush

This species is listed as irritant (Weber 1937).

Reference

Weber, L.F. (1937) External causes of Dermatitis. A list of irritants. Arch. Derm. Syph. 35, 129.

Colubrina

24 species have a disjunct distribution in tropical and subtropical regions, notably in America.

Colubrina ferruginosa
Bois pelé, snakebark

The wood of this species is said to be irritant (Sandermann and Barghoorn 1956).

This West Indian wood was listed as a cause of vomiting, diarrhoea and cramps (Vorreiter 1949/1958).

References

Sandermann, W. and Barghoorn, A.W. (1956) Gesundheitsschadigende Nutzholzer. Holz. Roh-Werkst. 14, 37.

Vorreiter, L. (1949) Holztechnologisches Handbuch. Wein, Fromme (later edition 1958).

Rhamnus

Perhaps 160 species are cosmopolitan. Some yield dyes.

Rahmnus sp.
Coffee Berry, Buck-thorn

The genus is said to contain species the sap and fruit of which can cause dermatitis (McCord 1962).

Rhamnus californica

Rhamnus cathartica

These species are listed as irritant (Pammel 1911).

Rhamnus purshiana
Bearwood

The bark, Cascara Sagrada, yields the anthraquinone derivative emodin (Merck Index 1968). Dermatitis from emodin is noted under Aloe.

References

McCord, C.P. (1962) The Occupational Toxicity of Cultivated Flowers. Ind. Med. Surg. 31, 365.

Merck Index (1968). An Encyclopedia of Chemicals and Drugs. ed. Stecher, P.G. 8th ed. Rahway, N.J. Merck and Co. Inc.

Pammel, L.H. (1911) A Manual of Poisonous plants. Torch Press. Cedar Rapids, Iowa. Reprinted Univ. Microfilms Inc. Ann Arbor, Mich. 1965. pp. 476-7.

Ziziphus
(syn. Zizyphus)

100 species are found in tropical America, Africa, the Mediterranean region, Indo Malaysia and Australia. Some yield edible fruit (lotus, jujube).

Ziziphus mucronata
Buffalo Thorn

The thorny branches are used on burial sites to discourage grave-spoilers (Irvine 1961).

Ziziphus spina-christa

Application of the powdered leaves is said to darken and lengthen women's hair (Irvine 1961). The tree is said to have furnished the Crown of Thorns of the New Testament but Paliurus spina-christi and Euphorbia splendens have also been considered for this role.

Reference

Irvine, F.R. (1961) Woody Plants of Ghana. Oxford University Press. London.

RHIZOPHORACEAE

120 species in 16 genera are found in tropical regions.

Chemistry is recorded by Hegnauer (1973).

Reference

Hegnauer, R. (1973) Chemotaxonomy of plants. Vol. 6. Basel, Birkhauser. pp. 77.

Anopysix and Rhizophora spp. (Mangroves) are used for astringent purposes in Africa and China respectively (Irvine 1961, Smith 1969).

References

Irvine, F.R. (1961) Woody Plants of Ghana. Oxford University Press. London.

Smith, F.P. (1969) Chinese Materia Medica. Vegetable kingdom. 2nd ed. Rev. by Hei, P.D. Taipei, Taiwan. Ku T'ing Book House.

ROSACEAE

2000 species in 100 genera are of cosmopolitan distribution.

Chemistry is recorded by Hegnauer (1973).

Reference

Hegnauer, R. (1973) Chemotaxonomy of plants. Vol. 6. Basel, Birkhauser. p. 84.

Alchemilla

250 species are found in temperate regions and on tropical mountains.

Alchemilla
Lady's Mantle

The plant is used to produce haemostasis (Wren 1968).

Reference

Wren, R.W. (1968) Potter's New Cyclopaedia of Botanical Drugs and Preparations by Wren, R.C. Re-edit. by Wren. R.W. Potter and Clarke Ltd. Health Science Press. Rustington, Sussex.

Agrimonia

Fifteen species are found in north temperate regions.

Agrimonia eupatoria
Beggars' Ticks,
Stickle Wort, Agrimony

The fruit is covered with hooks hence the first colloquial name. A decoction of the root and leaf is used as a blistering agent in Africa (Watt and Breyer-Brandwijk 1962). The plant was incriminated in Oppenheim's meadow dermatitis (O'Donovan 1942) but has, at the most, only slight photosensitising activity (Van Dijk and Berrens 1964, Van Dijk 1964) suggesting that irritation rather than photodermatitis can result from contact.

References

O'Donovan, W.J. (1942) Dermatitis Bullosa Striata Pratensis. Agrimony Dermatitis. A Brit. J. Derm. Syph. 54, 39.

Van Dijk, E. (1963) Phytophotodermatitis. Excerpta Medica 18, 371.

Van Dijk, E. and Berrens, L. (1964) Plants as an etiological factor in dermatitis venenata due to plants. Dermatologica 129, 321.

Watt, J.M. and Breyer-Brandwijk, M.G. (1962) The Medicinal and poisonous plants of Southern Africa. 2nd ed. Edinburgh. E.& S. Livingstone.

Amygdalus
(syn. Prunus)

40 species are found from the Mediterranean region to Central China.

Amygdalus amygdalus
(syn. Prunus amygdalus)
Almond

This species and Prunus spp. yield Oil of Bitter Almond. Perfumes, colognes and toilet water containing the oil can cause dermatitis in hypersensitive individuals (Tulipan 1938). An additional note is recorded under Prunus amygdalus.

Reference

Tulipan, L. (1938) Cosmetic irritants. Archs. Derm. Syph. 38, 906.

Cotoneaster

50 species are found in north temperate regions. C. vulgaris is visited solely by a wasp whose nests are often attached to the rocks where the plant grows.

Cotoneaster microphylla

Four cases of urticaria from cutting hedges of this plant were reported by Cooper (1900).

References

Cooper (1900) Australia Med. Gaz. 20th January, abstr. Brit. J. Derm. (1900) 12, 183, cited by White (1928).

White, R.P. (1928) The Dermatergoses or Occupational Affections of the Skin. 3rd ed. London. H.K. Lewis and Co. Ltd.

Crataegus

200 species are found in north temperate regions.

Crataegus spp.
Hawthorn

The hairs from the fruit can cause nodose conjunctivitis (Duke-Elder and MacFaul 1972). The thorns are particularly toxic to the eye. Corneal scratches led to loss of useful vision in 88 cases in 132 such accidents in Ireland (Smith 1940). The thorns are less injurious than those of Prunus spinosa.

References

Duke-Elder, S. and MacFaul, P.A. (1972) System of Opthalmology. Vol. XIV. Injuries Part 1. Mechanical Injuries. Extra-ocular foreign bodies. pp. 464-67 and Agricultural Injuries pp. 32-34. London. Henry Kimpton.

Smith, F.P.E. (1940) Eye injuries in agriculture. Trans. Lphthalm. Soc. U.K. 60, 252.

Cydonia

One species is found in eastern Asia Minor, the Caucasus, northern Persia and central Asia.

Cydonia oblonga
(syn. Pyrus cydonia)

A mucilage surrounding the seeds and used in pharmaceutical preparations is considered to be a known allergen and is therefore removed from certain brand-name cosmetics (Schieffelin 1973).

Reference

Schieffelin, and Co. (1973) Almay Hypo-allergenic cosmetics product formulary 8th ed. Pharmaceutical Laboratories Division, 562 Fifth Ave., New York, N.Y. 10036.

Cydonia vulgaris
Quince

A female cannery-worker developed severe hand eczema. Angelica was at first suspected to be the cause but a patch test to wet quince hair (tomentum) which she cleaned from the fruits produced a positive reaction; dry quince tomentum produced no reaction. A patch test to zinc chlorate used in the vats also produced a positive reaction (Stauffer 1931).

Reference

Stauffer, H. (1931) Die Ekzemprobem. Archs. f. Dermat. 162, 517.

Fragaria

15 species are found in North America, Chile and from Eurasia to southern India. Several species are cultivated for their edible fruit.

Fragaria sp.
Strawberry

A gardener developed eczema from contact with strawberries and from eating the fruit (Gougerot et al 1931). A confectionery factory worker (and one of 102 controls) showed a positive patch test reaction to a natural strawberry flavouring (Hegyi 1971).

References

Gougerot, R., Cohen and Ganot (1931) Eczema externe et interne dû aux fraises par sensibilisation. Bull. Soc. franc. Derm. (July) 1136, cited by White (1934).

Hegyi, E. (1971) Contact sensitivity to flavourings. Contact Dermatitis Newsletter, London, 9, 206.

White, R.P. (1934) The Dermatergoses or Occupational Affections of the Skin. 4th ed. London. H.K. Lewis.

Geum

40 species are found in north and south temperate regions and in the Arctic.

Species of this genus have hooked fruits which attach themselves to animals (Howes 1974).

Geum arbanum
Herb Bennet, Colewort

The seeds are covered with hairs which fix themselves on passing objects (Wren 1968).

References

Howes, F.N. (1974) A Dictionary of Useful and Everyday Plants and their Common Names. Cambridge University Press. pp. 290.

Wren, R.W. (1968) Potter's New Cyclopaedia of Botanical Drugs and Preparations by Wren, R.C. Re-edit. by Wren, R.W. Potter and Clarke Ltd. Health Science Press. Rustington, Sussex.

Malus

35 species are found in north temperate regions.

Malus pumila
Common Apple

Women employed in cleaning apples and pears (Pyrus) developed dermatitis and fissured eczema of the hands and paronychia (Szego 1966). Schwartz et al (1957) reviewed dermatitis in the fruit-canning industry. Albertin (1889) and Erhart (1925) reported dermatitis from fruit. Apple peel was found to be responsible for a case of periocular eczema (Hazen 1944).

2-chloro,6-phenyl phenol (Stopmold) is a fungicide which has been used on fruit. It has caused sensitization dermatitis and its vapours are irritating to the eyes (Scott 1949). Sodium bisulfite used as an antioxidant to prevent discoloration of fruit and vegetables caused allergic contact dermatitis in a salad-maker; patch test with sodium bisulfite 10% aqueous produced a positive reaction, negative in controls (Epstein 1970). Ethoxyquin produced dermatitis in apple-packers (Wood and Fulton 1972).

References

Albertin (1889) Note sur le mal des confiseurs. Gaz. hebdom. 15 March, cited by Touton (1932).

Epstein, E. (1970) Sodium bisulfite. Contact Dermatitis Newsletter, London, 7, 155.

Erhart (1925) Uber ein akute Gewerbedermatitis. Arch. f. Derm. 148, 516, cited by Touton (1932).

Hazen, H.H. (1944) Dermatitis of the eyelids. Archs. Derm. Syph. 49, 253.

Schwartz, L., Tulipan, L. and Birmingham, D.J. (1957) Occupational Diseases of the Skin. 3rd ed. Philadelphia. Lea and Febiger. pp. 637-672.

Scott, N. (1949) 'Leftarm dermatitis'. Industr. Hyg. Newsletter 9, 9.

Szego, L. (1966) Data on skin conditions caused by apples and pears in women working in canning factories. Borgyogy. Vener. Szle. 42, 117.

Wood, W.S and Fulton, R. (1972) Dermatitis from ethoxyquin in apple packers. Contact Dermatitis Newsletter, London 11, 295.

Touton, K. (1932) Hauterkrankungen durch phanerogamische Pflanzen und ihre Produkte (Toxicodermia et Allergodermia phytogenes), in Barnewitz, J. et al Angeborene Anomalien, Lichtdermatosen, Pflanzengifte, Thermische Schadidgungen, Einfluss Innerer Storungen auf die Haut. Berlin, Verlag von Julius Springer.

Mespilus

One species is found from south-eastern Europe to Central Asia.

Mespilus germanica
Medlar

The fruit is commonly eaten when partially decomposed. Genner and Bonnevie (1938) refer to a report of dermatitis from the leaves of Dwarf Medlar.

Reference

Genner, V. and Bonnevie, P. (1938) Eczematous eruptions produced by leaves of trees and bushes. Archs. Derm. Syph. 37, 583.

Photinia

60 species are found from the Himalayas to Japan and Sumatra, and in North America.

Photinia glabra

The pickled fruits, if eaten in excess, make the mouth and tongue rough and crack open (Smith 1969).

Reference

Smith, F.P. (1969) Chinese Materia Medica. Vegetable kingdom. 2nd ed. Rev. by Hei, P.D. Taipei, Taiwan. Ku T'ing Book House.

Potentilla

500 species are nearly cosmopolitan in distribution.

Potentilla spp.

Several species have astringent and styptic actions and were used to remove freckles and actinic keratoses (Gerard 1636, Wren 1968).

References

Gerard, J. (1636) The Herball or Generall Historie of Plantes. The essence thereof distilled by M. Woodward (1927) from the edition of Th. Johnson 1630. London. Gerald Howe.

Wren, R.W. (1968) Potter's New Cyclopaedia of Botanical Drugs and Preparations by Wren, R.C. Re-edit. by Wren, R.W. Potter and Clarke Ltd. Health Science Press. Rustington, Sussex.

Prunus

430 species are cosmopolitan in distribution.

Prunus amygdalus
Almond

The chemistry of Oil of Bitter Almond and Oil of Sweet Almond (Jordan Almond) is given by Merck (1968). Almond oil was considered to be an allergen for atopic individuals (Coca et al 1931). Tulipan (1938), Greenberg and Lester (1954) and Klarmann (1958) list Oil of Bitter Almond as capable of producing dermatitis. Oil of Almond and a major constituent of the oil, benzaldehyde, are considered to be known allergens and therefore removed from certain brand-name cosmetics (Schieffelin 1973). A report of contact sensitivity to almond flour but not to any other kind of flour was noted by White (1934), probably Molesworth (1930).

References

Coca, A.F., Walzer, M. and Thommen, A.A. (1931) Asthma and hayfever in theory and practice. Springfield, Ill. Charles C. Thomas.

Greenberg, L.A. and Lester, D. (1954) Handbook of Cosmetic Materials. New York. Interscience.

Klarmann, E.G. (1958) Perfume dermatitis. Ann. Allergy. 16, 425.

Merck Index (1968) An Encyclopedia of Chemicals and Drugs. ed. Stecher, P.G. 8th ed. Rahway, N.J. Merck and Co. Inc.

Molesworth, E.A. (1930) Allergy applied to Dermatology. Urol. Cutan. Rev. Oct. p. 647, cited by White (1934).

Schieffelin and Co. (1973) Almay Hypo-allergenic cosmetics product formulary 8th ed. Pharmaceutical Laboratories Division, 562 Fifth Avenue, New York, N.Y. 10036.

Tulipan, L. (1938) Cosmetic irritants. Archs. Derm. Syph. 38, 906.

White, R.P. (1934) The Dermatergoses or Occupational Affections of the Skin. 4th ed. London. H.K. Lewis.

Prunus avium

Hausen (1970) cites Brezina (1912) for an injurious effect of the wood.

References

Brezina, E. (1912 bis 1913) Internationale Ubersicht uber Gewerbekrankheiten. in: Teleky: Wiener Arbeiten aus dem Gebiet der sozialen Medizin. Verlag A. Holder. Wien.

Hausen, B.M. (1970) Untersuchungen uber Gesundheitsschadigende Holzer. Thesis, Hamburg.

Prunus cerasus
Cherry

In 289 women employed in making cherry preserves, cases of dermatitis, conjunctivitis, and respiratory disorders were found to be due to exposure to sulphur dioxide fumes. Skin lesions were constantly present in those affected (Fimiani et al 1963).

Reference

Fimiani, R., Boccalatte, F. and Napolitano, S. (1963) Morbidity of women workers of a factory making cherry conserves. Folia. Med. (Napoli) 46, 1038.

Prunus domestica
Plum (when dried forms Prune)

Sorters, shellers and packers of prunellas and sloes (Prunus spinosa) can become infested with a mite (Fuhs 1923, cited by White 1934, Rasch, cited by O'Donovan 1921). Molds on prunes can cause dermatitis

(White 1934). Spitzer (1927) reported dermatitis from prunes. Belisario (1948) referred to similar findings.

References

Belisario, J.C. (1948) Some aspects of occupational dermatitis in Australia. Proc. Brit. Med. Ass. Excerpta Medica Sect. 13 (1948) 3. Abstr. 1908, pp. 590.

Fuhs, H. (1923) cited by White (1934).

O'Donovan, W.J. (1921) Dermatitis due to *Carpoglyphus passularum*. Brit. J. Derm. Syph. 32, 297.

Rasch, cited by O'Donovan (1921).

Spitzer, E. (1927) Dermatitis papulovesiculosa durch Beschaftigung mit mibigen Dorrpflaumen. Zb. Hautkrkh. 22, 310, cited by Touton (1932).

Touton, K. (1932) Hauterkrankungen durch phanerogamische Pflanzen und ihre Produkte (Toxicodermia et Allergodermia phytogenes), in Barnewitz, J. et al Angeborene Anomalien, Lichtdermatosen, Pflanzengifte, Thermische Schadidungen, Einfluss Innerer Storungen auf die Haut. Berlin, Verlag von Julius Springer.

White, R.P. (1934) The Dermatergoses or Occupational Affections of the Skin. 4th ed. London. H.K. Lewis.

Prunus laurocerasus

Massage to the skin with cherry-laurel oil produced dermatitis (Rayer 1835).

Reference

Rayer (1835) Traité Théor. et Prat. des Mal de la Peau Paris p. 262, cited by Morrow, Prince (1887) Drug eruptions. A clinical study of the irritant effects of drugs upon the skin. New York. Wm. Wood and Co.

Prunus persica
Peach

Peaches have often caused dermatitis both among those who pick them and because of the sharp fuzz on many varieties and among those who can them (Schwartz et al 1957). The canners develop dermatitis from the juice of the peach which contains much sugar and is hygroscopic and irritating to the skin (Schwartz et al 1957). The 'fur' on the skin of peaches was considered to cause erythema and papules on the face, neck, forearms and elbow flexures of workers in the fruit canning industry (Foreign Letter 1929).

Positive Type I hypersensitivity skin reactions to juice of fresh peaches and melons (*Cucumis*) were reported by Tuft and Blumstein (1942). Dry fruit extracts produced negative reactions.

The fuzz of the peach acts as a mechanical irritant and later true sensitisation of the skin may appear (Weber 1949).

References

Foreign Letter (Australia)(1929) A survey of women in industry. JAMA 93, 931.

Schwartz, L., Tulipan, L. and Birmingham, D.J. (1957) Occupational Diseases of the Skin. 3rd ed. Philadelphia. Lea and Febiger. pp. 637-672.

Tuft, L. and Blumstein, G.I. (1942) Studies in food allergy: sensitization to fresh fruits; clinical and experimental observations. J. Allergy 13, 574.

Weber, L.F. (1949) Diseases of the skin due to foods. Med. Clin. North America (January) p. 239.

Prunus spinosa
Blackthorn, Sloe Tree

'The thorns have something of a poisonous nature in them' (Withering 1787). 'From some effects which I have repeatedly observed to follow the prick of the thorns, I have reason to believe there is something poisonous in them' (Withering 1801). Thorn injuries of the hands from this plant in 10 patients required nearly four times longer outpatient treatment than did thorn injuries from hawthorn (*Crataegus*), and gooseberry (*Ribes*) (Buhr 1960).

Shrikes (birds) often impale their "kills" i.e. small birds or insects, on the thorns of the blackthorn; the fly-infested putrefying bodies might be a source of infection (Uteau and Bouget 1928). Buhr (1960) recovered no 'unusual bacteria' from his patients. Probably the tip of the rough long brittle thorn of the blackthorn snaps off more readily in the skin than the short sharp needle-sharp point of hawthorn and retention of blackthorn tissues in the subcutaneous tissues is responsible for the disability. Dermatitis from Sloes is noted under *Prunus domestica*.

References

Buhr, A.J. (1960) The thorn in the flesh. Lancet 1, 309.

Uteau, R. and Bouget, J. (1928) Bull. Soc. Chir. Paris 20, 715, cited by Buhr (1960).

Withering, W. (1787), cited by Buhr (1960).

Withering, W. (1801), cited by Buhr (1960).

Pyracantha

Ten species are found from southeastern Europe to central China and IndoChina.

Pyracantha sp.

McCord (1962) noted the availability of a commercial extract for patch-testing. Apparently there are no reports of dermatitis from the plant.

Reference

McCord, C.P. (1962) The occupational toxicity of cultivated flowers. Ind. Med. Surg. 31, 365.

Pyrus

30 species are found in temperate Eurasia.

Pyrus communis
Common Pear

Dermatitis from pears is noted under *Malus*. In addition, women working with pears developed a painful oedematous swelling with hyperkeratosis, fissuring and immobility of the flexed finger (Szego 1966).

Pyrus chinensis
(syn. *Cydonia vulgaris*, according to Smith 1969)

The fruit is soaked in oil and used to darken grey or red hair (Smith 1969).

References

Smith, F.P. (1969) Chinese Materia Medica. Vegetable kingdom. 2nd ed. Rev. by Hei, P.D., Taipei, Taiwan. Ku T'ing Book House.

Szego, L. (1966) Data on skin conditions caused by apples and pears in women working in canning factories. Borgyogy. Vener. Szle. 42, 117.

Quillaja

Three species are found in temperate South America.

Quillaja saponaria
Soap Tree

The powdered bark lathers with water, is sternutatory and was formerly used as an external irritant (Merck Index 1968). The bark contains crystals of calcium oxalate and saponin. A splash of a solution of Quillaja saponin into the eye of a chemist caused irritation (Bakker 1940).

References

Bakker, A. (1940) Klin u. experimentelle Untersuchungen uber Augenveiletzungen durch Saponin. Opthalmologica 99, 356.

Merck Index (1968) An Encyclopedia of Chemicals and Drugs. ed. Stecher, P.G. 8th ed. Rahway, N.J. Merck and Co. Inc.

Rosa

250 species are found in north temperate regions and on tropical mountains.

Rosa
Rose

In 1645, Sir Kenelme Digby wrote: - '...Lady Hennage (who was of the bed-chamber to the late Queen Elizabeth)...had her cheeke blistered by laying a rose upon it whiles shee was asleepe, to try if her antipathy against that flower were so great as she used to pretend' (Macalpine and Hunter 1956). Malten (1972) thinks this is the "very oldest report on contact investigations and incidentally carried out with psychological precautions".

Contact dermatitis from rose or positive patch test reactions to the plant were reported by Harrison (1906), Niedziella (1930), Curtis (1960), Dorsey (1962) and Hjorth (1968).

A woman, aged 66 years, showed a positive patch test to the petal of a red rose; patch tests to a green leaf from the red rose, and to the petal and green leaf from a white rose were negative. The patient was also contact sensitive to Iris (Hjorth 1961).

Contact dermatitis was observed by van Ketel (1974) in four individuals, two culturists of roses and two florists especially handling roses (Rosa sorina). The dermatitis was traced to an organic phosphorus anti-mildew agent "Plondrel" (o.o. diethyl-phtalimido phosphothioate). This material is very stable and leaves a residue in the leaves and petals. Five days after spraying with Plondrel 9.2 ppm were found in the leaves, 0.45 ppm in the petals, by gas liquidchromatography. In two patients he could not exclude contact sensitivity to the rose itself. He classified contact dermatitis from the plants as arising: -

1. from products of the flowers only.
2. from pesticides only.
3. simultaneously from plant products and added pesticides.
4. from other materials too (polyvalent allergy).

Sulphur, used on roses, produced dermatitis in a gardener (Wilkinson 1975). Malathion which is often used on roses can cause contact dermatitis (Milby and Epstein 1964). Contact dermatitis from pesticides was reported by Sicherer (1965) and reviewed by Cronin and Wilkinson (1973).

A rose thorn which penetrated the skin produced an osteolytic lesion simulating a bone tumour (Maylahn 1952).

Kedes et al (1964) reported a case of sporotrichosis from the thorn of a rose-bush. Its victim was a gardener who often fell asleep at work after drinking wine.

In 1565, Botallus reported an individual who, after smelling roses, would have a violent attack of sneezing, rhinorrhoea and headache (Biederman 1937).

The pollen is a rare cause of hayfever (Wodehouse 1971). The scent of roses causes some persons to sneeze.

References

Biederman, J.B. (1937) Sensitivity to flowers. Laryngscope 47, 825.

Cronin, E. and Wilkinson, D.S. (1973) Contact Dermatitis in Recent Advances in Dermatology. ed. Rook, A. Edinburgh. Churchill Livingstone, p. 180.

Curtis, G.H. (1960) Plant dermatitis. Virgin. Med. Month 87, 301.

Dorsey, C.S. (1962) Plant dermatitis in California. Calif. Med. 96, 412.

Harrison, A.J. (1906) Dermatitis from without and dermatitis from within. Bristol. Med. Chir. J. 24, 325.

Hjorth, N. (1961) Eczematous allergy to Balsams, Allied perfumes and flavouring agents. Copenhagen. Munksgaard.

Hjorth, N. (1968) at Finsen Institute. Personal communication.

Kedes, L.H., Siemienski, J. and Brande, A.I. (1964) The syndrome of the alcoholic gardener. Ann. Intern. Med. 61, 1139.

Macalpine, I. and Hunter, R.A. (1956) A case of true allergy established by patch testing and reported by Sir Kenelme Digby in 1645. Brit. J. Derm. 68, 61.

Malten, K.E. (1972) The gap between clinical observation and scientific explanation. Nijmegen. Dekker and Van de Vegt.

Maylahn, D.J. (1952) Thorn-induced "Tumors" of Bone. J. Bone and Joint Surgery. 34-A, 386.

Milby, T.H. and Epstein, W.L. (1964) Allergic contact sensitivity to malathion. Arch. Environ. Health 9, 434.

Niedziella, F. (1930) Milliches uber Kunstunger in der Rosenchule Rosen-Skg 45(4) 85, cited by Touton (1932).

Sicherer, C.A.F.W. (1965) Kunstmeststoffen en Bestrjdingsmiddelen, Thesis, cited by van Ketel (1974).

van Ketel, W.G. (1974) Contact eczema by a new fungicide. Symposium on Contact Dermatitis Gentofte, Denmark, October 26, 27.

Wilkinson, D.S. (1975) Sulphur sensitivity. Contact Dermatitis 1, 58.

Touton, K. (1932) Hauterkrankungen durch phanerogamische Pflanzen und ihre Produkte (Toxicodermia et Allergodermia phytogenes), in Barnewitz, J. et al Angeborene Anomalien, Lichtdermatosen, Pflanzengifte, Thermische Schadidgungen, Einfluss Innerer Storungen auf die Haut. Berlin, Verlag von Julius Springer.

Wodehouse, R.P. (1971) Hayfever Plants. 2nd rev. edition. New York, Hafner.

Rosa damascena

Rosa gallica

Oil of Rose derived from these and other Rosa spp. was reported to cause dermatitis in hypersensitive individuals (Zundel 1936, Flandin et al 1937, Tulipan 1938, Tzanck et al 1938, 1939). Geraniol is contained in Oil of Rose. 2/15 patients contact sensitive to Balsam of Peru (Myroxylon) showed a positive patch test reaction to geraniol (Hjorth 1961). Merck Index (1968) gives other botanical sources of geraniol. Geraniol is isomeric with linalool (Bursera).

References

Flandin, C., Rabeau, H. and Ukrainczyk (1937) L'intolerance a la terebenthine et aux substances du groupe des terpenes. Bull. Soc. franc. Derm. Syph. 44, 315.

Hjorth, N. (1961) Eczematous allergy to Balsams, Allied perfumes and Flavouring agents. Copenhagen, Munksgaard.

Merck Index (1968) An Encyclopedia of Chemicals and Srugs. ed. Stecher, P.G. 8th ed. Rahway, N.J. Merck and Co. Inc.

Tulipan, L. (1938) Cosmetic irritants. Archs. Derm. Syph. 38, 906.

Tzanck, A., Sidi, E. and Dobkevitch (1938) Contribution a l'etude des tests d'intolerance. Bull. Soc. franc. Derm. Syph. 45, 400.

Tzanck, A., Sidi, E. and Dobkevitch (1939) Histamine et tests. Bull. Soc. franc. Derm. Syph. 49, 879.

Zundel, W. (1936) Erfahrungen mit Haufgunktionsprufungen an 2000 Patienten. Archs. Derm. Syph. (Wien) 173, 435.

Rubus

250 species are of cosmopolitan distribution.

Rubus spp.

Some e.g. R. fructisosus (Blackberry) are capable of producing mechanical injury by their thorns.

Sorbus

100 species are found in north temperate regions.

Sorbus aucuparia

The fruits are used to make jellies, etc, and in brandy (Germany), in vodka (Russia) and a substitute for coffee. The leaves are used as a tea and as an adulterant of tea (Camellia) (Usher 1974).

Sorbic acid may be obtained from the berries of this plant, where it occurs as the lactone, called parasorbic acid. Sorbic acid may cause slight skin irritation. The chemistry is given by Merck Index (1968). Sorbic acid in industrial accidents has given rise to a necrotic lesion of the corneal epithelium which has healed rapidly (Duke-Elder and MacFaul 1972). 0.5% of 200 eczematous patients showed positive patch test reactions to sorbic acid (Schorr 1971). 0.6% of 736 eczematous patients showed positive patch test reactions to sorbic acid (Klaschka and Beiersdorff 1965). 0.3% of 1,489 patients with skin diseases showed positive patch test reactions to sorbic acid (Hjorth and Trolle-Lassen 1963). At that time (1961) sorbic acid was not used as a preservative in dermatological creams in Denmark. The only other exposure they were able to trace was plants or berries known to contain sorbic acid. Guinea pigs could be sensitized to sorbic acid (Klaschka and Beiersdorff 1965).

References

Duke-Elder, S. and MacFaul, P.A. (1972) System of Opthalmology. Vol. XIV. Injuries Part 2. Non-mechanical injuries. Irritant Regetable Products. pp. 1180-1196. and Self-inflicted injuries. pp. 1016-1018. London. Henry Kimpton.

Hjorth, N. and Trolle-Lassen, K. (1963) Skin reactions to ointment bases. Trans. St. John's Hosp. Derm. Soc. (Lond.) 49, 127.

Klaschka, F. and Beiersdirff, H.U. (1965) Allergic eczematous reaction from sorbic acid used as a preservative in external medicaments. Munch. Med. Wschr. 107, 185.

Merck Index (1968) An Encyclopedia of Chemicals and Drugs. ed. Stecher, P.G. 8th ed. Rahway, N.J. Merck and Co. Inc.

Schorr, W.F. (1971) Cosmetic Allergy. Archs. Derm. 104, 459.

Usher, G. (1974) A Dictionary of plants used by man. London, Constable.

Spiraea

100 species are found in north temperate regions, south to the Himalayas and Mexico.

Spiraea spp.
Meadowsweet

The plant is a source of salicylaldehyde and in turn of salicylic acid. Aspirin is a word formulated from Spiraea (Shelley 1964). Spiraea or possibly Astilbe (Spirea) were noted as available in a commercial extract for patch-testing (McCord 1962). There do not appear to be any reports of dermatitis from the plant.

References

McCord, C.P. (1962) The Occupational Toxicity of Cultivated Flowers. Ind. Med. Surg. 31, 365.

Shelley, W.B. (1964) Birch pollen and aspirin psoriasis: a study in salicylate hypersensitivity. JAMA 189, 985.

RUBIACEAE

6000 species in 500 genera constitute one of the largest families of plants. Most are tropical but a number are temperate and there are a few Arctic species. Several are myrmecophilous (inhabited by ants). Randia spinosa and Vanqueria spinosa make spiny hedges. Asperula odorata provides aroma chemicals. Genera assigned to Naucleaceae (syn. Rubiaceae) (Shaw 1973) are included here.

Chemistry is recorded by Hegnauer (1973).

References

Hegnauer, R. (1973) Chemotaxonomy of plants. Vol. 6. Basel. Birkhauser. p. 130.

Shaw, H.K.A. (1973) A Dictionary of the Flowering Plants and Ferns. (the late J.C. Willis) 8th ed. Cambridge University Press.

Adina

20 species are found in tropical and subtropical Africa and Asia.

Adina cordifolia

The wood is said to be irritant to the respiratory tract (Orsler 1973).

Reference

Orsler, R.J. (1973) Personal communication from Forest Products Research Laboratory, Princess Risborough, Bucks, England.

Asperula

Over 200 species are found in Europe and Asia especially in the Mediterranean region; sixteen species are found in eastern Australia and Tasmania. Species of this genus have hooked fruits which attach themselves to animals (Howes 1974).

Reference

Howes, F.N. (1974) A Dictionary of Useful and Everyday Plants and their Common Names. Cambridge. University Press.

Bertiera

30 species are found in tropical America and Africa.

Bertiera racemosa

The leaves have styptic properties (Irvine 1961).

Reference

Irvine, F.R. (1961) Woody plants of Ghana. Oxford University Press.

Borreria

150 species are found in warm regions.

Borreria compacta

A paste of the leaf is used in Africa as a counter-irritant in the way that a mustard leaf or plant (Brassica) has been used by Europeans. There is a considerable degree of the itch from the application which is followed by scaling (Bally 1937, 1938, cited by Watt and Breyer-Brandwijk 1962).

Reference

Bally (1937, 1938) cited by Watt, J.M. and Breyer-Brandwijk, M.G. (1962) The Medicinal and poisonous plants of Southern Africa. 2nd ed. Edinburgh. E.& S. Livingstone.

Canthium

200 species are found in paleotropical regions.

Canthium coprosmoides

After grazing on this plant for three days, animals died in agony after the skin had blistered and the hair peeled off (Communication from an Australian stockowner in 1933 to Hurst 1942).

Reference

Hurst, E. (1942) The Poison Plants of New South Wales. N.S.W. Poison Plants Committee; Sydney.

Catesbaea

10 species are found in the Florida Keys and West Indies.

Catesbaea melanocarpa

The plant is listed as a cause of mechanical injury (Oakes and Butcher 1962).

Reference

Oakes, A.J. and Butcher, J.P. (1962) Poisonous and injurious plants of the U.S. Virgin Islands. Misc. Publ. 882. U.S. Department of Agriculture, Washington, D.C.

Cephaelis

180 species are found in tropical regions.

Cephaelis ipecacuanha

The root provides medicinal ipecacuanha. The dust or effluvium of the root produces inflammation of the air-passages and conjunctivitis, and applied to the skin in the form of an ointment, it excites a pustular eruption similar to that caused by tartar emetic (Dispensatory 1884). Acute kerato-conjunctivitis follows instillation of the powder into the eye. More chronic contamination may lead to the development of a granular conjunctivitis resembling trachoma. These reactions are sometimes seen in pharmacists who handle the powder either of ipecacuanha or of emetine but the most dramatic incidents have been self-inflicted by malingerers (Duke-Elder and MacFaul 1972). The particles of ipecac have a distinctive microscopical appearance which permits their identification if malingering is suspected (Grant 1962). Dermatitis from ipecacuanha was reported by Benjamin (1903), Robert (1922), Galewsky (1926), Hirszfeldowa and Prokopowicz-Wierzbowska (1924) and Lortat-Jacob et al (1930). Erythema, papules and intensive pruritus leading to crusted excoriations followed topical exposure to the drug (Bazin cited by White 1887). Vesicular (Piffard 1881) and pustular reactions (Duchworth, personal communication to White 1887) have been observed.

Emetine, the principal alkaloid of ipecacuanha, produced redness, papules, vesicles, pustules and urticaria on the forearms and arms of pharmacists (Peshkin 1924). A chemist, a boiler and a sorter developed eczematous dermatitis from contact with emetine, while making a preparation of ipecac (Schwartz et al 1957).

References

Bazin cited by White (1887).

Benjamin (1903) Schmidts Jb 278, 133, cited by Touton (1932).

Dispensatory (United States) 1884, cited by White (1887).

Duchworth, personal communication to White (1887).

Duke-Elder, S. and MacFaul (1972). System of Opthalmology Vol. XIV. Injuries Part 1. Mechanical Injuries. Extra-ocular foreign bodies, pp. 464-67, and Agricultural Injuries, pp. 32-34. London. Henry Kimpton.

Galewsky (1926) Uber die gewerbliche Schadigung durch Emetin. Wien. med. Wschr. 76, 17, 10 July, cited by Touton (1932).

Grant, W.M. (1962) Toxicology of the Eye. Springfield, Ill. Charles C. Thomas.

Hirszfeldowa and Prokopowicz-Wierzboska (1924) Uber das Wesen der Idiosynkrasie bei Kindern. Pedjatr. polska 4, 360, cited by Touton (1932).

Lortat-Jacob, Flandrin and Poumeau-Delille (1930) Un cas d'anaphylaxie cutanee a l'emetine. Bull. Soc. franc. Derm. Syph. 36, 1088, cited by Touton (1932).

Peshkin, M.M. (1924) Bronchial asthma and other allergic manifestations in pharmacists. JAMA 82, 1854.

Piffard, H.G. (1881) A treatise on the Materia Medica and Therapeutics of the skin. New York. Wm. Wood and Co.

Robert (1922) Un cas d'anaphylaxie locale a l'emetine. Bull. Soc. Path. exot. Paris 15, 680, cited by Touton (1932).

Schwartz, L., Tulipan, L., and Birmingham, D.J. (1957) Occupational Diseases of the Skin. 3rd ed. Philadelphia. Lea and Febiger.

Touton, K. (1932) Hauterkrankungen durch phanerogamische Pflanzen und ihre Produkte (Toxicodermia et Allergodermia phytogenes), in Barnewitz, J. et al Angeborene Anomalien, Lichtdermatosen, Pflanzengifte, Thermische Schadigungen, Einfluss Innerer Storungen auf die Haut. Berlin, Verlag von Julius Springer.

White, J.C. (1887) Dermatitis venenata: An account of the Action of External irritants upon the Skin. Boston. Cupples and Hurd.

Cinchona

40 species are found as trees in the Andes. Several species are cultivated for their bark which yields quinine and related alkaloids.

Cinchona spp.

Stripping of Cinchona bark and handling of the powdered bark and quinine produced dermatitis in pharmaceutical workers. The eyelids, face, neck, elbow flexures, genital area and upper thighs were principally affected (Chevallier 1852, Dold 1925, Blamoutier and Joannon 1922). Touton (1932) and White (1934) provide an extensive bibliography. Quinine can cause allergic contact dermatitis in factory workers (White 1887, Werz 1949) and when used in dandruff cream (Johnson 1935), hair tonic (Kissmeyer 1937, Peterkin 1953), aftershave lotion (Burgess and Usher 1930) and contraceptive pessaries (Danbolt 1931, Peterkin 1953, Zheltakov and Somov 1963, Guriev and Monakhova 1968). Ingestion of quinine, as in tonic water, can produce a focal flare of dermatitis (Kissmeyer 1937, Sulzberger and Baer 1948). Cross-sensitivity to related alkaloids has been observed and appears to be dependent on a quinoline ring (Bloch 1924, Ford 1934, Dawson and Garbade 1930). Contact dermatitis from the isomer, quinidine (Frenstrom 1965), and from the synthetic antimalarial, chloroquin (Hermann and Schulz 1965) is rare. Immediate hypersensitivity was reported by Gray (1929). Quinine sulphate, 2% aqueous, is suitable for patch testing (Calnan and Caron 1961). In Denmark, the incidence of sensitivity to quinine steadily declined from 1938 to 1961 and at the latter date was distinctly rare (Hjorth, personal communication to Calnan and Caron 1961).

References

Blamoutier and Joannon (1922) Quinine sickness of occupational origin. Rev. d'Hyg. 44, 521, cited by White (1934).

Bloch, B. (1924) Archs. Derm. Syph. (Berl.), cited by Calnan and Caron (1961).

Burgess, J.F. and Usher, B. (1930) On hypersensitiveness to quinine. Canad. Med. Ass. J. 23, 45.

Calnan, C.D. and Caron, G.A. (1961) Quinine sensitivity. Brit. Med. J. 2, 1750.

Chevalier, A. (1852) Essay upon the health of workers who prepare sulphate of quinine. Ann. k'Hygiene 48, 95, cited by White (1934).

Danbolt, N. (1931) Eczema due to suppositories in persons hypersensitive to quinine. Norsk. mag. f. laegervidensk. 92, 623.

Dawson, W.T. and Garbade, F.A. (1930) Idiosyncrasy to quinine, cinchonidene and ethylhydrocupreine. JAMA 94, 704.

Dold, H. (1925) Quinine idiosyncrasy of the skin in industrial workers. Arch. f. Hyg. 96, 167, cited by White (1934).

Fernstrom, A.I.B. (1965) Occupational quinidine contact dermatitis. Acta derm.-venereol. 45, 129.

Ford, W.K. (1934) Drug eruption due to quinine: recurrence following use of contraceptive. JAMA 103, 483.

Gray St., G.B.D. (1929) Idiosyncrasy to quinine injections. Brit. Med. J. 1, 200.

Guriev, L.N. and Monakhova, A.P. (1968) Contact-allergic dermatitis of sexual organs in men due to quinine. Vestn. Derm. Vener. 42, 87.

Hermann, W.P. and Schulz, K.H. (1965) Allergic contact eczema from resochin. Dermatologica (Basel) 130, 216.

Hjorth, N. Personal communication to Calnan, C.D. and Caron, G.A. (1961).

Johnson, D.W. (1935) Dermatitis due to application of dandruff cream. Urol. Cutan. Rev. 39, 173.

Kissmeyer, A. (1937) Trois cas d'intolerance a la quinine. Abstr. Acta Derm.-venereol. 19, 153.

Peterkin, G.A.G. (1953) Drug eruptions in the tropics. In Handbook of Tropical Dermatology and Medical Mycology. ed. Simons, R.D.G. Ph. Amsterdam. Elsevier. pp. 1453.

Sulzberger, M.B. and Baer, R.L. (1948) Eczematous eruptions of the hands, in Year Book of Dermatology. Chicago. Year Book Publishers.

Touton, K. (1932) Hauterkrankungen durch phanerogamische Pflanzen und ihre Produkte (Toxicodermia et Allergodermia phytogenes), in Barnewitz, J. et al Angeborene Anomalien, Lichtdermatosen, Pflanzengifte, Termische Schadigungen, Einfluss Innerer Storungen auf die Haut. Berlin, Verlag von Julius Springer.

Werz, J.F.C. (1949) Contact dermatitis in workers in quinine plant. Ned. T. Geneesk 93, 170.

White, J.C. (1887) Dermatitis venenata: An account of the action of external irritants upon the skin. Boston. Cupples and Hurd.

White, R.P. (1934) The dermatergoses or occupational affections of the skin. 4th ed. London. H.K. Lewis.

Zheltakov, M.M. and Somov, B.A. (1963) Allergic quinine dermatitis caused by contraceptives. Vestn. Derm. I Vener. 12, 8.

Levantine, A. and Almeyda, J. (1974) Cutaneous reactions to food and drug additives. Brit. J. Derm. 91, 359.

Coffea

40 species are found in palaeotropical regions especially in Africa. Several species are cultivated for their seeds, coffee beans.

Coffea arabica

Workers employed in sorting, milling or roasting coffee beans developed dermatitis, urticaria, rhinitis and asthma. Patch tests to the chaff produced positive results (Chopra et al 1949, Layton et al 1966). A role of chlorogenic acid in the respiratory symptoms suggested by Freedman et al (1962) was discounted by Layton et al (1966). Employees in a coffee-roasting plant developed allergic manifestations from castor-bean dust (*Ricinus*) which contaminated the burlap bags in which the coffee was transported (Figley and Rawling 1950). Cheilitis was attributed to coffee drinking; liquid coffee produced a positive patch test reaction but controls were not recorded (Lupton 1953). None of 691 persons patch tested to an ether extract of coffee showed positive reactions (Fregert and Hjorth 1968).

Inhalation of coffee bean dust can produce coffee worker's lung, a form of allergic alveolitis (Morgan and Seaton 1975).

References

Chopra, R.N., Badhwar, R.L. and Ghosh, S. (1948) Poisonous Plants of India. Monograph No. 17. Delhi. Indian Council of Agricult. Res.

Figley, K.D. and Rawling, F.A.A. (1950) Castor bean: industrial hazard as contaminant of green coffee dust and used burlap bags. J. Allergy 21, 545.

Freedman, S.O. et al (1962) Identification of a simple chemical compound (chlorogenic acid) as an allergen in plant materials causing human atopic disease. Am. J. Med. Sci. 244, 548.

Fregert, S. and Hjorth, N. (1968) Results of standard patch tests with substances abandoned. Contact Dermatitis Newsletter 5, 85.

Kaplan, R.J., Daman, L., Shereff, R. Rosenberg, E.W. and Robinson, H. (1976) Letter: treatment of atopic dermatitis with topically applied caffeine. Arch. Dermatol. 112, 880 and letter 113, 107.

Layton, L.D., Panzani, R. and Corse, J.W. (1966) Non-diffusable allergenic contaminant from samples of chlorogenic acid causing allergic reaction: Pure chlorogenic acid not an allergen. J. Allergy 38, 268 and correspondence p. 276.

Lupton, E.S. (1953) Cheilitis due to coffee. Arch. Derm. Syph. 68, 333.

Morgan, W.K.C. and Seaton, A. (1975) Occupational Lung Diseases. Philadelphia, Saunders.

Coryanthe

8 species are found in tropical Africa.

Coryanthe johimbe

This plant yields yohimbine, an adrenergic blocking agent formerly used as a local anaesthetic (Merck Index 1968).

Coryanthe pachyceras (syn. C. paniculata)

The bitter, astringent bark has a local anaesthetic action from alkaloids related to yohimbine (Dalziel 1937, Irvine 1961).

References

Dalziel, J.M. (1937) The Useful Plants of West Tropical Africa. London. Crown Agents for the Colonies.

Irvine, F.R. (1961) Woody plants of Ghana. Oxford University Press, quoted by Menninger (1967).

Menninger, E.A. (1967) Fantastic trees. New York. The Viking Press.

Merck Index (1968) An Encyclopedia of Chemicals and Drugs. ed. Stecher, P.G. 8th ed. Rahway, N.J. Merck and Co. Inc.

Craterispermum

17 species are found in tropical Africa, one species in the Seychelles.

Craterispermum laurinum

The powdered root or bark is used as a rubefacient in Central Africa (Watt and Breyer-Brandwijk 1962).

Reference

Watt, J.M. and Breyer-randwijk, M.G. (1962) The Medicinal and Poisonous Plants of Southern Africa. 2nd ed. Edinburgh. E.& S. Livingstone.

Diodia

50 species are found in tropical and subtropical regions.

Diodia teres

An extract of this plant produced a positive patch test reaction in one of 50 patients who had 'weed dermatitis' (Shelmire 1939).

Reference

Shelmire, B. (1939) Contact dermatitis from weeds: Patch testing with their oleoresins. JAMA 113, 1085 (and unpublished table accompanying reprints, courtesy of Dr. David Shelmire).

Duroia

20 species are found in South America.

Duroia hirsuta

The bark, when tied on the arm, causes blisters to form (Altschul 1973). The swollen stem of the plant regularly houses ants (Shaw 1973).

References

Altschul, S. von R. (1973) Drugs and foods from little-known plants. Cambridge, Mass. Harvard University Press.

Shaw, H.K.A. (1973) A Dictionary of the Flowering Plants and Ferns. (the late J.C. Willis) 8th ed. Cambridge University Press.

Exostema (syn. Exostemma)

50 species are found from Mexico to Brazil, Peru and the West Indies. Febrifugal alkaloids are contained in the bark.

Exostemma caribaeum

The wood yields a 4-phenylcoumarin, exostemin, related to those of *Dalbergia* spp.(Seshadri 1972).

Reference

Seshadri, T.R. (1972) Polyphenols of *Pterocarpus* and *Dalbergia* woods. Phytochemistry 11, 881.

Galium

400 species are of cosmopolitan distribution. Small reflexed hooks are present on the stem of *G. sparine*.

Species of this genus have hooked fruits which attach themselves to animals (Howes 1974).

Galium sparine

Dermatitis was reported from contact with the stem of this plant; a patch test produced a positive result (Fujita 1966).

Galium triflorum
Sweet-scented Bedstraw

For chest pains, this plant was rubbed on the skin, sometimes enough to draw blood, and then hellebore (*Veratrum viride*) was applied. North American Indians rub the body with the plant for its perfume, mash it and put it in the hair (Gunther 1945).

Galium verum
Lady's Bedstraw

The plant is astringent and bitter and the flowers are used for making cheese instead of rennet (Wren 1968).

References

Fujita, E. (1966) Jap. J. Derm. 76, 703, cited by Ito (1972).

Gunther, E. (1945) Ethnobotany of Western Washington. Seattle. University of Washington Press.

Howes, F.N. (1974) A Dictionary of Useful and Everyday Plants and their Common Names. Cambridge University Press. pp. 290.

Ito, K. (1972) Personal communication.

Wren, R.W. (1968) Potter's New Cyclopaedia of Botanical Drugs and Preparations by Wren, R.C. Re-edit. by Wren, R.W. Potter and Clarke Ltd. Health Science Press. Rustington, Sussex.

Gardenia

250 species are found in palaeotropical regions.

The odor of gardenia can cause hayfever (Biederman 1937).

Gardenia spp.

The fruits are used for haemostasis, apparently by ingestion, and for dyeing. The flowers are used to flavor tea which is then known as jasmine tea (Smith 1969, Kariyone 1971).

References

Biederman, J.B. (1937) Sensitivity to flowers. Larynogoscope 47, 825.

Kariyone, T. (1971) Atlas of Medicinal Plants. Osaka, Japan. Takeda Chemical Industries.

Smith, F.P. (1969) Chinese Materia Medica. Vegetable kingdom. 2nd ed. Rev. by Hei, P.D. Taipei, Taiwan. Ku T'ing Book House.

Paederia

50 species are found in tropical regions as climbing shrubs.

Paederia foetida

The plant has an offensive odour when bruised or even if slightly disturbed (Pope 1968) and the foul-smelling stems and leaves are used to stimulate moribund persons (Smith 1969).

References

Pope, W.T. (1968) Manual of Wayside Plants of Hawaii. Rutland, Vermont. Charles E. Tuttle Co.

Smith, F.P. (1969) Chinese Materia Medica. Vegetable kingdom. 2nd ed. Rev. by Hei, P.D. Taipei, Taiwan. Ku T'ing Book House.

Rothmannia

20 species are found in tropical and southern Africa.

Rothmannia longiflora

The fruits yield a black dye which is used in Nigeria for making blue-black markings on the face or body (Oliver 1961).

Reference

Oliver, B. (1961) Nigeria's Useful Plants. Nigerian Field, Part V. 26, 170-180.

Rubia

60 species are found in western and central Europe, the Mediterranean region, eastern tropical and southern Africa, temperate Asia, the Himalayas and from Mexico to tropical South America. Several species yield dyes.

Rubia tinctorum
Madder

The plant was formerly cultivated for its root which yields the dye alizarin. Alizarin is a sensitizer (Greenberg and Lester 1954) and on that account is removed from certain brand-name cosmetics (Schieffelin 1973).

References

Greenberg, L.A. and Lester, D. (1954) Handbook of Cosmetic Materials. New York. Interscience.

Schieffelin and Co. (1973) Almay Hypo-allergenic cosmetics product formulary. 8th ed. Pharmaceutical Laboratories Division. 562 - 5th Avenue, New York, N.Y. 10036.

Spermacoce

100 species are found in warm regions of America.

Spermacoce compacta

The leaf is used as a rubefacient (Watt and Breyer-Brandwijk 1962).

Reference

Watt, J.M. and Breyer-Brandwijk, M.G. (1962) The Medicinal and Poisonous Plants of Southern Africa. 2nd ed. Edinburgh. E.& S. Livingstone.

Uncaria

60 species are found in tropical regions. This genus has been placed in a family, Naucleaceae.

Uncaria gambir
Gambier

This species yields Gambir catechu or pale catechu, a dried aqueous extract of the leaves used for dyeing fabric brown or black. Sensitisation to vegetable dyes is rare (Schwartz et al 1957). Catechu is noted under Acacia.

Reference

Schwartz, L., Tulipan, L. and Birmingham, D.J. (1957) Occupational Diseases of the skin. 3rd ed. Philadelphia. Lea and Febiger, pp. 637-672.

RUTACEAE

900 species in 150 genera are found in tropical and temperate regions especially in southern Africa and Australia.

Chemistry is recorded by Hegnauer (1973).

Reference

Hegnauer, R. (1973) Chemotaxonomy of plants. Fol. 6. Basel, Birkhauser. P. 174.

This family is the source of some phototoxic chemical compounds. Phototoxicity may possibly explain some conflicting earlier reports of variable episodes of dermatitis from the woods e.g. from Fagara and Zanthoxylum.

Aegle

Three species are found in Indo-Malaysia.

Aegle Marmelos
Bael Tree

The tree is sacred in some parts of India. A mucilage which oozed from the bark of broken branches tastes sweet at first and then irritates the throat (Burkill 1935). The plant yields 8-methoxypsoralen (Pathak et al 1962).

References

Burkill, I.H. (1935) A dictionary of the economic products of the Malay Peninsula. 2 Vols. London. Crown Agents for the Colonies.

Pathak, M.A., Daniels, F. Jr. and Fitzpatrick, T.B. (1962) Presently known distribution of furocoumarins (Psoralens) in plants. J. Invest. Derm. 39, 225.

Amyris

30 species are found in warm regions of America and in the West Indies.

Amyris balsamifera
(syn. A. toxifera)
West Indian Sandalwood

West Indian Sandalwood oil is derived from this species. East Indian Sandalwood oil is derived from Santalum. Hausen (1970) cites Gougerot and Delzant (1940) for contact sensitivity to the oil.

Amyris simplicifolia and
Amyris spp.

Amyris spp. used to be considered one of the main sources of rosewood (Holtzapffel and Royle 1843, Burn, not dated, cited by Woods and Calnan 1976) but now provide very little timber (Record and Hess 1943). Amyris oil, known as West Indian Sandalwood oil, was formerly extracted from the wood. Grossmann (1920) stated that working with Amyris and some other rosewoods (Aniba) but improbably Convolvulus caused headache, weakness, drowsiness, dyspnoea and sometimes dermatitis.

Amyris opobalsamum

This plant is the source of Balm of Mecca (Genders 1972). According to Woods and Calnan (1976) the balm was a favourite beauty preparation in the Middle East but could produce alarmingly violent reactions on the face (Montagu 1717).

References

Burn, R.S. (n.d.) The New Guide to Carpentry. London, Fullarton (circa 1870), cited by Woods and Calnan (1976).

Genders, R. (1972) A History of Scent. London, Hamilton.

Gougerot, H. and Delzant, O. (1940) Sensibilisation au santal. An. Fac. med. (Montevideo) 25, 35.

Grossmann, J. (1920) Gesundheitsschadliche Holzarten. Der Holzkaufer (Leipzig) 17, 529, 540 and 545.

Hausen, B.M. (1970) Untersuchungen uber Gesundheitsschadigende Holzer. Thesis, Hamburg.

Holtzapffel, C. and Royle (1943) Descriptive catalogue of the woods commonly employed in this country for the mechanical and ornamental arts. An extract from: Turning and mechanical manipulation. London, Holtzapffel, cited by Woods and Calnan (1976).

Montagu, Lady M.W. (1717) Complete Letters. ed. Halsband, R. Oxford University Press (1965). Letter to Lady Rich of 17. 6. 1717, cited by Woods and Calnan (1976).

Record, S.J. and Hess, R.W. (1943) Timbers of the New World. New Haven, Yale.

Woods, B. and Ca.nan, C.D. (1976) Toxic Woods. Brit. J. Derm. 94, Suppl. 13, June.

Balfourodendron

One species is found in Southern Brazil, Paraguay and northern Argentina.

Balfourodendron riedelianum
Guatambú

The wood has been reported to cause dermatitis (Hausen 1970).

Reference

Hausen, B.M. (1970) Untersuchungen uber Gesundheitsschadigende Holzer. Thesis, Hamburg.

Casimiroa

Six species of central America yield edible fruit.

Casimiroa sp.

A species of this genus yields 5-methoxypsoralen (Dean 1963).

Casimiroa edulis
White Sapote

This tree, which is known in horticulture, yields furanocoumarins (Dean 1963).

Reference

Dean, F.M. (1963) Naturally occurring oxygen ring compounds. London. Butterworths.

Citrus

12 species are native to southern China, south-east Asia and Indo Malaysia. A nomenclature of the cultivated species is provided by Usher (1974); he gives botanical authors the names of whom are omitted here.

Citrus aurantifolia (syn. C. medica var. acida)	Lime
Citrus aurantifolia var. limetta	Sweet Lime
Cirtus aurantium	Bigarade, Seville Orange, Sour Orange
Citrus aurantium var. bergamia (syn. C. bergamia)	
Citrus aurantium x C. sinensis	Bitter Sweet Orange
Citrus bergamia (syn. C. aurantium var. bergamia)	Bergamot Orange
Citrus limetta	Sweet Lemon
Citrus limon	Lemon
Citrus limonia	Canton Lemon
Citrus medica	Citron
Citrus paradisi	Grapefruit
Citrus reticulata	Mandarin Orange (Tangerine)
Citrus sinensis	Sweet Orange

Shaw (1973) gives

Citrus aurantium var. aurantium (bigaradia or amara)	Seville or bitter orange

Citrus spp.

Fruit canners are subject to paronychia and loss of nails (Kingery and Thienes 1925, White 1941). 10% of cases of dermatitis of the eyelids were attributed to contact sensitivity to fruit peel (Hazen 1944). Atopic allergy of the hands from transepidermal penetration of agents of fruits and also by ingestion of fruits was postulated by Rowe (1946). The subject of contact urticaria was discussed by Maibach and Johnson (1975).

References

Hazen, H.H. (1944) Dermatitis of the eyelids. Arch. Derm. Syph. 49, 253.

Kingery, L.B. and Thienes, C.H. (1925) Mycotic paronychia and dermatitis. A hitherto undescribed condition apparently peculiar to fruit canners. Archs. Derm. Syph. 11, 186.

Maibach, H.I. and Johnson, H.L. (1975) Contact urticaria syndrome. Archs. Derm. 111, 726.

Rowe, A.H. (1946) Atopic dermatitis of the hands due to food allergy. Archs. Derm. Syph. 54, 683.

Shaw, H.K.A. (1973) A dictionary of the flowering plants and ferns. (the late J.C. Willis) 8th ed. Cambridge University Press.

Usher, G. (1974) A dictionary of plants used by man. London. Constable.

White, C. (1941) Contact dermatitis: Occupational importance, diagnosis, management, prevention. Mississippi Valley Med. J. 63, 120 and 154.

Mycotic infection of fruit canners known as 'fruit poisoning' was treated by application of thymol, oil of cinnamon (Cassia) and oil of clove (Syzygium) (Myers and Thienes 1925). Paronychia of orange-workers was attributed to the fungus of the family Mucoraceae (Sutherland-Campbell 1929).

References

Myers, H.B. and Thienes, C.H. (1925) The fungicidal activity of certain volatile oils and stearoptens. JAMA 84, 1985.

Sutherland-Campbell, H. (1929) Paronychia. An attempt to prove the etiologic factor in an epidemic among orange workers. Archs. Derm. Syph. 19, 233.

d-limonene is found in orange oil and in many other essential oils. Sensitization by limonene is probably due to autooxidation products (Opdyke 1974).

Reference

Opdyke, D.L.J. (1974) Monographs on fragrance raw materials. Fd. Cosmet. Toxicol. 12, 919.

Citral produced irritant reactions under hot conditions (Rothenborg et al 1977).

Reference

Rothenborg, H.W. et al (1977) Temperature dependent primary irritant dermatitis from lemon perfume. Contact Dermatitis 3, 37.

Dermatitis and asthma from the wood of Citrus spp.

Citrus limon
Lemonwood, zitroneholz

Citrus aurantium
Orangewood

Citrus medica
Citron, citronnier

Orangewood sawdust used for polishing jewels was said to cause asthma (Walker 1921) and Janson (1953) referred to a case of wood dermatitis in a paper on citrus fruit dermatitis. Grossman (1920) doubted whether genuine Citrus wood ever caused skin irritation.

According to Woods and Calnan (1976), citronnier used to be popular with french cabinet-makers (Hinckley 1960) but in Germany the name zitronenholz has been much more widely applied. According to these authors, it seems to have referred mainly to satinwoods, such as Fagara flava and Chloroxylon swietenia with a lemon scent (Gayer 1928) which were probably responsible for most if not all the reported cases of zitronenholz dermatitis.

References

Gayer, S. (1928) Die Holzarten und ihre Verwendung in der Technik. 3rd ed. Leipzig, Janecke, cited by Woods and Calnan (1976).

Grossmann, J. (1920) Gesundheitsschadliche Holzarten. Der Holzkaufer (Leipzig) 17, 529, 540 and 545.

Hinckley, F.L. (1960) Directory of the historic cabinet woods. New York. Bonanza, cited by Woods and Calnan (1976).

Janson, P. (1953) Citrusfruchte und Hauterkrankungen Zeitschrift fur Haut - und Geschlechtskrankheiten 14, 144.

Walker, I.C. (1921) Bronchial Asthma. In: The Oxford Medicine. ed. Christian, H.A. Vol. 2., p. 231. Oxford (1921-1947) looseleaf.

Woods, B. and Calnan, C.D. (1976) Toxic woods. Brit. J. Derm. Suppl. 13, June.

Citrus aurantifolia
(syn. C. medica var. acida)
Lime

The oil of the fruit peel was observed to be photosensitising. Oils from different kinds of lime varied in their activity (Sams 1941). The furanocoumarins of the species are given by Pathak et al (1962); C. acida yields 5-methoxypsoralen. The role of photoallergy versus phototoxicity requires clarification (Sams 1956).

References

Pathak, M.A., Daniels, F. Jr. and Fitzpatrick, T.B. (1962) Presently known distribution of furocoumarins (Psoralens) in plants. J. Invest. Derm. 39, 225.

Sams, W.M. (1941) Photodynamic action of Lime oil (Citrus aurantifolia). Arch. Derm. Syph. 44, 571.

Sams. W.M. (1956) Contact photodermatitis. Arch. Derm. 73, 142.

Citrus aurantium
Bigarade, Seville or Sour orange

Early reports of dermatitis from oranges were reviewed by Touton (1932), White (1934) and Schwartz (1938).

The outer-most orange-coloured layer of the fruit containing oil glands is named the exocarp, the white cottony layer the mesocarp and the fruit sac the endocarp.

Orange pickers suffer pricks and scratches from the thorns of the plant and secondary infection (Pardo-Castello 1962).

In growing oranges, dermatitis from insecticides and fertilizers can occur: in packing, splinters from boxes, dermatitis from washing solutions and from citrus oils: in canning, dermatitis and paronychia due to citrus oils and juices (Schwartz 1938). There are two reports of dermatitis attributed to sensitivity to dyes used for dyeing the skins of Florida oranges (Schwartz 1938, Traub 1936, Baer et al 1948).

A man who had contact dermatitis from dyed socks was contact-sensitive to Citrus Red 3 used for dyeing oranges; ingestion of Citrus Red 3 caused recurrence of the dermatitis (Mitchell 1972).

Carnauba wax (Copernicia) and paraffin wax are used for waxing the skins of oranges. Contact sensitivity attributed to carnauba has been reported (Greenberg and Lester 1954).

Cheilitis and stomatitis were reported from eating oranges (Zakon et al 1947). Persons who suck citrus fruits can develop circumoral dermatitis and hyperpigmentation, and cheilitis (Behl et al 1966). Cheilitis was attributed to the volatile oil of oranges (Sutton and Sutton 1953). Dermatitis of the hands from oranges was reported by Michel (1953).

Anaphylactoid reaction from ingestion of orange was reported by Bendersky and Lupas (1960) and contact urticaria from orange, grapefruit juice (C. paradisi) and lemon peel (C. limon) by Urbach (1931), Urbach and Gottlieb (1949). Beerman et al (1938), Horner (1931), Mayers (1932), Seidmann (1946), Schwartz et al (1957), Fanburg and Kaufman (1931), Djerassi et al (1967), Morris (1954), Rantuccio et al (1967), Rivasseau (1956), White (1941), Hazen and Washington (1944), Janson (1953), Kesten and Lyons (1932) and White (1887) refer to dermatitis from oranges.

Orange peel 25% in petrolatum produced seven positive reactions in 310 persons investigated for hand eczema (Agrup 1969). Orange peel produced positive patch test reactions in 19 of 590 patients tested (Menghini et al 1971). Hjorth (1961) observed 16 patients with a significant positive patch test to orange peel. 5 of 11 patients contact sensitive to orange peel also showed positive patch test reactions to Balsam of Peru (Myroxylon). 5 of 8 patients contact sensitive to Balsam of Peru showed positive patch test reactions to an ether extract of orange peel (Hjorth 1961).

Hjorth (1971) described a man with severe hand eczema for 10 years who, because he reacted to Balsam of Peru on patch testing, was told to avoid orange peel. To test the validity of this advice, the patient ate a jar of orange marmalade and in 12 hours had his worst attack of hand eczema. He then avoided "perfumes, cola drinks, vermouth, throat tablets, cinnamon and other items" and his hand eczema cleared.

One patient who was strongly contact sensitive to orange peel showed a positive patch test reaction to carotene (Hjorth 1961). Carotene was reported allergenic in a case of sensitivity to oranges and carrots (Daucus) (Sulzberger 1936). Citric acid has been reported to cause contact sensitivity (Stauffer 1948, Walsh 1975). Orange blossom can cause respiratory symptoms (Rebhun 1966).

Sensitization to limonene has been considered responsible for dermatitis from oranges but some cases of contact sensitivity to orange peel show no sensitivity to lemon peel which also contains limonene (Bonnevie 1939).

C. aurantium has been reported to evoke photodermatitis (Pathak et al 1962, van Dijk and Berrens 1964). Oil of Orange derived from orange peel has been reported to produce dermatitis (Greenberg and Lester 1954). Oil of Orange Flowers (Oil of Neroli) derived from orange flowers has been reported to produce dermatitis and photosensitivity (Greenberg and Lester 1954). Oil of Petitgrain distilled from the leaves has been reported to cause contact dermatitis and photosensitivity (Greenberg and Lester 1954). Contact sensitivity to Orange sweet terpeneless was reported by Larsen (1975).

Patch testing with oranges and lemons

Schwartz (1938a,b) reviewed the literature concerning dermatitis from citrus fruits and some chemical information on the oils of the rinds. The oil in the peel of citrus fruit is contained in the few layers of oil cells on the surface of the peel. Citrus oils are exceedingly irritating to the skin and will produce positive reactions when used in patch tests on the normal skin in less than an hour. α-Limonene and citral are also irritant by patch test. The juice of the fruit is generally not irritant by patch test. Lemon juice is said to be more irritant than orange or grapefruit juice because of its greater content of citric acid. Lemon peel may appear more often irritant than orange peel because lemons are seldom waxed. It is necessary to read these reports before attributing allergic contact dermatitis to citrus fruits and some reports of patch testing as indicating sensitivity must be discarded. However, it is considered that such sensitivity can occur in industry and that dermatitis could result from the use of oils of orange and lemon and limonene in perfumery.

Statements that the white under-surface of the peel (the mesocarp) is allergenic and that the outer surface of the peel (the exocarp) produced no reaction must be accepted with caution. It is possible to patch test with the mesocarp contaminated with citrus oil and to obtain a positive reaction; and to patch test with the exocarp which is unbroken and therefore with intact oil cells and to obtain a negative reaction. These apparently paradoxical results depend on the materials used and the technique used for obtaining samples of the fruit.

There is a great difference in patch testing with citrus fruit gathered directly from the tree and with citrus fruit obtained from stores. Before the citrus fruit finally reaches the consumer's market, it receives various treatments, among which is a wax finish on the surface of the peel. Patch testing with waxed citrus peel will not allow the actual peel to touch the skin, or if it does touch the skin, it will do so imperfectly. The thickness of the coat of wax on the peel will determine whether the peel will come in contact with the skin. When the peel is removed from the fruit for the purpose of patch testing, the wax coating may or may not have been cracked; the oil in the oil cells of the peel may or may not touch the skin, depending on whether the peel itself has been cracked. The number of days that the orange has been kept in storage will have some bearing on how dry the peel is and how much oil there is left in it. All these things have a marked bearing on the results of patch tests and may account for many of the negative results obtained by authors from testing with orange and grapefruit peel .

"I believe, from the experiments which I made, that oil of lemon, oil of orange and oil of grapefruit will irritate by far the larger proportions of skins if allowed to remain on in the form of a patch test" (Schwarts 1938, in discussion of Beerman et al 1938).

Summary of the above reports leads to the conclusion that patch testing with citrus fruit rind (peel) named exocarp, applied as is, does not produce reliable or meaningful information concerning sensitivity.

A suitable patch test concentration of orange peel is perhaps 10% or 25% w/w in petrolatum.

Orange oil produced positive patch test reactions in 3/60 and lemon oil (C. limon) in 1/60 perfumery workers who had dermatitis (Gutman and Somov 1968).

Dyes used for oranges were reported to cause contact dermatitis (Traub et al 1937).

References

Agrup, G. (1969) Hand eczema and other hand dermatoses in South Sweden. Acta derm.-venereol. 49, Suppl. 61.

Baer, R.L., Leider, M. and Mayer, R.L. (1948) Possible eczematous cross-hypersensitivity between paraphenylenediamine and azo-dyes certified for use in foods, drugs and cosmetics. Proc. Soc. Exper. Biol. Med. 67, 489.

Beerman, H., Fondé, G.H. and Callaway, J.L. (1938) Citrus fruit dermatoses. Archs. Derm. Syph. 38, 225.

Behl, P.N., Captain, R.M., Bedi, B.M.S. and Gupta, S. (1966) Skin-irritant and sensitizing plants found in India, New Delhi. P.N. Behl, Irwin Hospital.

Bendersky, G. and Lupas, J. (1960) Anaphylactoid reaction to ingestion of orange. JAMA 173, 255.

Bonnevie, P. (1939) Aetiologie und Pathogenese der Ekzemkrankheiten. Leipzig. Barth.

Djerassi, L.S., Kleinhaus, U. and Hefetz, G. (1967) Epidemiological data on occupational dermatitis in the Haifa area. Dapim. Refuiim 26, 4.

Fanburg, S.V. and Kaufman, J.G. (1931) Eczema due to lemon peel. JAMA 97, 390.

Greenberg, L.A. and Lester, D. (1954) Handbook of Cosmetic Materials. New York. Interscience.

Hazen, H.H. (1944) Dermatitis of the eyelids. Archs. Derm. Syph. 49, 253.

Hjorth, N. (1961) Eczematous allergy to Balsams, Allied Perfumes and Flavouring Agents. Copenhagen. Munksgaard.

Hjorth, N. (1971) Allergy to balsams. Spectrum. 8, 97.

Horner, S.G. (1931) Dermatitis from Oranges and Lemons. Lancet 2, 961.

Janson, P. (1953) Citrus fruits and skin diseases. Z. Haut. u. Geschlkr. 14, 144.

Kesten, B.M. and Lyons, R. (1932) Dermatitis due to contact with orange peel. J. Allergy 3, 552.

Larsen, W.G. (1975) Cosmetic dermatitis due to a perfume. Contact Dermatitis 1, 142.

Mayers, M.R. (1932) Occupational dermatitis due to handling plants, vegetables and fruits. Industr. Bull. (N.Y.) 11, 342.

Menenghini, C.L., Rantuccio, F. and Lomuto, M. (1970) Additives, vehicles and active drugs of topical medicaments as causes of delayed-type allergic dermatitis. Dermatologica 143, 137.

Michel, P.J. (1953) Dermite des mains récidivante par contacts avec des oranges. Bull. Soc. franc. Derm. Syph. 63, 86.

Mitchell, J.C. (1972) Allergic contact dermatitis from a certified food dye presenting as 'sock dermatitis'. Contact Dermatitis Newsletter, London 11, 247.

Morris, G.E. (1954) Dermatoses among food handlers. Industr. Med. Surg. 23, 343.

Pardo-Castello, V. (1962) Common dermatoses in agricultural workers in the Caribbean area. Industr. Med. Surg. 31, 305.

Pathak, M.A., Daniels, F. Jr. and Fitzpatrick, T.B. (1962) Presently known distribution of furocoumarins (Psoralens) in plants. J. Invest. Derm. 39, 225.

Rantuccio, F., Meneghini, C.L. and Bonifazi, E. (1967) Rilieve sui tests epicutanei con serie fisse di allergeni in soggetti eczematosi. Folia allerg. 14, 46.

Rebhun, J. (1966) A study of the orange. J. Allergy 24, 238.

Rivasseau, J. (1956) A propos des sensibilisations de groupe. Bull. Soc. franc. Derm. Syph. 63, 83.

Schwartz, L. (1938a) Cutaneous Hazards in the citrus fruit industry. Archs. Derm. Syph. 37, 631.

Schwartz, L. (1938b) in discussion of Beerman et al (1938) Citrus fruit dermatoses. Archs. Derm. Syph. 38, 225.

Schwartz, L., Tulipan, L. and Birmingham, D.J. (1957) Occupational Diseases of the Skin. 3rd ed. Philadelphia. Lea and Febiger.

Seidmann, M. (1946) Dermatitis among workers employed in the citrus by-product industry. J. Palestin. Jewish Med. Ass. 2 (Nov), cited by Schwartz et al (1957).

Stauffer, H. (1948) A case of citric acid dermatitis. Dermatologica 97, (Suppl.) 121.

Sulzberger, M.B. (1936) in discussion of Traub (1936).

Touton, K. (1932) Hauterkrankungen durch phanerogamische Pflanzen und ihre Produkte (Toxicodermia et Allergodermia phytogenes), in Barnewitz, J. et al Angeborene Anomalien, Lichtdermatosen, Pflanzengifte, Thermische Schadigungen, Einfluss Innerer Storungen auf die Haut. Berlin, Verlag von Julius Springer.

Traub, E.F. (1936) Dermatitis in food handler. Archs. Derm. Syph. 34, 1054.

Urbach, E. (1931) Citronendermatitis. Zentralbl. Haut. Geschlechtskr. 37, 787.

Urbach, E. and Gottlieb, P.M. (1949) Allergy. New York. Grune and Stratton.

Van Dijk, E. and Berrens, L. (1964) Plants as an etiological factor in dermatitis venenata due to plants. Dermatologica 129, 321.

Walsh, W.E. (1975) Food allergy in atopic dermatitis. Minnesota Med. 58, 310.

White, C. (1941) Contact dermatitis: Occupational importance, diagnosis, management, prevention. Mississippi Valley Med. J. 63, 120 and 154.

White, J.C. (1887) Dermatitis venenata: An account of the action of external irritants upon the skin. Boston. Cupples and Hurd.

White, R.P. (1934) The Dermatergoses or Occupational Affections of the Skin. 4th ed. London. H.K. Lewis.

Zakon, S.J., Goldberg, A.L. and Kahn, J.B. (1947) Lipstick cheilitis: Common dermatosis. Report of 32 cases. Archs. Derm. Syph. 56, 499.

Traub, E.F., Gordon, R.E. and Van Dyke, L.S. (1937) Dermatitis from dyes and otherwise treated citrus fruit. JAMA 108, 872.

Gutman, S.G. and Somov, B.A. (1968) Allergic reactions caused by components of perfumery preparations. Vestn. Derm. Vener. 42, 62.

Citrus aurantium
var. aurantium
Seville or bitter orange
(bigaradia or amara)
(Shaw 1973)

Citrus bigaradia
(syn. C. vulgaris)

Oil of Petitgrain derived from this species can produce irritation and photosensitisation (Greenberg and Lester 1954, Klarmann 1958).

According to Fenaroli (1971) Oil of Petitgrain is derived from C. aurantium ssp. amara.

Dermatitis from bitter orange was reported by Murray (1921); patch tests were not recorded.

References

Fenaroli, G. (1971) Fenaroli's Handbook of Flavor Ingredients. ed. Furia, T.E. and Bellanca, N. Cleveland, Ohio. The Chemical Rubber Co.

Greenberg, L.A. and Lester, D. (1954) Handbook of Cosmetic Materials. New York. Interscience.

Klarmann, E.G. (1958) Perfume dermatitis. Ann. Allergy 16, 425.

Murray, F.A. (1921) Dermatitis caused by bitter oranges. Brit. Med. J. 1, 739.

Shaw, H.K.A. (1973) A Dictionary of the Flowering Plants and Ferns. (the late J.C. Willis) 8th ed. Cmabridge University Press.

Citrus aurantium
var. bergamia
(syn. C. bergamia)
Bergamot orange

Oil of Bergamot can produce photodermatitis. The fruit yields furanocoumarins, including 5-methoxypsoralen (Pathak et al 1962). The name Bergamot dates from 1696 from the town of Bergamo in Italy.

Freund (1916) described a skin disease in necklace or berlock-form in four patients who applied eau de cologne to their skin, directly after which they exposed themselves to sunshine. Dermatitis was followed by hyperpigmentation. He suspected that oil of bergamot was responsible.

In modern German berlocke is the word for a pendant (a kind of necklace). The French equivalent is berloque. In present-day dermatologic literature one sees berloque and berlock which are reasonable and berlocque and Berloque (suggesting an eponym by its initial capital) which are incorrect (Harber et al 1964).

Eau de Cologne, containing Oil of Bergamot, is the commonest cause of berloque pigmentation which may or may not be accompanied by visible dermatitis (Espersen 1952). He reviewed the literature and noted that Kuske (1940) had found more than 100 publications on the subject. Goodman (1931), Klaber (1942), Greenberg and Lester (1954) and Pathak (1974) also reviewed the subject.

Erythema and vesicles appear at the skin site of contact following exposure to sunlight; the reaction is often present on the neck, hence the pendant-like distribution (Gross and Robinson 1930, Rogin and Sheard 1935, Lane and Strauss 1930, Downing 1932, Klarman 1958). The dermatitis is more severe in natural blondes but the residual pigmentation is more severe in brunettes. Only some persons are susceptible to photosensitisation by Oil of Bergamot and these only at certain times and/or certain sites (Harber et al 1964). They discuss four hypotheses and it seems possible that photoallergy is involved as well as phototoxicity from furanocoumarins. Bergamot oil produced positive patch test reactions in 3/590 (0.5%) of patients tested (Menighini et al 1971).

Samples of Bergamot oil can vary in their phototoxic capacity (Zaynoun et al 1974).

References

Downing, J.G. (1932) Pigmentation from perfume, Berlock "Dermatitis". N. Eng. J. Med. 207, 660.

Espersen, E. (1952) Berloque Dermatitis. Acta Dermatovener. 32, 91.

Freund, E. (1916) Uber bisher noch nicht beschriebene kunstliche Hautverfarbungen. Derm. Wschr. 63, 931.

Goodman, H. (1931) Perfume dermatitis: case report with review of literature and bibliography. Brit. J. Derm. 43, 177.

Greenberg, L.A. and Lester, D. (1954) Handbook of Cosmetic Materials. New York. Interscience.

Gross, P. and Robinson, L.C. (1930) Berlock dermatitis: unusual dermatitis and pigmentation following use of perfume. Arch. Derm. Syph. 21, 637.

Harber, L.C., Holloway, R.M. and Moragne, M. (1964) Polymorphous light eruption: office diagnosis and management. N.Y. State Med. J. 64, 619.

Klaber, R. (1942) Phyto-photodermatitis. Brit. J. Derm. Syph. 54, 193.

Klarmann, E.G. (1958) Perfume dermatitis. Ann. Allerg. 16, 425.

Kuske, H. (1940) Perkutane Photosensibilisierung durch pflanzliche Wirkstoffe. Dermatologica 82, 273.

Lane, J.E. and Strauss, M.J. (1930) Toilet Water Dermatitis, with special reference to Berlock Dermatitis. JAMA 95, 717.

Menighini, C.L., Rantuccio, F. and Lomuto, M. (1971) Additives, vehicles and active drugs of topical medicaments as causes of delayed type allergic dermatitis. Dermatologica 143, 137.

Pathak, M.A., Daniels, F. Jr. and Fitzpatrick, T.B. (1962) Presently known distribution of furocoumarins (Psoralens) in plants. J. Invest. Derm. 39, 225.

Rogin, J.R. and Sheard, C. (1935) Factors affecting color of skin: Their significance in Berlock Dermatitis. Arch. Derm. Syph. 32, 265.

Zaynoun, S., Hall, I., Johnson, B.E. and Frain-Bell, W. (1974) A study of bergamot sensitivity. Brit. J. Derm. 91 (Suppl. 10), 14.

Additional references

Marzulli, F.N. and Maibach, H.I. (1970) Perfume phototoxicity. J. Soc. Cosm. Chem. 21, 695.

Zaynoun, S.T., Johnson, B.E. and Frain-Bell, W. (1977) A study of oil of bergamot and its importance as a phototoxic agent. I. Characterization and quantitation of the photoactive component. Brit. J. Derm. 96, 475.

Zaynoun, S.T., Johnson, B.E. and Frain-Bell, W. (1977) A study of oil of bergamot and its importance as a photoxic agent. II. Factors which affect the phototoxic reaction induced by bergamot oil and psoralen derivatives. Contact Dermatitis 3, 225.

Early history of berlock dermatitis (from Goodman 1931)

In 1916 Freund reported a number of patients, observed some years earlier, who had a peculiar pigmentation of the skin of the neck, which was supposedly due to the application of toilet-water to the exposed parts followed immediately by sunlight. Freund made a number of experiments, and was convinced that oil of bergamot was the ingredient responsible.

Eight years later, Rosenthal (1924), unaware of the work of Freund, reported a patient before the Berlin Dermatological Society with a skin-eruption which he named "Berlocque dermatitis". The description which Rosenthal gave is an excellent one, for it serves for other reported cases, and explains some of the other names listed for the affliction. Rosenthal's description, as given by Lane and Strauss (1930), is as follows:

"Two or three dark yellowish streaks of pigmentation are seen running down from the front or back of the neck. Their upper portions are hardly visible and are poorly outlined, but farther down, and especially at the lower margin, they become more evident and darker. The streaks may also appear on the face, on the arms and on the trunk. The shape, outline, and the increase of pigment towards the lowest part of the streaks is especially characteristic. They give the appearance of being caused by a dark-coloured fluid running down. In the region of the pigmentation, by the use of a magnifying glass, distinct signs of inflammation are seen, also dilation of the capillaries and prominence of the openings of the hair-follicles."

The true nature of the disease was not recognized at the Berlin meeting and many guesses were made. A month after Rosenthal's presentation, Fischer (1925) presented two similar cases, and although no diagnosis was made, the possibility of external irritation was suggested.

In 1925 Hoffmann and Schmidtz rediscovered the cause of the condition and unearthed the work of Freund. In 1926 reports were published by Galewsky and by Falkenstein. In 1927 Samek, Linser, Freund and Brito reported cases. In 1928 Posso, Langer, Zurhelle, Uhrbach and others reported cases.

Gross and Robinson (1930), Lane and Strauss (1930) and Goodman (1931) reported cases from the United States.

Axmann, in 1925, claimed that he produced pigmentation on spots of depigmented skin (vitiligo) after rubbing eau de cologne on the areas. Du Bois, in 1927, found no increase of pigmentation following the application of pure alcohol, and thought that the eruption was due to essential oils and sensitization to light. Uhlmann, in 1927, exposed areas of depigmented skin to the beam from a quartz mercury vapour lamp, protecting the normal skin, and found no increase in pigmentation, although the vitiligo areas became red. The experiment was repeated, but he applied eau-de-Cologne to the depigmented spots before radiation with the mercury vapour arc. He was enabled by this means to produce pigmentation in the previously pigment-free areas. Uhlmann reported that the oil of bergamot alone did not produce the colour change, but that it required oil of bergamot in alcohol.

Freund, also in 1927, applied eau-de-Cologne to a boy's forearm and exposed the surface to sun and sea-water. The boy developed an inflammation on the site followed by pigmentation. Freund then used the oil of bergamot followed by sun exposure, and produced a blister which was followed by pigmentation. The attempt to pigment unpigmented areas of vitiligo was not successful.

Zurhelle, in 1928, reported that he considered perspiration to be one of the factors in the production of the dermatitis. He stated that the inflammatory process was strongest in blondes, but that the tendency for the formation of pigment was stronger in brunettes. Szanto, in 1928, used oil of bergamot in alcohol on depigmented skin and claimed eighteen successes in twenty-two trials. Bonnet, in 1928, reported negative results for production of pigment in depigmented areas by this method. Phipps, in 1929, reported the return of pigment in a case of vitiligo after the use of oil of bergamot and ultra-violet radiation. Gross, reporting in 1930, had one success and several failures.

References

Axmann (1925) "Behandlung der Pigmentatrophie mittels lichtsensibiler Stoffe", Munch. med. Wochenschr. 72, 1918 and 73, 90 (1926).

Bonnet, L.M. (1928) "Pigmentations cervicales 'en coulees' ou 'en breloques'", Lyon Med. 142, 153.

Brito, F. (1927) "Durch Koelnisches Wasser Hervergerufenee erythemato-pigmentierte Flecken" abstr. Zentrabl Haut Geschel. 23, 549.

Du Bois, C. (1927) "Dermite pigmentee en forme de coulees produite par des applications d'eau de Cologne", Ann. de Derm. et de Syph. 8, 539.

Falkenstein (1926) "Eau de Cologne Pigmentierung", Zentrabl. Haut. Geschel. 21, 400.

Fischer, W. (1925) "Fleckformige, Hautpigmentierung unbekannter Aetiologie", Derm. Seitschr. 43, 58.

Freund, E. (1916) "Ueber bisher noch nicht beschriebene keunstliche Hautverfaerbungen", Derm. Wochenschr. 63, 931.

Freund, E. (1927) "Hautverfaerbung durch Meerbaeder, Koelnische Wasser und Sonnenbaeder", Zentralbl. f. Haut u. Geschlechtskrankheiten 25, 61.

Galewsky (1926) "Demonstration zweier Moulagen der Berlocque Krankheit", Zentralbl. f. Haut-u. Geschlechtskrankheiten, 20, 273.

Goodman, H. (1931) Perfume dermatitis: case report, with a review of the literature and bibliography. Brit. J. Derm. Syph. 43, 177.

Gross, P. and Robinson, L.B. (1930) "Berlock Dermatitis", Archs. Derm. Syph. 21, 637.

Hoffmann, E. and Schmidtz, H. (1925) "Ueber lineaer und tropfenartig bergrenzte Pigmentierung nach starker Besonnung und Anspritzen mit parfumierten Spiritus (Koelnisch Wasser)", Munch. med. Wochenschr. 72, 1414.

Lane, J. and Strauss, M.J. (1930) "Toilet-Water Dermatitis", Journ. Amer. Med. Assoc. 95, 717.

Langer (1928) Presentation of case, Zentralbl. f. Haut-u. Geschlechtskrankheiten 25, 515.

Linser (1927) "Berloque Krankheit", Derm. Wochenschr. 84, 376.

Phipps, M. (1929) "Cas de vitiligo traite par les rayons ultra violets apres frictions, a l'essence de bergamote", Bull de la Soc. Franc. de Derm. et de Syph. 26, 1065.

Pozzo, A. (1928) "Pigmentazioni da aqua de Colonia e da raggi Solari", Policlinico 35, 86.

Rosenthal, O. (1924) "Hauterkrankung in Berlock Form", Derm. Zeitschr 42, 295. Published in 1925.

Samek (1927) "Pigmentation nach Koelnisch Wasser", Zentralbl. f. Haut-u. Geschlechtskrankheiten 23, 615.

Stein, R.P. (1925) "Hauterkrankung in Berlock Form", Zentralbl. f. Haut-u. Geschlechtskrankheiten 18, 510.

Szanto, J. (1928) "Uber Pigmentierungen nach Sensibilisierung der Haut mit aetherischen Oelen", abstr. Zentrabl. Haut. Geschl. 28, 451.

Uhrbach (1928) "Ueber die Berloque Krankheit", Zentrabl. Haut. Geschl. 28, 404.

Zurhelle, E. (1928) "Demonstration klinischer und histologische Befunde bei experimentellen Untersuchungen ueber die Einwirkung von Koelnischen Wasser", Zentrabl. Haut. Geschl. 27, 728.

Additional References

Opdyke, D.L.J. (1973) Monographs on fragrance raw materials. Bergamot oil expressed. Fd. Cosmet Toxicol. 11, 1031.

Meyer, J. (1970) Accidents due to tanning cosmetics with a base of bergamot oil. Bull. Soc. fr. Derm. Syph. 77, 881.

Additional References

Rosenthal, F. (1925) Berliner Dermatologische Gesselschaft. Dermatol. Zh. 42, 295; Der Berlock-dermatitis. Dermatol. Wochenschr. 86, 242, cited by Marzulli and Maibach (1970).

Marzulli, F.N. and Maibach, H.I. (1970) Perfume phototoxicity. J. Soc. Cosmet. Chem. 21, 695.

Citrus hystrix

The wood is said to be injurious to wood-workers (Vonkennel cited by Hausen 1970).

References

Hausen, B.M. (1970) Untersuchungen uber Gesundheitsschadigende Holzer. Thesis, Hamburg.

Vonkennel (1929) Teakholzdermatitis. Zbl. Haut-Geschlkrkh. 30, 14 and 691, cited by Hausen (1970).

Citrus limon
Lemon

Citrus limonia
Canton lemon

Citrus medica var. limonum
(Greenberg and Lester 1954)

Oil of Lemon (Oil of Cedro) derived from the last named variety has been reported to cause dermatitis (Greenberg and Lester 1954, Klarmann 1958). C. limonum yields 5-methoxypsoralen (Pathak et al 1962). Lemons have been reported to cause dermatitis (Fanburg and Kaufman 1931, Puglisi 1951). Lemon peel is frequently irritant by patch test. Lemon juice appears to be more irritant than orange juice since it has a higher content of citric acid. Lemon peel is irritant by patch test (Beerman et al 1938).

Keil (1947) observed a patient with contact dermatitis from Oil of Lemon: the patient was also contact sensitive to Oil of Citronella (Ceylon), Oil of Citronella (Java) (Cymbopogon) and to turpentine (Pinaceae). Further patch tests demonstrated contact sensitivity to dipentine (d-l-limonene), alpha-pinene and beta-pinene. The principal allergen appeared to be limonene present in these materials.

Lemon and lime (C. aurantifolia) pickers at times are seen with bands or lines of brown or black skin pigmentations caused by the oil from the skin of these fruits (Pardo-Castello 1962). Patch-testing to lemon is noted under C. aurantium.

Citrus limon

Workers handling lemons developed chronic dermatitis, hyperkeratosis and nail changes (Lacroix 1940).

Lemon juice or lemon peel applied to the face to make the skin smooth caused dermatitis of the face in four women. Patch tests were not recorded (Minami 1968).

References

Beerman, H., Fonde, G.H. and Callaway, J.L. (1938) Citrus fruit dermatoses. Archs. Derm. Syph. 38, 225.

Fanburg, S.V. and Kaufman, J.G. (1931) Eczema due to lemon peel. JAMA 97, 390.

Greenberg, L.A. and Lester, D. (1954) Handbook of Cosmetic Materials. New York. Interscience.

Keil, H. (1947) Contact dermatitis due to oil of citronella. Report of 3 cases with experimental studies on ingredients and related substances. J. Invest. Derm. 8, 327.

Klarmann, E.G. (1958) Perfume dermatitis. Ann. Allergy. 16, 425.

Pardo-Castello, V. (1962) Common dermatoses in agricultural workers in the Caribbean area. Industr. Med. Surg. 31, 305.

Pathak, M.A., Daniels, F. Jr. and Fitzpatrick, T.B. (1962) Presently known distribution of furocoumarins (Psoralens) in plants. J. Invest. Derm. 39, 225.

Puglisi, V. (1951) Dermatoses due to lemons. G. ital. Derm. Sif. 92, 237.

Minami, S. (1968) Dermatitis caused by lemons. Jap. J. Clin. Exp. Med. 45, 11.

Lacroix, G. (1940) Injuries of workers handling lemons. Folia. med. 26, 223.

Citrus paradisi
Grapefruit

Men who wore few clothes tore the fruit open and the juice spattered on their skin; hyperpigmentation of the skin of the abdomen resulted (Simons 1952). Oil of grapefruit did not have any photosensitizing activity (Sams 1941).

References

Sams, W.M. (1941) Photodynamic action of lime oil (Citrus aurantifolia). Archs. Derm. Syph. 44, 571.

Simons, R.D.G. (1952) Handbook of Tropical Dermatology. New York. Elsevier.

Clausena

30 species are found in palaeotropical regions. Some have edible fruit.

Clausena platyphylla

The glands of the plant have a caustic secretion (Altschul 1973).

Reference

Altschul, S. von R. (1973) Drugs and foods from little-known plants. Cambridge, Mass. Harvard Univ. Press.

Dictamnus

Six species are found from central and southern Europe to eastern Siberia and northern China.

Dictamnus spp.
Creosote Bush

A worker developed dermatitis after two weeks exposure to the wood dust which he was cooking and evaporating to prepare nordihydroguaiaretic acid (NDGA) used as an antioxidant for lard (Weber 1953). This chemical which occurs in the resinous exudates of many plants is commonly derived from Larrea.

A worker in a pharmaceutical factory, and a pharmacist, developed dermatitis of the face and hands from handling Vitamin AD tablets and lanoline cream respectively. Patch tests to NDGA, contained in these preparations, was positive 2% in vaseline. In the pharmaceutical worker, a patch test to hydrogenated Oil of Soybean (Glycine) containing 0.15 per cent NDGA was positive. The compound was not irritant at a concentration of 5% in vaseline. Many of the fats and oils used for local therapy contain stabilisers but the contents of these are not indicated (Jorgenson and Hjorth 1970).

References

Jorgenson, G. and Hjorth, N. (1970) Dermatitis from nordihydroguaiaretic acid, an antioxidant in fats. Contact Dermatitis Newsletter, London 7, 151.

Weber, L.F. (1953) Dermatitis venenata from native woods. Archs. Derm. Syph. 67, 388.

Dictamnus albus
(syn. D. fraxinella)
Dittany, Candle-plant,
Gas Plant, Burning Bush

The plant is cultivated as an ornamental shrub or hedge. Volatile and inflammable oil is excreted, so that on hot calm days the air around the plant may sometimes be ignited, hence the colloquial name, Burning Bush.

Dermatitis from contact with this plant was reported by Baronovysky (1929), Cummer and Dexter (1937), Muenscher and Brown (1944), Chopra et al (1949), Szego et al (1955), Shalupenko (1962), Voborova and Chmelova (1965) and Engel and Horn (1972).

The human skin is more susceptible if wetted. The seed pod is the most injurious part of the plant, next the leaves. Somner and Jillson (1967) clearly defined the role of sunlight in evoking photodermatitis from the plant and they tabulated the clinical features which enable a distinction from poison-ivy (Toxicodendron) dermatitis to be made.

References

Baronovsky, V. (1929) Einige beobachtungen uber die, durch "Dictamnus fraxinella". Russk. Vestnik. dermat. 7, 58.

Chopra, R.N., Bhadwar, R.L. and Ghosh, S. (1949) Poisonous Plants of India. The Indian Council of Agricultural Research. Delhi.

Cummer, C.L. and Dexter, R. (1937) Dermatitis caused by *Dictamnus albus* (gas plant). An example of photosensitisation. JAMA 109, 495.

Engel, S. and Horn, K. (1972) Phytodermatosen durch *Dictamnus alba*, *Sanicula europaea* and *Phyllodendron consanguineum*. Dermatol. Monatsschr. 158, 22.

Muenscher, W.C. and Brown, B.I. (1944) Dermatitis and photosensitisation produced by *Ptelea angustifolia*. Madrono 7, 184.

Shalupenko, V.N. (1962) Dermatitis caused by contact with *Dictamnus albus*. Vestn. Derm. I. Vener. 10, 82.

Somner, R.G. and Jillson, O.F. (1967) Phytophotodermatitis - Gas Plant and the wild parsnip. New Eng. J. Med. 276, 1484.

Szego, L. and Tamas, M. (1955) Untersuchungen uber die Rolle ker physikalischen Factoren bei durch *Ruta graveolens* verursachten dermatitis. Berufsdermatosen 3, 84.

Voborova, A. and Chmelova, M. (1965) Photodermatitis phytogenica. Cs. Derm. 1, 43.

Dictamnus albus
(syn. *D. fraxinella*)
var. *caucasicus*

Linear bullous dermatitis followed by hyperpigmentation resulted from contact with the fresh plant; old dried plant was inactive (Gorodinsky 1938).

Reference

Gorodinsky, M. (1938) Linear bullous dermatitis caused by *Dictamnus fraxinella caucasicus*. Sovet. vestnik. venereol. i. dermat. 1, 27.

Dictamnus dasycarpus

Bullous dermatitis from contact with this species was most commonly observed at the time of its blossoming when 3-5% of all dermatological out-patients were affected (Stekhun and Kurnakov 1962).

Reference

Stekhun, F.I. and Kurnakov, B.A. (1962) Dermatitis caused by *Dictamnus dasycarpus*. Vestn. Derm. i. Vener. 1, 67.

Esenbeckia

38 species are found in tropical America and the West Indies. The bark of some Brazilian species is used like angostura (*Galipea*) as a bitter for gin.

Esenbeckia leiocarpa
Guaranta

See *Euxylophora*.

Euxylophora

One species is found in the Amazon region and in Brazil.

Euxylophora paraensis
Amarelo, pau setim, boxwood

Esenbeckia leiocarpa
Guarantá

Raputia magnifica
Arapoca

Raputia alba
Arapoca branca

Balfourodendron riedelianum
Guatambú

Freise (1936) described fifteen cases of dermatitis caused by these satinwood or boxwood substitutes, and two similar cases from *Fagara flava*. Most of the eruptions were mild and confined to the finger-webs and other exposed areas, as the sawdust of fresh wood is coarse and does not penetrate under the clothes. Some were more severe, however, with widespread oedema accompanied by general symptoms, usually going on to vesicular dermatitis and often gangrenous ulcers which in three cases proved fatal. Freise confirmed the irritant action of the sawdust on his own skin and on laboratory animals.

E. leicarpa and E. paraensis contain the photosensitizer xanthotoxin, and B. riedelianum contains balfourodin and other alkaloids (Hausen 1970).

References

Freise, F.W. (1936) Vergiftungen durch Brasiliansiche Werkholzer I. II. Sammlund der Vergiftungsfallen. 7C, 1 and 61.

Hausen, B.M. (1970) Untersuchungen uber Gesundheitsschadigende Holzer. Thesis, Hamburg.

Fagara

250 species are found in tropical regions.

Fagara capensis

The berry is acrid and tastes strongly of lemon (Citrus) leaving a persistent burning sensation in the mouth (Watt and Breyer-Brandwijk 1962).

Fagara caribea

According to Woods and Calnan (1976) this species is one of a number of woods called zebrawood and not the only one likely to cause dermatitis. They index woods named zebrawood as Astronium, fagara caribaea and (possibly incorrectly) Baphia and as African zebrawood, Microberlinia.

Fagara daviji
Horse's Teats

The sharp thorns which usually tip the knobs which stud the trunk (Menninger 1967) are capable of causing mechanical injury.

Fagara flava
(syn. Zanthoxylum flavum)

This species is noted under Zanthoxylum flavum.

Fagara heitzii
Olon

The wood is said to be capable of producing dermatitis (Hausen 1970, Orsler 1973).

Fagara leprieurii
(syn. F. angolensis)

The pulverized bark is used as a counter-irritant (Irvine 1961).

Fagara macrophylla
Olon

This species can cause dermatitis and upper respiratory sumptoms in wood-workers (Rochaix and Vieux 1936, Zafiropoulo et al 1968). The bark makes part of a mixture, with Diospyros xanthochlamys and Mansonia altissima which is used for irritant and blistering purposes (Irvine 1961).

Fagara oilanthoides, F. schinofolia and F. xanthoxyloides (Artar Prickly Ash) yield furanocoumarins. The last named yields 8-methoxypsoralen and is therefore potentially phototoxic (Pathak et al 1962).

References

Hausen, B.M. (1970) Untersuchungen uber Gesundheitsschadigende Holzer. Thesis, Hamburg.

Irvine, F.R. (1961) Woody plants of Ghana. Oxford University Press. London.

Menninger, E.A. (1967) Fantastic Trees. New York. The Viking Press.

Orsler, R.J. (1973) Personal communication from Forest Products Research Laboratory, Princess Risborough, Bucks, England.

Pathak, M.A., Daniels, F. Jr. and Fitzpatrick, T.B. (1962) Presently known distribution of furocoumarins (Psoralens) in plants. J. Invest. Derm. 39, 225.

Rochaix and Vieux (1936) A dermatitis due to Olon wood. Rev. Hyg. 58, 590.

Watt, J.M. and Breyer-Brandwijk, M.G. (1962) The Medicinal and poisonous plants of Southern Africa. 2nd ed. Edinburgh. E.& S. Livingstone.

Zafiropoulo, A., Audibert, A. and Charpin, J. (1968) A propos des accidents dus a la manipulation des bois exotiques. Rev. Franc. Allerg. 8, 155.

Woods, B. and Calnan, C.D. (1976) Toxic Woods. Brit. J. Derm. 94, Suppl. 13, June.

Fagara macrophylla
Africa satinwood, olonvogo, olon dur

Fagara heitzii
Olon

Fagara inaequalis

Dermatitis and coryza affected all eight men present when a dried tree trunk of olon was sawn up producing much fine dust. A wetter section of the same trunk was sawn elsewhere without any trouble (Pillon and Martinez 1935). Rochaix and Vieux (1936) tried experimentally to sensitize rabbits with olon sawdust but could demonstrate only a primary irritant effect. Orsler (1973) and Hausen (1970) received trade reports of irritation by olon wood. Freise (1937) found xanthotoxin and an alkaloid in the wood. More recently, suberosin and the coumarins, psoralen and xanthotoxin have been found in Fagara spp. (King et al 1954). Earlier workers reported pungent resins from the wood (Auld and Pickles 1912).

References

Auld, S.J.M. and Pickles, S.S. (1912) The constituents of West Indian Satinwood. J. Chem. Soc. 101, 1052.

Hausen, B.M. (1970) Untersuchungen uber Gesundheitsschadigende Holzer. Thesis, Hamburg.

King, F.E., Housley, J.R. and King, T.J. (1954) Coumarin constituents of Fagara macrophylla, Zanthoxylum flavum and Chloroxylon swietenia. J. Chem. Soc. 1392.

Orsler, R.J. (1973) Personal communication from Forest Products Research Laboratory, Princess Risborough, Bucks, England.

Pillon, and Martinez (1935) Sur huit cas de dermite par bois exotique. Bull. Soc. franc. Derm. Syph. 42, 380.

Rochaix, A. and Vieux, G. (1936) Sur une dermatose provoquée par le 'bois d'olon'. Rev. Hyg. 58, 590.

Galipea

13 species are found in Central and South America.

Galipea officinalis

The bark is used in Herbal Medicine (Wren 1968) and is a source of angostura bitters used in gin. Cusparia of this family is used for the same purpose.

Reference

Wren, R.W. (1968) Potter's New Cyclopaedia of Botanical Drugs and Preparations by Wren, R.C. Re-edit. by Wren, R.W. Potter and Clarke Ltd. Health Science Press. Rustington, Sussex.

Glycosmis

60 species are found in Indo Malaysia. Some species yield edible fruit.

Glycosmis pentaphylla

This species yields furanocoumarins (Pathak et al 1962).

Reference

Pathak, M.A., Daniels, F. Jr. and Fitzpatrick, T.B. (1962) Presently known distribution of furocoumarins (Psoralens) in plants. J. Invest. Derm. 39, 225.

Halfordia

Four species are found in New Guinea, eastern Australia and New Caledonia.

Halfordia scleroxyla
Ghittoe Saffron-heart,
Kerosene wood

The wood is very inflammable even in a green state, hence the name kerosene tree. Splinters of the wood, when they penetrate the skin, cause festering. When chewed, or used to clean the teeth, as is the habit sometimes of men working in saw-mills, the splinters cause trouble with the gums (Webb 1948).

Reference

Webb, L.J. (1948) Guide to the medicinal and poisonous plants of Queensland. Bulletin No. 232. Council for Scientific and Industrial Research. Melbourne, Australia.

Haplophyllum
(syn. Ruta)

70 species are found from the Mediterranean region to eastern Siberia.

Haplophyllum tuberculatum

Possibly this species has been reported to cause facial dermatitis and oedema in the Sudan (Chalmers and Pekkloa cited by Simons 1953).

Reference

Simons, R.D.G. (1953) Jungle-Dermatitis (Dermatoses caused by tropical plants and woods) in Handbook of Tropical Dermatology and Medical Mycology, ed. Simons, R.D.G. Amsterdam. Elsevier Publ. Co. Vol. II. p. 1444.

Limonia

One species is found from India to Java.

Limonia acidissima
Elephant-apple,
Wood-apple

The wood is useful and yields a gum. The edible fruit is used in Japan as a substitute for soap.

Luvunga
(syn. Lavanga)

12 species are found in Indo Malaysia.

Luvunga scandens

This evergreen plant is sometimes grown for ornamental purposes in the citrus belt; the fruit has a lemon-like rind. The plant is potentially phototoxic from a yield of 8-methoxypsoralen (Pathak et al 1962).

Reference

Pathak, M.A., Daniels, F. Jr. and Fitzpatrick, T.B. (1962) Presently known distribution of furocoumarins (Psoralens) in plants. J. Invest. Derm. 39, 225.

Melicope

70 species are found in Indo Malaysia, in warm regions of Australia, in New Zealand and the Pacific area.

Melicope erythrocca
Tingle-Tongue

The plant is irritant to the tongue (Everist 1972).

Reference

Everist, S.L. (1972) Queensland Herbarium, Brisbane, Australia. Personal communication concerning plants recorded in Australia as having caused dermatitis or other contact injury to man or livestock.

Orixa

One species is found in Japan.

Orixa japonica

This tree causes dermatitis among agricultural workers (Ishibashi 1937). It is used as a fertilizer in Japan and is a type of Stink Tree or Stink wood. Ocotea (Lauraceae), Zieria (Rutaceae), Foetidia (Foetidiaceae) and Nyssa (Nyssaceae) are also called Stink Woods (Schwartz et al 1957).

References

Ishibashi, T. (1937) Dermatitis caused by Orixa japonica Thunb. Jap. J. Derm. Urol. 42, 135.

Schwartz, L., Tulipan, L. and Birmingham, D.J. (1957) Occupational Diseases of the Skin. 3rd ed. Philadelphia. Lea and Febiger. pp. 637-672.

Pelea

75 species are found in the Pacific region, mostly in the Hawaiian Islands.

Pelea anisata
Mokihana

The fresh plant when applied in the form of a lei (neck-garland) to the bare, perspiring neck for half an hour, can make the wearer very uncomfortable for a week or so afterward (Arnold 1968).

Reference

Arnold, H.L. (1968) Poisonous plants of Hawaii. Rutland, Vermont. Charles E. Tuttle.

Phebalium

40 species are found in Australia and New Zealand.

Phebalium anceps
Blister Bush

Contact with the plant can cause phytophotodermatitis (Aplin 1976).

Phebalium argenteum
Western Australian
Blister Plant

The plant is a small shrub about 1m high with white flowers and silvery scurfy leaves which grows in south-western Australia, and has been adapted to cultivation in California. Yellow flowers also occur. The plant blisters the human skin if handled (Morrison 1899, Maiden 1909). Cleland (1914) rubbed the dew-laden leaf on the back of his hand. No irritation was noted immediately. Erythema was first observed at 24 hours and within 48 hours bulla formation occurred at the site. Hyperpigmentation surrounding an area of leucoderma persisted for about 5 years. On several other occasions, he tried to produce similar results, apparently with the same plant, but failed. Francis and Southcott (1967) do not mention a role of sunlight for evoking reactions but since the plant yields psoralen (Finlayson 1928, Bose and Finlayson 1938) phytophotodermatitis seems to be possible for contact with the plant.

References

Aplin, T.E.H. (1976) Poisonous garden plants and other plants harmful to man in Australia. Western Australian Dept. of Agriculture Bull. 3964.

Bose, P.K. and Finlayson, H.H. (1938) Occurrence of psoralen in Phebalium argenteum. J. Indian Chem. Soc. 15, 516.

Cleland, J.B. (1914) Plants, including fungi, poisonous or otherwise injurious to man in Australia. Australasian Med. Gaz. 35, 569. idem. Tasmanian Ag. Gaz. 32, 361 and 401.

Finlayson, H.H. (1928) Essential oil of Phebalium argenteum Smith. Trans. Roy. Soc., S. Australia 52, 235.

Francis, D.F. and Southcott, R.V. (1967) Plants harmful to man in Australia. Misc. Bull. No. 1. Botanic Garden, Adelaide, Australia.

Maiden, J.H. (1904) Two more new weeds. Noxious weeds. Weeds of New South Wales. The Buffalo Burr (Solanum rostratum Dunal). Ag. Gaz. New South Wales. 15, 246, 316, 541.

Maiden, J.H. (1909) On some plants which cause inflammation or irritation of the skin. Ag. Gaz. New South Wales 20, 111 and 1073.

Morrison, A. (1899) Chemist and Druggist 8th July, pg. 63, cited by Maiden (1909).

Pilocarpus

22 species are found in tropical America and the West Indies.

Pilocarpus jaborandi
Pernambuco Jacorandi

This and other Pilocarpus species yield the alkaloid pilocarpine which can cause allergic kerato-conjunctivitis (Duke-Elder 1965). High concentrations of pilocarpine in hair preparations can produce irritant effects (Greenberg and Lester 1954).

Pilocarpus pennatifolius
Jaborandi

The leaves form officinal 'folia Jaborandi'. Prolonged contact with the powder can cause irritation of the skin (Dispensatory 1884).

References

Dispensatory, The National (1884) Philadelphia. Stille and Maisch, cited by White (1887).

Duke-Elder, S. (1965) System of Opthalmology. Vol. VIII. Diseases of the outer eye. Part 1. Allergic kerato-conjunctivitis. pp. 451. London. Henry Kimpton.

Greenberg, L.A. and Lester, D. (1954) Handbook of Cosmetic Materials. New York. Interscience.

White, J.C. (1887) Dermatitis venenata: An account of the Action of External irritants upon the Skin. Boston. Cupples and Hurd.

Ptelea

Three species are native to the United States and Mexico.

Ptelea spp.

The taxonomy of the genus is confused (Bailey and Bailey 1941) and phytochemical differences are known in sub-species and varieties (Szendrei et al 1973). P. isophylla and P. trifoliata are known in horticulture as ornamental shrubs.

Ptelea angustifolia
(syn. P. lutescens)
Hop Tree

This species grown as an ornamental shrub in New York State was observed to evoke photodermatitis (Muenscher and Brown 1944).

Ptelea aptera

This species yields psoralen (Dreyer 1969).

Ptelea baldwinii
(syn. P. angustifolia)
Wafer Ash, Hop Tree

Contact reactions to this plant have been reported (Muenscher and Brown 1944).

Ptelea crenulata

This species yields psoralen and bergapten (Dreyer 1969).

Ptelea trifoliata

Positive photopatch test reactions to an alcoholic solution of the leaves of this shrub could not be confirmed on re-testing with the stored solution (Lynne-Davies and Mitchell 1973, unpublished observations).

References

Bailey, L.H. and Bailey, E.Z. (1941) Hortus Second. New York. Macmillan.

Dreyer, D.L. (1969) Coumarins and alkaloids of the genus Ptelea. Phytochemistry 8, 1013.

Muenscher, W.C. and Brown, B.I. (1944) Dermatitis and photosensitisation produced by Ptelea angustifolia. Madrono 7, 184.

Szendrei, K., Novak, I., Petz, M. et al (1973) Coumarins and alkaloids from Ptelea trifoliata ssp. pallida var. confinis. Lloydia 36, 333.

Raputia

Ten species are found in the West Indies and in tropical South America.

Raputia alba
Arapoca branca

Raputia magnifica
Arapoca

See Euxylophora.

Ruta

Seven species are found in the Canaries, etc. and from the Mediterranean region to south-western Asia.

Ruta spp.
'Ruta sylvestris'

The vapour of rue raises up blisters, wheals and other accidents on the face (Gerard 1636).

Rue oil had phototoxic activity but was not found to be sensitizing (Opdyke 1975).

Ruta chalepensis

This species yields 8-methoxypsoralen (Pathak et al 1962).

Ruta graveolens
Common Rue

The plant was known by the Ancients to produce a pustular eruption of the hands in those who gathered it (Dispensatory 1884). The plant is irritant (Bigelow 1817, Oesterlen 1856) and vesicant (Soubeiran cited by Piffard 1881). Handling of the flowers and fruit produced erythema, burning, itching and vesication (Van Hasselt 1862). While the fresh leaves have vesicant effects, much of this activity is dissipated by drying (Loudon 1855). Bazin (cited by White 1887) reported the case of a druggist who developed itching, grouped vesicles then large bullae on the hands after gathering rue. On a second occasion, he was careful to take the branch only between the finger and thumb and to cut it below with scissors; however, an eruption developed, still more intense, and covered the whole surface of the right hand. Photodermatitis from the plant with positive photopatch tests was reported by Garat et al (1948) and Muenscher and Brown (1944). Klauder and Kimmich (1956) refer to dermatitis from the plant.

The plant yields 5-methoxypsoralen and 8-methoxypsoralen (Pathak et al 1962).

Ruta graveolens
var. augustifolia
Countryman's treacle

The moist foliage of the plant is irritant and vesicant to some individuals, especially in the heat of summer (Behl et al 1966).

Ruta montana

This species is irritant (Schwartz et al 1957). The plant yields 8-methoxypsoralen (Pathak et al 1962).

References

Behl, P.N., Captain, R.M., Bedi, B.M.S. and Gupta, S. (1966) Skin-irritant and sensitizing plants found in India, New Delhi. P.N. Behl, Irwin Hospital.

Bigelow (1817) American Medical Botany. Boston: (1824) Florula Bostoniensis. Boston cited by White (1887).

Dispensatory, The National (1884) Philadelphia. Stille and Maisch, cited by White (1887).

Garat, B.R. et al (1948) Dermatitis bullosa, striate dermatitis: 8 cases provoked by Ruta graveolens (rue). Rev. Argent. dermatosif. 32, 15.

Gerard, J. (1636) The Herball or Generall Historie of Plantes. The essence thereof distilled by M. Woodward (1927) from the edition of Th. Johnson 1630. London. Gerald Howe.

Klauder, J.V. and Kimmich, J.M. (1956) Sensitisation dermatitis due to carrots. Arch. Derm. 74, 149.

Loudon (1855) Encyclopedia of Plants. London. Cited by White (1887).

Muenscher, W.C. and Brown, B.I. (1944) Dermatitis and photosensitisation produced by Ptelea angustifolia. Madrono 7, 184.

Oesterlen (1856) Handbuch der Heilmittellehre. Tubingen cited by White (1887).

Opdyke, D.L.J. (1975) Monographs on Fragrance Raw Materials. Fd. Cosmet. Toxicol. 13, 455.

Pathak, M.A., Daniels, F. Jr. and Fitzpatrick, T.B. (1962) Presently known distribution of furocoumarins (Psoralens) in plants. J. Invest. Derm. 39, 225.

Piffard, H.G. (1881) A treatise on the Materia Medica and Therapeutics of the skin. New York. Wm. Wood and Co.

Schwartz, L., Tulipan, L. and Birmingham, D.J. (1957) Occupational Diseases of the Skin. 3rd ed. Philadelphia. Lea and Febiger. pp. 637-672.

Van Hasselt (1862) Handbuch der Giftlehre Braunschweig cited by White (1887).

White, J.C. (1887) Dermatitis venenata: an account of the Action of External irritants upon the skin. Boston. Cupples and Hurd.

Skimmia

Seven or eight species are native to the Himalayas, eastern Asia and the Philippine islands. The plants are dioecious. An oil from the leaves of S. laurifolia is used for scenting soap (Usher 1974). Several species are known in horticulture.

Skimmia laureola
Neera

This species yields 5-methoxypsoralen (Pathak et al 1962).

References

Pathak, M.A., Daniels, F. Jr. and Fitzpatrick, T.B. (1962) Presently known distribution of furocoumarins (Psoralens) in plants. J. Invest. Derm. 39, 225.

Usher, G. (1974) A dictionary of plants used by man. London. Constable.

Thamnosa

Eight or nine species are found in the southern United States, south-western Africa, the island of Socotra and Arabia.

Thamnosa montana
Turpentine Broom

This strongly scented shrub, which is known in horticulture, yields furanocoumarins (Pathak et al 1962, Bennett and Bonner 1953).

References

Bennett, E.L. and Bonner, J. (1953) Isolation of growth inhibitor from Thamnosa montana. Amer. J. Bot. 40, 29.

Pathak, M.A., Daniels, F. Jr. and Fitzpatrick, T.B. (1962) Presently known distribution of furocoumarins (Psoralens) in plants. J. Invest. Derm. 39, 225.

Zanthoxylum

20 or perhaps 30 species are found in temperate and subtropical regions of eastern Asia, in the Philippines, eastern Malaysia and in North America.

Zanthoxylum spp.

Some species can produce mechanical injury by their prickles (Oakes and Butcher 1962). The bark and berries are used in Herbal Medicine for treating skin diseases (Wren 1968).

Zanthoxylum caribeum

The wood is said to be irritant (Martinez 1969, Hausen 1970).

Zanthoxylum caribrosum

The wood is said to be irritant (Schwartz et al 1957).

Zanthoxylum flavum
(syn. Fagara flava, Xanthoxylum flavum)
West Indian satinwood

Dermatitis from Fagara spp., mainly F. flava, was well known among labourers in the West Indies (Grabham 1905). This author reported that he himself had had such dermatitis. A joiner who worked with Fagara flava developed dermatitis; a patch test to the sawdust of this wood alone produced a positive reaction (Wechselmann 1909).

This author stated that he found chloroxylonine (the sensitizing alkaloid of Chloroxylon swietenia) in F. flava and obtained positive patch test reactions with it on his patient and himself, but not on two volunteers. The colloquial names of Z. flavum (syn. Fagara flava) include West Indian satinwood, Jamaica or San Domingo satinwood, espenille, yellow sanders, atlaswood, citronwood and zitronenholz.

Many of the colloquial and trade names are used for other woods. Several other species of Zanthoxylum and related New World genera furnish satinwoods of poorer quality and some of these have been reported to produce ill-effects (Smith 1920, Lewin 1928). Freise (1936) described fifteen cases of dermatitis caused by satinwood or boxwood substitutes (Euxylophora paraensis; Esenbeckia leiocarpa; Raputia magnifica; R. alba; Balfourodendron riedelianum) and two similar cases from Zanthoxylum flavum (syn. Fagara flava). The dermatitis was usually mild and confined to the finger-webs and other exposed areas. He noted that the sawdust of fresh wood was usually coarse; it did not penetrate under the clothing. Some cases had more severe dermatitis, with widespread swelling and constitutional symptoms, usually proceeding to vesicular dermatitis and often gangrenous ulcers which in three cases proved fatal. He confirmed the irritant action of the sawdust on his own skin and on laboratory animals. The species Esenbeckia leiocarpa and Euxylophora paraensis contain the phototoxic compound, xanthotoxin (Hausen 1970).

Satinwood was found to cause dermatitis by Siegheim (1909) and Volk (1911) but the botanical species responsible were uncertain and the patch test results equivocal.

The reports of dermatitis from satinwoods by Oppenheim (1909), Brezina (1913), Noll (1931) named as satinwood, atlaswood, citronwood or zitronenholz may have referred to Z. flavum (Fagara flava) or to some other species.

References

Brezina, E. (1913) Internationale Ubersicht uber Gewerbekrankheiten uber des Jahr 1913. ed. Teleky, L. and Brezine, E. Berlin, Springer.

Freise, F.W. (1936) Verfigtungen durch Brasilianische Werkholzer I, II. Samm. Vergift. 7C, 1 and 61.

Grabham, M. (1905) Satinwoods and Dermatitis. Brit. med. J. 1, 822.

Hausen, B.M. (1970) Untersuchungen uber Gesuncheitsschadigende Holzer. Thesis, Hamburg.

Lewin, L. (1928) Gifte im holzgewerbe. Berlin. Stilke.

Noll, R. (1931) Citronenholzmehl - Uberempfindlichkeit. Zentrab. Haut. Geschl. 38, 437.

Oppenheim (1909) Satinholzdermatitis. Arch. Derm. u. Syph. 96, 97.

Siegheim (1909) Ueber Satinholzdermatitis. Berlin Klin. Woch. 46, 2020.

Smith, E.P. (1920) Plant Dermatitis. J. Bot. 58, 130.

Volk, R. (1911) Das Uberempfindlichkeits problem in der Dermatologie. Arch. Derm. u. Syph. 109, 163.

Wechselmann (1909) Uber satinholzdermatitis, eine Anaphylaxie der Haut. Deutsch. med. Woch. 35, 1389.

Fagara flava

The wood is slightly irritant by patch test (Cash 1911). The problem concerning the botanical origin of satinwood is noted under Chloroxylon.

This species is potentially phototoxic from a content of 8-methoxypsoralen (Pathak et al 1962).

Zanthoxylum fraxineum
Prickly Ash, Toothache-tree

The bark is used in America as a toothache remedy.

Zanthoxylum hirtellum

The bark is prickly. The bark is pounded to knock off the prickles and put into a hollow tooth as a counter-irritant (Burkill 1935).

Zanthoxylum myricanthum
Thorny Ivy-Rue

The common name is derived from a resemblance to Ivy, *Hedera*, and Rue (*Ruta*). The species name indicates 'thousands of thorns' (Menninger 1967).

Zanthoxylum piperitum
Japanese Pepper

The fruit is used as a condiment. The plant is chewed and the resulting saliva is applied to the face: the skin of the face is then said to be unaffected by 'varnish poisoning' (*Rhus vernicifera*) (Smith 1969).

References

Burkill, I.H. (1935) A Dictionary of the Economic Products of the Malay Peninsula. 2 Vols. London. Crown Agents for the Colonies.

Cash, J.T. (1911) The dermatitis produced by East Indian Satinwood (*Chloroxylon swietenia*). Brit. Med. J. 2, 784.

Grabham, M. (1905) Satinwoods and dermatitis. Brit. Med. J. 1, 822.

Hausen, B.M. (1970) Untersuchungen uber Gesundheitsschadigende Holzer. Thesis, Hamburg.

Martinez, M. (1969) The Medicinal Plants of Mexico. 5th ed. Mexico City. Andres Botas.

Menninger, E.A. (1967) Fantastic Trees. New York. The Viking Press.

Schwartz, L., Tulipan, L. and Birmingham, D.J. (1957) Occupational Diseases of the Skin. 3rd ed. Philadelphia. Lea and Febiger.

Smith, F.P. (1969) Chinese Materia Medica. Vegetable kingdom. 2nd ed. Rev. by Hei, P.D. Taipei, Taiwan. Ku T'ing Book House.

Wren, R.W. (1968) Potter's New Cyclopaedia of Botanical Drugs and Preparations by Wren, R.C. Re-edit. by Wren, R.W. Potter and Clarke, Ltd. Health Science Press. Rustington, Sussex.

Oakes, A.J. and Butcher, J.O. (1962) Poisonous and injurious plants of the U.S. Virgin Islands. Misc. Publ. 882. U.S. Department of Agriculture, Washington, D.C.

Pathak, M.A., Daniels, F. Jr. and Fitzpatrick, T.B. (1962) Presently known distribution of furocoumarins (Psoralens) in plants. J. Invest. Derm. 39, 225.

Zanthoxylum veneficum
Thorny yellow-wood

The bark possesses a peculiar tingling hot taste like aconite (*Aconitum*) (Webb 1948). The plant derives its specific name from its poisonous property.

Reference

Webb, L.J. (1948) Guide to the medicinal and poisonous plants of Queensland. Bulletin No. 232. Council for Scientific and Industrial Research. Melbourne, Australia.

SALICACEAE

530 species in three genera are distributed chiefly in north temperate regions.

Chemistry is recorded by Hegnauer (1973).

Populus

35 species are found in north temperate regions.

Populus sp.
Poplar

Dermatitis from poplar was noted by Senear (1933).

Dermatitis of the hands and forearms followed by exfoliative dermatitis and lymphadenopathy resembling lymphoma occurred in a wood-worker from the sawdust. Positive patch test reactions to dry and moistened wood dust were observed (Weber 1953). This author noted that closed patch test with moistened wood-dust of various woods often produced irritant reactions and he questioned some of his own findings as to the allergenicity of some native woods. A cabinet-maker developed dermatitis from poplar saw-dust which was derived from a factory situated above his workplace (Caro 1953). Cross-sensitivity has been observed between poplar (Populus), aspen (Populus) and willow (Salix) (Tan and Mitchell 1968). Two woodmen who had dermatitis had been in contact with resin of white poplar buds showed positive patch test reactions to purified balsamic resins and essential oils derived from the tree and to bee-glue (propolis) derived from the tree by honey-bees (Winkler 1956). There was no history of contact with bee-hives in these patients.

Poplar is one of the trees listed as a cause of wood-cutters' eczema (Schulmann and Detouillon 1932) now known to be caused by Frullania and lichens.

Bee-glue
(Propolis)

Beeswax was suspected as a cause of dermatitis in a man who worked inside a barrel which contained resin and beeswax (Queries and Monor Notes 1931).

Dermatitis from bee-glue was reported by Umansky in 1934. Bee-glue is a dark yellowish-brown substance with a fragrant smell suggestive of cinnamon (Cinnamomum). The composition of bee-glue varies according to its plant source and includes wax, crude resins, essential oils, colouring matters and esters of cinnamic alcohol (Bunney 1968, Hjorth 1961). Trees given by common name for their particular areas as sources of bee-glue are Populus, horse-chestnut (Aesculus), spruce (Picea), willow (Salix), lime (Tilia), sycamore (Platanus) and fruit trees (Ribbands 1953): and fir (Abies), alder (Alnus) and birch (Betula) (Rothenborg 1967).

In 14 cases of bee-keepers' dermatitis, positive patch test reactions were observed to samples of bee-glue obtained from various parts of the United Kingdom and in all of 7 and 6 patients tested to resins extracted from the buds of Balsam Poplar (P. balsamifera) and Lombardy Poplar (query P. nigra) respectively. Additional sensitivity was observed to extracts of buds of spruce (Picea), willow (Salix), horse-chestnut (Aesculus), lime (Tilia) and apple (Pomus) (Bunney 1968).

She concluded that once a patient has become sensitized by the more potent or abundant allergen in bee-glue derived from poplar, he may then react to the weaker or less abundant allergens in the resins of some other trees from which bee-glue is derived. The allergenic fraction of bee-glue is found in the volatile oil derived from it by distillation.

Patients contact sensitive to Populus and to bee-glue derived from Populus have been observed to show positive patch test reactions to Balsams of Peru and Tolu (Myroxylon) (Rothenborg 1967). Benzyl salicylate and cinnamic acid derivatives may be mutually responsible. According to Rothenborg (1967) allergic contact dermatitis from unpurified beeswax contaminated by bee-glue can occur in patients who have no contact with bees but who become sensitized by beeswax in cosmetics and medications or who are cross-sensitized by balsamic resins derived from other plants.

Early reports of dermatitis from beeswax (Greenberg and Lester 1954) probably refer to raw or unpurified beeswax. Patch test reactions to purified beeswax were negative in 2,634 patients who had dermatitis (Rothenborg 1967). It seems, therefore, that purified beeswax is unlikely to be a significant source of cosmetic dermatitis.

A bibliography is provided by Rothenborg (1967), Bunney (1968). Bee-keepers' dermatitis has been reported from Hungary (Racz 1960).

Beeswax has been reported to produce untoward reactions when used as an injection vehicle (Fernstrom 1957) and injection of honey produced a state of shock (Mazzi 1964). Beeswax used for art work caused dermatitis in a woman who was employed in making mouldings (Camarasa 1975).

References

Bunney, M.H. (1968) Contact dermatitis in beekeepers due to propolis (bee-glue). Br. J. Derm. 80, 17.

Camarasa, G. (1975) Occupational dermatitis from beeswax. Contact Dermatitis 1, 124.

Caro, M.R. (1953) in discussion of Weber (1953).

Fernstrom, A.I.B. (1957) Studies on procaine allergy with reference to urticaria due to procaine penicillin treatment. Acta Derm.-venereol. 39, 443.

Hegnauer, R. (1973) Chemotaxonomy of Plants. Vol. 6. Basel. Birkhauser. p. 241.

Hjorth, N. (1961) Eczematous Allergy to Balsams. Munksgaard, International Booksellers and Publishers Ltd. Copenhagen.

Mazzi, R. (1964) Detection of common antigens in pollen of anemophilic and entomophilic plants by the gell-diffusion method. Dermatologica (Basel) 129, 479.

Queries and Minor Notes (1931) Possible dermatitis from resin or beeswax. JAMA 97, 661.

Racz, L. (1960) Propolis eczema in bee-keepers as an occupational disease. Borgyrogy Vener Szemle 36, 24.

Ribbands, R. (1953) Behaviour and Social Life of Honey Bees. London: Bee Research Assoc. Ltd. p. 205.

Rothenborg, H.W. (1967) Occupational dermatitis in beekeeper due to poplar resins in beeswax. Archs. Derm. 95, 381.

Tan, K.S. and Mitchell, J.C. (1968) Patch and photopatch tests in contact dermatitis and photodermatitis. Canad. Med. Assoc. J. 98, 252.

Umansky, G.I. (1934) A professional dermatitis caused by the resin propolis from the bee. Dermat. Wchnschr. 98, 177.

Weber, L.F. (1953) Dermatitis venenata due to native woods. Arch. Derm. Syph. 67, 388.

Winkler, A. (1956) Dermatitis due to poplar resin. Derm. Wschr. 133, 81. (Germ.)

Schulmann, E. and Detouillon, P. (1932) L'eczéma du bois et al sensibilisation sylvestre. Paris Med. 1, 55.

Propolis in creams

Perioral dermatitis from propolis (bee-glue) in creams was reported by Wanscher (1976). In these patients Balsam of Peru (*Myroxylon*) produced negative patch test reactions. She states that propolis is collected by bees from resinous exudations of horse-chestnut (*Arbor castanea*, sic) (?*Castanea* or *Aesculus*), spruce (*Abies nobilis*), willow (*Salix*), larch (*Larix*), fir (*Pinus*) and especially poplar (*Populus*).

The horse-chestnut tree is *Aesculus hippocastanum*.

Reference

Wanscher, B. (1976) Contact dermatitis from Propolis. Brit. J. Derm. 94, 451.

Populus alba

The "cotton" of the seeds of pistillate trees can be drawn into the nose, eyes and mouth. This nuisance can be avoided by planting only cuttings from staminate trees (Standley and Steyermark 1952).

Populus balsamifera

The flowers are used as a styptic (Smith 1969).

Populus canadensis

Bee-glue derived from this species caused dermatitis in a beekeeper (Rothenborg 1967). Positive patch test reactions were observed to the leaf and bud of the tree and to raw beeswax from his hives.

Populus candicans
(syn. P. gileadensis,
P. balsamifera)
Balm of Gilead Poplar

Fragrant resinous leaf-buds from this tree preserved in rum or alcohol were a popular household remedy for external use in New England (White 1887). The application produced a smarting sensation. He noted that dermatitis from Balm of Gilead remained localized to the site of application whereas dermatitis from Tincture of Arnica (Arnica) became disseminated. He observed one or two cases of bullous dermatitis each year from this source. Balm of Gilead, in England, refers to Abies balsamea. Four of 14 patients contact sensitive to Balsam of Peru (Myroxylon) showed positive patch test reactions to Balm of Gilead U.S.P. (Hjorth 1961).

Populus carolensis

The allergens of Frullania present on the bark of 'carolins d'Italie' (query this species) penetrate into the wood and can cause dermatitis in match-makers (LeCoulant et al 1966).

Populus deltoides

The resin glands were described by Curtis and Lersten (1974).

Populus tremuloides
Aspen

Chemical derivatives of this species were studied by Mathes (1963).

Populus trichocarpa
Black Cotton Wood

North American Indians rub the sticky sweet-smelling buds on the face to prevent sunburn. The hairy fruit pods can irritate the hands (Turner and Bell 1973).

References

Mathes, M.C. (1963) Antimicrobial substances from aspen tissue (Populus tremuloides) grown in vitro. Science 140, 1101.

Rothenborg, H.W. (1967) Occupational dermatitis in Beekeeper due to poplar resins in beeswax. Archs. Derm. 95, 381.

Hjorth, N. (1961) Eczematous allergy to Balsams, Allied Perfumes and Flavouring Agents. Copenhagen. Munksgaard.

Smith, F.P. (1969) Chinese Materia Medica. Vegetable kingdom. 2nd ed. Rev. by Hei, P.D. Taipei, Taiwan. Ku T'ing Book House.

Standley, P.C. and Steyermark, J.A. (1952) Flora of Guatemala. Fieldiana. Botany. Vol. 24 P.V. 3. Chicago Natural History Museum. Chicago, Ill.

Turner, N.C. and Bell, M.A.M. (1973) The ethnobotany of the southern Kwakiutl Indians of British Columbia. Economic Botany, in press.

White, J.C. (1887) Dermatitis venenata: An account of the Action of External irritants upon the Skin. Boston. Cupples and Hurd.

LeCoulant, P., Texier, Maleville et al (1966) L'allergie au frullania: son role dans la 'dermite du bois de chene'. Bull. Soc. franc. Derm. Syph. 73, 440.

Curtis, J.D. and Lersten, N.R. (1974) Morphology, seasonal variation, and function of resin glands of buds and leaves of Populus deltoides (Salicaceae). Amer. J. Bot. 61, 835.

Additional reference

Wanscher, B. (1976) Contact dermatitis from propolis. Brit. J. Derm. 94, 451.

Salix

500 species are chiefly north temperate in distribution.

Salix alba and

Salix discolor
Willow

The bark has long been used in Herbal Medicine (Wren 1968). Contact sensitivity to Salix is noted under Populus.

Reference

Wren, R.W. (1968) Potter's New Cyclopaedia of Botanical Drugs and Preparations by Wren, R.C. Re-edit. by Wren, R.W. Potter and Clarke, Ltd. Health Science Press. Rustington, Sussex.

SALVADORACEAE

12 species in three genera are found in dry hot regions, particularly on the coasts of Africa and Asia.

Chemistry is recorded by Hegnauer (1973).

Salvadora

Four or five species are found in warm regions of Africa and Asia.

Salvadora oleoides

The bruised root-bark has a vesicant effect and the sweet fruit, which is eaten in Northern India, irritates the mouth producing tingling and ulceration (Behl et al 1966). The seeds contain a thioglucoside, glucotropaeolin, related to mustard oils of Cruciferae (Kjaer 1963).

Salvadora persica

On a hot, sunny day the plant gives off an acrid odour. The leaves taste like mustard (Brassica). This species has been thought by some, probably erroneously, to be the mustard of the Bible. A paste of the powdered root is used like a 'mustard plaster' for an irritant effect and can produce vesication (Watt and Breyer-Brandwijk 1962, Behl et al 1966).

References

Behl, P.N., Captain, R.M., Bedi, B.M.S. and Gupta, S. (1966) Skin-irritant and sensitizing plants found in India, New Delhi. P.N. Behl, Irwin Hospital.

Hegnauer, R. (1973) Chemotaxonomy of Plants. Vol. 6. Basel. Birkhauser. p. 259.

Kjaer, A. (1963) The distribution of sulphur compounds. In: Chemical Plant Taxonomy (ed. T. Swain), chap. 16, p. 453. Academic Press, London.

Watt, J.M. and Breyer-Brandwijk, M.G. (1962) The Medicinal and poisonous plants of Southern Africa. 2nd ed. Edinburgh. E.& S. Livingstone.

SAMBUCACEAE

40 species in one genus are almost cosmopolitan. A wine is made from elder-berries.

Chemistry is recorded by Hegnauer (1973).

Reference

Hegnauer, R. (1973) Chemotaxonomy of Plants. Vol. 6. Basel. Birkhauser. p. 261.

Sambucus nigra
Elder

The leaves and bark are used in Herbal Medicine as an ointment (Grieve 1970). Green elder leaves are said to be powerfully irritant (Crichton 1897). He ordered an application of elder-flower ointment. The druggist, having no elder flowers at the time, used the green leaves instead and a very violent irritation resulted.

References

Crichton (1897) in discussion of Johnson (1897).

Grieve, M. (1970) A Modern Herbal. Darien, Conn. Hafner Publ. Co.

Johnson, J.Y. (1897) Proc. Linn. Soc. 21st Jan. quoted by Maiden (1909).

Maiden, J.H. (1909) On some plants which cause inflammation or irritation of the skin. Agr. Gaz. New South Wales 20, 111 and 1073.

SANTALACEAE

400 species in 30 genera are found in tropical and temperate regions. Some are semi-parasitic on other plants.

Chemistry is recorded by Hegnauer (1973).

Reference

Hegnauer, R. (1973) Chemotaxonomy of Plants. Vol. 6. Basel. Birkhauser. p. 261.

Santalum

25 species are found in eastern Malaysia and from Australia to eastern Polynesia.

Santalum album

The oil has been found to irritate some animal skins experimentally (Opdyke 1974). The wood is said to be toxic (Doerr 1913, Grossmann 1920, Hanslian and Kadlec 1966) perhaps because the oil taken internally can produce eruptions. No clinical case reports of dermatitis from the wood were found (Hausen 1970, Woods and Calnan 1976).

The heartwood, cultivated in India, furnishes East Indian Sandalwood oil (Oil of Santal). The oil is sometimes adulterated with West Indian Sandalwood Oil derived from Amyris balsamifera. Australian Sandalwood Oil is derived from Eucarya of this family. Oral administration of Oil of Sandalwood produced a morbilliform eruption (Skin Gallery 1963). Oil of Sandalwood can produce dermatitis in some persons especially if present in high proportions in perfume (Greenberg and Lester 1954). The complexities of perfumery are demonstrated in a case of suspected photo allergy reported by Starke (1967). A male patient developed photodermatitis after using an after-shave lotion containing commercial Sandalwood Oil. The sample tested contained several essential oils and the findings were ambiguous.

References

Greenberg, L.A. and Lester, D. (1954) Handbook of Cosmetic Materials. New York. Interscience.

Hausen, B.M. (1970) Untersuchungen uber Gesundheitsschadigende Holzer. Thesis, Hamburg.

Skin Gallery (1963) Skin 2, 327.

Starke, J.C. (1967) Photoallergy to Sandalwood OIl. Archs. Derm. 96, 62.

Doerr, R. (1913) Allergie und Anaphylaxie in: Handbuch der pathogenen Mikroorganismen. ed. Kolle, W. and Wassermann, 2nd ed. Vol. 2 (11) p. 954. Fischer, Jena, Berlin, cited by Woods and Calnan (1976).

Grossmann, J. (1920) Gesundheitsschadliche Holzarten Der Holzkaufer (Leipzig) 17, 529, 540, 545.

Hanslian, L. and Kadlec, K. (1966) Wood from the standpoint of hygiene VII. Species with a highly aggressive biological effect. Drevo 21, 157.

Opdyke, D.L. (1974) Monographs on Fragrance Raw Materials. Fd. Cosm. Tox. 12, 807.

Woods, B. and Calnan, C.D. (1976) Toxic Woods. Brit. J. Derm. 94, Suppl. 13, June.

Thesium

325 species found in Europe, Africa, Asia and Australia are herbaceous root-parasites.

Thesium hystrix

The volatile oil of the resin is irritant (Watt and Breyer-Brandwijk 1962).

Reference

Watt, J.M. and Breyer-Brandwijk, M.G. (1962) The Medicinal and poisonous plants of Southern Africa. 2nd ed. Edinburgh. E.& S. Livingstone.

SAPINDACEAE

2000 species in 150 genera are found in tropical and subtropical regions. Litchi chinensis furnishes edible fruit (litchi).

Chemistry is recorded by Hegnauer (1973).

Reference

Hegnauer, R. (1973) Chemotaxonomy of Plants. Vol. 6. Basel. Birkhauser. p. 271.

Cardiospermum

15 species are found in tropical regions especially in America.

Cardiospermum halicacabum
Blister creeper

The leaf and root are irritant and are used for rubefacient purposes (Quisumbing 1951, Watt and Breyer-Brandwijk 1962, Behl et al 1966).

References

Behl, P.N. Captain, R.M., Bedi, B.M.S. and Gupta, S. (1966) Skin-irritant and sensitizing plants found in India, New Delhi. P.N. Behl, Irwin Hospital.

Quisumbing, E. (1951) Medicinal Plants of the Philippines. Tech. Bull. 16. Manila, Philippine Islands, Manila Bureau of Printing. 1234 pp.

Watt, J.M. and Breyer-Brandwijk, M.G. (1962) The Medicinal and poisonous plants of Southern Africa. 2nd ed. Edinburgh. E.& S. Livingstone.

Hippobromus

One species is native to southern Africa.

Hipporbomus pauciflorus

A decoction of the plant is used as a sternutatory. Frothing of the roots, when mixed with water, may indicate the presence of saponins (Watt and Breyer-Brandwijk 1962).

Reference

Watt, J.M. and Breyer-Brandwijk, M.G. (1962) The Medicinal and poisonous plants of Southern Africa. 2nd ed. Edinburgh. E.& S. Livingstone.

Melicoccus

Two species are found in tropical America and the West Indies.

Melicoccus bijugatus

This species which provides timber and edible fruit was reported to cause contact dermatitis by Pardo Castello and Reaud (1941).

Reference

Pardo Castello, V. and Reaud, B. (1941) Eczemas y Dermatitis Anais Bras. de Dermat. e Sifilog 17(1); 11.

Paullinia

180 species are found in warm regions of America. P. cupana (Guarana) is cultivated for its edible seeds.

Paullinia pinnata

The root and root bark are applied for rubefacient purposes (Watt and Breyer-Brandwijk 1962).

Paullinia sorbilis
Guarana

Ingestion of the plant caused urticaria and pruritus (Piffard 1881).

References

Piffard, H.G. (1881) A treatise on the Materia Medica and Therapeutics of the skin. New York. Wm. Wood and Co.

Watt, J.M. and Breyer-Brandwijk, M.G. (1962) The Medicinal and poisonous plants of Southern Africa. 2nd ed. Edinburgh. E.& S. Livingstone.

Sapindus

Thirteen species are found in tropical and subtropical Asia, the Pacific region (but not Australia) and America.

Sapindus drummondii
Soap berry

Dermatitis can result from handling of the fruits (Schwartz et al 1957).

Sapindus mukorossi
Soap-Nut Tree

The fruits have a slightly irritant effect on the mucous

membrane. The pulp of the fruit forms a lather which is used as a shampoo (Behl et al 1966). The fruit juice is used for removing freckles (Smith 1969).

Sapindus oblongifolius

A foam is produced by shaking the plant tissues with water (Watt and Breyer-Brandwijk 1962).

Sapindus saponaria
Soap berry

The berries form a lather with water and may be used as soap. The fruit contains an irritant (Allen 1943, Blohm 1962, Morton 1962).

References

Allen, P.H. (1943) Poisonous and Injurious Plants of Panama. Am. J. Trop. Med. Suppl. 23, 1.

Behl, P.N., Captain, R.M., Bedi, B.M.S. and Gupta, S. (1966) Skin-irritant and sensitizing plants found in India, New Delhi. P.N. Behl, Irwin Hospital.

Blohm, H. (1962) Poisonous Plants of Venezuela. Cambridge, Mass. Harvard University Press.

Morton, J.F. (1962) Ornamental Plants with Poisonous Properties. II. Proc. Florida Hort. Soc. 75, 484.

Schwartz, L., Tulipan, L. and Birmingham, D.J. (1957) Occupational Diseases of the Skin. 3rd ed. Philadelphia. Lea and Febiger. pp. 637-672.

Smith, F.P. (1969) Chinese Materia Medica. Vegetable kingdom. 2nd ed. Rev. by Hei, P.D. Taipei, Taiwan. Ku T'ing Book House.

Watt, J.M. and Breyer-Brandwijk, M.G. (1962) The Medicinal and poisonous plants of Southern Africa. 2nd ed. Edinburgh. E.& S. Livingstone.

Schleichera

One species, native to Indo Malaysia, is cultivated in other areas, notably Ceylon.

Schleichera trijuga
Kussum, Paka, Ceylon oak, Zeepboom

Shellac is a resinous excretion of an insect which sucks the juices of this and other trees (Hicks 1961). This tree yields Mirzapore lac and also, useful timber, edible seed and seed oil. Macassar oil (Kusum oil) is derived from the seed kernels (Merck 1968). Macassar oil is also a name for Ylang-ylang oil from Cananga. Macassar oil may contain additives such as Safflower oil from Carthamus tinctorius, Compositae family. Harry (1948) referred to two papers concerning dermatitis or allergy from the oil but considered it innocuous. Shellac is said to have irritant or sensitizing properties (Greenberg and Lester 1954) and is removed from certain brand-name cosmetics (Schieffelin 1973). Hausen (1970) refers to Wehmer (1929) and Anon (1940) for injurious effects of the plant products. The oil of Macassar wood, possibly of this species, caused dermatitis in a planer (Buschke and Joseph 1927). Shellac is noted under Acer.

References

Anon (1940) Giftige en voor de gezondheid nadeelige houtsoorten. Hout 20, 184.

Buschke, A. and Joseph, A. (1927) Uber Hautentzundung, Hervorgerufen durch Makassarholz mit Berucksichtigung gewerbehygienischer Fragen. Deutsch. med. Wchnschr. 53, 1641.

Greenberg, L.A. and Lester, D. (1954) Handbook of Cosmetic Materials. New York. Interscience.

Harry, R.G. (1948) Cosmetic Materials. Vol. 2. London. Leonard Hill.

Hausen, B.M. (1970) Untersuchungen uber Gesundheitsschadigende Holzer. Thesis, Hamburg.

Hicks, E. (1961) Shellac, its origin and applications. Chemical Publ. Co., New York.

Merck Index (1968) An Encyclopedia of Chemicals and Drugs. ed. Stecher, P.G. 8th ed. Rahway, N.J. Merck and Co. Inc.

Schieffelin, and Co. (1973) Almay Hypo-allergenic cosmetics produce formulary 8th ed. Pharmaceutical Laboratories Division, 562 Fifth Avenue, New York, N.Y. 10036.

Wehmer, C. (1929) Die Pflanzenstoffe. Verlag G. Fischer. Jena. 2. Aufl.

Serjania

215 species are found from the southern United States to tropical South America.

Serjania lethalis

The plant yields poisonous honey (Morton 1964).

Reference

Morton, J.F. (1964) Honeybee plants of South Florida. Proc. Florida State Horticult. Soc. 77, 415.

SAPOTACEAE

800 tropical species occur in 35 to 75 ill-defined genera. Many furnish useful products, especially gutta-percha and balata.

Poisoning by several Brazilian woods of this family causes alopecia (Friese 1932 cited by Senear 1933).

Chemistry is recorded by Hegnauer (1973).

References

Friese, F.W. (1932) Gesundheiteschadigengen durch Arbeiten mit giftingen Holzern. Beobachtungen aus brasilianischen Gewerbebetrieben Arch. Gewerbepath.-hyg. 3, 1.

Hegnauer, R. (1973) Chemotaxonomy of Plants. Vol. 6. Basel. Birkhauser. p. 287.

Senear, F.E. (1933) Dermatitis due to woods. JAMA 101, 1527.

Achras

Four species are native to the West Indies and tropical America.

Achras zapota
Sapodilla plum

This species is cultivated for its edible fruit and the latex is extracted to form Chicle, a chewing gum. The wood-dust is irritant to the nasal passages (Burkill 1935).

Reference

Burkill, I.H. (1935) A Dictionary of the Economic Products of the Malay Peninsula. 2 Vols. London. Crown Agents for the Colonies.

Autranella
(syn. Mimusops)

One species is native to tropical Africa.

Autranella congolensis
(syn. Mimusops congolensis)

The wood-dust is irritant to the respiratory tract (Orsler 1973). Hausen (1970) cites Anon (1954) for mucosal irritation from the wood.

References

Anon (1954) Bois et forets des tropiques 36, 25.

Hausen, B.M. (1970) Untersuchungen uber Gesundheitsschadigende Holzer. Thesis, Hamburg.

Orsler, R.J. (1973) Personal communication from Forest Products Research Laboratory. Princess Risborough, Bucks, England.

Baillonella

One species is native to west equatorial Africa.

Baillonella toxisperma
(syn. Mimusops djave)
Moabi

The wood is said to be injurious (Bois Tropicaux 1966, Helig 1957, cited by Hausen 1970).

References

Bois Troipcaux (1966) 3rd ed. Publ. No. 12. Centre Technique Forestier Tropical. 94-Nogent-sur Marne, France.

Hausen, B.M. (1970) Untersuchungen uber Gesundheitsschadigende Holzer. Thesis, Hamburg.

Heilig, P.M. (1957) Ziekten veroorsaakt door bewerking van zekere houtsoorten. Vakbl. meubelind 38, 1440.

Bassia
(syn. Illipe)

The genus is noted under Madhuca.

Bassia
(Madhuca)

see Paratecoma, Bignoniaceae re confused nomenclature (Woods and Calnan 1976).

Reference

Woods, B. and Calnan, C.D. (1976) Toxic Woods. Brit. J. Derm. 94, Suppl. 13, June.

Calocarpum

Six species are found from Mexico to tropical South America.

Calocarpum mammosum

The sap of the entire plant is caustic and vesicant to the skin and eyes (Allen 1943).

Reference

Allen, P.H. (1943) Poisonous and Injurious Plants of Panama. Am. J. Trop. Med. Suppl. 23, 1.

Chrysophyllum

150 species are found in tropical regions, especially in America. C. cainito is cultivated for its edible fruit, Star Apple.

Chrysophyllum sp.

A Brazilian species of this genus was reported to produce dermatitis from the fine dust produced in making veneers (Friese 1932).

References

Friese, F.W. (1932) cited by Hausen, B.M. (1970).

Hausen, B.M. (1970) Untersuchungen uber Gesundheitsschadigende Holzer. Thesis, Hamburg.

Illipe
(Madhuca)

see Paratecoma, Bignoniaceae for confused nomenclature (Woods and Calnan 1976).

Reference

Woods, B. and Calnan, C.D. (1976) Toxic Woods. Brit. J. Derm. 94, Suppl. 13, June.

Lucuma
(syn. Pouteria)

100 species are found in Malaysia, Australia, the Pacific region and tropical America. The fruit of L. bifera is edible.

Lucuma sp.
Abiuranda

Lucuma procera
Massaranduba

These Brazilian species were reported to cause dermatitis from the fine dust produced in making veneers (Friese 1932, Gottwald 1958).

References

Friese, F.W. (1932) Gesundheiteschadigungen durch Arbeiten mit Giftingen Holzern. Beobachtungen aus brasilianischen Gewerbebetrieben. Arch. Gewerbepath.-hyg. 3, 1: cited by Hausen (1970).

Gottwald, H. (1958) Handelsholzer. F. Hamburg. F. Holzmann Verlag: cited by Hausen (1970).

Hausen, B.M. (1970) Untersuchungen uber Gesundheitsschadigende Holzer. Thesis, Hamburg.

Madhuca J.F. Gmel.
(syn. Bassia Koen. ex. L.,
syn. Illipe)

85 species are native to IndoChina, Indo Malaysia and Australia. The botanical name Bassia All refers to a genus of Chenopodiaceae. The botany is complex (Hausen 1970); he confused the genus with another genus, Bassia, of the Chenopodiaceae.

Madhuca spp.
(syn. Bassia,
syn. Illipe)
Butter-nut tree,
Moah wood

The wood was reported to produce dermatitis in all woodworkers who were exposed, suggesting an irritant effect (Pflanz 1908, Matthes and Schreiber 1914).

According to Record (1925) the moah-wood or edelteak which Matthes and Schreiber (1914) identified as Illipe longifolia (or I. latifolia) was actually Paratecoma peroba. All the lists which include Bassia, Illipe and Madhuca as toxic woods appear to result from Matthes and Schreiber's error. Woods and Calnan (1976) suggest that the wood named moah (Pflanz 1908) may have been Flindersia.

The gummy juice from the bark can cause dermatitis, however, and the residue after expression of edible oil from the flower-meal irritates wounds and mucosal surfaces (Lewin 1962).

Thomson (1971) does not accept reports that the wood yields lapachol, a sensitizer of Tectona.

Madhuca betis

The powdered bark is sternutatory (Quisumbing 1951).

References

Lewin, L. (1962) Gifte und Vergiftungen, Haug, Ulm cited as Lewis (1962) by Woods and Calnon (1976).

Pflanz, V. (1908) Interessante Falle von 'dermatitis venenata'. Med. Klin. 4, 832.

Record, S.J. (1925) Lapachol. Tropical Woods 1, 7.

Woods, B. and Calnan, C.D. (1976) Toxic Woods. Brit. J. Derm. 94, Suppl. 13, June.

Hausen, B.M. (1970) Untersuchungen uber Gesundheitsschadigende Holzer. Thesis, Hamburg.

Matthes, H. and Schreiber, E. (1914) Uber Hautreizende Holzer. Ber. dtsch. pharm. Ges. 24, 385.

Quisumbing, E. (1951) Medicinal Plants of the Philippines. Philipp. Dep. Agr. and Nat. Resources Tech. Bull. No. 16. Manila. Bureau of Printing. 1234 pp.

Senear, F.E. (1933) Dermatitis due to Woods. JAMA 101, 1527.

Thomson, R.H. (1971) Naturally Occurring Quinones. 2nd ed. London. Academic Press.

Madhuca indica
(syn. Bassia latifolia)
Mahwa

The juice from the bark is irritant and is used as a rubefacient (Behl et al 1966). The wood is said to be irritant (Schwartz et al 1957).

Madhuca longifolia
(syn. Bassia longifolia)
Mahua, Mahwa, Mowa

The flowers are edible and are distilled to make a liquor. The leaves yield an essential oil. Schwartz et al (1957) list the wood as irritant. The thick sticky juice from the bark is irritant and workers with a meal derived from the plant can develop cellulitis of the hands and feet (Behl et al 1966).

The above statements of irritation re M. indica and M. parkii are possibly irrelevant by reason of the error noted in the report of Matthes and Schreiber (1914).

Madhuca parkii
(syn. Bassia parkii)
Illipe

The wood is said to be irritant (Schwartz et al 1957).

References

Matthes, H. and Schreiber, E. (1914) Uber hautreizende Holzer. Ber. dtsch. pharm. Ges. 24, 385.

Behl, P.N., Captain, R.M., Bedi, B.M.S. and Gupta, S. (1966) Skin-irritant and sensitizing plants found in India, New Delhi. P.N. Behl, Irwin Hospital.

Schwartz, L., Tulipan, L. and Birmingham, D.J. (1957) Occupational Diseases of the Skin. 3rd ed. Philadelphia. Lea and Febiger. pp. 637-672.

Manilkara

70 species are found in tropical regions. M. zapota is cultivated for its edible fruit, Sapodilla Plum.

Manikara bidentata
Balata rouge

This West Indies species is reported to be injurious (Heilig 1957). Mimusops balata which yields a gutta-percha is now referred to this genus.

Manilkara bidentata
Balata rouge, assapookoo

M. huberi
(syn. Mimusops spp.)

The fine dust produced in making veneers produced dermatitis (Freise 1932). Woods and Calnan (1976) cite an incompletely referenced report that the wood of assapookoo is very poisonous.

References

Freise, F.W. (1932) Gesundheitsschadigungen durch Arbeiten mit giftingen Holzern. Beobachtungen aus brasilianischen Gewerbebetrieben Achiv fur Gewerbepathologie und Gewerbehygiene 3, 1.

Woods, B. and Calnan, C.D. (1976) Toxic Woods. Brit. J. Derm. 94, Suppl. 13, June.

Hausen, B.M. (1970) Untersuchungen uber Gesundheitsschadigende Holzer. Thesis, Hamburg.

Heilig, P.M. (1957) Ziekten veroor zaakt door bewerking van mekere houtsoorten. Vakbl. meubslind. 38, 1440 cited by Hausen (1970).

Mimusops

57 species are found in tropical Africa; one species from Malaysia to the Pacific region.

Mimusops sp.
Sapodilla

The wood is injurious (Hanslian and Kadlec 1966).

Mimusops balata

This species is now referred to Manilkara.

Mimusops heckelii
Makore, Baku, Douka

This species is noted under Tieghemella.

Mimusops toxisperma
African Pearwood

The wood is injurious (Hanslian and Kadlec 1966).

Conjunctivitis, possibly allergic, occurred in 80 per cent of workers with the wood of this species (Kubena et al 1968).

Manilkara appears to be the preferred name for Mimusops spp. Woods and Calnan (1976), and the above reports appear to stem from Freise's (1932) report of dermatitis from this group of woods.

References

Hanslian, L. and Kadlec, K. (1966) Wood from the standpoint of hygiene VII. Species with a highly aggressive biological effect. Drevo. 21, 157.

Hanslian, L. and Kadlec, K. (1966) Wood from the standpoint of hygiene VIII. Species with some or little biological effect. Drevo. 21, 229.

Freise, F.W. (1932) Gesundheitsschadigungen durch Arbeiten mit giftengen Holzern. Beobachtungen aus brasilianischen Gewerbebetrieben Achiv fur Gewerbepathologie und Gewerbehygiene 3, 1.

Woods, B. and Calnan, C.D. (1976) Toxic Woods. Brit. J. Derm. 94, Suppl. 13, June.

Kubena, K., Kadlec, K. and Hanslian, L. (1968) Poskozeni oka drevnym prachem. Klin. oczna. leden cited by Heinc and Kubena (1969).

Heinc, A. and Kubena, K. (1969) Maladies oculaires externes par action directe d'elements exterieurs. Ophthalmologica 158, 181.

Palaquium

More than 115 species are found in Formosa, south-eastern Asia, Indo Malaysia and the Solomon Islands.

Palaquium sp.

Gutta-percha, a trans isomer of rubber, is derived from P. gutta, in cultivation, and from other species (Shaw 1973).

Reference

Shaw, H.K.A. (1973) A Dictionary of the Flowering Plants and Ferns. (the late J.C. Willis) 8th ed. Cambridge University Press.

Synsepalum

Ten species are native to tropical Africa.

Synsepalum dulcificum

After eating the fruit pulp, everything, even lemon juice, tastes deliciously sweet (Fairchild 1930, Menninger 1967).

References

Fairchild, D. (1930) Exploring for Plants. New York. Macmillan.

Menninger, E.A. (1967) Fantastic Trees. New York. The Viking Press.

Tieghemella
(syn. Dumoria)

Two species are native to west tropical Africa.

Tieghemella africana
Douka, Makore

Nasal and respiratory irritation with haemoptysis occurred in men sawying woods from Spanish Guinea probably mainly T. africana (Dantin-Gallego et al 1957). This wood is less often exported than T. heckelii but equally irritant (Anon 1955, Subiza Martin 1971).

References

Anon (1955) Douka. Bois et Forets des Tropiques 42, 37.

Dantin-Gallego, J. and Armayor, A.F. (1952) Some new toxic woods: Some new manifestations of toxicity. Ind. Med. Surg. 21, 41.

Subiza Martin, E. (1971) Etudes experimentales avec le bois d'Oukola (Dumoria africana). Les Bronches (Paris) 21, 517.

Tieghemella heckelii
(syn. Dumoria heckelii,
syn. Mimusops heckelii)
Makore

The wood dust can produce respiratory symptoms and dermatitis in wood-workers (Bois Tropicaux 1966) which have tended to discourage its use.

The wood can cause dermatitis, conjunctivitis and respiratory symptoms (Malespini 1935, Turc et al 1950, Sandermann and Barghoorn 1955). The wood contains a glycoside of bassic acid (Sandermann and Barghoorn 1955, King et al 1955).

References

Bois tropicaux (1966) 3rd ed. Publ. No. 12. Centre Technique Forestier Tropical. 94-Norgent-sur Marne, France.

King, F.E., Baker, J.A. and King, T.J. (1955) A saponin constituent of Malore (Mimusops heckelii). J. Chem. Soc. 1338.

Malespini, E. (1935) L'eczema du bois. Annales d'hygiene publique, industrielle et sociale 13, 313.

Sandermann, W. and Barghoorn, A.W. (1955) Uber die Inhalstoffe von Makore-und Peroba-Holz sowie ihre gesundheitschadigende Wirkung. Holzforschung 9, 112.

Turc, H., Brunel, R. and Tolot, F. (1950) Accidents allergiques dus au bois de Makore. Arch. Mal. Prof. 11, 490.

SAURURACEAE

Five genera are recognized. The family is related to Piperaceae and is similar to Polygonaceae.

Chemistry is recorded by Hegnauer (1973).

Reference

Hegnauer, R. (1973) Chemotaxonomy of plants. Vol. 6. Gasel. Birkhauser. p. 304.

Houttuynia

One species is found from the Himalayas of Japan.

Houttuynia cordata

The plant has properties like those of Piper and is used for an astringent effect (Smith 1969).

Reference

Smith, F.P. (1969) Chinese Materia Medica. Vegetable kingdom. 2nd ed. Rev. by Hei, P.D. Taipei, Taiwan. Ku T'ing Book House.

SAXIFRAGACEAE

580 species in 30 genera are found chiefly in north temperate regions, a few in south temperate regions and on tropical mountains. The family is botanically related to Ranunculaceae.

Chemistry is recorded by Hegnauer (1973).

Reference

Hegnauer, R. (1973) Chemotaxonomy of plants. Vol. 6. Basel. Birkhauser. p. 306.

Astilbe

25 species are found in eastern Asia and North America.

Astilbe japonica

McCord (1962) noted that a commercial extract was available for patch testing. No reports of dermatitis from the plant have been found.

Reference

McCord, C.P. (1962) The Occupational Toxicity of Cultivated Flowers. Ind. Med. Surg. 31, 365.

Heuchera

50 species are found in North America.

Heuchera americana

Use of the plant for obstinate ulcers (Piffard 1881) may indicate an irritant effect.

Reference

Piffard, H.G. (1881) A treatise on the Materia Medica and Therapeutics of the skin. New York. Wm. Wood and Co.

Saxifraga

370 species are found in north temperate regions, the Arctic and the Andes.

Saxifraga sarmentosa

The plant is dried in the shade and then set fire to in a bucket, and used to steam or smoke painful haemorrhoids (Smith 1969).

Reference

Smith, F.P. (1969) Chinese Materia Medica. Vegetable kingdom. 2nd ed. Rev. by Hei, P.D. Taipei, Taiwan. Ku T'ing Book House.

Tolmiea

One species, native to Pacific North America, is a popular rock-garden and house plant. The botanical name represents Dr. Tolmie, surgeon of the Hudson's Bay Company and Dr. Menzies, ship's surgeon to Captain Vancouver.

Tolmiea menziesii
Pickaback Plant,
Thousand Mothers

The plant is a glandular-hairy perennial. Hjorth (1965) from consideration of 28 positive patch test reactions to the plant at the Finsen Institute from 1935-1962 and from four positive patch test reactions in 93 consecutive cases, concluded that the plant is a sensitizer. A woman presented pruritic vesicles on the palms and fingers with erythema and pruritus of the eyelids and neck. A patch test to the plant was positive, negative in controls (Calnan 1969).

References

Calnan, C.D. (1969) Tolmiea menziesii. Contact Dermatitis Newsletter, London 5, 98.

Hjorth, N. (1965) Contact sensitivity to plants and balsams in Symposium on Allergic Contact Eczema in Theory and Practice. ed. Skog, E. (Europ. Congr. Allergy) Acta derm.-venereol. and Contact Dermatitis Newsletter 6, 126, 1969.

SCROPHULARIACEAE

3000 species in 220 genera are cosmopolitan.

Chemistry is recorded by Hegnauer (1973).

Reference

Hegnauer, R. (1973) Chemotaxonomy of plants. Vol. 6. Basel. Birkhauser. p. 343.

Antirrhinum

42 species are found in Pacific North America and the western Mediterranean region.

Antirrhinum sp.
Snapdragon

McCord (1962) noted that a commercial extract of the plant was available for patch-testing. No clinical reports of dermatitis from the plant have been found but Hjorth (1968) recorded one positive patch test reaction in a series of tests to the plant, suggesting allergenicity.

References

Hjorth, N. (1968) at Finsen Institute. Personal communication.

McCord, C.P. (1962) The Occupational Toxicity of Cultivated Flowers. Ind. Med. Surg. 31, 365.

Calceolaria

Between three and four hundred species are found from Mexico to South America. Some are cultivated and provide popular green-house and house plants.

Calceolaria integrifolia

Two male gardeners noted irritation of the eyes after taking cuttings of the plant. In one of them, patch tests to the leaf and stem sap produced negative reactions suggesting that the plant is a mild irritant for the conjunctiva (Mitchell 1973).

Reference

Mitchell, J.C. (1973) unpublished observations.

Digitalis

20 to 30 species are found in Europe, the Mediterranean region and the Canary Islands. D. purpurea provides digitalis.

Digitalis sp.
Foxglove

Contact sensitivity to Foxglove was reported by Whitfield (cited by White 1934). Untoward reactions to digitalis were reviewed by Brauner and Greene (1972).

Powdered Digitalis leaf is occasionally adulterated; the following leaves have been substituted for the true drug: mullein, Verbascum thapsus, Scrophulariaceae: comfrey, Symphytum officinale, Boraginaceae: primrose, Primula vulgaris, Primulaceae: ploughman's spikenard, Inula conyza, Compositae: Urtica dioica, Urticaceae (British Pharmaceutical Codex 1934).

References

Brauner, G.J. and Greene, M.H. (1972) Digitalis allergy: Digoxin-induced Vasculitis. Cutis 10, 441.

British Pharmaceutical Codex (1934) London. Pharmaceutical Society of Great Britain.

White, R.P. (1934) The Dermatergoses or Occupational Affections of the Skin. 4th ed. London. H.K. Lewis.

Gratiola

20 species are found in north and south temperate zones and on tropical mountains.

Gratiola officinalis

The dried plant was formerly officinal. Use of this plant in homeopathic Medicine caused itching and burning of the scalp, pustules on the forehead and chest and blisters on the hands and fingers (Schulz 1929).

References

Schulz, H. (1929) Vorlesungen uber Wirkung und Anwendyng der deutschen Arzneipflanzen. 2 Aufl. Leipzig cited by Touton (1932).

Touton, K. (1932) Hauterkrankungen durch phanerogamische Pflanzen und ihre Produkte (Toxicodermia et Allergodermia phytogenes), in Barnewitz, J. et al Angeborene Anomalien, Lichtdermatosen, Pflanzengifte, Thermische Schadigungen, Einfluss Innerer Storungen auf die Haut. Berlin. Verlag von Julius Springer.

Linaria

150 species are found in the Northern Hemisphere, excluding tropical regions, and especially in the Mediterranean region.

Linaria vulgaris

This species is listed as irritant by Pammel (1911). Linaria, Scrophularia and Veronica are used in Herbal Medicine, apparently for astringent effects (Wren 1968).

References

Pammel, L.H. (1911) A manual of poisonous plants. Torch Press. Cedar Rapids, Iowa. Reprinted Univ. Microfilms Inc. Ann Arbor, Mich. 1965. pp. 476-7.

Wren, R.W. (1968) Potter's New Cyclopaedia of Botanical Drugs and Preparations by Wren, R.C. Re-edit. by Wren, R.W. Potter and Clarke, Ltd. Health Science Press. Rustington, Sussex.

Verbascum

300 species are found in northern temperate Eurasia.

Verbascum thapsus
Moth-Mullein, Flannel plant

The leaves, which are thickly covered with wooly hairs that are irritant to the skin, are often applied externally to the throat in some parts of the United States to produce a rubefacient effect (White 1887). Dermatitis of the face and left wrist from contact with the plant was reported by Steiner-Wourlisch (1930). The plant does not seem to be notably irritant to field-workers (Behl et al 1966).

References

Behl, P.N., Captain, R.M., Bedi, B.M.S. and Gupta, S. (1966) Skin-irritant and sensitizing plants found in India, New Delhi. P.N. Behl, Irwin Hospital.

Steiner-Wourlisch, A. (1930) Unusual cases of dermatitis venenata. Klin. Wchnschr. 9, 205.

White, J.C. (1887) Dermatitis venenata: An account of the Action of External irritants upon the skin. Boston. Cupples and Hurd.

SIMABOUBACEAE

120 species in 20 genera are found in tropical and subtropical regions.

Chemistry is recorded by Hegnauer (1973).

Many species of the family contain bitter principles such as quassine. Quassia (Surinam quassia) and Aeschrion (syn. Picraena, Picrasma) (Jamaica quassia) have been used medicinally.

Reference

Hegnauer, R. (1973) Chemotaxonomy of plants. Vol. 6. Basel. Birkhauser. p. 387.

Aeschrion
(syn. Picrasma,
syn. Picraena)

Five species are native to the West Indies and southern Brazil.

The genus is also noted under Picrasma.

Aeschrion excelsa
(syn. Picrasma excelsa)
Jamaica quassia

Barham (1794) said that workmen disliked working with Jamaica quassia because it 'bittered' their mouths and throats and Stone (1921) quoted an account of temporary paralysis in a dog's legs after its ulcers had been bathed with a decoction of the wood. According to Woods and Calnan (1976) these reports hardly seem to justify Moll's (1950) claim that it is the 'most-feared' wood in South America for which he quotes no evidence. According to these authors P. excelsa should be referred to Aeschrion excelsa.

References

Barham, H. (1794) Hortus americanus. Kingston, Jamaica, cited by Woods and Calnan (1976).

Moll, F. (1950) Giftiges Holz und Gewerbekrankheiten Holz (Munchen) 4, 76.

Stone, H. (1921) A textbook of wood. London, Rider, cited by Woods and Calnan (1976).

Woods, B. and Calnan, C.D. (1976) Toxic Woods. Brit. J. Derm. 94, Suppl. 13, June.

Ailanthus

Ten species are found in Asia and Australia.

Ailanthus altissima
(syn. A. glandulosa)
Tree of Heaven,
Chinese Sumac

The odour of the foliage is intensely disagreeable and can cause headache and nausea (Ellis 1757) rhinitis and conjunctivitis (Blumstein 1943). The disagreeable odour of the male flowers is said to be carried by the pollen but the leaves and twigs are malodorous if rubbed or bruised only slightly (Swingle 1916). The pollen can cause hayfever (Wodehouse 1971). White (1887) remembered a case-report of dermatitis of the face from the plant but he could not find the reference. He also received a personal communication of the case of a lady who was poisoned by contact with the tree. Numerous authors have recorded these notes and some have added to them but further case-reports are lacking.

White (1887) may have been referring to a report of Cornevin (1887) that gardeners pruning the Tree of Heaven may get vesicular eruptions on the face and hands.

References

Blumstein, G.I. (1943) Sensitivity to Ailanthus pollen. J. Allergy 14, 329.

Ellis, J. (1757) Phil. Trans. Roy. Soc. 49, 870, cited by Swingle (1016).

Swingle, W.T. (1916) The early European history and the botanical name of the Tree of Heaven, Ailanthus altissima. J. Washington Acad. Sci. 6, 490.

White, J.C. (1887) Dermatitis venenata: An account of the action of external irritants upon the skin. Boston. Cupples and Hurd.

Wodehouse, R.P. (1971) Hayfever Plants. 2nd rev. edition. New York, Hafner.

Cornevin, C. (1887) Des plantes veneneuses. Paris, Firmin-Didot.

Ailanthus malabarica
(syn. A. imberbiflora)
White bean

The various forms of this species furnish a quantity of resin which, according to Dr. Lauterer, makes a good ointment for chronic ulcers. Fresh cuts and sores, however, should not be treated with this resin, on account of the acrid oil (Webb 1948).

Reference

Webb, L.J. (1948) Guide to the medicinal and poisonous plants of Queensland. Bulletin No. 232. Council for Scientific and Industrial Research. Melbourne, Australia.

Harrisonia

Four species are found in tropical Africa, south-eastern Asia, Indo Malaysia and tropical Australia.

Harrisonia abyssinica

The root is used as a topical application for bubonic plague, apparently for a rubefacient effect (Watt and Breyer-Brandwijk 1962).

Reference

Watt, J.M. and Breyer-Brandwijk, M.G. (1962) The Medicinal and poisonous plants of Southern Africa. 2nd ed. Edinburgh. E.& S. Livingstone.

Picrasma

Six species are found from the western Himalayas to Japan, Malaysia and Fiji. The bitter wood and bark are used as a substitute for Quassia (Quassia).

Picrasma excelsa
(syn. Picraena excelsa)
Bitter Wood,
Jamaica Quassia

The wood and bark are used as a substitute for Quassia. A benzoquinone is derived from the tree (Polonsky and Lederer 1959).

Cups turned out of the log are sold as Bitter Cups, the water standing in them for a short while acquiring the bitterness of the wood (Wren 1968). Hausen (1970) cites Moll (1950) for an injurious effect of the wood.

References

Hausen, B.M. (1970) Untersuchungen uber Gesundheitsschadigende Holzer. Thesis, Hamburg.

Moll, F. (1950) Giftiges Holz und Gewerbekrankheiten "Holz" 4, 77.

Polonsky, J. et Lederer, E. (1959) Note sur l'isolement de la dimethoxy-2,6-benzoquinone des ecorces et du bois de quelques Simaroubacees et Meliacees. Bull. Soc. chim. France 1157-58.

Wren, R.W. (1968) Potter's New Cyclopaedia of Botanical Drugs and Preparations by Wren, R.C. Re-edit. by Wren, R.W. Potter and Clarke, Ltd. Health Science Press. Rustington, Sussex.

Quassia
(syn. Simaba)

40 species are found in tropical regions, especially in America.

Quassia amara
(syn. Simarouba)

The bark of Simarouba amara and Khaya senegalensis and the wood of Picarasma crenata contain 2,6-dimethoxybenzoquinone (Polonsky and Lederer 1959). This was one of the quinones which produced positive patch test reactions in Heyl's (1966) case of dermatitis from Bowdichia. Woods and Calnan (1976) refer to a report of Prefontaine (1763) that negroes stripping the root-bark of simarouba (perhaps not S. amara) wore protective clothing because the sap would cause gale severe enough to prevent them walking for some days.

Quassia amara yields Surinam Quassia (Merck Index 1968). An extract of Quassia wood, used as an insecticide, caused dermatitis (Arton 1959, Semmola 1963).

Quassia cedron
(syn. Simaba cedron)

The seeds are intensely bitter (Wren 1968).

References

Heyl, V. (1966) Kontaktekzem bei Uberempfindlichkeit gegen Sucupira-und Palisanderholz. Berufsdermatosen 14, 239.

Polonsky, J. and Lederer, E. (1959) Note sur l'isolement de la dimethoxy-2,6-benzoquinone des ecorces et du bois de quelques Simarubacees et Meliacees. Bull. Soc. Chim. France 1157.

Prefontaine, de (1763) Maison rustique, a l'usage de Cayenne. pp. 139, 152, 208-209, Paris, Bauche.

Woods, B. and Calnan, C.D. (1976) Toxic Woods. Brit. J. Derm. 94, Suppl. 13, June.

Artom, M. (1959) Some occupational dermatoses of agricultural workers. Minerva Derm. (Torino) 34, 77.

Merck Index (1968) An Encyclopedia of Chemicals and Drugs. ed. Stecher, P.G. 9th ed. Rahway, N.J. Merck and Co. Inc.

Semmola, L. (1963) The juridical limitations of the list of occupational risks and industrial dermatoses without protection by insurance. Rass. Derm. Sif. 16, 57.

Wren, R.W. (1968) Potter's New Cyclopaedia of Botanical Drugs and Preparations by Wren, R.C. Re-edit by Wren, R.W. Potter and Clarke Ltd. Health Science Press. Rustington, Sussex.

SMILACACEAE

375 species in four genera are found in tropical and temperate regions.

Smilax

350 species are found in tropical and subtropical regions. The dried roots of several species form Sarsaparilla (Merck Index 1968).

Smilax havanensis

The tough stems and the leaves which are set with sharp thorns can cause mechanical injury particularly about the ankles of walkers. This species is a common weed in Miami, Florida.

Reference

Merck Index (1968) An Encyclopedia of Chemicals and Drugs. ed. Stecher, P.G. 8th ed. Rahway, N.J. Merck and Co. Inc.

SOLANACEAE

More than 2000 species in 90 genera are found in tropical and temperate regions. Central and South America are the chief centres of distribution.

Chemistry is recorded by Hegnauer (1973).

Reference

Hegnauer, R. (1973) Chemotaxonomy of Plants. Vol 6. Basel. Birkhauser. p. 403.

Acnistus

50 species are native to tropical America.

Acnistus arborescens

The leaves, which have been used for many years to treat cancerous growths, yield a tumor-inhibitory lactone (Kupchan 1970).

Reference

Kupchan, S.M. (1970) Recent advances in the chemistry of tumor inhibitors of plant origin. Trans. N.Y. Acad. Sci. (Series II) 32, 85.

Atropa

Four species are distributed from the Mediterranean region to central Asia and the Himalayas.

Atropa bella-donna
Deadly Nightshade

The sap of the plant can cause dermatitis of the hands and face of labourers who cut it and persons handling the berries can develop vesico-pustular eruptions on the face with disorders of visual accommodation (Schwartz et al 1957, Behl et al 1961, McCord 1962).

Ingestion of the plant can produce persistent erythema, urticaria, vesicular eruptions and hyperhidrosis (Brooks 1958). Atropine was recognized as a cause of dermatitis by Collins in 1888. Atropine, used in the eye, can produce allergenic kerato-conjunctivitis; allergy to homatropine is rare (Duke-Elder 1965). Apparent conjunctival allergy can result from old solutions of atropine in which irritant degradations products occur (Theodore 1953).

Belladonna plaster is applied for an irritant effect (Gardiner 1922). It cannot be assumed that Belladonna plasters, as purchased, contain only extractives of this plant since rubefacient materials may be added. The skin of pharmacists and chemists is sometimes affected by atropine (*dl*-hyoscyamine) (Herxheimer 1912, Dobkewitsch and Sidi 1948, Schwartz et al 1957).

References

Behl, P.N., Captain, R.M., Bedi, B.M.S. and Gupta, S. (1966) Skin-irritant and sensitizing plants found in India, New Delhi. P.N. Behl, Irwin Hospital.

Brooks, V.J. (1958) Poisons: their properties, chemical identification, symptoms and emergency treatments. Ed. 2. New York. Van Nostrand.

Collins, E.T. (1888) Atropine irritation. Royal Ophth. Hosp. Rept. 12, 164.

Dobkewitsch, S. and Sidi, E. (1948) Excema de la face provoque par un collyre au sulfate d' atropine. Bull. Soc. Franc. de dermat. et syph. 55, 60.

Duke, Elder, S. (1965) System of Ophthalmology. Vol. VIII. Diseases of the outer eye. Part 1. Allergic kerato-conjunctivitis. pp. 451. London. Henry Kimpton.

Gardiner, F. (1922) Occupational dermatitis. Brit. J. Derm. Syph. 34, 297.

Herxheimer, K. (1912) Uber die gewerblichen Erkrankungen der Haut. Deutsch. med. Wchnochr. 38, 1822.

McCord, C.P. (1962) The occupational toxicity of cultivated flowers. Ind. Med. Surg. 31, 365.

Schwartz, L., Tulipan, L. and Birmingham, D.J. (1957) Occupational Diseases of the Skin. 3rd ed. Philadelphia. Lea and Febiger. pp. 637-672.

Theodore, F.H. (1953) Drug sensitiveness and irritation of the conjunctiva. JAMA 151, 25.

Browallia

Six species, native to tropical America and the West Indies, are cultivated as greenhouse or house plants.

Browallia speciosa var. *major*

A woman who was contact sensitive to *Streptocarpus* showed a positive patch test reaction to this plant (Agrup and Fregert 1968).

Reference

Agrup, G. and Fregert, S. (1968) Patch test reactions to *Streptocarpus*. Contact Dermatitis Newsletter, London 4, 72.

Capsicum

50 species are native to central and South America.

Capsicum annuum
Cayenne Pepper, Paprika, Chilli, Tabasco

The fruit furnishes the pepper of the New World. *Piper* also furnishes pepper. Workers handling wet chilli beans developed dermatitis of the hands; the irritant appeared to penetrate rubber gloves (Cleland 1931). The fruit, even when dried, can have a vesicant effect. The smoke of burning chillies is irritant to the mucous membrane and was used for torture (Burkill 1935). Red pepper, marketed as a nostrum for rheumatism produced dermatitis (Report of Bureau of Investigation 1929). Submucous fibrosis of the palate and fauces has been observed in India where a high intake of chilli occurs. Recurrent oral ulceration can also occur. Smith et al (1970) studied the irritant effects of capsaicin on the human skin. Capsicum was used as a home-remedy producing a rubefacient effect and, if its application were continued, vesication could occur (White 1887).

Inhalation of paprika can produce paprika splitter's lung, a form of allergic alveolitis (Morgan and Seaton 1975).

Capsicum fastigiatum (syn. C. frutescens)

The plant has rubefacient properties (Perrot and Paris 1971).

References

Burkill, I.H. (1935) A Dictionary of the Economic Products of the Malay Peninsula. 2 Vols. London. Crown Agents for the Colonies.

Cleland, J.B. (1931) Plants including fungi, poisonous or otherwise injurious to man in Australia III. Med. J. Australia 2, 775.

Morgan, W.K.C. and Seaton, A. (1975) Occupational Lung Diseases. Philadelphia, Saunders.

Perrot, E. and Paris, R. (1971) Les plantes medicinales. 2 vols. Paris. Presses Universitaires de France. 245 (+XXVI (indec)) pp.

Report of Bureau of Investigation (1929) Mizar again. JAMA 93, 1240.

Smith, J.G. Jr., Crounse, R.G. and Spence, D. (1970) The effects of capsaicin on human skin, liver and epidermal lysosomes. J. Invest. Derm. 54, 170.

White, J.C. (1887) Dermatitis venenata: An account of the Action of External irritants upon the Skin. Boston. Cupples and Hurd.

Cestrum

150 species are native to warm regions of America and the West Indies.

Cestrum spp.

Some can produce mechanical injury (Oakes and Butcher 1962).

Cestrum nocturnum

The fragrant nocturnal emanations of the flowers can cause irritation of the nose and throat, headache, nausea and dizziness (Morton 1962).

Respiratory symptoms can occur from proximity to the plant (Morton 1969).

References

Morton, J.F. (1962) Ornamental Plants with Poisonous Properties II. Proc. Florida Hort. Soc. 75, 484.

Morton, J.F. (1969) Some ornamental plants excreting respiratory irritants. Proc. Florida State Hort. Soc. 82, 415.

Oakes, A.J. and Butcher, J.O. (1962) Poisonous and injurious plants of the U.S. Virgin Islands. Misc. Publ. 882. U.S. Dept. of Agriculture, Washington, D.C.

Datura

Ten species are found in tropical and warm temperate regions.

Datura spp.

Some, notably D. stramonium, yield poisonous honey. Contact with the plants can irritate the skin of 'sensitive' individuals (Morton 1958).

Datura candida

Systemic symptoms can occur from proximity to the plant (Morton 1969).

Datura cornigera

The wood-dust can produce mydriasis (Cleland 1925).

Datura ferox

The plant has spines capable of producing mechanical injury (Verdcourt and Trump 1958).

Datura knightii
(syn. Brugmansia)

The juice produced mydriasis (Cleland 1925).

Datura metel

Scopolamine, derived from the plant, can produce dermatitis of the eyelids (Duke-Elder 1965).

References

Cleland, J.B. (1925) Plants including fungi, poisonous or otherwise injurious to man in Australia (Series II). Med. J. Australia 2, 443.

Duke-Elder, S. (1965) System of Ophthalmology. Vol. VIII. Diseases of the outer eye. Part 1. Allergic kerato-conjunctivitis. pp. 451. London. Henry Kimpton.

Morton, J.F. (1958) Ornamental plants with poisonous properties. Proc. Florida State Hort. Soc. 71, 372.

Morton, J.F. (1969) Some ornamental plants excreting respiratory irritants. Proc. Florida State Hort. Soc. 82, 415.

Verdcourt, B. and Trump, E.C. (1958) Common Poisonous Plants of East Africa. London, Collins.

Datura stramonium
Thorn Apple

The fruit-capsule is covered with small sharp spines. A number of aklaloids, including atropine, hyoscyamine and hyoscine are present in all parts of the plant especially in the capsule and seeds (Francis and Southcott 1967). The seeds may be present as contaminants of edible seed mixtures and the leaves are used to make tea for asthma (Francis and Southcott 1967). Ocular effects can result from entry of seeds into the conjunctival sac of farmers at harvest-time (Simmons 1957). The plant causes swelling of the eyelids of those who collect it (Cheney 1887). Numerous authors have referred to dermatitis in gardeners, farmers and pharmacists from all parts of the plant but case-reports are lacking. Blohm (1962) noted no ill-effect from rubbing the leaf in his hands. Dermatitis from atropine is noted under Atropa. Hyoscine (Scopolamine) can cause allergic kerato-conjunctivitis (Duke-Elder 1965).

Dust from the weed can produce mydriasis (Goldey et al 1966). Tomato (Lycopersicon) grafted onto the plant produced adverse effects from a content of alkaloids (Miller 1975) which are hallucinogenic (Mahler 1975).

References

Blohm, H. (1962) Poisonous Plants of Venezuela. Cambridge, Mass. Harvard University Press.

Cheney (1887) Personal communication to White (1887). Cheney was a dealer in vegetable drugs.

Duke-Elder, S. (1965) System of Ophthalmology: Vol. VIII. Diseases of the outer eye. Part 1. Allergic kerato-conjunctivitis. pp. 451. London. Henry Kimpton.

Francis, D.F. and Southcott, R.V. (1967) Plants harmful to man in Australia. Misc. Bull. No. 1. Botanic Garden, Adelaide, Australia.

Goldey, J.A., Dick, D.A. and Porter, W.L. (1966) Cornpicker's pupil. A clinical note regarding mydriasis from Jimson weed dust (stramonium). Ohio State Med. J. 69, 921.

Mahler, D.A. (1975) Jimson weed seeds. Ann. Int. Med. 83, 905.

Miller, R.W. (1975) Jimson weed seeds. Ann. Int. Med. 83, 905.

Simmons, F.H. (1957) Jimson weed mydriasis in farmers. Am. J. Ophth. 41, 109.

White, J.C. (1887) Dermatitis venenata: An account of the Action of External irritants upon the skin. Boston. Cupples and Hurd.

Datura suaveolens

Systemic symptoms can occur from proximity to the plant (Morton 1969).

Reference

Morton, J.F. (1969) Some ornamental plants excreting respiratory irritants. Proc. Florida State Hort. Soc. 82, 415.

Duboisia

Two species are native to Australia and New Caledonia.

Duboisia sp.

A pharmaceutical worker, engaged in processing the leaf for extraction of hyoscyamine-atropine and hyoscyine, developed dermatitis of the finger webs, dorsa of hands, neck and shins. A similar attack occurred when he was put to work extracting Heliotropium spp., Boraginaceae. Patch tests were not recorded. The alkaloids of these plants are chemically distinct but both are tertiary bases containing one nitrogen atom in alicylic rings and at least one esterified hydroxy group. This structure was suggested as the common denominator in the causation of the dermatitis from the botanically unrelated plants (Trautner 1949).

Reference

Trautner, E.M. (1949) A contribution to the causation of atropine allergy. Med. J. Australia 2, 17.

Hyoscyamus

20 species are found in Europe and from North Africa and the Sahara to south-western and central Asia.

Hyoscyamus niger
Black Henbane

The roots can be mistaken for parsnips (Pastinaca) with untoward effects (Forsyth 1954). Inunction of the skin with Oil of Henbane can cause painful blistering (Schwartz et al 1957). Agrup et al (1970) observed positive patch test reaction to methscopolamine, its nitrate and scopolamine hydrobromide. Dermatitis from scopolamine (hyoscyine) is noted under Datura.

References

Agrup, G., Dahlquist, I., Fregert, S. et al (1970) Value of history and testing in suspected contact dermatitis. Archs. Derm. 101, 212.

Forsyth, A.A. (1954) British Poisonous Plants. Ministry of Agriculture, Fisheries and Food (London). Bull. 161.

Schwartz, L., Tulipan, L. and Birmingham, D.J. (1957) Occupational Diseases of the Skin. 3rd ed. Philadelphia. Lea and Febiger. pp. 637-672.

Lycium

Perhaps 90 species are found in temperate and tropical regions. Many are thorny. L. afrum, L. ferocissimum and L. horridum can produce mechanical injury. The thorns are said to be poisonous and injuries from them are said to be slow to heal (Ewart 1909, Hurst 1942, Howes 1946).

References

Ewart, A.J. (1909) The Weeds, Poison Plants and Naturalized Aliens of Victoria, Melbourne. Gov't Printer, cited by Hurst (1942).

Howes, F.N. (1946) Fence and barrier plants in warm climates. Kew. Bull. 2, 51.

Hurst, E. (1942) The Poison plants of New South Wales. N.S.W. Poison Plants Committee; Sydney.

Lycopersicon
(syn. Lycopersicum)

Seven species are native to the Pacific coast of South America and the Galapagos.

Lycopersicon lycopersicum
(syn. L. esculentum)
Tomato

Dermatitis has been reported from handling the plants, especially when wet. The reports suggest the possibility of an allergic effect from the leaves and stems rather than from the fruits but detailed patch tests are lacking (Lain 1918, Washburn 1918, Shelmire 1940, O'Donovan 1927, Sneid 1955, Zakon et al 1947, Schwartz et al 1957).

Workers processing the fruits can develop dermatitis (Foa 1927, White 1934, Semmola 1963). Templeton (1945) reported a patient who had dermatitis from handling and from ingestion of the fruit. From patch testing farmers, Szego (1965) concluded that heat-stable and heat-labile allergens are present in the plant. Szego (1970) reported additional cases.

Tomato can produce immediate hypersensitivity reactions by 20 minute patch test taking the form of vesiculation within 20 minutes on previously affected but presently non-eczematous skin (Hjorth and Roed-Petersen 1976).

References

Foa, G. (1927) Professional eczema. Il. Policlinico 34, 675 (Italian).

Lain, E.S. (1918) Dermatitis Lycopersicum exculentum (Tomato Plant). JAMA 71, 1114.

O'Donovan, W.J. (1927) Exogenic dermatitis. Lancet 1, 1128.

Schwartz, L., Tulipan, L. and Birmingham, D.J. (1957) Occupational Diseases of the Skin. 3rd ed. Philadelphia. Lea and Febiger. pp. 637-672.

Semmola, L. (1963) The juridical limitations of the list of occupational risks and industrial dermatoses without protection by insurance. Rass. Derm. Sif. 16, 57.

Shelmire, B. (1940) Contact dermatitis from vegetation. South Med. J. 33, 338.

Sneid, P. (1955) Occupational health on the farm. Indust. Med. 24, 117.

Szego, L. (1965) Sensitisation by agricultural crops and crop-protection preparations I. Studies of plant (leaf) extracts. Acta Med. Acad. Sci. Hung. 21, 19. (Excerpta Medica. XVII, 13, 3468)

Szego, L. (1970) Cases of occupational contact dermatitis from carrot and tomato. Borgy. Vener. Szemle. 46, 74 (Hungarian)

Templeton, H.J. (1945) Epidermal and dermal sensitisation (co-existing in the same individual). JAMA 127, 908.

Washburn, R.G. (1918) in discussion of Lain (1918).

White, R.P. (1934) The Dermatergoses or Occupational Affections of the Skin. 4th ed. London. H.K. Lewis.

Zakon, S.J., Goldberg, A.L. and Kahn, J.B. (1947) Lipstick cheilitis: common dermatosis. Report of 32 cases. Archs. Derm. Syph. 56, 499.

Hjorth, N. and Roed-Petersen, J. (1976) Occupational protein contact dermatitis in food handlers. Contact Dermatitis 2, 28.

Nicotiana

21 species are native to Australia and Polynesia, 45 to North and South America. Several furnish Tobacco.

Chemistry is reviewed by Schmeltz (1972), historical aspects by Redmond (1970).

References

Redmond, D.E. (1970) Tobacco and Cancer. The first Clinical Report, 1761. New Eng. J. Med. 282, 51.

Schmeltz, I. (1972) The chemistry of Tobacco and Tobacco smoke. New York. Plenum.

Nicotiana tabacum
Tobacco

Agricultural chemicals such as fertilizers and insecticides which are used in the field and chemical additives during processing must be considered as possible causes of dermatitis from the plant and its products. From patch testing farmers Szego (1965), Szego and Szilvassy (1966) concluded that the leaf of the plant contains heat-stable and heat-labile allergens.

Early reports of dermatitis from tobacco processing were reviewed by White (1934). Mechanical trauma and irritant dermatitis of the hands particularly of the thumb and index finger, hyperkeratosis and nail dystrophy are reported (Nasution et al 1973).

Waterers and sorters of the leaves in cigar-making tend to develop skin infection unless great cleanliness is observed; the mucous membranes may be affected by fragments of leaf most severly near the lower front teeth (White 1934). Dust in tobacco-factories causes skin infection and paronychia from mechanical or frictional injury by angular fragments of tobacco leaf (White 1934). A woman sorting out the pressed leaves of tobacco in a cigarette factory developed blisters on the hands, face and uncovered parts of the neck. She recovered on leaving this work but, on return to it, she relapsed (Karrenberg 1927, 1928). Dermatitis is fairly common in the process of stripping tobacco. Tobacco twist is lubricated with olive oil which is irritating (White 1934). Dermatitis was due to chemicals used in tobacco processing or by the fermenting process itself (Schwartz et al 1957).

During a nine year period, (1941-1949) 1065 cases of hand eruptions were reported in one large plant where cigars were manufactured. Patch tests to tobacco were negative. Wet work and alkali exposure appeared responsible. One per 1000 patients is susceptible to the smell of tobacco; nausea and vomiting are noted within the first 24 to 48 hours (Samitz et al 1949).

Vero and Genovese (1941) in an observation made over a period of 25 years state that the dermatoses encountered among cigar workers were chiefly due to infections, injuries and chemicals rather than to hypersensitivity to tobacco. They reported 3 cases of hypersensitivity to tobacco in cigar makers. Positive patch tests were obtained to both filler and wrapper in one case, and to the filler in two other cases. In 60 cases of hand dermatitis in cigar-workers observed by Franchi (1937) irritation from gum and tobacco rather than contact allergy was considered to be responsible. Davis (1924) reported dermatitis in a cigar salesman of seasonal occurrence and attributed to handling tobacco.

Patch tests with maceration and decoction products of fresh tobacco leaves and with powdered dry leaves produced positive reactions in four of 19 women employed in tobacco fermentation work (Szego and Szilvassy 1968). Two patients with vesicular dermatitis who were employed in the tobacco industry had positive patch tests to tobacco leaves (Panconesi 1954).

Dermatitis in the tobacco industry is uncommon (Gross 1931, Samitz et al 1949, Thiers et al 1965, Shanon and Tas 1958, Panconesi 1954, Silvette et al 1957). Tests were positive to wet tobacco leaf and negative to dry leaf (White 1934) and to old partially fermented leaves but not to new leaves (Vero and Genovese 1941). Contact with raw tobacco leaves, dry tobacco and cigars appeared to be innocuous (Vero and Genovese 1941).

Karrenberg (1928) obtained a positive patch test and Vero and Genovese (1941) negative patch tests in workers who had dermatitis attributed to tobacco. Cured and fermented leaf, but not the raw leaf could occasionally cause dermatitis. Dermatitis of the hands followed tobacco-smoking; a patch test was negative, an intradermal test positive (Cormia and de Gara 1965). Allergic dermatitis was found to be rare in tobacco workers; only three persons showed positive patch test reactions to the leaf (Samitz et al 1949). Nine cases were reported by Chanial et al (1970). Injections of tobacco extract produced generalized eczema (Harkavy 1939).

Smoking cigarettes with the lighted end inside the mouth produced palatal changes (Jensen and Williams 1964). Pipe-smoking and retention of tobacco snuff in the mouth can produce premalignant changes in the mucous membrane and cancer (Forsey and Sullivan 1961, Stecker et al 1964). Chewers of betel (*Piper*) can develop oral cancer probably from *Nicotiana* added to the quid (Muir and Kirk 1960). The leaf of *Diospyros* melanoxylon is used in Inda to roll tobacco (Behl et al 1966); this plant is irritant. Formaldehyde and menthol may be present in tobacco smoke. Dermatitis has been attributed to dyes, fungicides, antibiotics, coumarin derivatives, menthol and vanilla (Vanilla) in tobacco rather than the alkaloids of the plant (Gross 1931, Franchi 1937). Dermatitis was attributed to diethylene glycol in tobacco (Newman 1938) and to triacetin in a cigarette filter (Unna and Schulz 1963).

Arsenical dermatitis from tobacco has been reported (Barksdale 1940). Workers in tobacco sheds developed parasitic bites (Szego and Balogh 1965). Workers who have dermatitis in the tobacco industry can become desensitised (hardened) (Szego and Szilvassy 1968).

Cigarette paper made from flax (Linum) may cause dermatitis (Franchi 1937). Cross-reaction of tobacco with Balsam of Peru has been observed.

Certain foods may be involved in unexplained exacerbations of eczema in a patient sensitive to Balsam of Peru. The pertinent foods may be synthetic food flavors, but may also be spices, orange peel, and resinoids or essential oils in alcoholic and non-alcoholic beverages. The significance of tobacco flavours for patients with eczema is entirely unknown, but worthy of attention, as many of the ingredients, such as coumarins, oil of cinnamon and resinoids are well-known sensitizers (Hjorth 1961).

A laboratory worker had chronic urticaria which was traced to exposure to formaldehyde, tobacco smoke (both from the patient's own smoking and that of others in his environment) and certain fried and broiled foods (Rappaport and Hoffman 1941). Investigation showed that the cross-sensitisation extended to aliphatic nonconjugated aldehydes ranging from formaldehyde to an eighteen chain aldehyde. The reaction-producing concentration ranged from 1:1,000,000 for formaldehyde to 1:1 for the aldehyde containing eighteen carbon atoms, indicating that the shorter the carbon chain the more marked was the reaction. Aliphatic conjugated and aromatic aldehydes failed to produce urticarial skin reactions with the exception of acrolein. This case is reviewed by Baer (1954).

A machinist, aged 20 years, had chronic eczematoid dermatitis of the index and middle fingers of both hands; patch tests were positive to tobacco smoke residues deposited on the cigarette filter and to crude coal tar. This case was carefully investigated and the details may be found in the original paper which suggests that patients with hand eczema who show positive patch test reactions to coal tar should be investigated for tobacco contactants (Weary and Wood 1969).

Nicotine does not play any part in sensitisation to tobacco (Sulzberger 1933a,b). Reports provide clinical evidence that alkaloids of tobacco are absorbed through mucous membranes, damaged and even intact skin (Deacon 1926, Wilson 1930, Lockhart 1933, Burkill 1935) in a quantity sufficient to produce adverse effects. Nicotine addicts do not appear to have tried this route of administration which would seem preferable to inhalation of smoke, provided that the rate of absorption could be controlled. Sporotrichosis of the hands occurred in a cigar maker (Seilin 1919).

Blepharitis and conjunctivitis in workers with tobacco were reported by Jensi and Iserle (1949), Simko (1950) and reviewed by Heinc and Kubena (1969).

Handling of uncured tobacco leaves can cause systemic symptoms when the skin is wet with dew possibly from obsorption of nicotine (Gehlbach et al 1974).

A Japanese gardener who did not smoke was affected by nausea, vomiting, greenish pallor and shock twenty minutes after the application of a patch test to a spray containing 40 per cent nicotine sulphate. This resembled the reaction seen in persons inhaling the smoke from their first cigar (Schoch 1976).

References

Baer, R.L. (1954) Cross sensitisation phenomena in Modern Trends in Dermatology. (Second Series) ed. MacKenna, R.M.B. London. Butterworth.

Barksdale, E.E. (1940) Arsenical dermatitis from tobacco. Virg. Med. Monthly 67, 393.

Behl, P.N., Captain, R.M., Bedi, B.M.S. and Gupta, S. (1966) Skin-irritant and sensitizing plants found in India, New Delhi. P.N. Behl. Irwin Hospital.

Burkill, I.H. (1935) A Dictionary of the Economic Products of the Malay Peninsula. 2 Vols. London. Crown Agents for the Colonies.

Chanial, G., Joseph, J. Colin, L. et al (1970) Dermatitis in tobacco workers (9 cases). Bull. Soc. franc. Derm. Syph. 77, 281 (French).

Cormia, F.E. and de Gara, P.F. (1965) Vesiculobullous dermatitis from tobacco smoke. JAMA 193, 391.

Davis, W.D. (1924) A case of sensitisation dermatitis. Archs. Derm. Syph. 10, 112.

Deacon, J.N. (1926) Poisoning by tobacco applied to the skin. Brit. Med. J. 2, 61.

Forsey, R.R. and Sullivan, T.J. (1961) Stomatitis nicotina. Archs. Derm. 83, 945.

Franchi, F. (1937) Dermatite professionale delle sigaraie. Gior. ital. di dermat. e sif. 78, 475.

Gehlbach, S.H., Williams, W.A. and Perry, L.D. (1974) Green-tobacco sickness: Illness of tobacco harvesters. JAMA 229, 1880.

Gross, H. (1931) Uber Staubinkalationen and sonstige gesundheitliche Schadigungen der Tabakarbeiter. Mschr. Unfallheillk. 38, 151.

Harkavy, J. (1939) Tobacco skin reactions and their clinical significance. J. Invest. Derm. 2, 257.

Heinc, A. and Kubena, K. (1969) Maladies oculaires externes par action directe d'elements exterieurs. Ophthalmologica 158, 181.

Hjorth, N. (1961) Eczmatous allergy to Balsams, Allied Perfumes and Flavouring Agents. Copenhagen: Munksgaard.

Jensen, O.C. and Williams, R.M. (1964) Palatitis ab igne. Case due to unusual smoking habits. Archs. Derm. 89, 467.

Jensi, V. and Iserle, J. (1949) Vliv prace s tabakem na zrak. Cs. oftal 5, 161.

Karrenberg, C.L. (1927) Fall von Tabakdermatitis. Zbl. Hautkrkh 24, 594.

Karrenberg, C.L. (1928) Causation of occupational dermatoses: Dermatitis from tobacco leaves. Derm. Ztschr. 52, 31 (German).

Lockhart, L.P. (1933) Nicotine poisoning. Brit. Med. J. 1, 246.

Muir, C.S. and Kirk, R. (1960) Betel, Tobacco and Cancer of the Mouth. Brit. J. Cancer 14, 597.

Nasution, D., Klokke, A.H. and Nater, J.P. (1973) A survey of occupational dermatoses in indonesia. Berufsdermatosen 21, 215.

Newman, B.A. (1938) Diethylene glycol in tobacco. Dermatitis caused by diethylene glycol in tobacco. JAMA 111, 25.

Panconesi, E. (1954) Occupational skin diseases due to tobacco Rass. Derm. Sif. 7, 85.

Rappaport, B.Z. and Hoffman, M.M. (1941) Urticaria due to aliphatic aldehydes; clinical and experimental study. JAMA 116, 2656.

Samitz, M.H., Mori, P. and Long, C.F. (1949) Dermatological hazards in the cigar industry. Ind. Med. Surg. 18, 434.

Schoch, A.G. (1976) Patch test hazards. The Schoch Letter 26 (No. 7), 11.

Schwartz, L., Tulipan, L., and Birmingham, D.J. (1957) Occupational Diseases of the Skin. 3rd ed. Philadelphia. Lea and Febiger. pp. 637-672.

Seilin, J. (1919) Report of a case of dermatitis coccidiora. Med. Rec. 95, 360.

Shanon, T. and Tas, J. (1958) Dermatitis of the nose due to snuff tobacco. Ann Allergy 16, 156.

Silvette, H., Larson, P.S. and Haag, H.B. (1957) Immunological aspects of tobacco and smoking. Amer. J. Med. Sci. 234, 561.

Simko, S. (1950) Shodnotenie ocynych prehliadok v tabakovych tovarnach na Slovensku Slov. Lek 12, 619.

Stecker, R.H., Devine, K.D. and Harrison, E.G. (1964) Verrucose "Snuff Dipper's" carcinoma of the oral cavity. JAMA 189, 838.

Sulzberger, M.B. (1933a) Studies in tobacco hypersensitivity - a comparison between reactions to nicotine and to denicotinized tobacco extract. J. Immunol. 24, 87.

Sulzberger, M.B. (1933b) Recent immunological experiments in tobacco hypersensitivity. Bull. New York Acad. Med. 9, 294.

Szego, L. (1965) Sensitisation by agricultural crops and crop-protection preparations. I. Studies of plant (leaf) extracts. Acta Med. Acad. Sci. Hung. 21, 19 (Excerpta Medica XVII 13, 3468).

Szego, L. and Balogh, L. (1965) A form of occupational dermatitis due to the handling of reed matting. Borgyogy Vener Szle 41, 219.

Szego, L. and Szilvassy, I. (1966) Untersuchungen der chemischen Sensibilisierung tabakfermentierender Arbeiter mit Hilfe eines auf dem Transport der Makromolekule beruhenden Testvefahrens. Berufsdermatosen 14, 189.

Szego, L. and Szilvassy, I. (1966) Untersuchungen bei Werktatigen in einem Tabakfermentierungs-Betrieb. Berufsdermatosen 14, 151.

Szego, L. and Szilvassy, I. (1968) The 'hardening effect' in tobacco workers. Berufsdermatosen 16, 43 (Hungarian).

Thiers, H., Chanial, G. et Joseph, J. (1965) Les dermatoses professionnelles dans la region lyonnaise d'apres les statistiques de la Clinique Dermatologique. Rev. Med. (Paris) 6, 525.

Unna, P.J. and Schulz, K.H. (1963) Allergic contact-eczema due to Triacetin (Glycerine triacetate). Hautarzt 14, 423.

Vero, F. and Genovese, S. (1941) Occupational dermatitis in cigar makers due to contact with tobacco leaves. Archs. Derm. Syph. 43, 257.

Weary, P.E. and Woods, B.T. (1969) Allergic contact dermatitis from tobacco smoke residues. JAMA 208, 1905.

White, R.P. (1934) The Dermatergoses or Occupational Affections of the Skin. 4th ed. London. H.K. Lewis.

Wilson, J.B. (1930) Nicotine poisoning by absorption through the skin. Brit. Med. J. 2, 601.

Additional reference

Andre, Ichuk, I.E. (1975) Tobacco dermatitis. Vestn. Dermatol. Venerol. 4, 57.

Petunia

40 species are native to South America and to warm regions of North America.

Petunia spp.

This popular garden plant was found to be a minor sensitizer by Shelmire (1940). Detailed reports are lacking (McCord 1962).

References

McCord, C.P. (1962) The Occupational Toxicity of cultivated flowers. Ind. Med. Surg. 31, 365.

Whelmire, B. (1940) Contact dermatitis from vegetation. South Med. J. 33, 338.

Scopolia

Six species are found from central and southern Europe to India and Japan.

Scopolia carniolica

The rhizome has a mydriatic action (Wren 1968). Dermatitis from scopolamine derived from this plant is noted under Datura.

Reference

Wren, R.W. (1968) Potter's New Cyclopaedia of Botanical Drugs and Preparations by Wren, R.C. Re-edit. by Wren, R.W. Potter and Clarke Ltd. Health Science Press, Rustington, Sussex.

Solandra

Ten species are found from Mexico to tropical America.

Solandra spp.
Chalice vine

The sap is irritant to the eye (Aplin 1976).

Solandra longiflora
Trumpet Flower,
Chalice vine

The sap from pruning the shrubs is said to have caused temporary loss of sight in humans from full dilatation of the pupil suggesting an atropine-like effect (Cleland 1925).

Solandra nitida

The sap has a mydriatic action for gardeners (Morton 1958). Systemic symptoms can occur from proximity to the plant (Morton 1969).

References

Aplin, T.E.H. (1976) Poisonous garden plants and other plants harmful to man in Australia. Western Australian Dept. of Agriculture Bull. 3964.

Cleland, J.B. (1925) Plants including fungi, poisonous or otherwise injurious to man in Australia (Series II) Med. J. Australia 2, 443.

Morton, J.F. (1958) Ornamental plants with poisonous properties. Proc. Florida State Hort. Soc. 71, 372.

Morton, J.F. (1969) Some ornamental plants excreting respiratory irritants. Proc. Florida State Hort. Soc. 82, 415.

Solanum

Some 1700 species are found in tropical and temperate regions. S. melongena is the Egg-Plant.

Solanum spp.
Turkeyberry,
Cachalakaberry

Some can produce mechanical injury (Oakes and Butcher 1962) and the wounds are said to be 'poisoned' and slow to heal (Howes 1946).

References

Howes, F.N. (1946) Fence and barrier plants in warm climates. Kew. Bull. 2, 51.

Oakes, A.J. and Butcher, J.O. (1962) Poisonous and injurious plants of the U.S. Virgin Islands. Misc. Publ. 882. U.S. Department of Agriculture, Washington, D.C.

Solanum aculeastrum

The thorny stems and leaves are capable of producing mechanical injury (Williamson 1956).

Reference

Williamson, J. (1956) Useful Plants of Malasi. ed. Greenway, P.J. Zomba, Malasi. The Government Printer. Previously published as Useful Plants of Nyasaland.

Solanum asperrimum

The seeds have a caustic action (Altschul 1973).

Reference

Altschul, S. von R. (1973) Drugs and foods from little-known plants. Cambridge, Mass. Harvard University Press.

Solanum auriculatum

Vesicular dermatitis occurred in a gardener who handled this plant (Watt and Breyer-Brandwijk 1962).

Reference

Watt, J.M. and Breyer-Brandwijk, M.G. (1962) The Medicinal and poisonous plants of Southern Africa. 2nd ed. Edinburgh. E.& S. Livingstone.

Solanum carolinense
Horsenettle, Bullnettle

Slender prickles are present on the leaves (Gray's Manual 1970). The coloquial names suggest an irritant effect.

Reference

Gray's Manual of Botany (1970) 8th ed. ed. Fernald, M.L. New York. Van Nostrand.

Solanum dulcamara

This plant which has been used to treat cancers and warts from the time of Galen (c. A.D. 180) yields a tumour-inhibitory principle, the steroid alkaloid glycoside beta-solamarine (Kupchan 1970).

Reference

Kupchan, S.M. (1970) Recent Advances in the Chemistry of Terpenoid tumor inhibitors. Pure Applied Chem. 21, 227.

Solanum elaeagnifolium
White Horse Nettle,
Silver-leaved Nightshade

Some forms are prickly. In an investigation of 'weed dermatitis' an extract of this species produced a positive patch test reaction in one of 50 patients tested (Shelmire 1939).

Reference

Shelmire, B. (1939) Contact dermatitis from Weeds; Patch testing with their oleoresins. JAMA 113, 1085.

Solanum laciniatum
Kangaroo Apple

The ripe fruits are eaten. The unripe fruits are irritant to the mouth and throat (Ewart 1930).

Reference

Ewart, A.J. (1930) Flora of Victoria. Melbourne, quoted by Hurst (1942)

Hurst, E. (1942) The Poison Plants of New South Wales. N.S.W. Poison Plants Committee; Sydney.

Solanum incarnum

An 'exanthematous' form of poisoning is recognized in animals who ingest the plant. Vesicular scurfy eczema occurs on the legs, udder and scrotum with conjunctivitis and ulcerative stomatitis (Verdcourt and Trump 1969).

Reference

Verdcourt, B. and Trump, E.C. (1969) Common Poisonous Plants of East Africa. London. Collins.

Solanum lycopersicum
Tomato

This name previously referred to Lycopersicon.

Solanum macroscolum

This species was suspected of producing urticaria in a child who ate the fruits (Watt and Breyer-Brandwijk 1962).

Reference

Watt, J.M. and Breyer-Brandwijk, M.G. (1962) The Medicinal and poisonous plants of Southern Africa. 2nd ed. Edinburgh. E.& S. Livingstone.

Solanum mauritianum

This tree was suspected of causing dermatitis in a woman who handled it (Mair 1968).

Reference

Mair, K. (1968) Director, Royal Botanic Gardens, Sydney, Australia, personal communication from records of the Herbarium.

Solanum rostratum
Kansas Thistle

The prickle-covered burrs can produce mechanical injury (Watt and Breyer-Brandwijk 1962).

Reference

Watt, J.M. and Breyer-Brandwijk, M.G. (1962) The Medicinal and poisonous plants of Southern Africa. 2nd ed. Edinburgh. E.& S. Livingstone.

Solanum sodomaeum
Apple of Sodom

The fruit is irritant to the throat (Hurst 1942).

Reference

Hurst, E. (1942) The Poisonous plants of New South Wales. N.S.W. Poison Plants Committee; Sydney.

Solanum sisymbrifolium

The prickles can cause mechanical injury (Watt and Breyer-Brandwijk 1962).

Reference

Watt, J.M. and Breyer-Brandwijk, M.G. (1962) The Medicinal and poisonous plants of Southern Africa. 2nd ed. Edinburgh. E.& S. Livingstone.

Solanum tuberosum
Potato

Cattle and pigs, if fed large amounts of raw and cooked potato can develop 'potato disease' which includes a vesicular eruption of the lower parts of the limbs and alopecia. Contact with the leaf and stalk, used as litter, can produce a similar disorder (Watt and Breyer-Brandwijk 1962). Shelmire (1940) observed contact dermatitis of the hands of housewives from Irish potatoes. Potatoes are said to cause dermatitis in farmers (Sneid 1955). The plant is said to cause dermatitis but only at certain phases of its blossoming (Schwartz et al 1957). Irritation from handling potatoes can occur; evidence of sensitisation was lacking (Peck and Clare 1945).

Contact urticaria from handling and scraping potatoes occurred in housewives; prick tests with fresh raw potato juice were positive (Pearson 1966). Cronin (1973) reported aggravation of hand eczema in an atopic housewife from peeling raw potato; scratch tests with raw potato were positive; patch tests were negative. Contact urticaria was reviewed by Warin and Champion (1974) and Maibach and Johnson (1975).

Nater and Zartz (1967) reported a case of a woman aged 24 years who had atopic allergic reactions from inhalation of finely dispersed particles of raw potatoes. Besides upper respiratory symptoms, flares of localized atopic dermatitis followed inhalation. Scratch and intradermal tests with raw potato were positive, negative with cooked potato. Separation of potato proteins was carried out by agar gel electrophoresis. Scratch tests were carried out using some of the fractions. Positive reactions were obtained with both anionic and cationic fractions but predominantly with two cationic protein compounds.

References

Cronin, E. (1973) Immediate type hypersensitivity to potato. Contact Dermatitis Newsletter, London 13, 358.

Nater, J.P. and Zartz, J.A. (1967) Atopic allergic reactions due to raw potato. J. Allergy 40, 202.

Pearson, R.S.B. (1966) Potato sensitivity, an occupational allergy in housewives. Acta Allergol. 21, 507.

Peck, S.M. and Clare, H.C. (1945) Dermatitis from dehydration of potatoes. Arch. Derm. Syph. 52, 9.

Schwartz, L., Tulipan, L. and Birmingham, D.J. (1957) Occupational Diseases of the Skin. 3rd ed. Philadelphia. Lea and Febiger. pp. 637-672.

Shelmire, B. (1940) Contact dermatitis from vegetation. South Med. J. 33, 338.

Sneid, P. (1955) Occupational health on the farm. Indust. Med. 24, 117.

Watt, J.M. and Breyer-Brandwijk, M.G. (1962) The medicinal and poisonous plants of Southern Africa. 2nd ed. Edinburgh. E.& S. Livingstone.

Maibach, H.I. and Johnson, H.L. (1975) Contact Urticaria Syndrome. Archs. Derm. 111, 726.

Warin, R.P. and Champion, R.H. (1974) Urticaria. London. W.B. Saunders. p. 161-164.

Solanum xantii

Contact with the plant causes eruptions on delicate skins (Davidson 1899).

References

Davidson, A. (date uncertain, quoted 1899) Therap. Gaz. 22, 86 quoted in Pharm. Journ. 4th series 8, 335. Apr. 15, 1899, quoted by Maiden (1909).

Maiden, J.H. (1909) On some plants which cause inflammation or irritation of the skin. Ag. Gaz. New South Wales 20, 111 and 1073.

SONNERATIACEAE

Seven species in two genera are found from tropical East Africa and Asia to Australia and the western Pacific region.

Chemistry is recorded by Hegnauer (1973).

Reference

Hegnauer, R. (1973) Chemotaxonomy of plants. Vol. 6. Basel. Birkhauser. p. 452.

Sonneratia

Five species, found on coastal areas of tropical East Africa and the Pacific region, are of mangrove habit.

Sonneratia apetala
Kambala

The wood of this tree was listed as irritant (Schwartz et al 1957).

Reference

Schwartz, L., Tulipan, L. and Birmingham, D.J. (1957) Occupational Diseases of the Skin. 3rd ed. Philadelphia. Lea and Febiger. pp. 637-672.

SPIGELIACEAE

90 species in 30 genera are found from Madagascar and tropical Asia to northern Australia and warm regions of North and South America.

Spigelia

50 species are found in warm regions of America.

Spigelia anthelmia

Spigelia glabrata

These species were noted as irritant (Pammel 1911).

Reference

Pammel, L.H. (1911) A Manual of poisonous plants. Torch Press. Cedar Rapids, Iowa. Reprinted Univ. Microfilms Inc. Ann Arbor, Mich. 1965. pp. 467-7.

STACKHOUSIACEAE

27 species in 3 genera are found in Malaysia, Australia and New Zealand.

Chemistry is recorded by Hegnauer (1973).

Reference

Hegnauer, R. (1973) Chemotaxonomy of plants. Vol. 6. Basel. Birkhauser. p. 455.

Stackhousia

25 species are found in Australia and New Zealand, one species extending north-west to Sumatra, the Philippines and Micronesia.

Stackhousia monogyna

Horses can lose their hair and sheep their wool from eating this plant (Hurst 1942).

Reference

Hurst, E. (1942) The Poison Plants of New South Wales. N.S.W. Poison Plants Committee; Sydney.

STERCULIACEAE

700 species in 60 genera are chiefly found in tropical regions. The nuts of Cola spp. (Kola) which are used in flavoured drinks contain caffeine and theobromine (Irvine 1961, Wren 1968).

Chemistry is recorded by Hegnauer (1973).

Reference

Hegnauer, R. (1973) Chemotaxonomy of plants. Vol. 6. Basel. Birkhauser. p. 458.

Abroma is noted under Theobroma.

Brachychiton

Eleven species are found in Australia.

Brachychiton populneum
Kurrajong

Handling of the seeds caused irritation of the fingers and eyes (Hurst 1942).

References

Hurst, E. (1942) The poison plants of New South Wales. N.S.W. Poison Plants Committee; Sydney.

Irvine, F.R. (1961) Woody Plants of Ghana. Oxford University Press. London.

Wren, R.W. (1968) Potter's New Cyclopaedia of Botanical Drugs and Preparations by Wren, R.C. Re-edit. by Wren, R.W. Potter and Clarke Ltd. Health Science Press. Rustington, Sussex.

Byttneria

70 species are found in tropical regions.

Byttneria catalpifolia
spp. africana
(syn. B. africana)

The long spines on the fruits are a hazard for persons who drink the water from the stems (Irvine 1961).

Byttneria aculeata
(syn. Buettneria aculeata)

Cuts and scratches from the thorns on the canes become inflamed and heal slowly (Allen 1943).

References

Allen, P.H. (1943) Poisonous and Injurious Plants of Panama. Am. J. Trop. Med. Suppl. 23, 1.

Irvine, F.R. (1961) Woody plants of Ghana. Oxford University Press. London.

Cardiospermum

Twelve species are found in tropical regions, especially America.

Cardiospermum halicacabum
Balloon-vine

The leaf appears to be irritant. An infusion of the leaf and stalk is used for sores in southern Africa (Webb 1948).

Reference

Webb, L.J. (1948) Guide to the medicinal and poisonous plants of Queensland. Bulletin No. 232. Council for Scientific and Industrial Research. Melbourne, Australia.

Heritiera

35 species are found in West tropical Africa, Indo Malaysia, tropical Australia and the Pacific region.

Heritiera cochinchinensis
(syn. Tarrietia cochinchinensis)
Chumprak

The sawdust irritates the throat and nose (Timber Development Association 1963/64, personal communication to Woods and Calnan 1976).

Heritiera utilis
(syn. Tarrietia utilis)

The wood can produce dermatitis in construction workers (Raymond 1959).

Heritiera simplifolia

The wood is said to be irritant (Orsler 1973).

References

Orsler, R.J. (1973) Personal communication from Forest Products Research Laboratory, Princess Risborough, Bucks, England.

Raymond, V. (1959) Dermatoses professionneles dans le batiment. Rev. Prat. (Paris) 9, 2638.

Woods, B. and Calnan, C.D. (1976) Toxic Woods. Brit. J. Derm. 94, Suppl. 13, June.

Mansonia

Five species have a botanically disjunct distribution being found in West, Central and East Africa and in Assam and Burma.

Mansonia altissima
Bété, African Black Walnut

The wood was introduced from Nigeria into the world market in the thirties and its irritant properties were soon recognized (Bridge 1935). The fine dust from working the wood produced sneezing, sore throat, nosebleeds, headache and dermatitis (Horner and Wigley 1936, Bourne 1956, Salamone et al 1969). Handbook of Hardwoods (1956), Hublet et al (1972), Orsler (1969), Reinl (1965) and Zafiropoulo et al (1968) refer to dermatitis from the wood. Salamone et al (1969) found skin irritation with a follicular eruption in a minority of their patients; patch tests to the wood produced negative reactions. Mucosal irritation affected many more.

Hand-sanding of the wood was responsible for dermatitis in seven workers; the fine dust was responsible; cabinet-makers, sawyers and planers were not affected (Bourne 1956).

In 27 workers in the furniture industry who developed dermatitis, patch tests to aqueous extracts of the wood produced positive reactions in 70% of cases, alcoholic extracts in only 26% (Hanslian and Kadlec 1965). Species of this genus are among the six commoner causes of contact dermatitis from woods in France (Zafiropoulo et al 1968).

Borrie (1956) investigated 283 cases of dermatitis of the eyelids and found contact dermatitis to represent the third largest group (47 cases). Of these two cases were caused by Mansonia wood, one by teak wood (Tectona), two by Chrysanthemum and one by turpentine (Pinaceae).

Woods and Calnan (1976) reported four patients contact sensitive to mansonia wood. One was a female cleaner who only swept up sawdust and had dermatitis of the feet while the three men were a joiner, a cabinet-maker and a sawmill grinder. Positive patch test reactions were observed to mansonia wood dust. Tectona produced a positive patch test reaction in one of the cases, weakly positive (±) in another. Cross-sensitivity to Dalbergia was observed in one case and to Entandrophragma in another.

Chemistry

Mascré and Paris (1939) found in the bark a cardiac glycoside which they called mansonine. Several other glycosides related to strophanthin have since been found in the bark and heartwood (Frerejacque 1951, Sandermann and Dietrichs 1959). Sandermann and Dietrichs isolated a quinone, mansonia-quinone from the heartwood and showed by patch tests that it was the skin-sensitizer in their case. Schulz (1962) obtained positive patch tests with mansonia-quinone in three more patients who gave negative results with the glycosides and other constituents. At least nine quinones have now been isolated, and shown to have a sesquiterpenoid structure (Marini-Bettolo et al 1965, Galeffi et al 1969).

References

Handbook of Hardwoods (1956) Forest Products Research. Ministry of Technology. London. HMSO.

Hublet, P., Sporcq, J., Oleffe, J. et al (1972) Etude sur les accidents cutanes et muqueux provoques par les bois tropicaux dans l'industrie du bois en Belgique. Arch. Belges. Med. Social. 30, 314.

Orsler, R.J. (1969) The effects of irritant timbers. Woodworking Industry 26, 28.

Reinl, W. (1965) Erkrankungen durch tropische Holzer und kasuistischer Beitrag zur Erkrankung durch Mansonia altissima. Zbl. Arbeitsmed. Arbeitsschutz (Darmstad) 15, 101.

Sandermann, W. and Dietrichs, H. (1959) Chemische studien an Tropenholzern-3. Mitteilung: uber die Inhaltsstoffe von Mansonia altissima und ihre Gesundheitsschadigende. Wirkung Holz alz Roh-u. Werkstoff. 17, 88.

Schulz, K.H. (1962) Studies on Sensitizing Effect of Components of Tropical Woods. Berufsdermatosen 10, 17.

Zafiropoulo, A., Audibert, A. and Charpin, J. (1968) A propos des Accidents dus a la manipulation des bois exotiques. Rev. Franc. Allerg. 8, 155.

Borrie, P. (1956) Eczema of the eyelids. Brit. J. Ophthal. 40, 742.

Hanslian, L. and Kadlec, K. (1965) A contribution to the problem of the eczematogenic effect of Mansonia-wood. Pracov. Lek. 17, 392.

Mascré. M. and Paris, R. (1939) Sur l'ecorce de do et ses proprietes digitaliques. Bull. Scienc. Pharmacol. 46, 145.

Frèrejacque, M. (1951) La mansonine, Heteroside digitalique de Mansonia altissima. Comptes rendus de l'Academie des Sciences 233, 1220.

Marini-Bettolo, G.B., Casinovi, C.G. and Galeffi C. (1965) A new class of quinones: sesquiterpene quinones of Mansonia altissima Chev. Tetrahed. Lett. 42, 4857.

Woods, B. and Calnan, C.D. (1976) Toxic Woods. Brit. J. Derm. 94, Suppl. 13, June.

Bourne, L.B. (1956) Dermatitis from Mansonia wood. Brit. J. Industr. Med. 13, 55.

Bridge, J.C. (1935) Reports of the Chief Inspector of Factories and Workshops, London.

Galeffi, C., Delle Monache, E.M., Casinovi, C.G. et al (1969) A new Quinone from the heartwood of Mansonia altissima Chev: Mansonone L. Tetrahedron Letters 40, 3583.

Horner, S. and Wigley, J.E.M. (1936) A case of dermatitis venenata due to Mansonia wood (Sterculiacea altissima). Brit. J. Derm. 48, 26.

Salamone, L., Blasi, S. Di and Coniglio, L. (1969) Rilieve sulla patologia da legno di Mansonia. Folia medica (Napoli) 52, 427.

Mansonia nymphaeifolia
Bete

The wood can produce dermatitis (Bois Tropicaux 1966).

Reference

Bois Tropicaux (1966) 3rd ed. Publ. No. 12. Centre Technique Forestier Tropical. 94-Nogent-sur Marne, France.

Nesogordonia

Seventeen species are found in tropical Africa and Madagascar.

Nesogordonia papaverifera
(syn. Cistanthera papaverifera)
Danta

Woods and Calnan (1976) received a personal communication that some complaints of irritation by wood were received by the Forestry Department of Ibadan, Nigeria.

Reference

Woods, B. and Calnan, C.D. (1976) Toxic Woods. Brit. J. Derm. 94, Suppl. 13, June.

Pterospermum

40 species are found in the eastern Himalayas, southeastern Asia and western Malaysia.

Pterospermum indicum

Hausen (1970) cites Lewin (1928) for an injurious effect from the wood.

According to Woods and Calnan (1976) Pterospermum indicum is an incorrect name given by Lewin (1928) to Amboina wood, which is in fact Pterocarpus indicus. He mentions another Pterospermum sp. used as a fish poison, but it produces no commercial timber.

Pterospermum diversifolium

The wood is listed as injurious by Sandermann and Barghoorn (1956).

References

Hausen, B.M. (1970) Untersuchungen uber Gesundheitsschadigende Holzer. Thesis, Hamburg.

Lewin, L. (1928) Gifte in Holzgewerbe. Beitrage zur Giftkunde Heft 1. Berlin. Georg Stilke Verlag.

Sandermann, W. and Barghoorn, A.W. (1956) Gesundheitsschadigende Nutzholzer. Holz Roh-Werkst 14, 37.

Woods, B. and Calnan, C.D. (1976) Toxic Woods. Brit. J. Derm. 94, Suppl. 13, June.

Pterygota

20 tropical species are recognized chiefly from the Old World.

Pterygota macrocarpus

A sawyer who had dermatitis showed a weak positive patch test reaction to the sawdust of this species and reactions to Spondias and Terminalia (Woods and Calnan 1976). Control tests were not recorded.

Reference

Woods, B. and Calnan, C.D. (1976) Toxic Woods. Brit. J. Derm. 94, Suppl. 13, June.

Sterculia

300 species are found in tropical regions.

Sterculia spp.

The seed pods of several species possess small hairs which

cause intense itching on penetration of the skin (Allen 1943, Watt and Breyer-Brandwijk 1962).

<u>Sterculia caribaea</u>
Mahoe

Toe wood dust is irritant (Anon 1957). MacKenna and Horner (1954), Zafiropoulo et al (1968), Woods and Calnan (1976) could find no case reports to support the inclusion by MacKenna and Horner (1954) of the wood among those woods whose 'chief, if not only effect, is on the skin.'

<u>Sterculia urens</u>

Irritant hairs are present on the stems and fruits (Arnold 1968). The dried exudate of the tree forms Karaya Gum (Indian Tragacanth) which is often used to adulterate Tragacanth from <u>Astragalus</u> (Wren 1968, Smith and Montgomery 1959). Hog or Caramaria gum is an inferior grade mixed with fragments of bark. The resin of <u>Anacardium occidentale</u> is used as a substitute for karaya gum and gum arabic (<u>Acacia</u>) (Figley 1940). Karaya gum can cause atopic symptoms and urticaria (Figley 1940, Bowen 1939, Feinberg and Schoenkermah 1940, Greenberg and Lester 1954). According to Schwartz et al (1957) Karaya Gum in hand cream can cause contact dermatitis.

<u>References</u>

Allen, P.H. (1943) Poisonous and Injurious Plants of Panama. Am. J. Trop. Med. Suppl. <u>23</u>, 1.

Anon (1957) Wood dust and the woodworker. Timber Technology <u>65</u>, 205.

Arnold, H.L. (1968) Poisonous plants of Hawaii. Rutland, Vermont. Charles E. Tuttle.

Bowen, R. (1939) Karaya gum as a cause of urticaria. Archs. Derm. Syph. <u>39</u>, 506.

Figley, K.D. (1940) Karaya gum hypersensitivity. JAMA <u>114</u>, 747.

Greenberg, L.A. and Lester, D. (1954) Handbook of Cosmetic Materials. New York. Interscience.

Schwartz, L., Tulipan, L. and Birmingham, D.J. (1957) Occupational Diseases of the Skin. 3rd ed. Philadelphia. Lea and Febiger. pp. 637-672.

Smith, F. and Montgomery, R. (1959) The Chemistry of plant gums and mucilages. New York. Reinhold Publ. Corp.

Watt, J.M. and Breyer-Brandwijk, M.G. (1962) The Medicinal and poisonous plants of Southern Africa. 2nd ed. Edinburgh. E.& S. Livingstone.

Wren, R.W. (1968) Potter's New Cyclopaedia of Botanical Drugs and Preparations by Wren, R.C. Re-edit by Wren, R.W. Potter and Clarke Ltd. Health Science Press. Rustington, Sussex.

Feinberg, S.M. and Schoenkerman, B.B. (1940) Karaya and related gums as causes of atopy. Wisconsin Med. J. <u>39</u>, 734-736 and 786.

MacKenna, R.M.B. and Horner, S. (1954) Occupational skin diseases in Industrial Medecine and Hygiene. ed. Merewether, E.R.A. London, Butterworth.

Woods, B. and Calnan, C.D. (1976) Toxic Woods. Brit. J. Derm. <u>94</u>, Suppl. 13, June.

Zafiropoulo, A., Audibert, A. and Charpin, J. (1968) A propos des accidents dus a la manipulation des bois exotique. Rev. Franc. Allerg. <u>8</u>, 155.

Theobroma

30 species are found in tropical America. Several provide cacao, cocoa or chocolate. Cocoa butter is formed by pressing the seeds (beans).

Chemistry

Theobromine is present in the beans (Merck Index 1968).

Reference

Merck Index (1968) An Encyclopedia of Chemicals and Drugs. ed. Stecher, P.G. 8th ed. Rahway, N.J. Merck and Co. Inc.

Theobroma augusta (syn. Abroma augusta) Devil's Cotton

The bark yields a fibre. The plant possesses irritant hairs (Burkill 1935, Watt and Breyer-Brandwijk 1962) which affect gardeners and those who prepare indigenous drugs (Behl et al 1966).

Theobroma cacao Chocolate

Early reports of dermatitis in chocolate-makers were reviewed by White (1934). Gardiner (1922) reported six cases. Schwartz et al (1957), Samitz (1950), Queries and Minor Notes (1921), Weber (1937), Key (1961) provide additional reports. Morris (1954) reported a positive patch test reaction to chocolate. Dermatitis in a chocolate factory and subsequent 'hardening' were observed by Goldsmith and Hellier (1954). Greenberg and Lester (1954) reviewed reports of irritation by cocoa butter and considered it innocuous. Cocoa Butter is considered to be a known allergen and is therefore removed from certain brand-name cosmetics (Schieffelin 1973).

References

Behl, P.N., Captain, R.M., Bedi, B.M.S. and Gupta, S. (1966) Skin-irritant and sensitizing plants found in India, New Delhi. P.N. Behl, Irwin Hospital.

Burkill, I.H. (1935) A Dictionary of the Economic Products of the Malay Peninsula. 2 Vols. London. Crown Agents for the Colonies.

Gardiner, F. (1922) Occupational dermatitis. Brit. J. Derm. Syph. 34, 297.

Goldsmith, W.M. and Hellier, F.F. (1954) Recent Advances in Dermatology. 2nd ed. London. Churchill.

Greenberg, L.A. and Lester, D. (1954) Handbook of Cosmetic Materials. New York. Interscience.

Key, M.M. (1961) Some unusual reactions in industry. Archs. Derm. 83, 3.

Morris, G.E. (1954) Dermatoses among food handlers. Industr. Med. Surg. 23, 343.

Queries and Minor Notes (1921) Chocolate Dipper's Dermatitis. JAMA 77, 1199.

Samitz, M.H. (1950) Dermatitis in the making of chocolate candy. Industr. Med. Surg. 19, 35.

Schieffelin and Co. (1973) Almay Hypo-allergenic cosmetics produce formulary. 8th ed. Pharmaceutical Laboratories Division, 562 Fifth Avenue, New York, N.Y. 10036.

Schwartz, L., Tulipan, L. and Birmingham, D.J. (1957) Occupational Diseases of the Skin. 3rd ed. Philadelphia. Lea and Febiger. pp. 637-672.

Watt, J.M. and Breyer-Brandwijk, M.G. (1962) The Medicinal and poisonous plants of Southern Africa. 2nd ed. Edinburgh. E.& S. Livingstone.

Weber, L.F. (1937) External causes of dermatitis. A list of irritants. Archs. Derm. Syph. 35, 129.

White, R.P. (1934) The Dermatergoses or Occupational Affections of the Skin. 4th ed. London. H.K. Lewis.

Triplochiton

Two or three species are found in tropical Africa.

Triplochiton scleroxylon

Colloquial names: Wawa, Samba, Obeche, African Whitewood, Abachi. The wood was formerly sold in Liverpool as Satinwood (Irvine 1961).

Bridge (1937) reported a case of asthma due to the sawdust, skin tests being positive to this wood and negative to other woods. Oehling (1963) described 3 cases of asthma from the wood, one also sensitive to Terminalia. Contact urticaria could be produced by rubbing obeche wood on the skin. Orsler (1973) received trade reports of asthma and general symptoms from the wood-dust. Woods and Calnan (1976) received a personal communication of dermatitis from a lavatory seat made of the wood, with a positive patch test reaction. Hausen (1970) found no alkaloids or quinones in the wood. Hublet et al (1972) reported unspecified muco-cutaneous effects from the wood in Belgium. The wood seems to be less noxious than Mansonia (Zafiropoulo et al 1968).

References

Hublet, P., Sporcq, J., Oleoffe, J. et al (1972) Etude sur les accidentes cutanes et muquex provoques par les bois tropicaux dans l'industrie du bois en Belgique. Arch. Belges. Med. Social. 30, 314.

Irvine, F.R. (1961) Woody plants of Ghana. Oxford University Press. London.

Orsler, R.J. (1972) Personal communication from Forest Products Research Laboratory, Princess Risborough, Bucks England.

Zafiropoulo, A., Audibert, A. and Charpin, J. (1968) A propos des accidents dus a la manipulation des bois exotiques. Rev. Franc. Allerg. 8, 155.

Bridge, J.C. (1937) Reports of the Chief Inspector of Factories and Workshops. London.

Hausen, B.M. (1970) Untersuchungen uber Gesundheitsschadigende Holzer. Thesis, Hamburg.

Oehling, A. (1963) Berufsallergie um Holzgewerbe. Allergic u. Asthma 9, 312.

Woods, B. and Calnan, C.D. (1976) Toxic Woods. Brit. J. Derm. 94, Suppl. 13, June.

STILAGINACEAE

170 species in one genus are found in tropical and subtropical regions of Africa and Asia.

Antidesma
(syn. Stilago)

The genus was formerly included in Euphorbiaceae.

Antidesma bunius
Bignay

Contact with the sap can cause acute dermatitis (Souder 1963).

Reference

Souder, P. (1963) Poisonous plants on Guam. In Venomous and Poisonous Animals and Noxious Plants of the Pacific Region. Ed. Keegan, H.L. and Macfarlane, W.V. Oxford. Pergamon Press. pp. 15-29.

STRELITZIACEAE

Seven species in three genera are found in tropical South America, South Africa and Madagascar.

Strelitzia

Five species are native to South Africa.

Strelitzia reginae
Bird of Paradise

No clinical reports of dermatitis from this popular greenhouse plant have been found although McCord (1962) noted a commercial extract of the plant used for patch-testing. The seed hastens the souring of milk (Watt and Breyer-Brandwijk 1962).

References

McCord, C.P. (1962) The Occupational Toxicity of Cultivated Flowers. Ind. Med. Surg. 31, 365.

Watt, J.M. and Breyer-Brandwijk, M.G. (1962) The Medicinal and poisonous plants of Southern Africa. 2nd ed. Edinburgh. E.& S. Livingstone.

STRYCHNACEAE

250 species in four genera are found in tropical and subtropical regions.

Strychnos

200 species are found in tropical regions. Some have thorns. The related Fagraea yields an irritant alkaloid.

Strychnos nux-vomica

The plant is native to India and Ceylon. The fruit is a berry; the flesh is harmless but the seeds are exceedingly poisonous, owing to the presence of strychnine in the seed coats (Shaw 1973).

Dermatitis in a pharmaceutical worker was attributed to dust from the beans; a patch test to the flesh of the bean was negative (Gardiner 1922).

Strychnos potatorum
Clearing nut

The seeds are used to purify the water for drinking. They are rubbed on the inside of the vessel, and cause precipitation (Shaw 1973).

Strychnos toxifera

This South American species yields wourali or curare poison used for poisoning arrows; it is obtained from the bark by scraping and maceration in water (Shaw 1973).

References

Gardiner, F. (1922) Occupational dermatitis. Brit. J. Derm. Syph. 34, 297.

Shaw, H.K.A. (1973) A Dictionary of the Flowering Plants and Ferns. (the late J.C. Willis) 8th ed. Cambridge University Press.

STYRACACEAE

180 species in 12 genera are recognized in 3 centres of distribution: eastern Asia to western Malaysia; south-eastern United States; Mexico to tropical South America.

Chemistry is recorded by Hegnauer (1973).

Reference

Hegnauer, R. (1973) Chemotaxonomy of plants. Vol. 6. Basel. Birkhauser. p. 473.

Styrax

130 species are found in warm regions of Eurasia, Malaysia and America. S. benzoin yields the fragrant resin gum-benzoin which is used medicinally and for incense.

Styrax tonkinensis and other *Styrax* species yield Siam Benzoin. Benzoin - not gum benzoin - is the name for an unrelated material, bitter almond oil camphor (Merck Index 1968). Compound Tincture of Benzoin (Friar's Balsam, Balsam Traumatic) is composed of gum benzoin, storax (*Liquidambar*), Balsams of Tolu and Peru (*Myroxylon*), aloe (*Aloe*), myrrh (*Commiphora*) and angelica (*Angelica*).

Styrax officinale, a Mediterranean species, provided a storax used in Ancient Egypt. Storax (styrax) of more recent time is provided by *Liquidambar*.

Allergic contact dermatitis from Compound Tincture of Benzoin has been reported following local application in the treatment of fissured nipples (Eades 1934), following its use as a supportative dressing in rhinoplasty (Luria 1967), under plaster cases (Spott and Shelley 1970, Cullen et al 1974), under adhesive tape (Steiner and Leifer 1949), following its use as an antiseptic (James 1930) and in a hair preparation (Garnier 1950).

Cross-sensitivity has been observed to aloe (*Aloe*), Storax (*Liquidambar*), Balsam of Peru (*Myroxylon*), benzoic acid and cinnamic acid (James 1930, Steiner and Leifer 1949, Hjorth 1961, Mitchell and Dupuis 1972). Rockl and Bandmann (1957) reported that 4% of 230 patients who had eczema showed positive patch test reactions to benzoin. Two of ten patients who had skin disease were actively sensitized by patch testing with Compound Tincture of Benzoin (Steiner and Leifer 1949).

Friar's Balsam used for inhalations is derived from Sumatra benzoin (*Styrax benzoin* and *S. paralleoneurus* and other species) (Howes 1974).

References

Cullen, S.I., Tonkin, A. and May, F.E. (1974) Allergic contact dermatitis to Compound Tincture of Benzoin spray. J. Trauma. 14, 348.

Garnier, G. (1955) Dermatitis bullosa due to wave set containing tincture of benzoin. Bull. Soc. franc. derm. syph. 57, 397.

Hjorth, N. (1961) Eczematous allergy to balsams. Munksgaard. International Booksellers and Publishers Ltd. Copenhagen.

Howes, F.N. (1974) A dictionary of useful and everyday plants and their common names. Cambridge University Press. pp. 290.

James, B.M. (1930) Dermatitis produced by Compound Tincture of Benzoin. J. Med. Soc. New Jersey 27, 259.

Merck Index (1968) An Encyclopedia of Chemicals and Drugs. ed. Stecher, P.G. 8th ed. Rahway, N.J. Merck and Co. Inc.

Mitchell, J.C. and Dupuis, G. (1972) Allergic contact dermatitis from storax (Styrax). Contact Dermatitis Newsletter, London 11, 274.

Rockl, H. and Bandmann, H.J. (1957) Benzoin, a relatively frequent contact allergen. Hautarzt 8, 416.

Spott, D.A. and Shelley, W.B. (1970) Exanthem due to contact allergen (benzoin) absorbed through the skin. JAMA 214, 1881.

Steiner, K. and Leifer, W. (1949) Investigation of contact-type dermatitis due to Compound Tincture of Benzoin. J. Invest. Derm. 13, 351.

TAXACEAE

20 species in five genera are found in the northern hemisphere south to Celebes and Mexico, one species in New Caledonia.

Taxus

10 species are found in north temperate regions south to the Himalayas, Phillipines, Celebes and Mexico.

Taxus sp.

Grossmann (1920) had experienced mild headache and discomfort while working with yew, as had other workers with him. The wood was said to irritate the respiratory passages and the skin (Moll 1950).

Most parts of the tree contain poisonous alkaloids, taxines and also an irritant volatile oil (Forsyth 1968). Wine from hip-flasks made of yew wood was said by Pliny to poison travellers (Woods and Calnan 1976).

Taxus Baccata
Common Yew, English Yew

Senear (1933) reported dermatitis in a man who scraped his archery bow made of yew wood imported from England. Attacks followed several exposures to the dust of the wood, which produced a positive patch test reaction. Tests in controls were not recorded. The patient applied the patch test on his own initiative and therefore deserves a place in the history of Patch Testing. Irritant effects of yew wood have been ascribed to oil of yew and formic acid (Long 1938). Hausen (1970) cites Powetz (1949) for an injurious effect of the wood.

Miliary eruptions were reported from sleeping under the tree (Piffard 1881).

Taxus cuspidata
Japanese Yew

The wood is said to be irritant (Schwartz et al 1957).

References

Schwartz, L., Tulipan, L., Birmingham, D.J. (1957) Occupational Diseases of the skin. 3rd ed. Philadelphia. Lea and Febiger.

Senear, F.E. (1933) Dermatitis due to woods. JAMA 101, 1527.

Hausen, B.M. (1970) Untersuchungen uber Gesundheitsschadigende Holzer. Thesis, Hamburg.

Long, H.C. (1938) Poisonous plants on the farm. Bull. Ministry Agriculture London 75.

Powetz, J. (1949) Vergiftungen durch die Eibe. Allg. Forst-holzwirtsch. Z. 60, 59.

Forsyth, A.A. (1968) British Poisonous Plants. 2nd ed. Bull. 161. Ministry of Agriculture, Fisheries and Food. London. HMSO.

Grossmann, J. (1920) Gesundheitsschadliche Holzarten Der Holzkaufer (Leipzig) 17, 529, 535, 540 and 545.

Moll, F. (1950) Giftiges Holz und Gewerbekrankheiten. Holz (Munchen) 4, 76.

Woods, B. and Calnan, C.D. (1976) Toxic Woods. Brit. J. Derm. 94, Suppl. 13, June.

Piffard, H.G. (1881) A treatise on the Materia Medica and Therapeutics of the skin. New York. Wm. Wood and Co.

TAXODIACEAE

16 species in 10 genera are found in eastern Asia, Tasmania and North America.

Sequoia

This genus is found in California.

Sequoiadendron

Is represented by one species in California.

Sequoia sempervirens
California Red Wood, Sequoia

Oliver (1902) described coryzal symptoms in men sawing and chipping sequoia wood. They complained of running at the nose, sneezing, coughing, laboured breathing, oppression at the pit of the stomach and smarting in the eyes and were noted to have tachycardia. The symptoms were worst on the first exposure and lasted about 24 hours but tolerance later developed except in asthma subjects. Cabinet-makers developed similar symptoms (MacPherson 1925). Cohen et al (1967) described a case of pneumonitis (sequoiosis) with circulating antibodies to redwood sawdust (or possibly to an associated fungus) in a sawmill worker.

Inhalation of fungi of red wood sawdust can produce sequoiosis, a form of allergic alveolitis (Morgan and Seaton 1975).

References

Cohen, H.I., Merigan, T.C., Kosek, J.C. et al (1967) Sequoiosis: a granulomatous pneumonitis associated with redwood sawdust inhalation. Am. J. Med. 43, 785.

MacPherson, J. (1925) Dermatitis caused by Queensland Maple. Med. J. Australia. 2, 542.

Oliver, T. (1902) Dangerous Trades. Chap. 59. London. J. Murray.

Morgan. W.K.C. and Seaton, A. (1975) Occupational Lung Diseases. Philadelphia, Saunders.

THEACEAE

500 species in sixteen genera are found in tropical and subtropical regions. Chemistry is recorded by Hegnauer (1973).

Camellia (syn. Thea)

82 species are found in Indo Malaysia, China and Japan.

Camellia sinensis
Tea Plant

Young shoots consisting of buds and two or more leaves are picked and dried to form tea. For scenting Chinese teas, the petals of Chloranthus and Jasminum are used; the leaves of Salix (Willow) and Populus (white Poplar) are sometimes used to adulterate tea (Smith 1969). Dermatitis in a "tea-boy" whose occupation was the carrying of tea to workers on a construction site was found to be due to alkali dust from the work site (O'Donovan 1927).

'Water-itch', a vesicular eruption affecting the feet of coolies in the tea gardens of Assam during the wet season, is caused by a mite Rhizoglyphus (White 1934). Simons (1952) refers to the bites R. parasiticus as the cause of "tea dermatosis". Caterpillars (Limacodidae) on the tea-plants can cause contact dermatitis (Van Thiel 1953). Workers in tea-plantations suffer wounds on the legs from cut branches of the tea-shrubs, hyperkeratosis of the skin of the index finger from the chemical effect of tea-juice and dew, and vesicular dermatitis of the feet attributed to nitrogenous fertilizers in the soil (Sturua 1957). Processed tea contains small amounts of essential oil which constitutes the odour. The constituents of the oil include geraniol, linalool, benzyl alcohol, phenylethyl alcohol and methylsalicylate (Kariyone 1971). Reactions to salicylate are noted under Betula. Theophylline is present in small amounts in tea. Aminophylline which consists of theophylline and ethylenediamine can cause reactions in ethylenediamine sensitive individuals (Baer et al 1959, Epstein and Maibach 1968).

References

Baer, R.L., Cohen, J.H., Neideroff, A.H. (1959) Allergic eczematous sensitivity to aminophylline. Arch. Derm. 79, 647.

Epstein, E. and Maibach, H.I. (1968) Ethylenediamine allergic contact dermatitis. Arch. Derm. 98, 476.

Hegnauer, R. (1973) Chemotaxonomy of Plants. Vol. 6. Basel, Birkhauser Verlag, p. 487.

Kariyone, T. (1971) Atlas of Medicinal Plants. Osaka, Japan. Takeda Chemical Industries.

O'Donovan, W.J. (1927) Exogenic dermatitis. Lancet 1, 1128.

Simons, R.D.G. (1952) Handbook of Tropical Dermatology. New York. Elsevier.

Smith, F.P. (1969) Chinese Materia Medica. Vegetable kingdom. 2nd ed. Rev. by Hei, P.D., Taepei, Taiwan. Ku T'ing Book House.

Sturua, G.A. (1957) Occupational skin diseases among tea pickers. Batumi 48pp (Russian) abstr. Excerpta Medica.

Van Thiel, P.H. (1953) Arthropods and other animals in relation to Dermatology in Handbook of Tropical Dermatology and Medical Mycology ed. Simons, R.D.G. Amsterdam. Elsevier Publ. Co. Vol. II, p. 908.

White, R.P. (1934) The Dermatergoses of Occupational Affections of the Skin. 4th ed. London. H.K. Lewis.

Schima

15 species are found from the eastern Himalayas to Formosa and western Malaysia.

Schima noronhae

The sap of this large evergreen tree is said to be irritating to the skin (Corner 1952).

Schima wallichii

This tree, which provides good timber, is known to produce dermatitis in Malaya (Kochummen 1972). Mechanical injury occurs from glistening white needles on the bark (Behl et al 1966).

References

Behl, P.N., Captain, R.M., Bedi, B.M.S. and Gupta, S. (1966) Skin-irritant and sensitizing plants found in India, New Delhi. P.N. Behl, Irwin Hospital.

Corner, E.J.H. (1952) Wayside Trees of Malaysia. Singapore, Government Printer.

Kochummen, K.M. (1972) Forest Botanist. Forest Research Institute. Kepong, Selangor, Malaya. Personal communication.

THYMELAEACEAE

500 species in 50 genera are found in temperate and tropical regions especially in Africa. Aquilaria (Aloe-Wood) provides a perfume material. Many members of the family have a vesicatory effect on the skin and cause excessive pain in the mouth when chewed (Anon 1891). Many species contain a strong poison which blisters the skin (Ewart 1930).

Chemistry is recorded by Hegnauer (1973). The irritant principles of some species are chemically related to those of Croton.

Reference

Hegnauer, R. (1973) Chemotaxonomy of plants. Vol. 6. Basel. Birkhauser Verlag, p. 508.

Arthrosolen

15 species are found in tropical and Southern Africa.

Arthrosolen polycephalus

The root is exceedingly bitter. The dust produced irritation of the respiratory tract, nausea and headache in technicians who examined the wood (Watt and Breyer-Brandwijk 1972).

References

Anon (1891) cited by Hurst (1942).

Ewart, A.J. (1930) Flora of Victoria. Melbourne quoted by Hurst (1942).

Hurst, E. (1942) The Poison Plants of New South Wales. N.S.W. Poison Plants Committee, Sydney.

Watt, J.M. and Breyer-Brandwijk, M.G. (1962) The Medicinal and Poisonous Plants of Southern Africa. 2nd ed. Edinburgh. E. and S. Livingstone.

Daphne

70 species are found in Europe, North Africa, temperate and sub-tropical regions of Asia, Australia and the Pacific region. The bark is used for paper in India.

Daphne cannabina

Systemic symptoms can occur from proximity to the plant (Morton 1969).

Daphne genkwa

The buds are used in Chinese Medicine. Old buds which have been stored for several years are used because fresh buds are irritating.

Crushed root-bark is applied to boils to produce vesication (Kariyone 1971).

Daphne gnidium

The bark is irritant (De Candolle 1904)

Dermatitis from this species was reported by Gouin (1921).

Daphne laureola
Spurge Laurel, Wood Laurel

The berries contain an acrid resin and the properties are similar to those of D. mezereum (White 1887).

Daphne mezereum
Dwarf Laurel, Spurge Olive, Wild Pepper

All parts of the plant produce irritation on contact (Oesterlen 1856). The bark, when applied to the skin, produces erythema, vesiculation and ulceration (Dispensatory 1884). Mezereum bark was formerly official. The berries if eaten produce burning in the mouth and swelling of the tongue and lips (North 1967).

References

Dispensatory, The National (1884) Philadelphia. Stille and Maisch. Cited by White (1887).

Gouin, (1921) Dermites par l'écorce de garou (Daphne Gnidium). Arch. Méd. et mil. 1, 71.

Kariyone, T. (1971) Atlas of Medicinal Plants. Osaka, Japan. Takeda Chemical Industries.

North, P.M. (1967) Poisonous Plants and Fungi in Colour. London. Blandford Press Ltd.

Oesterlen (1856) Handbuch der Heilmittellehre. Tubingen cited by White (1887).

White, J.C. (1887) Dermatitis venenata: An account of the Action of External irritants upon the Skin. Boston. Cupples and Hurd.

DeCandolle, A.P. (1804) Esşai sur les proprietes medicales des plantes, etc. Paris cited by Piffard (1881).

Piffard, H.G. (1881) A treatise on the Materia Medica and Therapeutics of the skin. New York. Wm. Wood & Co.

Morton, J.F. (1969) Some ornamental plants excreting respiratory irritants. Proc. Florida State Hort. Soc. 82, 415.

Daphnopsis

46 species are found from Mexico and the West Indies to eastern Argentina.

Daphnopsis gnidium

Daphnopsis oleoidies

These species are irritant (Pammel 1911).

Reference

Pammel, L.H. (1911) A Manual of Poisonous Plants. Torch Press. Cedar Rapids, Iowa. Reprinted Univ. Microfilms Inc. Ann Arbor, Mich. 1965.

Dirca

Two species are found in North America.

Dirca palustris
Leatherwood, Moosewood

Application of the fresh bark to the skin causes redness, vesication and sores which are very difficult to heal (Dispensatory 1884).

Reference

Dispensatory, The National (1884) Philadelphia. Stille and Maisch, cited by White (1887).

White, J.C. (1887) Dermatitis venenata: An account of the Action of External irritants upon the Skin. Boston. Cupples and Hurd.

Gnidia

100 species are found in tropical and southern Africa, Madagascar, south-western Arabia and

the west coast of India and Ceylon.

Gnidia spp.

The plants contain an irritating resinous principle, mezereine, which has a vesicant action (Watt and Breyer-Brandwijk 1962).

Gnidia vatkeana

The root was used as a vesicant in India (Watt and Breyer-Brandwijk 1962).

Reference

Watt, J.M. and Breyer-Brandwijk, M.G. (1962) The Medicinal and Poisonous Plants of Southern Africa. 2nd ed. Edinburgh. E. and S. Livingstone.

Gonystylus

30 species are found in Malaysia, the Solomon Islands and Fiji.

Gonystylus affinis

The wood is known to produce dermatitis in Malaya (Kichummen 1972).

Gonystylus spp.
principally G. bancanus
Ramin, Malawis

The fibrous portion of the inner bark (bast) causes skin and eye irritation in wood-workers (Burgess 1966). Workers handling logs can develop skin irritation which is thought to be due to sharp pointed fibres of the inner bark which remain on the logs after the logs have been peeled (Handbook of Hardwoods 1959).

The sawdust produced dermatitis and a patch test gave a positive reaction (Wilkinson 1973, cited by Woods and Calnan 1976).

Oehling (1963) reported a case of 'sensitivity' to the wood without clinical details. Ramin was said to be one of the more toxic woods (Salamone et al 1969) but they gave no details. Hausen (1970) quoted trade reports of asthma and skin irritation from the sawdust and bark.

A carpenter who had dermatitis showed positive patch test reactions to the wood dust of ramin, Araucaria and Tectona and to epoxy resin (Woods and Calnan 1976).

The inner bark must be completely removed from logs before sawing because it contains sharp-pointed fibers that may cause skin irritation. Goggles are recommended for sawyers. The logs, green lumber, and lumber not completely air dried often exhibit a stong, unpleasant odor. This disappears as the wood is thoroughly dried but may appear again if the wood is rewet (McMillen 1967).

Reference

McMillen, J.M. (1967) Seasoning and handling of ramin. U.S. Forest Research Note FPL-0172. U.S. Department of Agriculture Forest Products Laboratory. Madison, Wis.

Handbook of Hardwoods (1956) Forest Products Research. Ministry of Technology. London. HMSO.

Hausen, B.M. (1970) Untersuchungen uber Gesundheitsschadigende Holzer. Thesis, Hamburg.

Oehling, A. (1963) Berufsallergie im Holzgewerbe. Allergie und Asthma 9, 312.

Salamone, L., Blasi, S. Di and Coniglio, L. (1969) Rilievi sulla patologia da legno di Monsonia. Folia medica (Napoli) 52, 427.

Woods, B. and Calnan, C.D. (1976) Toxic Woods. Brit. J. Derm. 94, Suppl. 13, June.

Burgess, P.F. (1966) Timbers of Sabah (Sabah Forest Records No. 6). Sabah, Malaysia.

Kochummen, K.M. (1972) Forest Botanist. Forest Research Institute. Kepong, Selangor, Malaya. Personal communication.

Lasiosiphon

50 species are found from tropical and southern Africa and Madagascar to western peninsular India and Ceylon.

Lasiosiphon anthylloides

Lasiosiphon burchella

The roots of these species produced irritation of the respiratory tract in laboratory workers (Watt and Breyer-Brandwijk 1962).

Lasiosiphon capitatus

The root, at first tasteless, ultimately becomes very hot when chewed (Watt and Breyer-Brandwijk 1962).

Lasiosiphon eriocephalus
Wooly-Headed Gnidia

The leaves of this species are used as a rubefacient (Behl et al 1966). The bark and leaves are irritant often producing vesication. The dust of the dried bark irritates the eyes, nostrils and faces of persons who handle it (Chopra et al 1958).

Lasiosiphon kraussianus

A tiny pinch of the plant, when brought into contact with the tongue, produces an intense sensation of burning with irritation of the throat lasting several hours (Watt and Breyer-Brandwijk 1962).

Lasiosiphon meisnerianus

The root and root-bark are irritant to the mouth (Watt and Breyer-Brandwijk 1962).

References

Behl, P.N., Captain, R.M., Bedi, B.M.S. and Gupta, S. (1966) Skin-irritant and sensitizing plants found in India, New Delhi. P.N. Behl, Irwin Hospital.

Chopra, R.N., Chopra, I.C., Handa, K.L. and Kapur, L.D. (1958) Chopra's Indigenous Drugs of India, Ed. 2, Calcutta, U.N. Dhur and Sons Ltd.

Watt, J.M. and Breyer-Brandwijk, M.G. (1962) The Medicinal and Poisonous Plants of Southern Africa. 2nd ed. Edinburgh. E. and S. Livingstone.

Pimelea

80 species are found in South Pacific islands and Australasia.

Pimelea sp.

A species of this genus, when tasted, gave rise to a burning sensation in the mouth (Cleland 1931).

Pimelia laevigata and
Pimelia spp.
Strathmore weed

The bark when chewed produces after a few minutes an intense burning sensation in the mouth. All parts of the plants are acrid and poisonous, especially the bark and berries (Aston 1923).

References

Aston, B.C. (1923) The poisonous, suspected and medicinal plants of New Zealand. New Zealand J. Agricult. 26, 78 and 149.

Cleland, J.B. (1931) Plants including fungi, poisonous or otherwise injurious to man in Australia. II. Med. J. Austr. 2, 775.

Thymelaea

20 species are found in the Mediterranean region and temperate Asia.

Thymelaea tartonraira

This species is irritant (Pammel 1911).

Reference

Pammel, L.H. (1911) A Manual of Poisonous Plants. Torch Press. Cedar Rapids, Iowa. Reprinted Univ. Microfilms Inc. Ann Arbor, Mich. 1965.

Wikstroemia

70 species are found in southern China, Indo China, Australia and the Pacific region.

Wikstroemia spp.

Arnold (1968) noted that the sap and bark were said to be irritant and caustic by other authors. He did not find this to be so on his own skin.

Reference

Arnold, H.L. (1968) Poisonous Plants of Hawaii. Rutland, Vermont. Charles E. Tuttle.

TILIACEAE

450 species in 50 genera are found in tropical and temperate regions especially in south-eastern Asia and Brazil.

Sloanea was formerly included in this family.

Chemistry is recorded by Hegnauer (1973).

Berrya

Six species are found in Indo Malaysia and Polynesia.

Berrya cordifolia
(Syn. B. ammonilla)
Trincomali wood

This timber tree is said to have irritating qualities (Zschokke cited by Arnold 1968).

References

Arnold, H.L. (1968) Poisonous Plants of Hawaii. Rutland, Vermont. Charles E. Tuttle.

Hegnauer, R. (1973) Chemotaxonomy of plants. Vol. 6. Basel. Birkhauser. p. 518.

Corchorus

100 species are found in warm regions.

Corchorus capsularis
Jute

Corchorus olitorius

These species furnish the chief supply of the fibre jute or gunny. The stems are cut and retted in water and the fibre is beaten out. Oils are used for softening the fibre. Burlap is a coarsely-woven textile made from jute fibre.

Mineral oil used in the processing can produce folliculitis and oil-acne. In contrast to jute, flax (Linum) requires no added oil in its manufacture and oil-acne is less commonly observed in flax-workers. Fish oil used for softening jute fibre can liberate irritating fatty acids as it decomposes. Potassium hydroxide, used as an additive, can produce irritation (White 1887, Curjel and Acton 1924, Stevens and Jordani 1938, Schwartz et al 1957, Simons 1952). Eczema with ulceration of the skin of the legs from standing in water and respiratory symptoms can occur in jute-workers (Bhar 1952). Burlap can also produce respiratory symptoms (Stevens and Jordani 1938). Kinner et al (1955) found no evidence of sensitisation to jute; skin cancer can result from exposure to oil used to treat the jute.

References

Bhar, B. (1952) Hazards in jute industry in India with special reference to jute dermatitis. Proc. Soc. Industr. Med. (Jemeshedpur) 4, 106.

Curjel, D.F. and Acton, H.W. (1924) Jute Dermatitis. Indian J. Med. Res. 12, 257.

Kinnear, J., Rogers, J., Finn, O.A. and Mair, A. (1955) Dermatoses in jute-workers. Brit. J. Industr. Med. 12, 36.

Schwartz, L., Tulipan, L. Birmingham, D.J. (1957) Occupational Diseases of the skin. 3rd ed. Philadelphia. Lea and Febiger.

Simons, R.D.G. (1952) Handbook of Tropical Dermatology. New York. Elsevier.

Stevens. F.A. and Jordani, L. (1938) Sensitisation to Jute. J. Allergy 9, 610.

White, J.C. (1887) Dermatitis venenata: An account of the Action of External irritants upon the Skin. Boston. Cupples and Hurd.

Sparmannia

Seven species are found in tropical and southern Africa and in Madagascar.

Sparmannia africana
Indoor Linden, African Hemp

The hairs of the leaf have an irritant effect on the skin. Patch tests to the leaf produced positive reactions in 90% of 511 patients but extracts of the leaf produced negative reactions (Schulze 1940). He concluded that contact sensitivity was not involved but Kuske and Bandi (1958) observed that a small number of persons tested showed eczematous reactions to the leaves.

References

Kuske, H. and Bandi, B. (1958) Dermatitis and eczema caused by an indoor linden. Dermatologica (Basel) 116, 308.

Schulze, W. (1940) Investigation of the irritative action of the leaves of African hemp. Arch. f. Dermat. u. Syph. 181, 63.

Tilia

50 species are found in north temperate regions, south to Indo China and Mexico.

Tilia spp.
Lime, Linden

The upper surfaces of the leaves are usually covered with honey-dew. Effects of Aphis which produce honey-dew are noted under Acer.

The pollen of some species has been suspected of causing hay-fever (Wodehouse 1971).

Tilia americana
Bass-Wood

This species is said to produce dermatitis (Schwartz et al 1957).

It is possible that this statement results from an incorrect listing of Bassia (see Madhuca) as a cause of dermatitis.

References

Schwartz, L., Tulipan, L., Birmingham, D.J. (1957) Occupational Diseases of the skin. 3rd ed. Philadelphia. Lea and Febiger.

Wodehouse, R.P. (1971) Hayfever Plants. 2nd rev. edition. New York, Hafner.

Triumfetta

150 species are found in tropical regions. The fruits possess hooked spines.

Triumfetta spp.

The burrs cling to the wool of sheep (Watt and Breyer-Brandwijk 1962).

Triumfetta rhomboidea

The seeds stick on touch to clothes and animal skin.

Triumfetta semitriloba
Mahoe

This species can produce mechanical injury (Oakes and Butcher 1962).

References

Oakes, A.J. and Butcher, J.O. (1962) Poisonous and injurious plants of the U.S. Virgin Islands. Misc. Publ. 882. U.S. Dept. of Agriculture, Washington, D.C.

Watt, J.M. and Breyer-Brandwijk, M.G. (1962) The Medicinal and Poisonous Plants of Southern Africa. 2nd ed. Edinburgh. E. and S. Livingstone.

TRILLIACEAE

53 species in four genera are found in temperate Eurasia and North America

Paris

20 species are found in north palaeotemperate regions.

Paris quadrifolia

This species is irritant (Pammel 1911).

Reference

Pammel, L.H. (1911) A Manual of Poisonous Plants. Torch Press. Cedar Rapids, Iowa. Reprinted Univ. Microfilms Inc. Ann Arbor, Mich. 1965.

TROPAEOLACEAE

92 species in two genera are found from Mexico to temperate South America.

Chemistry is recorded by Hegnauer (1973).

All parts of the plant contain 'mustard oil' as in Cruciferae (Shaw 1973).

Reference

Hegnauer, R. (1973) Chemotaxonomy of Plants. Vol. 6. Basel. Birkhauser Verlag, p. 538.

Tropaeolum
Nasturtium

90 species are found from Mexico to temperate South America. About 14 species are known in horticulture. The pickled seeds are used as a condiment having a mustard-like taste. The common name is from the Latin nasi tortium (distortion of the nose) referring to the pungent quality of the plant.

Tropaeolum majus
Garden Nasturtium

White (1887) reported two female patients in whom the plant repeatedly produced dermatitis. In the first case both hands were affected. In the second case, the right hand in which she carried the plants was affected and the left hand which had been gloved was unaffected. The plant has rubefacient properties (Burkill 1935). The plant contains a thioglucoside, glucotropaeolin (Kjaer 1963). Contact sensitivity to mustard oil is noted under Raphanus.

References

Burkill, I.H. (1935) A Dictionary of the Economic Products of the Malay Peninsula. 2 Vols. London. Crown Agents for the Colonies.

Kjaer, A. (1963) The distribution of sulphur compounds in Chemical Plant Taxonomy. ed. Swain, T. London. Academic Press. p. 453.

Shaw, H.K.A. (1973) A Dictionary of the Flowering Plants and ferns. (the late J.C. Willis) 8th ed. Cambridge University Press.

TYPHACEAE

Ten species in one genus are found in temperate and tropical regions.

Typha

The distribution of the genus is that of the family. The plants are found in ponds and still water.

Typha spp.
Cattail, Cattail Flag

The pollen of some species occasionally causes hayfever (Wodehouse 1971).

Typha latifolia
False Bulrush

A widespread papular eruption occurred in workers who contacted the plant. The bites of Chilacis typhae were incriminated on circumstantial evidence (Laszlo and Balogh 1965).

Typha orientalis

The pollen is used for an astringent and styptic effect. It is inflammable like Lycopodium powder (Smith 1969).

Reference

Laszlo, and Balogh, (1965) Gyekeny Felhasznalase Kapcsan Keletkezett foglalkozasi dermatitis. Borgzogy. Vener. Szem. (Hung.) 41 219.

Smith, F.P. (1969) Chinese Materia Medica. Vegetable kingdom. 2nd ed. Rev. by Hei, P.D. Taipei, Taiwan. Ku T'ing Book House.

Wodehouse, R.P. (1971) Hayfever Plants. 2nd rev. edition. New York, Hafner.

ULMACEAE

200 species in 15 genera are found in tropical and temperate regions.

Chemistry is recorded by Hegnauer (1973).

Aphananthe

One species is found in Madagascar, one species from India and Ceylon to Japan, Indo China, the Phillipines, Celebes, Java and eastern Australia, one species in Mexico.

Aphananthe aspera

The hard, rough leaves are used as 'sandpaper' to polish wood (Uphof 1959).

References

Hegnauer, R. (1973) Chemotaxonomy of Plants Vol. 6. Basel. Birkhauser Verlag, p. 545.

Uphof, J.C. (1959) Dictionary of Economic Plants. New York. Hafner Publ. Co.

Celtis
Hackberry, Nettle tree

80 species are found in the northern hemisphere and southern Africa. About 17 species are known in horticulture.

The pollen of some species is suspected of causing hayfever (Wodehouse 1971).

Celtis africana
(syn. C. kraussiana)

The yellow wood has an unpleasant odour (Irvine 1961).

Celtis australis
Nettle Tree

The fruit is edible, the wood useful for turning and the plant is used as fodder in India. The common name possibly refers to the effects of the hairy leaves.

Celtis brieyi
Diania

Mucocutaneous reactions from this species in the wood working industry were reported by Hublet et al (1972).

Celtis cinnamomea
Stinkwood, Hackberry

The heartwood has an unpleasant odour and a recently felled tree can be smelt for many days at a long distance (Menninger 1967).

Celtis durandii

The wood is irritant to the respiratory tract (Orsler 1973).

References

Hublet, P., Sporcq, J., Oleffe, J. et al (1972) Étude sur les accidents cutanes et muqueux provoques par les bois tropicaux dans l'industrie du bois en Belgique. Arch. Belges. Med. Social. 30, 314.

Irvine, F.R. (1961) Woody Plants of Ghana. London. Oxford University Press.

Menninger, E.A. (1967) Fantastic Trees. New York. The Viking Press.

Orsler, R.J. (1973) Personal communication from Forest Products Research Laboratory, Princess Risborough, Bucks, England.

Wodehouse, R.P. (1971) Hayfever Plants. 2nd rev. edition. New York, Hafner.

Planera

One species found in the southern United States, is a useful timber tree.

Planera aquatica
Water Elm

The pollen can cause hayfever (Wodehouse 1971).

Reference

Wodehouse, R.P. (1971) Hayfever Plants. 2nd rev. edition. New York, Hafner.

Trema

30 species are found in

tropical and subtropical regions.

Trema aspera
Peach-leaved Poison Bush

The leaves act as a mechanical irritant to animals or cause impaction of the stomach owing to the tough nature of the fibre. Dermatitis and photodermatitis in cattle has been ascribed to the plant (Hurst 1942).

Trema guineensis
Ficalho

The rough leaves are used as a substitute for 'sand-paper' (Williamson 1956).

References

Hurst, E. (1942) The poison Plants of New South Wales. N.S.W. Poison Plants Committee, Sydney.

Williamson, J. (1956) Useful Plants of Malawi. ed. Greenway, P.J. Zomba, Malawi. The Government Printer. Previously published as Useful Plants of Nyasaland.

Ulmus
Elm

45 species are found in north temperate regions south to the Himalayas, Indo China and Mexico.

The pollen of some species can cause hayfever (Wodehouse 1971).

Reference

Wodehouse, R.P. (1971) Hayfever Plants. 2nd rev. edition. New York, Hafner.

Ulmus campestris
Elm

Ulmus montana

A man, who contacted elm trees at work, developed acute eczema of the hands and face during the summer. A patch test to elm leaf produced a positive reaction. Two persons developed dermatitis of the hands and forearms after trimming an elm hedge. A patch test to elm leaf produced a positive reaction in one of them who was tested. Patch tests to elm leaves produced irritant reactions in 17 of 67 controls (Genner and Bonnevie 1938). The irritant reaction may depend on the occasional penetration of the skin by the small hairs on the leaf producing mechanical and chemical effects (Woods 1962). Elm pollen was reported to produce a positive patch test reaction in a patient who had hand eczema (Agrup 1969). Elm was incriminated in wood-cutters' eczema (Schulman and Detouillon 1932) now known to be caused by lichens and Frullania.

Ulmus fulva
Oohooska (It slips)
North American Indian
Slippery Elm

The inner bark is used as a demulcent and for soothing application to inflamed skins in Herbal Medicine (Wren 1968).

Ulmus procera
English Elm

This species is listed as injurious (Woods 1968).

References

Agrup, G. (1969) Hand eczema and other hand dermatoses in South Sweden. Acta derm.-venereol. 49, suppl. 61.

Genner, B. and Bonnevie, P. (1938) Eczematous eruptions produced by leaves of trees and bushes. Arch. Derm. Syph. 37, 583.

Schulman, E. and Detouillon, P. (1932) L'eczema du bois et al sensibilisation sylvestre. Paris. med. 83, 55.

Woods, B. (1968) Principal timbers causing dermatitis in Textbook of Dermatology ed. Rook, A., Wilkinson, D.S. and Ebling, F.J.G. Oxford. Blackwell Scientific Publ.

Wren, R.W. (1968) Potter's New Cyclopaedia of Botanical Drugs and Preparations by Wren, R.C. Re-edit. by Wren, R.W. Potter and Clarke Ltd. Health Science Press. Rustington, Sussex.

UMBELLIFERAE
(syn. APIACEAE)

2850 species in 275 genera are of cosmopolitan distribution

but chiefly found in north temperate regions.

Chemistry is recorded by Hegnauer (1973), Nielsen (1970, 1971).

References

Hegnauer, R. (1973) Chemotaxonomy of plants. Vol. 6. Basel. Birkhauser p. 554.

Nielsen, B.E. (1970) Coumarins of Umbelliferous plants. Copenhagen. Royal Danish School of Pharmacy.

Nielsen, B.E. (1971) Coumarin patterns in the Umbelliferae, in The Biology and Chemistry of the Umbelliferae. ed. Heywood, V.H. Suppl. 1 to Bot. J. Linnaean Soc. Vol. 64. London. Academic Press.

Photosensitisation by umbelliferous plants.

Of about 200 coumarins isolated from plants, about 125 have been isolated from 161 umbellifer species, representing 33 genera of the family. Coumarins have only been isolated from the sub-family Apioideae especially from members of the tribes Smyrnieae, Ammineae and Peucedanae (Nielsen 1971).

Of the coumarins, linear furanocoumarins have the capacity to evoke photodermatitis. Soine (1964) listed furanocoumarins which had been tested in guinea-pig and man. Some 18 compounds showed some effect on guinea-pig skin, some 22 compounds on human skin.

Compounds with a linear tricyclic structure resembling that of psoralen are capable of evoking photosensitisation e.g. 4-methylpsoralen, 4,4'-dimethylpsoralen, 4,5'-dimethylpsoralen, 4,8'-dimethylpsoralen, 4,5',8-trimethylpsoralen, 8-methoxypsoralen, 5-methoxypsoralen. Compounds with a nonlinear structure (e.g. isopsoralens and isopseudopsoralens) are without any photosensitising activity. Inactive structures include isopsoralens, pseudopsoralen, pseudoisopsoralen, 3-methylpsoralen, 4',5'-dihydropsoralens, coumarins, furans, benzodifurans, furanochromones, oxazolocoumarins, naphthofurans and naphtho-alpha-pyrones (Pathak et al 1971).

For the purpose of this review plants have been recorded as yielding 5-methoxypsoralen, 8-methoxypsoralen and other furanocoumarins. Further information is provided by Nielsen (1970, 1971). The wave-lengths which most effectively evoke photodermatitis are in the range between 320 and 380nm with maximum effectiveness between 330 and 360nm(Pathak 1974).

References

Nielsen, B.E. (1970) Coumarins of Umbelliferous Plants. Copenhagen. The Royal Danish School of Pharmacy.

Neilsen, B.E. (1971) Coumarin patterns in the Umbelliferae in The Biology and Chemistry of the Umbelliferae. ed. Heywood, B.H. London. Academic Press.

Pathak, M.A. (1974) Phytophotodermatitis. Chapter 32 in Sunlight and Man ed. Pathak, M.A. et al. University of Tokyo Press. p. 495.

Pathak, M.A., Toda, K. and Fitzpatrick, T.B. (1971) Psoralens and cutaneous photosensitisation. Scientific Exhibit. American Academy of Dermatology. Chicago. December.

Soine, T.O. (1964) Naturally occurring coumarins and related physiological activities. J. Pharm. Sci. 53, 231.

Introduction

Of 36 furocoumarin and 42 coumarin derivatives tested for phototoxicity, none was found to have greater potency than unsubstituted, linearly annulated psoralen (Pathak et al 1967).

Reference

Pathak, M.A., Worden, L.R. and Kaufman, K.D. (1967) Effect of structural alterations on the photosensitising potency of furocoumarins (psoralens) and related compounds. J. Invest. Derm. 48, 103.

Photosensitisation of the eye has been reported in animals (Cloud et al 1960, 1961, Cogan 1961, Freeman 1966) but not in man (Grant 1962).

References

Cloud, T.M., Hakim, R. and Griffen, A.C. (1960) Photosensitization of the eye with Methoxsalen. Arch. Ophthal. 64, 346.

Cloud, T.M., Hakim, R. and Griffen, A.C. (1961) Photosensitization of the eye with Methoxsalen. II. Chronic effects. Arch. Ophthal 66, 689.

Cogan, D.G. (1961) Photosensitization and cataracts. Arch. Ophthal. 66, 612.

Freeman, R.G. (1966) Morphologic changes resulting from photosensitization of the eye with 8-methoxy-psoralen: a comparison with conventional ultraviolet injury. Texas Rep. Biol. Med. 24(4), 588.

Grant, W.M. (1962) Toxicology of the eye. Springfield, Ill. Charles C. Thomas.

Mutagenesis for microorganisms from psoralen and ultraviolet light was reported by Clarke (1974), Ingali et al (1970) and Townsend et al (1971).

References

Clarke, C.H. (1974) Giant Hogweed sap: another environmental mutagen. Mutation Research 31, 63.

Igali, S., Bridges, B.A., Ashwood-Smith, M.J. and Scott, B.R. (1970) Mutagenesis in Escherichi coli, IV. Photosensitisation to near ultraviolet light by 8-methoxypsoralen. Mutation Research 9, 21.

Townsend, M.E., Wright, H.M. and Hopwood, D.A. (1971) Efficient mutagenesis by near ultraviolet light in the presence of 8-methoxypsoralen in streptomyces. Journal of Applied Bacteriology 34, 799.

Aciphylla

35 species are found in Australia and New Zealand.

Aciphylla squarrosa
Bayonet Grass

The spiny leaves (Howes 1974) are capable of producing mechanical injury.

Reference

Howes, F.N. (1974) A Dictionary of Useful and Everyday Plants and their Common Names. Cambridge University Press. pp. 290.

Tribe: Apieae

Aegopodium

Seven species are found in Europe and temperate regions of Asia.

Aegopodium podagraria
Gout Weed

The leaves are used for a counter-irritant effect (Grieve 1970).

Reference

Grieve, M. (1970) A Modern Herbal. Darien, Conn. Hafner Publ. Co.

Tribe: Apieae

Aethusa

One species is native to Europe, North Africa and western Asia.

Aethusa cynapium
Fool's Parsley

This poisonous plant has an irritant effect (Pammel 1911).

Reference

Pammel, L.H. (1911) A manual of poisonous plants. Torch Press. Cedar Rapids, Iowa. Reprinted Univ. Microfilms Inc. Ann Arbor, Mich. 1965.

Tribe: Ammineae

Ammi

Ten species are found in the Azores, Madeira, the Mediterranean region and temperate western Asia.

Ammi majus
Aatrillal (Egypt),
Bishop's Weed

The seeds of this plant which grows abundantly in the Nile Valley have been used in Egypt for the treatment of vitiligo since the 13th Century (El Mofty 1968). Photodermatitis is evoked by application of an extract of the seeds to the skin. Severe blistering can follow application of the plant to the skin and exposure to light: hyperpigmentation of the skin is a prominent aftermath (Cheymol 1958). According to Behl et al (1966) the plant has rarely been a sensitizer in addition to evoking photodermatitis. Five linear furanocoumarins, which include 5-methoxypsoralen and 8-methoxypsoralen, are derived from the fruits (Nielsen 1971).

Ammi visnaga

Ingestion of the seeds can produce photosensitization in chickens (Trenchi 1960). Coumarins of the plant recorded by Nielsen (1971) are not known to be photosensitizing for man.

References

Behl, P.N., Captain, R.M., Bedi, B.M.S. and Gupta, S. (1966) Skin-irritant and sensitizing plants found in India, New Delhi. P.N. Behl, Irwin Hospital.

Cheymol, J. (1958) Ammi majus and skin darkening. Therapie (Paris) 13, 974.

El Mofty, A.M. (1968) Vitiligo and psoralens. Oxford Pergamon Press.

Nielsen, B.E. (1971) Coumarin patterns in the Umbelliferae in The Biology and Chemistry of the Umbelliferae. ed. Heywood, V.H. London. Academic Press.

Trenchi, H. (1960) Ingestion of Ammi visnaga seeds and photosensitization - the cause of vesicular dermatitis in fowls. Avian Disease 4, 275.

Tribe: Ammineae

Anethum

One species is native to North Africa, three to western Asia.

Anethum graveolens
Dill

The fruit is used as a condiment. A positive patch test reaction to Dill was observed in a sandwich-maker who had contact dermatitis (Hjorth and Weisman 1972).

Dill was noted as a source of furanocoumarins (Klaber 1942) and listed as a plant implicated in causing phytophotodermatitis by Pathak et al (1962) but other clinical reports of dermatitis from the plant appear to be lacking. A coumarin derived from the plant (Nielsen 1971) is not known to be photosensitizing. Oil of Dill has been reported to be sensitizing (Urbach 1942). Carvone which is derived from the oil of this and other plants (Fenaroli 1971) has produced contact sensitivity when used in toothpaste (Hjorth 1967).

References

Fenaroli, G. (1971) Fenaroli's Handbook of Flavor Ingredients. ed. Furia, T.E. and Bellanca, N. Cleveland, Ohio. The Chemical Rubber Co.

Greenberg, L.A. and Lester, D. (1954) Handbook of Cosmetic Materials. New York. Interscience.

Hjorth, N. (1967) Toothpaste sensitivity. Contact Dermatitis Newsletter, London 1, 14.

Hjorth, N. and Weismann, K. (1972) Occupational dermatitis in chefs and sandwich makers. Contact Dermatitis Newsletter. London. 11, 301.

Klaber, R. (1942) Phyto-photo-dermatitis. Brit. J. Derm. Syph. 54, 193.

Nielsen, B.E. (1971) Coumarin patterns in the Umbelliferae in The Biology and Chemistry of the

Umbelliferae. ed. Heywood, V.H. London. Academic Press.

Urbach, E. (1942) Odors (osmyls) as allergenic agents. J. Allergy 13, 387 cited by Greenberg and Lester (1954).

Pathak, M.A., Daniels, F. Jr. and Firzpatrick, T.B. (1962) Presently known distribution of furocoumarins (Psoralens) in plants. J. Invest. Derm. 39, 225.

Tribe: Peucedanae

Angelica

80 species are found in the northern hemisphere and New Zealand.

Angelica sp.

A confectioner had recurrent vesicular dermatitis of the forearm flexures after gathering the plant for preserving as candy; a friend who assisted him was similarly affected (Walsh 1897). Oil of Angelica root can produce dermatitis in hypersensitive individuals (Greenberg and Lester 1954). 29 species of the genus which were investigated yielded 16 linear furanocoumarins (Nielsen 1971).

Contact sensitivity to Angelica root was reported by Larsen (1975).

Angelica acutiloba

Kariyone (1971) sneezed repeatedly and suffered from nasal haemorrhages when he studied the active principles of this species.

Angelica anomala

The plant is used as a sternutatory in Chinese Medicine (Smith 1969). The roots yield 5-methoxypsoralen (Nielsen 1970).

Angelica archangelica (syn. Archangelica officinalis)
Engelwurz, Angelica

The leaf stalks are candied and used in confectionery. The plant has been reported to evoke photodermatitis (Pathak 1974, Van Dijk and Berrens 1964). This species yields 5-methoxypsoralen and 8-methoxypsoralen (Nielsen 1970).

Angelica brevicaulis

This species yields 5-methoxypsoralen (Nielsen 1970).

Angelica formosana

This species yields 5-methoxypsoralen (Nielsen 1970).

Angelica glabra
Byakusi (Japanese Ivy)

This species yields furanocoumarins (Pathak et al 1962).

Angelica hirsutiflora

This species yields 5-methoxypsoralen and 8-methoxypsoralen (Nielsen 1970).

Angelica japonica

This species yields 5-methoxypsoralen (Nielsen 1970).

Angelica keiskeri

This species yields 5-methoxypsoralen and 8-methoxypsoralen (Nielsen 1970).

Angelica officinalis

This species yields furanocoumarins (Pathak et al 1962, Dean 1963).

Angelica polymorfa

This species yields 5-methoxypsoralen (Nielsen 1970).

Angelica pubescens

This species yields 5-methoxypsoralen (Nielsen 1970).

Angelica sylvestris

This species has been reported to evoke photodermatitis (Bogdanovitch et al 1933). A paste of the fruit is used to kill headlice (Usher 1974).

References

Larsen, W.G. (1975) Cosmetic dermatitis due to a perfume. Contact Dermatitis 1, 142.

Bogdanovitch, I.I. et al (1933) Vestn. Derm. Ven. 389, cited by Klaber (1942).

Dean, F.M. (1963) Naturally occurring oxygen ring compounds. London. Butterworths.

Greenberg, L.A. and Lester, D. (1954) Handbook of Cosmetic Materials. New York. Interscience.

Kariyone, T. (1971) Atlas of Medicinal Plants. Osaka, Japan. Takeda Chemical Industries.

Klaber, R. (1942) Phyto-photo-dermatitis. Brit. J. Derm. Syph. 54, 193.

Nielsen, B.E. (1970) Coumarins of Umbelliferous Plants. Copenhagen. The Royal Danish School of Pharmacy.

Nielsen, B.E. (1971) Coumarin patterns in the Umbelliferae in The Biology and Chemistry of the Umbelliferae. ed. Heywood, V.H. London. Academic Press.

Pathak, M.A., Daniels, F. Jr. and Fitzpatrick, T.B. (1962) Presently known distribution of furocoumarins (Psoralens) in plants. J. Invest. Derm. 39 225.

Pathak, M.A. (1974) Phytophotodermatitis. Chapter 32 in Sunlight and Man. ed. Pathak, M.A. et al. University of Tokyo Press. P. 495.

Smith, F.P. (1969) Chinese Materia Medica. Vegetable kingdom. 2nd ed. Rev. by Hei, P.D. Taipei, Taiwan. Ku T'ing Book House.

Usher, G. (1974) A dictionary of plants used by man. London. Constable.

Van Dijk, E. and Verrens, L. (1964) Plants as an etiological factor in phytophotodermatitis. Dermatologica (Basel) 129, 321.

Walsh (1897) Case report. Brit. J. Derm. 9, 287.

Tribe: Scandiceae

Anthriscus
(syn. Antriscus)

20 species are found in Europe and temperate regions of Asia.

Anthriscus cerefolium
(syn. Antriscus cerefolium)
Chervil

A case of occupational dermatitis from this plant and from Lagurus ovatus was reported by Benini et al (1970).

Anthriscus sylvestris
Cow Parsley, Wild Chervil

The plant was reported to evoke photodermatitis (Bell-Ringer 1949); photopatch tests produced positive results. Extracts of this plant exhibit a weak phototoxic activity (Van Dijk and Verrens 1964).

References

Bell-Ringer, H.E. (1949) Phyto-photo-dermatitis. Brit. Med. J. 1, 984

Benini, et al (1970) A case of occupational phytodermatitis caused by Lagurus ovatus and Antriscus cerefolium. Arcisp. S Anna Ferrara 23, 427.

Van Dijk, E. and Berrens, L. (1964) Plants as an etiological factor in phytophotodermatitis. Dermatologica (Basel) 129, 321.

Tribe: Apieae

Apium

One species is found in regions from Europe to India, North and South Africa.

Apium graveolens
Celery

Varieties and cultivars are known.

Apium graveolens var. dulce
Blanching Celery

Apium graveolens
var. rapaceum
Celeriac

Apium graveolens
var. silvestre
(Usher 1974)

Legraine and Barthe (1926) reported the case of a celery-gatherer who developed a pruritic papulo-vesicular dermatitis on the hands and face and commented that the eruption closely resembled that produced by Cow-Parsnip (Heracleum). Henry (1933, 1938) reported dermatitis in 22 workers preparing celery for canning. In a case of celery dermatitis, Gelfand (1936) obtained positive patch test reactions to oil of celery. The oil was also implicated by Wiswell et al (1948) and Palumbo and Lynn (1953). Klaber (1942) suspected a role of sunlight in dermatitis among workers who handled celery. 5-methoxypsoralen was isolated from A. graveolens var. dulce by Musajo et al (1954). Birmingham et al (1961) investigated dermatitis in celery-workers in Michigan and confirmed the opinion of field-workers that pink rot celery, that is celery infected with the fungus Sclerotinia sclerotiorum, evoked photodermatitis. The infected celery contained a photoreactive furanocoumarin: Scheel et al (1963) isolated 8-methoxypsoralen and 4,5',8-trimethylpsoralen from celery infected with this fungus. Perone et al (1963) obtained negative photo-patch test reactions with uninfected celery and positive reactions with infected celery. Normal green Pascal celery contains 5-methoxypsoralen and the diseased celery contains potent photosensitizing agents, 8-methoxypsoralen and 4,5',8-trimethylpsoralen (Pathak 1974). According to Nielsen (1970) A. graveolens yields 5-methoxypsoralen and also 2',4,8-trimethylpsoralen. Dark-skinned labourers appeared to be immune whereas over one-third of the whites were affected (Wiswell et al 1948).

Phototoxicity from fungus-infected celery appears to be the principal cause of celery dermatitis but probably allergic contact dermatitis can also occur as indicated by the patch test results of Wiswell et al (1948) and Palumbo and Lynn (1954). Professional dermatitis from celery and parsley (Petroselinum) was found in 10% of 182 persons in a rural population (Luppi and Bucchi 1970).

Three of three women contact sensitive to carrot (Daucus) showed positive patch test reactions to turnip-rooted celery; three of three also reacted to parsnip (Pastinaca) (Klauder and Kimmich 1956). Agrup (1969) observed a positive patch test reaction to celery. Alleged cross-sensitivity to orange and lemon (Citrus) appears to be anecdotal (Birmingham et al 1961). The aromatic ingredient of celery is sedanolide, which is an isomer of cnidilide (Kariyone 1971).

Variety or cultivar-specific allergenicity has been observed, the variety of celery named Pascal green being the most active sensitiser (Wiswell et al 1948, Palumbo and Lynn 1954). The latter authors did not state the concentration of the extracted oil which was used for patch-testing.

References

Agrup, G. (1969) Hand eczema and other hand dermatoses in South Sweden. Acta derm.-venereol. 49 Suppl. 61. pp. 1-91.

Birmingham, D.J., Key, M.M., Tubich, G.E. et al (1961) Phototoxic bullae among celery harvesters. Arch. Derm. 83, 127.

Gelfand, H.H. (1936) Hypersensitiveness to celery. J. Allergy 7, 590.

Henry, S.A. (1933) Celery itch. Dermatitis due to celery in vegetable canning. Brit. J. Derm. 45, 301.

Henry, S.A. (1938) Dermatitis due to celery in vegetable canning. Brit. J. Derm. 50, 342.

Kariyone, T. (1971) Atlas of Medicinal Plants. Osaka, Japan. Takeda Chemical Industries.

Klaber, R. (1942) Phyto-photodermatitis. Brit. J. Derm. Syph. 54, 193.

Klauder, J.V. and Kimmich, J.M. (1956) Sensitisation dermatitis to carrots. Arch. Derm. 74, 149.

Legraine, M.M. and Barthe, R. (1926) Dermite professionelle des mains et des avant-bras chez un remasseur de celeris. Bull. Soc. franc. dermat. et syph. 33, 662.

Luppi, A. and Bucci, G. (1970) Epidemiological research on the morbosity in a rural district. Note III. A professional dermatosis in horticulture from celery and parsley. Ig. Med. 63, 617.

Musajo, L., Caporale, G. and Rodighiero, G. (1954) Gazz. Chim. Ital. 84, 870, cited by Pathak et al 1962.

Nielsen, B.E. (1970) Coumarins of Umbelliferous Plants. Copenhagen. The Royal Danish School of Pharmacy.

Palumbo, J.F. and Lynn, E.V. (1954) Dermatitis from celery. J. Am. Pharm. Assoc. 42, 57.

Pathak, M.A., Daniels, F. Jr. and Fitzpatrick, T.B. (1962) Presently known distribution of furocoumarins (Psoralens) in plants. J. Invest. Derm. 39, 225.

Pathak, M.A. (1974) Phytophotodermatitis in Sunlight and Man. ed. Pathak, M.A. et al. University of Tokyo Press. p. 495.

Scheel, L.D., Perone, B.V., Larkin, R.L. et al (1963) Biochemistry 2, 1127, cited by Pathak 1975.

Usher, G. (1974) A dictionary of plants used by man. London. Constable.

Wiswell, J.G., Irwin, J.W., Guba, E.F. et al (1948) Contact dermatitis of celery workers. J. Allergy 19, 396.

Tribe: Peucedanae

Archangelica
(syn. Angelica)

Twelve species are found in north temperate regions. The petiole of A. officinalis is used in confectionery.

Archangelica sp.

Angelica is previously noted.

Archangelica decurrens

This species yields 5-methoxypsoralen (Nielsen 1970).

Reference

Nielsen, B.E. (1970) Coumarins of Umbelliferous plants. Copenhagen. The Royal Danish School of Pharmacy.

Tribe: Apieae

Athamanta

15 species are found in the Mediterranean region.

Athamanta oreoselinum

This species yields furanocoumarins (Dean 1963) which are not known to be phototoxic.

Reference

Dean, F.M. (1963) Naturally occurring oxygen ring compounds. London. Butterworths.

Tribe: Apieae

Carum

30 species are found in temperate and subtropical regions.

Carum carvi
Caraway

The fruits provide caraway seeds. The fruit and seeds were used by the Ancient Greeks and Romans as a condiment and are recorded in 1552 B.C. in the medical Papyrus of Thebes. Oil of Caraway may cause cutaneous irritation in hypersensitive individuals (Greenberg and Lester 1954). The plant is listed as a photosensitiser (Pathak et al 1962). Carvone derived from this and other oils (Fenaroli 1971) has produced contact sensitivity (Hjorth 1967).

Carum copticum

This species yields Ajowan oil (Merck Index 1968).

References

Fenaroli, G. (1971) Fenaroli's Handbook of Flavor Ingredients. ed. Furia, T.E. and Bellanca, N. Cleveland, Ohio. The Chemical Rubber Co.

Greenberg, L.A. and Lester, D. (1954) Handbook of Cosmetic Materials. New York. Interscience.

Hjorth, N. (1967) Toothpaste sensitivity. Contact Dermatitis Newsletter, London. 1, 14.

Merck Index (1968) An Encyclopedia of Chemicals and Drugs. ed. Stecher, P.G. 8th ed. Rahway, N.J. Merck and Co. Inc.

Pathak, M.A., Daniels, F. Jr. and Fitzpatrick, T.B. (1962) Presently known distribution of furocoumarins (Psoralen) in plants. J. Invest. Derm. 39, 225.

Centella

40 species are found in Africa, Australia, New Zealand and America.

Centella asiatica

A glycoside terpene, asiaticoside, derived from this plant causes cicatrization and stimulates growth in the skin (Laerum and Iversen 1972).

Reference

Laerum, O.D. and Iversen, O.H. (1972) Reticuloses and epidermal tumours in hairless mice after topical skin applications of cantharidin and asiaticoside. Cancer res. 32, 1463.

Cnidium

20 species are found in northern palaeotemperate regions and in southern Africa.

Cnidium dubium

Cnidium monnieri

These species yield linear furanocoumarins (Nielsen 1971)

Reference

Nielsen, B.E. (1971) Coumarin patterns in the Umbelliferae in The Biology and Chemistry of the Umbelliferae ed. Heywood, V.H. London. Academic Press.

Tribe: Smyrnieae

Conium

Four species are found in northern Eurasia and southern Africa.

Conium maculatum
Poison Hemlock

Dermatitis from the plant was reported by several authors cited by Touton (1932). Massey (1941) and Hardin and Arena (1969) list the plant as capable of producing dermatitis. The plant yields two linear furanocoumarins (Nielsen 1971). The plant is sometimes sold as an ornamental under the name of California fern (Massey 1941). Application of the plant to the skin produces a burning feeling followed by paralysis of sensation (Piffard 1881).

References

Hardin, J.W. and Arena, J.M. (1969) Human Poisoning from Native and cultivated plants. Durham, North Carolina. Duke University Press.

Massey, A.B. (1941) Plant poisoning. Merck Reports 50. 24

Nielsen, B.E. (1971) Coumarin patterns in the Umbelliferae in The Biology and Chemistry of the Umbelliferae. ed. Heywood, V.H. London. Academic Press.

Piffard, H.G. (1881) A treatise on the Materia Medica and Therapeutics of the Skin. New York. Wm. Wood and Co.

Touton, K. (1932) Hauterkrankungen durch phanerogamische Pflanzen und khre Produkte (Toxicodermia et allergodermia phytogenes), in Barnewitz, J. et al Angeborene Anomalien, Lichtdermatosen, Pflanzengifte, Thermische Schadigungen, Einfluss Innerer Storungen auf die Haut. Berlin, Verlag von Julius Springer.

Tribe: Coriandreae

Coriandrum

Two species are found in the Mediterranean region.

Coriandrum sativum
Coriander

The fruits provide coriander seeds used in flavouring. The seeds were found in Egyptian tombs of 960-880 B.C. and the plant was recorded in the medical Papyrus of Thebes in 1552 B.C. Loveman (1938) observed a positive patch test reaction to Oil of Coriander. Oil of Coriander is considered to be a known allergen and therefore removed from certain brand-name cosmetics (Schieffelin 1973).

References

Loveman, A.B. (1938) Stomatitis venenata. Archs. Derm. Syph. 37, 70.

Schieffelin, and Co. (1973) Almay Hypo-allergenic cosmetics product formulaty. 8th ed. Pharmaceutical Laboratories Division, 562 Fifth Avenue, New York, N.Y. 10036.

Tribe: Apieae

Cuminum

Two species are found from the Mediterranean region to the Sudan and central Asia.

Cuminum cyminum
Cummin

The seeds were used as a condiment by the Ancient Greeks and in the Middle Ages. Oil of Cumin used in perfumery is said to have some of the properties of other essential oils but has not been implicated in dermatitis (Greenberg and Lester 1954). Distinct phototoxic effects were reported for undiluted cumin oil but none from its principal ingredient, cuminaldehyde (Opdyke 1974).

References

Greenberg, L.A. and Lester, D. (1954) Handbook of Cosmetic Materials. New York. Interscience.

Opdyke, D. (1974) Monographs on fragrance raw materials. Fd. Cosmet. Toxicol. 12, 807.

Daucus

60 species are found in Europe, Africa, Asia and America.

Daucus spp.

The fruits are burred and adhere to animals. D. carota is the wild carrot.

Daucus carota var. sativa
Carrot

The plant is more or less bristly, bearing stiff strong hairs. The volatile oil contained in the leaves and fruits varies greatly from one kind of carrot to another (Burkill 1935, Watt and Breyer-Brandwijk 1962). Pammel (1911) reported that handling the foliage of carrots, especially when wet, produced irritation, even vesication, in some persons. Prolonged exposure to carrots in canning factories can produce irritation of the skin and mechanical injury from the hairs (Peck et al 1944). In seven cases of occupational dermatitis from carrots, the eruption was localized to the hands in five cases but in two cases the forearms, neck and face were also affected (Vickers 1941). Peck et al (1944) described acute or chronic dermatitis affecting the hands and forearms and in some persons, the neck and face. 15 of 17 persons showed positive patch test reactions to slices of raw carrot. Aqueous extracts of carrot, the dried residue of this extract, ether and acetone extracts, carrot juice and heated carrot produced positive patch test reactions.

Allergic contact dermatitis from carrots was reported by Klauder and Kimmich (1956) affecting 13 employees in a food-processing plant. The incubation period was usually about two weeks. Vesicular dermatitis affected the fingers and dorsa of the hands. All 13 patients showed positive patch test reactions to carrot slices, stronger to the cut surface than to the outer intact surface. In one of two patients tested, boiled carrot produced a positive reaction.

Two of 77 (Peck et al 1944) and three of 55 controls (Vickers 1941) showed irritant reactions to raw carrot slices.

Cross-sensitivity was observed to parsnip (Pastinaca) and celery (Apium); negative reactions were observed to some other umbelliferous plants (Klauder and Kimmich 1956). Dermatitis from carrots is an industrial problem (Henry 1933, Vickers 1941, Peck et al 1944, Klauder and Kimmich 1956) but is considered significant in housewife's eczema (Shelmire 1940, Agrup 1969).

Spitzer (1937) observed a case of meadow dermatitis; besides the erythema there was an exact copy of a leaf of wild carrot (D. carota) on the skin of the patient who had lain undressed in a meadow; he considered this copy of a leaf to be due to mechanical irritation by hairs of the plant. Vickers (1941) suggested a photosensitizing effect of carrots. Extracts of the plant had a weak phototoxic activity (Van Dijk and Berrens 1964). Pathak (1975) lists the plant as implicated in causing phytophotodermatitis. Carrots have been reported to cause contact urticaria (Urbach and Gottleib 1949). Oil of carrot seed has been suspected as an agent of contact dermatitis (Greenberg and Lester 1954, Klarmann 1958). Contact sensitivity to carotene is noted under Citrus.

References

Agrup, G. (1969) Hand eczema and other hand dermatoses in South Sweden. Acta derm.-venereol. 49, Suppl. 61. pp. 1-91.

Burkill, I.G. (1935) A dictionary of the economic products of the Malay Peninsula. 2 Vols. London. Crown Agents for the Colonies.

Greenberg, L.A. and Lester, D. (1954) Handbook of Cosmetic Materials. New York. Interscience.

Henry, S.A. (1933) Celery itch. Dermatitis due to celery in vegetable canning. Brit. J. Derm. 45, 301.

Klarmann, E.G. (1958) Perfume dermatitis. Ann. Allergy 16, 425.

Klauder, J.V. and Kimmich, J.M. (1956) Sensitisation dermatitis to carrots. Arch. Derm. 74, 149.

Pammel, L.H. (1911) A manual of poisonous plants. Torch Press. Cedar Rapids, Ilwa. Reprinted Univ. Microfilms Inc. Ann Arbor, Mich. 1965. pp. 476-7.

Pathak, M.A. (1975) Phytophotodermatitis in Sunlight and Man. Chap. 32. ed. Pathak, M.A. et al. University of Tokyo Press. p. 495.

Peck, S.M., Spolyar, L.W. and Mason, H.S. (1944) Dermatitis from carrots. Arch. Derm. Syph. 49, 266.

Shelmire, B. (1940) Contact dermatitis from vegetation. South Med. J. 33, 338.

Spitzer, E. (1937) Meadow dermatitis due to Daucus carota. Oesterreichische dermat. Gesellsch. Wien. Apr. 17.

Urbach, E. and Gottlieb, P.M. (1949) Allergy. New York. Grune and Stratton.

Van Dijk, E. and Berrens, L. (1964) Plants as an etiological factor in dermatitis venenata due to plants. Dermatologica 129, 321.

Vickers, H.R. (1941) The carrot as a cause of dermatitis. Brit. J. Derm. 53, 52.

Watt, J.M. and Breyer-Brandwijk, M.G. (1962) The Medicinal and poisonous plants of Southern Africa. 2nd ed. Edinburgh. E.&S. Livingstone.

Tribe: Apieae

Elaeoselinum

Ten species are found in the western Mediterranean region.

Elaeoselinum asclepium

Elaeoselinum foetidum

These species were noted as irritant (Pammel 1911).

Reference

Pammel, L.H. (1911) A manual of poisonous plants. Torch Press. Cedar Rapids, Iowa. Reprinted Univ. Microfilms Inc. Ann Arbor, Mich. 1965. pp. 476-7.

Tribe: Peucedanae

Ferula

133 species are found from the Mediterranean region to central Asia.

Ferula communis (syn. F. abyssinica)

The root contains a toxic principle which, like dicoumarol from Trifolium, leads to lowering of the prothrombin level of the blood and haemorrhages in animals who ingest the plant (Verdcourt and Trump 1969).

Ferula galbaniflua

Ferula rubicaulis

These species are sources of medicinal gum galbanum which is rubefacient and irritant (Dioscorides 1st Cent. A.D., Dispensatory 1884, Piffard 1881). Three of 15 individuals who were contact sensitive to Balsam of Peru (Myroxylon) showed positive patch test reactions to galbanum (Hjorth 1961).

References

Dioscorides, The Greek Herbal of: Englished by John Goodyer: A.D. 1655. Edited and first printed A.D. 1933 by R.T. Gunther 1959. New York. Hafner Publishing Co. 2, 206.

Dispensatory, The National (1884) Philadelphia. Stille and Maisch, cited by White (1887).

Hjorth, N. (1961) Eczematous Allergy to Balsams. Munksgaard, International Booksellers and Publishers Ltd. Copenhagen.

Piffard, H.G. (1881) A treatise on Materia Medica and Therapeutics of the skin. New York. Wm. Wood and Co.

Verdcourt, B. and Trump. E.C. (1969) Common poisonous plants of East Africa. London. Collins.

White, J.C. (1887) Dermatitis venenata: An account of the action of external irritants upon the skin. Boston. Cupples and Hurd.

Tribe: Apieae

Foeniculum

Five species are found in the Mediterranean region and Europe.

Foeniculum vulgare
Fennel

The young blanched leaves provide a vegetable and the fruit a condiment. Fennel tea infusions applied to inflamed skin increased the inflammation. Oil of Fennel is reported to produce dermatitis in sensitive individuals (Greenberg and Lester 1954). Cross-sensitivity with Oil of Anise (Pimpinella) was reported by Loveman (1938). The plant has been implicated in causing phytophotodermatitis (Pathak et al 1962). Ingestion of fennel and fennel seed were implicated in a case of bronchial asthma (Levy 1948).

References

Greenberg, L.A. and Lester, D. (1954) Handbook of Cosmetic Materials. New York. Interscience.

Levy, S.B. (1948) Bronchial asthma due to ingestion of fennel and fennel seed. Ann. Allergy 6, 415.

Loveman, A.B. (1938) Stomatitis venenata. Report of a case of sensitivity of the mucous membranes and the skin to oil of anise. Arch. Derm. Syph. 37, 70.

Pathak, M.A., Daniels, F. Jr. and Fitzpatrick, T.B. (1962) Presently known distribution of furocoumarins (Psoralens) in plants. J. Invest. Derm. 39, 225.

Tribe: Peucedanae

Heracleum

70 species are found in north temperate regions and on tropical mountains.

Heracleum spp.
Cow-parsnip, Berce (French)

Chemistry is recorded by Molho et al (1971), Mielsen (1970). Of 29 species investigated, all were found to yield linear furanocoumarins.

References

Molho, D., Jossang, P., Jarreau, M.C. and Carbonnier, J. (1971). Derives furannocoumariniques du genre Heracleum in The Biology and Chemistry of the Umbelliferae. ed. Heywood, V.H. London. Academic Press.

Nielsen, B.E. (1970) Coumarins of Umbelliferous plants. Copenhagen. Royal Danish School of Pharmacy.

The outer rind and the root of the cow-parsnip (berce) contain an acrid sap sufficiently strong to inflame and ulcerate the skin (Chaumton 1815). Persons handling or weeding the plants developed papulo-vesicular or bullous dermatitis (Bulletin 1926). The roots and rind of certain Heracleum species contain an acrid irritant sap (Behl et al 1966). Cases of dermatitis from the plants were reported by Imschenetzky (1928), Colomb et al (1969), Sokolova (1968), Klepov (1960), Leonenko (1962), Krauskoff and Belek (1972). Camm et al (1976) note the difficulties of botanical identification for phytochemical study, numerous synonyms for plant species and the absence of a botanical monograph of the genus.

References

Behl, P.N., Captain, R.M., Bedi, B.M.S. and Gupta, S. (1966) Skin-irritant and sensitizing plants found in India, New Delhi. P.N. Behl, Irwin Hospital.

Bulletin Soc. franc. Derm. Syph. 33, 663, (Nov.) 1926 cited White (1934).

Camm. E., Buck, H.W.L. and Mitchell, J.C. (1976) Phytophotodermatitis from Heracleum mantegazzianum. Contact Dermatitis 2, 68 and letter 2, 230.

Chaumton, F.P. (1815) Flore Med. Paris 2, 32 cited by White (1934)

Colomb, D., Perrot, H. and Beyvin, A.J. (1969) Oppenheim's dermatitis of the meadows doubtlessly due to "cow parsnips". Lyon. Med. 221, 1095.

Imschenetzky, A. (1928) Dermatitis from Heracleum and Geranium. Russk. Vestn. Dermat. 6, 3.

Klepov. I.D. (1960) Vesicular dermatitis caused by cow parsnip. Vestn. Derm. Vener. 34, 55.

Krauskoff, J. and Bilek, J. (1972) Phytodermatoses. Cesk. Dermatol. 41, 136.

Leonenko, P.M. (1962) On the clinical aspects and prevention of dermatitis caused by cow parsnip. Zdravookhr. Beloruss. 8, 83.

Sokolova, E.M. (1968) Occupational bullous dermatitis caused by the cow parsnip plant. Vestn. Derm. Vener. 42, 64.

White, R.P. (1934) The Dermatergoses or Occupational affections of the skin. 4th ed. London. H.K. Lewis.

Heracleum alpinum

This species yields furanocoumarins (Molho et al 1971).

Reference

Molho, D., Jossang. P., Jarreau, M.-C. and Carbonnier, J. (1971) Derives furannocoumariniques du genre Heracleum in The Biology and Chemistry of the Umbelliferae. ed. Heywood, V.H. London. Academic Press.

Heracleum antasiaticum

This species yields 5-methoxypsoralen from the roots (Nielsen 1970).

Reference

Nielsen, B.E. (1970) Coumarins of Umbelliferous Plants. Copenhagen. The Royal Danish School of Pharmacy.

Heracleum asperum

This species yields 5-methoxypsoralen from the fruits (Nielsen 1970).

Reference

Nielsen, B.E. (1970) Coumarins of Umbelliferous Plants. Copenhagen. The Royal Danish School of Pharmacy.

Heracleum candicans

This species yields 5-methoxypsoralen from the fruits (Nielsen 1970).

Reference

Nielsen, B.E. (1970) Coumarins of Umbelliferous Plants. Copenhagen. The Royal Danish School of Pharmacy.

Heracleum ceylanicum

This species yields furanocoumarins (Molho et al 1971).

Reference

Molho, D., Jossang. P., Jarreau, M.-C. and Carbonnier, J. (1971) Derives furannocoumariniques du genre Heracleum in The Biology and Chemistry of the Umbelliferae. ed. Heywood, V.H. London. Academic Press.

Heracleum concanense

This species yields 5-methoxypsoralen from the fruits (Nielsen 1970).

Reference

Nielsen, B.E. (1970) Coumarins of Umbelliferous Plants. Copenhagen. The Royal Danish School of Pharmacy.

Heracleum cyclocarpum

This species yields 5-methoxypsoralen from the roots (Nielsen 1970).

Reference

Nielsen, B.E. (1970) Coumarins of Umbelliferous Plants. Copenhagen. The Royal Danish School of Pharmacy.

Heracleum dissectum

This species yields 5-methoxypsoralen from the roots (Nielsen 1970).

Reference

Nielsen, B.E. (1970) Coumarins of Umbelliferous Plants. Copenhagen. The Royal Danish School of Pharmacy.

Heracleum dulce

357 cases of photodermatitis from this species were reported by Efremov (1961); he noted a requirement for sunlight in evoking the dermatitis since inunction of the juice of the plant without exposure to sunlight was harmless.

Reference

Efremov, A.I. (1961) The photodermatitis caused by Sweet Cow Parsnip (Heracleum dulce) (Russian). Vestn. Derm. Vener. 4, 64.

Heracleum flavescens

This species yields furanocoumarins (Molho et al 1971).

Reference

Molho, D., Jossang, P., Jarreau, M.-C. and Carbonnier, J. (1971) Derives furannocoumariniques du genre Heracleum in The Biology and Chemistry of the Umbelliferae. ed. Heywood, V.H. London. Academic Press.

Heracleum hypoleucum

This species yields 5-methoxypsoralen from the fruits (Nielsen 1970).

Reference

Nielsen, B.E. (1970) Coumarins of Umbelliferous Plants. Copenhagen. The Royal Danish School of Pharmacy.

Heracleum giganteum

According to Bailey and Bailey (1941) this name is a synonym for H. villosum.

Contact with the young shoots of the plant caused acute dermatitis of the hands and forearms of a gardener (Stowers 1897). Harrison (1906) listed the plant as a cause of dermatitis.

Straton (1912) reported that he had occasionally seen, in summer, contact dermatitis affecting the hands and arms of gardeners who had handled the cut stems of this plant which was largely used in the arrangement of perennial borders. In the worst case, the patient had cut down about 200 plants and the hands and arms had become smeared with the sap. Wherever it touched, it produced a glow which was soon followed by intense itching and burning; then an erythemato-vesicular eruption appeared. However he said, unlike that produced by Toxicodendron, it never spread to other parts of the body but was limited to the areas actually touched by the sap. He further observed that the acridity of the sap of Heracleum, Angelica and similar plants varied with the season of the year and all skins were not equally susceptible to its action.

Heracleum giganteum Fisch. yields 5-methoxypsoralen from the fruits (Nielsen 1970).

References

Bailey, L.H. and Bailey, E.Z. (1941) Hortus. Second. New York. Macmillan.

Harrison, A.J. (1906) Dermatitis from without and dermatitis from within. Bristol Med. Chir. J. 24, 325.

Nielsen, B.E. (1970) Coumarins of Umbelliferous Plants. Copenhagen. The Royal Danish School of Pharmacy.

Stowers, J.H. (1897) Case exhibited at Annual meeting of Dermatological Society of Great Britain and Ireland. Brit. J. Derm. Syph. 9, 285.

Straton, C.R. (1912) Dermatitis venenata. Brit. Med. J. 2, 1139.

Heracleum laciniatum

This species yields 5-methoxypsoralen from the fruits (Nielsen 1970).

Reference

Nielsen, B.E. (1970) Coumarins of Umbelliferous Plants. Copenhagen. The Royal Danish School of Pharmacy.

Heracleum lanatum
Masterwort, Cow-parsnip

The young leaf-stalks and young stems, before the expanding of the flowers, are eaten like stewed celery (Apium). The northern Indians of the United States ate the peeled stalks either raw or cooked (Fernald and Kincey 1943). This plant was the most widely used native umbellifer in North America, being employed in numerous ways (French 1971). The blossoms were steeped in oil and rubbed on the body to keep off flies and mosquitoes by North American Indians (Smith 1928). The plant is used for rubefacient purposes (Courchet 1882). The leaves are used as a counterirritant and may produce vesication (Dispensatory 1884). Portions of the leaf and stem using the method of Daniels (1965) were phototoxic for Candida albicans (Camm et al, 1976). The fruits yield 5-methoxypsoralen (Molho et al 1971).

Extracts of the plant inhibit DNA repair in UV-irradiated cultured human fibroplasts (Stich et al 1975).

References

Camm. E., Buck, H.W.L. and Mitchell, J.C. (197) Phytophotodermatitis from Heracleum mantegazzianum. Contact Dermatitis 2, 68.

Courchet, L. (1882) Les Ombelliferes en general et les especes usitees en pharmacie en particulier. Montpellier: Imprimerie Cristin, Serre and Ricome, 221 (+10) pp.

Daniels, F. Jr. (1965) A simple microbiological method for demonstrating phototoxic compounds. J. Invest. Derm. 44, 259.

Dispensatory, The National (1884) Philadelphia, Stille and Maisch, cited by White (1887).

Fernald, M.L. and Kincey, A.D. (1943) Edible Wild Plants of North America. Cornwall, N.Y. Idlewild Press.

French, D.H. (1971) Ethnobotany of the Umbelliferae in The Biology and Chemistry of the Umbelliferae. ed. Heywood, V.H. Supp. 1 to Bot. J. Linnaean Soc. Vol. 64. London. Academic Press. pp. 385-412.

Stich, H.F., Lam, P. Lo, L.W. et al (1975) The search for relevant short term bioassays for chemical carcinogens. Canad. J. Genet. Cytol. 17, 471.

Molho, D., Jossang, P., Jarreau, M.-C. and Carbonnier, J. (1971) Derives furannocoumariniques du genre Heracleum in The Biology and Chemistry of the Umbelliferae. ed. Heywood, V.H. London. Academic Press.

Smith, H.I. (1928) Materia Medica of the Bella-Coola and neighbouring tribes of British Columbia. Bull. No. 56. National Museum of Canada. Ottawa. King's Printer pp. 47-68.

White, J.C. (1887) Dermatitis venenata: An account of the Action of the External irritants upon the Skin. Boston. Cupples and Hurd.

Heracleum lanatum var. asiaticum

This variety yields 5-methoxypsoralen from the fruits (Nielsen 1970).

Reference

Nielsen, B.E. (1970) Coumarins of Umbelliferous Plants. Copenhagen. The Royal Danish School of Pharmacy.

Heracleum lanatum var. nipponicum

This variety yields 5-methoxypsoralen from the roots and fruits (Nielsen 1970).

Reference

Nielsen, B.E. (1970) Coumarins of Umbelliferous Plants. Copenhagen. The Royal Danish School of Pharmacy.

Heracleum lehmannianum

This species yields 5-methoxypsoralen from the fruits (Nielsen 1970).

Reference

Nielsen, B.E. (1970) Coumarins of Umbelliferous Plants. Copenhagen. The Royal Danish School of Pharmacy.

Heracleum leucocarpum

This species yields furanocoumarins (Molho et al 1971).

Reference

Molho, D., Jossang. P., Jarreau, M.-C. and Carbonnier, J. (1970) Derives furannocoumariniques du genre Heracleum in The Biology and Chemistry of the Umbelliferae. ed. Heywood, V.H. London. Academic Press.

Heracleum mantegazzianum
Giant Hogweed, Wild parsnip, Wild Rhubarb (Canada)

This species is a native of the Caucasus and has been introduced into horticulture. Dermatitis from the plant was reported by Miescher and Burckhardt (1937) who suspected the possibility of light sensitisation. Kuske (1938, 1940) elicited bullous reactions 48 to 72 hours after applying fresh plant juice to the skin and following this with 40 minutes exposure to sunlight. The subsequent English and German literature concerning this plant was reviewed by Drever and Hunter (1970) who reported 13 cases of dermatitis from Scotland. Additional reports were provided by Jones and Russell (1968), Smellie (1968), Kvicalova and Stava (1962), Camm et al 1976).

Hinterman (1962) reported dermatitis from the plant in a dog. A woman had phytophotodermatitis of the skin of the jaw-line from contact with her cat which had been playing with her garden specimen of the plant (Champion, R.H. 1974, pers. comm. to Camm et al 1976).

The plant was reported to be running slightly wild in central Europe (Schulz and Spier 1951). Naturalization and spread of the plant has occurred in the United Kingdom in the past sixty years (Drever and Hunter 1970).

The plant was introduced to Kew Gardens, England for ornamental purposes but has now become a frank weed, usually found near water. The plant can grow to nearly 4m during its growing season and has large hollow stems. Those affected are most often fishermen and bathers and children who use the hollow stems for a telescope or pea-shooter and for blowing noises as with a trumpet. The hands are usually affected and also the back of those who have been hit with the stem in children's play. Cutting of plants for the intended purpose of eradication may result in dispersal since the dried stems and flower heads readily float downstream to reach the lower reaches (Editorial 1970).

The botanical taxonomy of the plant is complex, in that two authored species and a 'Kew species' are known (Molho et al 1971). The Causasian species has been divided into three species (Mandenova 1950). The plant yields 5-methoxypsoralen and 8-methoxypsoralen (Nielsen 1970). Chemovars i.e. biochemical varieties within a species are reported (Molho et al 1971). The essential oil from the plant contains chemicals (Jain 1969) which give rise to a notion that allergic contact dermatitis from the plant is a possibility.

References

Camm, E., Buck, H.W.L. and Mitchell, J.C. (1976) Phytophotodermatitis from Heracleum mantegazzianum. Contact Dermatitis 2, 68 and letter 2, 230.

Drever, J.C. and Hunter, J.A.A. (1970) Giant Hogweed dermatitis. Scottish medical Journal 15, 315.

Editorial (1970) The Giant Hogweed. Lancet 2, 32.

Hinterman, J. (1962) Dermatosis in a dog due to Heracleum mantegazzianum. Schweizer Archiv fur Tierheilkunde 109, 654.

Jain, S.R. (1969) Investigations on the essential oil of Heracleum mantegazzianum L. Planta Medica 17, 230.

Jones, J.G. and Russell, D.G. (1968) Giant Hogweed dermatitis. Practitioner 200, 704.

Kuske, H. (1938) Experimental investigations on photodermatitis caused by plant juices. Archiv fur Dermatologie und syphilis 178, 112.

Kuske, H. (1940) Percutaneous photosensitization by plant juices. Dermatologica (Basel) 82, 273.

Kvicalova, E. and Stava, Z. (1962) Dermatitis bullosa phytogenes post Heracleum mantegazzianum. Ceskoslovenska derm. 37, 31.

Mandenova, I.P. (1950) Causasian species of the genus Heracleum. U.R.S.S.: Academy Sciences of Georgia, Tbilissi. pg. 103.

Miescher, G. and Burckhardt, W. (1937) Herakleum Dermatitis: Case Presentation, Swiss Dermatologic Association, Oct. 3-4, 1936. Schweizer Medizinische Wochenschrift (Basel) 67, 82.

Molho, D., Jossang, P., Jarreau, M.-C. and Carbonnier, J. (1971) Derives furannocoumariniques du genre Heracleum in The Biology and Chemistry of the Umbelliferae. ed. Heywood, V.H. London. Academic Press. pp. 337.

Nielsen, B.E. (1970) Coumarins of Umbelliferous Plants. Copenhagen. The Royal Danish School of Pharmacy. pp. 191.

Schulz, K.H. and Spier, H.W. (1951) Dermatitis venenata due to photosensitization by Heracleum mantegazzianum. Hartarzt. 2, 77.

Smellie, J.H. (1968) Giant Hogweed. Brit. Med. J. 3, 123.

Heracleum montanum

This species yields furanocoumarins (Molho et al 1971).

Reference

Molho, D., Jossang. P., Jarreau, M.-C. and Carbonnier, J. (1971) Derives furannocoumarninques du genre Heracleum in The Biology and Chemistry of the Umbelliferae. ed. Heywood, V.H. London. Academic Press.

Heracleum nepalense

The roots and rind contain an acrid irritant sap (Behl et al 1966). This species yields 5-methoxypsoralen from the fruits (Nielsen 1970).

References

Behl, P.N., Captain, R.M., Bedi, B.M.S. and Gupta, S. (1966) Skin-irritant and sensitizing plants found in India, New Delhi. P.N. Behl, Irwin Hospital.

Nielsen, B.E. (1970) Coumarins of Umbelliferous Plants. Copenhagen. The Royal Danish School of Pharmacy.

Heracleum olgae

This species yields 5-methoxypsoralen from the fruits (Nielsen 1970).

Reference

Nielsen, B.E. (1970) Coumarins of Umbelliferous Plants. Copenhagen. The Royal Danish School of Pharmacy.

Heracleum palmatum

This species yields furanocoumarins (Molho et al 1971).

Reference

Molho, D., Jossang, P., Jarreau, M.-C. and Carbonnier, J. (1970) Derives furannocoumariniques du genre Heracleum in The Biology and Chemistry of the Umbelliferae. ed. Heywood, V.H. London. Academic Press.

Heracleum panaces

This species yields 5-methoxypsoralen from the roots (Nielsen 1970).

Reference

Nielsen, B.E. (1970) Coumarins of Umbelliferous Plants. Copenhagen. The Royal Danish School of Pharmacy.

Heracleum pastinacifolium

This species yields 5-methoxypsoralen from the fruits (Nielsen 1970).

Reference

Nielsen, B.E. (1970) Coumarins of Umbelliferous Plants. Copenhagen. The Royal Danish School of Pharmacy.

Heracleum persicum

This species is listed as a source of phytophotodermatitis (Van Dijk and Berrens 1964).

Reference

Van Dijk, E. and Berrens, L. (1964) Plants as an etiological factor in phytophotodermatitis. Dermatologica (Basel) 129, 321.

Heracleum platytaenium

This species yields furanocoumarins (Nielsen 1970).

Reference

Nielsen, B.E. (1970) Coumarins of Umbelliferous Plants. Copenhagen. The Royal Danish School of Pharmacy.

Heracleum pubescens

This species yields 5-methoxypsoralen from the fruits (Nielsen 1970).

Reference

Nielsen, B.E. (1970) Coumarins of Umbelliferous Plants. Copenhagen. The Royal Danish School of Pharmacy.

Heracleum pyrenaicum

This species yields furanocoumarins (Molho et al 1971).

Reference

Molho, D., Jossang, P., Jarreau, M.-C. and Carbonnier, J. (1971) Derives furannocoumarniques du genre Heracleum in The Biology and Chemistry of the Umbelliferae. ed. Heywood, V.H. London. Academic Press.

Heracleum sibiricum

This species is treated as H. sphondylium spp. sibiricum by Tutin et al (1968) Flora Europaea Vol. 2. p. 366.

The bark and roots of this plant are corrosive and vesicant (Courchet 1882). This species yields 5-methoxypsoralen from the fruits (Nielsen 1970).

References

Courchet, L. (1882) Les Ombelliferes en general et les especes usitees en pharmacie en particulier. Montpellier: Imprimerie Cristin, Serre and Ricome, 221 (+10) pp.

Nielsen, B.E. (1970) Coumarins of Umbelliferous Plants. Copenhagen. The Royal Danish School of Pharmacy.

Heracleum sosnowskyi

This species yields 5-methoxypsoralen and 8-methoxypsoralen from the stalks, leaves and fruits (Nielsen 1970).

Reference

Nielsen, B.E. (1970) Coumarins of Umbelliferous Plants. Copenhagen. The Royal Danish School of Pharmacy.

Heracleum sphondylium
European Cow-parsnip,
Hogweed, Heltrot,
Cow Parsley, Bibernell

This species is reported to evoke phytophotodermatitis (Van Dijk and Berrens 1964, Pathak et al 1962). Michon et al (1956) reported purpuric dermatitis from the plant. This species yields 5-methoxypsoralen and 8-methoxypsoralen from the roots and fruits (Nielsen 1970).

References

Michon, P. et al (1956) Purpuric dermatitis from plant Heracleum spondylium. Rev. med. Nancy 81, 924.

Nielsen, B.E. (1970) Coumarins of Umbelliferous Plants. Copenhagen. The Royal Danish School of Pharmacy.

Pathak, M.A., Daniels, F. Jr. and Fitzpatrick, T.B. (1962) Presently known distribution of furocoumarins (Psoralens) in plants. J. Invest. Derm. 39, 225.

Van Dijk, E. and Berrens, L. (1964) Plants as an etiological factor in phytophotodermatitis. Dermatologica (Basel) 129, 321.

Heracleum sprengelianum

This species yields furanocoumarins (Molho et al 1971).

Reference

Molho, D., Jossang. P., Jarreau, M.-C. and Carbonnier, J. (1971) Derives furannocoumariniques du genre Heracleum in The Biology and Chemistry of the Umbelliferae. ed. Heywood, V.H. London. Academic Press.

Heracleum stevenii

This species yields 5-methoxypsoralen from the fruits (Nielsen 1970).

Reference

Nielsen, B.E. (1970) Coumarins of Umbelliferous Plants. Copenhagen. The Royal Danish School of Pharmacy.

Heracleum trachyloma

This species yields 5-methoxypsoralen from the fruits (Nielsen 1970).

Reference

Nielsen, B.E. (1970) Coumarins of Umbelliferous Plants. Copenhagen. The Royal Danish School of Pharmacy.

Heracleum transcaucasicum

This species yields 5-methoxypsoralen from the fruits (Nielsen 1970).

Reference

Nielsen, B.E. (1970) Coumarins of Umbelliferous Plants. Copenhagen. The Royal Danish School of Pharmacy.

Heracleum villosa

This species yields 8-methoxypsoralen (Nielsen 1970).

Reference

Nielsen, B.E. (1970) Coumarins of Umbelliferous Plants. Copenhagen. The Royal Danish School of Pharmacy.

Heracleum wilhelmsii

This species yields furanocoumarins (Molho et al 1970).

Reference

Molho, D., Jossang, P., Jarreau, M.-C. and Carbonnier, J. (1971) Derives furannocoumariniques du genre Heracleum in The Biology and Chemistry of the Umbelliferae. ed. Heywood, V.H. London. Academic Press.

Tribe: Smyrnieae

Hippomarathrum

12 species are found from the Mediterranean region to the Caucasus. The genus may have affinities with Seseli.

Hippomarathrum capsicum

The leaves, stalks and fruits yield 5-methoxypsoralen and 8-methoxypsoralen (Nielsen 1970).

Hippomarathrum microcarpum

The fruits yield 5-methoxypsoralen and 8-methoxypsoralen (Nielsen 1970).

Reference

Nielsen, B.E. (1970) Coumarins of Umbelliferous Plants. Copenhagen. The Royal Danish School of Pharmacy.

Hydrocotyle

This genus is noted under family Hydrocotylaceae.

Tribe: Peucedanae

Levisticum

Three species native to south-western Asia are cultivated and naturalized in North America and Europe. Two species yielded linear furanocoumarins (Nielsen 1971).

Levisticum officinale
(syn. Ligusticum officinale, Angelica levisticum)
Lovage

The plant was used as a condiment and eaten like celery (Apium). A laboratory technician developed dermatitis of the wrist and elbow flexures after making extracts of Lovage and cleaning out vats containing Oil of Lovage. Patch tests were positive to Lovage concentrate, negative in eight controls (Calnan 1969). Oil of Lovage is used in perfumery (Greenberg and Lester 1954).

Levisticum scoticum
Scotch Lovage

The root is hot and disagreeable to the taste; it was sometimes chewed in Scotland as tobacco (Nicotiana).

References

Calnan, C.D. (1969) Lovage sensitivity. Personal communication. Contact Dermatitis Newsletter, London 5, 99.

Greenberg, L.A. and Lester, D. (1954) Handbook of Cosmetic Materials. New York. Interscience.

Nielsen, B.E. (1971) Coumarin patterns in the Umbelliferae in The Biology and Chemistry of the

Umbelliferae. ed. Heywood, V.H. London. Academic Press.

Tribe: Ammineae

Libanotis
(syn. Seseli)

15 species are found in temperate Eurasia.

Libanotis buchtormensis

This species yields 5-methoxypsoralen and 8-methoxypsoralen (Nielsen 1970).

Reference

Nielsen, B.E. (1970) Coumarins of Umbelliferous Plants. Copenhagen. The Royal Danish School of Pharmacy.

Tribe: Ammineae

Ligusticum

60 species are found in the northern hemisphere. L. scoticum is sometimes used as a pot-herb. Some are cultivated and some used as vegetables (French 1971).

Ligusticum acutilobum

This species yields 5-methoxypsoralen (Nielsen 1970).

References

French, D.H. (1971) Ethnobotany of the Umbelliferae in The Biology and Chemistry of the Umbelliferae. ed. Heywood, V.H. Sull. 1 to Bot. J. Linnaean Soc. ol. 64. London Academic Press. pp. 385-412.

Nielsen, B.E. (1970) Coumarins of Umbelliferous Plants. Copenhagen. The Royal Danish School of Pharmacy.

Tribe: Apieae

Oenanthe

40 species are found in temperate Eurasia and on mountains of tropical Africa.

Oenanthe sp.

The whole genus is acrid (Bowie cited by Watt and Breyer-Brandwijk 1961).

Oenanthe crocata

Oenanthe fistulosa

Oenanthe phellandrium
Water Fennel

These species are described as irritant (Pammel 1911). O. phellandrium is used in Herbal Medicine.

References

Pammel, L.H. (1911) A Manual of Poisonous plants. Torch Press. Cedar Rapids, Iowa. Reprinted Univ. Microfilms Inc. Ann Arbor, Mich., 1965.

Watt. J.M. and Breyer-Brandwijk, M.G. (1962) The Medicinal and poisonous plants of Southern Africa. 2nd ed. Edinburgh. E.& S. Livingstone.

Oenanthe crocata

Applications of the plant 'excoriate' the skin (Piffard 1881).

Reference

Piffard, H.G. (1881) A treatise on the Materia Medica and Therapeutics of the skin. New York. Wm. Wood and Co.

Tribe: Peucedanae

Opopanax

Three species are found from the Balkans to Persia. Gum opopanax, used in perfumery, was obtained from the roots. Recently, c.opanax or Sweet Myrrh is obtained from Commiphora (Fenaroli 1971).

Opopanax sp.

Six of eleven patients who were contact sensitive to Balsam of Peru (Myroxylon) showed positive patch test reactions to opopanax (Hjorth 1961).

References

Fenaroli, G. (1971) Fenaroli's Handbook of Flavor Ingredients. ed. Furia, T.E. and Bellanca, N. Cleveland, Ohio. The Chemical Rubber Co.

Hjorth, N. (1961) Eczematous Allergy to Balsams. Munksgaard, International Booksellers and Publishers Ltd., Copenhagen.

Tribe: Peucedanae

Pastinaca

15 species are native to temperate Eurasia. *P. sativa* L. is the parsnip, a biennial, often cultivated for its edible root. The plant has been cultivated in Europe since Roman times and was introduced to America during the 17th century.

According to Bailey (1971) *P. sativa* L. is the cultivated parsnip and *P. sativa* L. var. *sylvestris* DC is the wild parsnip which is extensively naturalized in North America. According to Clapham et al (1962) *P. sativa* L. is the wild parsnip which is native to Great Britain found at roadsides and in grassy waste places. In Scotland and Ireland, it is found only as an escape from cultivation. The plant is found in Europe except in the extreme North and Portugal and is found eastwards to the Caucasus. It has been introduced to North and South America, Australia and New Zealand. Somner and Jillson (1967) refer to the cultivated parsnip as *P. sativa* var. *hortensis* and to the wild parsnip as *P. sativa* var. *pratensis*. The wild variety reverts to the edible variety with appropriate horticulture and vice versa.

In Great Britain the wild variety is colloquially named Heeltrot, Hockweed, Bird's Nest, Hart's Eye and Madnip (Klaber 1942). The wild parsnip can be identified in early summer by the clusters of yellow flowers arising from a main stalk on stems arranged like the spines of an everted umbrella (Somner and Jillson 1967). The plant which is established as a weed in fields, waste places and roadsides throughout the United States looks somewhat like the wild carrot or Queen Anne's Lace (*Daucus*) but has yellow flowers (Hardin and Arena 1969).

Phytochemistry

Three *Pastinaca* species which were investigated yielded linear furanocoumarins (Nielsen 1971).

Dermatitis from parsnips was recognized at the end of the 19th century (White 1887, Jamieson 1897, Stowers 1897). The dermatitis can affect gardeners (Lee 1946), market-gardeners (Lengyel and Palicska 1965), farmers (Edel 1916), factory-workers employed in processing parsnips (Dicker 1935, Strack 1945, Henry 1933) and troops in the field (Fantl 1917, McKinlay 1938) and soldiers who peeled the vegetable (Belisario 1952). In the case of soldiers the lesions have been mistaken for self-induced lesions or mustard-gas burns. Reports were contributed by Freche and Plissomeau (1908), Nestler (1912), Straton (1912), Cleland (1925), Hartmann and Briel (1927), Heye (1929), Hirschberger and Fuchs (1936), Whittle et al (1946), Gruebel (1946), Lee (1946), Stevanovic (1959), Young (1964), Voborova et al (1965), Federico (1957), Andreichuk (1960) and Binnie (1964).

The active spectral band for evoking phytophotodermatitis from the plant was found to be 320-360nm (Jensen and Hansen 1939). Wetness of the skin on contact with the plant is important in the pathogenesis of the lesions and residual hyperpigmentation is characteristic (Somner and Jillson 1967). These authors noted that phytophotodermatitis from the plant was invariably misdiagnosed as poison ivy (*Toxicodendron*) dermatitis. Lying on plants in grass can cause Meadow-dermatitis (Charpy 1939). Both wild and cultivated parsnip can evoke phytophotodermatitis. It is possible that allergic contact dermatitis can also occur.

Parsnip was found to be not irritant by patch test (Starck 1945).

The plant yields 5-methoxypsoralen and 8-methoxypsoralen (Nielsen 1970).

Pastinaca urens

The plant can evoke phytophotodermatitis (Van Dijk and Berrens 1964). During the spring and beginning of the summer, Pastinaca sylvestris and during the summer P. urens evoke phytophotodermatitis in France (Gougerot and Charteaud 1952). The plant yields 5-methoxypsoralen and 8-methoxypsoralen (Nielsen 1970).

References

Andreichuk, I.E. (1960) Pastinaca dermatitis. Vestn. Derm. Vener. 34, 81.

Bailey, L.H. (1971) Manual of cultivated plants. New York. Macmillan Co.

Belisario, J.C. (1952) Parsnip dermatitis in the tropics under active service conditions. Australian J. Dermat. 1, 3.

Bellringer, H.E. (1949) Phyto-photodermatitis. Brit. Med. J. 1, 984.

Binnie, G.A. (1964) Wild parsnips. Lancet 2, 533.

Charpy, A. (1939) Les formes jardinieres de dermite striee des pres k'Oppenheim et leurs sequelles verruciformes. Bull. Soc. franc. Derm. Syph. p. 247, cited by Gougerot and Carteaud (1952).

Clapham, A.T., Tutin, T.G. and Warburg, E.F. (1962) Flora of the British Isles. Cambridge University Press.

Cleland, J.B. (1925) Plants including fungi, poisonous or otherwise injurious to man in Australia. (series II) Med. J. Australia 2, 443.

Dicker, S. (1935) Occupational bullous dermatitis caused by Pastinaca sativa (parsnip). Rev. med. de la Suisse Rom. 55, 310.

Edel, K. (1916) Ned. T. Geneesk. 2, (12) 1024, cited by White (1934).

Fantl, G. (1917) Feldarztliche Blatter der K. K. s Armee 1917. No. 5. Ref. Dermat. Wschr. 67, 347, cited by Touton (1932).

Federico, G.P. (1957) Phytodermatitis caused by Pastinaca sativa. Arcisped. S. Anna di Ferrara. Riv. 9, 111.

Freche and Plissomeau (1908) Pastinaca sylvestris. J. Med. Bordeaux 791, cited by White (1934).

Gougerot, H. and Carteaud, A. (1952) Les dermatoses professionelles. Paris. Norbert Maloine.

Grubel, L.H. (1946) Dermatitis bullosa striata pratensis. Proc. Roy. Soc. Med. 40, 14.

Hardin, J.W. and Arena, J.M. (1969) Human Poisoning from native and cultivated plants. Durham, North Carolina. Duke University Press.

Hartmann, E. and Briel, J. (1927) Derm. Z. 50, 205, cited by Bellringer (1949).

Henry, S.A. (1933) Celery itch. Dermatitis due to celery in vegetable canning. Brit. J. Derm. 45, 301.

Heye, R.G.H. (1929) Uber die Dermatitis durch Pastinaca sativa, Beitrag zur Atiologie der beim Freibaden entstehenden Hautausschlage Dtsch. med. Wschr 42 (Sep. abdr) cited by Touton (1932).

Hirschberger, A. and Fuchs, H. (1936) Munch med Wschr. 83, 1965, cited by Bellringer (1949).

Jamieson, (1897) Edinburgh Med. J. 2, 601, cited by White (1934).

Jensen, T. and Hansen, K.G. (1939) Active spectral range for phytogenic photodermatitis produced by Pastinaca sativa. Archs. Derm. Syph. 40, 566.

Klaber, R. (1942) Phyto-photodermatitis. Brit. J. Derm. Syph. 54, 193.

Lee, H.G. (1946) Dermatitis bullosa striata pratensis. Proc. Roy. Soc. Med. 40, 14.

Lengyel, B. and Palicska, J. (1965) Dermatite due au panais, affection professionnelle des maraichers. in Pemphigus. Occupational Dermatoses due to Chemical Sensitisation ed. Liebner, E. and Florian, E. Budapest. Hungarian Derm. Soc. (Apr. 65).

McKinlay, R. (1938) J. Roy. Army Med. Corps. 71, 401, cited by Bellringer (1949).

Nestler, A. (1912) lst Pastinak, hautreizend. Ber. dtsch. bot. Ges. cited by Touton (1934).

Nielsen, B.E. (1970) Coumarins of Umbelliferous Plants. Copenhagen. The Royal Danish School of Pharmacy.

Nielsen, B.E. (1971) Coumarin patterns in the Umbelliferae in The Biology and Chemistry of the Umbelliferae. ed. Heywood, V.H. London. Academic Press.

Somner, T.G. and Jillson, O.F. (1967) Phytophotodermatitis - Gas Plant and the wild parsnip. New Eng. J. Med. 276, 1484.

Starck, V. (1945) Percutaneous photosensitization due to handling of parsnips. Acta derm.-venereol. 25, 179.

Stevanovic, D. (1959) Photodynamic action of the sun rays, with reference to a case of dermatitis pratensis. Vojno-Sanit. Pregl. 16, 601.

Stowers, J.H. (1897) Case exhibited at Annual meeting of Dermatological Society of Great Britain and Ireland. Brit. J. Derm. Syph. 9, 285.

Straton, C.R. (1912) Dermatitis venenata. Brit. Med. J. 2, 1139.

Touton, K. (1932) Hauterkrankungen durch phanerogamische Pflanzen und ihre Produkte (Toxicodermia et Allergodermia phytogenes), in Barnewitz, J. et al, Angeborene Anomalien, Lichtdermatosen, Pflanzengifte, Thermische Schadigungen, Einfluss Innerer Storungen auf die Haut. Berlin, Verlag von Julius Springer.

Touton, K. (1934) Hauterkrankungen durch phanerogamische Pflanzen und ihre Produkte in Jadassohn, J. (1934) Handbuch der Haut- und Geschlechtkrankheiten. Berlin. Julius Springer. Vol. 4: pt. 2, pg. 486.

Van Dijk, E. and Berrens, L. (1964) Plants as an etiological factor in dermatitis venenata due to plants. Dermatologica 129, 321.

Voborova, A. and Chmelova, M. (1965) Photodermatitis phytogenica. Cesk. Derm. 40, 43.

White, J.C. (1887) Dermatitis venenata: An account of the action of external irritants upon the skin. Boston. Cupples and Hurd.

White, R.P. (1934) The Dermatergoses or Occupational affections of the skin. 4th ed. London. H.K. Lewis.

Whittle, C.H., Hellier, F.F. and Lee, H.G. (1946) Proc. Roy. Soc. Med. 40, 14, cited by Bellringer (1949).

Young, J. (1964) A list of photosensitizing agents of interest to the dermatologist. Bull. Assoc. Military Dermat. 13, 33.

Tribe: Ammineae

Petroselinum
Parsley

The majority of female workers who prepared parsley in a canning factory developed vesicular inflammation and purple discolouration of the skin and hands and forearms followed by purulent folliculitis and carbuncles (Heubschmann and Cupik 1941). Occupational dermatitis from parsley and celery (*Apium*) was found in 10% of 182 persons in a rural population (Luppi and Bucci 1970). A positive patch test to parsley was observed in a sandwich-maker who had dermatitis (Hjorth and Weissman 1972). Oil of parsley used in perfumery is said to cause dermatitis (Greenberg and Lester 1954). Evidence that the plant can evoke phytophotodermatitis is scanty (Klaber 1942). 5-methoxypsoralen is derived from the plant (Nielsen 1970).

References

Greenberg, L.A. and Lester, D. (1954) Handbook of Cosmetic Materials. New York. Interscience.

Hjorth, N. and Weissman, K. (1972) Occupational dermatitis in Chefs and Sandwich makers. Contact Dermatitis Newsletter, London 11, 301.

Huebschmann, K. and Cupik, J. (1941) Allergic dermatitis with small and large vesicles caused by parsley. Derm. Wchnschr. 113, 725, 744 and 766.

Klaber, R. (1942) Phyto-photodermatitis. Brit. J. Derm. Syph. 54, 193.

Luppi, A. and Bucci, G. (1970) Epidemiological research on the morbosity in a rural district. Note III. A professional dermatosis in horticulture, from celery and parsley. Ig. Mod. 63, 617.

Nielsen, B.E. (1970) Coumarins of Umbelliferous Plants. Copenhagen. The Royal Danish School of Pharmacy.

Petroselinum sativum

The furocoumarins of the plant were investigated and were found to be increased in amount in the summer hot weather (Innocenti et al 1976).

Reference

Innocenti, G., Dall-acqua, F. and Caporale, G. (1976) Investigation of the content of furocoumarins in Apium graveolens and Petroselinum sativum. Planta medica 29, 165.

Tribe: Peucedanae

Peucedanum

120 species are found in temperate Eurasia, tropical and southern Africa. A few species are cultivated.

Phytochemistry

Seventeen species which were investigated yielded eight linear furanocoumarins (Nielsen 1970, 1971). These compounds appear to be of a type which is not known to evoke phytophotodermatitis.

Peucedanum galbanum
Blister Bush

In South Africa, this plant can cause severe blistering of the skin as many who ascend Table Mountain and accidentally brush against the plants will know (Howes 1974). The plant produces dermatitis and blisters 40-50 hours after contact with the bare skin; the vesicant effects vary with the weather (Greshoff 1913, Marloth 1913-1932, Wicht 1918 cited by Watt and Breyer-Brandwijk 1962).

Peucedanum officinale
Sulphur root, Masterwort

This species which is used in veterinary medicine yields furanocoumarins (Dean 1963).

Peucedanum oreoselinum
Mountain Parsley

The plant is said to evoke phytophotodermatitis (Pathak et al 1962).

Peucedanum ostruthium
(syn. Imperatoria ostruthium)
Masterwort

This species which is used in Herbal Medicine is reported to evoke phytophotodermatitis (Kuske 1938, 1940, cited by Pathak et al 1962).

Peucedanum sativum
Parsnip

This species which is reported to cause dermatitis (Hurst 1942) is apparently a synonym of Pastinaca sativa. In a feeding experiment, two ducks which were fed parsnip seed and placed in the sun developed dermatitis (Hurst 1942).

Peucedanum tenuifolium

This species apparently blisters the skin (Wicht 1918, cited by Watt and Breyer-Brandwijk 1962).

References

Dean, F.M. (1963) Naturally occurring oxygen ring compounds. London.

Butterworths.

Greshoff, M. (1913) Beutenzorg Med. Dep. Landb. 17 Batavia. Kolff. cited by Watt and Breyer-Brandwijk (1962).

Howes, F.N. (1974) A dictionary of useful and everyday plants and their common names. Cambridge University Press. pp. 290.

Hurst, E. (1942) The Poison plants of New South Wales. N.S.W. Poison Plants Committee; Sydney.

Kuske, H. (1938) Arch. Derm. u. Syph. 178, 112, cited by Pathak et al (1962).

Kuske, H. (1940) Dermatologica 82, 273, cited by Pathak et al (1962).

Marloth, R. (1913-1932) The Flora of South Africa. London. Wesley, cited by Watt and Breyer-Brandwijk (1962).

Nielsen, B.E. (1970) Coumarins of Umbelliferous Plants. Copenhagen. The Royal Danish School of Pharmacy.

Nielsen, B.E. (1971) Coumarin patterns in the Umbelliferae in The Biology and Chemistry of the Umbelliferae. ed. Heywood, V.H. London. Academic Press.

Pathak, M.A., Daniels, F. Jr. and Fitzpatrick, T.B. (1962) Presently known distribution of furocoumarins (Psoralens) in plants. J. Invest. Derm. 39, 225.

Watt, J.M. and Breyer-Brandwijk, M.G. (1962) The medicinal and poisonous plants of Southern Africa. 2nd ed. Edinburgh. E.&S. Livingstone.

Wicht, J. (1918) S. Afr. Med. Rec. 16, 306, cited by Watt and Breyer-Brandwijk (1962).

Tribe: Peucedanae

Phellopterus
(syn. Cymopterus)

Five species are native to the south-western United States. One of the species is cultivated.

Phellopterus littoralis

This species yields a furanocoumarin (Nielsen 1971).

Reference

Nielsen, B.E. (1971) Coumarin patterns in the Umbelliferae in The Biology and Chemistry of the Umbelliferae. ed. Heywood, V.H. London. Academic Press.

Tribe: Apieae

Pimpinella

150 species are found in Eurasia, one species in Pacific North America, a few species in South America. P. magna is cultivated.

Phytochemistry

Pimpinella heyneana, P. magna and P. saxifraga yield 5-methoxypsoralen (Nielsen 1970).

Pimpinella anisum
Anise (Aniseed)

The condiment, aniseed, was taxed by Edward I (1239-1307) for revenue to repair London Bridge. The oil of the plant inflames the skin (Piffard 1881).

In a case of dermatitis from denture cream and gum-drops, Oil of Anise 1.1%, produced a positive patch test reaction, negative in the same vehicle in controls (Loveman 1938). Since Oil of Anise contains about 90% anethole, the patient was patch tested with anethole; a positive reaction was observed, negative in controls. Positive patch test reactions were also observed from Oil of Fennel (Foeniculum), which contains about 60% anethole and with Oil of Coriander (Coriandrum) which does not contain anethole. Loveman (1938) suggested that the patient showed multiple specific sensitivity to Coriandrum from eating dill pickles (Anethum) which are flavoured with Oil of Coriander. In the patient who was tested, Oil of Caraway (Carum) produced a negative reaction. A volatile component of Oil of Anise appeared to be responsible for the dermatitis. Anethole, used to flavour toothpaste, was reported to produce contact sensitivity (Hjorth

1967) and aniseed was listed as an agent of cheilitis and stomatitis (Zakon et al 1947). Oil of Aniseed and anethole appear to be both irritant and sensitizing (Greenberg and Lester 1954). Hypersensitivity to Oil of Aniseed was observed in candy workers (Schwartz 1934).

Pimpinella saxifraga
Cow Parsnip

This species yields linear furanocoumarins (Nielsen 1971).

References

Greenberg, L.A. and Lester, D. (1954) Handbook of Cosmetic Materials. New York. Interscience.

Hjorth, N. (1967) Toothpaste sensitivity Contact Dermatitis Newsletter, London 1, 14.

Loveman, A.B. (1938) Stomatitis venenata. Report of a case of sensitivity of the mucous membranes and the skin to oil of anise. Arch. Derm. Syph. 37, 50.

Nielsen, B.E. (1970) Coumarins of Umbelliferous Plants. Copenhagen. The Royal Danish School of Pharmacy.

Nielsen, B.E. (1971) Coumarin patterns in the Umbelliferae in The Biology and Chemistry of the Umbelliferae. ed. Heywood, V.H. London. Academic Press.

Piffard, H.G. (1881) A treatise on the Materia Medica and Therapeutics of the skin. New York. Wm. Wood and Co.

Schwartz, L. (1934) Skin hazards in American industry. Pt. 1. U.S. Publ. Health Bull. No. 215.

Zakon, S.J., Goldberg, A.L. and Kahn, J.B. (1947) Lipstick cheilitis: Common dermatosis: Report of 32 cases. Arch. Derm. Syph. 56, 499.

Tribe: Smyrnieae

Prangos

30 species are found from the Mediterranean region to central Asia.

Phytochemistry

Six species yield linear furanocoumarins (Nielsen 1971).

Prangos pabularia

The leaves and blossoms of this plant which grows wild in central Asia were observed to produce a pruritic papular dermatitis followed by hyperpigmentation which persisted for three to six months; patch tests to alcoholic extracts of the leaves and flowers produced positive reactions; to the seeds and stems, negative reactions (Bocharov et al 1963).

References

Bocharov, A.P., Guzina, G.G., Moroz, L.I. et al (1963) A dermatitis caused by the plant *Prangos*. Vestn. Derm. Vener. 37, 73.

Nielsen, B.E. (1971) Coumarin patterns in the Umbelliferae in The Biology and Chemistry of the Umbelliferae. ed. Heywood, V.H. London. Academic Press.

Tribe:

Sanicula

37 species are cosmopolitan except in New Guinea and Australasia.

Sanicula europaea
Butterwort

This species which has been used to lubricate chapped hands in Herbal Medicine has been reported to cause dermatitis (Engel and Horn 1972).

Reference

Engel, S. and Horn, K. (1972) Phytodermatosen durch *Dictamnus alba*, *Sanicula europaea* and *Phyllodendron consanguineum*. Derm. Mschr. 158, 22.

Tribe: Apieae

Seseli

80 species are found from Europe to central Asia.

Seseli spp.
Hog Celery

Four species yield linear furanocoumarins (Nielsen 1971).

Reference

Nielsen, B.E. (1971) Coumarin patterns in the Umbelliferae in The Biology and Chemistry of the Umbelliferae. ed. Heywood, V.H. London. Academic Press.

Tribe: Apieae

Sium

Ten or perhaps 15 species are cosmopolitan except in South America and Australia. S. sisarum is cultivated for its tuberous roots.

Sium erectum

This species is said to have irritant properties (Pammel 1911).

Sium latifolium
Water Parsnip

From Australia, Hurst (1942) states that the plant is reported to produce skin irritation in the United States.

References

Hurst, E. (1942) The poison plants of New South Wales. N.S.W. Poison Plants Committee; Sydney.

Pammel, L.H. (1911) A Manual of poisonous Plants. Torch Press. Cedar Rapids, Iowa. Reprinted Univ. Microfilms Inc. Ann Arbor, Mich. 1965.

Tribe: Ammineae

Sphenosciadium

One species is found in the western United States.

Sphenosciadium capitelulatum

The root was used for medicinal purposes (French 1971). Nielsen (1971) records six linear furanocoumarins from S. capitellatum (sic),

References

French, D.H. (1971) Ethnobotany of the Umbelliferae in The Biology and Chemistry of the Umbelliferae. ed. Heywood, V.H. Supp. 1 to Bot. J. Linnaean Soc. Vol. 64 London. Academic Press. pp. 385-412.

Nielsen, B.E. (1971) Coumarin patterns in the Umbelliferae in The Biology and Chemistry of the Umbelliferae. ed. Heywood, V.H. London. Academic Press.

Tribe: Laserpitieae

Thapsia

Six species are found in the Mediterranean region.

Thapsia sp.

Various forms of this plant from which a plaster is made have produced dermatitis of the hands and face (White 1934).

Thapsia garganica

Theophrastus (370-285? B.C.) noted that druggists and herb-diggers recommended standing to windward when cutting this plant, 'for that one's body will swell up if one stands the other way.' The juice irritates and causes swelling of the hands and face of workmen employed in making an extract of the plant. Its acrid principle is a resin which causes severe itching vesication and ulceration with scarring when applied to the skin (Dispensatory 1884 cited by White 1887). An alcoholic solution of the resin is strongly rubefacient (Courchet 1882). Irritation by medicinal applications was noted by three authors cited by Piffard (1881), by Sabouraud (1900) and Lacassagne and Joly (1927).

Thapsia villosa

This species is irritant (Pammell 1911).

References

Courchet, L. (1881) Les Ombelliferes en general et les especes usitees en pharmacie en particulier.

Montpellier: Imprimerie Cristin, Serre and Ricome, 221 (+10) pp.

Dispensatory, U.S. cited by White (1887).

Lacassagne, J. and Joly, H. (1927) La Jambe de Dieu. - Les ulceres des gueux au XVI siecle. J. Med. Lyon 8, 177, 197.

Pammel, L.H. (1911) A Manual of Poisonous plants. Torch Press. Cedar Rapids, Iowa. Reprinted Univ. Microfilms Inc. Ann Arbor, Mich. 1965.

Piffard, H.C. (1881) A treatise on the Materia Medica and Therapeutics of the Skin. New York. Wm. Wood and Co.

Theophrastus (370-285? B.C.) Enquiry into Plants. English transl. by Hort, A. (1916) 2 vols. London. Wm. Heinemann Lts.

Sabouraud (1900) Etude clinique et bacteriol. de l'impetigo. Ann. de Dermat. cited by Touton (1932).

Touton, K. (1932) Hauterkrankungen durch phanerogamische Pflanzen und ihre Produkte (Toxicodermia et Allergodermia phytogenes), in Barnewitz, J. et al, Angeborene Anomalien, Lichtdermatosen, Pflanzengifte, Thermische Schadigungen, influss Innerer Storungen auf die Haut. Berlin, Verlag von Julius Springer.

White, J.C. (1887) Dermatitis venenata; An account of the action of external irritants upon the skin. Boston. Cupples and Hurd.

White, R.P. (1934) The Dermatergoses or Occupational Affections of the Skin. 4th ed. London. H.K. Lewis.

Tribe: ?

Torilis

15 species are found in the Canary Islands and from the Mediterranean region to eastern Asia.

Torilis japonicus

The plant is known to cause a skin rash in 'susceptible' persons when wet (Altschul 1973).

Reference

Altschul, S. von R. (1973) Drugs and foods from little-known plants. Cambridge, Mass. Harvard Univ. Press.

Tribe: ?

Umbellularia

One species is found in California.

Umbellularia californica
California Bay, Laurel or Olive

Inhalation of the pungent emanations of this plant produces violent sneezing (Wodehouse 1971).

Reference

Wodehouse, R.P. (1971) Hayfever plants. 2nd Rev. ed. New York. Hafner Publ. Co.

URTICACEAE

550 species in 45 genera are found in tropical and temperate regions. Stinging hairs are found in genera of the tribe Urticeae.

Airy Shaw (1973) gives the following classification:

A. With stinging hairs.
   1. Urticeae (Urereae): Urtica, Urera, Laportea.

B. No stinging hairs.
   2. Procrideae. Pilea, Pellionia, Elatostema.
   3. Boehmerieae: Boehmeria, Maoutia.
   4. Parietarieae: Parietaria.
   5. Forskohleeae: Forskohlea.
   6. Conchocephaleae: Poikilospermum, Cecropia.

Chemistry is recorded by Hegnauer (1966).

Boehmeria

100 species are found in tropical and northern subtropical regions. *B. nivea* is cultivated for fibre.

Boehmeria platyphylla

This species yields cryptopleurine which has vesicant properties (Johns et al 1970). This chemical has also been isolated from *Cryptocarya*.

Cecropia

100 species are native to tropical America.

Cecropia spp.

The plants possess stinging hairs, a milky caustic sap and are often inhabited by stinging ants (Allen 1943, Martinez 1969). Shaw (1973) states that this genus belongs to a tribe without stinging hairs.

References

Allen, P.H. (1943) Poisonous and Injurious Plants of Panama. Am. J. Trop. Med. Suppl. 23, 1.

Hegnauer, R. (1966) Chemotaxonomy of plants. Vol. 4. Basel, Birkhauser.

Johns. S.R., Lamberton, J.A., Sioumis, A.A. and Willing, R.I. (1970) New alkaloids from *Cryptocarya pleurosperma* (Lauraceae). Aust. J. Chem. 23, 353.

Martinez, M. (1969) The Medicinal Plants of Mexico. 5th ed. (Quinta edicion 5th Mexican language). Mexico City. Andres Botas.

Shaw, H.K.A. (1973) A Dictionary of the Flowering Plants and Ferns. (the late J.C. Willis) 8th ed. Cambridge University Press.

Dendrocnide

70 species are found in tropical and subtropical regions.

Dendrocnide spp.

Several species are known to sting violently producing urticaria and shock (Everist 1972).

Fleurya (syn. *Laportea*)

Several species are known to possess stinging hairs (Pardo-Castello 1923, Allen 1943, Watt and Breyer-Brandwijk 1962, Behl et al 1966).

Girardinia

Eight species native to tropical Africa, Madagascar, eastern Asia and Indo Malaysia possess stinging hairs (Shaw 1973, Behl et al 1966). *G. heterophylla* yields histamine and 5-hydroxytryptamine (Saxena et al 1964) and acetylcholine' (Saxena et al 1966).

Girardinia zeylanica

The plant yields a fibre which has been used for making clothes, with unpleasant results, owing to the extreme difficulty experienced in entirely removing the stinging principles, even in the severe processes to which the plant is subjected in order to extract the fibre (Smith 1920).

Gyrotaenia

Six species are found in the West Indies.

Gyrotaenia spp.

Stinging hairs are known in species of this genus (Thurston and Larsten 1969).

Hesperocnide

Two species native to Hawaii and California possess stinging hairs (Hardin and Arena 1969, Abrams 1955).

Stinging hairs are known in species of this genus (Thurston and Lersten 1969).

References

Abrams, L. (1955) Illustrated Flora of the Pacific States. Stanford, Calif. Stanford University Press.

Allen, P.H. (1943) Poisonous and Injurious Plants of Panama. Am. J. Trop. Med. Suppl. 23, 1.

Behl, P.N., Captain, R.M., Bedi, B.M.A. and Gupta, S. (1966) Skin-irritant and sensitizing plants found in India, New Delhi. P.N. Behl, Irwin Hospital.

Everist, S.L. (1972) Queensland Herbarium, Brisbane, Australia. Personal communication concerning plants recorded in Australia as having caused dermatitis or other contact injury to man or livestock.

Hardin, J.W. and Arena, J.M. (1969) Human Poisoning from native and cultivated plants. Durham, North Carolina. Duke University Press.

Pardo-Castello, V. (1923) Dermatitis venenata. Arch. Derm. Syph. 7, 80.

Saxena, P.R., Kishor, K., Pant, M.C. and Bhargava, K.P. (1964) Pharmacologically active constituents of Girardinia heterophylla (Dcne) J. Pharm. Pharmacol. 16, 361.

Shaw, H.K.A. (1973) A Dictionary of the Flowering Plants and Ferns. 8th ed. (the late J.C. Willis) Cambridge University Press.

Watt, J.M. and Breyer-Brandwijk, M.G. (1962) The Medicinal and poisonous plants of Southern Africa. 2nd ed. Edinburgh. E.& S. Livingstone.

Saxena, P.R., Tangri, K.K. and Bhargava, K.P. (1966) Identification of acetylcholine, histamine, and 5-hydroxytryptamine in Girardinia heterophylla Canad. J. Physiol.Pharmacol. 44, 621.

Smith, E.P. (1920) Plant Dermatitis. I. Journal of Botany 58, 130: II, 58, 173.

Thurston, E.L. and Lersten, N.R. (1969) The morphology and toxicology of plant stinging hairs. Botan. Rev. 35, 393.

Laportea

23 species are found in tropical and subtropical regions and in temperate eastern Asia, north-eastern America, southern Africa and Madagascar.

Laportea spp.
Nettle Tree

Some species become bushes to 8m high or trees to 40m high. The stinging hairs can affect animals or humans. Airborne hairs from the dried leaves can produce respiratory symptoms. Dead plants 60 years old have been reported to be capable of producing urtication. The hairs have siliceous tips which break off under the skin. Macfarlane (1963) reviewed the literature and his own work on the physiochemical properties of the pharmacologically active substances of Laportea and other plants of this family. Laportea differs from Urtica in producing intense pain which persists for weeks or months. Skin effects were described by Uchida and Norikane (1936) and Imschenetzky (1928).

The pain-producing substance is not acetylcholine, histamine or 5-hydroxytryptamine but a non-dialysable substance of unknown composition.

References

Macfarlane, W.V. (1963) The stinging properties of Laportea. Econ. Bot. 17, 303.

Urchida, C. and Norikane, S. (1936) The pathology of dermatitis caused by 'Iranoki" (Laportea pterostidua weed), Indigenous plant of Formosa. J. Med. Ass. Formosa. 35, 1958.

Imschenetzky, A. (1928) Laportea dermatitis. Experimentelle Untersuchungen Dermat. Wschr. 89, 1087-1094.

The following species have been reported to produce stinging:

Laportea canadensis
(Wood Nettle)
Eastern North America

L. cordifolia
Australia

L. crenulata
(Devil Nettle)
India

L. gigas
(Giant Stinging Tree)
Australia

L. moroides
(Gympie Bush)
Eastern Austraila

L. photiniphylla
(Stinging Tree)
Eastern Australia

L. pterostidua
(Man biting Dog)
Formosa

L. pustulosa
Malaysia

L. stimulans
Java

L. subclausa

L. terminalis
India

The locations are those of the authors.

Nanocnide

Four species are found in eastern Asia.

Nanocnide spp.

Stinging hairs are known in species of this genus (Thurston and Lersten 1969).

Reference

Thurston, E.L. and Lersten, N.R. (1969) The morphology and toxicology of plant stinging hairs. Botan. Rev. 35, 393.

Obetia

Five species are found in tropical Africa, Madagascar and Reunion.

Obetia spp.

Stinging hairs are known in species of this genus (Thurston and Lersten 1969).

Reference

Thurston, E.L. and Lersten, N.F. (1969) The morphology and toxicology of plant stinging hairs. Botan. Rev. 35, 393.

Parietaria

30 species are found in temperate and tropical regions.

Parietaria officinalis

The pollen is reported to cause hayfever in Europe (Wodehouse 1971).

Reference

Wodehouse, R.P. (1971) Hayfever Plants. 2nd. rev. edition. New York, Hafner.

Scepocarpus
(syn. Urera)

Scepocarpus spp.

Stinging hairs are known in species of this genus (Thurston and Lersten 1969).

Reference

Thurston, E.L. and Lersten, N.R. (1969) The morphology and toxicology of plant stinging hairs. Botan. Rev. 35, 393.

Sceptrocnide
(syn. Laportea)

Sceptrocnide spp

Stinging hairs are known in species of this genus (Thurston and Lersten 1969).

Reference

Thurston, E.L. and Lersten, N.R. (1969) The morphology and toxicology of plant stinging hairs. Botan. Rev. 35, 393.

Urera

35 species are found in Hawaii, warm America, tropical and southern Africa and Madagascar.

The following species have been reported to produce stinging:

Urera baccifera
(Ortiga)
Central America, Virgin Islands.

U. cameroonensis
East Africa

U. caracasana
Venezuela

U. dominguensis
Central America

U. mannii
East Africa

U. oblongifolia
East Africa

U. obovata
East Africa

U. repens
East Africa

U. rigida
(syn. U. elliotii)
East Africa

U. robusta
East Africa

U. tenax
South Africa

The locations are those of the authors.

Urtica

Most of 50 species are found in north temperate regions, a few in tropical and south temperate regions. The American and European species produce less severe stinging than those growing in the East Indies. Urtication was practiced for the treatment of certain diseases and consisted of beating the skin with a bunch of nettles. The result was erythma and whealing but after the third or fourth successive application, the skin ceased to react under fresh contact (White 1887). The literature of the physico-chemical properties of the pharmacologically active substances was reviewed by Macfarlane (1962). Acetylcholine, histamine and 5-hydroxytryptamine have been implicated in itching from the stinging hairs (Emmelin and Feldburg 1947, Pilgrim 1959, Saxena et al 1965). The hairs are described by Thurston and Lersten (1969), Uphof and Hummeh (1962).

The stinging hairs consist of a long stiff shaft, narrowing towards the point, and provided with a small bulbous tip. The portion of the shaft immediately under this tip is not thickened and silicified like the rest, so that a very slight touch is sufficient to break off the bulbous end. The tip breaks off at a slant, leaving a finely pointed hollow shaft, like the needle of a hypodermic syringe, which makes a puncture in the skin through which the secretion can enter (Smith 1920).

Reference

Smith, E.P. (1920) Plant Dermatitis. I. Journal of Botany 58, 130: II, 58, 173.

The following species have been reported to cause stinging:

Urtica chamaedryoides
United States

U. crenulata
United States

U. dioica
(common Nettle)
United States, Australia, South Africa, India

U. echinata

U. ferox
New Zealand

U. gracilis
United States

U. holosericea
Australia

U. hyperborea
India

U. incisa
Australia

U. lobulata
South Africa

U. lyallii
North America

U. parviflora
India

U. pilulifera
India, South Africa

U. purpurascens
United States

U. stimulans
United States

U. urens
Europe, United States, Australia, South Africa

U. urentissima
United States

The locations are those of the authors. Some have been introduced elsewhere, e.g. U. dioica and U. urens, common nettles of Europe.

References

Emmelin, N. and Feldburg, W. (1947) The mechanism of the sting of the common nettle (Urtica dioica). J. Physiol. 106, 440.

Macfarlane, W.V. (1963) The stinging properties of Laportea. Econ. Bot. 17, 303.

Pilgrim, R.L.C. (1959) Some properties of the sting of the New Zealand nettle (Urtica ferox). Proc. Roy. Soc. London Ser. B. 151, 48.

Saxena, P.R., Pant, M.C., Kishar, K. and Bhargava, K.P. (1965) Pharmacologically active constituents of Urtica parviflora (Roxb.) Can. J. Physiol. Pharmacol. 43, 869.

Thurston, E.L. and Lersten, N.L. (1969) The morphology and toxicology of plant stinging hairs. Botan. Rev. 35, 393.

Uphof, J.C. and Hummeh, K. (1962) Plant hairs in Encyclopedia of Plant Anatomy. volume 4, part 5. ed. W. Zimmerman and P.G. Ozenda. Gebruden Borntraeger. Berlin-Nikolassee.

White, J.C. (1887) Dermatitis venenata: An account of the Action of External irritants upon the Skin. Boston. Cupples and Hurd.

Urtica dioica

The structure of the stinging hairs was described by Thurston (1974).

Reference

Thurston, E.L. (1974) Morphology, fine structure, and ontogeny of the stinging emergence of Urtica dioica. Amer. J. Bot. 61, 809.

VALERIANACEAE

400 species in 13 genera are found in Europe, Asia, Africa and America.

Chemistry is recorded by Hegnauer (1973).

Valeriana

Over 200 species are found in Eurasia, southern Africa, temperate North America and the Andes.

Valeriana capensis

The root is used externally as an irritant (Watt and Breyer-Brandwijk 1962).

Valeriana officinalis
Valerian, Setwall, All-Heal

The root has a strong disagreeable flavour. Oil of Valerian is derived from the plant which has been used in Herbal Medicine from ancient times (Wren 1968, Merck Index 1968). Bateman (1817) observed vesicular and pustular reactions from the local irritation of Valerian root.

Valeriana septentrionalis

Valeriana sitchensis

The plants mixed with bear grease are used for a hair-perfume (Smith 1928).

References

Bateman, T. (1817) Delineations of cutaneous diseases: exhibiting the characteristic appearance of the principal genera and species comprised in the classification of the late Dr. Willan; and completing the series of engravings begun by that author. London, Longman, Hurst, Rees & Co. viii, 721 p 72 col plates.

Hegnauer, R. (1973) Chemotaxonomy of Plants. Voo. 6. Basel. Birkhauser Verlag, p. 638.

Merck Index (1968) An Encyclopedia of Chemicals and Drugs. ed. Stecher, P.G. 8th ed. Rahway, N.J. Merck and Co. Inc.

Smith, H.I. (1928) Materia Medica of the Bella Coola and neighbouring tribes of British Columbia. Bull. No. 56 National Museum of Canada. Ottawa. King's Printer.

Watt, J.M. and Breyer-Brandwijk, M.G. (1962) The Medicinal and Poinsous Plants of Southern Africa. 2nd ed. Edinburgh. E.& S. Livingstone.

Wren, R.W. (1968) Potter's New Cyclopaedia of Botanical Drugs and Preparations by Wren, R.C. Re-edit. by Wren, R.W. Potter and Clarke Ltd. Health Science Press. Rustington, Sussex.

VERBENACEAE

3000 species in 75 genera are almost all tropical and subtropical. Some are armed with thorns.

Aloysia citriodora provides an oil used in perfumery (Wren 1968).

Chemistry is recorded by Hegnauer (1973).

References

Hegnauer, R. (1973) Chemotaxonomy of Plants. Vol. 6. Basel. Birkhauser Verlag, p. 658.

Wren, R.W. (1968) Potter's New Cyclopaedia of Botanical Drugs and Preparations by Wren, R.C. Re-edit. by Wren, R.W. Potter and Clarke Ltd. Health Science Press. Rustington, Sussex.

Clerodendrum
(syn. Clerodendron)

400 species are found in tropical and subtropical regions.

Clerodendron

Some species of this genus are said to yield poisonous honey (Pammel 1911).

Clerodendron aculeatum
Crab Prickle

This species produces mechanical injury (Oakes and Butcher 1962).

Clerodendrum fistulosum

The hollow internodes are inhabited by ants (Shaw 1973).

References

Oakes, A.J. and Butcher, J.O. (1962) Poisonous and injurious plants of the U.S. Virgin Islands. Misc. Publ. 882, U.S. Dept. of Agriculture, Wash., D.C.

Pammel, L.H. (1911) A Manual of Poisonous Plants. Torch Press. Cedar Rapids, Iowa. Reprinted Univ. Microfilms Inc. Ann Arbor, Mich. 1965.

Shaw, H.K.A. (1973) A Dictionary of the Flowering Plants and Ferns. (the late J.C. Willis) 8th ed. Cambridge University Press.

Gmelina

Two species are found in tropical Africa and Madagascar, 33 species in eastern Asia, Indo-Malaysia and Australia.

Gmelina elliptica
(syn. G. villosa)
Common Bulang

This species which finds several uses in Malayan native medicine (Corner 1952) is capable of producing mechanical injury by its thorns.

Reference

Corner, E.J.H. (1952) Wayside Trees of Malaysia. Singapore, Government Printer.

Lantana

150 species are found in America, the West Indies and

southern Africa. Some species have edible fruit.

Lantana camara
Common Lantana, Yellow Sage

This species forms a garden shrub or hedge in Australia and is grown as an annual in colder climates. Acute poisoning by ingestion in animals, takes the form of 'pink-nose' with reddening of the muzzle and conjunctivitis, and severe gastroenteritis with death in as short a time as 3-5 days (Hurst 1942). In chronic poisoning, signs of photosensitisation appear if the animal is exposed to sunlight. One pound of dried mature leaves can produce sensitisation in a 400 lb. steer. Non pigmented skin without hair shows the first evidence of the disease; pigmented skin covered with black hair may never become involved. The skin of the muzzle, ear, neck, shoulders, legs, or other parts of the body becomes yellow, swollen, hard, cracked, and painful. The skin often peels, leaving large exposed raw areas. Areas of inflammation extend to the adjacent mucous membranes of the mouth and nasal passages. Affected animals refuse food, drool saliva from the mouth, and lose weight. The skin and membranes surrounding the eyes may become affected, as well as the eyeball itself (Oakes and Butcher 1962).

The compound responsible is a polycyclic triterpenoid named lantadene A identical in structure with rehmannic acid, the active principle in Lippia. Hepatogenous photosensitisation results from liver damage by lantadene A leading to accumulation of phylloerthrin (a normal breakdown product of chlorophyll) in the blood. Phylloerythrin has photosensitising properties (Kingsbury 1964).

In humans, contact with the prickly plant is reported to cause dermatitis (Morton 1962). The aromatic leaves are used to make a tea (Watt and Breyer-Brandwijk 1962).

References

Hurst, E. (1942) The Poison Plants of New South Wales. N.S.W. Poison Plants Committee, Sydney.

Kingsbury, J.M. (1964) Poisonous Plants of the United States and Canada. Englewood Cliffs, New Jersey. Prentice-Hall Inc.

Morton, J.F. (1962) Ornamental Plants with poisonous Properties II. Proc. Florida Hort. Soc. 75, 484.

Oakes, A.J. and Butcher, J.O. (1962) Poisonous and injurious plants of the U.S. Virgin Islands. Misc. Publ. 882. U.S. Dept. of Agriculture, Washington, D.C.

Watt, J.M. and Breyer-Brandwijk, M.G. (1962) The Medicinal and Poisonous Plants of Southern Africa. 2nd ed. Edinburgh. E.& S. Livingstone.

Lippia

220 species are found in tropical America and Africa.

The leaves of L. citriodora yield an aromatic oil used in perfumery under the name Verbena Oil. Verbena oil is also a name for Lemongrass oil (Cymbopogon).

The dried leaves of Lippia (as well as Origanum, Labiatae, and other genera) enters into the composition of the spice Oregano which is an ingredient of curry powder. The increased consumption of pizza has stimulated the use of Oregano which was practically unknown in the United States until after World War II (Collins 1969).

Lippia spp.
especially L. rehmanni

Several species have been reported to evoke hepatogenous photosensitisation in animals. The active principle is rehmannic acid which causes liver damage and the accumulation of phylloerythrin (a normal breakdown product of chlorophyll) in the blood. Phylloerythrin has photosensitising properties. The symptoms in animals are similar to those of the photosensitisation syndrome produced by ingestion of Lantana and Tribulus (Watt and Breyer-Brandwijk 1962).

These authors reviewed the plant species which have been incriminated and suspected. Photosensitisation may appear in shorn animals on the second or third day after experimental feeding.

Lippia javanica

The leaf and stem have been used to make a tea in southern Africa; the leaf is variously described as having the odour of vanilla or of mint. The Zulu drink an infusion of the leaf for medicinal purposes. Ingestion results in photosensitisation in animals (Watt and Breyer-Brandwijk 1962). Photosensitisation has not been reported in man.

Lippia nodiflora

The seeds stick on touch to clothes and animal skin.

Lippia scaberimma

An infusion of the leaf which is lemon scented is taken as a tonic by the Zulu people. Among Dutch people in South Africa, brandy in which the leaf has been soaked is used as a stomachic and tonic. A cloth dipped in a decoction of the plant is applied as a counter-irritant for backache, the application producing a severe and painful dermatitis (Watt and Breyer-Brandwijk 1962).

References

Collins, M. (1969) Spices of the World Cookbook. Baltimore, Maryland. McCormick.

Watt, J.M. and Breyer-Brandwijk, M.G. (1962) The Medicinal and Poisonous Plants of Southern Africa. 2nd ed. Edinburgh. E.& S. Livingstone.

Tectona

Three species are native to Indo Malaysia.

Chemistry is recorded by Thomson (1971) and Sandermann and Simatupang (1966).

Tectona grandis
Teak, teck, djati

This tree is grown in India and Java etc. for its timber. T. grandis found in south-eastern Asia and Malaysia is the true teak; two lesser species T. tenuifolia found in Burma and T. philippinensis found in the northern Phillipine Islands are also named teak. The wood sinks in water unless thoroughly dried; this is effected in India by the process of 'girdling' which consists in removing a ring of bark and sapwood from the tree near its base. It soon dies and is left standing for two years (Shaw 1973). The tree possesses an essential oil which fills the pores of the wood and makes it extremely durable. The wood has been found well preserved in temples in western India that have been standing for over 2000 years (Garratt 1922). Teak leaves are rough and are used for polishing wood in Java (Burkill 1935). Afrormosia and Chlorophora are sometimes named teak (Krogh 1962).

Teak was reported as a cause of dermatitis in 1896 (Anon 1896), and Evans (1905) described the case of a carpenter who had dermatitis of the exposed skin after working with teak and relapsed on using it again 10 years later. Other workers exposed to the fine dust were affected. John (1913) described dermatitis in six patients and obtained positive patch test reactions with the sawdust and an alcoholic extract, negative reactions in control subjects. Many subsequent reports were reviewed by Hoffman (1926). A shipwright developed vesicular dermatitis of the hands, forearms, neck and genitals. He was given a piece of freshly sawn Rangoon teak to hold in his hand for one hour and developed dermatitis of the dorsa of the hands and subsequently disseminated dermatitis (Hunt 1931). Krogh (1962, 1964) gave a detailed report of an outbreak of dermatitis in a furniture factory, and showed that patch tests with moist teak sawdust often gave false positive reactions. Mechanical and chemical irritation seemed to play a part, as well as allergic sensitisation. Installation of adequate dust extraction reduced the incidence of dermatitis from 20 to 8% in the factory he studied.

Lapachol and lapachonone, known as sensitizers of Tabebuia and Paratecoma, were found in

Tectona wood (Sandermann and Dietrichs 1959, Sandermann and Simatupang 1961, 1962, 1966) and Schulz (1962) showed that teak-sensitive patients reacted to lapachol. Tectoquinone produced negative reactions but the possibility of other sensitizers in the wood could not be ruled out. Later, Schulz (1965, 1967) found that desoxylapachol gave much stronger patch test reactions and was probably the principal sensitizer in teak and in Tabebuia. Indonesian natives have long distinguished three grades of the wood, the poorest (Djati sempoerna) being liable to cause skin irritation (Altona 1924) and Hausen (1970) noted that local races of teak and even individual trees vary greatly in desoxylapachol content. Teak is among the six commoner causes of dermatitis from woods in France (Zafiropoulo et al 1968) and the commonest wood to produce dermatitis at St. John's Hospital, London (Woods and Calnan 1976). They reported 44 cases of dermatitis from teak; most were wood-workers, one a butcher who handled teak sawdust at work and did woodwork as a hobby, another a painter who rubbed down some teak wood with sandpaper.

Some of the in patients reacted to other woods. Contact sensitivity in a cabinet-maker to teak, and to Turreanthus and Juglans (Calnan 1970) probably indicated multiple specific sensitivity. Krogh (1964) found that 9 of 13 furniture makers who had contact dermatitis from teak showed positive patch test reactions to lapachol 2% in acetone; seven reacted to lapachol 1% in acetone. Teak wood dust is often irritant by patch test; for patch testing 1 gramme of dust in methyl ethyl ketone is satisfactory (Morgan et al 1968).

References

Altona, T. (1924) Djati en Hindoes. Tectona 17, 865.

Anon (1896) A skin affection produced by working in teak. Lancet 1, 1113, 1193 and 1265.

Hausen, B.M. (1970) Untersuchungen uber Gesundheitsschadigende Holzer. Thesis, Hamburg.

Hoffmann, H. (1926) Uber Hautentzundungen nach Teakholzbearbeitung Zentralblatt fur Gewerbehygiene, NF 3, 333.

John (1913) Dermatitis nach Teakholzbearbeitung Aerzliche Sachverstandigen-Zeitung 8, 170.

Sandermann, W. and Dietrichs, H.H. (1959) Ueber die Inhalsstoffe von Mansonia altissima und ihre gesundheitsschadigende Wirkung. Holz als Roh-und Werkstoff 17, 88.

Sandermann, W. and Simatupang, M.H. (1961) Zur chemie der Teaks, eines ungewohnlichen Holzes. Chemikerzeitung 85, 38.

Sandermann, W. and Simatupang, M.H. (1962) Ein toxisches Chinon aus Teakholz. Angewandte Chemie 74, 782.

Schulz, K.H. (1965) Allergische Kontaktdermatitis durch tropische Holzer. Dermatologica Internationalis 4, 121.

Schulz, K.H. (1967) Berufsdermatosen -ausgewahlte Kapitel. Zeit, Haut. Geschlech. 42, 499.

Woods, B. and Calnan, C.D. (1976) Toxic Woods. Brit. J. Derm. 94, Suppl. 13, June.

Burkill, I.H. (1935) A dictionary of the Economic Products of the Malay Peninsula. 2 Vols. London. Crown Agents for the Colonies.

Calnan, C.D. (1970) Avodiré wood sensitivity. Contact Dermatitis Newsletter (London) 8, 190.

Evans, W. (1905) A note on Teak dermatitis. Brit. J. Derm. 17, 447.

Garratt, G.A. (1922) Poisonous Woods. J. Forestry 20, 479.

Hausen, B.M. (1973) Holzarten mit gesundheitsschadigenden Inhaltsstoffen. DRW-Verlags-GmbH. Stuttgart.

Hoffman, H. (1926) Ueber Teakholz-Dermatitis. Klin. Wchnschr. 5, 578.

Hunt, E. (1931) A case of teakwood dermatitis. Lancet 1, 75.

Krogh, H.K. (1962) Contact eczema caused by true teak (Tectona grandis). Brit. J. Industr. Med. 19, 42.

Krogh, H.K. (1964) Contact eczema caused by true teak (Tectona grandis). A follow-up study of a previous epidemiological investigation, and a study into the sensitizing effect of various teak extracts. Brit. J. Indust. Med. 21, 65.

Morgan, J.W.W., Orsler, R.J. and Wilkinson, D.S. (1968) Dermatitis due to the wood dusts of Khaya anthotheca and Macherium scleroxylon. Br. J. Ind. Med. 25, 119.

Sandermann, W. and Simatupang, M.H. (1966) Zur Chemie und Biochemie des Teakholzes (Tectona grandis L). Holz Roh-Werkst. 24, 190.

Schulz, K.H. (1962) Untersuchung uber die sensibilisierende Wirkung von Inhaltsstoffen exotischer Holzer. Berufsderm. 10, 17.

Schulz, K.H. (1962) Chemische Struktur und allergene Wirking. Aulendorf i. Wurtt. Editio Cantor, K.G.

Shaw, H.K.A. (1973) A Dictionary of the Flowering Plants and Ferns. (the late J.C. Willis) 8th ed. Cambridge University Press.

Thompson, R.H. (1971) Naturally occurring Quinones. 2nd ed. London Academic Press.

Zafiropoulo, A., Audibert, A. and Charpin, J. (1968) A propos des accidents dus a la manipulation des bois exotiques. Rev. Franc. Allerg. 8, 155.

Teijsmanniodendron (syn. Teysmanniodendron)

Fourteen species are found in Southern Indo China and Malaysia.

Teysmanniodendron pteropodium

The wood ashes cause itching (Altschul 1973).

Reference

Altschul, S. von R. (1973) Drugs and foods from little-known plants. Cambridge, Mass. Harvard Univ. Press.

Verbena

250 species are found in tropical and temperate regions of America, two or three species in the old World. Oil of Verbena is derived from Lippia.

Verbena hastata

This species can produce dermatitis (Pammel 1911).

Verbena officinalis
Vervain, Wild Vervena

The plant was formerly used for eye diseases (Wren 1968). The fresh leaves are used as a rubefacient (Quisumbing 1951). The statement that the plant has irritant properties (Pammel 1911) is open to doubt (Watt and Breyer-Brandwijk 1962). Shelmire (1939) states that the plant can cause acute dermatitis similar to that caused by Toxicodendron. An extract of the plant produced a positive patch test reaction in one of 50 patients who had 'weed dermatitis' (Shelmire 1940).

Verbena venosa

This species can produce dermatitis (Pammel 1911).

References

Pammel, L.H. (1911) A Manual of Poisonous Plants. Torch Press. Cedar Rapids, Iowa. Reprinted Univ. Microfilms Inc. Ann Arbor, Mich., 1965.

Shelmire, B. (1939) Contact Dermatitis from Weeds; Patch Testing with Their Oleoresins. JAMA 113, 1085.

Shelmire, B. (1940) Contact dermatitis from vegetation. South Med. J. 33, 338.

Watt, J.M. and Breyer-Brandwijk, M.G. (1962) The Medicinal and Poisonous Plants of Southern Africa. 2nd ed. Edinburgh. E.& S. Livingstone.

Wren, R.W. (1968) Potter's New Cyclopaedia of Botanical Drugs and Preparations by Wren, R.C. Re-edit. by Wren, R.W. Potter and Clarke Ltd. Health Science Press. Rustington, Sussex.

Vitex

250 species are found in tropical and temperate regions.

Vitex trifolia and var. variegata

These aromatic plants, commonly planted as hedges in South Florida, cause respiratory irritation, especially when being trimmed and afterward while the cuttings still are lying on the ground. Some people suffer not only asthma-like symptoms but also dizziness, headaches and nausea. Children sometimes chew the leaves but desist because of the burning taste (Morton 1962).

Vitex littoralis
Puriri, New Zealand teak

The splinters penetrating the hands and feet cause severe inflammation (Aston 1923).

References

Aston, B.C. (1923) The poisonous, suspected and medicinal plants of New Zealand. N.Z. Agricult. J. 26, 78, 149 and 230.

Morton, J.F. (1962) Ornamental Plants with Poisonous Properties II. Proc. Florida Hort. Soc. 75, 484, and (1969) 82, 415.

VIOLACEAE

900 species in 22 genera are cosmopolitan. Chemistry is recorded by Hegnauer (1973).

Viola

500 species are cosmopolitan chiefly north temperate but many Andine.

Viola spp.

Oil of violet derived from V. odorata, V. tricolor and V. pedata can produce dermatitis in hypersensitive individuals (Greenberg and Lester 1954).

Viola odorata
Sweet Violet

Poultices of the leaves are used in Herbal Medicine (Wren 1968). The plant contains a glycoside, gaultherin, which on hydrolysis yields methylsalicylate (Watt and Breyer-Brandwijk 1962). Reactions to salicylate are noted under Betula.

Viola Tricolor
Pansy, Heart's Ease

Piffard (1881) described the use of a decoction of the plant for topical application and occasional irritation from its use.

A decoction of the plant produced dermatitis (Leclerc 1930). The plant is used in Herbal Medicine for moist skin eruptions in children. Preparations of the plant give an offensive odour to the urine and irritation of the skin of the genital area can ensue (Wren 1968). The plant yields methylsalicylate (Watt and Breyer-Brandwijk 1962).

Methyl heptine carbonate used for the production of artificial violet odours is a sensitizer (Tulipan 1938, Whitacre and Parsil 1950, Greenberg and Lester 1951, Klarmann 1958).

References

Greenberg, L.A. and Lester, D. (1954) Handbook of Cosmetic Materials. New York. Interscience.

Hegnauer, R. (1973) Chemotaxonomy of plants. Vol. 6. Basel. Birkhauser Verlag, p. 681.

Klarmann, E.G. (1958) Perfume dermatitis. Ann. Allergy 16, 425.

Leclerc, H. (1930) La pensee sauvage (Viola tricolor L.) dans le traitment des dermatoses. Presse med. No. 76, 1283 cited by Touton (1932).

Touton, K. (1932) Hauterkrankungen durch panerogamische Pflanzen und ihre Produkte (Toxicodermia et Allergodermia phytogenes), in Barnewitz J. et al Angeborene

Anomalien, Lichtdermatosen, Pflanzengifte, Thermische, Schadigungen, Einfluss Innerer Storungen auf die Haut. Berlin. Verlag von Julius Springer.

Tulipan, L. (1938) Cosmetic irritants. Arch. Derm. and Syph. 38, 906.

Watt, J.M. and Breyer-Brandwijk, M.G. (1962) The Medicinal and Poisonous Plants of Southern Africa. 2nd ed. Edinburgh. E.& S. Livingstone.

Whitacre, F.M. and Parsil, R.C. (1950) Cosmetic sensitizers. Ann. Allergy 8, 670.

Wren, R.W. (1968) Potter's New Cyclopaedia of Botanical Drugs and Preparations by Wren, R.C. Re-edit by Wren, R.W. Potter and Clarke Ltd. Health Science Press. Rustington, Sussex.

Piffard, H.G. (1881) A treatise on the Materia Medica and Therapeutics of the skin. New York. Wm. Wood and Co.

VITIDACEAE

700 species in 12 genera are mostly found in tropical and subtropical regions.

Chemistry is recorded by Hegnauer (1973).

Reference

Hegnauer, R. (1973) Chemotaxonomy of Plants. Vol. 6. Basel. Birkhauser Verlag, p. 689.

Ampelocissus

95 species are found in tropical regions.

Ampelocissus arnottiana
(syn. Vitis indica)
Indian Grape Vine

The tubers are acrid when fresh and the fruits are inedible possibly from the presence of calcium oxalate crystals (Behl et al 1966).

Reference

Behl, P.N., Captain, R.M. Bedi, B.M.S. and Gupta, S. (1966) Skin-irritant and sensitizing plants found in India, New Delhi. P.N. Behl, Irwin Hospital.

Ampelopsis

Two species are found in temperate and subtropical regions of Asia and America.

Ampelopsis quinquefolia
Virginia Creeper

Dermatitis from Virginia creeper was reported by Burd (1891) and Palm (1891). It is possible that the plant incriminated was actually poison ivy (Toxicodendron) (Harrison 1906, Walker 1911, White 1928, Davies 1939), or Hedera (Turton 1925).

According to Smith (1920), Toxicodendron (Rhus toxicodendron) was put on the market in recent years as an ornamental plant under the trade-name of "Ampelopsis Hoggii," owing to a general resemblance to the North American Ampelopsis quinquefolia, Virginian Creeper, of commerce, from which it can be distinguished at once by having three instead of five leaflets in its compound leaf. Masquerading under this name, the plant was employed as a decorative climber by many unfortunate people, some of whom suffered severely for their ignorance.

References

Burd, E.L. (1891) Eczema caused by Virginia creeper. Lancet 1, 17.

Davies, J.H.T. (1939) Contact dermatitis. Practitioner 142, 636.

Harrison, A.J. (1906) Dermatitis from without and dermatitis from within. Bristol Med. Chir. J. 24, 325.

Palm, W.S. (1891) Eczema caused by Virginian Creeper. Lancet 1, 142.

Turton, P.H.J. (1925) Poisoning by ivy. Brit. Med. J. 2, 294.

Walker, N. (1911) An introduction to Dermatology. 5th ed. Toronto. Macmillan.

White, R.P. (1928) The Dermatergoses or Occupational Affections of the Skin. 3rd ed. London. H.K. Lewis and Co. Ltd.

Cissus

350 species are found in tropical, rarely in subtropical regions.

Cissus antartica

The berries are astringent with a slightly irritative effect (Altschul 1973). Hjorth (1968) recorded three positive patch test reactions to this species; negative reactions were observed in 61 consecutive cases.

Cissus cirrhosa

The fruit is astringent or irritant but nevertheless is eaten by children who seem to become habituated to the astringency (Watt and Breyer-Brandwijk 1962).

Cissus crameriana

Chewing a fragment of leaf produced a burning sensation and dysphagia (Steyn 1949). The fresh leaf yields about 7% oxalic acid but this author was of the opinion that the symptoms which he experienced could not be due to the oxalic acid alone.

Cissus rhombifolia

The sap is said to produce blisters on the skin (Altschul 1973).

Cissus setosa
(syn. Vitis setosa)
Hardy wild-vine

The plant is covered with glandular bristly hairs. Every part of the plant is acrid and the juice is irritant. The macerated leaves are used as a poultice to promote suppuration and to aid in the extraction of the guinea worm (Behl et al 1966).

Cissus unguiformifolius

The fruit is juicy and sweet but produces an unpleasant sensation in the mouth and throat similar to those resulting from chewing a leaf of Colocasia. Oxalates are thought to be responsible for these symptoms (Watt and Breyer-Brandwijk 1962).

References

Altschul, S. von R. (1973) Drugs and foods from little-known plants. Cambridge, Mass. Harvard Univ. Press.

Behl, P.N., Captain, R.M., Bedi, B.M.S. and Gupta, S. (1966) Skin-irritant and sensitizing plants found in India, New Delhi. P.N. Behl, Irwin Hospital.

Hjorth, N. (1968) at Finsen Institute. Pers. communication.

Steyn (1949) cited by Watt and Breyer-Brandwijk (1962).

Watt, J.M. and Breyer-Brandwijk, M.G. (1962) The Medicinal and Poisonous Plants of Southern Africa. 2nd ed. Edinburgh. E.& S. Livingstone.

Parthenocissus

15 species are found in temperate regions of Asia and America.

Parthenocissus quinquefolia
(syn. Ampelopsis quinquefolia)
Virginia Creeper

This plant was reported to cause dermatitis by Grinden (1895) and Harrison (1906). The foliage of this vine, especially in autumn, frequently causes a smarting of the skin in gardeners: cases have been observed in which vesicular eczema has resulted from contact with the plant (Schwartz et al 1957). Probably Toxicodendron was responsible, see Ampelopsis.

This species is also recorded under Vitis hederacea, see Ampelopsis.

References

Grinden (1895) J. of Cutan. Dis April cited by Touton (1932).

Harrison, A.J. (1906) Dermatitis from without and Dermatitis from within. Bristol Med. Chir. J. 24, 325.

Schwartz, L., Tulipan, L. and Birmingham, D.J. (1957) Occupational Diseases of the skin. 3rd ed. Philadelphia. Lea and Febiger.

Touton, K. (1932) Hauterkrankungen durch phanerogamische Phlanzen und ihre Produkte (Toxicodermia et Allergodermia phytogenes), in Barnewitz, J. et al Angeborene Anomalien, Lichtdermatosen, Pflanzengifte, Thermische Schadigungen, Einfluss Innerer Storungen auf die Haut. Berlin. Verlag von Julius Springer.

Rhoïcissus

12 species are found in tropical and southern Africa.

Rhoïcissus sp.

Hjorth (1968) recorded five positive patch test reactions to members of this genus; negative reactions were recorded in 69 consecutive cases.

Reference

Hjorth, N. (1968) at Firsen Institute. Pers. communication.

Vitis

Between 60 and 70 species are found in the northern hemisphere.

Vitis spp.

The leaves and sometimes the roots of various species, used for poulticing in Herbal Medicine, act as slight irritants (Burkill 1935). Some of the Australian species contain calcium oxalate and the fruits have caused severe irritation in the mouths of people who have accidentally eaten them (White 1935).

Vitis hederacea
(syn Ampelopsis quinquefolia)

This species is irritant (Pammel 1911). (see Ampelopsis)

Vitis indica

This species is noted under Ampelocissus arnottiana.

Vitis repens

The fruits are very acid and leave a stinging sensation in the mouth which lasts for 24 hours (Burkill 1935).

Vitis serjanfolia

Dried slices of the roots are used for poulticing in Chinese Medicine (White 1935).

Vitis setosa

This irritant species is noted under Cissus setosa.

Vitis vinifera
Grape vine

The leaf and stem of the grape vine has astringent properties. Shelmire (1940) observed contact dermatitis of the hands in housewives from grapes. The resin on the skin of ripe grapes has been observed in France to cause acute conjunctivitis in those who tend vineyards (Duke-Elder and McFaul 1972). A case of dermatitis from grapes with positive patch test reaction was recorded by Ramirez and Eller (1930). Anderson (1935) reported a case of dermatitis caused by washing grapes. Patch tests with the inside of the grape skin were positive only after the patient had eaten grapes. Spillman and de Lavergne (1926) observed dermatitis from this species. Dermatitis has been reported from insecticides used on grapes (Schwartz et al 1957, Coricciati 1960). Zinc diethyldithiocarbaniate used for this purpose can evoke photodermatitis (Coricciati 1960).

Van Ketel and Tan-Lim (1975) reviewed the literature of dermatitis from alcohol and reported allergic contact dermatitis to ethanol, some lower alphatic alcohols, acetone and some alcoholic drinks.

References

Anderson, J.M. (1935) Dermatitis from Grapes. Arch. Derm. Syph. 31, 658.

Burkill, I.H. (1935) A Dictionary of the Economic Products of the

Malay Peninsula. 2 Vols. London. Crown Agents for the Colonies.

Coricciata, L. (1960) Associated intolerance to anticryptogamic agents in rural workers. Minerva Derm. 35, 65.

Pammel, L.H. (1911) A Manual of Poisonous Plants. Torch Press. Cedar Rapids, Iowa. Reprinted Univ. Microfilms Inc. Ann Arbor, Mich., 1965.

Ramirez, M.A. and Eller, J.J. (1930) The "patch test" in "contact Dermatitis" (Dermatitis venenata). J. Allergy 1, 489.

Schwartz, L., Tulipan, L. and Birmingham, D.J. (1957) Occupational Diseases of the skin. 3rd ed. Philadelphia. Lea and Febiger.

Shelmire, B. (1940) Contact dermatitis from vegetation. South Med. J. 33, 338.

Spillman, and de Lavergne (1926) Presse Med. 81, 1345 Ref. Derm. Swchr. 82, 628 cited by Touton (1932).

Van Ketel, W.G. and Tan-Lim (1975) Contact dermatitis from ethanol. Contact Dermatitis 1, 7.

White, C.T. (1935) Answers to correspondents. Queensland Agr. Jour. 43, 414.

WINTERACEAE

120 species in seven genera are found from Malaysia to the Pacific region, eastern Australia, New Zealand and in Central and South America.

Chemistry is recorded by Hegnauer (1973).

Reference

Hegnauer, R. (1973) Chemotaxonomy of Plants. Vol. 6. Basel. Birkhauser Verlag, p. 700.

Drimys

70 species are used in Borneo, New Guinea, New Caledonia, Australia, Tasmania, New Zealand and South America.

Drimys insipida

Drimys lanceolata

The leaves of these species have an acrid taste causing a burning sensation of the tongue. The seeds and bark are used as a native pepper in Australia (Hurst 1942).

Drimys winteri
Winter's Bark

The bark is known as 'pepper bark' and is very pungent to the taste and astringent (wren 1968). False Winter's Bark is noted under Canella.

References

Hurst, E. (1942) The Poison Plants of New Wouth Wales. N.S.W. Poison Plants Committee; Sydney.

Wren, R.W. (1968) Potter's New Cyclopaedia of Botanical Drugs and Preparations by Wren, R.C. Re-edit. by Wren, R.W. Potter and Clarke Ltd. Health Science Press. Rustington, Sussex.

XANTHORRHOEACEAE

66 species in eight genera are found in Australia, New Caledonia and New Zealand.

Xanthorrhoea

15 species are found in Australia.

Xanthorrhoea hastilis
Black Boy, Grass Tree

A thick yellow sap which exudes around the bases of the old leaves is used in the manufacture of sealing wax, varnish, dyes and picric acid (Menninger 1967). Picric acid, which is also made synthetically, is an irritant and sensitizer.

Reference

Menninger, E.A. (1967) Fantastic Trees. New York. The Viking Press.

ZINGIBERACEAE
Ginger Family

700 species in 45 genera native to tropical regions especially Indo Malaysia are perennial aromatic herbaceous plants with fleshy or tuberous roots. The seeds and oil of Aframomum melegueta (Guinea Grains) are used in flavourint (Fenaroli 1971) and as a condiment (Wren 1968). The ripe fruits of Elettaria cardamomum are known as Cardomums and the seeds provide a spice and perfume known to the Ancient World.

Alpinia
(syn. Languas)

250 species are native to warm regions of Asia and Polynesia.

Alpinia galanga
(syn. Languas galanga)

Contact sensitivity to Laos which is made from the root was observed in a cook who had hand dermatitis. This material is frequently used in Indonesian cooking to prepare "Sateh" (roasted meat on sticks prepared with a special sauce). Positive patch tests in this case were also found with Rhizoma galanga, Djahe (ginger) Rhizoma zingiberis, as well with Balsam of Peru (Myroxylon) (Neering and van Ketel 1974).

Alpinia officinarum
Chinese Ginger

The root of this plant named Galanga root, is officinal. The chemistry is given by Merck (1968). The powdered root is used as a snuff and as a spice (Burkill 1935, Wren 1968). A druggist who accidentally splashed a preparation of Galanga root into his eyes developed keratitis and iritis (Hartmann 1955).

References

Burkill, I.H. (1935) A Dictionary of the Economic Produces of the Malay Peninsula. 2 Vols. London. Crown Agents for the Colonies.

Fenaroli, G. (1971) Fenaroli's Handbook of Flavor Ingredients. ed. Furia, T.E. and Bellanca, N. Cleveland, Ohio. The Chemical Rubber Co.

Hartmann, K. (1955) Corneal injury due to Rhizoma galangae. Klin. Mbl. Augenb. 127, 97.

Mercl Index (1968) An Encyclopedia of Chemicals and Drugs. ed. Stecher, P.G. 8th ed. Rahway, N.J. Merck & Co. Inc.

Neering, H. and van Ketel, W.G. (1974) Allergy from some spices used in Indonesian cooking, symposium on Contact Dermatitis. Gentofte, Denmark. Oct. 26, 27.

Wren, R.W. (1968) Potter's New Cyclopaedia of Botanical Drugs and Preparations by Wren, R.C. Re-edit. by Wren, R.W. Potter and Clarke Ltd. Health Science Press. Rustington, Sussex.

Amomum

150 species are found in tropical regions.

Amomum xanthoides

The plant was observed to have irritant effects (Tsirch 1913). According to Burkill (1935) the species described may have been A. krervanh.

References

Burkill, I.H. (1935) A Dictionary of the Economic Products of the Malay Peninsula. 2 Vols. London. Crown Agents for the Colonies.

Tsirch (1913) Hand b.d. Pharmakogn. 2, 1086 cited by Burkill (1935).

Curcuma

Five species are native to Indo Malaysia and China. The tubers of C. angustifolia provide East Indian Arrowroot. C. zedoaria (Zedoary) is used in the East in perfumery.

Curcuma longa

The dried ground rhizomes provide a spice, turmeric, which gives a yellow colour to pickles and curry. The pungent taste and yellow colour of turmeric are attributed to curcumin which is chemically related to zingerone (Zingiber). Turmeric is harmless as a hair-dye (Greenberg and Lester 1954) but is said to have caused dermatitis when used as a fur dye (Schwartz et al 1957). The aromatic oil derived from the rootstock is irritant to the mucous membranes and intact skin (Behl et al 1966).

References

Behl, P.N., Captain, R.M., Bedi, B.M.S. and Gupta, S. (1966) Skin-irritant and sensitizing plants found in India, New Delhi. P.N. Behl, Irwin Hospital.

Greenberg, L.A. and Lester, D. (1954) Handbook of Cosmetic Materials. New York. Interscience Publishers Inc.

Schwartz, L., Tulipan, L. and Birmingham, D.J. (1957) Occupational Diseases of the Skin. 3rd ed. Philadelphia. Lea and Febiger, pp. 637-672.

Elettaria

Seven species are native to Indo Malaysia.

Elettaria cardamomum
Cardamoms

The plant is cultivated in the mountains of Ceylon and southern India. The ripe fruits are picked and dried; the seeds form a strongly flavoured spice, mainly used in India.

Contact sensitivity to cardamom and to certain terpenoid compounds present in the dried seeds was reported by Mobacken and Fregert (1975).

No evidence has been presented of irritation from Oil of Cardamom in perfumes (Greenberg and Lester 1954).

References

Greenberg, L.A. and Lester, D. (1954) Handbook of Cosmetic Materials. New York. Interscience.

Mobacken, H. and Fregert, S. (1975) Allergic contact dermatitis from cardamom. Contact Dermatitis 1, 175.

Zingiber

80 or 90 species are native to eastern Asia, Indo Malaysia and northern Australia.

Chemistry. The root yields gingerol and gingerone (Merck 1968).

Zingiber amaricans

The rhizome has rubefacient and irritant properties (Burkill 1935).

Zingiber officinalis
Ginger

The rhizomes provide Ginger which can cause dermatitis in workers who prepare it (Behl et al 1966), and in pharmacists (Schwartz et al 1957). When applied to a wound, the rhizome is irritant (Burkill 1935). The dust can cause mechanical irritation (Greenberg and Lester 1954). Oil of Ginger is irritant (Watt and Breyer-Brandwijk 1962) and allergenic (Zundel and Jentsch 1939, Greenberg and Lester 1954). Hjorth (1961) observed that 7 of 20 patients contact sensitive to Balsam of Peru (Myroxylon) showed positive patch test reactions to ginger resinoid, a material stated to be similar to oleoresin of ginger.

Low level phototoxic effects reported for ginger oil are not considered significant (Opdyke 1974).

References

Behl, P.N., Captain, R.M., Bedi, B.M.S. and Gupta, S. (1966) Skin-irritant and sensitizing plants found in India, New Delhi. P.N. Behl, Irwin Hospital.

Burkill, I.H. (1935) A Dictionary of the Economic Products of the Malay Peninsula. 2 Vols. London. Crown Agents for the Colonies.

Greenberg, L.A. and Lester, D. (1954) Handbook of Cosmetic

Materials. New York. Interscience Publishers Inc.

Hjorth, N. (1961) Eczematous Allergy to Balsams, Allied Perfumes and Flavouring Agents. Copenhagen: Munksgaard.

Merck Index (1968) An Encyclopedia of Chemicals and Drugs. ed. Stecher, P.G. 8th ed. Rahway, N.J. Merck & Co. Inc.

Schwartz, L., Tulipan, L. and Birmingham, D.J. (1957) Occupational Diseases of the Skin. 3rd ed. Philadelphia. Lea and Febiger, pp. 637-672.

Watt, J.M. and Breyer-Brandwijk, M.G. (1962) The Medicinal and Poisonous Plants of Southern Africa. 2nd ed. Edinburgh. E.& S. Livingstone.

Zundel, W. and Jentsch, M. (1939) Die allergischen Vorgange beim Backerekzem und ihre Deutung. Arch. Derm. Syph. (Berlin) 178, 469.

Opdyke, D. (1974) Monographs on fragrance raw materials. Fd. Cosmet. Toxicol. 12, 807.

ZYGOPHYLLACEAE

240 species in 25 genera are found in tropical and subtropical regions.

Chemistry is recorded by Hegnauer (1973).

Reference

Hegnauer, R. (1973) Chemotaxonomy of plants. Vol. 6. Basel. Birkhauser. p. 707.

Guaiacum

Six species are found in warm regions of America and the West Indies.

Guaiacum arboreum

The sawdust caused sneezing and was called in French piquenіz (Guibort 1849).

Guaiacum officinale
Lignum vitae

This species yields Lignum vitae wood from which is obtained the medicinal resin guaiacum. The heart-wood has an aromatic and irritating taste. The wood is used to make bowling woods and brush-backs, etc. Frei (1932) described a case of dermatitis which began around a minor finger wound contaminated with lignum vitae sawdust, and spread to the hands and arms. Patch tests to the sawdust gave positive reactions, negative to some other woods and in controls. A case of contact dermatitis from application of tincture of guaicum was reported by White (1897). Guaicol derived from guaiacum has irritant properties (Greenberg and Lester 1954). The resin of the wood yields guaiaretic acid. Sensitivity to nordihydroguaiaretic acid is noted under Larrea.

Guaiacum sanctum
Lignum sanctum

This species has properties similar to those of G. officinale (Wren 1968). Oil of Guaiac wood is derived from Bulnesia (Greenberg and Lester 1954).

References

Greenberg, L.A. and Lester, D. (1954) Handbook of Cosmetic Materials. New York. Interscience.

Schwartz, L., Tulipan, L. and Birmingham, D.J. (1957) Occupational Diseases of the Skin. 3rd ed. Philadelphia. Lea and Febiger. pp. 637-672.

Senear, F.E. (1933) Dermatitis due to woods. JAMA 101, 1527.

White, J.C. (1897) Notes on dermatitis venenata. Boston Med. Surg. J. 136, 77.

Wren, R.W. (1968) Potter's New Cyclopaedia of Botanical Drugs and preparations by Wren, R.C. Re-edit. by Wren, R.W. Potter and Clarke Ltd. Health Science Press. Rustington, Sussex.

Zafiropoulo, A., Audibert, A. and Charpin, J. (1968) A propos des accidents dus a la manipulation des bois exotizues. Rev. Franc. Allerg. 8, 155.

Frei, (1932) Pockholzekzem infolge Sensibilisrierung nach Trauma. Zentralblatt fur Haut-und Geschlechtskrankheiten 41, 29.

Guibort, M.J.-B.G. (1849) Histoire naturelle des Drigues simples. Paris, ailliere cited by Woods and Calnan (1976).

Woods, B. and Calnan, C.D. (1976) Toxic Woods. Brit. J. Derm. 94, Suppl. 13, June.

Kallstroemia

Seven species are found in northern Australia, 16 species from the southern United States and West Indies to Argentina.

Kallstroemia maxima
Greater Caltrop

In an investigation of 'weed dermatitis' in the southern United States, positive patch test reactions to an extract of this plant were observed in three of 50 consecutive patients tested (Shelmire 1939).

Reference

Shelmire, B. (1939) Contact dermatitis from weeds; patch testing with their oleoresins. JAMA 113, 1085.

Larrea
(syn. Covillea)

Two species are found in temperate South America.

Larrea divaricata
(syn. Covillea tridentata)
Creosote Bush

This common native shrub of the deserts of the south-western United States is also cultivated. A gummy secretion makes the leaves look varnished and imparts a distinctive creosote-like odour, especially after rain. A tea is made from the root (Reemtsa and Maloney 1974).

Covillea glutinosa
Creosote Bush

A male developed dermatitis of the face, neck and hands a few hours after gathering the plant. A patch test to the leaf produced a positive reaction, negative in controls (Smith 1937). A man who was employed in preparing the wood for extraction of nordihydroguairetic acid developed dermatitis two weeks after he was first exposed (Weber 1953).

Nordihydroguairetic acid, used as an antioxidant of fats, can cause allergic contact dermatitis (Jorgenson and Hjorth 1970, Hjorth and Roed-Petersen 1976).

The Zygophyllaceae family is closely related to the Rutaceae which contains a Creosote Bush (Dictamnus).

Greasewood noted as a cause of contact dermatitis by Dorsey (1962) may refer to Larrea divaricata but, in California, Sarcobatus vermiculatus and Adenostoma fasciculata are also colliquially named Greasewood (Ayres, S. Jr. 1973, pers. comm.).

References

Dorsey, C.S. (1962) Plant dermatitis in California. Calif. Med. 96, 412.

Jorgensen, G. and Hjorth, N. (1970) Dermatitis from nordihydroguaiaretic acid, an antioxidant in fats. Contact Dermatitis Newsletter, London 7, 151.

Reemtsma, K. and Maloney, J.V. Jr. (1974) The Economics of instant medical news. New Eng. J. Med. 290, 439.

Smith, L.M. (1937) Dermatitis caused by Creosote Bush. J. Allergy 8, 187.

Weber, L.F. (1953) Dermatitis venenata from native woods. Arch. Derm. Syph. 67, 388.

Hjorth, N. and Roed-Petersen, J. (1976) Contact dermatitis from antioxidants. Hidden sensitizers in tropical medications and foods. Brit. J. Derm. 94, 233.

Neoschroetera
(syn. Larrea)

Four species are found as xerophytic plants in subtropical

North and South America.

Neoschroetera tridentata
(syn. Larrea mexicana)
Creosote plant

Its strong smell prevents it from being eaten by animals.

Tribulus

20 species are found in tropical and subtropical regions.

Tribulus spp.
Caltrop

The mericarps have sharp rigid spines which can stick into the foot of an animal. The name, caltrop, refers to the form of the fruit and indicates an iron ball armed with sharp prongs used on the battlefield in former times to impede cavalry-horses. Centaurea is also known as Caltrop.

Tribulus species, especially
T. terrestris

Photodermatitis similar to that described under Lippia can occur in aminals which eat the plant (Watt and Breyer-Brandwijk 1963). The toxic principles of the plant cause liver damage and accumulation of phylloerythrin in the blood. Phylloerythrin which is a breakdown product of chlorophyll acts as a photosensitising agent. A suggestion of photodermatitis in man from the plant (Mathews 1937) lacks confirmation.

Tribulus cestoides

This native weed of Hawaii known as Carpet Weed, since it covers large areas, can cause mechanical injury to the hands and feet (Pope 1968).

Tribulus terrestris
Puncture Vine

The thorns can cripple the hoof of animals by rotting the frog and ingestion of the spiny fruit in hay can cause internal injury (Maiden 1895).

For homicidal purposes, the poisonous juice of Acokanthera venenata is smeared on a suitable prickly fruit such as that of T. terrestris and strewn on a path which is likely to be used by the victim (watt and Breyer-Brandwijk 1962).

References

Maiden, J.H. (1895) The Weeds of New South Wales. Supplementary Notes No. 1. Ag. Gaz. New South Wales 6, 671.

Mathews, F.P. (1937). Photosensitisation and the photodynamic diseases of man and the lower animals. Arch. Path. 23, 399.

Pope, W.T. (1968) Manual of Wayside Plants of Hawaii. Rutland, Vermont. Charles E. Tuttle Co.

Watt, J.M. and Breyer-Brandwijk, M.G. (1962) The medicinal and poisonous plants of Southern Africa. 2nd ed. Edinburgh. E.& S. Livingstone.

Zygophyllum

100 species are found from the Mediterranean region to central Asia and in southern Africa and Australia in deserts and steppes.

Zygophyllum foetidum

The leaf forms a lather when crushed in water and is used as soap (Watt and Breyer-Brandwijk 1962).

Reference

Watt, H.M. and Breyer-Brandwijk, M.G. (1962) The Medicinal and poisonous plants of Southern Africa. 2nd ed. Edinburgh. E.& S. Livingstone.

Zygophyllum fabago

The flower buds are used as a substitute for capers (Capparis).

"The solution of our problems does not principally lie in an exchange of opinions, but in investigation".

Spinoza (1632-1677)

Perfume, flavorings and essential oil dermatitis

Perfumes (fragrances) and flavourings, collectively known as aroma chemicals, can cause contact dermatitis. Historically, these products were mainly obtained from plants and now many are synthesized. Relevant essential oils and aroma chemicals have been indexed. Dr. Alexander Fisher provides the following information and recommendations for patch-testing with perfume ingredients:

"There are about 5,000 odoriferous substances in use today. The approximate concentration of perfume oils used in cosmetics generally is 0.5%, in colognes and toilet water 4% and in perfumes as much as 20%. A complete perfume compound may consist of from 10 to more than 60 basic components in three basic classifications: natural products from flowers, plants, roots, herbs, woods and gums; animal products and their extracts; and the synthetic aromatic chemicals, which may account for as much as 90% of the perfume compositions.

Pinpointing the specific sensitizer in a perfume is a formidable task. Certain perfumes are both sensitizers and photosensitizers; others are solely photosensitizers. Patch tests with perfumes must be done not only by the usual closed patch test method, but also by the open method with exposure to light. Photosensitization is associated with a number of essential perfume oils, especially bergamot, lavender, cedarwood, neroli and petitgrain.

Benzyl alcohol, a perfume solvent, and gum benzoin as well as various balsams added to perfumes to retard evaporation, may be the actual sensitizers in perfumes. The significance of these perfume additives as the causes of perfume dermatitis is illustrated by the fact that in my recent series of 16 patients with perfume allergy, three had positive patch reactions to benzyl alcohol and eight to balsam of Peru.

The following lists of perfume ingredients and their concentration and vehicle for patch test purposes have been formulated through personal experience, and with the help of the North American Contact Dermatitis Research Group and the Food and Drug Administration".

Perfume ingredients, patch test concentrations and vehicles

Key to abbreviations

acet.	-	acetone
alc.	-	alcohol 70%
aq.	-	aqueous
as is	-	undiluted
BA	-	benzyl alcohol
BL	-	butyrolactone*
c.o.	-	castor oil
DE	-	detyl extra (isopropyl palmitate)
o.o.	-	olive oil
pet.	-	petrolatum
sol.	-	solution

*Butyrolactone is a cyclic ester that is not volatile. It is non-irritating and non-sensitizing and is useful not only as a vehicle for certain cosmetic ingredients, but is also an unreactive solvent suitable for testing many liquid resins. It is available from Antara Chemicals, a division of General Aniline and Film Corp., 435 Hudson Street, New York, N. Y. 10014.

Cosmetic ingredient	Concentration and vehicle
Acacia (gum arabic)	as is
Acrylic monomer	10% o.o.
Aldehyde C-10	10% DE
Aldehyde C-11	Und. 10% DE
Aldehyde C-12	Lauric 10% DE
Almond Oil	as is
Alpha-amyl cinnamaldehyde	1% pet.
Alpha-methyl ionone	1% pet.
Alpha-pinene	1% pet.
Alpha-terpineol	5% o.o.
Aluminum chlorhydroxide	10% aq. sol.
Anise oil	25% c.o.
Balm, oil of	1% pet.
Balsam of Peru	10% pet.
Balsam of Tolu	1% alc.
Bay, oil of	1% pet.
Bay rum	as is
Benzildyene acetone	5% pet.
Benzoic acid	5% pet.
Benzoin	10% alc.

Benzoyl peroxide	1% pet.
Benzyl acetate	as is
Benzyl alcohol	5% pet.
Benzyl benzoate	5% pet.
Benzyl salicylate	2% pet.
Bergamot, oil of	10% pet.
Beta-myrcene	1% pet.
Beta-phenyl ethyl acetate	1% pet.
Beta-phenyl ethyl alcohol	1% pet.
Bitter almond, oil of	10% o.o.
Blancophore	0.1% pet.
p-Butyl-hydroxy-anisol	5% pet.
p-Butyl-hydroxytoluene	10% pet.
Butylated hydroxy toluene	10% DE
Cananga oil	2% pet.
Carnation oil	10% aq. sol.
Carophyllene	5% pet.
Cassie synthetique	10% DE
Cedartone V	as is
Cedarwood oil	10% o.o.
Cetavlon	5% pet.
Cetyl alcohol	30% pet.
Cinnamates (2-ethoxy-ethyl-p-methoxy)	1% pet.
Cinnamic acid	5% pet.
Cinnamic alcohol	1% pet.
Cinnamic alcohol styrax type	5% pet.
Cinnamic aldehyde	2% pet.
Cinnamon oil	0.5% pet.
Cinnamyl alcohol	1% pet.
Cis-beta-terpineol	25% in BL
Citracetal parento	10% DE
Citral oil	1% pet.
Citric acid	1% aq. sol.
Citron, oil of	1% pet.
Citronella, oil of	1% pet.
Citronellol	1% pet.
Citronellyl oxyacet-aldehyde	1% pet.
Clove oil	1% pet.
Coniferyl benzoate	1% pet.
Coumarin	5% pet.
Delta cadinene	1% pet.
Deltylextra	5% pet.
Diethyl phthalate	2% pet.
3,7 Dimethyl-1-octanol	2% pet.
Dimethyl phthalate	2% pet.
Essential oils	1% alc. or 2% pet.
Estradiol	5% pet.
Ethyl alcohol	as is
Ethyl vanillin	10% pet.
Eucalyptus, oil of	1% pet
Eugenol	5% pet.
Geraniol	2% pet.
Geranium oil	2% pet.
Ginger, oil of	1% pet.
Gum (s)	as is
Gylan	as is
Hamamelis Virg.	5% aq. sol.

Hexyl cinnamic aldehyde	2% pet-
Hibitane dibluc.	1% pet.
4-Hydroxy azobenzene carboxillic acid	2% pet.
Hydroxycitronellal	1% pet.
Irisone alpha	as is
Isoamyl salicylate	5% pet.
Isobutyl salicylate	
Isopropyl myristate	10% alc. or 2% pet.
Isopropyl quinolone	as is
Jasmin oil	2% pet.
Jasmin 9140	as is
Laurel oil	2% pet.
Lauryl alcohol	5% pet.
Lauryl gallate	5% pet.
Lauryl sulphate (ammonium)	5% pet.
Lavender, oil of	1% pet.
Lemon, oil of	1% pet.
Lemon grass, oil of	1% pet.
Limonene, oil of	1% alc.
Linalool, oil of	10% pet.
Linayl acetate	1% pet.
Mahogonate Dragoco	as is
Menthanyl acetate	as is
Methoxycitronellal	1% pet.
Methyl ionone gamma pure IFF	as is
Methyl salicylate	1% pet.
Mint oil	1% pet.
Mirbane oil (nitro-benzene)	25% c.o.
Musk ambrette	2% pet.
Musk Ketone	10% pet.
Myristyl alcohol	5% pet.
Neroli, oil of	10% o.o.
Orange, oil of	1% pet.
Orange peel, oil of	1% alc.
p-anisaldehyde	1% pet.
Patchouli, oil of	1% pet.
p-Cymene	1% pet.
Peppermint oil	1% pet.
Perfumes	as is (open and closed)
Petitgrain oil	10% o.o.
Petitgrain rectified	as is
Phenylacetaldehyde	2% pet.
Pine oil	pure
Piperonal (methyl ionone)	1% pet.
Rhodamin	5% pet.
Rose, oil of	1% alc.
Rose oil Bulgaria	2% pet.
Rose 62 ter	as is
Sandalwood oil	1% pet.
Sandela 10	as is
Sassafras, oil of	1% pet.
Sesame oil	50% o.o.
Spice, oil of	5% pet.
Styrax essence GD	5% pet.
Terpineol extra	25% in BL
Terpinolene	1% pet.
Tetra hydromuguol	as is

Thioglycollate (calcium)	5% aq. sol.
Thyme, oil of	25% c.o.
Trans-cinnamaldehyde	2% pet.
Trienthanolamine	5% pet.
Vanilla (alcohol extract)	10% acet.
Versalide prime	10% pet.
Verbena, oil of	1% pet.
Vetivert rectified	as is
Ylang Ylang oil	5% pet.

References

Fregert, S. (1970) Sensitization to Phenylacetaldehyde. Dermatologica 141, 11-14.

Harry, R.G. (1956) Cosmetics: Their Principles and Practices. New York: Chemical Publishing Co.

Klarmann, E.G. (1958) Perfume dermatitis. Annals of Allergy 16, 425-430.

Laymon, C.W. (1960) Cutaneous reactions to cosmetics and related substances. Minnesota Medicine 43, 4-8.

March, C.H. & Fisher, A.A. (1965) Cutaneous cosmetic reactions. General Practitioner 31, 89-93.

Masters, B.J. (1960) Allergies to cosmetic products. New York Journal of Medicine 60, 1934-1939.

Middleton, A.W. (1959) Cosmetic Science. London: Butterworths Scientific Publications.

Nakayama, H. Personal communication. Saiseikai Central Hospital, Tokyo, Japan.

Osbourne, R.A. et al (1956) Dermatological evaluation of perfumes of low sensitizing index. Proceedings of the Scientific Section of the Toilet Goods Association 17, 80 89.

Rothborg, H.W. & Hjorth, N. (1968) Allergy to perfume from toilet soaps and detergents in patients with dermatitis. Archives of Dermatology 97, 417-420.

Sagarin, B. (1957) Cosmetics, Science and Technology. New York: Interscience Publisher, Inc.

Schwartz, L. & Peck, S. (1960) Cosmetics and dermatitis. New York Journal of Medicine 60, 1940-1944.

Schorr, W.F. (1970) Allergic skin reactions from cosmetic preservatives. American Perfumery and Cosmetics 23, 64-68.

Wells, F.V. & Lubowe, I.I. (1964) Cosmetics and the Skin. New York: Rheingold Publishing Co.

Ill-effects to the eye from contact with plants

Contact with plants can cause ill-effects to the eye, usually associated with skin irritation and often with respiratory ill-effects. Reports are indexed under Eye, ill-effects.

Respiratory ill-effects of contact with plants

Contact with plants can cause injurious effects to the lips, mouth, throat and the respiratory tract. Such reports, including those of allergic alveolitis, are indexed under Respiratory ill-effects.

Hayfever plants, causing allergic rhinitis

Major, minor and suspect hayfever plants have been included in this review and are indexed under Hayfever plants.

Tree, wood, sawdust dermatitis

The key to investigation of industrial dermatitis from these sources is identification of the botanical species responsible. No reliance whatever can be obtained from trade, commercial, colloquial or common names. Some principal timbers of commerce are listed below, by common name:

Common names of commercial woods

(Kukachka 1970)

Abura (*Mitragyna ciliata*)

Acapu (*Vouacapoua americana*)

Aceituno (*Simarouba amara*)

"African mahogany" (*Khaya spp.*)

Afrormosia (*Pericopsis elata*)

Agba (*Gossweilerodendron balsamiferum*)
Aiele (*Canarium schweinfurthii*)
Albizia (*Albizia spp.*)
Alerce (*Fitzroya cupressoides*)
Alstonia (*Alstonia boonei* & *congensis*)
Amaranth (*Peltogyne* spp.)
Andiroba (*Carapa* spp.)
Angelique (*Dicorynia guianensis*)
Apamate (*Tabebuia rosea*)
Apitong (*Dipterocarpus* spp.)
Avodire (*Turraeanthus africanus*)
Ayan (*Distemonanthus benthamianus*)
Azobe (*Lophira alata*)
Bagtikan (*Parashorea plicata*)
Balsa (*Ochroma pyramidale*)
Basra locus (*Dicorynia guianensis*)
Batai (*Albizia falcataria*)
Benge (*Guibourtia arnoldiana*)
Bete (*Mansonia altissima*)
Bilinga (*Nauclea diderrichii*)
Blackwood, African (*Dalbergia melanoxylon*)
Bosse (*Guarea cedrata* & *thompsonii*)
Bubinga (*Guibourtia* spp.)
Capirona (*Calycophyllum spruceanum*)
Capomo (*Brosimum-Alicastrum* group)
Caribbean pine (*Pinus caribaea*)
Cativo (*Prioria copaifera*)
Cedro (*Cedrela* spp.)
Cedro macho (*Carapa* spp.)
Ceiba (*Ceiba pentandra*)
Chenchen (*Antiaris africana* & *welwitschii*)
Cocal (*Brosimum* spp.) utile group
Cocobolo (*Dalbergia retusa*)
Coubaril (*Hymenaea courbaril*)
Crabwood (*Carapa* spp.)
Degame (*Calycophyllum candidissimum*)
Determa (*Ocotea rubra*)
Ebony, African (*Diospyros* spp.)
Ebony, East Indian (*Diospyros* spp.)
Edinam (*Entandrophragma angolense*)
Ehie (*Guibourtia ehie*)
Ekki (*Lophira alata*)
Emeri (*Terminalia ivorensis*)
Encino (*Quercus* spp.)
Espave (*Anacardium excelsum*)
Framire (*Terminalia ivorensis*)
Freijo (*Cordia* spp.)
Fuma (*Ceiba pentandra*)
Goncalo alves (*Astronium* spp.)
Greenheart (*Ocotea rodiaei*)
Guanacaste (*Enterolobium cyclocarpum*)
Guapinol (*Hymenaea courbaril*)
Guarea (*Guarea* spp.)
Gumbo-limbo (*Bursera simaruba*)
Gurjun (*Dipterocarpus* spp.)
Indigbo (*Terminalia ivorensis*)
Ilomba (*Pycanthus angolensis*)
Imbuia (*Phoebe porosa*)
Ipe (*Tabebuia - Lapacho* group)
Ipil (*Intsia* spp.)
Iroko (*Chlorophora* spp.)
Jabillo (*Hura crepitans*)
Jacaranda (*Dalbergia nigra*)
Jarrah (*Eucalyptus marginata*)
Jelutong (*Dyera costulata*)
Kambala (*Chlorophora* spp.)
Kapur (*Dryobalanops* spp.)
Karri (*Eucalyptus diversicolor*)
Keladan (*Dryobalanops* spp.)
Kempas (*Koompassia malaccensis*)
Keruing (*Dipterocarpus* spp.)
Kevazingo (*Guibourtia* spp.)
Khaya (*Khaya* spp.)
Kokko (*Albizia lebbek*)
Kokrodua (*Pericopsis elata*)
"Korina" (*Terminalia superba*)
Kosipo (*Entandrophragma candollei*)
Lapacho (*Tabebuia - Lapacho* group)
Lauan, Dark red (*Shorea* spp.)
Lauan, Light red (*Shorea*, *Parashorea*, *Pentacme* spp.)
Laurel (*Cordia* spp.)
Lignum vitae (*Guaiacum sanctum*)
Limba (*Terminalia superba*)

Louro vermelho (Ocotea rubra)
Lovoa (Lovoa trichilioides)
Lumbayau (Tarrietia spp.)
Lupuna (Ceiba samauma)
Mahogany (Swietenia macrophylla)
Makore (Tieghemella heckelii)
Mansonia (Mansonia altissima)
Maria (Calophyllum brasiliense)
Marupa (Simarouba amara)
Mayflower (Tabebuia rosea)
Menkulang (Tarrietia spp.)
Merbau (Intsia spp.)
Mora (Mora excelsa)
Morabukea (Mora gonggrijpii)
Movingui (Distemonanthus benthamianus)
Muninga (Pterocarpus angolensis)
Narra (Pterocarpus indicus)
Nato (Mora megistosperma)
Niangon (Tarrietia utilis)
Nogal (Juglans spp.)
Oak, tropical (Quercus spp.)
Obeche (Triplochiton scleroxylon)
Ocote pine (Pinus oocarpa)
Ojoche (Brosimum-Alicastrum group)
Okoko (Sterculia oblonga)
Okoume (Aucoumea klaineana)
Okwen (Brachystegia spp.)
Omu (Entandrophragma candollei)
Opepe (Nauclea diderrichii)
Oriental wood (Endiandra palmerstonii)
Padauk, African (Pterocarpus soyauxii)
"Parana pine" (Araucaria angustfolia)
Pau amarello (Euxylophora paraensis)
Peroba de campos (Paratecoma peroba)
Peroba rosa (Aspidosperma spp.)
Peterebi (Cordia spp.)
"Philippine mahogany" (Shorea, Parashorea, Pentacme)
Pine, Caribbean (Pinus caribaea)
Pine, ocote (Pinus oocarpa)
Possumwood (Hura crepitans)
Purpleheart (Peltogyne spp.)
Ramin (Gonystylus spp.)
Ramon (Brosimum-Alicastrum group)
Rauli (Nothofagus procera)
Red peroba (Aspidosperma spp.)
Roble (Quercus spp.)
Rosewood, Brazilian (Dalbergia nigra)
Rosewood, Indian (Dalbergia latifolia)
Samauma (Ceiba samauma)
Samba (Triplochiton scleroxylon)
Sande (Brosimum-Utile group)
Santa Maria (Calophyllum brasiliense)
Sapele (Entandrophragma cylindricum)
Satinwood, East India (Chloroxylon swietenia)
Seraya, white (Parashorea plicata)
Sipo (Entandrophragma utile)
Siris (Albizia lebbek)
Spanish-cedar (Cedreia spp.)
Tchitola (Oxystigma oxyphyllum)
Teak (Tectona grandis)
Tiama (Entandrophragma angolense)
Tigerwood (Lovoa trichilioides)
Tola (Gossweilerodendron balsamiferum)
Utile (Entandrophragma utile)
Walnut, Tropical (Juglans spp.)
Wana (Ocotea rubra)
Wawa (Triplochiton scleroxylon)
Whismore (Tarrietia utilis)
Yang (Dipterocarpus spp.)
Yellow sterculia (Sterculia oblonga)

Reference

Kukachka, B.F. (1970) Properties of imported tropical woods. U.S.D.A. Forest Service Research Paper FPL125. Forest Products Laboratory, Madison, Wis.

Weed dermatitis

Of a dozen definitions of a 'weed', there are:

'A plant out of place'

'A plant for which no use has yet been found'

No attempt has been made to index 'weeds' as opposed to horticultural or agricultural plants. The key to investigation of 'weed dermatitis' is to identify the botanical species responsible and to use the index for reports of ill-effects. No reliance can be obtained from colloquial names of weed and botanical identification is essential. The Compositae family provides the bulk of allergenic weeds.

Reference

King, L.J. (1966) Weeds of the World. Biology and Control. London. Leonard Hill.

Phytophotodermatitis

Phytophotodermatitis is evoked by contact with plants containing furanocoumarins, notably psoralens, and exposure to long wave ultraviolet light (UVA). During the search for causes of Oppenheim's meadow dermatitis, many plants which are not known to contain psoralens were incorrectly implicated. In the case of some plants e.g. Ranunculus, irritant contact dermatitis actually occurred or a combination of irritation and sunburn (UVB). Reports of phytophotodermatitis from plants which are not known to contain psoralens should be treated with caution. Recently, phototoxic dermatitis has been reported from alpha-terthienyl and polyacetylenics of Compositae (Towers et al 1977, Chan et al 1977). There are distinctive differences between photodermatitis from alpha-terthienyl and from psoralen. Photodermatitis from polyacetylenics has, so far, hardly been evaluated.

References

Chan, G.F.Q., Prihoda, M., Towers, G.H.N. and Mitchell, J.C. (1977) Phototoxicity evoked by alpha-terthienyl. Contact Dermatitis 3, 215-16.

Towers, G.H.N., Wat, Chi-Kit, Graham, E.A., Chan, G.F.Q., Bandoni, R.J., Mitchell, J.C. and Sam, J. (1977) Ultraviolet-Mediated Antibiotic Activity of Species of Compositae caused by Polyacetylenic Compounds. Lloydia, 40, 487.

Contact Urticaria

Whealing of the skin from contact with plants can be pharmacologically mediated (e. g. nettle rash, Urtica), allergic or of ill-defined cause. We have deliberately restricted the review to contact urticaria since urticaria from ingestion (e.g. from eating strawberries) is dealt with in other works.

References

Maibach, H.I. and Johnson, H.L. (1975) Contact Urticaria syndrome. Archs. Derm. 111, 72b.

Odom, R.B. and Maibach, H.I. (1976) Contact urticaria: a different contact dermatitis. Cutis 18, 672.

Agricultural chemicals, pesticides, etc.

Irritant and allergic effects from chemicals applied to plants or to the soil, etc. have been indexed by name.

Recent Advances

The Supplement consists of material which has accumulated recently. During the course of publication, it was found possible to incorporate most of the material into the text.

SUPPLEMENT I

ALGAE: Eating of certain dried algae can produce carotinemia (Tanikawa et al 1961).

Reference: Tanikawa, K. et al (1961) Aurantiasis cutis due to overeating of dried Laver (Nori). J. Jap. Soc. Intern. Med. 50, 414.

Additional References:
Mynderse, J.S. et al (1977) Antileukemia activity in the Osillatoriaceae: isolation of Debromoaplysiatoxin from Lyngbya. Science 196, 538.

Richard, J.L. (1973) Mycotoxin photosensitivity. J. Am. Vet. Med. Assoc. 163, 1298.

Shilo, M. (1972) Toxigenic algae. Prog. Ind. Microbiol. 11, 233.

ALGAE - CHARACEAE: The Characeae have been classified as algae.

Chara spp. and Nitella spp.: These aquatic plants (Cook 1974) can have irritant effects (Behl et al 1966).

References: Behl, P.N. et al (1966) Skin-irritant and sensitizing plants found in India, New Delhi. P.N. Behl, Irwin Hospital.

Cook, C.D.K. (1974) Water Plants of the World. The Hague. W. Junk.

ALGAE - Cladophora: The fresh water green alga C. nitida is eaten in Hawaii (Usher 1974). Contact with species of the genus can produce intense itching and a papulo-vesicular eruption occurring 7-10 hours after contact from staying in sluggish water in marshy places (Pashkevich 1975).

References: Pashkevich, Y.A. (1975) The clinical pattern, treatment and prophylaxis of dermatitis developing after contact with Cladaphara. Vestn. Derm. Venereol. 7, 68.

Usher, G. (1974) A dictionary of plants used by man. London. Constable.

ALGAE - CHROOCOCCACEAE - Microcystis toxica: Ingestion of the alga produces hepatogenous photosensitisation in cattle (Wild 1961).

Reference: Wild, H. (1961) Harmful aquatic plants in Africa and Madagascar. Kirkia 2, 1.

ALLIACEAE - Allium:
Additional Reference:
van Ketel, W.G. and de Haan, P. (1978) Occupational eczema from garlic and onion. Contact Dermatitis 4, 53.

AMARANTHACEAE -?Amaranthus retroflexus: Keratitis attributed to entry into farmers' eyes of the pollen of pigweed-red root (Anneberg 1938). Pigweed is also a colloquial name for Chenopodium. Photosensitivity attributed to ingestion of the plant is noted under Atriplex.

Reference: Anneberg, A.R. (1938) Corneal reaction to weed pollen. Am. J. Ophthalm. 21, 1265.

Amaranthus spp.(Amaranthus Pigweed): The pollen of some species can cause hayfever (Wodehouse 1971).

Reference: Wodehouse, R.P. (1971) Hayfever Plants. 2nd rev. edition. New York, Hafner.

Chemistry is recorded by Hegnauer (1964).

Reference: Hegnauer, R. (1964) Chemotaxonomy of Plants. Vol. 3. Basel. Birkhauser. p. 81.

ANACARDIACEAE - Anacardium excelsum: This tree provides timber but Woods and Calnan (1976) found no reference to dermatitis from it.

Reference: Woods, B. and Calnan, C.D. (1976) Toxic woods. Brit. J. Derm. 94, Suppl. 13, June.

Anacardium occidentale: An early report of dermatitis from the shell of the cashew nut was that of Prefontaine (1763). The wood perhaps causes dermatitis (Lewin 1928).

References: Lewin, L. (1928) Gifte im Holzgewerbe. Berlin, Stilke.

Prefontaine, de (1763) Maison rustique, a l'usage de Cayenne. pp. 139, 152, 108-109. Paris, Bauche, cited by Woods and Calnan (1976).

Woods, B. and Calnan, C.D. (1976) Toxic Woods. Brit. J. Derm. 94, Suppl. 13, June.

Small amounts of antigen, transferred from the shell to the nuts during shelling, produced dermatitis when the fresh nuts were ingested in large amounts by five Toxicodendron sensitive individuals. Its antigenicity disappeared in a few days so that "stale" raw cashews like the commercially available dry-roasted variety were harmless (Ratner et al 1974).

Reference: Ratner, J.H. et al (1974) Cashew nut dermatitis, an example of internal-external contact-type hypersensitivity. Arch. Dermatol. 110, 921.

A woman who put one half of a bean in her ear to relieve a toothache and pain in the face developed a violent vesicular dermatitis and oedema of the ear, eyelid, cheek and neck (Schwerin undated). A bean, divided longitudinally, was placed upon a string hung around the neck in such a manner that it lay over the manubrium sterni. Two days later vesicular dermatitis appeared on the upper anterior trunk (Lewin 1882).

References: Lewin, L. (1882) The Incidental Effects of Drugs. New York, cited by Morrow, Prince (1887) Drug eruptions. A clinical study of the irritant effects of drugs upon the skin. New York. Wm. Wood and Co.

Schwerin (undated) cited by Lewin, L. (1882) The Incidental Effects of Drugs. New York, cited by Morrow, Prince (1887) Drug eruptions. A clinical study of the irritant effects of drugs upon the skin. New York. Wm. Wood and Co.

Occupational dermatitis from cashew nut shell liquid was discussed by Schwartz et al (1945).

Reference: Schwartz, L. et al (1945) Skin hazards. Ind. Med. Surg. 14, 500.

Comocladia dentata: Lunin (1969) observed 330 patients with dermatitis from this species on the steppes of Russia and from Metopium toxiferum in coastal regions.

Reference: Lunin, M.M. (1969) Burns caused by the tropical plant Huao. Vestn. Khir. Grekov. 102, 96.

Gluta renghas: "The poisonous character of Gluta renghas was known to Rumphius (Herb. Amboin. ii. 259, t. S6; 1750). The exhalations of this tree are considered noxious, and the people of Macassar and other parts of Celebes in particular, entertain such dread of it, that they dare not remain long under it, much less repose beneath its shade; they say that whoever receives the droppings from it will have his body swell and be affected with malignant sores."

Linnaeus published the species as G. benghas, evidently with the intention of employing the vernacular name as a trivial. As the Malay name is "rengas", and "benghas" is meaningless, it seems desirable to alter the specific name to G. renghas.

"Not only are the fruit, leaves and twigs of the Rengas trees (species of Gluta and Melanorrhoea) poisonous, but the timber also, even after long keeping, is apt to produce injury. Dr. Brown says that he was informed that after years of seasoning, when the wood is cut up, it gives rise to painful and intractable eruptions on the hands and bodies of the workmen. The timber is a very handsome red wood, streaked more or less with black, and was formerly known as Singapore mahogany and much valued as a cabinet wood or for buildings. The Kedah Malays, on felling a tree, would leave it lying in the forest till the bark and sap-wood was rotted away or removed by termites, after which they said it was safe to move. As a furniture wood, however, it went out of fashion, as even after being made up it was said to seriously affect many persons living in the room with it, producing great irritation of the mouth, nose and throat, especially when it began to get old, worn-out and dusty." (Ridley 1911, cited by Sprague 1921).

Reference: Sprague, T.A. (1921) Plant dermatitis. Journal of Botany 59, 308.

Rhus:

Reference: Gorbovitski, I.S.E. et al (1974) Sumac dermatitis (Review of the literature). Vestn. Dermatol. Venerol. 48, 16.

Rhus juglandifolia: "Humboldt and Bonpland were skeptical as to the alleged ill-effects of remaining under the tree without actual contact taking place. 'Lac aquosum, quod arbor stillat, in cute post 2 vel 3 dies ejicit pustulas similes variolis, quamobrem incolae non solum succum sed etiam umbram arboris metuunt, fabulantes eam noxiam esse, praesertim quando post pluvias sol arborem calefecit. Sunt tamen, qui nec post contactum, nec post tritum allum sentiunt effectum adversum' (Sprague 1921).

Triana, on the other hand, was satisfied that the popular idea of the 'shade' of the tree being dangerous was well-founded. 'Le Rhus juglandifolia exerce une actione curieuse sur l'homme: l'ombre suelement de l'arbre ou ses émanations, son contact, son approche, la fumee de son bois, produisent... irritation... gonflement... démangeaisons. L'intensité de ces accidents est presque nulle pour certaines personnes, plus ou moins grave pour d'autres. L'un de nous (Triana) a éprouvé ces effects en récoltant et en desséchant la plante; même action sur une autre personne qui l'avait touchée. Les gens du pays combattent ces affections en faisant des frictions avec de la graisse ou avec de la crème' (Ann Sc. Nat. ser. 5, xiv. 289; 1872). Triana's evidence as to the poisonous nature of Rhus juglandifolia seems to have been overlooked (Kew Bull. 1898, 100." (Sprague 1921).

Reference: Sprague, T.A. (1921) Plant dermatitis. Journal of Botany 59, 308.

Rhus metopium: Lifting and carrying the branches on the shoulders caused vesicular dermatitis of the hands, neck and shoulders. The sap of the plant in Jamaica is pale yellow but changes to a deep brown colour on the skin (Grabham 1899).

Reference: Grabham, M. (1899) Acute dermatitis caused by handling Rhus. Brit. Med. J. 1, 1140.

Rhus (Toxicodendron) succedaneum - Japanese wax tree: Plants of Japanese wax tree were voluntarily withdrawn from sale by several South Australian nurserymen, when six or seven workers in one nursery were affected through handling the plant (Aplin 1976).

Reference: Aplin, T.E.H. (1976) Poisonous garden plants and other plants harmful to man in Australia. Western Australian Dept. of Agriculture Bull. 3964.

Schinopsis quebracho-colorado: This plant has been implicated in causing phytophotodermatitis (Pathak 1974), but psoralens are not known from the plant.

Reference: Pathak, M.A. (1974) Phytophotodermatitis. Chapter 32 in Sunlight and Man, ed. Pathak, M.A. et al. University of Tokyo Press. p. 495.

Semecarpus anacardium: The sensitizers are semecarpol and bhilawanol (Pillay and Siddiqui 1931).

Reference: Pillay, P.P. and Siddiqui, S. (1931) Chemical examination of the marking nut (Semecarpus anacardium L.). J. Ind. Chem. Soc. 8, 517.

Swintonia floribunda - Merpeau: Mucocutaneous reaction from this species in the wood working industry was reported by Hublet et al (1972).

Reference: Hublet, P. et al (1972) Etude sur les accidents cutanes et muqueux provoques par les bois tropicaux dans l'industrie du bois in Belgique. Arch. Belges. Med. Social. 31, 314.

Toxicodendron:

Hyposensitization: Hyposensitization to Poison Ivy. Med. Lett. Drugs Ther. 17, 52, June 1975.

Antibodies to urushiol were found in a patient who had nephrosis attributed to dermatitis from poison oak (Devich et al 1975).

Reference: Devich, K.B. et al (1975) Renal lesions accompanying poison oak dermatitis. Clinical Nephrology 3, 106.

ANNONACEAE - Cananga odorata: Ylang Ylang oil had sensitizing properties in Draize test but showed no sensitizing properties by several other methods (Opdyke 1974).

Reference: Opdyke, D.L.J. (1974) Monographs on fragrance raw materials. Fd. Cosmet. Toxicol. 12, 1015.

APOCYNACEAE - Carissa spectabilis (syn. Toxicophloea spectabilis, Acokanthera spectabilis) - Winter Sweet: Contact with the plant has caused irritation to eyes, skin and throat (Aplin 1976).

Reference: Aplin, T.E.H. (1976) Poisonous garden plants and other plants harmful to man in Australia. Western Australian Dept. of Agriculture Bull. 3964.

ARACEAE - Dieffenbachia: Irritation of the mouth from the plant was observed by Faivre et al (1974).

Reference: Faivre, M. et al (1974) Toxicity of an ornamental plant. A case of poisoning by Dieffenbachia picta. Nouv. Presse Med. 3, 1313.

Rhaphidophora (syn. Pothos, Scindapsus): The nomenclature is as above (Mitchell and Rook 1976).

Reference: Mitchell, J.C. and Rook, A.J. (1976) Scindapsus Dermatitis. Contact Dermatitis 2, 125.

ARALIACEAE - Echinopanax:
Reference: Lopatin, A.I. and Kolesnikova, N.P. (1974) Skin Diseases caused by the use of extracts of Echinopanax elatum Naici. Vestn. Dermatol. Venerol. 48, 83

ASCLEPIADACEAE - Asclepias tuberosa: The powdered root, when applied to the skin, has an escharotic effect (Piffard 1881).

Reference: Piffard, H.G. (1881) A treatise on the Materia Medica and Therapeutics of the Skin. New York. Wm. Wood and Co.

BETULACEAE - Betula sp.: A cabinet maker who had dermatitis showed positive patch test reactions to Swedish birch, teak (Tectona), deal (?Pinus) and to lapachol (see Tabebuia) and to anthothecol (see Khaya)(Woods and Calnan 1976).

Reference: Woods, B. and Calnan, C.D. (1976) Toxic Woods. Brit. J. Derm. 94, Suppl. 13, June.

Betula - Birch: Oleum Betulae and Oleum Fagi (Fagus) (of each 5%) produced positive patch test reactions in 3% of patients with stasis dermatitis (Rudski and Baranowska 1974).

Reference: Rudski, E. and Baranowska, E. (1974) Contact sensitivity in stasis dermatitis. Dermatologica 148, 352.

Betula spp. - Birches: The pollen of some species can cause hayfever (Wodehouse 1971). See also Carpinus.

Reference: Wodehouse, R.P. (1971) Hayfever Plants. 2nd rev. edition. New York, Hafner.

Betula sp.: Salicylic acid is derived from Betula and other plants. The foods most likely to contain salicylates were listed by Noid et al (1974). A list of products containing aspirin was provided by Leist and Banwell (1974).

References: Leist, E.R. and Banwell, J.G. (1974) Products containing aspirin. New Eng. J. Med. 291, 711.

Noid, H.E., Schulz, F.W. and Winkelmann, R.K. (1974) Diet Plan for patients with salicylate-induced urticaria. Archs. Derm. 109, 866.

Betula: Apple (Malus), carrot (Dauca), parsnip (Pastinaca) and potato (Solanum), less often than other vegetables, produced immediate type hypersensitivity reactions in persons who were hypersensitive to birch pollen (Hannuksela and Lahti 1977).

Reference: Hannuksela, M. and Lahti, A. (1977) Immediate reactions to fruit and vegetables. Contact Dermatitis 3, 79.

BIGNONIACEAE - Tabebuia spp.(Lapacho series) - Lapacho, ipe: The lapacho group or series of the genus Tabebuia consists of about 20 species of trees and occurs in practically every Latin American country except Chile. The common name adopted there is lapacho, which is derived from the yellow-green compound lapachol which occurs in the heartwood vessels of this group. Lapachol is usually visible on planed surfaces confined to the vessel lines, or in some specimens may cover the entire surface during sawing. In the presence of alkaline solutions the lapachol turns a bright red (Kakuchka 1970).

Reference: Kukachka, B.F. (1970) Properties of imported tropical woods. USDA Forest Service research paper. FPL125 March. U.S. Dept. Agric. Forest Service. Forest Products Laboratory. Madison, Wis. U.S.A.

BLEPHAROCARYACEAE:
Reference: Mitchell, J.C. and Maibach, H.I. (1977) Absence of cross sensitivity between Toxicodendron (syn. Rhus) and Blepharocarya. Contact Dermatitis 3, 169.

BROMELIACEAE - Ananas sativus: Ethyl acrylate, found in the fruits, produced sensitisation in 10 of 24 subjects by a maximisation test. The compound is used in soap, detergent, creams, lotions, perfumes and food (Opdyke 1974).

Reference: Opdyke, D.L.J. (1974) Monographs on fragrance raw materials. Fd. Cosmet. Toxicol. 12, 919.

CANNABINACEAE - Cannabis:
Reference: Silverstein, M.J. and Lessin, P.J. (1974) Normal skin test responses in chronic marijuana users. Science 186, 740.

CARPINACEAE - Carpinus spp. - Hornbeam, Ironwood: The pollen appears to be a complicating factor in Birch (Betula) hayfever (Wodehouse 1971).

Reference: Wodehouse, R.P. (1971) Hayfever Plants. 2nd rev. edition. New York, Hafner.

CHENOPODIACEAE - Chenopodium anthelminticum - Wormseed: The plant is cultivated for its anthelmintic volatile oil which caused an irritating itch to a person who handled the plant (Aplin 1976).

Reference: Aplin, T.E.H. (1976) Poisonous garden plants and other plants harmful to man in Australia. Western Australian Dept. of Agriculture Bull. 3964.

COMPOSITAE:

Additional Reference:
Heywood, V.J. et al (1977) The Biology and Chemistry of the Compositae. 2 vols. London. Academic Press.

Biological activities of sesquiterpene lactones (Rodriquez et al 1976).

Reference: Rodriguez, E. et al (1976) Biological activities of sesquiterpene lactones. Phytochemistry 15, 1573.

Phytotoxicity by Compositae.

Reference: Towers, G.H.N. et al (1977) Ultraviolet-mediated antibiotic activity of species of Compositae caused by polyacetylenic compounds. Lloydia 40, 487.

Six patients in Denmark were contact sensitive to Compositae plants (Bergh 1975).

Reference: Bergh, M. (1975) Dermatitis from weeds detected by patch testing with oleoresins (Hollister-Stier). Contact Dermatitis 1, 61.

Ambrosia:
Reference: Samo Ilov, A.V. and Terekhova-Uvarova, N.A. (1974) Immediate and delayed allergic reactions in experimental sensitization with Ambrosia pollen. Vestn. Akad. Med. Nauk. SSSR 11, 16.

Hjorth, N. et al (1976) Airborne contact dermatitis from Compositae dermatitis simulating photodermatitis. Brit. J. Derm. 95, 613.

Anthemis nobilis: This species is now named Chamaemelum nobile (McClintock 1977).

Reference: McClintock, D. (1977) 'Treneague chamomile' The Garden. Journal of the Royal Horticultural Society 102(5) (May) 224, cites Mrs. Martell (Feb. p. 70).

Arnica:
References: Schleicher, H. (1974) Uber phytogene allergische Kontaktekzeme. Dermatologische Monatsschrift 160, 433.

Willuhn, G. and Hermann, H.D. (1976) Swei Sesquiterpenelaktone aus des Bluten von Arnica longifolia. Archiv. der Pharmazie 309, 333.

Hausen, B.M. et al (1978) The sensitizing capacity of Compositae plants 1. Occupational contact dermatitis from Arnica longifolia Eaton. Contact Dermatitis 4, 3. (carabron and helenalin allergenic)

Chamaemelum: see Anthemis.

Chrysanthemum: External washing with organic solvents released major amounts of sesquiterpene lactones of some Compositae species e.g. Chrysanthemum (Hausen 1977).

Reference: Hausen, B.M. (1977) A simple method for extracting crude sesquiterpene lactones from Compositae plants for skin tests, chemical investigations and sensitizing experiments in guinea pigs. Contact Dermatitis 3, 58.

Scabiosa of the Dipsacaceae family produced a negative patch test reaction in a patient who had Chrysanthemum dermatitis (Liepold 1936).

Reference: Liepold (1936) Dermatitis of the hands and face due to hypersensitivity to chrysanthemum and camomile. Report: 62 Tagund d. Vereinig. Suedwest deutsch Dermat. Heidelberg. Nov. 14.

Cultivar specificity: Instances of contact sensitivity to some cultivars and lack of sensitivity to others were reported by Olivier and Renkin (1954), Rook (1961), Malten (1973) and Mitchell (1974). This finding can be of importance to a flower grower who may be able to continue growing cultivars to which he is not reactive.

References: Malten, K.E. (1973) Chrysanthemum contact hypersensitivity. Contact Dermatitis Newsletter (London) 13, 357.

Mitchell, J.C. (1974) Applied chemotaxonomy of plants I. A biological model. Contact Dermatitis Newsletter (London) 16, 494.

Olivier, J. and Renkin, A. (1954) Eczema par sensibilite a une seule variete de chrysanthemes. Arch. Belg. Derm. 10, 296.

Rook, A. (1961) Plant dermatitis. Botanical aspects. Trans. St. John's Hosp. Derm. Soc. 46, 41.

Rook, A. (1961) Plant dermatitis. The significance of variety specific sensitisation. Brit. J. Derm. 73, 283.

Chrysanthemum coreanum: A florist had dermatitis from this plant; patch tests produced positive reactions in the patient, negative in two controls. The patient also reacted to C. sinensis, cultivar C. Turner (Sertoli and Fabbri 1974).

Reference: Sertoli, A. and Fabbri, P. (1974) Firenza, Italy. personal communication.

Cosmos: The odour of Cosmos caused hayfever in a patient. Tagetes had a similar effect in this patient (Biederman 1937).

Reference: Biederman, J.B. (1937) Sensitivity to flowers. Laryngoscope 47, 825.

Cynara: Artichokes contain a potentially allergenic sesquiterpene lactone, cynaropicrin (Schneider and Thiele 1974).

Reference: Schneider, von G. and Thiele, Kl. (1974) Eigenschaften und bestimmung des artischoken-bitterstoffen, cynaropicrin. Planta Medica 25, 149.

Dahlia:
Reference: Calnan, C.D. (1978) Sensitivity to dahlia flowers. Contact Dermatitis 4, 168.

Helenium:
Reference: Calnan, C.D. (1978) Dermatitis from helenium. Contact Dermatitis 4, 115.

Inula helenium: Piyankova and Nugmanova (1975) described cases of allergic contact dermatitis due to contact with elecampane. This medicinal herb is apparently widely used in the Soviet Union for self treatment of skin ailments.

Reference: Piyankova, Z.P. and Nugmanova, M.L. (1975) Dermaitis due to elecampane. Vestn. Derm. Vener. 51, 52, Dec.

Additional Reference:
Opdyke, D.L.J. (1976) Monographs on fragrance raw materials. Allantroot oil. Fd. Cosmet. Toxicol. 14, 307. (found to be strong sensitizer)

Lactuca: Lactuca sativa and Cichorium produced immediate and delayed hypersensitivity (Krook 1977).

Reference: Krook, G. (1977) Occupational dermatitis from Lactuca satica and Cichorium (endive). Contact Dermatitis 3, 77.

Matricaria:
Reference: Beetz, D. et al (1971) Zur Haufigkeit der epidermalen Allergie gegenuber Kamille in kamillehaltigen Arzneimitteln und Kosmetika. Dermatologische Monatsschrift 157, 505.

Krauskopf, J. and Ad Amkov, A.D. (1975) 3 cases of simultaneous contact hypersensitivity to wild chamomile (Matricaria chamomilla) and Frullania tamarisci. Cesk. Dermatol. 50, 299.

Parthenium: The trichomes (plant hairs) of the plant contain sesquiterpene lactones (Rodriquez et al 1977).

Reference: Rodriquez, E. et al (1977) Dermatologically active sesquiterpene lactones in trichomes of Parthenium hysterophorus L. (Compositae). Experientia 32, 236.

The major allergen in Parthenium hysterophorus is parthenin (Lonkar et al 1976).

Reference: Lonkar, A. et al (1976) An antigen from Parthenium hysterophorus L. Contact Dermatitis 2, 151.

Additional Reference:
Doley, D. (1977) Parthenium weed (Parthenium hysterophorus L.) gas exchange characteristics as a basis for prediction of its geographical distribution. Aust. J. Agric. Res. 28, 449.

Picris: 40 to 50 species are found in Eurasia, the Mediterranean region and Abyssinia.

Picris heiracroides: The plant or its oil causes skin eruptions in those who handle it (Towers, G.H.N. personal communication).

Saussurea: Lactone free costus oil and hydrogenated costus oil lost their sensitizing capacity (Opdyke 1974).

Reference: Opdyke, D.L.J. (1974) Monographs on fragrance raw materials. Fd. Cosmet. Toxicol. 12, 867.

Tagetes: The odour of marigolds caused hayfever and asthma in two patients respectively. Cosmos had a similar effect in one of them.

Crown of Gold marigold which had odourless foliage, had no ill-effect (Biederman 1937).

Reference: Biederman, J.B. (1937) Sensitivity to flowers. Laryngoscope 47, 825.

CRUCIFERAE:
Additional Reference:
Vaughan, J.G. et al (1976) The Biology and Chemistry of the Cruciferae. Academic Press, New York.

Armoracia:
Reference: Straus, W. (1974) Immunocyto immunocytochemical observations on hypersensitivity skin reactions to horseradish peroxidase gammaglobulin. J. Histochem. Cytochem. 22, 303.

Brassica - Brassica oleraceae var. botrytis 10% - Cauliflower: Extraction was performed by homogenization of 10 grams of fresh plant parts with 100ml of water or ethanol (Ultra-Turax type 18/2) followed by cold maceration for 3 hours. Filtrates were used for patch testing. The patient reacted strongly to all cauliflower extracts (van Ketel 1975).

Reference: van Ketel, W.G. (1975) A cauliflower allergy. Contact Dermatitis 1, 324.

EUPHORBIACEAE - Croton tiglium: The irritant activity of the seed oil is due to the occurrence of 12,13-diesters of the tetracyclic diterpene phorbol (Hecker and Schmidt 1974).

Reference: Hecker, E. and Schmidt, R. (1974) Phorbolesters - the irritants and cocarcinogens of Croton tiglium L. In Progress in the Chemistry of Organic Natural Products 31, 377. ed. Werz, H. et al. Vienna, Springer-Verlag.

Additional References:
Hecker, E. (1975) Cocarcinogens and cocarcinogenesis. In Handbuch des allgemeinen Pathologie. Vol. 6, Pt. 6, p. 651. Berlin, Springer.

Hergenhahn, M. et al (1974) Diterpene esters from 'Euphorbium' and their irritant and cocarcinogenic activity. Experientia 30, 1438.

Euphorbia: The latex contains tetracyclic triterpenes (euphol, euphorbol, cycloartenol and others) and other substances (Ponsinet and Ourisson 1968).

Reference: Ponsinet, G. and Ourisson, G. (1965,1968). Etudes chimiotaxonomiques dans la famille des Euphorbiacees. Phytochemistry 4, 813 and 7, 89.

Euphorbia spp. produced a hydrocarbon similar to crude oil which might be used as an energy source (Dr. Melvin Calvin, University of California at Berkeley, Newspaper item, undated.)

References: Samochval, G.T. and Krivak, G.G. (1974) Durch buntblattrige Wofsmilch verusachte Dermatitis. Vestn. Derm. Vener. 48, 85.

Smirnov, L.D. and Efremov, A.I. (1970) Durch harte Wolfsmilch vernsachte Dermatitis. Vestn. Derm. Vener. 44, 67.

Euphorbia ingens: The latex produces irritation and blistering of the skin and a single drop in the conjunctival sac produces intense pain and temporary blindness or even loss of the eye. Cattle driven through dense bush, where the tree is growing, can develop severe burns of the lips, face and eyes; death of the animal can result from these caustic effects. Honey containing the nectar of the plant is irritant (Watt and Breyer-Brandwijk 1962). Roe and Field (1965) found the latex to be irritant.

References: Roe, F.J.C. and Field, W.E.H. (1965) Chronic toxicity of essential oils and certain other products of natural origin. Fd. Cosmet. Toxicol. 3, 311.

Watt, J.M. and Breyer-Brandwijk, M.G. (1962) The medicinal and poisonous plants of Southern Africa. 2nd ed. Edinburgh. E.& S. Livingstone.

Euphorbia peplus:
Reference: Flood, W.J. (1976) Home treatment of basal cell carcinoma. Med. J. Australia 2, 111 (Jul. 17) and Beardmore, G.L. same pg. and June 12 (Weedon and Check).

Hippomane mancinella: Colloquial names: Manchineel or manchineale (English); Mancenillier (French); Manzinellbaum (German); Manzanilla or manzanillo (Spanish) (Earle 1938).

Irritation of the penis followed handling the plant (Wedd 1937).

References: Earle, K.V. (1938) Toxic effects of Hippomane mancinella. Trans. Roy. Soc. Trop. Med. Hyg. 32, 363.

Wedd, G.D. (1937) The manchineel tree. J. Royal Naval Medical Services 23, 250.

Additional references:
Caddy, D.J. (1894) Poisoning by manchineal. Lancet 2, 1478.

Bodeau (1936) A propos de quelques accidents dus au mancenillier. Arch. Med. Pharm. nav. 126, 122, (cites older French Literature)

Perianal dermatitis followed the use of the leaves as toilet paper (Satulsky and Wirts 1943). Five sailors developed dermatitis after a beach barbeque under the trees (Lowe 1974).

References: Lowe, N.J. (1974) Primary irritant dermatitis from the manchineel tree (Hippomane mancinella) in the eastern Caribbean. J. Royal Naval Med. Service 60, 133.

Satulsky, E.M. and Wirts, C.A. (1943) Dermatitis venenata by manzillo tree. Archs. Derm. Syph. 47, 36 and 797.

Hippomane: The early literature of dermatitis from the plant was reviewed by Earle (1938).

Reference: Earle, K.V. (1938) Toxic effects of Hippomane mancinella. Trans. Roy. Soc. Trop. Med. Hyg. 32, 363.

Jatropha: All species with stinging hairs which were contained in Jatropha are regarded as belonging to Cnidoscolus (Thurston and Lersten 1969).

Reference: Thurston, E.L. and Lersten, N.R. (1969) The morphology and toxicology of plant stinging hairs. Botan. Rev. 35, 393.

Ricinus: 21 of 50 workers preparing castor oil had a pruritic papular eruption; the sharp husks of the seeds and some constituents of the oil was considered responsible (Korobow cited by White 1934).

Reference: White, R.P. (1934) The Dermatergoses or Occupational Affections of the Skin. 4th ed. London. H.K. Lewis.

FUNGI - Alternaria: Alternaria on logs used for wood pulp can produce hypersensitivity pneumonitis (Schlueter et al 1972).

Reference: Schleuter, D.P. et al (1972) Wood-pulp worker's disease: a hypersensitivity pneumonitis. Ann. Int. Med. 77, 907.

Contact sensitivity to antibiotics derived from fungi: Penicillin, streptomycin, neomycin and some other antibiotics derived from fungi can produce allergic contact dermatitis.

Fairy rings: The circular or arcuate shapes of fungous infections of grass known as fairy rings have a morphological resemblance to fungous infections of the skin (Jackson 1971).

References: Jackson, R. (1971) Fairy rings. Canad. Med. Ass. J. 105, 703.

Jackson, R. (1967) The shapes of infectious disease lesions in the integument of plants, animals and humans. Can. Med. Assoc. J. 97, 573.

Lebeau, J.B., Hawn, E.J. (1961) Fairy rings in Alberta, Canada. Plant Dis. Survey 41, 317.

Shantz, H.L. and Piemeisel, R.L. (1917) Fungus fairy rings in eastern Colorado. J. Agr. Res. 11, 191.

Hypogymnia:
Reference: Krauskopf, J. (1976) Contact hypersensitivity to Hypogymnia physodes. Cesk. Dermatol. 51, 217. (a lichen)

Additional References:
Fujisawa, S. et al (1966) Eczematous dermatitis produced by airborne molds. Archs. Derm. 94, 413.

Hellgren, L. and Vincent, J. (1976) Contact sensitizing properties of some fatty acids in dermatophytes. Sabouraudia 14, 243.

Elinov, N.P. et al (1975) The immune response to polysaccharides from yeast-like fungi in sensitized experimental animals. Mykosen 18(10), 407.

Lee, W.L. and Lloyd, K.O. (1975) Immunological studies on a yeast peptidogalactomannan. Nature of antigenic determinants reacting with rabbit antisera and those involved delayed hypersensitivity in guinea pigs. Arch. Biochem. Biophys. 171, 624.

Rifkind, D. et al (1976) Delayed hypersensitivity to fungal antigens in mice. 1. Use of the intradermal skin and footpad swelling tests as assays of active and passive sensitization. J. Infect. Dis. 133, 50.

GERANIACEAE - Pelargonium: Cosmetics containing oil of geranium may cause dermatitis in hypersensitive individuals (Flandin, Rabeau and Ukrainczyk 1937, Schwartz and Peck 1946, Schwartz, Tulipan and Peck 1947, Sezary and Horowitz 1937, Tulipan 1938).

References: Flandin, C. et al (1937) L'intolerance a la terebenthine et aux substances du groupe des terpenes. Bull. Soc. fr. Derm. Syph. 44, 315.

Schwartz, L. and Peck, S.M. (1946) Cosmetics and Dermatitis. Hoeber, New York.

Schwartz, L. et al (1947) Occupational Diseases of the Skin. Lea and Febiger. Philadelphia.

Sezary, A. and Horowitz, A. (1937) La cheilite du rouge. Presse med. 45, 137.

Tulipan, L. (1938) Cosmetic irritants. Arch. Derm. Syph. 38, 906.

Pelargonium crispus: A case of contact dermatitis from this plant was observed by Kirton (1974). The patient pinched the leaves because she liked the smell of the plant.

Reference: Kirton, V. (1974) personal communication.

GINKOACEAE - Ginkgo: Contact with ginko-nuts during harvesting produced dermatitis (Minami 1969). Other cases were reported by Aoki and Shingawa (1960), Okawa et al (1954). The pollen has been suspected of causing hayfever (Wodehouse 1971).

References: Aoki and Shingawa (1960) Jap. J. Derm. 70, 589.

Minami, S. (1969) Studies on dermatitis due to Ginkgo nut. Jap. J. Clin. Exp. Med. 46, 1381.

Okawa et al (1954) Jap. J. Derm. 64, 41.

Wodehouse, R.P. (1971) Hayfever Plants. 2nd rev. edition. New York, Hafner.

Peeling, breaking and washing ginkgo nuts produced dermatitis in 7 patients during October and November (Minami 1969). The author stated that Aoki and Shinagawa (1960) reported that dermatitis is caused by immature nuts but some insist that old nuts can also produce dermatitis. He cited other references in the Japanese literature (Okawa et al 1954, Saito 1928, 1929, Tabayashi 1927).

Reference: Aoki and Shinagawa (1960) Japan J. Derm. 70, 589: Okawa et al (1954) 64, 41: Saito (1928) 28, 579 and 29, 105: Tabayaski (1927) 27, 962 cited by Minami, S. (1969) Studies on dermatitis due to Ginkgo-nut. Jap. J. Clin. Exper. Med. 46, 1381.

GRAMINEAE - Cymbopogon:
Reference: Opdyke, D.L.J. (1973) Monographs on fragrance raw materials. Citronella oil. Fd. Cosmet. Toxicol. 11, 1067.

Hydroxycitronellal:
Reference: Mathias, C.G.T. et al (1978) Contact dermatitis caused by spouse's perfume and cologne. Canad. Med. Ass. J. 119, 257.

Hordeum: Inhalation of fungi of moldy barley can produce malt worker's lung, a form of allergic alveolitis (Morgan and Seaton 1975).

Reference: Morgan, W.K.C. and Seaton, A. (1975) Occupational Lung Diseases. Philadelphia, Saunders.

Contact sensitivity to barley is noted under Beta.

Oryza:
References: Grant, J.B., Davies, J.D., Jones, J.V. et al (1976) The immunogenicity of starch glove powder and talc. Brit. J. Surg. 63 (Nov), 864.

712 cases of yellow rice borer dermatitis. Chin. Med. J. 5, 295, 1974.

Spiked hairs from the husks of paddy-grain can produce corneal reactions in rice threshers (Joseph 1968).

Reference: Joseph, T. (1968) Paddy grain injury of the eye. Brit. J. Ophthal. 52, 191.

The scale hairs of the hair of a rice insect Schoenobius incertellus produced positive patch test reactions in rice farmers and also in school-children (Anon 1974).

Reference: Anon (1974) 712 cases of yellow rice borer dermatitis. Chinese Medical Journal 5 (May), 295. Abstracted by Mitchell, J.C. (1976) An aspect of contact dermatitis in China. Contact Dermatitis 2, 122.

Saccharum: Inhalation of a fungus of moldy bagasse can produce bagassosis, a form of allergic alveolitis (Morgan and Seaton 1975).

Reference: Morgan, W.K.C. and Seaton, A. (1975) Occupational Lung Diseases. Philadelphia, Saunders.

The pollen causes hayfever in Hawaii (Wodehouse 1971).

Reference: Wodehouse, R.P. (1971) Hayfever Plants. 2nd rev. edition. New York, Hafner.

Vetiveria zizanioides: Vetiver acetate prepared from vetiver oil had sensitizing properties; the oil itself did not (Opdyke 1974).

Reference: Opdyke, D.L.J. (1974) Monographs on fragrance raw materials. Fd. Cosmet. Toxicol. 12, 1012 and 1013.

Cereals: Occupational asthma in cereal workers was discussed by Morgan and Seaton (1975).

Reference: Morgan, W.K.C. and Seaton, A. (1975) Occupational lung diseases. Philadelphia, W.B. Saunders.

Grain dust:
Reference: Chan-Yeung, M. et al (1978) Grain dust and the lungs. Canad. Med. Ass. J. 118, 1271.

Grass: Boys rolling in St. Augustine grass often show urticaria-like lesions (Grater, W.C. 1975. personal communication).

Hay and Straw: Packing straw (Gonzalez 1956) and Kansas prairie hay (Tosh 1972) were sources of sporotrichosis.

References: Gonzalez, B.J. (1956) Sporotrichosis as an occupational disease in workers in the pottery industry. Bol. Soc. Cubana Derm. Sif. 13, 89.

Tosh, F.E. (1972) Children affected in Sporotrichosis outbreak from hay. Dermatology in Practice 5, 7.

Hay-fungi: Inhalation of fungi of mouldy hay can produce farmers' lung, a form of allergic alveolitis (Morgan and Seaton 1975).

Reference: Morgan, W.K.C. and Seaton, A. (1975) Occupational Lung Disease. Philadelphia, Saunders.

Reeds:
Reference: Ferraud, Laval and Stengauer (1954) A propos de 10 cas de maladies allergiques, d'origine professionelle chez des ouvriers manipulant des roseaux. Maroc Medical 33.

Straw: Inhalation of a fungus of moldy straw can produce "dog house disease" a form of allergic alveolitis (Morgan and Seaton 1975).

Reference: Morgan, W.K.C. and Seaton, A. (1975) Occupational Lung Diseases. Philadelphia, Saunders.

HIPPOCASTANACEAE - Aesculus: 'Mano-Vausse', a proprietary 'Horse Chestnut Extract Compound' sold in Ottawa, Canada, produced acute dermatitis; the patient was both taking the pills and applying the ointment (Jackson, R.J. 1977. personal communication).

JUBULACEAE - Frullania:
Reference: Fernandez de Corres, L. and Corrales Torres, J.L. (1976) Contact dermatitis by Frullania dilatata (L) Dum. Allergol. Immunopathol. (Madr.) 4, 229.

Asakawa, Y. et al (1974) Editorial: Cross-sensitisation between Frullania and Laurus nobilis: The allergen laurel. Arch. Dermatol. 110, 957.

deCorres, F. and Torres, C. (1978) Dermatitis from Frullania, Compositae and other plants. Contact Dermatitis 4, 175.

Krauskopf, J. and Ad Amkov, A.D. (1975) 3 cases of simultaneous contact hypersensitivity to wild chamomile (Matricaria chamomilla) and Frullania tamarisci. Cesk. Dermatol. 50, 299.

LABIATAE - Mentha - Menthol:
Reference: Camarasa, G. and Alomar, A. (1978) Menthol dermatitis. Contact Dermatitis 4, 169.

LAURACEAE - Cinnamomum: Cinnamic aldehyde is an important sensitizer in perfumes (Schorr 1975). Cinnamon in an ointment produced dermatitis (Calnan 1976).

References: Calnan, C.D. (1976) Cinnamon dermatitis from an ountment. Contact Dermatitis 2, 167.

Schorr, W.F. (1975) Cinnamic aldehyde allergy. Contact Dermatitis 1, 108.

In the course of maximization testing in human subjects, three instances arose in which an individual aldehyde (phenylacetaldehyde, citral or cinnamic aldehyde) occurring widely in nature proved to be a skin sensitizer. However, the essential oil in which the aldehyde occurred naturally did not induce sensitization reactions, although the aldehyde was present in concentrations as high as 85%. It appeared that some other component(s) of the natural oil inhibited the induction or expression of sensitization. As a test of this hypothesis, several terpenes and alcohols, found along with the particular aldehyde in the natural composition, were combined with each of the aldehydes in question. It appears now to be a consistent finding that each of these aldehydes, although producing sensitization reactions when applied alone, produces no sensitization reactions in selected simple mixtures with other compounds (Opdyke 1976).

References: Opdyke, D.L.J. (1976) Inhibition of sensitization reactions induced by certain aldehydes. Fd. Cosmet. Toxicol. 14, 197.

Drake, T.E. and Maibach, H.I. (1976) Allergic contact dermatitis and stomatitis caused by a cinnamic aldehyde-flavored toothpaste. Archs. Derm. 112, 202.

Cinnamomum cassia: A maximization test with Cassia oil was carried out on 25 volunteers. The material was tested at a concentration of 4% in petrolatum and produced two sensitisation reactions (Opdyke 1975). Cinnamon bark oil, "Ceylon" 8 per cent in petrolatum was strongly sensitizing, producing sensitization in 18 and 20 of 25 volunteers.

Reference: Opdyke, D.L.J. (1975) Monographs on fragrance raw materials. Fd. Cosmet. Toxicol. 13, 109 and 111.

Cinnamomum tamala: This plant and also Berberis and oleander oil (Nerium) are used topically in indigenous Indian medicine (Behl 1967).

Reference: Behl, P.N. (1967) Ancient Indian Dermatology. Probe 6, 137.

Laurus nobilis: The dried leaves are used for flavouring the dish 'bouillabaise' (Howes 1974).

Reference: Howes, F.N. (1974) A dictionary of useful and everyday plants and their common names. Cambridge University Press.

Laurus:

Reference: Asakawa, Y. et al (1974) Editorial: Cross-sensitization between Frullania and Laurus nobilis: The allergen laurel. Arch. Dermatol. 110, 957.

Opdyke, D.L.J. (1976) Monographs on fragrance raw materials. Laurel leaf oil. Fd. Cosmet. Toxicol. 14, 307.

LEGUMINOSAE - ?Acacia - Mimosa tree of southern States: The caterpillar of the flannel moth, called the asp, which frequents mimosa trees, can cause a painful severe contact dermatitis (Grater 1975).

Reference: Grater, W.C. (1975) Hypersensitivity dermatitis from American weeds other than poison ivy. Ann. Allergy 35, 159.

Dalbergia spp.: Natural dalbergenones (dalbergiquinones) of these species were reviewed by Seshadri (1972).

Reference: Seshadri, T.R. (1972) Polyphenols of Pterocarpus and Dalbergia woods. Phytochem. 11, 881.

Dalbergia:

Reference: Holst, R. et al (1976) Sensitization to tropical woods giving erythema multiforme-like eruptions. Contact Dermatitis 2, 295.

Dalbergia retusa - Cocabolla: Respiratory allergy occurred from the wood (Eaton 1973).

Reference: Eaton, K.K. (1973) Respiratory allergy to exotic wood dust. Clinical Allergy 3, 307.

Mansonia:

Reference: Nava, C. et al (1975) Mansonia altissima disease (study of 30 cases). Med. Lav. 66, 574.

Myrocarpus: Four species of southern Brazil and Paraguay yield a balsam like Balsam of Peru (Myroxylon).

Myrocarpus frondosus: The wood of this Brazilian species yields Cabreuva oil from which is derived nerolidol and hence, the sesquiterpene alcohol, farnesol. Man himself uses farnesol, which occurs in his own surface lipid, as a perfume (Nicolaides 1965).

Reference: Nicolaides, N. (1965) Skin lipids IV. Biochemistry and Function. American Oil Chemists Society Journal 42, 708.

Myroxylon:

Reference: Temesvari, E. et al (1978) Contact urticaria provoked by Balsam of Peru. Contact Dermatitis 4, 65.

Olholm-Larsen, P. and Heydenreich, G. (1976) Allergy to Balsam of Peru and wood tars: an increasing problem? Contact Dermatitis 2, 293.

Ingestion of materials related to Balsam of Peru.

Hjorth (1961) reported 2 children who were sensitive to Balsam of Peru and orange peel and whose excema flared after eating fruits and ices. He has also described (1971) a man with severe hand eczema for 10 years who, because he reacted to Balsam of Peru on patch testing, was told to avoid orange peel. To test the validity of this advice the patient ate a jar of orange marmalade and in 12 hours had his worst attack of hand eczema. He then avoided "perfumes, cola drinks, vermouth, throat tablets, cinnamon, and other items" and his hand eczema cleared. Eating vanilla sugar has also caused a flare of eczema in a patient sensitive to Balsam of Peru (Pirila 1970).

References: Hjorth, N. (1961) Eczematous allergy to balsams. Copenhagen: Munksgaard.

Pirila, V. (1970) Endogenic contact eczema. Allergie Asthma 16, 15.

Immediate reactions to Balsam of Peru were cited by Rudzki and Grzywa(1976) and Friis and Hjorth (1973).

References: Friis, B. and Hjorth, N. (1973) Immediate reactions to patch tests with Balsam of Peru. Contact Dermatitis Newsletter 13, 389.

Rudzki, E. and Grzywa, Z. (1976) Immediate reactions to Balsam of Peru, cassia oil and ethyl vanillin. Contact Dermatitis 2, 360.

4.8% of patients with leg ulcers were contact sensitive to Balsam of Peru (Angelini et al 1975).

Reference: Angelini, E. et al (1975) Contact dermatitis in patients with leg ulcers. Contact Dermatitis 1, 81.

Pisum: In the Pels-Mach phytopharmacological test for pemphigus, white pea seedlings were grown in affected patients serum and the rootlets studies (Birt, A. 1978, personal communication) for peculiarities of growth.

Ricinus - Castor oil: Examinations for hypersensitivity to extract of castor oil seeds made amongst the workers in the 'Banat' works and the inhabitants of Nova Crnja, indicate that the incidence of sensitization and of allergic manifestations to extracts of castor oil seeds is considerable, that the incidence of allergic manifestations is greater among the population cultivating the castor oil plant than amongst operatives working in the factory for the extraction of the castor oil; this difference in the appearance of allergic manifestations between the workers in the 'Banat' factory and the population cultivating the castor oil plants, may be explained by the more unfavorable working conditions for the cultivators than those for the factory workers (Spoujitch et al 1966).

Reference: Spoujitch, V. et al (1966) Allergic manifestations provoked by the allergen of seeds of the castor oil plant among the inhabitants of Nova Crnja in the Banat (Cyrillic). GL. Srpske Akad. Nauka. Od. Med. Nauka 267/19 (73-77).

Additional References:

DeLaet, M. (1946) An industrial accident due to ricin. Arch. Belg. Med. Soc. Med. Trav. et Med. Leg.

Figley, K.D. and Elrod, R.H. (1928) Endemic asthma due to castor bean dust. JAMA 90, 79.

Figley, K.D. and Rawling, F.F.A. (1950) Castor bean: industrial hazard as contaminant of green coffee dust and used burlap bags. J. Allergy 21, 545.

Kathren, R.L. et al (1959) Airborne castor bean pomace allergy: new solution to old problem. Arch. Indust. Health 19, 486.

Mendes, E. and Citra, U.S. (1954) Collective asthma, simulating an epidemic, provoked by castor-bean dust. J. Allergy 25, 253.

Ordman, D. (1955) Outbreak of bronchial asthma in South Africa, affecting more than 200 persons caused by castor bean dust from a processing factor. Internat. Arch. Allergy 7, 10.

Panzani, R. (1958) Les formes cliniques de l'allergie respiratoire des poussieres de ricin. Presse med. 66, 1788.

Rejsek, K. (1948) Allergic reactions in workers employed in plants processing castor oil beans. Med. Deporte y Trab. 13, 2082.

Snell, M.A. (1952) Castor bean pomace exposure. Arch. Indust. Health 6, 113.

Spies, J.R. et al (1944) Chemistry of allergens. IX. Isolation and properties of active, carbohydrate-free protein from castor beans. J. Am. Chem. Soc. 66, 748.

LICHENS:

References: Krauskopf, J. (1974) Phytodermatoses caused by lichens. Cesk. Dermatol. 49, 383.

Thune, P. (1977) Contact allergy due to lichens in patients with a history of photosensitivity. Contact Dermatitis 3, 267.

MYRTACEAE - Eugenia caryophyllata: Sensitisation of human skin reported to be caused by clove oil was attributed to the presence of eugenol (Woeber and Kromback 1969).

Reference: Woeber, K. and Kromback, M. (1969) Zur Frage der Sensibilisierung durch atherische Ole Vorlaufige Mittielung. Berufsdermatosen 17, 320.

Eugenol: This chemical can cause contact stomatitis in patients and in dental personnel (Goransson et al 1967).

Reference: Goransson, L. et al (1967) Some cases of eugenol hypersensitivity. Derm. Venereol. Tandlak. T. 60, 545.

PEDALIACEAE - Sesamum:
Reference: Neering, H. et al (1975) Allergens in sesame oil contact dermatitis. Acta Derm. Venereol. (Stockh.) 55, 31.

PINACEAE - Abietic acid: Two patients had contact dermatitis from dehydroabietic acid in the resin of an adhesive plaster. Allergic reactions to adhesive are often related to plant products (balsams, colophony, turpentine) but antioxidants and preservatives have also been implicated. Abietic acid and its derivatives are composed of isoprene units which helps to explain their structural and antigenic relation to balsams, colophony and turpentine (Rasmussen and Fisher 1976).

Reference: Rasmussen, J.E. and Fisher, A.A. (1976) Allergic contact dermatitis due to a salicylic acid plaster. Contact Dermatitis 2, 237.

Coal:
Reference: Mumford, P.B. and Auckland, G. (1947) Sensitivity to burnt coal-gas. Brit. J. Derm. Syph. 59, 169.

Rosin: Rosin used for application to a belt surface to increase friction, contaminated honing oil and produced dermatitis in an engineer (Wilkinson and Calnan 1975).

Reference: Wilkinson, D.S. and Calnan, C.D. (1975) Rosin used for belt drive machine. Contact Dermatitis 1, 64.

Hydroabeityl alcohol prepared from hydrogenated rosin acids has sensitizing properties. Three of 25 persons were sensitized by a maximisation test (Opdyke 1974).

Reference: Opdyke, D.L.J. (1974) Monographs on fragrance raw materials. Fd. Cosmet. Toxicol. 12, 919.

Colophony:
References: Kirk, J. (1976) Colophony collar dermatitis. Contact Dermatitis 2, 294.

Wahlberg, J.E. (1978) Abietic acid and colophony. Contact Dermatitis 4, 55.

Calnan, C.D. (1978) Diethyldithiocarbamate in adhesive tape. Contact Dermatitis 4, 61.

Cronin, E. and Calnan, C.D. (1978) Allergy to hydroabietic alcohol in adhesive tape. Contact Dermatitis 4, 57.

Colophony caused dermatitis in 6 patients in a spinal injuries centre (Walshe 1975) and in two patients from contaminated physiotherapy wax (Hambly and Wilkinson 1975).

References: Hambly, E.M. and Wilkinson, D.S. (1975) Dermatitis from contaminated physiotherapy wax. Contact Dermatitis 1, 53.

Walshe, M.M. (1975) Contact dermatitis in a spinal injuries centre. Contact Dermatitis 1, 3.

Gasoline:
References: Biederman, J.B. A case of contact dermatitis produced at a distance by a sensitizing agent. JAMA 106, 2236.

Whitfield, A. (1937) Lancet 132, 265.

Turpentine:
Reference: Calnan, C.D. (1978) Turpentine in paint brush cleaner. Contact Dermatitis 4, 57.

Turpentine produced a positive patch test reaction in a man who was contact sensitive to a hair piece adhesive (Kanof 1977).

Reference: Kanof, N.B. (1977) Eczematous contact dermatitis to turpentine signalled by a reaction to a hair piece adhesive. Contact Dermatitis 3, 108.

Pinus canarensis and Pinus halepensis: These trees, in Israel, harbour caterpillars, Thaumatopoea pinivora, which cause urticarial dermatitis resembling scabies (Katzenellenbogen 1955), and eye damage (Cheverton 1936). Pine forests also support irritant processionary caterpillars. Living and dead caterpillars alike can cause the dermatitis.

References: Cheverton, R.L. (1936) Irritation caused by contact with processionary caterpillar (larva of Thaumetopoea wilkinsoni Tams) and its nest. Trans. Roy. Soc. Trop. Med. 29, 555.

Katzenellenbogen, I. (1955) Caterpillar dermatitis as an occupational disease. Dermatologica 111, 99.

PIPERACEAE - Piper methysticum - Kawa, Yangona: The powdered root of this plant, prepared so as to form a beverage, is drunk on festive occasions among the Polynesians and Fijians. Overindulgence induces a state of exhilaration with loss of power in the legs. Chronic addiction induces a marked coarsening and roughening of the skin, with wasting and debility (Cilento 1944).

Reference: Cilento, R. (1944) Some poisonous plants, sea and land animals of Australia and New Guinea. Brisbane. W.R. Smith and Patterson Pty. Ltd. (University of Queensland Library Q.L. 100 C5. 1944. 3. Biol.)

PLANTAGINACEAE - Plantago spp. - Plantain: The pollen of some species, especially P. lanceolata (English plantain) can cause hayfever (Wodehouse 1971).

Reference: Wodehouse, R.P. (1971) Hayfever Plants. 2nd rev. edition. New York, Hafner.

Plantago psyllium (syn. Psyllium sp.): The seeds are used in silk and cotton manufacture and as a cosmetic.

A male pharmaceutical worker who demonstrated a laxative containing ground psyllium seeds developed vasomotor rhinitis and gastrointestinal allergy; scratch and intradermal tests to psyllium seed produced strong positive reactions. Ingestion of the seed produced gastrointestinal allergy in a female patient who had hayfever and 2 others of 342 allergic persons gave positive reactions to tests with the seed (Ascher 1941).

Reference: Ascher, M.S. (1941) Psyllium seed sensitivity. A case report. J. Allergy 12, 607.

PLATANACEAE - Platanus spp.: The pollen of some species can cause hayfever (Wodehouse 1971).

Reference: Wodehouse, R.P. (1971) Hayfever Plants. 2nd rev. edition. New York, Hafner.

PODOPHYLLACEAE - Podophyllum:
Reference: Perez-Figaredo, R.A. and Baden, H.P. (1976) The pharmacology of Podophyllum. Progress in Dermatology 10, (no. 1) (Feb) 1. Dermatology Foundation 1700 Walnut Street, Philadelphia, Pa.

POLYGONACEAE - Fagopyrum esculentum: Inhalation of buckwheat flour has been reported to cause vasomotor rhinitis and asthma; the pollen is suspected of causing hayfever (Wodehouse 1971).

Reference: Wodehouse, R.P. (1971) Hayfever Plants. 2nd rev. edition. New York, Hafner.

Additional Reference:
Nakamura, S. and Yamaguchi, M.Y. (1974-75) Studies on the buckwheat allergose report 2: Clinical investigation on 169 cases with the buckwheat allergose gathered from the whole country of Japan. Allerg. Immunol. (Leipz) 20-21(4), 457.

Rumex spp. - Dock: The pollen of some species can cause hayfever (Wodehouse 1971).

Reference: Wodehouse, R.P. (1971) Hayfever plants. 2nd rev. edition. New York, Hafner.

PROTEACEAE - Cardwellia sublimis: Sawyers and others handling the fresh timber may contract dermatitis (H.C. Whibley, Cairns, personal communication to Webb 1948).

Reference: Webb, L.J. (1948) Guide to the medicinal and poisonous plants of Queensland. Bulletin No. 232. Council for Scientific and Industrial Research. Melbourne, Australia.

ROSACEAE - Malus:
Reference: Michel, F.B. et al (1977) Allergy to the apple tree parasite Panonychus ulmi (Koch). Rev. Fr. Allergol. 17, 93.

Prunus armeniaca - Apricot: A woman who had sores in the mouth and hives, as a child, from eating apricots developed pruritis ani and vulvae from an apricot soap (Yaffee 1978).

Reference: Yaffee, H.S. (1978) Apricot allergy. Schoch Letter 28, July, Item 46.

Malus: Quinones, which darken on exposure to air, are formed during the enzymatic browning reaction that occurs when cut or bruised surfaces of certain fruits and vegetables when exposed to air; the subject was reviewed by Friedman and Shibko (1969).

Reference: Friedman, L. and Shibko, S.I. (1969) Adventitious Toxic Factors in Processed Foods in Toxic Constituents of Plant Foodstuffs. ed. Liener, I.E. New York, Academic Press.

RUBIACEAE - Cinchona:
References: Levantine, A. and Almeyda, J. (1974) Cutaneous reactions to food and drug additives. Brit. J. Derm. 91, 359.

Hardie, R.A. et al (1978) Quinine dermatitis: Investigation of a factory outbreak. Contact Dermatitis 4, 121.

Calnan, C.D. (1978) Photodermatitis and quinine sensitivity. Contact Dermatitis 4, 58.

SALICACEAE - Populus:
Additional References:
Steinbrink, H. (1973) Poplar spinner caterpillars injurious to health in a nursery school. Angew Parasitol. 14(4), 224.

Wanscher, B. (1976) Contact dermatitis from propolis. Brit. J. Derm. 94, 451.

SCROPHULARIACEAE - Digitalis: The external application of the fresh leaves of foxglove in the form of an ointment excites an irritation of the skin which may result in an erythema, or an eruption papular in character (Morrow 1887).

Reference: Morrow, Prince (1887) Drug eruptions. A clinical study of the irritant effects of drugs upon the skin. New York. Wm. Wood and Co.

SOLANACEAE - Capsicum:
Reference: Temesvari, E. et al (1978) Contact urticaria provoked by balsam of Peru. Contact Dermatitis 4, 65.

Datura stramonium:
References: Goldey, J.A. et al (1966) Cornpicker's pupil. Ohio State Med. J. 62, 921.

Miller, R.W. (1975) Jimson weed seeds. Ann. Intern. Med. 83, 905.

Mikolich, J.R. et al (1975) Acute anticholinergic syndrome due to Jimson seed ingestion. Ann. Intern. Med. 83, 321.

Lycopersicon: Tomatoes from stalks grafted into a Jimson weed plant (Datura) poisoned five persons (Roueche 1967).

Reference: Roueche, B. (1967) Something a little unusual. in Annals of Epidemiology. ed. Roueche, B. Boston. Little Brown. p. 285.

Nicotiana:
Reference: Tulebaev, R.K. et al (1975) Allergic changes of the skin and mucous membranes in workers of the tobacco industry. Vestn. Dermatol. Venerol. (7), 63.

TAXODIACEAE - Sequoia:
Reference: Chan-Yeung, M. and Abboud, R. (1976) Occupational asthma due to California redwood (Sequoia semperivirens) dusts. Amer. Rev. Resp. Dis. 114, 1027.

UMBELLIFERAE - Carum:
Reference: Hegyi, E., Dole Zalov, A.A. (1976) Urticarial reaction after patch tests of toothpaste with a subshock condition. Hypersensitivity to caraway seed (Author's transl.) Cesk. Dermatol. 51(1), 19.

Foeniculum vulgare: Fennel oil has sensitizing properties (Opdyke 1976).

Reference: Opdyke, D.L.J. (1976) Monographs on fragrance raw materials. Fennel oil, bitter. Fd. Cosmet. Toxicol. 14, 309.

Pastinaca: Parsnip dermatitis was described by Lengyel et al (1965).

Reference: Lengyel, B. et al (1965) Konyhakerteszeti dolgozokon tomegesen fellepo pasztinak dermatitisek es megelozesiik Munkavedelem Budapest 21, 29.

Pastinaca sativa: Photoallergic reactions to furocoumarins have been reported (Sidi and Bourgeois-Gavardin 1953, Fulton and Willis 1968, Ljunggren 1977) but seem to be rare.

References: Fulton, J.E. and Willis, I. (1968) Photoallergy to methoxsalen. Archs. Derm. 98, 445.

Ljunggren, B. (1977) Psoralen photoallergy by plant contact. Contact Dermatitis 3, 85.

Sidi, E. and Bourgeois-Gavardin, J. (1953) Mise au point du traitment du vitiligo par L'ammi majus. Presse Med. 61, 436.

In addition to phototoxic reactions, four psoralens can produce photoallergic contact dermatitis (Ljunggren 1977).

Reference: Ljunggren, B. (1977) Psoralen photoallergy caused by plant contact. Contact Dermatitis 3, 85.

URTICACEAE - Laportea:
Reference: Francis, W.D. (1956) Australian stinging trees. Queensland Naturalist 15, 66. (C.T. White Memorial Lecture for 1955).

VERBENACEAE - Tectona:
Reference: Schmidt, H. (1978) Contact urticaria to teak with systemic effects. Contact Dermatitis 4, 176.

Animal Food-additive:
Reference: Tennstedt, D. et al (1978) Virginiamycin (food additive, pigs, poultry). Contact Dermatitis 4, 133.

Coal tar:
Reference: Kaidbey, K.H. and Kligman, A.M. (1977) Clinical and Histological Study of Coal Tar Phototoxicity in Humans. Arch. Dermatol. 113, 592.

Occupational mark - violin and viola:
Reference: Peachey, R.D.G. and Matthews, C.N.A. (1978) 'Fiddler's neck'. Brit. J. Derm. 98, 669.

Occupational stigmata - White finger: In Ontario, a disorder known as white-finger occurs in forest-workers using vibration tools mostly in winter (Jackson, R. 1978, personal communication), a form of induced Raynaud's phenomenon.

Mechanical injury: A thorn prick was followed by erythema chronicum migrans (Bessiere 1966).

Reference: Bessiere, M.L. (1966) Erythema chronicum migrans par piqure d'epine. Bull. Soc. fr. Derm. Syph. 73, 455.

Wood:
References: Nava, C. (1974) Pathology caused by wood-dust. Med. Lav. 65, 1.

Shevliakov, L.V. (1974) Occupational skin diseases in the wood industry abroad and in the USSR (Review). Gig. Tr. Prof. Zabol. 18, 33.

Varnish:
Reference: Cirla, A.M. and Zedda, S. (1974) Pathology of varnish products. Med. Lav. 65, 8.

Tocopherols in Plants: Among the eight naturally occurring tocopherols, Vitamin E or alpha-tocopherol has the greatest biological activity. It occurs in plants and can be synthesized industrially. Contact dermatitis from tocopherols was discussed by Hjorth and Roed-Petersen (1976).

Reference: Hjorth, N. and Roed-Petersen, J. (1976) Contact dermatitis from antioxidants. Hidden sensitizers in topical medications and foods. Brit. J. Derm. 94, 233.

Foods:
Reference: Speer, F. (1975) Multiple food allergy. Ann. Allergy 34, 71.

Polysaccharides of Plants: Polysaccharides of decaying plants trapped in new houses can be allergenic ('construction dust') (Loeb 1967).

Reference: Loeb, L. (1967) cited in Dead Plants Cause Allergy. Medical Post. Dec. 5, p. 31.

Perfume: Fisher and Dooms-Goossens (1976) point out that an ingredient of a perfume which is a sensitizer may become hypo-allergenic by interacting with other ingredients during the ageing process of the perfume. There are several theories as to why cinnamic aldehyde can become a non-sensitizer in a perfume mixture. Testing with a mature perfume may for such reasons be much more significant than testing with individual ingredients.

Reference: Fisher, A.A. and Dooms-Goossens, A. (1976) The effect of perfume "ageing" on the allergenicity of individual perfume ingredients. Contact Dermatitis 2, 155.

Pseudophytodermatitis: Psocide insects (Stenopscocus or Psocus) of the Copoegnata in wood dust produced a varicelliform eruption in members of a family (Teodoresco et al 1959).

Reference: Tsodoresco, St., et al (1959) Varicelliform skin rashes due to a collective re-actogen (carious Psocidoea wood dust) in a family. Derm. Vener. (Bucuresti) 4, 103.

Food Dyes: Some food dyes were found to be allergenic (Grater 1976).

Reference: Grater, W.C. (1976) Hypersensitive skin reactions to F.D. and C. Dyes. Cutis 17, 1163.

Foods - additives:

Reference: Roed Petersen, J. and Hjorth, N. (1976) Contact dermatitis from antioxidants. Hidden sensitizers in topical medications and foods. Brit. J. Derm. 94, 233.

Ethoxyquin:

Reference: Zachariae, H. (1978) Ethoxyquin dermatitis. Contact Dermatitis 4, 117.

Colophony:

Reference: Ducombs, G. (1978) Allergy to colophony. Contact Dermatitis 4, 118.

Contact urticaria from plants: Immediate hypersensitivity to fruits, edible roots and vegetables has been well known for decades. Oranges, tomatoes, strawberries, melons and nuts are said to be the most common such allergens. Reactions to potatoes, carrots and celery have been reported to be common but reactions to other roots are rare. Legumes are allergenically more active than other vegetables. However, asparagus, onion, chive and cabbage are also allergenic vegetables. The reactions are usually immediate, appearing within minutes of ingestion of these foods. Urticaria is the most common reaction but anaphylactic shock, gastrointestinal symptoms and a worsening of atopic dermatitis can also occur.

Handling of foods can aggravate hand eczema (Maibach 1976, Hjorth and Roed-Petersen 1976). Apple, carrot, parsnip and potato elicit positive scratch test reactions in persons allergic to birch pollen (Hannuksela and Lahti 1977)

References: Hannuksela, M. and Lahti, A. (1977) Immediate reactions to fruits and vegetables. Contact Dermatitis 3, 79.

Hjorth, N. and Roed-Petersen, J. (1976) Occupational protein contact dermatitis in food handlers. Contact Dermatitis 2, 28.

Maibach, H. (1976) Immediate hypersensitivity in hand dermatitis. Archs. Derm. 112, 1289.

Thrips: Thrips in a bouquet of flowers may cause an arthropod infestation (Waldron 1972).

Reference: Waldron, W.G. (1972) Entomologist and illusions of parasitosis. Calif. Med. 117, 76.

Agricultural chemicals:

References: Burry, H.N. (1976) Contact dermatitis from agricultural fungicide in South Australia. Contact Dermatitis 2, 289.

van Ketel, W.G. (1976) Sensitivity to the pesticide benomyl. Contact Dermatitis 2, 289.

Pesticides - Sulphur: Sulphur caused contact sensitivity in a gardener (Wilkinson 1975).

Reference: Wilkinson, D.S. (1975) Sulphur sensitivity. Contact Dermatitis 1, 58.

Herbicides: Carbyne(R) a herbicide produced contact dermatitis and depigmentation (Brancaccio and Chamales 1977).

Reference: Brancaccio, R.R. and Chamales, M.H. (1977) Contact dermatitis and depigmentation produced by the herbicide Carbyne(R). Contact Dermatitis 3, 108.

Pesticide: Picking the leaves of plants can produce dermatitis from pesticide residues either on or in certain plants (van Ketel 1975, 1976).

References: van Ketel, W.G. (1975) Allergic dermatitis from a new pesticide. Contact Dermatitis 1, 297.

van Ketel, W.G. (1976) Sensitivity to the pesticide benomyl. Contact Dermatitis 2, 290.

Fungicide:

References: Matsushita, T. et al (1976) Experimental study on contact dermatitis caused by dithiocarbamates maneb, zineb, and their related compounds. Int. Arch. Occup. Environ. Health 37, 169.

Shelley, W.B. (1964) Golf-course dermatitis due to thiuram fungicide. JAMA 188, 415.

Herbicides:

Reference: Iden, D.L. and Schroeter, A.L. (1977) Allergic contact dermatitis to herbicides. Archs. Derm. 113, 983.

Pesticides: Difolatan can produce allergic contact dermatitis (Groundwater 1977).

Reference: Groundwater, J.R. (1977) Contact Dermatitis 3, 104.

Hazard of patch testing with agricultural chemical - rotenone: A patient tested with rotenone developed nausea, vomiting, diarrhoea, "etc." mimicking poisoning from ingestion of this pesticide (Schoch 1976).

Reference: Schoch, A.G. (1976) Patch test hazards. The Schoch Letter 26 (No. 7), 11.

Toxic constituents of plant food stuffs:

Haemagglutinins were reviewed by Jaffe (1969).

Goitrogens were reviewed by Van Etten (1969).

Cyanogens were reviewed by Montgomery (1969).

Saponins were reviewed by Birk (1969).

Lathyrogens were reviewed by Sarma and Padmanaban (1969).

Estrogenic factors were reviewed by Liener (1969).

Favism was reviewed by Mager, Razin and Hershko (1969).

General:

Jaffe, W.G. (1969) Haemagglutinins;
Van Etten, C.H. (1969) Goitrogens;
Montgomery, R.D. (1969) Cyanogens;
Sarma, P.S. and Padmanaban, G. (1969) Lathyrogens;
Mager, J., Razin, A. and Hershko, A. (1969) Favism;
Liener, I.E. (1969) Miscellaneous Toxic Factors; in Toxic Constituents of Plant Foodstuffs, ed. Liener, I.E. New York, Academic Press.

Minerals in Foods: The levels of trace elements found in foods can vary considerably in amount from region to region; they are dependent on soil composition, contamination, storage and techniques of preparation.

Cadmium: Oysters, canned anchovies, lamb, chicken.

Calcium: Milk, cheeses, fish (eaten with bones), dark green leafy vegetables.

Chloride: Common salt, animal products.

Chromium: Brewers yeast (dried), black pepper, liver (calf), American cheese, wheat germ, whole wheat bread. NOTE: These foods are those with highest chromium biological values (i.e. highest chromium glucose tolerance factor) rather than those with highest total chromium.

Cobalt: Fish, bran, molasses, cocoa, green leafy vegetables.

Copper: Liver, shellfish (esp. oysters), nuts, legumes, whole grains (wheat, barley and corn), cocoa.

Fluorine: Fluoridated water.

Iodine: Iodized salt, seafoods.

Iron: Organ meats (esp. liver), muscle meats, egg yolk, legumes, whole grain and enriched bread and cereals, green vegetables, bran and molasses. NOTE: Oxalic acid in spinach binds its iron, preventing adequate absorption by the body.

Magnesium: Nuts, whole grain bread and cereals, legumes, green leafy vegetables, sesame seeds, cocoa.

Manganese: Nuts (esp. pecans, brazils and almonds), whole grain cereals and breads (esp. those of wheat, buckwheat, rye and barley), legumes, tea.

Molybdenum: Legumes, cereal grains, leafy vegetables, liver, kidney.

Nickel: Whole grains (esp. buckwheat, rye, oats, corn, rice, wheat), legumes, green leafy vegetables, fresh oysters, herring (canned), tea, cocoa.

Phosphorus: Milk, poultry, fish, meats, eggs, cheese, nuts, whole grain cereals and breads, legumes.

Potassium: Fruits (esp. oranges, bananas, apricots, dried fruits), fruit juice, vegetables (esp. potatoes, squash).

Selenium: Kidney, liver, seafoods, wheat (esp. that grown in Western Canada).

Sodium: Table salt, processed foods.

Sulfur: Protein foods.

Zinc: Meat, fish, shellfish (esp. oysters), poultry, egg yolk, dairy products, legumes, bran and germ of wheat, cocoa.

References:

Arthur, D. (1972) Selenium content of Canadian foods. Can. Inst. Food Sci. Techol. J. 5, 165.

Church, C.F. and Church, H.N. (1975) Food Values of Portions Commonly Used, 12 edition. J.B. Lippencott Co., Toronto.

Freeland, J.H. and Cousins, R.J. (1976) Zinc content of selected foods. J. Am. Diet. Assoc. 68, 526.

Gormican, A. (1970) Inorganic elements in foods used in hospital menus. J. Am. Diet. Assoc. 56, 397.

Guthrie, Belen (1975) Introductory Nutrition - 3rd edition. The C.V. Mosby Co., St. Louis.

Haeflein, K.A. and Rasumssen, A.I. (1977) Zinc content of selected foods. J. Am. Diet. Assoc. 70, 610.

Lagua, R.T. et al (1974) Nutrition and Diet Therapy Reference Dictionary, 2nd Edition. The C.V. Mosby Co., St. Louis.

Mitchell, H.S. et al (1976) Nutrition in Health and Disease, 16th edition. J.B. Lippencott Co., Toronto.

Morris, V.C. and Levander, O.A. (1970) Selenium content of foods. J. Nutri. 100, 1383.

Murphy, E.W. et al (1975) Provisional tables on the zinc content of foods. J. Am. Diet. Assoc. 66, 345.

Pennington, J.T. and Calloway, D.H. (1973) Copper content of foods. J. Am. Diet. Assoc. 63, 143.

Schroeder, H.A. et al (1962) Abnormal trace elements in man - nickel. J. Chron. Dis. 15, 51.

Schroeder, H.A. et al (1966) Essential trace elements in man: Manganese. J. Chron. Dis. 19, 545.

Schroeder, H.A. et al (1967) Essential trace metals in man: Zinc. Relation to environmental cadmium. J. Chron. Dis. 20, 179.

Schroeder, H.A. et al (1967) Essential trace elements in man: Cobalt. J. Chron. Dis. 20, 869.

Schroeder, H.A. et al (1970) Essential trace metals in man: Selenium. J. Chron. Dis. 23, 227.

Thomas, B. et al (1974) Cobalt, chromium and nickel content of some vegetable food stuffs. J. Sco. Fd. Agric. 25, 771.

Toepfer, E.W. et al (1973) Chromium in foods in relation to biological activity. J. Agr. Food Chem. 21, 69.

Underwood, E.J. (1971) Trace Elements in Human and Animal Nutrition - 3rd edition. Academic Press, New York.

Vought, R.L. and London, W.T. (1964) Dietary sources of iodine. Am. J. Clin. Nutri. 14, 186.

Watt, B. K. and Merrill, A. L. (1963) Composition of Foods - Agriculture Handbook No. 8, U. S. Government Printing Office, Washington, D. C.

Zook, E. G. and Lehmann, J. (1968) Mineral composition of fruits. II. Nitrogen, calcium, magnesium, phosphorus, potassium, aluminum, boron, copper, iron, manganese and sodium, J. Am. Diet. Assoc. 52, 225.

Zook, E. G. et al (1970) Nutrient composition of selected wheats and wheat products. VI. Distribution of manganese, copper, nickel, zinc, magnesium, lead, tin, cadmium, chromium and selenium as determined by atomic absorption spectroscopy and coloriemtry. Cereal Chemistry 47, 720.

Malingering by use of plants

To induce dermatitis artefacta, a patient first made a small incision in the skin then inserted a chick-pea or garbanzo and covered the site with a cabbage leaf. The edema and localized necrosis so produced was intended to simulate industrial dermatitis (Downing 1950).

Zacchia, in 1674 listed irritant plants used by beggars to mortify the flesh and stimulate philanthropy: Thapsia, Clematis, Bryonia and Euphorbia and also turpentine, (Woods 1962). Sapium is used by small boys to raise blisters and Buttercups (Ranunculus) have been used to produce leg ulcers. Malingering by self-inflicted injury to the eye in war-time tends to run in epidemics. Thus in W. W. I, malingerers in the French Army specialized in ipecacuanha, the Italians in tobacco, ipecacuanha and croton oil, the Austrians in pepper and tobacco and the Indians in jequirity, castor oil and croton oil (Duke-Elder and MacFaul 1972). Other examples are indexed under Malingering. The use of plants against others is indexed under Criminal Poisoning.

References

Duke-Elder, S. and MacFaul, P. A. (1972) System of Ophthalmology. Vol. 14, p. 1016, London, Kimpton.

Woods, B. (1962) Irritant plants. Trans. St. John's Hosp. Derm. Soc. 48, 75.

Downing, J. G. (1950) Simulation and self-infliction as encountered in Industrial Dermatology. Arch. Ind. Hyg.and Occup. Med. 1, 271

The End